Essentials of General Surgery and Surgical Specialties

SEVENTH EDITION

Essentials of General Surgery and Surgical Specialties

SEVENTH EDITION

Senior Editor

PETER F. LAWRENCE, MD

Chief of Vascular and Endovascular Surgery, Emeritus
Director, Gonda (Goldschmied) Vascular Center, Emeritus
Department of Surgery
David Geffen School of Medicine at UCLA
Los Angeles, California

Editors

JESSICA BETH O'CONNELL, MD

Chief of Surgery, Greater Los Angeles VA Healthcare System
Professor of Clinical Surgery
Vice Chair for Veterans Affairs
Division of Vascular and Endovascular Surgery
David Geffen School of Medicine at UCLA
Los Angeles, California

MATTHEW R. SMEDS, MD

Professor of Surgery
Division of Vascular and Endovascular Surgery
Department of Surgery
Saint Louis University
St. Louis, Missouri

Student Editor

NAKEISHA FAVORS, MPH

Medical Student
Charles R. Drew University of Medicine and Science
Los Angeles, California

Wolters Kluwer

Philadelphia • Baltimore • New York • London
Buenos Aires • Hong Kong • Sydney • Tokyo

Acquisitions Editor: Matt Hauber
Development Editor: Deborah Bordeaux
Editorial Coordinator: Erin E. Hernandez
Editorial Assistant: Parisa Saranj
Marketing Manager: Kirsten Watrud
Production Project Manager: Kirstin Johnson
Art Director, Illustration: Jennifer Clements
Manager, Graphic Arts & Design: Stephen Druding
Manufacturing Coordinator: Margie Orzech
Prepress Vendor: S4Carlisle Publishing Services

Seventh Edition

9 8 7 6 5 4 3 2 1

Printed in Mexico

Library of Congress Cataloging-in-Publication Data

ISBN-13: 978-1-975197-52-0

Library of Congress Control Number: 2024925751

shop.lww.com

QUADM0325

Preface

This seventh edition of the textbook, *Essentials of General Surgery and Surgical Specialties*, was written to address the following question: "What do *all* medical students need to know about surgery to be effective clinicians in their chosen fields?" The clinical years of medical school focus on basic clinical training and are the foundation for a physician's clinical skills. In surgery, because of the length of time needed to completely train surgeons, surgical residents and fellows remain "students" for 3 to 9 years beyond medical school. As a result of this extensive training period, at most medical schools, resident and fellow training, rather than student education, makes up the bulk of their educational efforts. To address this issue, *Essentials of General Surgery and Surgical Specialties* is devoted exclusively to medical students.

NOT JUST FOR SURGEONS

This textbook was produced for medical students who are *not* planning a surgical career. We believe that all physicians need to have a fundamental understanding of the options provided by surgery to be competent clinicians. Rather than using traditional textbook-writing techniques, the editors and authors of this textbook, many of whom are members of the Association for Surgical Education, have conducted extensive research to define the content and skills needed for an optimal education program in surgery. Somewhat surprisingly, there has been consensus among practicing surgeons and internists (and even psychiatrists!) about the knowledge and skills in surgery needed by all physicians, and the information from this research has become the basis for this textbook.

SEVENTH EDITION ENHANCEMENTS

The seventh edition of this textbook has continued the approach that has resulted in its use by many medical students in the United States, Canada, and throughout the world:

1. This edition has been extensively revised to provide the most current and up-to-date information on all fields of surgery, including general surgery and surgical specialties.

2. Our authors are surgeons or surgical educators devoted to teaching medical students, and so they understand the appropriate depth of knowledge for a third-year student to master.

3. We do not attempt to provide an encyclopedia of surgery. We include only information that students need to know—and explain it well.

4. We intentionally limit the length of each section so that it can be read during the surgery clerkship.

5. We have added an online summary of each chapter that allows you to more efficiently prepare for the operating room, educational conferences, or simply read a shortened version of each chapter.

6. Through sample written exam questions, with explanations as to why the correct answer is the best one, and with links to the text, we provide numerous opportunities to practice test taking. We believe that this approach best prepares students to score highly on department of surgery exams and the National Board of Medical Examiners clinical examination. If you use this textbook to prepare, you should do well on both oral and written exams.

7. We have added an online summary of each chapter that allows you to more efficiently prepare for the OR, educational conferences, or exams, or simply read a shortened version of each chapter. This should not be considered a substitute for the main text but instead a refresher, memory jogger, or quick way to identify areas of the text to review.

SUCCESS!

You are entering an exciting and dynamic phase of your professional life. This textbook is designed to help you achieve your goal of becoming a great doctor. It should also help you get into the residency of your choice. Best wishes for success in your endeavor.

Acknowledgments

Many members of the Association for Surgical Education (ASE) provided advice and expertise in starting the first edition of this project nearly 40 years ago. Since that time, ASE members have volunteered to assist in writing chapters and editing the textbook. We would also like to extend our thanks to the many editors at Wolters Kluwer, our publisher, who helped in the production of this textbook and online shortened version of the textbook.

Contributors

Vatche G. Agopian, MD
Professor of Surgery
Department of Surgery
David Geffen School of Medicine at UCLA
Los Angeles, California

James B. Alexander, MD
Professor of Surgery
Department of Surgery
Sidney Kimmel Medical College at Thomas Jefferson
  University
Philadelphia, Pennsylvania

Adnan Alseidi, MD, EdM, FACS
Professor of Surgery
Vice Chair Education
Department of Surgery, Hepatobiliary, and Endocrine
University of California at San Francisco
San Francisco, California

Kwame S. Amankwah, MD, MSc
Professor and Chief of Vascular and Endovascular
  Surgery
Department of Surgery
University of Connecticut Health
Farmington, Connecticut

Peyman Benharash, MD
Associate Professor
Department of Surgery
David Geffen School of Medicine at UCLA
Los Angeles, California

Bennett Berning, MD
Assistant Professor of Surgery
Department of Surgery
University of Nebraska Medical Center
Omaha, Nebraska

Andreana Butter, MD, MSc, FACS, FRCSC
Chair/Chief, Division of Pediatric Surgery
Department of Surgery
Children's Hospital
London Health Sciences Centre
Western University
London, Ontario, Canada

Anthony G. Charles, MD, MPH
Professor of Surgery
Department of Surgery
University of North Carolina
Chapel Hill, North Carolina

David C. Chen, MD
Professor of Clinical Surgery
Department of Surgery
David Geffen School of Medicine at UCLA
Los Angeles, California

S. Ariane Christie, MD
Assistant Professor of Surgery in Residence
Department of General Surgery
David Geffen School of Medicine at UCLA
UCLA Health
Los Angeles, California

Jesse Clanton, MD
Associate Professor of Surgery
Department of Surgery
Prisma Health, Midlands
University of South Carolina School of Medicine at
  Columbia
Columbia, South Carolina

Brian J. Daley, MD, FACS
Professor of Surgery
Department of Surgery
University of Tennessee Health Science Center at
  Knoxville
Knoxville, Tennessee

Charity Evans, MD, MS
Chief, Division of Acute Care Surgery
Department of Surgery
University of Nebraska Medical Center
Omaha, Nebraska

Gregory R. D. Evans, MD
Distinguished Professor, Plastic Surgery and Biomedical
  Engineering
Founding Chair, Department of Plastic Surgery
Bruce F. Connell Endowed Chair in Plastic Surgery
Department of Plastic Surgery
The University of California at Irvine
Orange, California

Amy R. Evenson, MD, MPH
Transplant Surgeon
Department of Surgery
Beth Israel Deaconess Medical Center
Boston, Massachusetts

Steven Farley, MD
Vascular Surgeon
Department of Surgery
David Geffen School of Medicine at UCLA
Los Angeles, California

Abbey L. Fingeret, MD, MHPTT
Associate Professor
Department of Surgery
University of Nebraska Medical Center
Omaha, Nebraska

Gregory A. Greco, DO, FACS
Chairman, Division of Plastic Surgery
Department of Surgery
Monmouth Medical Center
Long Branch, New Jersey

O. Joe Hines, MD
Professor and Chair
Department of Surgery
David Geffen School of Medicine at UCLA
Los Angeles, California

Jared M. Huston, MD
Vice Chair for Education
System Chief, Division of Surgical Education
Department of Surgery
Zucker School of Medicine at Hofstra/Northwell
Hempstead, New York

Tess C. Huy, MD
Resident Physician
Department of Surgery
David Geffen School of Medicine at UCLA
Los Angeles, California

Benjamin C. James, MD, MS
Associate Professor of Surgery
Chief, Section of Endocrine Surgery
Department of Surgery
Harvard Medical School
Beth Israel Deaconess Medical Center
Boston, Massachusetts

Ted A. James, MD
Chief, Breast Surgical Oncology
Department of Surgery
Harvard Medical School
Beth Israel Deaconess Medical Center
Boston, Massachusetts

Adam S. Kabaker, MD
Associate Professor
Department of Surgery
Loyola University Medical Center
Maywood, Illinois

James N. Lau, MD, MHPE
Professor of Surgery and Medical Education
Department of Surgery
Stritch School of Medicine
Loyola University Chicago
Maywood, Illinois

Peter F. Lawrence, MD
Chief of Vascular and Endovascular Surgery, Emeritus
Director, Gonda (Goldschmied) Vascular Center, Emeritus
Department of Surgery
David Geffen School of Medicine at UCLA
Los Angeles, California

Patrick Lec, MD
Physician
Department of Urology
David Geffen School of Medicine at UCLA
Los Angeles, California

Jong Lee, MD
Professor of Surgery
Department of Surgery
University of Texas Medical Branch
Galveston, Texas

Seung Ah Lee, MD
Assistant Professor of Surgery
Division of Plastic and Reconstructive Surgery
University of California at San Francisco
San Francisco, California

Dan C. Little, MD
Chief of Surgery and Division Director of Pediatric
  Surgery
Department of Surgery
McLane Children's Hospital
Professor of Surgery
Texas A&M College of Medicine
Temple, Texas

Felix Y. Lui, MD
Associate Professor
Department of Surgery
Yale School of Medicine
New Haven, Connecticut

David Machado-Aranda, MD, FACS
HS Clinical Associate Professor of Surgery
Department of Surgery
David Geffen School of Medicine at UCLA
Los Angeles, California

Ian T. MacQueen, MD
Assistant Clinical Professor
Department of Surgery
David Geffen School of Medicine at UCLA
Los Angeles, California

James A. McCoy, MD
Clinical Professor
Medical Education and Surgery
Morehouse School of Medicine
Grady Memorial Hospital
Atlanta, Georgia

Patrick R. McGrew, MD
Assistant Professor
Department of Surgery
Tulane University School of Medicine
New Orleans, Louisiana

Jonathan Meisel, MD
Pediatric Surgeon
Department of Surgery
Emory University School of Medicine
Atlanta, Georgia

John J. Murnaghan, MD, MSc, MA, FRCSC
Staff Orthopedic Surgeon
Department of Surgery
Holland Orthopaedic and Arthritic Centre at Sunnybrook
   Health Sciences Centre
Toronto, Ontario, Canada

Roman Nowygrod, MD, MS
Professor
Department of Surgery
Columbia University
New York, New York

Jessica Beth O'Connell, MD
Chief of Surgery, Greater Los Angeles VA Healthcare System
Professor of Clinical Surgery
Vice Chair for Veterans Affairs
Division of Vascular and Endovascular Surgery
David Geffen School of Medicine at UCLA
Los Angeles, California

John T. Paige, MD
Professor of Clinical Surgery
Department of Surgery
Louisiana State University Health Sciences Center New
   Orleans
New Orleans, Louisiana

Tina Palmieri, MD, FACS, MCCM
Professor and Burn Division Chief
Department of Burn Surgery
Shriners Children's Northern California
University of California, Davis
Sacramento, California

Ho H. Phan, MD
Professor
Department of Surgery
University of California, Davis
Sacramento, California

Constantine Poulos, MD
Cardiothoracic Surgery Fellow
Department of Cardiothoracic Surgery
Tufts Medical Center
Boston, Massachusetts

Timothy A. Pritts, MD, PhD
Chief, Section of General Surgery
Department of Surgery
University of Cincinnati
Cincinnati, Ohio

Hadley E. Ritter, MD, FACS
Assistant Professor of Clinical Surgery
Adjunct Assistant Professor of Clinical Otolaryngology
Department of Surgery
Department of Otolaryngology
Indiana University School of Medicine
Indianapolis, Indiana

Sajani N. Shah, MD
Chief of Bariatric and Minimally Invasive Surgery
Department of Surgery
Tufts Medical Center
Boston, Massachusetts

Saad Shebrain, MD, MMM, FACS
Professor of Surgery
Program Director
Department of Surgery
Homer Stryker MD School of Medicine
Western Michigan University
Kalamazoo, Michigan

Joseph Shirk, MD
Assistant Professor of Urology, Chief of Urology
Department of Urology
David Geffen School of Medicine at UCLA
Greater Los Angeles VA Health System
Los Angeles, California

Matthew R. Smeds, MD
Professor of Surgery
Division of Vascular and Endovascular Surgery
Department of Surgery
Saint Louis University
St. Louis, Missouri

Meredith J. Sorensen, MD, MS
Assistant Professor of Surgery
Department of Surgery
Dartmouth Hitchcock Medical Center
Lebanon, New Hampshire

Emily Speer, MD
Foregut and Bariatric Surgeon
Department of Surgery
Lutheran Medical Center
Wheat Ridge, Colorado

Hayden W. Stagg, MD
Clinical Assistant Professor
Department of Surgery
Texas A&M College of Medicine
Pediatric Surgeon
Department of Surgery
Baylor, Scott & White Health
Temple, Texas

Nicole A. Stassen, MD, FCCS, FCCM
Professor of Surgery
Department of Surgery
University of Rochester
Rochester, New York

Christopher Steffes, MD
Professor of Surgery
Associate Dean of Clinical Education
Department of Surgery
Wayne State University School of Medicine
Detroit, Michigan

Veronica F. Sullins, MD
Assistant Clinical Professor of Surgery
Department of Surgery
David Geffen School of Medicine at UCLA
Los Angeles, California

Mediget Teshome, MD, MPH
Associate Clinical Professor
Department of Surgery
David Geffen School of Medicine at UCLA
Los Angeles, California

Areti Tillou, MD, MSEd
Professor of Clinical Surgery
Department of Surgery
David Geffen School of Medicine at UCLA
Los Angeles, California

Jacquelyn Seymour Turner, MD
Professor of Surgery
Department of Surgery
Tulane University
New Orleans, Louisiana

Andrew M. Vahabzadeh-Hagh, MD
Associate Professor
Department of Otolaryngology—Head and Neck Surgery
University of California, San Diego Health
La Jolla, California

Sanah Vohra, PhD, MPH
Medical Student
David Geffen School of Medicine at UCLA
Los Angeles, California

Justin P. Wagner, MD
Assistant Professor
Department of Pediatric Surgery
David Geffen School of Medicine at UCLA
Los Angeles, California

Isaac Yang, MD, FAANS, FACS
Professor
Department of Neurosurgery
David Geffen School of Medicine at UCLA
Los Angeles, California

Contents

1

Perioperative Evaluation and Management of Surgical Patients

David Machado-Aranda

PREOPERATIVE EVALUATION

Introduction

Surgery and anesthesia introduce biologic and psychological stresses impacting vital physiologic functions. To address the physiologic challenges associated with surgery, preoperative evaluation and anesthesia techniques that have been refined over time have led to the development of specialized fields such as Perioperative Medicine (POM) and the implementation of Enhanced Recovery After Surgery (ERAS) protocols, which have improved surgical outcomes.

Anesthesia has been essential in the advancement of modern surgery. Anesthesia helps to keep patients pain-free and immobile during procedures, allowing interventions in a relatively controlled physiologic state. Early inhalation-type anesthetics were effective in suppressing cortical stimulation; however, their delivery caused various unintended side effects such as hypoxia, hypercarbia, extreme blood pressure fluctuations, intravascular shifts, pulse changes, and irregular muscle relaxation. Fortunately, newer drugs, better organ monitoring and support, and better ways of delivering anesthesia, coupled with refinements of surgical technique, have resulted in lower complication rates and improved outcomes.

The goal of Perioperative Evaluation is to identify and manage risks associated with a patient's medical/surgical condition and procedure to ensure successful recovery and avoid complications. This involves understanding the patient's personalized risk profile, which then guides a tailored anesthesia approach, and a focused proactive postoperative plan geared toward the early identification and treatment of complications to ensure a smooth recovery.

Initial Preoperative Evaluation

Surgeons are typically consulted after another health care provider has identified a pathologic condition that requires surgery. It initiates a process that includes validating the need for an intervention, assessing whether such operation is feasible, and evaluating the patient's physical capacity to tolerate surgical and anesthetic stresses.

Surgeons abide by the guiding principle of "Primum Non-Nocere," which translates to "first, do no harm" in Latin. This serves as a reminder that surgery involves risks, may not necessarily result in the intended outcome, and may even cause additional harm. Therefore, prioritizing and ensuring that a patient will have clinically significant benefit from surgery is the primary step in the decision-making process. Better nonsurgical alternatives should be sought out and entertained when surgical risks

are higher than their real benefits. For instance, in some cases, this has led to the disappearance of highly morbid acid reduction surgery for peptic ulcer disease, as we came to understand and better treat the underlying causes.

The next step is to determine if surgery is viable. The decision varies depending on the patient's condition, the technical demands of the disease, and the available health care resources. A surgeon's experience and infrastructure (operating room [OR], blood bank, life support machinery, intensive care unit [ICU] capacity, specialty care consultants) should also be considered. If any of these technical requirements are not met, the patient may need to be transferred to another medical facility.

Risk Assessment

The last and most crucial step is to evaluate the patient's ability to undergo the surgery. This assessment is done by carefully reviewing the patient's medical history and conducting a thorough physical examination. It is the basis for all preoperative evaluations and cannot be replaced by routine screening tests. Understanding the patient's past medical conditions, medication usage, allergies, family medical history, and current physical state provides valuable insights to the surgical team. If not already done, pointed questions and physical examinations are carried out to understand the extent of the patient's cardiopulmonary and metabolic reserve, which the proposed surgery will soon stress. Previous surgeries can affect the current operation plan. Anticipating anatomic changes, scar tissue, and adhesions can prevent complications. This also guides in the diagnosis, incision placement, access routes, and the feasibility of minimally invasive approaches. It is important not to overlook social history as it can reveal potential somatic risks to a patient's health and issues that could hinder their recovery process once they leave the hospital, such as economic, familial, and social challenges, access to resources, and transportation.

Once all the necessary information is collected and considered, a personalized risk profile can be created to help guide decisions related to preoperative preparation, surgical readiness, anesthesia planning, postoperative management, and the anticipation of potential complications that may arise during or after surgery. This individualized profile can range from a minimal low-risk profile to an extremely high-risk profile that, with appropriate management, surgery can still be performed. This pairing of surgery and patient is dynamic and should be reevaluated each time a patient undergoes a procedure. For example, the risk profile for a young, healthy individual undergoing an elective hernia repair may be initially low. However, the risk profile will change if a complication arises and a second operation is required during the same hospitalization.

Any initial laboratory or imaging testing should be ordered to confirm or complement this risk profile. A one-size-fits-all model should be discouraged. Ordering a broad-side battery of preoperative screening tests on otherwise low-risk and asymptomatic patients does not improve patient safety and outcomes. There is a misconception that this shotgun approach may reveal medical issues that, while unrelated to the surgical pathology, may interfere with the surgical act, but this is often not the case. Abnormal test results without clinical correlation are frequently ignored and cause confusion. The confusion they create can lead to delays in necessary surgery, a false sense of security, or trigger unnecessary and risky presurgical procedures that could have negative consequences.

Diagnostic Tests Before Surgery

Depending on initially identified perioperative risks some of the laboratory adjuncts most commonly used include:

1. Complete blood count (CBC): A CBC provides information about a patient's red blood cells, white blood cells, and platelets. Anemia, leukocytosis, or thrombocytopenia can indicate potential bleeding or clotting risks.
2. Coagulation studies: Prothrombin time (PT), international normalized ratio (INR), and activated partial thromboplastin time (aPTT) assess the patient's clotting function. Abnormal results might indicate a bleeding tendency or risk of thrombosis.
3. Electrolyte and metabolic panel: This panel includes tests to assess electrolyte levels (sodium, potassium, chloride), kidney function (creatinine, blood urea nitrogen [BUN]), and glucose levels. Abnormalities can impact fluid balance and overall physiologic stability.
4. Liver function tests: These tests evaluate liver enzymes, bilirubin, and albumin levels, offering insights into liver health. Impaired liver function can affect drug metabolism and postoperative recovery.
5. Cardiac biomarkers: Troponin and brain natriuretic peptide (BNP) levels are indicators of cardiac stress or damage. Elevated levels might suggest a heightened risk of perioperative cardiac complications.
6. Hemoglobin A1c (HbA1c): HbA1c reflects long-term glucose control and is particularly relevant for patients with diabetes. Elevated levels could influence wound healing and infection risk.
7. Blood type and crossmatching: Determining blood type and performing crossmatching is crucial for ensuring compatibility during potential blood transfusions, thus important for procedures anticipating significant blood loss (>500 mL).
8. Urinalysis: Assesses information regarding kidney function, hydration status, and signs of urinary tract infections (UTIs).
9. Preoperative imaging: Depending on the procedure, imaging studies like x-rays, computed tomography (CT) scans, or magnetic resonance imaging (MRIs) may be performed to map anatomic structures and assess potential technical risks.

The need for emergency surgery, especially for patients who cannot provide historical data, obviously alters these recommendations. The distinction between emergency and elective surgery is striking. While both types aim to enhance the patient's well-being and restore their health, they differ in timing, preparation, surgical approach, postoperative care, and, most importantly, morbidity and mortality. Table 1-1 summarizes the implications for patients,

TABLE 1-1. General Characteristics and Differences Between Elective Versus Emergency Surgery		
Category	**Emergency Surgery**	**Elective Surgery**
Timing	Immediacy, often within minutes to hours	Scheduled at a convenient time
Flexibility	Cannot be scheduled or delayed	Can be postponed
Indications	Trauma, perforated viscus, necrotizing soft tissue infection	Hernia repairs, joint replacements, cancer resections
Patient physiologic status	Patients present usually in shock	Patients are in the usual state of preoperative health.
Preparedness	Limited preoperative assessment	Comprehensive preoperative workup
Risks of complications	Increased risks due to urgency	Managed risks through preoperative optimization
Assessing cardiac risks	Rapid assessment, basic ECGs	Comprehensive assessment with stress tests, echocardiograms
Assessing pulmonary risks	Limited evaluation, rely on clinical judgment	Advanced testing, pulmonary function tests
Intraoperative monitoring	Paramount due to limited preassessment	Also important but may be less critical
Informed consent	Limited scope, may have legal exceptions sometimes obtained via a surrogate or post hoc	Comprehensive, exhaustive
Resource allocation	Rapid allocation of available resources. It may require a system-wide approach.	Planned allocation that can bring additional resources when necessary
Mortality	Generally higher, baseline in lowest ASA category can be 3%-15% depending on condition, increases with each ASA category	Generally lower, approx. 0.5%-3% depending on procedure

ASA, American Society of Anesthesiologists; ECG, electrocardiogram;

surgeons, and health care systems. These differences are significant, and the mortality rate is notably higher in those who undergo emergency procedures. Table 1-2 shows the American Society of Anesthesiologists (ASA) classification system, a very early but still used, for surgical patients, guiding intraoperative management. An emergency surgery will be assigned a letter "E" to indicate this condition and upgrade the need for added measures.

Preoperative Consultations for Risk Mitigation and Optimization of the Surgical Patient

Specialty consultation may be required to optimize the patient's chance of a successful operation. Medical consultants should not be asked to "clear" patients for a surgical procedure; their primary value is in helping to define the degree of perioperative risk and making recommendations about how best to prepare the patient. Postoperative consultation should be sought when the patient has unexpected complications or does not respond to initial maneuvers commonly employed to address a specific problem. For example, a nephrology consultation is for a patient who remains oliguric despite appropriate intravascular volume repletion, particularly if the creatinine level is rising. Likewise, consultation should be obtained from specialists with expertise in areas where the treating physician does not have sufficient knowledge. In this case, a general surgeon would be well advised to obtain consultation from a cardiologist for a patient with a postoperative

myocardial infarction, no matter how benign the myocardial infarction appears.

Next, we will examine the main risk profiles and perioperative health conditions that must be assessed and closely monitored in patients undergoing surgery.

Cardiovascular Risk Assessment and Perioperative Management

Managing cardiovascular risk during the perioperative period is a complex task, especially in cases when patients have complex medical histories. As surgical procedures become more advanced, the need for accurate risk assessment and optimization of cardiovascular function has become even more critical. To meet these demands, ever-increasing methods for sophisticated evaluation are employed to ensure that patients receive the best possible assessment and appropriate care.

The concept of "cardiac clearance" is completely inaccurate. **Clinicians assess cardiovascular risk**. Since the 1970s, various scoring systems have been developed to measure the risk of cardiovascular disease starting with the initial Goldman criteria. Over time, with the advancement of cardiovascular sciences, better instruments like the Eagle Preoperative Risk Assessment Tool, the Revised Cardiac Risk Index (RCRI), the Myocardial Infarction or Cardiac Arrest (MICA) calculator, and from the surgical side, the American College of Surgeons Surgical Risk Calculator have been created. Factors such as patient

ASA Class	Description	Examples	Suggested Anesthesia Management
ASA I	A normal healthy patient	Healthy, nonsmoking, no or minimal alcohol use	Standard anesthesia protocols; lower risk for anesthesia-related complications
ASA II	A patient with mild systemic disease	Mild diseases without substantive functional limitations, such as controlled hypertension and diabetes	Standard protocols with slight modifications based on specific conditions; close monitoring of vitals and blood glucose levels if diabetic
ASA III	A patient with severe systemic disease that is not incapacitating	Poorly controlled diabetes, COPD, morbid obesity	Tailored anesthesia plan considering specific disease conditions; increased intraoperative monitoring; may require ICU postoperatively
ASA IV	A patient with severe systemic disease that is a constant threat to life	Recent myocardial infarction, congestive heart failure, severe sepsis	High-risk case; multidisciplinary approach including cardiology, pulmonology, etc; likely ICU postoperatively; consider regional anesthesia to minimize systemic effects
ASA V	A moribund patient who is not expected to survive without the operation	Ruptured abdominal/thoracic aneurysm, massive trauma, intracranial hemorrhage	Extreme caution; maximize all available resuscitative measures; multiple consultations with various specialties; almost certain ICU postoperatively
ASA VI	A patient who has been declared brain dead whose organs are being removed for donor purposes	–	Tailored anesthesia aimed at preserving organ function for transplantation
E	Emergency surgery	An addendum placed after the ASA score, for instance, ASA III-E	Increased risk; rapid assessment and intervention; consider regional anesthesia if feasible to minimize systemic effects.

TABLE 1-2. American Society of Anesthesiologists (ASA) Classification and General Recommendations

COPD, chronic obstructive pulmonary disease; ICU, intensive care unit.

age, medical history, functional capacity, relevant electrocardiogram (ECG), laboratory and echocardiographic data, and surgical urgency are used to estimate the risk of adverse cardiovascular events (Table 1-3). Clinicians can use these calculators in the preoperative evaluation to identify high-risk patients and adjust their management accordingly.

Patients with a higher cardiovascular risk may have their surgery delayed. They may undergo further cardiac-specific testing to check for correctable lesions of the coronary arterial anatomy, evaluate overall myocardial function, and given their common pathophysiology, additional unrecognized cardiovascular disease (Table 1-4). This can lead to the initiation of potentially life-saving cardiac interventions and procedures for conditions that might have been identified dramatically during a perioperative crisis (Table 1-5). It is essential to recognize that specific cardiovascular therapies, such as antiplatelet agents and anticoagulants, elevate the risk of surgical bleeding. However, with carefully management of these medications, adequate consultation, effective coordination, and meticulous planning, surgery can still be safely performed, thus constituting a fundamental aspect of the overall process.

Aside from these cardiac-specific plans and interventions, other strategies that should be used to reduce the risk of cardiovascular complications and boost heart function are:

1. Preoperative noncardiac medical optimization: Collaboration between surgical teams, anesthesiologists, primary care, and cardiologists is important to manage chronic conditions such as hypertension and diabetes (Table 1-5). Medications may need to be adjusted, and lifestyle changes may be necessary. Active coronary events and uncompensated heart failure (HF) need to be addressed before other elective surgical pathology.

2. Exercise and fitness enhancement: Cardiopulmonary exercise testing (CPET) can evaluate functional capacity and also detect high-risk patients. Customized exercise plans can improve cardiovascular fitness and decrease the risk of complications.

3. Smoking cessation: Quitting smoking before surgery is crucial for reducing the risk of cardiovascular complications. Programs, nicotine replacement therapy, and counseling can be effective.

4. Nutritional optimization: Poor nutrition can harm heart health, but assessing and optimizing vitamin and mineral levels can help improve cardiovascular function.

5. Stress relief: Stress and anxiety harm the heart. Relaxation techniques like mindfulness and meditation can help stabilize heart rate and blood pressure.

6. Medication management: Evaluate medications carefully to manage cardiovascular risk. Adjustments may be needed to address interactions or adverse effects. For instance, β-blockers may be prescribed during the perioperative period to minimize risk, while calcium channel blockers with pure vasodilatory effect may be suspended before surgery.

Some of these have been included as general overall strategies for all major surgeries, a novel concept called *prehabilitation*, with overall improvements in clinical outcomes, reduction of complications, better utilization of health care resources, and reduced costs.

TABLE 1-3. Categories of Cardiac Risk									
Cardiac Risk Category	History	Physical Examination	Metabolic Reserve	Exercise Tolerance	Echo-cardiography Findings	ECG Findings	CAC Score	Troponin	Other Laboratory
Low risk	No known heart disease	Normal	Good (>7 METs)	Good (>10 min)	Normal EF, no wall motion abnormality	Normal	0-10	Normal	Normal lipid panel
Moderate risk	Controlled hypertension	Mild abnormalities	Moderate (4-7 METs)	Moderate (7-10 min)	Mild LV dysfunction	Nonspecific changes	11-100	Slightly elevated	Abnormal lipid panel
High risk	Prior MI, uncontrolled HTN	Significant abnormalities	Poor (<4 METs)	Poor (<7 min)	Severe LV dysfunction	Pathologic changes	>100	Elevated	Elevated CRP, abnormal coagulation

Metabolic equivalent (MET) is a unit that quantifies the energy expenditure of physical activities, using 1 MET (sitting down quietly) as the baseline for resting metabolic rate. Activities like going up stairs, for instance, may require 4 to 8 METs, representing a 4 to 8-fold increase in energy expenditure compared to resting.

CAC, Cardiac Arterial Calcium Score, is a noninvasive imaging test that quantifies the amount of calcium deposits in coronary arteries using computed tomography (CT).

The score helps assess the risk of coronary artery disease and future cardiac events.

CRP, c-reactive protein; EF, ejection fraction; HTN, hypertension; LV, left ventricle; MI, myocardial infarction.

TABLE 1-4. General Recommendations for Preoperative Cardiac Risk Management

Patient Profile	Recommended Preoperative Tests	Timing	Additional Notes
Low-risk surgery (eg, cataract, skin biopsy)	None unless clinically indicated	N/A	Assess need based on symptoms, not type of surgery
Intermediate risk surgery (eg, abdominal, orthopedic)	**ECG, CBC, basic metabolic panel**	1-2 wk prior	ECG is recommended if patient has known heart disease, significant hypertension, or is >65 years old.
High-risk surgery (eg, cardiac, vascular, thoracic)	**ECG, CBC, basic metabolic panel, echocardiogram, stress test** (if indicated), **CAC Score** (if indicated)	2-4 wk prior	Consider cardiology consultation. Assess for cerebrovascular and peripheral vascular disease.
History of cardiac disease	**ECG—echocardiogram, cardiac stress test, CAC Score** (if indicated)	2-4 wk prior	Cardiology consultation is often warranted. Assess for cerebrovascular and peripheral vascular disease.
Multiple cardiovascular risk factors	**ECG—echocardiogram, cardiac stress test, CAC Score, cardiac MRI** (if indicated)	2-4 wk prior	A thorough assessment should be done to identify any need for intervention before surgery. Assess for cerebrovascular and peripheral vascular disease.
Age >65 with comorbid conditions	**ECG, CBC, basic metabolic panel, echocardiogram** (if indicated), **CAC Score** (if indicated)	1-3 wk prior	Older adults should be evaluated carefully, especially if comorbid conditions like hypertension, diabetes, etc, are present.
Asymptomatic but family history of cardiac issues	**ECG** (potentially), **CBC, basic metabolic panel, CAC Score** (if indicated)	1-2 wk prior	Consider more thorough tests if the patient's family history suggests increased risk.
Emergency surgery	**Focused cardiac ultrasound (FoCUS)** if available, **point-of-care ECG, rapid CBC** and **metabolic panel**	Immediately or within minutes	Cardiac evaluation should be as rapid as possible without delaying necessary surgical intervention.
Cardiac arrhythmia	**ECG, Holter monitoring, echocardiogram**—electrophysiology study (if indicated), **CAC Score** (if indicated)	2-4 wk prior	Cardiology consultation is essential; antiarrhythmic medication adjustments may be needed. Assess for cerebrovascular and peripheral vascular disease.

The inclusion of the CAC Score is primarily for those at risk for coronary artery disease (CAD) or those with a history of cardiac disease. It can help guide the need for more aggressive risk modification and the possible need for revascularization procedures before surgery.

CAC, coronary artery calcium; CBC, complete blood count; ECG, electrocardiogram; MRI, magnetic resonance imaging.

Pulmonary Risk Assessment and Perioperative Management

Next to cardiovascular events, perioperative pulmonary complications are the second most significant concern for morbidity and mortality in surgical patients, especially those with preexisting respiratory conditions. Volatile anesthetic agents may irritate the respiratory mucosa, potentially triggering reflex-mediated bronchoconstriction and inflammation of both the vocal cords and airways.

Positive pressure ventilation used during inhalational anesthesia can modify pulmonary dynamics to levels that may cause injury (either from pressure—barotrauma or volume—volutrauma). Mechanical ventilation can lead to the derecruitment of functional alveolar units, compromising gas exchange. Paralytic agents and steroids reduce diaphragm muscle strength, weakening spontaneous inspiratory effort after surgery. All these factors make it difficult to wean the patient off ventilatory support postoperatively.

TABLE 1-5. List of Tiered Cardiac Interventions

Preoperative Cardiac Risk	Tiered Approach of Recommended Cardiac Interventions
Low risk	• Lifestyle modifications • Statin therapy (in line with guidelines) • Routine postoperative monitoring
Moderate risk	• β-Blockers (if not contraindicated) • Comprehensive cardiac evaluation • Angiography/CT angiogram • Antiplatelet therapy (aspirin/clopidogrel) • Consider elective PCI for significant obstructions
High risk	• Immediate cardiac assessment • Inotropic support (eg, dobutamine) • Aggressive antiplatelet and anticoagulant therapy • Consider early coronary artery bypass graft (CABG) • Mechanical support (IABP, ECMO)

CT, computed tomography; ECMO, extracorporeal membrane oxygenation; IABP, intra-aortic balloon pump; PCI, percutaneous coronary intervention.

Clinical evaluation remains the most important tool in assessing the respiratory system. Taking a detailed medical history that focuses on tobacco use and on respiratory conditions such as chronic obstructive pulmonary disease (COPD), asthma, prior reactions to general inhalational anesthesia, issues with endotracheal intubation, or recent respiratory infections provides vital information for creating an anesthesia plan, which may involve regional or general techniques; developing a postsurgical respiratory treatment plan; and identifying potential interventions. On surgery day, a brief physical examination is conducted to listen to breath sounds and evaluate chest movements. This helps to identify any underlying respiratory issues that may require the surgical intervention to be canceled. Ongoing tobacco use may lead to the cancelation of elective surgery. Urine nicotine detection screening on the day of surgery may be used for this purpose.

Chest x-rays or CT scans are recommended for patients undergoing intrathoracic procedures and those with signs and symptoms of active cardiac or pulmonary disease. Specialized testing is indicated for patients who are expected to undergo an operation that carries a relatively high intrinsic risk of pulmonary complications.

Pulmonary function tests (PFTs) are used to measure ventilatory function through spirometry and lung volume measurements. The impact of neurodegenerative diseases can be measured with some of these tests. In addition, they measure gas exchange capacity through diffusing capacity of the lungs for carbon monoxide (DLCO). The values of the former can be improved dynamically with bronchodilators and other medications that should be scheduled as part of the perioperative treatment plan. On the other hand, the latter cannot be improved and, if significantly abnormal, it limits the amount of lung tissue removal during surgery or indicates a need for ventilatory support in the ICU after the operation.

Arterial blood gas (ABG) is a critical diagnostic tool to evaluate the physiologic status of oxygenation and acid-base balance. In patients with chronic respiratory insufficiency, ABGs should ideally exhibit compensatory mechanisms that counterbalance deficits in gas exchange and pH buffering. The absence of appropriate compensatory responses can be a warning sign, suggesting underlying issues in other crucial physiologic systems, including the cardiovascular, endocrine, and renal systems.

Risk indices, such as ARISCAT (assess respiratory risk in surgical patients in Catalonia), provide a measurable indicator of the pulmonary risk during the perioperative period, and their usage is becoming more widespread. These indices are continuously improved to provide increasingly accurate predictive models, which can guide adjustments in perioperative management.

Intraoperative and Postoperative Mitigation Strategies to Decrease Pulmonary Complications

With the exception for some genetic predispositions, many factors that contribute to pulmonary complications during surgery are like those causing cardiovascular issues. Fortunately, both types of complications can be mitigated by sharing mitigation strategies that have been already discussed in this chapter. Table 1-6 summarizes specific pulmonary considerations. Thoracic surgery has its own specific subcategory of risks, which will be discussed elsewhere in this textbook. Some beneficial perioperative pulmonary management strategies are as follows:

1. Lung-protective ventilation: Lower tidal volumes and positive end-expiratory pressures (PEEP) have decreased postoperative pulmonary complications.
2. Restrictive fluid management during surgery: Conservative fluid strategies can minimize pulmonary edema.
3. Positioning: Proper surgical positioning can optimize or compromise lung function. Thus, special attention should be provided when a patient is in a prone or Trendelenburg position.
4. Postoperative interventions:
   a. Early mobilization: Encouraging patients to walk and move can reduce atelectasis and respiratory infections.
   b. Incentive spirometry: Utilization postoperatively can improve lung function.
   c. Pharmacotherapy: appropriate use of bronchodilators, mucolytics, and occasionally corticosteroids. Postoperative pain management is very important as

TABLE 1-6. Pulmonary Risk Assessment and Mitigation Strategies

Risk Category	Clinical Indicators	Preoperative Assessment	Perioperative Consideration	Postoperative Measures
Low risk	ASA 1-2 No history of respiratory illness Nonsmoking or quit >6 mo	Baseline SpO_2 >94% Normal FEV1/FVC ratio	Standard anesthesia protocol Supplemental oxygen as needed	Routine postoperative care No specific respiratory monitoring required
Moderate risk	ASA 3 Mild to moderate COPD or asthma Current or recent smoker	Baseline SpO_2 90%-94% FEV1/FVC ratio moderately reduced	Lung-protective ventilation strategy Invasive monitoring as needed	Enhanced respiratory monitoring Early mobilization encouraged
High risk	ASA 4-5 severe COPD or restrictive lung disease Acute or recent pneumonia	Baseline SpO_2 <90% FEV1/FVC ratio severely reduced	Consult pulmonologist for advanced respiratory management Consider regional anesthesia if possible	ICU admission may be required. Close respiratory monitoring
Very high risk	Severe respiratory failure requiring mechanical ventilation Active pulmonary infection	Arterial blood gas analysis, comprehensive pulmonary function tests	Consult multidisciplinary team including pulmonologist and anesthesiologist. Strong consideration for postponing elective procedures	Likely ICU admission Ventilatory support may be required.

ASA, American Society of Anesthesiologists; COPD, chronic obstructive pulmonary disease; FEV1/FVC (forced expiratory volume in the first one second/forced vital capacity); ICU, intensive care unit.

some narcotics may induce respiratory depression. Use of regional anesthesia or axial blockade such as an epidural catheter can improve tremendously recovery by decreasing opioid use and consequent side effects and encouraging early mobility and its protective benefits (reduction of pneumonia and venous thromboembolic events).

c. ERAS Protocols: All the above can be protocolized in a streamlined approach that can standardize care and proactively prevent respiratory complications.

e. Telemedicine: remote monitoring of patient's respiratory status for early intervention

Perioperative Renal Risk Assessment and Management of Renal Dysfunction

Around 30% to 50% of surgical patients have some degree of preexisting chronic kidney disease (CKD). Conversely, 1% to 5% of perioperative patients will exhibit some form of acute renal impairment (acute kidney injury—AKI), but it can be as high as 20% in all hospitalized patients. Renal disease significantly impacts surgical outcomes, with a 2- to 4-fold increase in perioperative morbidity and mortality. Sepsis, hemorrhage, and cardiovascular events are common complications, with acute kidney disease and CKD being independent risk factors for their occurrence. Unfortunately, these risks do not diminish with renal replacement therapy. Therefore, it is paramount to avoid new-onset AKI or increased severity of CKD.

AKI is a sudden loss of renal function. Risk factors for its appearance include hypovolemia, severe infection, sepsis, and certain medications such as nonsteroidal anti-inflammatory drugs (NSAIDs) and antibiotics.

There are several classification systems for AKI based on urine output and laboratory markers such as BUN and creatinine, which can used to predict temporal or permanent impairment of glomerular filtration rate (GFR). CKD implies nephron loss and no eventual recovery of function. CKD is classified into five stages based on GFR. A decrease in GFR below 60 mL/min/1.73 m^2 indicates significant impairment and a need for medication adjustments that have renal clearance. Further decreases in GFR may indicate the need for dialysis.

As in other sections within this chapter, a multidisciplinary approach that incorporates the expertise of anesthesiologists, nephrologists, and surgeons is crucial for optimizing patient outcomes. Careful planning and evidence-based interventions can mitigate the risks associated with renal dysfunction, thereby improving the overall quality of care.

Anesthesia selection in patients with renal impairment is a delicate balancing act that requires consideration of multiple factors, including drug metabolism and excretion, hemodynamic stability, and potential nephrotoxic effects. Renal disease significantly affects both the pharmacokinetics and pharmacodynamics of anesthetic agents. Drugs such as morphine are primarily cleared by the kidney, thus can accumulate in the body and require dosage adjustments. Alterations in fluid balance can affect the volume of distribution for hydrophilic drugs, leading to altered drug concentrations failing to reach their effective receptor threshold or site of action.

Significant consideration should be given to the choice and use of anesthetic agents. While generally considered safe, propofol, by causing hypotension, can impact renal function. Sevoflurane can exacerbate existing renal dysfunction due to its fluoride metabolites. Desflurane has minimal renal clearance and is a reasonable choice in patients with renal impairment. Neuromuscular blockers exclusively cleared by the kidneys may remain in circulation longer than their predicted half-life and lead to prolonged residual effects of paralysis, especially of the diaphragm. Regional anesthesia utilization can avoid risks caused by a lack of renal drug clearance. Techniques such as epidurals or peripheral nerve blocks can assist in reducing overall anesthetic and analgesic drug usage.

Impaired renal clearance also influences the choice of analgesic medication. For instance, morphine should be used with caution as its metabolites (M3G and M6G) can accumulate in patients with renal failure, potentially causing neurotoxicity. Fentanyl and remifentanil are preferable as they are eliminated through nonrenal routes. On the other hand, NSAIDs should be avoided, as they may worsen renal dysfunction and affect the half-life of other drugs. Acetaminophen is a safer alternative in such cases.

Table 1-7 summarizes some of the recommendations for perioperative management in patients with chronic renal dysfunction. Surgical interventions should ideally employ minimally invasive or endovascular techniques whenever possible. These methods are generally associated with reduced blood loss and minimized shifts in bodily fluids, which lessen AKI. Maintenance of euvolemia and renal perfusion is the goal in the perioperative management of patients with CKD or AKI. A judicious use of balanced crystalloid solutions is recommended to avoid both hypo and hypervolemia, which exert undue stress on the kidneys. Electrolyte replacements and hypotonic or hypertonic solutions should be cautiously used, especially in patients with preexisting renal conditions. Avoidance of hypotension and careful administration of medications that can induce this can prevent exacerbation of renal failure.

The management of blood loss requires special attention in patients with CKD. CKD often leads to normochromic, normocytic anemia due to decreased erythropoietin production. Kidney-related coagulation disorders can arise from recent heparinization during dialysis, from the prolonged half-life of antiplatelet and anticoagulant medications, or from interference with the coagulation cascade during a uremic state. A coagulation profile and modern viscoelastic tests can help identify some of these intrinsic deficiencies. Intraoperative administration of D-Desmino arginine vasopressin (DDAVP) can help address some kidney disease–related coagulopathy by promoting the release of von Willebrand factor associated with endothelial cells. Excellent surgical technique, abundant use of topical

TABLE 1-7. General Recommendations for Perioperative CKD Risk Management

eGFR (mL/min/1.73 m^2)	CKD Stage	Perioperative Risk	Rate of Complications (%)	Mortality Rate	Perioperative Recommendations	Tiered Management Approach
>90	Stage 1	Low risk	1-3	<1	Routine monitoring, no special interventions	Monitor for other comorbidities.
60-89	Stage 2	Low-moderate risk	4-6	1-2	Closer monitoring, optimize fluid management.	Consult with nephrologist if necessary.
45-59	Stage 3a	Moderate risk	10-15	3-5	Preoperative nephrology consult, adjust medications, avoid nephrotoxic agents.	Potential for post-op AKI
30-44	Stage 3b	High risk	20-30	6-10	Comprehensive nephrology evaluation, consider postponing elective surgery.	Strict fluid and electrolyte management
15-29	Stage 4	Very high risk	30-50	11-20	Strongly consider postponing elective surgery, preoperative renal replacement therapy if needed.	High risk of AKI, renal failure
<15 (or on dialysis)	Stage 5	Extremely high risk	>50	>20	Only proceed with life-saving surgeries, pre- and postoperative dialysis.	Potential need for post-op ICU care, as they may need CRRT.

AKI, acute kidney injury; CKD, chronic kidney disease; CRRT, continuous renal replacement therapy; ICU, intensive care unit.

hemostatic agents, and energy devices such as electrocautery can be invaluable in controlling bleeding. These approaches can reduce the need for blood transfusions, which carry their own risks of exacerbating renal impairment.

After surgery, it is essential to keep a close eye on the patient's clinical condition and laboratory results to detect any signs of AKI or other renal problems at an early stage. This requires monitoring urine output, conducting appropriately scheduled laboratory tests, and possibly using renal ultrasound to evaluate the kidney's structure and function. It is crucial to maintain euvolemia and normal electrolyte values, as imbalances can lead to kidney stress, worsen existing renal impairment, or precipitate new-onset dysfunction. Daily weighing and accurate recording of intake and output are essential. The assistance of a clinical pharmacist is indispensable in providing advice on how to adjust the dosage and scheduled administration of medications to these patients. Renal function is monitored by accurate assessment of the fluid balance and periodic measurements of the markers of renal function (creatinine and BUN). Renal dialysis may be needed when the patient cannot manage their own fluid balance, or when the detoxification or excretory function of the kidney is not performing properly. Examples of this would include volume overload with overt congestive HF in a patient who have anuria, life-threatening hyperkalemia, and intractable acidosis. If postoperative renal dysfunction persists for more than 3 months, it is termed CKD.

Metabolic Risks for Surgery—The Impact of Diabetes and Blood Glucose Control in Perioperative Management

As of 2021, over 34 million Americans (about 10.5% of the U.S population) have diabetes according to the Centers for Disease Control and Prevention (CDC). The International Diabetes Federation (IDF) estimates that globally, around 463 million adults had diabetes in 2019, and this number is projected to rise to 700 million by 2045. Around 25% of patients with diabetes in the United States undergo some form of surgical procedure annually, which translates to roughly 8.5 million surgical cases involving patients with diabetes annually in the United States alone.

Diabetes mellitus (DM) is a complex metabolic disorder that has a significant impact on surgical pathophysiology. Patients suffering from DM pose unique challenges during perioperative management, including changes in the inflammatory response and an increased risk for complications such as poor wound healing, infections, and organ failure. DM affects individual cellular and whole-body homeostasis, leading to diverse adverse effects both during and after surgery. Conversely, stress from surgery triggers a hormonal response which makes it challenging to manage blood sugar levels, even for those who do not usually require insulin. Postoperative complications, especially those of infectious nature, increase dramatically blood glucose levels. Therefore, careful glucose monitoring and insulin management are crucial and part of the fundamental knowledge of a surgeon.

Elevated blood sugar levels and DM-associated conditions like hyperlipidemia have a significant impact on the development of surgical pathologies, particularly cardiovascular and renal diseases. DM is also considered to be a part of a larger metabolic syndrome, which is still not fully understood. When combined with obesity, hypertension, hyperlipidemia, sleep apnea, and cardiovascular dysfunction, this syndrome can cause adverse surgical and nonsurgical outcomes.

Diabetes disrupts the normal healing process by affecting collagen synthesis and maturation. High blood sugar impairs the ability of fibroblasts to produce and deposit collagen. The glycation of collagen also reduces its tensile strength, which can cause wounds to split open. Hyperglycemic conditions make it harder for new blood vessels to form, impairing the delivery of oxygen and nutrients to the healing tissues. Diabetes delays the initiation of the healing process by impairing macrophages' ability to migrate toward the wound site. In addition, diabetes favors an inflammatory environment that is less conducive to effective healing by the over selection of pro-inflammatory M1 macrophages over regulatory M2 macrophages. This hyperinflammatory response paradoxically suppresses appropriate immune function and defense mechanisms, which raises the risk of postoperative infections. Neutrophil migration and phagocytic functions are also compromised in the diabetic setting, which can further prolong the healing process.

Diabetic Ketoacidosis

Diabetic ketoacidosis (DKA) is a dangerous and potentially life-threatening complication of diabetes that can be particularly concerning during surgery. DKA can cause many problems, including electrolyte imbalances and metabolic acidosis, and pose significant risks to multiple organ systems. High levels of ketone bodies, especially β-hydroxybutyrate, produce myocardial depression decreasing cardiac output. This worsens an already fragile hemodynamic state during the perioperative period. The acidotic environment in DKA can impair vascular smooth muscle function, leading to peripheral vasodilation and hypotension. This can be particularly dangerous during and after surgery, as it may lead to total cardiovascular collapse if not managed promptly and effectively. DKA creates an acidic intracellular environment that can affect neuronal ion channels, potentially altering how patients respond to anesthesia and later cognitive recovery. In extreme cases, DKA may contribute to severe impairments like coma and seizures. The body's attempt to compensate for metabolic acidosis through hyperventilation can lead to respiratory muscle fatigue and respiratory failure. Electrolyte imbalances and volume depletion can lead to or aggravate AKI and eventually renal failure, requiring emergency renal replacement therapy and further complicating recovery from surgery. The resulting cascade of organ failures, along with other hepatic and hematologic dysfunctions, can ultimately result in death.

ICU admission with subsequent supportive care, insulin infusions, and close monitoring of metabolic values (such as acid-balance balance, anion gap closure, and ketone bodies) are the pillars of DKA management during the perioperative period.

Hypoglycemia

Hypoglycemia is a condition where the blood glucose levels drop below 70 mg/dL. This can create significant challenges and risks during the perioperative period. Although hyperglycemia is more commonly discussed, the dangers of hypoglycemia are equally alarming but often overlooked.

Hypoglycemia can trigger a sympathetic response, leading to the release of adrenaline and other catecholamines. This can cause tachycardia, palpitations, and even myocardial ischemia, which is particularly concerning for patients with preexisting cardiovascular disease and low physiologic reserve. Low levels of glucose in the blood can cause cognitive impairment, reduced reaction time, and in severe cases, coma, or seizures. These neurologic effects can be particularly dangerous when patients are under anesthesia, as they may not be noticed until permanent damage has already occurred. Hypoglycemia can affect liver enzyme function, changing the metabolism of anesthetic agents and other medications and making their effects unpredictable. It is also important to think about the long-term consequences of hypoglycemia. Repeated occurrences of low blood sugar levels have been linked with a gradual decline in cognitive function, which is especially concerning for older patients or those undergoing multiple surgical procedures. Frequent hypoglycemic occurrences can lead to a state of "unawareness" where the patient no longer experiences the typical warning signs of low blood sugar levels. This can be especially problematic during surgery as it is important to act quickly to avoid damage to glucose-dependent cells like neurons, myocytes, and renal tubular cells.

The NICE-SUGAR (normoglycemia in intensive care evaluation-survival using glucose algorithm regulation) trial is one of the most comprehensive randomized controlled studies (RCT [randomized controlled trial]) that have been conducted to date. It was designed to examine the impact of tight glucose control in an intensive care setting, including surgical patients. The study found that tight glucose control (81-108 mg/dL) led to a higher mortality rate than conventional glucose control (180 mg/dL or less), primarily due to a significant increase in severe hypoglycemia episodes. These results have ignited a debate on the optimal glucose control strategies during the perioperative period. It suggests that overly aggressive glycemic control may only sometimes be beneficial, emphasizing the need for a more nuanced, individualized approach to insulin management in surgical settings.

Glycemic Targets

The American Diabetes Association (ADA) suggests that individuals should maintain their blood glucose levels between 80 and 180 mg/dL before any surgery. If the glucose levels are higher than 200 mg/dL on the day of surgery, an elective operation may need to be postponed. This is because the patient's insulin responsiveness may be unpredictable in this highly stressful situation. During the surgery itself, both the ADA and the American Association of Clinical Endocrinologists (AACE) recommend that blood glucose levels should be within the same 80 to 180 mg/dL range. Maintaining blood glucose levels within this range has demonstrated a clear reduction in wound and infection complications, but importantly the risk of cardiovascular events and AKI. After surgery, the aim is generally to keep blood glucose levels within the range of 140 to 180 mg/dL during the first 48 hours. However, in certain cases, such as in cardiothoracic surgery, a tighter control of 110 to 140 mg/dL may be considered. Nonetheless, for all other surgeries, the risks of hypoglycemia must be weighed against the benefits before assigning the patient to a tight control regimen.

Insulin Protocols

Multiple recent studies have demonstrated that a basal-bolus insulin regimen is more effective than Insulin Sliding Scale (ISS) in managing perioperative hyperglycemia. However, it is important to exercise caution for all regimens when patients are nothing per os (NPO) and provide a carbohydrate source such as 5% solution of dextrose to prevent hypoglycemia. Continuous insulin infusion (insulin drip) is the most often recommended setting in critical care situations. However, it requires frequent glucose monitoring, thus decreasing patient satisfaction, as well as adjustments to the infusion rate, making it labor-intensive. One commonly cited protocol is the Yale Insulin Infusion Protocol. ISS regimens, although widely used, have been less effective and associated with a higher risk of both hyperglycemia and hypoglycemia than basal-bolus or continuous infusion regimens. This is a problem associated with the patient's food intake and compliance to diet, common in the postoperative period. Some protocols advocate for supplemental correctional insulin for glucose levels exceeding the target range's upper threshold. Given the heterogeneity in response to insulin sensitivity, a tailored approach that considers patient-specific factors such as insulin sensitivity, prior insulin responsiveness, and type of surgery is gaining traction. A specialized endocrinology consultation is often recommended to adjust insulin regimens and address any complications, such as in patients with brittle diabetes, prior hypoglycemia unawareness, or recurrent DKA episodes.

The Patient With Brittle Diabetes

Patients with brittle diabetes pose a significant challenge in surgical settings due to their rapidly fluctuating blood glucose levels. Surgical procedures such as total pancreatectomy can cause brittle diabetes, and pancreas transplantation may be the best solution. Continuous glucose monitoring (CGM) devices can provide health care providers with more detailed information on patient glucose patterns, and advanced CGM devices can automatically deliver insulin, providing tighter glycemic control. However, the effectiveness of these systems in the immediate postoperative period is still being studied. When it comes to anesthesia, techniques with less impact on glucose metabolism should be selected. Vigilant intraoperative monitoring is necessary, with frequent glucose monitoring (every 15-30 minutes) and microdosing of fast-acting insulin to help with rapid adjustments. Postsurgery, endocrinologists should be consulted to determine the best timing and method for transitioning back to subcutaneous insulin. Nutrition planning is crucial, and a return to normal eating patterns should be coordinated carefully with insulin management. Patients may benefit from meditation and other coping mechanisms during this period, as psychological stress can also impact blood sugar levels in these patients.

Risk Profile for Special Surgical Situations

Perioperative surgical risks also escalate significantly in patients with comorbidities such as liver disease, cancer, sepsis, and those who have undergone organ transplantation. The Model for End-Stage Liver Disease (MELD) score is a critical prognostic tool for patients with liver disease, aiding in the risk stratification before surgery. A high MELD score indicates severe liver dysfunction, potentially elevating risks related to drug metabolism, clotting abnormalities, perioperative bleeding, poor wound healing, and infection. Surgery on these extremely high-risk patients should only be performed in specialized centers with ample resources. Patients with cancer are inherently immunocompromised due to both the malignancy and adjuvant treatments like chemotherapy, posing greater susceptibility to postoperative infections and delayed wound healing. It is imperative to consider the timing of surgery to attain the best possible outcome in terms of cancer treatment and wound healing. Sepsis, an extreme systemic response to infection, can exacerbate perioperative complications by impairing multiple organ systems and amplifying the body's inflammatory response, sometimes leading to septic shock and multiple organ failure. Patients with recent bone marrow or solid organ transplants are particularly vulnerable as they are on potent immunosuppressive therapy to prevent organ rejection or graft-versus-host disease, rendering them highly susceptible to postoperative infections and poor wound healing. Many of these patients require a multidisciplinary approach that includes subspecialized anesthesiologists, hepatologists, oncologists, infectious disease specialists, and transplant teams to mitigate risks. Perioperative care in these groups involves meticulous preoperative screening, strategic choice of surgical technique, and vigilant postoperative monitoring to preempt and manage complications effectively. Given the complex interplay of these conditions, clinical decision-making should be highly individualized and based on a thorough risk-benefit analysis, considering the latest evidence and guidelines in the field.

Coagulopathy

Coagulopathy is a pathologic condition wherein the blood's coagulation ability is impaired. An unrecognized or inadequately managed coagulopathy in the perioperative setting can lead to excessive bleeding, necessitating transfusion, and potentially increasing morbidity and mortality. The clinical history remains the most essential tool in screening for coagulopathy. Traditional clotting tests such as PT, PTT, and INR are often used but may not capture the entire picture of a patient's coagulation status. Point-of-care tests like rotational thromboelastometry (ROTEM) or thromboelastography (TEG) provide a more comprehensive understanding and should be utilized more frequently. Addressing coagulopathy proactively through risk assessment, tailored prophylaxis, and vigilant monitoring is essential for preventing hemorrhagic complications.

Temperature Management

Perioperative hypothermia is a condition that is often underestimated in its potential to induce complications. Lowered body temperature impairs cellular function, leads to vasoconstriction, and can exacerbate coagulopathy—forming a part of what is commonly called the "lethal diamond of death," including acidosis and hypocalcemia. Active warming measures, such as forced-air warming systems or warm intravenous (IV) fluids, controlling operative environmental temperature are simple yet effective ways to maintain normothermia and mitigate associated

risks. Postsurgery fever (and hyperthermia) can be worrisome as it heightens the body's demand for oxygen and energy, without any true physiologic advantage. This can pose challenges since surgical patients may already be in a fasting state, have respiratory insufficiencies, and reduced gastrointestinal function. Inadequate aerobic adenosine triphosphate (ATP) production can impair the functioning of high energy-demand tissues (like the brain, heart, and certain parts of the nephron), prompting the use of anaerobic pathways and the accumulation of lactic acid and acid-base imbalance. Hormonal responses are triggered reflexively to mobilize energy sources, but this can hinder wound healing by prioritizing short-term glucose gain over protein synthesis.

The Lethal Diamond of Death

The concept of the lethal diamond of death encapsulates four interlinked physiologic aberrations that frequently occur in the perioperative and trauma settings: hypothermia, acidosis, coagulopathy, and hypocalcemia. These conditions often synergistically worsen each other, creating a vicious cycle that is difficult to break and irreversibly fatal. Management involves a multimodal approach targeting all four facets. Failing to address even one can unravel the efforts put into managing the others.

The significance of optimizing coagulopathy management, maintaining body temperature, and reducing bacterial colonization cannot be overstated. While the spotlight often falls on surgical technique and immediate postoperative care, these ancillary factors are crucial in determining patient outcomes. Recognizing and addressing these factors proactively can markedly improve the safety and efficacy of surgical interventions, ultimately serving the overarching goal of better patient care.

Reduction of Bacterial Colonization

Proper control of bacterial colonization is crucial to reduce the risk of surgical-site infections (SSI) during surgery. We are barely starting to understand the importance of the influence of a patient's microbiome (the community of bacteria living on and inside the individual) regarding surgical interventions and their outcomes. In the meantime, we try to reduce potentially pathogenic bacteria that could negatively impact the surgical process. Preoperative antibiotics are currently standard, and additional measures like chlorhexidine skin preparation and intraoperative antimicrobial irrigation can further decrease bacterial load. Preoperative antibiotic selection should be specific and tailored to achieve high peak concentrations in the anatomic areas about to be intervened.

For specific cases like colorectal surgeries, a bowel preparation regimen has also been proven effective. Careful surgical techniques with gentle tissue handling and separate instrument trays are equally important. In some cases, staged surgery or delays in primary closure may be necessary to allow the individual's immune system to control bacterial colonization before final reconstruction. Combining these strategies can minimize SSI risk and improve surgical outcomes. Medical devices like indwelling urine catheters, endotracheal tubes, and central venous access naturally form biofilms containing bacteria. Prompt removal of these devices once they are no longer needed is crucial to prevent other forms of hospital-acquired infections.

THE GERIATRIC SURGICAL PATIENT

The demographic shift toward an aging population poses new challenges for surgeons. Geriatric patients present a unique surgical landscape characterized by frailty, significant physiologic changes, and, often, complex medical histories. Managed appropriately, these should not represent contraindications for surgical care. As our population ages, the focus on optimizing surgical outcomes in this cohort will become increasingly pertinent, making research in this area both timely and essential.

Physiologic Changes in Aging Patients

Aging is accompanied by systemic physiologic changes that affect multiple organ systems. Reduced cardiovascular reserve, decreased lung function, and impaired renal clearance are some of the changes that can compromise a geriatric patient's resilience to surgical stress. These age-related shifts influence reactions to anesthesia, fluid balance, and potential for wound healing, necessitating tailored perioperative care. Apart from these changes in physiologic reserve, geriatric patients commonly have actual preexisting conditions, multiplying the degrees of risk and incidence of complications. Older patients who have already survived other life-threatening illnesses like heart disease, infections, bowel surgeries, and organ transplants may have lingering effects on their metabolism and immune system. This adds to the complexity of their surgical risk and their postoperative recovery, requiring a team effort from multiple specialists.

Frailty, characterized by reduced physiologic reserve and increased vulnerability to stressors, has emerged as a critical prognostic indicator in geriatric surgery. The assessment of frailty involves various domains, including physical performance, nutritional status, and cognitive function. Various clinical scores are available to evaluate the level of frailty in patients and identify when prehabilitation may be necessary. It is important to note that not all older patients are frail. Ongoing research is being conducted to enhance frailty assessment and develop comprehensive programs to improve surgical outcomes by modifying some of these functional domains.

Weighing the Benefits of Surgery Versus Its Inherent Risks

One of the conundrums that arise in the context of providing surgical care for an older patient is whether to proceed with an aggressive plan of intervention. The calculus of weighing benefits against risks in surgical interventions is a complex interplay of medical science, ethics, and individual patient factors. It is not merely a quantitative assessment but also involves qualitative judgments that account for patient values, life circumstances, and comorbidities. Surgeons and patients should openly discuss these factors, using language that is easy to understand and within the patient's system of values.

Repeated discussions with patients and their families should be held, beginning preoperatively and continuing in the postoperative phase. Generally, patients wish to feel that aggressive medical care will be rendered if there is a reasonable chance for meaningful survival. Newer

quantitative assessment tools have been introduced to eliminate subjectivity and bias. Still, with limitations, these models are becoming more relevant in some of these conversations. Some approaches include:

Predictive analytics: Machine learning algorithms and Artificial Intelligence can now integrate vast amounts of patient data—from lab results to imaging studies—to predict outcomes. These tools can provide a quantitative risk score juxtaposed with the expected benefits.

Validated Risk Assessment Scales: Tools such as the American Society of Anesthesiologists (ASA) Physical Status Classification System, National Surgical Quality Improvement Program (NSQIP), or the RCRI offer validated metrics to stratify perioperative risk. Although not flawless, these scales provide a framework for comparing procedural benefits to risks.

Graded evidence and artificial intelligence: Evidence-based medicine continues to hold a significant position. The most reliable evidence comes from RCTs, meta-analyses, and systematic reviews. However, in some cases, there may be limitations in the available evidence or its applicability to a specific patient, which may require a more personalized approach, relying on the expertise of clinicians. This raises interesting questions about the future use of machine learning and artificial intelligence in health care. Will these models be effective, and can they provide the humane touch that may decide whether a patient chooses to undergo surgery or not?

Within the construct of system of patient's values and beliefs, there are nonmedical circumstances worth mentioning and include:

Life circumstances: such as social determinants, including housing, employment, and family support, can affect postoperative recovery and thus must be factored into the decision-making process, resource allocation, and discharge plans.

Quality of life and patient preferences: The potential benefit is not solely defined by medical outcomes such as survival rates or complications but also by improving the patient's quality of life. Patient-reported outcome measures (PROMs) can be vital for gauging this aspect. In addition, patient preferences should be incorporated into the decision-making calculus, acknowledging that individuals may prioritize different outcomes (eg, pain relief over longevity).

Long-term versus short-term outcomes: Some surgical interventions may offer immediate relief but carry long-term risks, or vice versa. The time horizon for potential benefits and risks should be a part of the discussion. This consideration is especially pertinent in geriatric patients with limited life expectancy and functional reserve.

The Informed Consent Process

The relationship between a patient and their surgeon is one of the strongest in any professional endeavor. The patient comes to the surgeon with a problem, the solution to which may include alteration of the patient's anatomy while they are in a state of total helplessness. There is an immense duty on the part of the surgeon to merit this level of trust. Part of earning this trust involves honest discussions with patients and their families about available choices (including the choice not to operate) and their consequences.

After gathering sufficient information to identify the problem and its contributing factors, the surgeon will discuss various reasonable courses of action with the patient (and their family where necessary) in terms that they can understand. Together, they will select the best course of action. This process is *informed consent* and is not just a one-time event or a form. Informed consent may occur over multiple sessions as the patient has time to digest the information and formulate further questions.

There is an ongoing debate over whether this should shift to an *informed choice* model where physicians engage more fully with patients' values and preferences. Critics argue that the standard informed consent model can be paternalistic, while supporters of the informed choice model advocate for a more balanced doctor-patient relationship and a shared decision-making model. Sometimes, patients cannot speak for themselves. In these situations, the health care team will turn to those who might reasonably be thought to be able to speak on behalf of the patient. Usually, but not always, this is the next of kin. These individuals are known as surrogate decision-makers. Every jurisdiction will have codified how to define and identify these advocates.

Advance directives are legal documents that inform care providers and family members about the general wishes of the patient regarding the level of care to be delivered should the patient not be able to speak for themself. Most people wish to receive enough medical care to alleviate their suffering and give them a reasonable chance of enjoying the remainder of their lives in a functional manner. However, the definitions of "reasonable" and "functional" are up for interpretation and will vary among individuals. Similar to informed choice, these definitions should follow the patient's values and preferences, information that may be gathered sometimes indirectly from the patient's surrogates.

ON THE DAY OF SURGERY

Operative Suite Preparations

In each of the forthcoming chapters of this textbook, we will cover the necessary preparations and technical operative aspects for the anesthesia and surgical team to carry out successful operations. These preparations include, but are not limited to, positioning the patient on the operative table, familiarizing oneself with different equipment such as the anesthesia ventilator and fluoroscopy, selecting appropriate anesthesia, choosing surgical instrumentation, and positioning the surgeons around the patient. In the next section, we will discuss other important aspects of care inside the operating suite.

Intraoperative Checklist

Intraoperative checklists have become a cornerstone in the pursuit of surgical excellence and improve surgical outcomes. Their implementation is a testament to surgeons' commitment to reducing human error and enhancing the best outcomes in the OR. The concept of a preoperative checklist is not new. Historically, surgeons have always had informal checklists, to ensure they were prepared for the operation. However, these were often inconsistent and

widely variable among surgeons. The modern structured checklist has its roots in safety protocols from the aviation industry. The aviation sector's success in using checklists to prevent accidents in complex, high-risk environments inspired similar approaches in medicine.

The pivotal moment in the history of surgical checklists came with the development of the WHO Surgical Safety Checklist in 2008. Spearheaded by Dr Atul Gawande and a team of international experts, this initiative addressed the alarming rates of surgical complications and deaths worldwide. The checklist was designed to be simple, clear, and applicable in all surgical environments, regardless of the country's income level. It covered three critical phases of surgery: before anesthesia (Sign-In), before skin incision (Time-Out), and before the patient leaves the OR (Sign-Out). The results are reported in a landmark study published by Haynes et al (2009) titled "A Surgical Safety Checklist to Reduce Morbidity and Mortality in a Global Population," which showed that after its implementation across eight cities worldwide, there was a significant reduction in surgery-related complications and deaths by one-third. Since its success, it has become a standard of care in many health care systems, frequently mandated by surgical governing bodies and health administration accrediting bodies.

The components of an effective surgical checklist include verification of patient identification, confirmation of the type of surgery, side of surgery, clear site marking, antibiotic prophylaxis, and identification of fire risks, followed by general equipment checks and identification of possible needs outside the OR, such as an ICU placement. It encourages active participation and engagement from all OR personnel, fostering a safety and communication culture. The checklist's use symbolizes a move away from the outdated hierarchical structure of surgical teams to a more collaborative approach. Over time, checklists have evolved to include specific customization for surgical specialties (orthopedics, cardiac surgery, neurosurgery), ensuring that all the necessary instrumentation, equipment, and technical elements are present to complete the proposed operation.

There are several challenges that come with implementing surgical checklists. Compliance with them varies greatly among different hospitals and even teams within the same institution. Some surgical teams view checklists as bureaucratic and time-consuming, especially in emergency situations where time is of the essence. Checklists, by oversimplifying complex procedures, may also result in the omission of critical, case-specific steps or considerations. Overreliance on checklists can give staff a false sense of security, which might cause them to neglect nonlisted but critical aspects of patient care. The culture of safety that the checklist promotes is more important than the checklist itself. Using checklists repetitively for every procedure, regardless of its complexity or risk level, can lead to staff desensitization, reducing the checklist's effectiveness. Other implementation challenges include insufficient training and education, which result in superficial compliance and treating checklists as a formality rather than a critical safety tool. In addition, there is still a lack of reporting and feedback mechanisms, which can hold people accountable. Integrating checklists with the other elements of the medical record is another barrier and often leads to duplication of work. Finally, in resource-limited settings, implementing checklists can be difficult because of a lack of basic supplies and equipment, making some checklist items irrelevant or impossible to comply with. As a result, checklists need regular review and adaptation to remain relevant and effective, considering new surgical techniques, technologies, and evidence.

POSTOPERATIVE CARE

Perioperative Notes

It is important to carefully consider the information entered in the patient's records. The information must be clearly written and accurately represent the patient's diagnosis, current treatment plan, and any future requirements. The easy ability to copy and paste information in electronic medical records (EMR) should be used with caution to prevent the propagation of misinformation.

The **Surgical Admission History and Physical** (H&P) is the foundational clinical document of the patient's care. Starting with the chief complaint, followed by a brief narrative of the patient's present illness, provides the initial go-to information for any provider to understand the reason for the patient's current admission. Other elements in this note include all the prior medical, surgical, social, and familial history relevant to the patient's surgical condition. A review of current medications should be updated with accurate routes of administration, doses, and last dose taken. Also documented should be the patient's allergies or similar reactions to important medications (antibiotics, analgesics, and others) that could be used during the patient's surgical course. A focused physical examination will document the patient's presurgical physical condition, vital signs, and other clinical information that will be later used to compare the patient's postoperative state.

Immediately after the surgery, ideally, while the patient is still in the OR, record a **Brief Operative Note** including the essential elements of the operation, with consideration given to recording information that might be important in the immediate perioperative period, such as complications, blood loss, fluid replacement, and urine output. The **Operative Note** should be written and dictated as soon as possible, to ensure no information is missed. The operative note should provide a narrative that expands on all the elements of the brief operative note. This includes technical details, such as the surgical technique, the completeness of tumor resection, type of hardware or prosthetic material used. This information is not only relevant for the patient's present admission but also for future treatments and prognosis.

It is important to document the patient's condition after surgery or a **Postoperative Check** by taking notes on the night or right after recovery. This note should include the patient's comfort level and vital signs, fluid balance, pertinent examination findings, and any critical laboratory values caregivers need to know within the next few hours. The guiding principle should be to focus on relevant clinical information resulting from the patient's recent operation, following a general wellness examination. For instance, look for evidence of ongoing bleeding after trauma surgery, perform a pulse check after a vascular surgery, examine chest tube output after a thoracic intervention, or specific hormonal values from an endocrine operation.

Medical Orders

The order section within the medical record demands meticulous attention to detail. The impetus for transitioning to EMR was largely driven by the need to address the prevalent issue of errors arising from poorly handwritten or misinterpreted medical orders. EMR have been instrumental in enhancing safety, allowing for a more seamless integration with other evidence-based aspects of postoperative care that are crucial for improving patient outcomes.

ERAS protocols, in particular, exemplify the advancements in postoperative care. They have been progressively adopted across a wide range of surgical specialties, standing at the forefront of modern surgical practices. The integration of ERAS protocols into EMR facilitates adherence to best practices and allows for real-time monitoring and adjustments based on individual patient responses. Significantly, the adoption of ERAS within EMR has led to measurable improvements in patient care. These protocols have been associated with reductions in morbidity and mortality, as well as decreased lengths of hospital stay. By leveraging the structured and data-driven environment provided by EMR, ERAS protocols optimize the postoperative trajectory, supporting a patient's rapid return to health. This multifaceted approach not only streamlines the delivery of care but also ensures a patient-centered process that prioritizes the swift and safe recovery of surgical patients. In cases where no ERAS protocols are available, other important nonbundled Practice Management Guidelines (PMG) have been developed. These guidelines suggest the best care practices recommended by different surgery societies, some of which are supported by evidence-based medicine or the consensus opinion of experts. Institutions follow quality metrics tied to many of these guidelines, and deviations may need to be explained. PMG allows flexibility as some of the recommendations may not be applicable to a particular patient for different reasons, particularly when the risk/benefit profile is unfavorable. As in the case of ERAS, many of these PMG have been incorporated in EMR and may show as default options when orders are being selected.

The ordering sets, contents, and formats within the EMR can differ based on the type of medical or surgical admission, procedure, and overall status of the patient's care. Although a few companies dominate the EMR landscape, the general structure of orders should be the same for easy visualization and execution. A list of the important sections that relate to surgical care is as follows:

Admitting headline—Order sets begin with the admitting diagnosis, primary team, and level of monitoring. Surgeons may not be the first responders, as other physicians may possess more knowledge. In some cases, critical care specialists manage care, with surgeons comanaging. The admitting headline identifies the contact information for the team responsible for the patient.

Code status—"Code status" indicates the level of rescue agreed upon by the patient. A full resuscitation and life-sustaining effort will be initiated in case of an arrest. Patients may refuse treatments, known as "Partial Code" or "Do Not Resuscitate—DNR." Recently, "Limitations of Life-Sustaining Interventions (LSIs)" has been suggested as a replacement for DNR to allow patients to accept or refuse specific treatments. Regardless of the process, it should align with the patient's wishes and Advance Directives.

Nursing activities—Bedside nurses are crucial in managing a patient's care after surgery. Nursing order sets provide clear expectations for patient care, including monitoring vital signs, activity levels, outputs, and wound care. Nurses should communicate critical information to other health care providers, especially when anticipating major issues. It is important to note that nurses may have a high workload in certain wards due to varying patient-to-nurse ratios. Therefore, nursing tasks should be taken into account when selecting an appropriate ward for patient care.

Diet—Postoperative diet orders consider two things: a patient's ability to swallow and the type of nutrition they need. NPO means no food or drink for a period. A diet should be tailored to the patient's needs, including timing, amount, consistency, and nutrition. Not all diets meet caloric and protein requirements, for example, clear liquid diets offer little sustenance. Institutions have dietary specialists who offer recommendations for optimal nutrition.

Dietary management is a cornerstone of ERAS protocols, playing a vital role in optimizing surgical outcomes. The ERAS guidelines recommend a shift from traditional fasting practices to preoperative carbohydrate loading and the early reintroduction of oral nutrition postsurgery. This nutritional strategy is designed to minimize the body's fasting response, reduce insulin resistance, and promote better metabolic outcomes. By enabling patients to maintain muscle mass, improve wound healing, and enhance overall recovery, the implementation of a targeted dietary regimen within ERAS protocols significantly contributes to reducing the length of hospital stays and improving patient satisfaction.

Medications—The medication management section is perhaps the most complex of the postoperative order set. Medication orders can be systematically divided into several subsections. The initial category considers the time basis of administration. For example, it classifies medications as those that should be provided continuously such as IV fluids, the basal rates for epidurals, or patient-controlled analgesia; followed by those that require a timed-scheduled regimen such as antibiotics, venous thromboembolic events (VTE) prophylaxis, and oral analgesics; and finally those that are only given in responsive to a specific condition (PRN [pro re nata; as needed]) for example pain medication for breakthrough pain relief, antihypertensives for systolic blood pressure above 160 mm Hg.

A second category differentiates between acute inpatient medications specific to the surgical context and the patient's home medications for chronic conditions. This delineation is where the process of Medication Reconciliation becomes essential. It ensures that ongoing treatments do not adversely interact with surgical interventions, such as the potential complications arising from systemic anticoagulants. Medication Reconciliation involves a comprehensive review and alignment of all medications, harmonizing them with the patient's historical and current medical needs while preempting any harmful interactions or withdrawal issues. It also sets the stage for safe and effective outpatient medication management post-discharge.

The final classification within postoperative medication management addresses the specific classes of medications. A thorough examination of the various families of drugs, and the nuances of prescribing each within the context of different medical and surgical conditions, is a subject too extensive for this chapter's scope. It is important to note,

however, that the EMR often employ this classification strategy when physicians order medications. Such a system facilitates the orderly arrangement of prescriptions within the Medication Administration Record (MAR), ensuring a clear and organized approach to medication delivery.

While the precise ordering parameters for each medication class will be tailored to individual patient needs and specific surgical scenarios, there are overarching principles that should guide the clinician. These include considerations of drug-drug interactions, the patient's preoperative medication profile, and the pharmacokinetics and pharmacodynamics relevant to the surgical setting. In this intricate process, the expertise of inpatient pharmacists is invaluable. They play a pivotal role in enhancing medication safety for postoperative patients and should be consulted routinely to verify and optimize the pharmacologic regimen for all patients following surgery.

In integrating these classifications into EMR systems, we see a dual benefit: There is a standardization of orders that promotes safety and efficiency, and there is also the potential for customization within those standards to meet individual patient requirements. As the MAR reflects this structured ordering process, it becomes a crucial tool in the execution of safe pharmacotherapy, serving as a checkpoint for both the health care team and the patients they care for.

Ancillary staff orders—Additional health care staff orders are a critical component of postoperative care. Respiratory therapists manage ventilation, oxygen supplementation, and administer treatments. Physical and occupational therapists facilitate patient mobility and assess disabilities. Social workers and case managers address social and familial aspects of patient care.

Laboratory and studies—Laboratory studies and special diagnostic procedures should also be specified. Special procedures, such as radiographs, require additional thought. Orders for these studies should specifically state the presumptive diagnosis and the reason for the test. Personal consultation with the radiologist or technician avoids confusion and prevents delays or unnecessary repetition of procedures. Some procedures require special patient preparation; therefore, the orders must include these instructions. "Routine" or "daily" laboratory or radiology orders rarely contribute to care and should be avoided. In the occasional situation where serial studies are needed to follow some aspect of the patient's course, a stop time should be specified (eg, "Please draw hematocrit q6h $\times$ 24 hours"). Laboratory and diagnostic studies should be used to confirm clinical suspicions and not as a shotgun approach to reveal a diagnosis.

Consultations—While this is an order, it should not substitute actual direct communication among providers. When a consultation is requested, it should specify the nature of the question or problem to be addressed, the scope of management that will be permitted to this additional provider, and the time frame expected for response. Effective communication with medical specialists is crucial for making the best evidence-based decisions in perioperative management. As the conductor of a well-tuned orchestra, the surgeon ties in all the information to produce a beautiful symphony. Directly asking relevant questions about the specialist's expertise can help clarify any issues. It is vital to involve the patient in these discussions and allow them to ask questions, which fosters mutual trust and creates an environment for shared decision-making. Cooperation and compliance from all parties involved are essential for the successful execution of all phases of the perioperative process, which ultimately leads to positive outcomes.

Pain Management

Surgeons should take the pain management of their patients seriously. It is not uncommon for physicians to overlook pain, while closely monitoring other medical aspects of their patients. However, physicians have also been criticized for prescribing excessive amounts of potentially addictive medications, such as opioids, which have been associated with societal problems of epidemic proportions. It is important to know that pain can limit advancing the patient's healing process. Inability to get out of bed or ambulate limited by pain can produce consequences that slow the patient's progress or cause complications such as atelectasis, pneumonia, or VTE.

Asking patients about important characteristics of pain (level, duration, timing, triggers, mitigators) should be a routine part of the review of systems taken on daily rounds. For patients who cannot report pain (eg, those in the ICU, who may be mechanically ventilated and unable to speak), attention to their facial expressions and vital signs will give clues as to their level of discomfort. The nature of the patient's disease process and their comorbidities will determine the type of pain management strategy they require. Another central tenet of ERAS protocols involves using multimodal pain management strategies. This approach moves away from the traditional reliance on using opioids as the primary method for postoperative pain control, advocating instead for a variety of other analgesic medications and therapies that can be equally effective in providing relief. The use of axial and regional anesthesia/ analgesia options has also allowed a decrease in the usage of opioids. Many patients with thoracic or abdominal incisions are well served with epidural analgesia administered by the Anesthesia Pain Service. When opioids are necessary, prescribing them at the lowest effective dose will minimize the risk of adverse effects. Intravenous opioid-based patient-controlled analgesia can be used safely and effectively to relieve intense pain that accompanies the early postoperative state. Once the patient can tolerate oral intake, transitioning to oral analgesics is advisable due to their longer duration of action, contributing to sustained comfort and facilitation for recovery.

Surgeons must become familiar with safe practices of opioid usage. Except for patients with cancer, prolonged treatment of chronic pain with opioids has not shown significant clinical benefits. Therefore, a tapering plan should be in place to wean off opioids and avoid opioid use disorder (OUD). Numerous tables and corresponding applications have been developed to predict the necessary amount and duration of pain relief treatment after surgery, depending on the type of surgical procedure. It has been shown that with unthoughtful and indiscriminate prescription practices, many of these oral agents remain unused at home. This poses a risk of having tablets available for potential misuse. Many state programs have been developed for the safe return and disposal of these drugs and should be part of the prescription plan provided by the surgeon. For chronic users (and before surgery), it is recommended to have a consultation with chronic pain specialists before and after surgery to avoid the dangers of double prescribing, addiction, and drug overdose.

Deep Vein Thrombosis Prophylaxis

Without adequate prophylaxis, VTE can affect up to 25% of postoperative patients. Some surgical patients are at a higher risk of developing VTE due to the presence of all three of Virchow risk factors for venous thrombosis. These factors include stasis, hypercoagulability, and endothelial injury, further intensified by varying degrees of inflammation related to injury or underlying surgical pathology. For example, patients who are severely injured from polytrauma, who are immobile, who have congestive HF or malignancy, who undergo pelvic or joint replacement operations, or who have vertebral, pelvic, or long bone fractures are at highest risk. Over the last two decades, several VTE risk calculators have been developed, such as the Caprini score, to help identify patients at the highest risk. Low-molecular-weight heparin is the most effective drug for preventing VTE due to its reliable pharmacokinetic profile. However, its use may be limited in patients with renal failure as it can accumulate and cause bleeding. Unfractionated heparin is an alternative, but it requires more frequent dosing and may not achieve the intended action consistently. Recent experiences suggest that these drugs can be coupled with factor Xa monitoring and dose adjustments to improve chemoprophylaxis. Newer information also indicates that aspirin can be an option, particularly in orthopedic surgery. Early engagement in physical therapy is crucial in preventing VTE, as ambulation and mobilization are helpful measures. In the case of patients who have lower mobility or are unconscious, they can use stockings or pneumatic compression devices. These devices help promote the release and distribution of natural anticoagulants, but their effectiveness is much lesser than the protection provided by chemoprophylactic agents. The American College of Chest Physicians has published extensive guidelines for optimal thromboprophylaxis, which take into account the risks of VTE and potential bleeding complications. This allows for the creation of individualized patient care plans.

POSTOPERATIVE SURGICAL COMPLICATIONS

Surgeons require exceptional skills for successful outcomes, including analytical precision, artistic finesse, courage, and the ability to introspect. They must adapt to unforeseen challenges in real time, perform minimally invasive procedures, and accept and openly discuss surgery-related complications. Accepting complications is vital for professional growth and ethical practice and is the foundation of all surgical science. The most significant complications are summarized in Table 1-8, some of these will be discussed in the next section.

Cardiovascular Perioperative Complications

Cardiovascular complications are among the most severe and life-threatening postoperative events. Early recognition, effective monitoring, and prompt treatment are vital in reducing morbidity and mortality. While some patients are at greater risk due to existing comorbidities, these complications can also occur in previously healthy individuals, making vigilant postoperative care imperative for all surgical patients.

Statistical Data on Outcomes

Literature has shown that experiencing a heart attack or stroke after surgery can increase the risk of death within 30 days by up to 5 times the baseline for the procedure. In some studies, the mortality rate has been reported to be as high as 15% to 25%. Developing an irregular heartbeat, specifically atrial fibrillation (A-fib), after surgery is also linked to a higher risk of death. Some studies have reported a 2-fold increase in 30-day mortality rates. If not diagnosed and treated promptly, the mortality rate for pulmonary embolism (PE) can range from 25% to 50%. Cardiovascular complications make up around 20% to 30% of unexpected admissions to the ICU after surgery. Postoperative cardiovascular complications are associated with a significant extension in hospital length of stay and discharge to skilled nursing as opposed to home.

Major Cardiovascular Events

Myocardial ischemia after surgery is a common occurrence in patients who already have coronary artery disease. The risk is particularly high if the surgery is performed within a month after a major adverse cardiovascular event (MACE),

even if the patient had some form of revascularization and coronary stents. Postoperative myocardial infarction often presents with unusual symptoms and ECG changes. Similarly, patients may experience abnormal heart rhythms, which affect cardiac output and the stability of their blood flow. The most common type of arrhythmia that occurs after surgery is A-fib. Many factors related to surgery contribute to its appearance. A-fib increases myocardial oxygen demand and negatively impacts pumping by reducing the time it takes for the atria to contract and fill the ventricles. These factors can contribute to reduced blood flow to the heart muscle, impairing its function and decreasing blood supply to peripheral tissues. Another condition, HF, can worsen or occur for the first time, particularly in patients who undergo high-risk surgeries or those with preexisting cardiovascular disease. Left unchecked, the above conditions will evolve into cardiogenic shock. Although it is considered a less severe complication, blood pressure can be significantly affected by various factors such as pain, stress, blood loss, or drug interactions. These factors might be an unusual sign or a triggering cause of other MACE. Therefore, special attention and prompt treatment should be given to such cases.

Management Strategies

It can be difficult to identify classic symptoms of heart injury due to anesthesia, painkillers, or confusion after

TABLE 1-8. Compilation of Most Significant Postoperative Complications

Complication	Incidence After Surgery—Average (%)	Definition	Potential Risk Factors
Major adverse cardiovascular events (MACE)	3-5	Adverse cardiac events including heart attack, stroke, or cardiac death	Preexisting heart disease, hypertension, advanced age
Pneumonia	1-5	Inflammation of the lung tissue typically due to infection	Advanced age, smoking, chronic lung disease
Atelectasis	1-10	Partial or complete lung collapse	Poor pulmonary hygiene, preexisting lung disease
Anesthesia complications	0.1-0.4	Adverse effects related to anesthesia, eg, malignant hyperthermia, aspiration	History of adverse reactions, certain genetic factors, recent meals
Pulmonary embolism (PE)	0.1-0.5	Blood clot lodged in the pulmonary artery	Prolonged immobilization, hypercoagulable state
Deep vein thrombosis (DVT)	0.5-2	Blood clot in a deep vein, usually in the legs	Prolonged bed rest, smoking, oral contraceptives
Surgical-site infection (SSI)	2-5	Infection occurring at the site of surgical incision	Poor wound care, obesity, diabetes
Acute kidney injury (AKI)	1-5	Rapid loss of renal function	Hypotension, nephrotoxic drugs, dehydration
Postoperative bleeding	1-3	Excessive bleeding following a surgical procedure	Anticoagulation, technical error, liver dysfunction
Ileus	10-20	Temporary absence of bowel motility	Electrolyte imbalance, narcotics, recent surgery
Delirium	5-15	Acute confusion and altered mental status	Age, preexisting cognitive impairment, medications

the operation. Unusual signs such as hiccups, jaw pain, or paleness may be the only hints that something is wrong. Continuous ECG and pulse oximetry monitoring can help detect heart problems early by analyzing waveforms and telemetry data. In addition, biomarkers such as high-sensitivity troponin levels can quickly indicate whether there is any muscle injury or ischemia in the heart.

Pharmacologic interventions for postsurgical cardiovascular events may include the resumption of antiplatelet agents after consulting with the surgical team, especially in patients with coronary artery stents. Full systemic anticoagulation may be necessary for coronary interventions, as well as for the treatment of deep vein thrombosis (DVT) and PE. However, it may be problematic in the immediate postoperative period due to the increased risk of surgical bleeding. β-Blockers should be continued in patients who were already taking them and may be initiated in high-risk patients if there are no contraindications. Vasopressors and inotropes are used to manage hypotension or HF. Mechanical circulatory support devices such as intra-aortic balloon pumps and extracorporeal life support (ECLS/ECMO [extracorporeal membrane oxygenation]) may be required in cases of severe HF or refractory arrhythmias. Finally, electrical cardioversion may be necessary for severe or refractory arrhythmias.

There are other modifiable risk factors that are important to manage in cases of MACE after surgery. These include maintaining tight glycemic control in patients with diabetes and carefully monitoring fluid status to prevent volume overload, especially in patients with HF. Given the complexity of managing these risk factors, it is recommended that surgeons involve cardiology, pharmacology, and critical care teams to take a multidisciplinary approach to treatment.

Anesthetic Complications

Among the various anesthetic complications—such as allergic reactions, aspiration, or hemodynamic instability—one of the most serious and potentially life-threatening is malignant hyperthermia (MH).

Malignant Hyperthermia

MH is an uncommon but severe pharmacogenetic condition. It results in a hypermetabolic crisis that is most often triggered by exposure to volatile anesthetic agents such as halothane, desflurane, or sevoflurane or depolarizing muscle relaxants like succinylcholine. The underlying pathophysiology involves an abnormal release of calcium ions in skeletal muscle cells. This leads to muscle rigidity, metabolic acidosis, and a rapid increase in body temperature.

The early signs of MH may include unexplained irregular heart rhythms or a faster heartbeat than usual. The levels of carbon dioxide in the body may also rapidly increase despite proper ventilation, and muscle stiffness or spasms, specifically in the masseter muscle, may occur. Another potential indicator is unexpected metabolic acidosis. Elevated temperature may also be present, but this is often a late sign of MH.

In an MH crisis, take the following steps immediately:

1. Discontinue triggering agents: Stop the triggering anesthetic or muscle relaxant immediately.
2. Alert the team: Notify all surgical and anesthetic team members of the suspected MH crisis.
3. Administer dantrolene: Give dantrolene sodium as quickly as possible. The initial dose is 2.5 mg/kg, which can be repeated up to a maximum of 10 mg/kg.
4. Manage hyperthermia: Use cooling techniques like cold IV fluids, ice packs around large arteries, and cooling blankets to reduce the elevated body temperature.
5. Optimize ventilation: Increase minute ventilation to lower end-tidal CO_2 and counteract metabolic acidosis.
6. Provide hemodynamic support: Use IV fluids, vasopressors, or antiarrhythmics for circulatory support.
7. Monitor and assess: Continually monitor vital signs, end-tidal CO_2, blood gases, electrolytes, and coagulation parameters.
8. Transfer to ICU: Once stabilized, move the patient to an intensive care setting for ongoing monitoring and treatment.
9. Consider genetic counseling: Once the acute crisis is managed, consider genetic counseling for the patient and potentially affected family members.
10. Take future precautions: Patients who have experienced or are genetically predisposed to MH should carry medical identification. Anesthetic teams must exercise extreme caution and opt for MH-safe anesthesia protocols in these cases.

Aspiration Events

Aspiration during anesthesia is a serious complication that can result in life-threatening respiratory distress. It occurs when the contents of the stomach enter the trachea and subsequently the lungs. This usually happens during induction or emergence from anesthesia. Aspiration can cause aspiration pneumonia, acute respiratory distress syndrome (ARDS), and even death.

Patients who require emergency surgery and have not observed a reasonable fasting period are at risk of aspiration. Other factors that increase the risk of aspiration include the presence of gastrointestinal obstructions, esophageal dysfunction, pregnancy, obesity, history of prior aspiration events, and alcohol or drug intoxication.

The following preventive measures are often recommended to avoid aspiration events. Patients are advised to refrain from eating or drinking fluids for 6 to 8 hours before surgery. However, this recommendation has been somewhat controversial and challenged, as different populations may be negatively impacted, such as pediatric patients or those taking medications that require oral intake and a certain amount of fluids for their passage. Some drugs, like antacids such as H2 blockers, or gastric motility agents, can be used as prophylactic medication to decrease these events. Finally, anesthesia techniques such as rapid sequence intubation should be utilized in these high-risk patients.

In the event of aspiration related to anesthesia, immediate measures for respiratory support should be taken. To combat hypoxia, high-flow oxygen should be administered right away. This may require re-intubation either in the OR or in the Postanesthesia Care Unit (PACU). The airway must be cleared of any gastric contents through suction and if possible, a nasogastric tube should empty the stomach with antiemetics to avoid repeated episodes. If the patient is still intubated or requires re-intubation for respiratory support, a bronchoscopy should be performed to remove any particulate matter in the lower airway. Broad-spectrum antibiotics should be initiated promptly to prevent aspiration pneumonia, especially in cases of bowel obstruction or positive particulate matter present in the lower airway. In addition, lung-protective ventilation strategies, such as low tidal volume, should be employed to further minimize lung injury. Intensive monitoring will be necessary to detect and manage any complications.

Atelectasis

Atelectasis after surgery is a common problem, especially when general anesthesia is used. This condition causes the collapse or incomplete expansion of alveoli, which leads to difficulties in breathing and lower oxygen levels. Although it usually appears within the first 48 hours postoperation, factors such as the patient's health and the type of surgery can also affect its onset. More research is necessary to understand the condition better.

Management of postoperative atelectasis should begin preoperatively, under ideal conditions, by encouraging cessation of smoking for 8 weeks preoperatively and instituting inspiratory exercises. Chest physiotherapy may also begin, particularly for patients with productive cough or chronic bronchitis. Re-expansion techniques (incentive spirometry) are appropriate for all patients. The most important strategies involve adequate postoperative pain management, frequently obtained with epidural analgesia, and early mobilization. One of the advantages of minimally invasive surgery is the significant reduction in atelectasis as well as other more serious pulmonary problems.

Major Respiratory Complications

Respiratory complications are relatively common in the postoperative setting. Respiratory issues have far-reaching implications for patient outcomes, ranging from relatively minor events like the already mentioned atelectasis to severe complications like pneumonia and ARDS.

ARDS in the surgical population has been associated with mortality rates ranging from 35% to 45%. Aspiration pneumonia (see "Anesthetic Complications") also has mortality rates as high as 20%. Atelectasis, if left untreated, can progress to hospital-associated pneumonia. Organisms involved have higher antibiotic resistance than those causing community-acquired pneumonia. Complications deriving into respiratory failure account for an estimated 15% to 25% of the postoperative ICU population and are a leading diagnosis of unplanned ICU admission in the postoperative period. In surgical patients, respiratory failure is typically treated with supportive care such as intubation and mechanical ventilation, given that these patients often cannot breathe deeply and progress into severe hypoxia and hypercapnia, leading to cardiopulmonary arrest. Breathing treatments, aggressive and noninvasive positive pressure ventilation by face mask, should only be used selectively and with caution as they could induce a second hit injury by triggering an aspiration event. Not surprisingly, patients experiencing postoperative respiratory complications can expect an extended hospital stay, with estimates suggesting an additional 3 to 7 days on average. ICU stays are typically prolonged when patients are experiencing respiratory complications. PEs, as part of the cardiopulmonary spectrum of complications, are also considered highly lethal.

Dyspnea or shortness of breath is one of the initial signs of a respiratory problem. When respiratory centers in the medulla and other areas of the central nervous system detect local respiratory acidosis (low pH and high Pco_2), involuntary activation of the neck's secondary respiratory muscles and nasal flaring occurs. This mechanism also increases respiratory rate to eliminate the accumulation of CO_2 (hyperventilation). This response may be less effective in surgical patients due to pain, third spacing, and atelectasis. Decreased breath sounds may indicate a space-occupying lesion of the pleura, such as air (pneumothorax), fluid (effusion), or blood (hemothorax). Wheezing or stridor occurs when there is an obstruction of the airway (edema, foreign body, vocal cord paralysis) or a bronchoreactive response. With smaller tidal volumes and reduced gas exchange, respiratory acidosis worsens. This causes pulmonary vasoconstriction and $\dot{V}/\dot{Q}$ mismatch leading to hypoxia. There is now a reliance on anaerobic pathways to produce ATP, accumulating lactic acid. Confusion and agitation occur due to impaired oxygen delivery to the brain, and acidosis interferes with neuronal and myocardial activity. Finally, if left unchecked, it will lead to a cardiopulmonary arrest. Thus, clinicians must be mindful of any early indication of respiratory distress.

Many hospital systems have established Rapid Response Teams (RRTs) that can be activated quickly based on certain criteria, including the above clinical indicators. Recently, early warning detection systems powered by machine learning and artificial intelligence have emerged, offering physicians a better way to identify potential issues in postsurgical wards. With the help of these systems, RRTs can be activated at the right time, ensuring that patients receive prompt and appropriate care. In high-risk postsurgical patients, monitoring strategies such as continuous pulse oximetry provide real-time information about oxygenation. Capnography is useful for monitoring ventilation, especially in patients who are sedated or those receiving potent opioid analgesia.

To assess the degree of respiratory failure, aside from the above telltale clinical criteria, imaging such as chest x-ray can be used to detect atelectasis, pneumonia, or pneumothorax, while CT scans are better for PEs. Point-of-care ultrasound (POCUS) can detect pleural space abnormalities, pulmonary edema, diaphragmatic and accompanying heart function, ventricular failure, and volume overload. However, ABG provides the most direct information on respiratory function. Measuring levels of oxygen and carbon dioxide, as well as the pH of the blood and their trends, may indicate the trajectory toward severe respiratory failure and the need for further supportive care.

Invasive mechanical ventilation may be necessary in severe cases of respiratory distress and failure. Code status must be confirmed before intubating a patient. Intraoperative lung-protective strategies can reduce the incidence of postoperative pulmonary complications. Patients with chronic respiratory insufficiency (such as obstructive sleep apnea) may need to resume their continuous positive airway pressure (CPAP) mask. However, noninvasive techniques for respiratory support should be used in the short term only and closely monitored in postsurgical patients. When treating reactive airways, we may commonly prescribe bronchodilators even in non-COPD patients or patients with asthma. In cases where there is a suspected PE, thrombolytics and anticoagulants may be necessary. These treatments should be permitted and vetted by the operating surgeon. If a patient is experiencing third spacing or pulmonary edema, aggressive diuretic treatment can help. However, this can deplete intravascular volume and induce hypotension, so it should be used with caution. Patients are weaned from the ventilator when the underlying causes of respiratory failure have been addressed and the patient's own effort (work of breathing) and gas exchange are sufficient.

Urinary Tract Infection

A UTI can put a significant strain on health care resources. It is defined as an infection that affects any part of the urinary system, and it is the most commonly reported type of health care-associated infection to the National Healthcare Safety Network. During surgery, UTIs can occur due to various risk factors including surgical trauma, and changes in host defense mechanisms due to anesthesia or medications, but the majority of cases (over 75%) are associated with the prolonged use of a urine catheter (Foley catheter) that drains the bladder. Therefore, catheters should only be used for appropriate indications and removed as soon as they are no longer needed.

Symptoms of UTIs can vary from asymptomatic bacteriuria to severe sepsis, renal failure, and delayed wound healing. Management usually involves the use of antibiotics that are targeted based on culture sensitivity, supportive care, and the removal or replacement of urinary catheters, whenever possible.

Surgical-Site Infection

Surgical-site infections (SSIs) are the second most common nosocomial infection and will occur in 2% to 5% of all surgical patients. Per CDC definition, a surgical-site infection is an infection that occurs after surgery in the part of the body where surgery took place. These can be further categorized as:

Superficial incisional: infection that occurs only in the skin and subcutaneous tissue
Deep incisional: infection that occurs in deeper layers, such as fascia and muscles
Organ space: infection that extends to any part of the anatomy other than the incised body wall, such as a cavity that was opened and manipulated during the procedure

Factors contributing to SSIs are discussed in Chapter 6 and can be patient-related, procedure-related, and environmental. Signs of SSIs are those associated with inflammation: redness (rubor), swelling (tumor), localized heat and erythema (calor), and increased pain at the incision site (dolor). Deeper infections (deep incisional and organ space) manifest systemically, showing sepsis, abscess formation in deeper spaces and organs, and prosthetic implant infections. Tachycardia may be the first sign and fever may develop only later. Spontaneous drainage from the surgical wound indicates that there has been a delay in recognition of this postoperative problem. Delay in recognition leads to the destruction of the fascia and contributes to dehiscence or incisional hernias. Prompt drainage minimizes these sequelae, and antibiotics play a secondary role unless there are extenuating circumstances. Deeper infections may require additional axial imaging and radiologically guided interventions. Occasionally, the diagnosis is made by surgical exploration. Guidelines have been developed by the Centers for Disease Control to minimize the incidence of SSIs.

Central Line-Associated Bloodstream Infection

Central line-associated bloodstream infections (CLABSIs) are infections that occur when harmful bacteria enter a patient's bloodstream through a central line or catheter, which is a medical device that is inserted into a main vein. These infections can be very serious and even life-threatening. CLABSIs are usually caused by a lack of proper sterile techniques during insertion or maintenance of the catheter. Therefore, health care providers must always follow strict infection control practices to prevent these infections from occurring. The most effective way to prevent CLABSIs is to remove the catheter as soon as it is no longer necessary.

Preventive Measures

Aside from the removal of unnecessary devices, the following measures are provided specifically for surgical patients, some have been discussed already within this chapter.

Antibiotic prophylaxis: Administer appropriate antibiotics to achieve peak concentrations before the surgical incision.
Skin preparation: To prepare the skin, it is advised to use antiseptic solutions like chlorhexidine-alcohol. This can sometimes involve at-home kits and showers to reduce bacterial buildup, particularly in patients who carry harmful bacteria like methicillin-resistant *Staphylococcus aureus* (MRSA).
Glycemic control: For patients with diabetes, maintain strict glycemic control.
Sterile technique: It is vital to adhere to strict aseptic techniques while performing the procedure.
Surgical team hygiene: Ensure the surgical team follows the correct hand hygiene procedures and wears sterile clothing.
Instrument sterility: Double-check that all surgical instruments are properly sterilized.
Wound care: Patients must be educated on wound care, signs of infection, and seeking medical help to ensure their safety and well-being.
Follow-up: Schedule timely postoperative follow-up visits to monitor for signs of infection.

Postoperative Delirium

Postoperative delirium (POD) is a serious complication arising after surgical procedures. Its varying manifestations have led to several classification systems that aid in diagnosis and treatment. POD is a rising issue that continues to escalate in terms of morbidity and mortality rates. POD prolongs hospital stays, increases health care costs, and can lead to long-term cognitive impairments. Accurate classification can aid in timely diagnosis and targeted management. The prevalence of POD varies, affecting between 10% and 50% of general surgery patients and up to 70% in high-risk groups such as those undergoing major cardiothoracic or orthopedic surgeries. The incidence is particularly high among older patients and those with preexisting cognitive impairments. **Hyperactive Delirium** is characterized by agitation, hallucinations, and restlessness. **Hypoactive Delirium** manifests as lethargy, reduced alertness, and withdrawal. **Mixed Delirium** has fluctuating symptoms from both hyperactive and hypoactive categories. There are two types of risk factors that can lead to POD. Intrinsic risk factors are related to the patient and include older age, preexisting cognitive impairment, and the presence of comorbid conditions. Extrinsic risk factors are related to the surgery and associated medical treatments and include major surgeries, especially those involving cardiothoracic and abdominal regions. The use of deliriogenic medications such as benzodiazepines, antibiotics, and anticholinergic agents can also contribute to the development of POD.

Mitigation Strategies

Mitigation strategies include preemptive actions such as programmatic screening to identify important intrinsic risk factors and guide anesthetic and surgical technique selection that focuses on reducing extrinsic risk factors. Pharmacologic treatment strategies vary depending on the classification of delirium, existing comorbidities, and the risk of adverse effects. The two main classes of drugs discussed here are antipsychotics and α-2 agonists. Antipsychotics such as haloperidol are the most used antipsychotics for treating POD, especially in hyperactive delirium. It has a rapid onset but can have side effects like QT prolongation and extrapyramidal symptoms. Usually administered in small, frequent doses. Atypical antipsychotics such as quetiapine are used for both hyperactive and hypoactive delirium; it has a lower risk of extrapyramidal symptoms compared to haloperidol. Initiated at low doses, usually around 12.5 to 25 mg every 12 hours, and titrated as necessary. Olanzapine is another option for hyperactive delirium with a lower risk of extrapyramidal symptoms. However, it's associated with anticholinergic side effects. α-2 Agonists such as dexmedetomidine can be used for hypoactive delirium, it has been shown to have sedative properties without causing respiratory depression. However, it can lead to hypotension and bradycardia. Clonidine is less commonly used due to its less favorable side effect profile, including hypotension, and rebound hypertension upon abrupt discontinuation.

Nonpharmacologic interventions are recommended as the first line of treatment and can be effective for various types of delirium. The effectiveness and applicability of these interventions vary according to the individual patient's needs and circumstances. Reality orientation techniques such as using clocks, calendars, and frequent verbal reminders can help the patient understand the current time and place. Cognitive stimulation, which involves engaging the patient in simple mental exercises like recalling names, solving puzzles, or conversing on familiar topics, can also be helpful. Finally, family involvement is essential, as regular visits from family members can provide emotional anchoring, and they can bring in familiar objects or photos to help reorient the patient.

Early mobility is a crucial component in preventing postoperative delirium. This involves guided walking under supervision, where the patient is helped to walk within the room or ward as soon as it is medically feasible. Physical therapy involves targeted exercises to improve strength and balance, which can lead to a quicker recovery after surgery. These sessions should be tailored to the patient's physical condition and are usually initiated with short sessions of 5 to 10 minutes, gradually increasing as tolerated.

Sleep hygiene and controlling environmental factors can help ensure appropriate cerebral function in high-risk patients. It is recommended to have natural lighting during the day and dim or dark lighting at night to regulate the circadian rhythm. Exposure to certain types of light spectra, such as natural light or blue light, is believed to be beneficial. It is also helpful to reduce ambient noise through earplugs or white noise machines. Health care providers should encourage protocols that promote regular sleep schedules, avoid unnecessary naps that could interfere with nighttime sleep, and prevent unnecessary wake-up cycles at night. Hospital Elder Life Program (HELP) is an evidence-based approach that combines several of these interventions, customized to individual patient needs. ABCDE bundle is also a multicomponent strategy that stands for awakening and breathing coordination, delirium monitoring, and early exercise/mobility.

Fever

An elevation in a patient's core temperature postoperatively is so common that many mistakenly consider it a normal postoperative state. Next to requests for laxatives, analgesics, and sleep aids, calls from the nursing staff regarding temperature elevation are perhaps the most common.

The Society of Critical Care Medicine has adopted the guideline that a temperature elevation to 38.3 °C is the trigger to initiate an investigation. The evaluation process begins with a review of the circumstances surrounding the patient: patient location (ICU vs ward), length of hospitalization, presence of mechanical ventilation and its duration, instrumentation (eg, catheters, vascular lines, tubes in the nose or chest), duration of the instrumentation, medications, surgical sites and the reason for the surgical procedure (eg, elective, emergent, trauma, gastrointestinal tract), current treatments, and diagnosis. This first step, if performed carefully and thoughtfully, will indicate the direction the doctor should take to investigate the cause of the fever. Second, a directed physical examination is performed to look for clues and/or confirmation of a suspected source. Only after these two steps have been taken should consideration be given to ordering diagnostic studies. Undirected blanket ordering of laboratory tests, random cultures, and radiographs is appropriate only in very specific circumstances (eg, patients on prolonged mechanical ventilation, those who are immunosuppressed, or those with indwelling catheters or monitoring devices). For the majority of postoperative surgical patients, a selective approach to confirmatory testing is cost-efficient, effective, and high-quality medical practice. Once the diagnosis is established, appropriate therapeutic steps can be taken.

PERIOPERATIVE SAFETY

In 2000, the National Academy of Medicine (former Institute of Medicine) issued a report, *To Err Is Human*, which looked at population-based studies of medical error. The report concluded that between 44,000 and 98,000 Americans die yearly in hospitals from medical mistakes. This report brought the issue of medical safety to the forefront of our national consciousness.

It is essential to continuously monitor and manage patient risk profiles and postoperative complications within a structured, nonpunitive peer review system that prioritizes problem resolution and education. Closed-loop communication should be utilized, especially when addressing actionable items and correctible issues within the health care system. Both individual surgeon and collective institutional practices should be regularly reviewed and audited using established nonbiased standardized definitions. This allows for year-over-year evaluations and comparisons with other institutions with similar patient populations. Adoption of benchmarking processes can be typically conducted through specialty collaborative networks focused on performance improvement initiatives (CQIs [continuous quality improvements]). Surgeons and hospitals can voluntarily provide data in exchange for identifying individual strengths and areas for improvement.

In summary, POM stands as a multifaceted domain in which meticulous preoperative workup is instrumental in predicting and altering the trajectory of surgical care. Cardiopulmonary and other risk assessment series serve as a pivotal cornerstone, allowing clinicians to tailor perioperative risk mitigation strategies that have demonstrable impacts on clinical outcomes. Equally significant is the ethical imperative of informed consent, which assures that patients are cognizant of the risks and benefits associated with surgical interventions. Advancements in multimodal pain modalities and ERAS protocols have revolutionized postoperative care, significantly attenuating common postsurgical complications. However, the key to perpetual improvement lies in learning from complications, an exercise that imbues resilience and adaptability into surgical practice. Looking forward, machine learning and artificial intelligence hold unprecedented promise in these spheres. They have the potential to refine risk assessments, optimize resource allocation, and even predict clinical outcomes with increasingly high accuracy, paving the way for a new era in POM.

SUGGESTED READINGS

Altman AD, Helpman L, McGee J, et al. Enhanced recovery after surgery: implementing a new standard of surgical care. *CMAJ*. 2019;191(17):E469-E475. doi:10.1503/cmaj.180635

Douketis JD, Spyropoulos AC, Murad MH, et al. Perioperative management of antithrombotic therapy: an American College of Chest Physicians clinical practice guideline. *Chest*. 2022;162(5):e207-e243. doi:10.1016/j.chest.2022.07.025

Haynes AB, Weiser TG, Berry WR, et al. A surgical safety checklist to reduce morbidity and mortality in a global population. *N Engl J Med*. 2009;360(5):491-499. doi:10.1056/nejmsa0810119

Hobson C, Singhania G, Bihorac A. Acute kidney injury in the surgical patient. *Crit Care Clin*. 2015;31(4):705-723. doi:10.1016/j.ccc.2015.06.007.

Lawton JS, Tamis-Holland JE, Bangalore S, et al. 2021 ACC/AHA/SCAI guideline for coronary artery revascularization: a report of the American College of Cardiology/American Heart Association Joint Committee on Clinical Practice Guidelines. *Circulation*. 2022;145(3):e18-e114. doi:10.1161/CIR.0000000000001038

NICE-SUGAR Writing Group. Intensive versus conventional glucose control in critically ill patients. *N Engl J Med*. 2009;360(13):1283-1297. doi:10.1056/nejmoa0810625

Nijbroek SG, Schultz MJ, Hemmes SNT. Prediction of postoperative pulmonary complications. *Curr Opin Anaesthesiol*. 2019;32(3):443-451. doi:10.1097/ACO.0000000000000730

Thompson A, Fleischmann KE, Smilowitz NR, et al. 2024 AHA/ACC/ACS/ASNC/HRS/SCA/SCCT/SCMR/SVM Guideline for Perioperative Cardiovascular Management for Noncardiac Surgery: A Report of the American College of Cardiology/American Heart Association Joint Committee on Clinical Practice Guidelines. *Circulation*. 2024. doi:10.1161/CIR.0000000000001285

SAMPLE QUESTIONS

QUESTIONS

Choose the best answer for each question.

1. A 47-year-old woman is scheduled for elective laparoscopic cholecystectomy to treat symptomatic cholelithiasis. She is postmenopausal and takes a proton pump inhibitor for reflux symptoms and a thiazide diuretic for nonpitting edema of her lower extremities. She is otherwise healthy and is referred by her primary care provider after an evaluation of typical right upper quadrant symptoms revealed the presence of gallstones on ultrasound. Which of the following would be appropriate for her preoperative evaluation?

   A. Analysis of her hemoglobin concentration
   B. Urinalysis
   C. Serum electrolyte concentration measurement
   D. Scheduling a follow-up visit with the referring provider for clearance
   E. Chest x-ray

2. A 72-year-old man who has previously undergone lower extremity revascularization for disabling claudication is being considered for carotid endarterectomy because of symptomatic 85% stenosis of his left internal carotid artery. He quit smoking 5 years ago after smoking one and a half packs per day for 50 years. He no longer has claudication symptoms, but he admits to minimal physical activity. He cannot go up a flight of stairs without experiencing dyspnea. All of the following should be considered except:

   A. ECG
   B. Chest x-ray
   C. Cardiac stress test
   D. Formal evaluation by a cardiologist
   E. Denying surgery given the excessive risk

3. Which of the following is true regarding the pulmonary risk of a patient undergoing abdominal surgery for colon cancer and general anesthesia?

   A. Higher ASA classifications appear to predict a higher risk of postoperative pulmonary complications.
   B. Thromboprophylaxis is not indicated because the risks of bleeding outweigh the risk of VTE.

C. Pulmonary function testing is indicated because of the risk of metastatic disease to the lung.

D. Atelectasis in the postoperative period would be unlikely in this patient.

E. Increased age, chronic lung disease, congestive HF, and long-term tobacco use do not appear to increase the risk of perioperative pulmonary complications.

4. Which of the following is an accurate statement regarding AKI?

A. AKI is a common postoperative occurrence and usually results in permanent damage to the kidneys.

B. It is transitioned to the term CKD when the renal dysfunction persists for more than 6 months.

C. AKI is most commonly due to a prerenal cause.

D. AKI can be made more severe or prolonged by bleeding, sepsis, hypovolemia, or improper medication dosages.

E. Dialysis is not recommended for nonoliguric AKI, even with severe electrolyte imbalance or volume overload leading to congestive HF, as loop diuretics can increase urine production.

5. The following measures have proven to decrease the incidence of perioperative complications and improve patient satisfaction, except:

A. Administration of prophylactic antibiotics before surgery

B. Adequate patient warming to maintain normothermia

C. Using a surgical safety checklist to ensure all steps are followed

D. Appropriate risk assessment and optimization of comorbid conditions before surgery

E. Prescription of sufficient opioids for 30 days postoperation with additional refills

ANSWERS AND EXPLANATIONS

1. **Answer: C**

Serum electrolyte concentration measurement is appropriate, given the use of a thiazide diuretic. Hemoglobin concentration and chest x-ray would be expected to yield little information that would change management. Clearance is an inaccurate term and should be avoided. Risk stratification by the referring provider, which is a more appropriate term, would not be needed in this patient. Urinalysis would not be needed because the procedure does not involve the genitourinary tract. For more information on this topic, see section "Initial Preoperative Evaluation."

2. **Answer: E**

Denying surgery given the excessive risk. Although the patient does have substantial cardiac risk associated with surgery and anesthesia, the risks may be stratified and possibly mitigated by answers A through D. The surgery should not be categorically denied because of the substantial risks of stroke. For more information on this topic, see section "Cardiovascular Risk Assessment and Perioperative Management."

3. **Answer: A**

Higher ASA classifications appear to predict a higher risk of postoperative pulmonary complications. Thromboprophylaxis is important in all patients unless specifically contraindicated. This patient's risk for thrombotic events is elevated because of the planned procedure and the history of cancer. Metastatic lung disease should be identified before deciding on the need for PFTs and may alter treatment. Major abdominal surgery is a risk for the development of atelectasis. The listed patient-dependent factors do increase the risk of perioperative pulmonary complications. For more information on this topic, see sections "Initial Preoperative Evaluation," and "Pulmonary Risk Assessment and Perioperative Management."

4. **Answer: D**

AKI can be worsened by bleeding, sepsis, hypovolemia, or incorrect medication dosages. Therefore, it is important to pay close attention to avoid these issues during the perioperative period. Hobson et al (2015) provide a comprehensive review of AKI in surgical patients. Several initiatives have tried to establish consensus definitions for AKI. The "Risk, Injury, Failure, Loss, and End-stage Kidney" (RIFLE) criteria broadened the scope to include less severe AKI stages, based on changes in creatinine levels and urine output, and provided a structured classification for severity and recovery. The most recent and widely accepted guidelines are the "Kidney Disease: Improving Global Outcomes" (KDIGO), which have expanded the AKI criteria to include changes as small as 0.3 mg/dL. Given the changes in definition, the epidemiology of AKI has also changed. While prerenal causes were once the most common origin for AKI, recent data suggest that sepsis has become the most important cause of AKI in surgical patients. If renal dysfunction persists for more than 3 months, it is termed CKD. Dialysis may be necessary due to various physiologic reasons (such as acidosis, uremia, electrolyte imbalances, volume overload, and drug overdose), regardless of urine production level, even if it is not a prolonged or permanent need. For more information on this topic, see section "Perioperative Renal Risk Assessment and Management of Renal Dysfunction."

5. **Answer: E**

Options A, B, C, and D are established measures for reducing perioperative complications and enhancing patient satisfaction. However, option E, prescribing sufficient opioids for 30 days with additional refills, is not recommended as it may contribute to the risk of long-term opioid use, dependence, and potential overdose, thus not improving patient satisfaction in the context of perioperative care. Hence, option E is the correct answer to this question as it is the exception to measures that have been proven to decrease complications and improve satisfaction. For more information on this topic, see section "Pain Management."

2

Fluids, Electrolytes, and Surgical Nutrition

S. Ariane Christie and Areti Tillou

This chapter highlights the critical importance of maintaining fluid and electrolyte balance within a narrow physiologic window; reviews the causes and resultant pathology associated with fluid and electrolyte imbalance; summarizes the impact of surgical stress on nutritional status; discusses energy, macro- and micronutrient needs as well as methods to deliver nutrition; and describes principles of postoperative nutritional management to optimize patient outcomes.

FLUID AND ELECTROLYTE PHYSIOLOGY

Total Body Water and Compartments

Total body water (TBW) varies according to age, sex, and lean body mass. TBW is directly proportional to muscle mass and occupies intracellular and extracellular compartments. Intracellular fluid (ICF) represents approximately two-thirds of TBW (40% of body weight); extracellular fluid (ECF) represents one-third of TBW. ECF is further divided into intravascular (1/3 of the blood volume) and interstitial fluid compartments (2/3 of the ISF), which interact in osmotic equilibrium.

Electrolytes

Typical adult maintenance electrolyte needs are shown in Table 2-1. Careful daily monitoring of losses and serum concentrations should be done to guide supplemental replacement as needed.

TABLE 2-1. General Daily Electrolyte Recommendations

	Adults	Infants and Children
Sodium	50-250 mEq	2-4 mEq/kg
Potassium	30-200 mEq	2-3 mEq/kg
Chloride	50-250 mEq	2-3 mEq/kg
Phosphate	10-40 mmol	0.5-2 mmol/kg
Calcium	10-20 mEq	1-3 mEq/kg
Magnesium	10-30 mEq	0.25-0.5 mEq/kg

Sodium

Sodium and its anions represent 97% of the osmotically active particles present in the ECF. Extracellular osmolarity is estimated by the formula:

$$\text{Osmolarity} = 2 \times [\text{Na}^+] + \left[\frac{\text{glucose (mg/dL)}}{18}\right] + \left[\frac{\text{blood urea nitrogen (BUN)}}{2.8}\right],$$

where $[\text{Na}^+]$ is serum sodium concentration. Normal osmolarity is around 290 ± 10 mOsm/L. Humans require, on average, 1 to 3 mEq/kg/d of sodium.

Normal kidneys resorb and excrete sodium to maintain fluid and osmolar homeostasis. Extracellular volume reduction sensed in the glomerular hilum causes the juxtaglomerular apparatus to release renin into the blood stream. Renin cleaves angiotensinogen to produce angiotensin I. Angiotensin-converting enzyme (ACE) in the lung converts angiotensin I to angiotensin II, a potent stimulator of aldosterone secretion. Adrenocorticotropic hormone (ACTH) also directly stimulates aldosterone production from the adrenal cortex. Aldosterone acts on the distal tubule to resorb sodium in exchange for potassium and hydrogen ion excretion. Conversely, extracellular volume expansion, increased sodium concentration, and decreased potassium concentration suppress the secretion of aldosterone.

Decreased blood sensed by volume receptors in the heart, increased plasma osmolarity at intracranial osmoreceptors, and angiotensin II all stimulate the release of antidiuretic hormone (ADH, vasopressin) from the posterior pituitary gland. ADH increases the reabsorption of water from cells in the distal convoluted tubule and collecting ducts. This effect modulates fluid volume and osmolarity. ADH production occurs in a diurnal fashion, peaking between 2:00 and 4:00 AM and to a lesser extent in the early afternoon.

Potassium

Potassium is the predominant intravascular cation, with 98% in the ICF compared to only 2% of total body potassium in the ECF. Humans intake an average of 100 mEq/d of potassium; however, 95% is excreted in the urine, 5% is lost in feces and sweat, and only 0.5 to 1 mEq/kg/d of this electrolyte is required. In the kidney, most potassium is resorbed in the proximal tubular system. Potassium excretion is directly related to the circulating levels of aldosterone, cellular and extracellular potassium content, and tubular urine flow rates. Acid-base disturbances also affect potassium balance.

PERIOPERATIVE FLUIDS AND ELECTROLYTES

Normally, fluid and electrolyte balance is maintained by sufficient oral intake of water, sodium, potassium, and chloride to offset daily obligatory losses. In perioperative patients, restricted access to oral intake and abnormal electrolyte losses from pathophysiologic states often interfere with self-regulation. Frequent physical examination and laboratory monitoring help to identify fluid and electrolyte abnormalities. *Maintenance fluid* (5% dextrose in 1/2 normal saline [D5 1/2 NS] with 20 mEq KCl) can be administered to offset ongoing losses from urine, stool, lungs, and skin (Table 2-2) to prevent imbalance. In contrast, *replacement fluids* are administered to restore homeostasis after fluid or electrolyte imbalance has occurred and should reflect the composition of the loss (Table 2-3). Patients who have experienced excessive losses or are in hypovolemic or distributive shock require a rapid infusion of *resuscitation fluids* which approximate the ECF.

Fluid, electrolyte, and acid-base imbalances must be identified and treated promptly, particularly in the critically ill or in patients requiring urgent operation. History and physical examination should solicit information regarding the extent of the deficit, and laboratory data should be obtained immediately.

Third spacing refers to isotonic vascular volume depletion caused by the sequestering of fluid in the interstitial space. Third spacing is common in surgical diseases including sepsis, peritonitis, intestinal obstruction, soft tissue inflammation, and trauma. Resultant fluid shifts effectively reduce intravascular volume, leading to hemodynamic changes (tachycardia, narrowed pulse pressure, hypotension), decreasing urine output (<0.5 mL/kg/h), and laboratory evidence of isotonic volume contraction (rising hematocrit and serum BUN-to-creatinine ratio greater than 20:1, urine sodium concentrations <20 mEq/L). In response, fluid resuscitation must be undertaken promptly and should be monitored by correction of vital signs, improved laboratory parameters (pH, lactate, base deficit), and increased urine output. Hypervolemia increases demands on cardiac function and may predispose patients to pneumonia, respiratory failure, pleural effusions, and pulmonary edema. Gastrointestinal (GI) motility may be inhibited, prolonging postoperative ileus. Excess interstitial fluid may also reduce tissue oxygenation with implications for wound (anastomotic) healing. Particularly among critically ill patients, additional static and dynamic measures of volume evaluation including point-of-care ultrasound (right atrial fill and vena caval compression), passive leg raise, and pulse pressure variability can help with the evaluation of clinical status and response to therapy. It is critical to understand the limitations and appropriate interpretation of each test; the best evaluation involves multiple metrics and maintains appreciation of the patient's overall physiology and trajectory.

Intraoperatively, ongoing resuscitation priorities include maintaining circulating volumes and adequate tissue perfusion, acid/base, and electrolyte balance, and keeping up with ongoing blood product losses. Crystalloid solutions are often used throughout the operation to keep up with the dramatic fluid shifts associated with having an open viscous cavity (eg, 1 L/h insensible fluid loss per hour for an open abdomen). In general, we prefer the use of a buffered isotonic solution such as Lactate Ringer's (LR) or Plasmalyte to normal saline which can result in metabolic acidosis, but resuscitation should be tailored to the specific clinical scenario. There is less evidence to support routine resuscitation with colloid solutions, outside of use in specific hypoalbuminemic states such as end-stage liver disease. Although discussed more extensively elsewhere (see Chapter 3), crystalloid should not be used as the primary means of resuscitating actively bleeding patients as this results in dilutional coagulopathy, multiorgan system failure, and increased long-term mortality compared to resuscitation with a 1:1:1 balanced blood product ratio or whole blood. Ongoing discussion with the anesthesia team is critical to communicate fluid goals, projected volume losses, and case duration.

In the immediate postoperative period, patient fluid needs depend on the type and acuity of the procedure and may incorporate resuscitation (iso-osmolar fluids), replacement (loss-specific fluids), and maintenance fluids (daily losses). A guideline frequently cited in the literature for estimating normal daily fluid requirements is the 4:2:1 rule, which states that for normal maintenance fluids per hour, 4 mL is given for the first 10 kg, 2 mL for the second 10 kg, and 1 mL for the remainder of the weight. However, fluid and electrolyte needs should be calculated for each patient.

TABLE 2-2. Composition of Commonly Used Intravenous Solutions

	Glucose (g/L)	Na$^+$ (mEq/L)	K$^+$ (mEq/L)	Cl$^-$ (mEq/L)	Lactate[a] (mEq/L)	Ca^{2+} (mEq/L)
0.9% Sodium chloride ("normal" saline)		154		154		
Lactated Ringer's solution		130	4.0	109	28	3.0
5% Dextrose water	50					
5% Dextrose in 0.45% sodium chloride	50	77		77		
3% Sodium chloride		513		513		

[a]Converted to bicarbonate.

TABLE 2-3. Composition of Normal Body Fluids (mEq)

Fluid	Na$^+$	K$^+$	Cl$^-$	HCO$_3^-$
Plasma	135-150	3.5-5.0	98-106	22-30
Stomach	10-150	4-12	120-160	0
Bile	120-170	3-12	80-120	30-40
Pancreas	135-150	3.5-5.0	60-100	35-110
Small intestine	80-150	2-8	70-130	20-40
Colon	50-100	10-30	80-120	25-30
Perspiration	30-50	5	30-50	0

The composition of most gastrointestinal fluids and of perspiration varies according to the rate of secretion.

FLUID AND ELECTROLYTE DISORDERS IN THE SURGICAL PATIENT

Volume Depletion

Volume depletion may be caused by blood loss, ECF loss, or TBW reductions. Vomiting, diarrhea, nasogastric suction, or enteric fistulas result in ECF volume depletion. Most GI losses are isotonic and can be replaced with NS or LR. Gastric losses usually result in hypochloremic, hypokalemic metabolic alkalosis (contraction alkalosis) which needs to be treated with a higher chloride solution such as NS.

Excess urinary loss of water and electrolytes can lead to volume depletion, as is seen with diuretic therapy, high-output renal failure, or osmotic diuresis associated with nonelectrolyte hyperosmolar solute loading (eg, hyperglycemia or mannitol). Finally, there are volume depletions involving losses of water and excess of solute. These losses include excessive free-water excretion associated with the primary deficiencies of ADH, including diabetes insipidus. Diabetes insipidus can be either from severe head injury or from nephrogenic causes. These hypotonic losses create a hypernatremic, hyperosmolar state in the extracellular compartment that draws water out of the cell.

Volume loss from the extracellular space is usually more rapid than loss from the intracellular space. Neurologic and cardiovascular signs are more prominent with acute losses, whereas tissue signs may not be evident for up to 24 hours. In acute circumstances, changes in hemodynamic parameters will precede changes in renal perfusion. When faced with decreased urine output secondary to hypovolemia, the fractional excretion of sodium (Fe_{Na}) can be used to distinguish between prerenal and renal causes of low urine output:

$$Fe_{Na} = [(U_{Na} \times P_{Cr}) / (P_{Na} \times U_{Cr}) \times 100],$$

where U_{Na} is the urine sodium concentration, P_{Cr} the plasma creatinine concentration, P_{Na} the plasma sodium concentration, and U_{Cr} the urine creatinine concentration.

An Fe_{Na} of less than 1% is characteristic of prerenal azotemia, whereas greater than 2% is most common with renal injury. In acute renal failure, U_{Na} usually increases to more than 40 mEq/L because renal tubular absorption of sodium is impaired.

Isotonic extracellular deficits caused by intestinal, biliary, pancreatic, or third space losses are best treated with LR or NS if hyperchloremia is not a problem. For high-volume resuscitation, bear in mind that smaller-gauge intravenous (IV) needles restrict the amount of fluid that can be given rapidly. Poiseuille law states that the amount of resistance to flow through a system is dependent on the radius to the fourth power ($R = \eta L/\pi r^4$; η is the dynamic viscosity of the fluid, L the length of the pipe, r the radius of the pipe). A "large-bore" IV is a 16-gauge IV.

Determination of the end points of resuscitation continues to be debated. Vital signs such as pulse, blood pressure, and urine output can be used; adequate urine output is more than 0.5 mL/kg/h in adults or 1.0 mL/kg/h or children. In the critically ill, monitoring adjuncts as described previously can be used.

Volume Excess

Volume excess, for any or all fluid compartments, can occur from abnormal fluid retention, excessive or inappropriate fluid intake, or both. The clinical presentation of extracellular volume excess may range from simple weight gain, decreases in hemoglobin (hemodilution), modest elevation of peripheral and central venous pressure (CVP), and dependent sacral or lower extremity edema to extreme changes such as congestive heart failure, pleural effusions, pulmonary edema, anasarca, and hepatomegaly.

Treatment is adjusted according to the severity and rate of development of fluid compartment changes and related clinical findings. If it is determined that the patient has an increase in all fluid compartments, treatment might be as simple as fluid or sodium restriction. If symptoms are severe, the patient may need diuresis. If the patient is thought to have an intravascular volume deficit, then careful replacement with crystalloid or blood products may be needed, despite extravascular fluid overload.

Disorders of Sodium Balance

Sodium is the principal solute determining ECF osmolarity and fluid volume balance. Increased extracellular sodium creates an osmotic gradient that draws water out of cells. Decreased extracellular sodium does the reverse. As such, sodium balance and fluid balance disorders are usually linked.

Hyponatremia

Hyponatremia results from the presence of excess body water relative to total body sodium and the failure of the kidneys to excrete the excess water. Serum sodium concentration does not always reflect true total body sodium content or even osmolarity. For example, total body sodium may be increased in patients with chronic cardiac, hepatic, or renal disease, but hyponatremia persists because of a proportionally greater increase in water.

Hyponatremia may be associated with decreased, increased, or normal ECF volume, and each requires a different approach to correct the abnormality. In surgical patients, dilutional hyponatremia occurs most commonly when hypotonic fluids are used to replace significant isotonic GI or third space losses. Artifactually, very low serum sodium values are seen in the presence of severe hyperglycemia and hypertriglyceridemia, or after IV infusion of lipids. Hyponatremia has also been associated with necrotizing soft tissue infections.

The primary clinical manifestations of hyponatremia are the signs and symptoms of central nervous system (CNS) dysfunction because of cerebral and spinal cord swelling. Neurologic disturbances occur as a result. Serum sodium between 130 and 120 mEq/L may cause irritability, weakness, fatigue, increased deep tendon reflexes, and muscle twitches if the hyponatremia developed rapidly. If left untreated, severe hyponatremia may lead to seizures, coma, reflexia, and death.

In diagnosing hyponatremia, serum and urine sodium, serum and urine osmolality, and pH may be assessed. Blood tests can exclude associated electrolyte abnormalities (eg, hyperglycemia, liver diseases, and acid-base disorders). Volume status must be assessed by accurate history and physical examination.

The treatment of hyponatremia depends on the cause, severity, and nature of any associated volume abnormality. Psychogenic polydipsia is treated with water restriction. Most asymptomatic dilutional hyponatremia that is iatrogenically induced in the perioperative period is treated by simple fluid restriction. Thiazide diuretics cause hyponatremia by blocking the resorption of sodium and chloride in the cortical-diluting segment. The best treatment for this condition is discontinuation of the diuretic. Chronic hyponatremia correction must be done slowly. Disorders that involve total body sodium excess, in addition to disproportionate volume excess, are treated by a restriction of both sodium and water. Hyponatremia associated with volume contraction is treated with combined sodium and volume repletion, usually with normal saline solution (NSS) or LR solution. The rate of repletion is dictated by the degree of volume deficit.

Hypertonic saline solutions (2% or higher) are indicated *only* when hyponatremia causes life-threatening neurologic disturbances. To estimate the amount of sodium needed to correct the serum deficit, multiply the decrease in serum sodium (in milliequivalents) by TBW (in liters) as a percentage of total body weight:

$$\text{mEq Na}^+ \text{ needed} = (140 - \text{measured serum Na}^+) \times \text{TBW},$$

where TBW = estimated % of body water × body weight (kg). No more than one-half of the total calculated amount of sodium is given in the first 12 to 18 hours, and it is given at a maximum rate of 12 mEq/L of concentration per 24 hours to avoid central pontine myelinolysis.

The prognosis of hyponatremia usually depends on the prognosis of the underlying condition. Severe neurologic symptoms may have irreversible sequelae.

Hypernatremia

Hypernatremia results from excess body sodium content relative to body water. Clinically significant hypernatremia, serum sodium greater than 150 mEq/L, can be lethal if it is allowed to progress unchecked. Hypernatremia may result from the loss of water alone (eg, hypothalamic abnormalities, nonreplaced insensible losses), from the loss of water and salt together (GI losses, osmotic

diuresis, excessive diuretic use, central or nephrogenic diabetes insipidus, burns, excessive sweating), as a side effect of many drugs, or from increased total body sodium without any water loss (Cushing syndrome, hyperaldosteronism, ectopic production of ACTH, iatrogenic sodium administration, ingestion of seawater). Severe hypernatremia occurs only in situations in which a person cannot obtain water (infancy, disability, altered mental states).

The pathophysiologic consequences of hypernatremia reflect both extracellular volume losses and cellular dehydration that result from water shifts in response to osmotic pressure. The severity of the clinical manifestation is directly related to both the degree of hypernatremia and the rapidity with which it develops. Serum sodium concentrations more than 160 mEq/L may be associated with the signs and symptoms of dehydration, decreased tissue turgor, oliguria, fever, and tachycardia. The signs and symptoms also include those of neuromuscular and neurologic disorders, from twitching, restlessness, and weakness, to delirium, coma, seizures, and death. Intracranial hemorrhage is a common postmortem finding in patients who die of hypernatremia.

The treatment of hypernatremia consists of correcting the relative or absolute water deficit. If deficits are modest, they can be replaced orally or with IV D5W. If deficits are more severe, the TBW deficit is calculated according to the formula to estimate total body sodium. The relative water deficit (in liters) is equal to the milliequivalent change in serum $\text{Na}^+/140$. The water must be replaced slowly, with no more than one-half given over the first 12 to 24 hours. For pure water loss, D5W is infused intravenously.

The process of reversing hypernatremia requires close monitoring. If water is replaced too rapidly, osmotic shifts can produce cellular edema. Brain cells accumulate intracellular solutes slowly in response to slowly developing extracellular hypertonicity. A sudden decrease in extracellular osmolarity leads to a rapid swelling of brain cells, causing serious neurologic dysfunction.

Disorders of Potassium Balance

As the principal intracellular cation, potassium is a major determinant of intracellular volume. It is a significant cofactor in cellular metabolism. Extracellular potassium plays an important role in neuromuscular function.

Hypokalemia

Hypokalemia is defined as a serum potassium less than 3.5 mEq/L and may reflect deficiency that results from inadequate intake, GI tract losses, or renal losses. Hypokalemia may also reflect shifts from the extracellular to the intracellular compartment (eg, insulin administration or alkalosis). GI losses can be major factors in hypokalemia. The highest GI concentrations of potassium are found in the colon and the rectum. Prolonged vomiting or nasogastric aspiration causes hypokalemia through a combination of factors. In addition to the loss of potassium in the gastric fluid, the loss of hydrogen and chloride ions produces hypochloremic, hypokalemic metabolic alkalosis. The increase in extracellular pH causes the movement of potassium into the cells, which makes the hypokalemia worse. Paradoxical aciduria can contribute to the "contraction alkalosis" that ensues.

Hypokalemia usually does not become clinically significant until serum potassium decreases to less than 3.0 mEq/L. Hypokalemia may cause neuromuscular symptoms such as skeletal muscle weakness, fatigue, paresthesias, paralysis, and rhabdomyolysis. Deep tendon reflexes may be diminished or absent. Other symptoms include anorexia, polyuria, and nausea and vomiting associated with paralytic ileus. Total body potassium depletion produces cellular atrophy and negative nitrogen balance. Renal tubular function is impaired, which may result in polyuria and polydipsia because of reduced concentrating ability. Progressive electrocardiogram (ECG) abnormalities include low-voltage, flattened, or inverted T waves, with prominent U waves, depressed S-T segments, prolonged P-R intervals, and widened QRS complexes. A rapid decrease in serum potassium may lead to cardiac arrest.

If the deficiency is mild and the cause is clear from the history, serum potassium may be the only test required. Digoxin level should be measured when pertinent. If hypokalemia is more severe or refractory to treatment, other serum electrolytes, including calcium and magnesium, should be measured. The treatment of hypokalemia involves replacing potassium and correcting the underlying cause. Whenever possible, potassium is repleted orally. If the IV route is required, the rate should not exceed 10 mEq/h, with the dose repeated as often as necessary to increase the serum level to greater than or equal to 3.5 mEq/L. IV administration that is too rapid can cause hyperkalemia and fatal cardiac arrhythmias. Magnesium and calcium levels should be repleted concurrently.

Hyperkalemia

Hyperkalemia is a serum potassium level greater than 5.0 mEq/L, and the etiology is usually multifactorial. Endogenous loading can result from excessive intake in a patient with renal insufficiency, or it can occur post transfusion. Endogenous loading occurs whenever large amounts of intracellular potassium are released into the extracellular space (as in crush injuries, hemolysis, lysis, and the absorption of large hematomas, and in the catabolism of fat and muscle tissue). Hyperkalemia can also be caused by decreased renal excretion. Shifts of potassium from the intracellular to the extracellular compartment also cause hyperkalemia (eg, acute metabolic or respiratory acidosis, insulin deficiency, therapy with digitalis and related cardiotonic agents).

Numerous drugs cause hyperkalemia. Impaired renal excretion can be caused by diuretics (eg, spironolactone, triamterene, amiloride) and by nonsteroidal anti-inflammatory drugs, β-adrenergic antagonists, and ACE inhibitors. Digitalis preparations, arginine, β-adrenergic antagonists, and some poisons can also cause shifts of potassium out of the intracellular compartment, raising the serum level.

Although hyperkalemia causes peripheral muscle weakness that ultimately progresses to respiratory paralysis, the most important signs and symptoms are cardiac. The first ECG abnormality is peaked T waves, at serum concentrations between 6.0 and 7.0 mEq/L. Further elevations produce multiple ECG abnormalities. At elevations greater than 8.0 mEq/L, ventricular fibrillation and cardiac arrest are possible. Diagnosis is made by measuring the serum potassium level. If spurious hyperkalemia is suspected, blood should be redrawn, but the treatment of a very high serum potassium level should not be delayed while waiting for results.

The primary goal of the treatment of hyperkalemia is to reduce serum potassium to levels that are not life threatening. In mild hyperkalemia (<6 mEq/L), the simplest measures are to restrict potassium intake, eliminate causes such as potassium-sparing diuretics, and treat fluid volume or acid-base disorders. Potassium-wasting diuretics may be administered, and hormone deficiencies may be replaced. For higher potassium levels, 10 units of insulin are administered intravenously along with 25 g of glucose intravenously over 5 minutes. This therapy shifts potassium from the extracellular to the intracellular compartment. A similar shift may be created by administering bicarbonate. These compartment shifts last only a few hours. Sodium polystyrene sulfonate (Kayexalate), a cation-exchange resin, administered orally or rectally actually removes potassium from the body. Patients with evidence of cardiac toxicity should be treated with IV calcium gluconate given slowly over 5 minutes to reduce cardiac muscle electrical excitability. Hemodialysis and peritoneal dialysis also remove potassium from the body and may be necessary in patients with renal failure.

Hyperkalemia itself does not affect recovery from illness or surgery, and it is usually correctable. Cardiac events caused by hyperkalemia may be fatal if the hyperkalemia and its effects are not promptly treated.

Disorders of Calcium Balance

The normal range of total serum calcium is 8.0 to 10.5 mg/dL, and that of ionized calcium is 4.75 to 5.30 mg/dL. Most bound calcium is bound to albumin, and total serum calcium is dependent on serum albumin. Ionized calcium is a more accurate indicator of physiologic activity than total calcium. Overall calcium homeostasis, largely regulated by parathyroid hormone (PTH), is the result of intestinal absorption, renal excretion, and calcium exchange between bone and the ECF.

Hypocalcemia

Hypocalcemia is defined as total serum calcium less than 8 mg/dL. It is seen in many conditions common to surgical patients, several of which are acute problems. It is often seen in acute pancreatitis. Inadequate intestinal absorption of calcium may result from inflammatory bowel disease, pancreatic exocrine dysfunction, or malabsorption syndromes. Excessive fluid losses from chronic diarrhea or pancreatic or intestinal fistulas may also seriously deplete extracellular calcium. Low serum calcium levels are seen with severe soft tissue infections, such as necrotizing fasciitis. Artifactual hypocalcemia is seen when serum albumin is low and total calcium, rather than ionized calcium, is measured. Vitamin D deficiency may result from synthetic failure in renal or hepatic disease or from conversion to inactive metabolites caused by drugs such as phenytoin and phenobarbital. Hypocalcemia can also occur after blood transfusion as a result of citrate binding and dilution.

Another way to classify hypocalcemia is according to its relation to PTH, which may be (1) deficient or absent (eg, hypomagnesemia, any type of true hypoparathyroidism), (2) ineffective (eg, vitamin D disorders, chronic renal failure, pseudohypoparathyroidism), or (3) overwhelmed (eg, hyperphosphatemia).

The early symptoms of hypocalcemia include circumoral tingling, numbness and tingling of the fingertips, and muscle cramps. Hyperactive deep tendon reflexes develop, with a Chvostek sign (unilateral facial spasm when the facial nerve on the side is lightly tapped), tetany, and Trousseau sign (carpopedal spasm), eventually progressing to seizures. The patient may be confused or depressed. Prolonged Q-T intervals are seen on ECG.

Diagnosis is made by measuring serum calcium, along with serum potassium, magnesium, phosphate, and alkaline phosphatase. During physical examination, a search should be made for a transverse surgical scar on the anterior neck, which would suggest previous thyroidectomy or parathyroidectomy.

The treatment of symptomatic hypocalcemia is directed at correcting the calcium deficit, normalizing the relation between ionized and protein-bound calcium by correcting acid-base disorders and treating the underlying causes. When the need for correction is urgent (eg, severe, highly symptomatic hypocalcemia), calcium gluconate or calcium chloride is infused. Vitamin D supplements may be needed; the high doses required in hypoparathyroidism may be reduced if urinary calcium loss is decreased with thiazide diuretics.

Hypercalcemia

Hypercalcemia is defined as serum calcium greater than 10.5 mg/dL. In surgical patients, primary and secondary hyperparathyroidism and metastatic breast cancer are among the common causes. Malignancies cause hypercalcemia both by bony involvement and by the secretion of PTH-like substances that affect calcium metabolism. Malignancies that are sufficiently advanced to cause hypercalcemia are usually symptomatic. The mobilization of calcium from bone in bedridden patients can cause mild, asymptomatic hypercalcemia.

The initial clinical manifestations of hypercalcemia are nonspecific: weakness, fatigue, anorexia, nausea, and vomiting. As serum calcium increases, severe headaches, diffuse musculoskeletal pain, polyuria, and polydipsia develop.

The combination of decreased oral intake, vomiting, and polyuria leads to hypovolemia and dehydration, which may become pronounced. The ECG shows shortened Q-T intervals and widened T waves. With normal or elevated phosphate, calcification may develop in the kidneys as well as in unusual locations (eg, heart, skin). Pancreatitis and renal failure may develop as well. The renal failure has multiple causes, including volume depletion, nephrocalcinosis, and the deposition of nephrotoxic myeloma proteins or light chains. When serum calcium increases to 15 mg/dL and above, confusion and depression progress to somnolence, stupor, and coma. This degree of hypercalcemia results in death unless it is corrected promptly.

The presence of symptomatic bone metastasis may be the initial presentation of some malignancies, such as those originating in the prostate or breast.

Initially, calcium intake is restricted, hydration status is improved, and urinary calcium excretion is increased. If the patient is symptomatic or the calcium level is high, the patient should be hospitalized. Large volumes of IV NS or 1/2 NS are infused. Loop diuretics enhance calcium excretion. Great care must be taken during the process of vigorous hydration and diuresis, with close monitoring. Oral or IV phosphate supplements are sometimes used to form complexes with ionized calcium. Given intravenously, these supplements may produce a precipitous decrease in serum calcium.

Disorders of Magnesium Balance

Magnesium plays an important role in metabolism because it is a cofactor for many enzymes.

Hypomagnesemia

Hypomagnesemia is common in surgical patients, particularly the older adults, who are often in a starvation state, are experiencing GI loss, or have absorption defects. Severe hypomagnesemia also produces severe hypocalcemia by decreasing PTH secretion and by an apparent skeletal resistance and an impaired renal response.

The most common cause of hypomagnesemia is dietary deficiency combined with GI losses and deficiencies in other elements. Other causes include chronic alcoholism, malabsorption, acute pancreatitis, improperly constituted parenteral nutrition (PN), and endocrine disorders. Hypomagnesemia also occurs as a side effect of many therapeutic drugs.

Magnesium affects neuromuscular function. Symptoms develop insidiously, first as nonspecific systemic symptoms that include nausea, vomiting, anorexia, weakness, and lethargy. Neuromuscular symptoms including muscle cramps, fasciculations, tetany, carpopedal spasm, paresthesia, irritability, inattention and confusion, and cardiac arrhythmias follow. Diagnosis is made by testing serum values.

Primary attention must be given to correcting the cause. If hypomagnesemia is mild and does not result from an absorptive defect, oral supplements are given. If it is moderate or severe, then it is treated with IV magnesium sulfate.

Importantly, hypomagnesemia often leads to refractory hypocalcemia and hypokalemia.

Hypermagnesemia

Clinically significant hypermagnesemia is rare, especially if renal function is normal. Hypermagnesemia can result from renal failure, dehydration, severe metabolic acidosis, adrenal insufficiency, familial benign hypocalciuric hypercalcemia, or overdosage with magnesium salts in cathartics. In addition, in either mother or newborn, it can occur after the treatment of eclampsia. It also occurs in patients with renal failure who use magnesium-containing antacids. Renal excretion is decreased in metabolic alkalosis.

Symptomatic hypermagnesemia follows a progressive pattern, with increasing neuromuscular and CNS abnormalities as the serum level increases. Initial nausea is superseded by lethargy, weakness, hypoventilation, and decreased deep tendon reflexes. The condition then progresses to hypotension and bradycardia, skeletal muscle paralysis, respiratory depression, coma, and death. Diagnosis is made by testing serum values.

Mild hypermagnesemia is treated with oral hydration and by controlling magnesium intake. Severe symptoms are reversed temporarily by IV calcium, and the magnesium excess is treated with hydration and diuretics, or hemodialysis.

Disorders of Phosphate Balance

Phosphorus is a component of all body tissues, and it participates in virtually all metabolic processes. The intestine, influenced by vitamin D, absorbs approximately 70% of ingested soluble phosphorus. The normal range of serum phosphate is 2.5 to 4.5 mg/dL.

Hypophosphatemia

Hypophosphatemia is common in surgical patients. When phosphorus is deficient, there are also losses of potassium and magnesium, the other two major elements in cells. The causes of hypophosphatemia are categorized as (1) inadequate uptake as a result of inadequate dietary intake, malabsorption, GI losses, prolonged antacid use, improperly constituted PN, or vitamin D deficiency; (2) increased renal excretion as a result of diuretic use, hypervolemia, corticoid therapy, hyperaldosteronism, syndrome of inappropriate secretion of ADH, or hyperparathyroidism; or (3) compartmental shifts as a result of hormones, nutrients that stimulate insulin release, the treatment of diabetic ketoacidosis, recovery from hypometabolic states, rapidly growing malignancies, or respiratory alkalosis. It is also seen in chronic alcoholism, in burns, and after parathyroidectomy or renal transplantation.

Severe phosphorous deficiency causes anorexia, dizziness, osteomalacia, severe congestive cardiomyopathy, proximal muscle weakness, visual defects, ascending paralysis, hemolytic anemia, and respiratory failure. Inability to wean from the ventilator can be seen in critically ill patients with hypophosphatemia. Leukocyte and erythrocyte malfunction, rhabdomyolysis, hypercalciuria, and severe hypocalcemia are also seen. CNS dysfunction occurs and can progress to seizures, coma, and death. Diagnosis is made by testing serum values.

Severe hypophosphatemia should prompt an aggressive search for and treatment of the cause. Phosphate salts may be given orally or intravenously. Other associated electrolyte abnormalities must also be treated. Diuretics may be withdrawn. VIPomas should be surgically removed. Repletion of phosphorus corrects or decreases most abnormalities. Respiratory failure may not be reversed completely, and the ultimate outcome is likely to depend on the prognosis of the underlying deficiency.

Hyperphosphatemia

Hyperphosphatemia is relatively common in adults and is seen even in the presence of total body phosphate deficiency. The causes of hyperphosphatemia are categorized as (1) decreased renal excretion; (2) increased intestinal absorption as a result of sarcoidosis or tuberculosis (both of which produce vitamin D), or excess phosphate or vitamin D ingestion; (3) iatrogenic, as a result of IV infusion of phosphate-containing fluids; or (4) shifts from the intracellular to the extracellular compartment as a result of acidotic states, tumor lysis, hemolytic anemia, thyrotoxicosis, or rhabdomyolysis.

Hyperphosphatemia is associated with no symptoms, although in the presence of severe hypercalcemia, renal failure, or vitamin D intoxication, it may be accompanied by a deposition of calcium phosphate in abnormal locations. It is diagnosed by testing serum values.

Aluminum-based antacids decrease absorption by binding phosphate, and diuretics increase the rate of urinary phosphate excretion. Dialysis is used in patients with renal failure. It is often unnecessary to treat hyperphosphatemia, except by correcting excess intake and addressing associated problems.

Disorders of Acid-Base Balance

The pH disorders of blood can be grouped into two broad categories: respiratory and metabolic. Respiratory acid-base disorders are disorders of $Paco_2$. Metabolic acid-base disorders are disorders of bicarbonate. An arterial blood pH that is less than 7.35 signifies acidemia, whereas a pH greater than 7.45 signifies alkalemia. The normal limits of $Paco_2$ are 37 to 45 mm Hg. An arterial $Paco_2$ that is elevated above the normal range produces respiratory acidosis. Respiratory alkalosis occurs if the $Paco_2$ is below the normal range.

Bicarbonate concentration normally varies between 22 and 26 mEq/L. A plasma HCO_3^- concentration that is less than 22 mEq/L is defined as metabolic acidosis. Metabolic alkalosis is present when the bicarbonate level is above normal (26 mEq/L).

Simple acid-base disorders occur when there is a primary change either in the bicarbonate concentration or in the $Paco_2$ with an appropriate (normal) secondary change in the other parameter, as illustrated in the following equation:

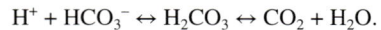

$$H^+ + HCO_3^- \leftrightarrow H_2CO_3 \leftrightarrow CO_2 + H_2O.$$

Normally, the CO_2 that is produced is eliminated rapidly by the lungs.

The presence of an isolated acid-base disorder is unusual. With normal kidney and lung function, compensation occurs. As a result, many disorders of acid-base are mixed. Two rules are helpful in assessing the degree to which the respiratory or bicarbonate component contributes to the change in pH.

1. An acute change in $Paco_2$ of 10 mm Hg is associated with a reciprocal change of 0.08 pH units from baseline pH.
2. An acute change in HCO_3 of 10 mEq/L is associated with a direct change of 0.16 pH units from baseline pH.

Respiratory Acidosis

Respiratory acidosis is the result of retention of CO_2 because of pulmonary alveolar hypoventilation. It can be acute or chronic. Acute causes are typically respiratory depression or caused by reduced respiratory effort. Chronic respiratory acidosis is most often caused by advanced lung diseases such as chronic obstructive pulmonary disease. This results in a compensated hypoventilation and can be well tolerated.

The acid-base disorder has a primary respiratory cause if the $Paco_2$ is abnormal and the $Paco_2$ and pH change in opposite directions. The clinical consequences of acute respiratory acidosis are caused by hypercapnia and the accompanying hypoxia. With more severe elevations of $Paco_2$ levels, confusion, somnolence, and ultimately coma can occur as a result of CO_2 narcosis. In combination with hypoxemia, cardiovascular dysfunction can occur, which may result in cardiac arrest and death. In patients with chronic hypoventilation and respiratory acidosis, the major threat is CO_2 narcosis. In chronic compensated respiratory acidosis, the stimulus to breathe is hypoxia, not hydrogen ion concentration in arterial blood. By adding oxygen, the stimulus to breathe is removed, and CO_2 narcosis ensues.

The treatment of respiratory acidosis requires the identification and correction of the underlying cause of reduced alveolar ventilation while maintaining oxygenation. This may be as simple as administering supplemental oxygen, instituting mechanical ventilation, or simply improving pain control because many patients have enough postoperative pain that their breathing is inhibited. Acute hypercapnia should not be overcorrected. An abrupt decrease in $Paco_2$ below normal levels can cause cerebral vasoconstriction and decrease cerebral blood flow, particularly in patients with acute brain injury.

Metabolic Acidosis

Metabolic acidosis can be acute or chronic. One cause of metabolic acidosis is the loss of bicarbonate from the extracellular space. This may be due to diarrhea, intestinal fistula, biliary fistula, or pancreatic fistula. Chronic bicarbonate losses occur with renal dysfunction, ureterointestinal anastomosis, decreased mineralocorticoid activity, and the use of the diuretic acetazolamide, which is also a carbonic anhydrase inhibitor. In burn patients, the use of mafenide acetate, which is also a carbonic anhydrase inhibitor, can result in metabolic acidosis.

The second major cause of metabolic acidosis is an increased acid load. Lactic acidosis occurs with shock whether hypovolemic, hemorrhagic, septic, or cardiogenic, and is due to the production of lactic acid as the body responds to the insult with anaerobic metabolism and/or increased accumulation in tissue of metabolites due to reduced cellular clearance. Ketoacidosis that occurs with untreated hyperglycemia is another cause of metabolic acidosis, as is the ingestion of toxins, including salicylates, methanol, and other toxins. Liver failure can result in metabolic acidosis when the liver decompensates to the point where lactate and citrate that are normally produced by the body cannot be metabolized. Renal failure can cause metabolic acidosis when the kidney fails to retain bicarbonate as a result of injury to the tubules.

Metabolic acidosis is the primary disorder if the pH is abnormal and the pH and the $Paco_2$ change in the same direction. Respiratory compensation occurs with both acute and chronic metabolic acidosis. The determination of the anion gap will help distinguish the loss of bicarbonate from the presence of additional acids as the cause of metabolic acidosis. The anion gap is the difference between the serum sodium concentration and the sum of the bicarbonate and chloride concentrations in serum.

Normal anion gap is approximately 12 ± 3 mEq/L. With the loss of bicarbonate, the chloride increases and the anion gap remains normal. With the addition of metabolic acids, the chloride levels do not increase and bicarbonate levels fall, thus causing an anion "gap."

Identifying the underlying disorder causing metabolic acidosis and correcting it expeditiously are critical. Hypovolemia must be corrected, bleeding must be stopped, sepsis must be controlled, and/or cardiac function must be improved to improve tissue perfusion in order to satisfy cellular metabolic needs. The administration of bicarbonate without correcting the underlying problem will not return the pH to normal.

Respiratory Alkalosis

Respiratory alkalosis is present when an increase in pH is related to alveolar hyperventilation and a reduced $Paco_2$. This is common in surgical patients and may be caused by apprehension, pain that does not impede respiratory effort, hypoxia, fever, brain injury, sepsis, and liver failure that results in elevated serum ammonia. Hypocapnia is also common in patients who are mechanically ventilated. The compensatory mechanism for respiratory alkalosis is renal excretion of bicarbonate.

Acute respiratory alkalosis may appear similar to hypocalcemia with paresthesias, carpopedal spasm, and Chvostek sign. Potassium, magnesium, calcium, and phosphate metabolism are all disturbed in alkalotic states. The acute hypocarbia can also cause cerebral vasoconstriction and decreased cerebral blood flow.

In the spontaneously breathing patient, the treatment is aimed at correcting the underlying cause of the hyperventilation.

Metabolic Alkalosis

Metabolic alkalosis occurs when the pH is elevated in association with an elevated serum bicarbonate level. It is one of the most common acid-base abnormalities in surgical patients. Renal and GI losses of potassium and chloride result in hypochloremic, hypokalemic metabolic alkalosis. The infusion of excess bicarbonate can also cause metabolic alkalosis. The administration of loop diuretics may also result in a contraction of extracellular volume and metabolic alkalosis. Hypoventilation may allow for the accumulation of CO_2 and correction of the metabolic alkalosis. The kidneys' response to metabolic alkalosis initially results in alkaline urine as bicarbonate is excreted. With hypochloremic, hypokalemic metabolic alkalosis, the loss of electrolytes and the kidney's mechanism of saving potassium, absorbing bicarbonate instead of chloride, and excreting hydrogen ions will result in paradoxical aciduria.

The clinical problems associated with metabolic alkalosis are manifestations of hypochloremia, hypokalemia, and intravascular volume deficiency. This may be caused by GI or renal losses and result in paralytic ileus, cardiac dysrhythmias, and digitalis toxicity.

The treatment of metabolic alkalosis requires the replacement of electrolytes (particularly chloride and potassium) and fluids specific to the type of loss, as well as control of ongoing losses. Once the kidney has adequate intravascular volume, and the electrolytes are replaced, the kidney will again excrete bicarbonate. The treatment is the administration of chloride as a balanced salt solution, for example, NSS. Chloride-unresponsive hypochloremic metabolic alkalosis is characterized by urinary chloride that is greater than 20 mEq/L. This does not usually respond to chloride administration and may require glucocorticoid administration even when the electrolytes are corrected.

OVERVIEW OF METABOLISM

Impact of Starvation and Stress

During the first 24 to 72 hours of nonstressed starvation, basal energy requirements are reduced and are supplied by liver and muscle glycogen stores. With persistent starvation and glycogen depletion, deamination of gluconeogenic amino acids, such as alanine and glutamine, accounts for an increasingly greater percentage of total glucose production to meet preferential needs for glucose by the brain, CNS, and red blood cells. Because of body protein structural and functional importance, they are not a long-term source of fuel, and protein depletion in excess of 20% is not compatible with life. With persistent starvation, fat mobilization, possibly resulting from decreased insulin levels, inhibits lipase and allows for intracellular hydrolysis of triglycerides, which decreases proteolysis and hepatic gluconeogenesis. Because of only partial hepatic oxidation of fatty acids, serum levels of acetoacetate, β-hydroxybutyrate, and acetone increase and can be oxidized to CO_2 and H_2O by tissues such as the kidney, muscle, and brain. Although the brain and CNS can convert to utilizing ketoacids for fuel during nonstressed starvation, these by-products of incomplete fatty acid metabolism eventually become toxic. During unstressed starvation, energy expenditure is decreased, and a change in the insulin:glucagon ratio to favor mobilization of stored fuels, glycogen, and adipose tissue and to minimize lean body tissue loss occurs.

The metabolic response to injury or infection is classically divided into the ebb and flow phase. The ebb phase begins immediately after injury and typically lasts between 12 and 24 hours, but it may last longer depending on injury severity and adequate resuscitation. This early phase is characterized by tissue hypoperfusion and hypometabolism. In order to compensate, catecholamines are released, with norepinephrine being the primary mediator. Released from peripheral nerves, norepinephrine binds to $\beta\beta_1$ receptors in the heart and to α and $\beta\beta_2$ receptors in peripheral and splanchnic vascular beds. This results in increased cardiac contractility, heart rate, and vasoconstriction in an attempt to restore blood pressure, increase cardiac performance, and maximize venous return.

The flow phase encompasses the catabolic and anabolic phases and is signaled by high cardiac output with the restoration of oxygen delivery and metabolic substrate. Although the duration of the flow phase depends on the severity of injury and illness, it typically peaks at 3 to 5 days and subsides by 7 to 10 days, merging with the anabolic phase over the next few weeks. During this hypermetabolic phase, although insulin levels are elevated, high levels of catecholamines, glucagon, and cortisol counteract most of insulin's metabolic effects. This hormonal imbalance results in the mobilization of amino acids and free fatty acids from peripheral muscles and adipose tissue. Some of these released substrates are used for energy production, as previously described. Other substrates contribute to the synthesis of proteins in the liver, where humoral mediators increase the production of acute-phase reactants, and in the immune system for healing damaged tissues. The net result is a significant loss of protein, characterized by negative nitrogen balance and decreased adipose stores, accompanied by enlarged extracellular water compartments.

Stress hyperglycemia is common and results from accelerated gluconeogenesis and relative insulin resistance. This can become quite exaggerated in patients with or without underlying diabetes. Glucose control (eg, blood glucose 80-150 mg/dL) is important in surgical patients to limit infectious complications, other morbidities, and mortality.

Determining Energy Requirements

Indirect calorimetry is the measurement of respiratory gas exchange to make inference about cellular gas exchange, which equates to metabolic rate and substrate utilization. The measured parameters of indirect calorimetry are oxygen consumption (Vo_2) and carbon dioxide production (VCO_2). From these measurements, respiratory quotient and metabolic rate can be calculated. Indirect calorimetry is valid only when respiratory and cellular gas exchange is equivalent. Because of several limitations in using indirect calorimetry, including availability and cost, predictive equations or simplistic weight-based formulas (20-30 kcal/kg/d) are used to estimate resting metabolic rate (RMR).

Various conditions (eg, trauma, burns, pregnancy, lactation) can increase basal metabolic rate (BMR) by 10% to 100%, so many predictive equations add factors for activity and/or injury above BMR. An estimated dry and lean body mass weight is to be used to avoid overfeeding.

In people who are obese, lean body and cell mass are very difficult to assess, making RMR difficult to predict. With obesity, achieving some degree of weight loss may increase insulin sensitivity, improve nursing care, and reduce the risk of comorbidities. To promote steady weight loss in this population and adequate healing, providing 65% to 70% of energy requirements as measured by indirect calorimetry or 11 to 14 kcal/kg actual body weight is recommended. Protein should be provided at a dose of 2.0 to 2.5 g/kg ideal body weight per day to approximate protein requirements and neutral nitrogen balance.

Macronutrient Requirements
Carbohydrate
Carbohydrates supply 4 kcal of energy/g, and glycogen is the principal storage form of glucose. The brain and red and white blood cells are primarily obligate glucose tissues; therefore, approximately 120 g/d is necessary to maintain CNS function. Liver glycogen stores are limited (180 g in a 70-kg person) and are usually exhausted within 24 hours in the unfed state. The maximal glucose oxidation rate is 4 to 7 mg/kg/min, roughly equivalent to 400 to 700 g/d in a 70-kg person. During hypermetabolism, oxidized glucose derived from amino acid substrates via gluconeogenesis can yield up to 2 to 3 mg/kg/min of glucose. Exogenous insulin delivery can increase cellular glucose uptake in critically ill patients; however, it is relatively ineffective in improving glucose oxidation. In order to limit the diabetogenic response, carbohydrates should comprise approximately 50% to 60% of total energy requirements, delivered at 3 to 4 mg/kg/min. Supplemental insulin can then be used to maintain normoglycemia.

Protein
Proteins provide 4.0 kcal/g and should account for 20% to 30% of the total daily caloric intake or 1.5 to 2 g/kg/d. In the nonstressed state, approximately 2.5% of total body protein is broken down and resynthesized every 24 hours. All protein in the body is functional and should not be considered a storage form of energy; therefore, any protein utilized for gluconeogenesis and acute-phase protein synthesis should be considered a loss of functional protein. Table 2-4 includes individual serum proteins and their half-life, normal range, and function.

TABLE 2-4. Select Serum Proteins: Classification and Functions

Serum Protein	Function	Half-Life	Normal Range	Interpreting Results
Positive				
C-Reactive protein	General marker of inflammation and infection	5 h	0.2-8 mg/dL	Synthesized by liver Rises during inflammation and infection Falls when infection or inflammation resolves
Negative				
Albumin	Maintains plasma on-cotic pressure; carrier for amino acids, zinc, magnesium, calcium, free fatty acids, drugs	21 d	3.5-5.0 mg/dL	Routinely available Synthesized in the liver; altered by liver disease Alterations occur in kidney disease with glomerular damage Elevated in dehydration Levels fall with protein-losing enteropathy; may be low in chronic, long-term unstressed malnutrition Negative acute-phase reactant, levels drop in inflammation, shock
Prealbumin (transthyretin)	Thyroxine transport, formation of a complex with retinol-binding protein	2-3 d	18-38 mg/dL	Synthesized in the liver Highly sensitive to dietary deprivation and refeeding Elevated in renal dysfunction Negative acute-phase reactant
Transferrin	Iron-binding protein	8 d	202-336 mg/dL	Decreased levels when diet deficient in protein Synthesized in the liver; altered by liver disease Elevated in iron deficiency, pregnancy, chronic blood loss Low levels in chronic diseases, cirrhosis, nephritic syndrome, protein-losing enteropathy Negative acute-phase reactant
Retinol-binding protein	Transports vitamin A; bound to prealbumin	12 h	2-6 mg/dL	Highly sensitive to acute changes in protein malnutrition and dietary intake Elevated in renal failure Decreased in vitamin A deficiency Negative acute-phase reactant

Glutamine, the most abundant amino acid and primary fuel source for small intestine enterocytes, comprises more than 50% of the free amino acid pool and is synthesized in most tissues of the body. During catabolic illness, glutamine uptake by the small intestine and immunologically active cells can exceed glutamine synthesis and release from the skeletal muscle, making glutamine a conditionally essential amino acid. Although glutamine is a major contributor to homeostasis in the surgical population, improved outcome benefit with exogenous glutamine provision is lacking.

Arginine is a nonessential amino acid in unstressed conditions because of adequate arginine synthesis for normal maintenance of tissue metabolism, growth, and repair. Growth hormone, glucagon, prolactin, and insulin release are all increased with supplemental arginine. Arginine is also the substrate for nitric oxide synthase, producing nitric oxide and citrulline. Nitric oxide is a ubiquitous molecule with significant roles in the maintenance of vascular tone, coagulation cascade, immunity, and GI tract function. Although positive effects on wound healing are noted with arginine supplementation, arginine is controversial and not recommended in severe sepsis, because it is believed to contribute to hemodynamic instability via its conversion to nitric oxide.

Pediatric amino acid solutions have altered amino acid profiles compared with the adult solutions. This is because infants have a number of immature enzymatic metabolic pathways, so that certain amino acids that are considered nonessential for adults are considered essential for infants.

Lipids

Lipids supply an average of 9.0 kcal/g and generally should account for 10% to 30% of the total daily caloric load with a minimum of 2% to 4% as essential fatty acids to prevent deficiency. Lipids are the main component in cellular and subcellular membranes. Linoleic and linolenic acids are essential fatty acids that serve as precursors for prostaglandin synthesis and are essential for cell signaling. Essential fatty acids are required for sterol-based hormone production including cortisol, gluconeogenic hormones, and growth hormone, which are important in wound healing and in the response to surgical stress.

Patients supported with PN should be monitored for tolerance of lipid delivery because long-chain triglyceride solutions may diminish immune function and cause hypertriglyceridemia. Complications may be minimized by infusing lipids continuously over 18 to 24 hours at a rate not to exceed 0.1 g/kg/h. Most patients tolerate lipid infusions when provided as an intermittent or continuous infusion. Standard IV lipids in the United States contain ω-6 fatty acid–rich soybean oil, which can lead to the generation and accumulation of linoleic and arachidonic acids that can exert pro-inflammatory effects. A newer formulation contains 30% soybean and medium-chain triglyceride (MCT) oil, 25% olive oil, and 15% fish oil, with the addition of α-tocopherol, and provides essential fatty acids including eicosapentaenoic acid (EPA) and docosahexaenoic acid (DHA), MCT, and a decreased ω-6:ω-3 fatty acid ratio. The use of SMOFlipid compared with soybean oil–based lipids reveals improvements in inflammatory markers, liver function, lipid profile, safety, tolerance, and clinical outcomes. It is acceptable not to give lipids during the first week of PN. Once initiated, lipids can be given 3 times weekly to daily, depending on nutritional needs. They may be combined with the other PN nutrients in the solution as part of a total nutrient admixture or given as a separate infusion.

Because of the anti-inflammatory profile of ω-3 fatty acids, they have been provided to critically ill patients as well as patients with chronic inflammatory processes. ω-3 Fatty acids EPA and DHA displace ω-6 fatty acids from the membranes of immune cells, thus reducing systemic inflammation through the production of biologically less inflammatory prostaglandins (prostaglandin E$_3$) and leukotrienes of the five-series. EPA and DHA (fish oils) have also been shown to reduce neutrophil attachment and transepithelial migration to modulate systemic and local inflammation, and they also help stabilize the myocardium and lower the incidence of cardiac arrhythmias. The use of enteral formulations containing ω-3 fatty acids and arginine is recommended perioperatively for enhanced postoperative recovery.

Vitamins and Minerals

Vitamins and minerals are essential for optimal postoperative recovery. The antioxidant vitamin C is required for collagen, carnitine, and neurotransmitter synthesis and for the immune-mediated and antibacterial functions of white blood cells. Iron is essential for producing hemoglobin and myoglobin, which are necessary for muscle iron storage, and cytochromes, which are necessary for the oxidative production of cellular energy. Vitamin K is required for blood clotting. Trace element deficiencies of zinc, copper, manganese, and selenium can lead to impaired wound healing, glucose metabolism, and protein sulfination. Supplemental vitamin A may assist wound healing in surgical patients requiring steroid medications by aiding in collagen cross-linking.

ASSESSMENT OF NUTRITIONAL STATUS

Increased postoperative morbidity and mortality are associated with preoperative malnutrition. It is estimated that approximately 30% to 50% of hospitalized patients are malnourished. Therefore, nutritional screening, assessment, and intervention are necessary components of patient evaluation.

Nutrition Risk Screening and Impact on Surgical Complications

A thorough history and physical examination remains a primary nutritional assessment tool. Surgical patients should be screened for risk factors including comorbidities, magnitude of the proposed surgical procedure, medications, body mass index (BMI), recent unexplained weight changes, cachexia, and unplanned changes in diet or appetite.

An accurate height and dry body weight are to be used for nutritional calculations. A nutrition-focused history and physical exam, including muscle and fat losses, can reveal the signs and symptoms of nutrient and vitamin deficiencies or toxicities (Table 2-5), and patients should be screened for nutrition risk within 24 hours of admission with referral to a dietitian for full nutrition assessment. Many medications have nutritionally related side effects or increase nutrient requirements. Recent unexplained lean body mass weight loss of 10% over 2 to 6 months or 5% in 1 month and a BMI greater than 30 or less than 18 are associated with increased postoperative complications. Although visceral proteins are not markers of nutritional status, albumin and total protein levels may reflect long-term nutritional adequacy in a nonstressed state and may be an additional marker for preoperative nutritional risk in nonhypermetabolic general surgical patients. These levels can be affected by fluid shifts and are thus not useful in the acute care setting. Serum prealbumin levels may be evaluated along with acute-phase proteins (eg, C-reactive protein [CRP]) to assist in the delineation of an inflammatory process but are not reflective of nutritional status (see below for further details).

Every surgical procedure carries some risk of postoperative complications, and this risk correlates linearly with the magnitude and complexity of individual procedures, as well as preoperative nutrition levels. There is a linear increase in complications in patients undergoing elective GI surgery because preoperative albumin decreases from normal to levels below 2.0 g/dL. Patients undergoing esophagectomy appear at risk if albumin drops below 3.75 g/dL. Complications increase in patients undergoing gastrectomy or pancreatic surgery when

TABLE 2-5. Nutrient Deficiencies Revealed by Physical Examination

Suspected Nutrient Deficiency	Physical Findings
General	
Protein, calories	Loss of weight, muscle mass, or fat stores; growth retardation; poor wound healing; infections
Protein, thiamine	Edema (ankles and feet; rule out sodium and water retention, pregnancy, protein-losing enteropathy)
Obesity	Excessive adipose tissue
Iron	Anemia, fatigue
Skin	
Protein, vitamin C, zinc	Poor wound healing, pressure ulcers; cellophane appearance
Protein, thiamine	Body edema, round swollen face (moon face)
Essential fatty acids, vitamin A, pyridoxine	Xerosis (rule out the environmental cause, lack of hygiene, aging, uremia, hypothyroidism); follicular hyperkeratosis; mosaic dermatitis (plaques of skin in the center, peeling at the periphery on shins)
Vitamin C	Slow wound healing, petechiae (especially perifollicular)
Niacin	Pigmentation, desquamation of sun-exposed areas
Zinc	Delayed wound healing, acneiform rash, skin lesions, hair loss
Vitamin K or vitamin C	Excessive bleeding, petechiae, ecchymoses; small red, purple, or black hemorrhagic spots
Iron	Pallor, fatigue
Dehydration (fluid)	Poor skin turgor
Excess β carotene	Yellow pigmentation of palms of hands with normal white sclera
Eyes	
Iron, folate, or vitamin B_{12}	Pale conjunctivae (anemia)
Vitamin A	Bitot spots, conjunctival xerosis, corneal xerosis, keratomalacia
Riboflavin, pyridoxine, niacin	Redness, fissuring in corners of eyes
Thiamine, phosphorus	Ophthalmoplegia
Hyperlipidemia	Corneal arcus, xanthelasma
Hair	
Protein	Hair lacks shine, luster; flag sign; easily plucked with no pain
Vitamin C, copper	Corkscrew hair; unemerged, coiled hairs
Protein, biotin, zinc	Sparse
Nose	
Riboflavin, niacin, pyridoxine	Seborrhea on nasolabial area, nose bridge, eyebrows, and back of ears (rule out poor hygiene)
Nails	
Iron	Koilonychia (considered normal if seen on toenails only)
Protein	Dull, lusterless with transverse ridging across the nail plate
Vitamins A and C	Pale, poor blanching, irregular, mottled
Protein, calories	Bruising, bleeding
Vitamin C	Splinter hemorrhages

(continued)

TABLE 2-5. Nutrient Deficiencies Revealed by Physical Examination (*continued*)

Suspected Nutrient Deficiency	Physical Findings
Lips and mouth	
Niacin, riboflavin, pyridoxine	Cheilosis, angular scars
Riboflavin, pyridoxine, niacin, iron	Angular stomatitis
Tongue	
Riboflavin, niacin, folate, iron	Atrophic filiform papillae
Vitamin B_{12}	Glossitis
Zinc	Taste atrophy
Riboflavin	Magenta tongue
Teeth	
Excess sugar, vitamin C	Edentia, caries
Fluorosis	Mottled tooth enamel
Gums	
Vitamin C	Swollen, bleeding gums; receding gums
Neck	
Iodine	Enlarged thyroid gland
Protein, bulimia	Enlarged parotid glands (bilateral)
Excess fluid	Venous distension, pulsations
Thorax	
Protein, calories	Reduced muscle mass and strength, shortness of breath, fatigue, reduced pulmonary function
Cardiac system	
Thiamine	Heart failure
Gastrointestinal system	
Protein, calories, zinc, vitamin C	Poor wound healing
Protein	Hepatomegaly
Urinary tract	
Dehydration	Dark, concentrated urine
Overhydration	Light-colored, diluted urine
Musculoskeletal system	
Vitamin D, calcium	Rickets, osteomalacia
Vitamin D	Persistently open anterior fontanel (after age 18), craniotabes (softening of skull across back and sides before age 1); epiphyseal enlargement (painless) at wrist, knees, and ankles; pigeon chest and Harrison sulcus (horizontal depression on lower chest border)
Protein	Emaciation, muscle wasting, swelling, pain, pale hair patches
Vitamin C	Swollen, painful joints
Thiamine	Pain in thighs, calves
Nervous system	
Protein	Psychomotor changes (listless, apathetic); mental confusion
Vitamin B_{12}, thiamine, vitamin B_6	Weakness, confusion, depressed reflexes, paresthesias, sensory loss, calf tenderness
Niacin, vitamin B_{12}	Dementia
Calcium, vitamin D, magnesium	Tetany

preoperative albumin levels drop below 3.25 g/dL. Patients undergoing elective colectomy have little increased risk unless preoperative albumin levels drop below 2.5 g/dL.

OPTIONS FOR NUTRITIONAL THERAPY

Patients unable to self-consume adequate nutrients orally (at least 80% of nutritional needs) require adjunctive nutritional therapy in the form of either enteral nutrition (EN) or PN.

Enteral Nutrition

Table 2-6 lists commonly used feeding tube access techniques for short-term and long-term enteral nutritional support. Critically ill patients often tolerate continuous infusion best, with bolus or intermittent infusion reserved for stable patients requiring long-term enteral feeding and gastric infusion.

The GI tract is the body's largest immunologic organ serving as a protective barrier against intraluminal toxins and bacteria. The body's immunoglobulin-producing cells line the GI tract, with 80% of the body's synthesized immunoglobulin being secreted here. Trillions of microbes inhabit the GI tract and are important for immune and barrier protection in addition to digestion and synthesis of vitamins and enzymes.

Current nutrition guidelines recommend that EN be started within the first 24 to 48 hours of intensive care unit (ICU) and hospital admission because there is a "window of opportunity" that exists following a hypermetabolic insult. Early feedings are associated with less gut permeability and diminished activation and release of inflammatory cytokines. The impact of early EN on patient outcome appears to be a dose-dependent effect. Low-rate feeding, often termed "trophic" feeds (10-30 mL/h), may be sufficient to prevent mucosal atrophy but is insufficient to achieve the usual end points desired from EN therapy.

All efforts should be made to achieve the goal EN feedings in hemodynamically stable patients, but if this is not feasible, initiation of PN should be considered to prevent excessive energy and protein deficits. The majority of patients can tolerate a standard enteral formula. Initiation of immune-modulated formulas perioperatively in GI surgery patients and those with trauma may help reduce infections and infectious complications.

Parenteral Nutrition

PN is an IV infusion of a hyperosmolar solution that contains macronutrients (dextrose, protein, lipids), micronutrients, electrolytes, and fluids. PN is given via a central venous catheter in order to accommodate its osmolarity. Table 2-7 lists PN indications.

PN increases the likelihood of hyperglycemia, even in patients without diabetes. PN should not be initiated if blood glucose levels are greater than or equal to 300 mg/dL; blood glucose should be treated to achieve an acceptable range (80-150 mg/dL) prior to initiating PN. Dextrose can be initiated at 150 to 250 g/d depending on the patient's expected glucose tolerance and/or tolerance to prior dextrose infusions (eg, IV dextrose). If after 24 hours glycemic control is acceptable, then the dextrose can be advanced to the goal over the next 24 to 48 hours as tolerated. Protein can be provided at the targeted patient goal but may need to be adjusted for patients with acute renal or liver failure. Lipids may be infused 3 to 4 times weekly or daily and for up to 24 hours, depending on a patient's nutritional needs. Prolonged lipid-based sedation needs to be considered in energy provision.

Peripheral Parenteral Nutrition

Peripheral parenteral nutrition (PPN) is generally not recommended, but if provided should be for only short periods (≤2 weeks) because it provides insufficient nutrients (800-1,200 kcal/d). Generally, decisions to use PPN are based on energy demands, anticipated duration of use, availability of peripheral IV access, and tolerance to large fluid volumes.

TABLE 2-6. Methods for Gaining Enteral Feeding Access

Short-Term Access (<4 wk)	Long-Term Access (>4 wk)
Naso/oroenteric access	**Percutaneous feeding tube**
Spontaneous passage	PEG
Active passage	PEG/J
• Bedside, assisted	DPEJ
• Endoscopic	**Laparoscopic**
• Fluoroscopic	Gastrostomy
• Operative (passed in the operating room)	Jejunostomy
	Surgical
	Gastrostomy
	Jejunostomy

DPEJ, direct percutaneous endoscopic jejunostomy; PEG, percutaneous endoscopic gastrostomy; PEG/J, percutaneous endoscopic transgastric jejunostomy.

TABLE 2-7. Indications and Contraindications for PN Therapy	
Indications	**Consensus**

Nonfunctional GI tract	Obstruction, ileus
	    Distal to the site of possible enteral access
	    Malnutrition awaiting surgery and needed for ≥7 d
	    Prolonged ileus (≥7 d) with poor nutritional status
	Intractable vomiting or diarrhea
	    For losses >500-1,000 mL/d
	    Unable to maintain adequate nutritional status
	Short bowel syndrome
	    Inability to absorb adequate nutrients enterally
	    <60 cm small bowel may require indefinite provision.

Inability to adequately utilize GI tract	Slow progression of enteral feeding
	    Unable to provide at least 60% of nutrient needs enterally for ≥7 d
	Enterocutaneous fistula
	    Fistula exhibits increased output with enteral feeding.
	    High-output fistula (>200 mL/d)
	Unable to safely gain enteral access
	    Patient at nutritional risk
	    Anticipated duration of need ≥7 d

Perioperative support	Preoperative
	    Severely malnourished and EN not feasible
	    Provide for at least 5-7 d preoperatively.
	Postoperative
	    If severely malnourished and initiated preoperative, begin as soon as
	        resuscitated.
	    Provide if therapy anticipated to be for ≥7 d.

Critical care	Unable to gain enteral access Resuscitated and hemodynamically stable Expected to remain NPO ≥7 d
Severe pancreatitis	If enteral feeding worsens the condition Provide if anticipate therapy to be for ≥7 d.
Contraindications	
No central venous access	Safe access not achievable
EN as an alternative therapy	All means of providing EN not attempted
Well nourished, short duration	No indication of nutritional risk Anticipated need ≤7 d
Postoperative provision only	If not provided preoperatively Provide postoperatively only after 7 d of EN not being feasible.
Grim prognosis when PN will be of no benefit	End-of-life issues preclude nutritional support.

EN, enteral nutrition; GI, gastrointestinal; NPO, nil per os; PN, parenteral nutrition.

Parenteral Nutrition: Advantages and Disadvantages

The advantages of PN are the following: A functional GI tract is not required; nutrients are delivered easily; and it provides an enhanced provision of nutritional requirements particularly if the patient is on high-dose vasopressor support that prevents enteric feeding. The disadvantages are the following: increased systemic hyperglycemia and hyperinsulinemia; increased metabolic complications; increased infectious complications and morbidity; and increased liver complications (eg, biliary stasis, cholecystitis, liver fibrosis), bacteremia, and gut mucosal atrophy. Table 2-8 lists the metabolic complications of PN.

Enteral Nutrition: Advantages and Disadvantages

The advantages of EN are as follows: attenuation of the metabolic response to stress, improved nitrogen balance, better glycemic control, increased visceral protein synthesis, increased GI anastomotic strength and increased collagen deposition, stimulation of the gut-associated lymphoid tissue, reduced nosocomial infections, enhanced visceral blood flow, increased variety of nutrients for delivery, and reduced risk of GI bleeding. Although a few studies have shown a differential effect on mortality, EN has consistently resulted in better outcomes generally by reducing infectious morbidity (pneumonia

TABLE 2-8. Metabolic Complications of PN

Complication	Possible Cause	Treatment
Hypovolemia	Inadequate fluid provision, overdiuresis	Increase free-water delivery.
Hypervolemia	Excess fluid delivery, renal dysfunction, congestive heart failure, hepatic failure	Fluid restriction, diuretics, dialysis
Hypokalemia	Refeeding syndrome, inadequate potassium provision, increased losses	Increase IV potassium.
Hyperkalemia	Renal dysfunction, too much potassium provision, metabolic acidosis, potassium-sparing drugs	Decrease potassium intake, potassium binders, and dialysis in extreme cases.
Hyponatremia	Excessive fluid provision, nephritis, adrenal insufficiency, dilutional states	Restrict fluid intake, increase sodium intake as indicated clinically.
Hypernatremia	Inadequate free-water provision, excessive sodium intake, excessive water losses	Decrease sodium intake, replete free-water deficit.
Hypoglycemia	Abrupt discontinuation of PN, insulin overdose	Dextrose delivery
Hyperglycemia	Rapid infusion of large dextrose load, sepsis, pancreatitis, steroids, diabetes, older adults	Insulin, decrease dextrose as indicated
Hypertriglyceridemia	Inability to clear lipid provision, sepsis, too much exogenous dextrose and insulin provision, multisystem organ failure, medications altering fat absorption, history of hyperlipidemia	Decrease lipid volume provided, increase infusion time, hold lipids up to 14 d to normalize levels.
Hypocalcemia	Decreased vitamin D intake, hypoparathyroidism, citrate binding of calcium resulting from excessive blood transfusion, hypoalbuminemia	Calcium supplementation
Hypercalcemia	Renal failure, tumor lysis syndrome, bone cancer, excess vitamin D delivery, prolonged immobilization-stress hyperparathyroidism	Isotonic saline, inorganic phosphate supplementation, corticosteroids, mithramycin
Hypomagnesemia	Refeeding syndrome, alcoholism, diuretic use, increased losses, medications, diabetic ketoacidosis, chemotherapy	Magnesium supplementation
Hypermagnesemia	Excessive magnesium provision, renal insufficiency	Reduce magnesium provision.
Hypophosphatemia	Refeeding syndrome, alcoholism, phosphate-binding antacids, dextrose infusion, overfeeding, secondary hyperparathyroidism, insulin therapy	Phosphate supplementation, discontinue phosphate-binding antacids, avoid overfeeding, initiate dextrose delivery cautiously.
Hyperphosphatemia	Renal dysfunction, excessive provision	Reduce phosphate delivery, phosphate binders.
Prerenal azotemia	Dehydration, excessive protein provision, inadequate nonprotein calorie provision with mobilization of endogenous proteins	Increase fluid intake, reduce protein delivery, increase nonprotein calories.
Essential fatty acid deficiency	Inadequate polyunsaturated long-chain fatty acid provision	Provide lipids.

IV, intravenous; PN, parenteral nutrition.

and central-line infections) in most patient populations and specifically by reducing abdominal abscess in patients with trauma. The disadvantages of EN are the inability to consistently provide adequate nutrition via the GI tract, difficulties obtaining GI feeding access, and increased intolerance to enteral feedings. Critically ill patients on high-dose vasopressor support should not be given full nutritional support through enteric feeds as this diverts blood flow from perfusing other organs and can increase the risk of bowel necrosis. The complications of EN are jejunal necrosis, aspiration, diarrhea, and respiratory compromise. In addition, the formulas themselves can induce problems related to their composition (Table 2-9).

TABLE 2-9. Common Complications Associated With Enteral Feeding

Complication	Possible Causes	Corrective Measures
Mechanical		
Obstructed feeding tube	Crushed medications administered through the tube	Give medications as an elixir.
	Formula coagulated in the tube because of contact with acidic medium (gastric contents, medications)	Flush the tube with water before and after each medication.
	Formula viscosity excessive for feeding tube	Use less viscous formula and a pump.
	Formula buildup inside the tube	Flush tube with water under pressure several times per day.
Metabolic		
Hyperglycemia	Metabolic stress, sepsis, trauma, diabetes mellitus	Treat the origin of stress and provide insulin needed to maintain blood glucose of 110–150 mg/dL.
		Avoid excessive carbohydrate delivery.
Altered serum electrolytes	Inadequate electrolytes in the formula	Change formula.
	Refeeding syndrome	Monitor electrolytes closely (K^+, Mg^{2+}, PO_4) and replace as indicated.
Dehydration	Osmotic diarrhea caused by rapid infusion of hyperosmolar formula	Avoid hyperosmolar formulas delivered into the small intestine.
	Excessive protein, electrolytes, or both	Increase fluid provision or reduce protein and electrolytes.
	Inadequate free-water provision	Ensure adequate free-water provision.
Overhydration	Excessive fluid intake	Assess fluid intake; monitor daily fluid intake and output.
	Rapid refeeding in malnourished patient	Use calorically dense formula to reduce free-water provision.
	Cardiac, hepatic, or renal insufficiency	Diuretic therapy
	Increased extracellular mass catabolism causing loss of body cell mass with subsequent potassium loss	Monitor serum electrolytes and body weight daily; weight change >0.2 kg/d reflects a decrease or increase in extracellular fluid.
Gradual weight loss	Inadequate calories	Ensure patient is receiving estimated calorie requirements.
	Malabsorption	Adjust nutrient delivery as indicated on the basis of patient monitoring.
		Adjust nutrient composition or add PN if there is malabsorption of nutrients.
Excessive weight gain	Excess calories	Ensure patient is receiving caloric needs.
	Volume overload	Rule out weight gain due to volume status.

Visceral protein depletion	Active inflammatory process	Treat the cause of inflammation.
	Inadequate calories or protein	Adjust calorie and protein provision if inflammatory markers are normal.
Essential fatty acid deficiency	Prolonged (>10 d) lack of sufficient lipid provision (LCT)	Include at least 4% of daily caloric needs as essential fatty acids.
Gastrointestinal		
Nausea and vomiting	Excessive formula volume or rate of infusion	Decrease the rate of infusion or volume infused.
	Hyperosmolar formula infusion (especially in the small intestine)	Change to isotonic formula.
	Delayed gastric emptying	Add prokinetic agent. Change to lower fat formula.
	Improper tube location	Reposition the tube if needed.
	Very cold formula provided	Provide formula at room temperature.
	Smell of enteral formulas	Use polymeric formula as less offensive odor.
Diarrhea	Excessive rate of infusion of formula	Decrease infusion rate.
	Bolus feedings into the small intestine	Only continuous feeds into small bowel
	Hyperosmolar formula infused	Change to isotonic formula.
	Hyperosmolar medication infused	Avoid hyperosmolar medications or dilute them with water prior to giving.
	Altered GI anatomy or short bowel syndrome Malabsorption	Change to hydrolyzed, free amino acid and MCT oil-containing formula.
	Lactose intolerance	Use lactose-free formula.
	GI bacterial overgrowth	Check stool for pathogens and treat accordingly.
	Antibiotic therapy	Consider prebiotics and/or probiotics.
Vomiting and diarrhea	Contamination	Check sanitation of formula and equipment and ensure proper handling technique.
Abdominal distension, bloating, cramping, gas	Rapid bolus or intermittent infusion with cold formula	Administer formula at room temperature.
	Rapid infusion with a syringe	Infuse continuously and gradually advance to the goal.
	Nutrient malabsorption or maldigestion	Hydrolyzed formula, MCT containing, lactose free
	Rapid administration of MCT	Administer MCT gradually as tolerated.

(continued)

TABLE 2-9. Common Complications Associated With Enteral Feeding (*continued*)

Complication	Possible Causes	Corrective Measures
Constipation	Lack of fiber	Add fiber formula.
	Inadequate free water	Ensure adequate free water.
	Fecal impaction, GI obstruction	Rectal exam, digital disimpaction
	Inadequate physical activity	Increase physical therapy if able to turn the patient.
	Medications	Stool softener
Aspiration or gastric retention of formula	Altered gastric motility, diabetic gastroparesis, altered gag reflex, altered mental status	Postpyloric nutrient delivery with continuous infusion
	Gastric, vagotomy surgery	Add prokinetic agent.
	Head of bed <30°	Elevate head of bed >30° if possible.
	Displaced feeding tube	Verify feeding tube placement and reposition as needed.
	Ileus or hemodynamic instability	For prolonged intolerance, may need PN
	Medications that slow gastric emptying (opiates, anticholinergics)	Evaluate medications and change if able to.

GI, gastrointestinal; LCT, long-chain triglycerides; MCT, medium-chain triglycerides; PN, parenteral nutrition.

Parenteral Nutrition Therapy Indications

Several organizations have developed practice guidelines to identify appropriate and inappropriate indications for PN (see Table 2-7). PN should be provided only in those patients where enteral nutrient provision is not feasible for 7 or more days. Malnourished surgical patients benefit most if PN is provided for a minimum of 7 to 10 days preoperatively and then continued throughout the perioperative period.

ASSESSMENT OF NUTRITIONAL EFFECTIVENESS

Catabolism to Anabolism Switch

Nutritional support does not convert a patient with septic catabolism into an anabolic state. Numerous hormonal and inflammatory factors that limit the effectiveness of exogenously administered nutritional substrates are present. Only the resolution of the underlying stress can reverse these effects. The switch from catabolism to anabolism is one of the signs that the hypermetabolic response of stress is resolving and the patient is improving.

Nitrogen Balance Studies

Nitrogen balance studies reflect the balance between exogenous nitrogen intake and renal removal of nitrogen-containing compounds. Nitrogen balance studies are not protein turnover studies that require labeled (stable isotope) protein methods. Nitrogen balance studies are most accurate in patients who receive a defined and consistent nutrient intake. For these calculations, proteins are assumed to be 16% nitrogen (6.25 g of protein = 1 g of nitrogen). Nitrogen balance is calculated by subtracting the excreted nitrogen (24-hour urine urea nitrogen collection plus insensible losses) from the nitrogen intake provided in the nutrition therapy. A positive nitrogen balance in the range of 2 to 4 g of nitrogen per day indicates an anabolic state. The validity of nitrogen balance is affected by severe nitrogen retention disorders (eg, creatinine clearance <50 mL/min, severe hepatic failure); massive diuresis; abnormal nitrogen losses through excessive diarrhea, large draining wounds, or fistulas; skin exfoliation as in burns; and the accuracy of protein and amino acid intake data.

Serum Proteins

During the acute-phase response to injury, a systemic response to stress and inflammation, the liver reprioritizes transport protein synthesis (eg, albumin, prealbumin), downregulating synthesis and upregulating the synthesis of acute-phase proteins (eg, CRP). Transport proteins become a marker of severity of illness and inflammation, not malnutrition. Altering the nutritional plan when a prealbumin level is low and a CRP is high will not result in improved nutritional status and may result in complications of overfeeding. However, once the inflammation resolves and CRP levels decrease, then it may be reasonable to alter the nutritional plan if prealbumin levels remain low. In addition, because of the long half-life of serum albumin and its depletion with large fluid volumes, it is not an accurate marker during acute illness, but rather a good prognostic indicator of surgical risk when evaluated in the preoperative, ambulatory care setting.

Other Biochemical Parameters

Other various laboratory assays exist that reflect a change in nutrition status, tolerance, or response to nutrition therapy. Electrolyte and micronutrients should be evaluated when deficiencies or toxicities are suspected. Hepatic, renal, and respiratory function strongly affects a patient's dietary prescription and should be included in the nutrition assessment and monitoring process. Iron levels, iron transport proteins, hemoglobin, and hematocrit with indices may determine an anemia of nutritional origin. Serum magnesium and calcium vary inversely with albumin levels. Correction of total serum levels of these elements should be made for serum albumin levels. Currently, only calcium has an accepted correction value calculated by the formula: $Ca_{(true)} = Ca_{(serum)} + 0.8(Alb_{(normal)} - Alb_{(actual)})$. Measurements of ionized calcium can also be used. In general, total magnesium levels greater than 1.5 mg/dL, even without albumin correction, rarely result in metabolic consequences.

COMPLICATIONS OF INITIATING NUTRITIONAL THERAPY

Refeeding Syndrome

Refeeding syndrome may be defined as a constellation of fluid, micronutrient, electrolyte, and vitamin imbalances that occur within the first hours to days following nutrient infusion in a chronically starved patient. Refeeding syndrome can include hemolytic anemia, respiratory distress, paresthesias, tetany, and cardiac arrhythmias. Typical laboratory findings include hypokalemia, hypophosphatemia, and hypomagnesemia. Reported risk factors for refeeding syndrome include prolonged inadequate nutrient intake, due to nausea or vomiting, as in a patient with an intestinal obstruction, as well as alcoholism, anorexia nervosa, marasmus, rapid refeeding, and excessive dextrose infusion. In these patients, proportional increases in the provision of carbohydrate-dependent electrolytes such as magnesium and phosphorus, protein-dependent electrolytes such as potassium, and volume-dependent electrolytes such as sodium should be made as the macronutrients are increased. Dextrose should be limited initially to 100 to 150 g/d. In addition, a careful observation and replacement of potassium, magnesium, and phosphorous levels are necessary because they may fall rapidly with refeeding.

Transition From Parenteral to Enteral Nutrition

Before discontinuing PN, assurance that the patient is consuming and absorbing adequate nutrients enterally is imperative. To avoid complications of overfeeding, PN should be sequentially decreased as the enteral intake and tolerance improves. PN may be discontinued once the patient is tolerating approximately 60% to 80% of goal nutrients via the enteral route and may be reduced and discontinued over a 24- to 48-hour period. If PN is inadvertently, but abruptly, discontinued in patients who are not eating, all insulin should be stopped and blood glucose levels should be monitored for 30 to 120 minutes after the discontinuation of PN, with the appropriate therapy for hypoglycemia implemented. Previously, most clinicians advocated the immediate initiation of 10% dextrose in water ($D_{10}W$) if PN was abruptly discontinued, but most clinicians now find that it is unnecessary and that patient monitoring is adequate. If PN was used as a vehicle for medication or electrolyte administration, an alternate plan should be made once it is discontinued.

NUTRITIONAL CONCERNS FOR PATIENTS UNDERGOING SURGERY

Digestive Tract Surgery

Various surgical interventions involving the GI tract can result in malabsorption and maldigestion that in turn lead to nutritional deficiencies (Tables 2-10 and 2-11). Understanding where nutrients are absorbed in the GI tract will aid in determining which nutrient may become deficient postoperatively (Figure 2-1). Dumping syndrome is a common complication of upper GI surgery, and therefore, an antidumping diet should be the first intervention to resolve the problem (Table 2-12).

Optimization of nutritional status and intervention is a component of enhanced recovery after surgery (ERAS) protocols. ERAS protocols are multimodal and address preoperative nutrition optimization, early postoperative diet delivery with regular foods and nutritional supplements, and gum chewing to reduce the incidence of postoperative ileus, expedite hospital discharge, and minimize postoperative complications.

LOOKING AHEAD

Nutritional assessment and support of surgical patients impact surgical outcomes. With increased pressure to reduce hospital stay and complications and prevent readmissions, the nutritional status of patients is closely scrutinized by regulatory agencies, our hospitals, and payers. The role of PN in the achievement of full nutritional support is undergoing renewed interest and investigation, as is tailored enteral nutritional support. Prevention of complications will likely become even more important, emphasizing the role and benefit of preoperative nutritional supplementation when possible.

TABLE 2-10. Nutritional Consequences of Gastrointestinal Surgery

Location/Procedure	Potential Consequence
Total gastric and truncal vagotomy	Impairs proximal and distal motor function of the stomach Digestion and emptying of solids are retarded. Emptying of liquids is accelerated.
Total gastrectomy	Early satiety, nausea, vomiting Weight loss Inadequate bile acids and pancreatic enzymes available because of anastomotic changes Malabsorption Protein-calorie malnutrition Anemia Dumping syndrome Bezoar formation Vitamin B_{12} deficiency Metabolic bone disease
Subtotal gastrectomy with vagotomy	Early satiety Delayed gastric emptying Rapid emptying of hypertonic fluids
Proximal small intestine	Malabsorption of vitamins (A, D) and minerals (calcium, magnesium, iron)
Gastric bypass	Protein-calorie malnutrition from malabsorption due to dumping, unavailability of bile acids, and pancreatic enzymes due to anastomotic changes Bezoar formation
Distal small intestine	Malabsorption of water-soluble vitamins (folate, vitamins B_{12}, B_1, B_2, C, pyridoxine) and minerals Protein-calorie malnutrition due to dumping Fat malabsorption Bacterial overgrowth if ileocecal valve is resected.
Colon	Fluid and electrolyte malabsorption—potassium, sodium, chloride

TABLE 2-11. Nutrient Deficiencies Associated With Gastric Surgery

Deficiency	Causes

Microcytic anemia	Iron malabsorption or deficiency
	 • Total and subtotal gastrectomy
	 • Achlorhydria leads to insufficient
	   ○ cleavage of iron from food to which it is bound.
	   ○ reduction and solubilization of ferric iron to the ferrous form.
	 • Bilroth II is more common as the primary sites of absorption are bypassed.
	 • Reduced intake of iron-rich foods due to intolerance and reduced gastric capacity
	 • Supplementation: 325 mg ferrous sulfate twice daily with the coadministration of vitamin C

Macrocytic anemia	Folate, vitamin B_{12} deficiency, or anemia • Achlorhydria leads to insufficient liberation of vitamin B_{12} from protein foods it is bound. • Reduced intrinsic factor leads to a reduced binding of vitamin B_{12}. • Reduced intake of protein-rich foods due to intolerance and reduced gastric capacity • Intramuscular vitamin B_{12} monthly injections (1,500 µg)
Metabolic bone disease	Calcium deficiency or malabsorption • Bilroth II (BII) is more common than BI procedure because of bypassing of the duodenum and proximal jejunum. • Rapid gastric emptying can reduce absorption. • Fat malabsorption can lead to insoluble calcium soap formation. • Vitamin D malabsorption may accompany fat malabsorption, which can impair calcium and phosphorous metabolism. • Daily supplementation: 1,500 mg calcium, 800 IU vitamin D

IU, international units.

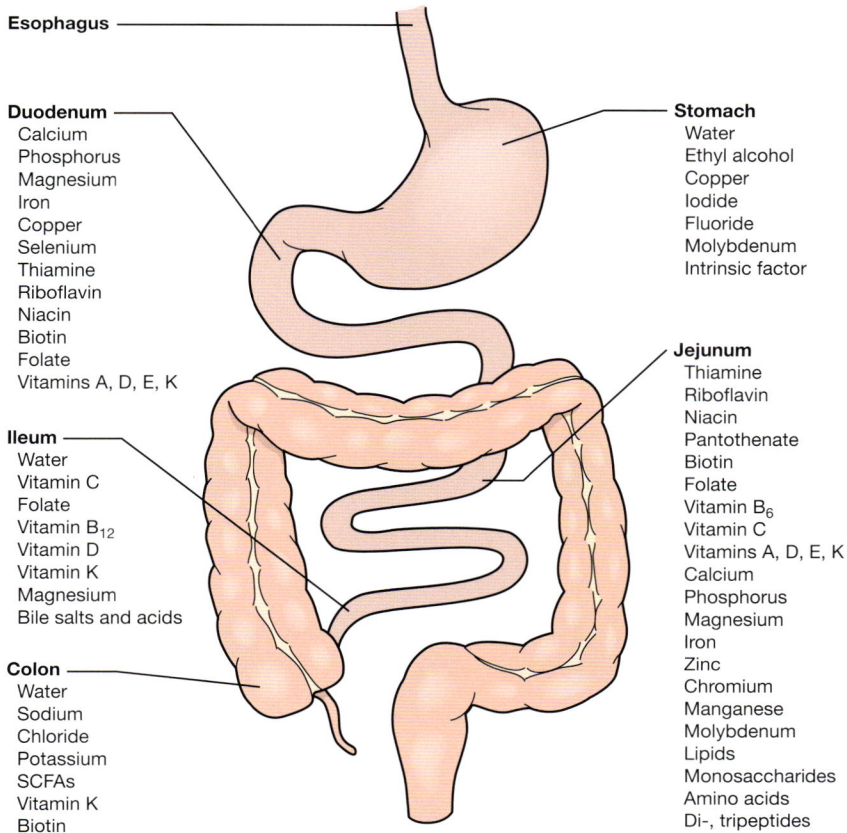

Figure 2-1. Nutrient absorption in the gastrointestinal tract. SCFA, short-chain fatty acids.

TABLE 2-12. Postgastrectomy/Antidumping Diet

Principles of Diet

Postoperatively, some discomfort (gas, bloating, cramping) and diarrhea may occur. To reduce the likelihood of these symptoms, a healthy, nutritionally complete diet should be followed. Every person may react to foods differently. Foods should be reintroduced into the diet slowly.

Diet Guidelines

1. Eat small, frequent "meals" per day.
2. Limit fluids to 4 oz (1/2 cup) at a meal. Just enough to "wash" food down.
3. Drink remaining fluids at least 30-40 min before and after meals.
4. Eat slowly and chew foods thoroughly.
5. Avoid extreme temperatures of foods.
6. Use seasonings and spices as tolerated (may want to avoid pepper, hot sauce).
7. Remain upright while eating and at least 30 min after eating.
8. Avoid simple sugars in foods and drinks.
9. Examples: fruit juice, Gatorade, PowerAde, Kool-Aid, sweet tea, sucrose, honey, jelly, corn syrup, cookies, pie, and doughnuts
10. Complex carbohydrates are unlimited.
11. Examples: bread, pasta, rice, potatoes, vegetables
12. Include a protein-containing food at every meal.
13. Limit fats (<30% of total calories). Avoid fried foods, gravies, fat-containing sauces, mayonnaise, fatty meats (sausage, hot dogs, ribs), chips, biscuits, and pancakes.
14. Milk and dairy products may not be tolerated because of lactose. Introduce these slowly into the diet if they were tolerated preoperatively. Lactose-free milk or soy milk is suggested.

SUGGESTED READINGS

Baggaley A, Ramsay G, Kumar M. Intravenous fluid therapy in the adult surgical patient. *Int J Surg*. 2016;36(1):S46.

McClave S, Taylor BE, Martindale RG, et al. Guidelines for the provision and assessment of nutrition support therapy in the adult critically ill patient: Society of Critical Care Medicine (SCCM) and American Society for Parenteral and Enteral Nutrition (A.S.P.E.N.). *JPEN J Parenter Enteral Nutr*. 2016;40:159-211.

Piper GL, Kaplan LJ. Fluid and electrolyte management for the surgical patient. *Surg Clin North Am*. 2012;92(2):189-205.

Semler MW, Self WH, Rice TW. Balanced crystalloids versus saline in critically ill adults. *N Engl J Med*. 2018;378(20):1951. doi: 10.1056/NEJMc1804294

Voldby AW, Brandstrup B. Fluid therapy in the perioperative setting—a clinical review. *J Intensive Care*. 2016;4:27.

Wischmeyer PE. Tailoring nutrition therapy to illness and recovery. *Critical Care*. 2017;21(suppl 3):316.

SAMPLE QUESTIONS

QUESTIONS

Choose the best answer for each question.

1. ADH works to increase intravascular volume by what mechanism?

   A. By direct vasoconstriction of the renal artery
   B. By decreasing capillary leak during sepsis
   C. By increasing water resorption in the distal convoluted tubules and collecting tubules
   D. By increasing aldosterone secretion
   E. By vasoconstriction of afferent arterioles in the kidney

2. Sodium resorption in exchange for potassium and hydrogen ion secretion in the distal tubules is a direct effect of which of the following?

   A. ADH
   B. Aldosterone
   C. ACTH
   D. Cortisol
   E. Testosterone

3. Appropriate maintenance intravenous fluid (IVF) for an 85-kg male who is nil per os (NPO) but not dehydrated is

   A. D5 LR at 200 mL/h.
   B. D10 NSS at 85 mL/h.
   C. LR at 150 mL/h.
   D. D5 1/2 NS with 20 mEq KCl/L at 125 mL/h.
   E. D5 NSS with 20 mEq KCl/L at 120 mL/h.

4. Optimal fluid resuscitation for acute fluid loss should always be done with which fluid?

   A. Any colloid solution
   B. Iso-osmotic crystalloid solutions that most closely match the source of loss
   C. LR
   D. Dextrose-containing fluids
   E. Hypertonic saline (3%)

5. In sepsis, increased fluid requirements are due to which of the following consequences?

   A. Vasoconstriction
   B. Increased ADH secretion
   C. Decreased capillary permeability
   D. Arteriole vasodilation and increased capillary permeability
   E. Aldosterone increase

6. A 27-year-old man is in the ICU 24 hours after an automobile collision. He has a left pneumothorax, multiple broken ribs, a ruptured spleen requiring splenectomy, a pelvic fracture, and bilateral femur fractures. He is intubated and is now hemodynamically stable. Which of the following reflects current nutrition guidelines?

   A. NPO for at least 72 hours
   B. Trophic feeds (10-30 mL/h) within 24 to 48 hours
   C. EN within 24 to 48 hours
   D. Total PN within 24 to 48 hours
   E. Total PN with trophic feed (10-30 mL/h) within 24 to 48 hours

7. A 45-year-old man was admitted to the hospital 3 days ago with nausea and vomiting due to a gastric outlet obstruction. Further studies have confirmed gastric cancer involving the antrum of the stomach. He has a history of alcohol misuse and being homeless. The patient is thin and has temporal wasting and exposed ribs. He has an albumin of 1.9 g/dL. A nasogastric tube was placed on admission, and he was started on total parenteral nutrition (TPN). Which of the following albumin levels are associated with an increased surgical risk?

   A. Esophagectomy less than 3.75 g/dL, gastrectomy less than 3.25 g/dL, colectomy less than 2.5 g/dL
   B. Esophagectomy less than 3.25 g/dL, gastrectomy less than 3.00 g/dL, colectomy less than 2.5 g/dL
   C. Esophagectomy less than 2.5 g/dL, gastrectomy less than 3.25 g/dL, colectomy less than 3.75 g/dL
   D. Esophagectomy less than 3.75 g/dL, gastrectomy less than 2.5 g/dL, colectomy less than 3.25 g/dL
   E. Esophagectomy less than 3.25 g/dL, gastrectomy less than 2.5 g/dL, colectomy less than 2.5 g/dL

8. A 48-year-old woman is in the hospital because of nausea, vomiting, and abdominal pain. She has a history of multiple abdominal surgeries for small bowel obstruction. On admission, she was quite thin with temporal and thenar muscle wasting. Her albumin level was 1.7 g/dL. A nasogastric tube was inserted, and she has been receiving TPN for 2 days. You are now called by her nurse because, in addition to nausea and abdominal pain, she's begun to feel short of breath and have tingling in her fingers. She suddenly goes into cardiac arrest. Laboratory values now show a potassium level of 2.4 mEq/L, a magnesium level of 1.3 mEq/L,

a phosphorus level of 1 mg/dL, and a glucose level of 350 mg/dL. What nutritional complication may have resulted in this patient's condition?

   A. Marasmus
   B. Refeeding syndrome
   C. Overfeeding
   D. Underfeeding
   E. Kwashiorkor

9. A 46-year-old man with an enterocutaneous fistula has been maintained on TPN for several weeks. The fistula has healed and prior to removing the central line, the patient is given a unit of packed red blood cells through his central line for his chronic anemia. Two hours into his red cell infusion, a rapid response is called when the nurse discovers the patient comatose and hypotensive. What is the most likely cause of the patient's condition?

   A. Hypokalemia
   B. Transfusion reaction
   C. Hypoglycemia
   D. Air embolus
   E. Catheter-related sepsis

10. A 58-year-old female is involved in a motor vehicle collision. She sustains multiple broken ribs, a grade 2 (nonsurgical) splenic laceration, and a stable pelvic fracture. Which of the following serum proteins is increased as a result of her traumatic injury?

   A. Albumin
   B. Transthyretin
   C. Transferrin
   D. Retinol-binding protein
   E. CRP

ANSWERS AND EXPLANATIONS

1. **Answer: C**

   ADH is released from the posterior pituitary gland. The production and release of ADH depends on the activity of intracranial osmoreceptors and volume receptors in the heart. ADH increases the reabsorption of water from cells in distal convoluted tubules and collecting tubules. For more information on this topic, see section "Sodium."

2. **Answer: B**

   Normal kidneys excrete sodium when intake is high to maintain homeostasis. Sodium resorption in exchange for potassium and hydrogen ion secretion in the distal tubules is a direct effect of the adrenal cortical hormone aldosterone. This action helps maintain both extracellular volume and osmolarity. Extracellular volume reduction causes renin release by the juxtaglomerular apparatus. Renin cleaves angiotensinogen to produce angiotensin I, which is then converted by ACE to angiotensin II, a potent stimulator of aldosterone secretion. For more information on this topic, see section "Sodium."

3. **Answer: D**

   Fluid and electrolyte balance is maintained by the intake of adequate amounts of water, sodium, potassium, and chloride to balance daily obligatory losses. Intake is calculated to balance outputs of urine, stool water, sweat, and combined insensible losses from the lungs and skin. This is called *maintenance fluid*. Given the average normal daily fluid and electrolyte losses, this makes D5 1/2 NS with 20 mEq KCl an ideal maintenance fluid. A guideline frequently cited in the literature for estimating normal daily fluid requirements is the 4:2:1 rule, which states that for normal maintenance fluids per hour, 4 mL is given for the first 10 kg, 2 mL for the second 10 kg, and 1 mL for the remainder of the weight (see Table 2-1). For more information on this topic, see section "Perioperative Fluids and Electrolytes."

4. **Answer: B**

   In the immediate postoperative period, the fluid, electrolyte, and acid-base needs of the patient are related to the need for ongoing resuscitation (iso-osmolar fluids), replacement (loss-specific fluids), and maintenance (daily losses). The fluid needs of the postoperative patient depend on the type and acuity of the procedure. Table 2-3 lists the relative composition of bodily fluids and can be used as a guide for what fluid to use for replacing losses. For more information on this topic, see section "Perioperative Fluids and Electrolytes."

5. **Answer: D**

   Isotonic vascular volume depletion caused by fluid sequestered into interstitial space—as seen in sepsis or locally such as with peritonitis (bacterial or chemical), intestinal obstruction, extensive soft tissue inflammation or trauma—is common. "Third spacing" is sometimes used to refer to this sequestration. Sepsis further decreases intravascular volume by causing vasodilation of arterioles. For more information on this topic, see section "Perioperative Fluids and Electrolytes."

6. **Answer: C**

   Current nutrition guidelines recommend that EN be started early, within the first 24 to 48 hours of ICU and hospital admission because there is a "window of opportunity" that exists following a hypermetabolic insult. Early feedings are associated with less gut permeability and diminished activation and release of inflammatory cytokines. The impact of early EN on patient outcome appears to be a dose-dependent effect. Low-rate feeding, often termed "trophic" feeds (10-30 mL/h), may be sufficient to prevent mucosal atrophy, but it is insufficient to achieve the usual end points desired from EN therapy. All efforts should be made to achieve the goal EN feedings in hemodynamically stable patients, but if this is not feasible, initiation of PN should be considered to prevent excessive energy and protein deficits. For more information on this topic, see section "Parenteral Nutrition: Advantages and Disadvantages."

7. **Answer: A**

   There is a linear increase in complications in patients undergoing elective GI surgery because preoperative albumin decreases from normal to levels below 2.0 g/dL. Patients undergoing esophagectomy appear at risk if albumin drops below 3.75 g/dL. Complications increase in patients undergoing gastrectomy or pancreatic surgery when preoperative albumin levels drop below 3.25 g/dL. Patients undergoing elective colectomy have little increased risk unless preoperative albumin levels drop below 2.5 g/dL. For more information on this topic, see section "Assessment of Nutritional Status."

8. **Answer: B**

   Refeeding syndrome occurs when chronically starved patients lose the ability to tolerate acute changes in volume or caloric load. This results in a constellation of fluid, micronutrient, electrolyte, and vitamin imbalances within the first hours to days following nutrient infusion. These patients are typically hypokalemic, hypophosphatemic, hypomagnesemic, and hyperglycemic. This may result in symptoms that include hemolytic anemia, respiratory distress, paresthesias, tetany, and cardiac arrhythmias including sudden cardiac death. For more information on this topic, see section "Complications of Initiating Nutritional Therapy."

9. **Answer: C**

   When long-term infusion of highly concentrated glucose solutions is suddenly discontinued, the increased endogenous insulin levels precipitate hypoglycemia. A blood transfusion would be more likely to elevate rather than depress potassium levels. Transfusion reactions cause fever, back pain, hemolysis, and hypotension, but not coma. The air embolus could cause both shock and unconsciousness and is unlikely to be associated with a blood transfusion. Catheter-related sepsis could induce fever and hypotension, but not coma. For more information on this topic, see section "Transition From Parenteral to Enteral Nutrition."

10. **Answer: E**

    CRP increases with stress (inflammation, infection, etc). Albumin, prealbumin (transthyretin), transferrin, and retinol-binding protein are negative acute-phase reactants. For more information on this topic, see section "Protein."

3

Surgical Bleeding: Bleeding Disorders, Hypercoagulable States, and Replacement Therapy in the Surgical Patient

Timothy A. Pritts

Bleeding may occur during any surgical procedure. Although the volume of blood lost is usually not large enough to create a major problem, certain operations are invariably associated with large blood losses that may impair the normal hemostatic process. In addition, some patients with congenital or acquired disorders of hemostasis require elective or emergency surgery. Therefore, surgeons must be prepared for significant blood losses that may have an adverse effect on patient recovery, and they must be able to manage blood loss and bleeding disorders in their patients. Careful screening for bleeding risks can detect bleeding disorders before surgery and allow for correction to avoid major bleeding problems during and after surgery (Table 3-1). In addition, surgeons must be knowledgeable about common bleeding disorders and causes of hypercoagulable states, the components of blood replacement, and the problems associated with the transfusion of blood products.

CAUSES OF SIGNIFICANT SURGICAL BLEEDING

Most patients are hemostatically normal before they enter the operating room. However, in some patients with significant intraoperative blood loss, generalized oozing may

be observed after a period of time. Some operations (eg, cardiopulmonary bypass, aortic surgery, liver transplant surgery, prostate surgery, construction of portacaval shunts, major trauma) are frequently associated with large blood losses.

Preexisting Hemostatic Defects

Preexisting hemostatic defects should be suspected when a prior history of bleeding exists or when abnormal bleeding begins within the first 30 minutes of the operative period. Bleeding disorders may be congenital (Table 3-2) or acquired (Table 3-3).

All anticoagulants and platelet-inhibiting drugs carry the risk of inducing bleeding in any patient. The most common anticoagulants that are currently in use include the vitamin K antagonist warfarin and heparins, both unfractionated and low-molecular weight. The use of newer classes of direct factor Xa inhibitors (eg, apixaban) is also common. Direct thrombin inhibitors, such as argatroban and bivalirudin, have limited indications and are often used to treat patients with heparin-induced thrombocytopenia (HIT). The most commonly used platelet-inhibiting drugs are aspirin and clopidogrel (Plavix), both of which cause irreversible inhibition of platelet function. Because of the increased risk of bleeding associated with all anticoagulants and platelet-inhibiting drugs, great care must be taken when using these drugs (Table 3-4).

Intraoperative Complications

Several common conditions contribute to bleeding during a surgical procedure. Shock may cause or aggravate consumptive coagulopathy. Massive transfusion of stored packed red blood cells (PRBCs) alone may lead to bleeding due to inadequate replacement of clotting factors. For this reason, the standard of care has become the administration of a balanced, 1:1:1 transfusion of PRBCs, platelets, and plasma, along with cryoprecipitate and calcium for patients receiving massive transfusion of red blood cells.

Intraoperative bleeding from needle holes, vascular suture lines, or extensive tissue dissection can often be controlled through the use of local hemostatic agents. These include gelatin sponge, oxidized cellulose, collagen sponge, microfibrillar collagen, topical thrombin (with or without topical cryoprecipitate or a gelatin matrix), topical ε-aminocaproic acid (EACA), and topical aprotinin.

TABLE 3-1. Preoperative Evaluation for Bleeding and Clotting Disorders	
Study	**When Performed**
History	In all patients as part of routine preoperative evaluation
Physical examination	As part of routine surgical evaluation
Laboratory studies: aPTT, PT, bleeding time (less commonly used) or whole blood platelet function, thrombin time, thromboelastography	In patients with history or evidence of bleeding disorders or in whom excessive bleeding is anticipated because of the nature of the surgery

aPTT, activated partial thromboplastin time; PT, prothrombin time.

TABLE 3-2. Congenital Bleeding Disorders

	Hemophilia A	von Willebrand Disease
Incidence	25 per 100,000 in the United States	1% of U.S. population
Pathophysiology	Reduced or absent factor VIII activity. Factor VIII molecule is present.	Reduced factor VIII activity and von Willebrand activity
Site of bleeding	Joints and intramuscular	Mucocutaneous
Inheritance	X-linked	Autosomal dominant
Patients	Only males	Males and females
Laboratory studies	Prolonged aPTT	Prolonged aPTT
	Normal PT	Normal PT
	Normal platelet function	Abnormal platelet function

aPTT, activated partial thromboplastin time; PT, prothrombin time.

Acute hemolytic blood transfusion reactions may lead to disseminated intravascular coagulation (DIC). When a patient is under general anesthesia, there may be no clues that incompatible blood has been infused until the onset of generalized bleeding as a result of DIC. The usual symptoms of an incompatible blood transfusion (eg, agitation, back pain) are not apparent under general anesthesia. Hemoglobinuria and oliguria provide additional clinical evidence of DIC.

Massive Hemorrhage and Damage-Control Resuscitation

Massive hemorrhage following injury is defined as bleeding requiring a transfusion of 10 or more units of PRBCs in 24 hours or more than four units in 1 hour, replacement of a patient's entire blood volume in 24 hours or more than 50% in 4 hours, or a rate of blood loss more than 150 mL/min with hemodynamic instability. Early recognition and treatment of patients with massive hemorrhage is critical to survival. Predictors of massive transfusion requirements include a systolic blood pressure of 90 mm Hg or less in the emergency room, a heart rate of 120 beats/min or more, positive focused assessment with sonography for trauma scan, and penetrating injury.

Treatment of massive hemorrhage has evolved dramatically over the past 20 years. The impetus for this change is a better understanding of acute traumatic coagulopathy (ATC), also known as trauma-induced coagulopathy. ATC is present on admission in approximately 25% of patients with major trauma, occurs independently of injury severity, and is associated with a 4-fold higher mortality rate. ATC results from inadequate tissue perfusion, not excessive consumption of circulating clotting factors. Elevated plasma thrombomodulin (a marker of endothelial damage) and decreased protein C concentrations result in hyperfibrinolysis.

Damage-control resuscitation (DCR) is a comprehensive strategy designed to guide the care of patients with trauma who are bleeding severely from critical injuries. Its main objective is to minimize blood loss until definitive hemostasis is achieved. Essential principles of DCR include early hemorrhage control during transport, limitation of non-blood fluids, and avoidance of delays in surgical or angiographic hemostasis. Damage-control surgery involves an abbreviated initial operation to stop bleeding and ongoing bacterial contamination, followed by a more definitive procedure after resuscitation and stabilization in the intensive care unit. This approach is the current standard of care for patients with severe abdominal, thoracic, pelvic, and extremity injuries, and it results in significantly improved survival. Other important principles include delayed aggressive volume resuscitation and targeted low-normal blood pressure (permissive hypotension), which can help avoid hypothermia and hemodilution stemming from excess crystalloid administration.

Massive transfusion protocols (MTPs) are perhaps the most widely studied DCR intervention. The optimal ratio of plasma, platelets, and PRBCs to achieve hemostasis and prevent death from exsanguination is 1:1:1. Supplementary calcium should be given with every two units of PRBCs. Evidence suggests that the implementation of MTPs improves patient survival, reduces blood product usage, and lowers treatment costs. Adjuncts to MTPs include recombinant factor VIIa (rVIIa) to augment clot formation, tranexamic acid (TXA) to inhibit fibrinolysis, and functional laboratory measures of coagulation to guide resuscitation, such as thromboelastography. Administration of rVIIa may reduce the need for massive transfusions, but there is no significant mortality benefit. Because of a favorable side effect profile when used within

TABLE 3-3. Causes of Acquired Bleeding Disorders

Advanced liver disease
Anticoagulation therapy
Acquired thrombocytopenia
Platelet-inhibiting drugs
Uremia
Over-the-counter medications, eg, herbal supplements
DIC
Primary/secondary fibrinolysis

DIC, disseminated intravascular coagulation.

TABLE 3-4. Mechanism of Action and Monitoring of Anticoagulants

Mechanism of Action	Anticoagulant	Laboratory Monitoring
Xa inhibition and thrombin inhibition	Unfractionated heparin	aPTT or anti-Xa activity
Xa inhibition	Low-molecular-weight heparin (Lovenox), apixaban (Eliquis), edoxaban (Lixiana), rivaroxaban (Xarelto), fondaparinux (Arixtra)	Anti-Xa activity
Production of inactive vitamin K–dependent clotting factors IX, X, VII, II	Warfarin (Coumadin)	PT, INR
Thrombin inhibition	Argatroban (Acova), dabigatran (Pradaxa), bivalirudin (Angiomax)	aPTT, TCT

aPTT, activated partial thromboplastin time; INR, international normalized ratio; PT, prothrombin time; TCT, thrombin clotting time.

3 hours after injury, TXA is conditionally recommended for adult patients with trauma who are severely bleeding. TXA competitively inhibits the activation of plasminogen to plasmin, resulting in its antifibrinolytic activity. More recent clinical studies have begun to evaluate the use of whole blood for resuscitation in patients with trauma, with results indicating that whole blood is effective in this setting. This remains an area of active research.

Postoperative Bleeding

Fifty percent of postoperative bleeding is caused by inadequate hemostasis during surgery. Residual heparin that remains after cardiopulmonary or peripheral vascular bypass surgery can cause significant oozing or overt bleeding. Shock due to any cause that results in consumptive coagulopathy can lead to significant postoperative bleeding. Altered liver function after partial hepatectomy may be associated with bleeding as the remaining liver may need 3 to 5 days to increase its production of clotting factors sufficiently to support hemostasis. Acquired deficiency of the vitamin K–dependent clotting factors (II, VII, IX, and X) can develop in patients who are poorly nourished and are receiving antibiotics. Supplementation with vitamin K in postoperative patients who are not able to adequately nourish themselves is essential to avoid the development of these clotting factor deficiencies. Factor XIII deficiency is an uncommon disorder but must be considered as a possible cause for delayed postoperative bleeding. In this case, bleeding occurs 3 to 5 days after surgery. The diagnosis of this deficiency is confirmed by a factor XIII assay.

Disseminated Intravascular Coagulation

In any patient with postoperative bleeding, DIC must be considered as a possible cause. This is particularly true if there is severe infection or shock. DIC is characterized by intravascular coagulation and thrombosis that is diffuse rather than localized at the site of injury. This process results in the systemic deposition of platelet-fibrin microthrombi that cause diffuse tissue injury. Some clotting factors may be consumed in sufficient amounts to eventually lead to diffuse bleeding. DIC may be acute or clinically asymptomatic and chronic. The etiology of DIC may be any of the following: (1) the release of tissue debris into the bloodstream after trauma or an obstetrical catastrophe; (2) the introduction of intravascular aggregations of

platelets as a result of activation by various materials, including adenosine diphosphate (ADP) and thrombin (which may explain the occurrence of DIC in patients with severe septicemia or immune complex disease); (3) extensive endothelial damage, which denudes the vascular wall and stimulates coagulation and platelet adhesion (as seen in patients with widespread burns or vasculitis); (4) hypotension that leads to stasis and prevents the normal circulating inhibitors of coagulation from reaching the sites of the microthrombi; (5) blockage of the reticuloendothelial system; (6) some types of operations that involve the prostate, lung, or malignant tumors; (7) severe liver disease; and (8) brain trauma or surgery because the brain is rich in thromboplastin, which activates clotting if released into the circulation.

The diagnosis of DIC is established by the detection of diminished levels of coagulation factors and platelets. The following laboratory results may be useful in diagnosing DIC: (1) prolonged activated partial thromboplastin time (aPTT); (2) prolonged prothrombin time (PT); (3) hypofibrinogenemia; (4) thrombocytopenia; and (5) the presence of fibrin and fibrinogen split products and positive D-dimers. The presence of fibrin and fibrinogen split products is caused by activation of the fibrinolytic pathway in response to activation of the clotting pathway. The D-dimer is a product of fibrin digestion by the fibrinolytic process.

The most important aspect of the treatment of DIC is to remove the precipitating factors (eg, treating septicemia). If DIC is severe, replacement of coagulation factors is required to correct the coagulation defect. Cryoprecipitate is the best method for the replacement of a profound fibrinogen deficit. Platelet transfusions may also be required. Fresh frozen plasma (FFP) is useful for replacing other deficits that are identified, but it must be used judiciously if volume overload is a potential problem.

Bleeding Disorders Caused by Increased Fibrinolysis

Postsurgical bleeding may also be caused by disorders leading to increased fibrinolysis. Primary fibrinolysis is a disorder that occurs when the fibrinolytic pathway is activated, leading to the production of plasmin without antecedent activation of the coagulation pathways. Most commonly, primary fibrinolysis occurs after fibrinolytic therapy with drugs such as tissue plasminogen activators, which are used to lyse coronary artery or peripheral artery thromboses. Primary fibrinolysis is also seen in conjunction with surgical procedures on the prostate, which is rich in urokinase. It also occurs in patients with severe liver failure. Very rare disorders of inhibitors of the fibrinolytic pathway (eg, congenital deficiencies of α_2-antiplasmin) can also cause primary fibrinolysis. The treatment of these disorders is best accomplished by eliminating the precipitating cause, such as discontinuing lytic therapy. Because the half-life of lytic agents is short (in minutes), bleeding usually stops rapidly.

If primary fibrinolysis becomes severe, EACA can be used for therapy. This drug must be used cautiously because it blocks the fibrinolytic pathway and may predispose the patient to thrombotic events.

Secondary fibrinolysis is most often seen in response to DIC. The coagulation pathways are activated, followed by the fibrinolytic pathway. Manifestations of this activation in laboratory tests include hypofibrinogenemia, the presence of fibrin split products, and positive D-dimers. As the DIC is corrected, the secondary fibrinolysis resolves.

Hypercoagulable States in the Surgical Patient

Thromboembolism may occur for a number of reasons during the course of surgery and in the postoperative period (Table 3-5). Both congenital and acquired disorders can put surgical patients at risk for venous thromboembolism (VTE). The evaluation of patients for surgery must include an assessment of the degree of risk the patient has for a VTE event. Virtually all operations carry varying degrees of risk for VTE, from minimal to highly significant. A number of steps are essential in the assessment of the degree of risk in a patient.

The most important first step in the assessment of VTE risk is the medical history of the patient. The information to be obtained should address the following points: Has the patient suffered a VTE event before the age of 40 or had an unprovoked VTE event at any age? A recurrent VTE event at any age can be a harbinger of a hypercoagulable state, as can a thrombosis occurring at an unusual site (eg, mesenteric vein thrombosis). Perhaps

one of the most important points in history is the family history, which can provide helpful clues about the risks for VTE in any patient. A significant positive family history can guide one to evaluate patients for inherited hypercoagulable risk factors.

A positive history of thrombosis associated with pregnancy, oral contraceptives, or hormone replacement therapy should alert practitioners to the possibility of an underlying hypercoagulable state. The specific complications of pregnancy that one must address in the history include recurrent fetal loss, fetal growth retardation, preeclampsia, or eclampsia. Each of these disorders can be an indicator of any underlying hypercoagulable state.

Management of Hypercoagulable States

Therapy for hypercoagulable states is primarily directed at (1) interfering with the coagulation pathways (with heparin, warfarin, or both) and (2) interfering with platelet function (with aspirin, clopidogrel, or other platelet-inhibiting drugs). Therapy must be individualized both to the patient and to the site and severity of the thromboembolism. Great caution must be exercised when using warfarin in patients with protein C deficiency. These patients may develop "coumadin-induced skin necrosis" if a long overlap period with heparin is not allowed. This long overlap allows the metabolism of all vitamin K–dependent proteins to reach a steady state. The duration of anticoagulation therapy requires careful consideration, and the risks and benefits of protracted anticoagulation therapy must be weighed against potential benefits.

During the perioperative period, therapy for patients with a history of thromboembolism and a documented hypercoagulable state must be planned carefully by both the surgeon and the hematologist. Low-dose heparin (5,000 international units), subcutaneously administered, provides adequate protection from thromboembolism for short periods without compromising surgical hemostasis. Alternatively, low-molecular-weight heparin prophylaxis may be used. For patients with a documented hematologic risk factor for thrombosis who have never had a thromboembolic event, prophylaxis with pneumatic compression boots or low-dose

TABLE 3-5. Differential Diagnosis of Hypercoagulable States by Site of Thrombosis	
Arterial Thrombosis (eg, Myocardial Infarction)	**Venous Thrombosis (eg, VTE)**
Common: antiphospholipid syndrome	Common: factor V Leiden
Prothrombin 20210 mutation	Prothrombin 20210
HIT syndrome	Protein C deficiency
Uncommon: elevated PAI-1 activity	Protein S deficiency
Hyperhomocysteinemia (strokes in children)	Antithrombin deficiency
tPA deficiency	Uncommon: hyperhomocysteinemia (patients with uremia)
Anomalous coronary arteries	Factor XII deficiency
Vasculitis	Trauma
	Immobilization
	Pregnancy, oral contraceptive therapy, or hormone replacement therapy

HIT, heparin-induced thrombocytopenia; PAI, plasminogen activator inhibitor; tPA, tissue plasminogen activator; VTE, venous thromboembolism.

heparin is adequate. Deep vein thrombosis prophylaxis is also covered in detail in Chapter 1.

Special Populations

Several subgroups of commonly encountered patients have unique needs with regard to bleeding and clotting. Pregnant females experience an expansion of circulating blood volume with a relative anemia, but elevated levels of factor VIII, fibrinogen, and other clotting factors. Clotting and pulmonary embolism are the leading causes of death in pregnant females. This risk is highest during the third trimester and after delivery. Low-molecular-weight and unfractionated heparins are the preferred modalities of anticoagulation therapy in pregnant women.

Physiologically, healthy children and adolescents differ only slightly from their adult counterparts. Aging does not bring about any major changes to the hemostatic system; however, it is associated with increasing disease burden and decreased physiologic reserves. For this reason, when hemorrhage and coagulopathy do occur in older individuals, the event is typically more serious and associated with worse outcomes.

Patients with cirrhosis, acute liver failure (including "shock liver" and hepatitis), and other liver dysfunctions have a metabolic coagulopathy as a result of decreased protein production. The international normalized ratio (INR) test is the modality of choice for measuring synthetic liver function. Bilirubin, ammonia, and transaminase levels are not useful measurements in determining coagulopathy for patients with liver disease. Paradoxically, patients with liver disease may experience inappropriate bleeding or clotting, or even both simultaneously, because of a derangement of both anticoagulant and procoagulant processes.

Patients with renal failure are more prone to bleeding events primarily because of platelet malfunction secondary to uremia. Anticoagulants used during the dialysis process, a buildup of medications because of decreased renal drug elimination, and dilutional anemia also play a role in the increased risk of bleeding for these patients. Dialysis may help correct these issues but cannot ultimately eliminate them. Patients on dialysis are also at risk for thrombotic events because of chronic platelet activation caused by platelet contact with synthetic surfaces within the dialysis machine or the surgical graft for venous access.

In rare instances, after exposure to any type or amount of heparin, a patient can develop HIT. HIT is a hypercoagulable state manifested by arterial and venous thromboses. It occurs as a result of antibody formation to heparin-platelet complexes and results in thrombocytopenia because of intravascular platelet activation and aggregation. There is no indication of platelet transfusion. Patients must be anticoagulated with an alternate agent such as argatroban or fondaparinux.

BLOOD COMPONENT THERAPY

Typing and Crossmatching of Blood Components

There are over 600 known red blood cell antigens organized into 22 blood group systems. Only two groups have immunologic relevance: the ABO and Rhesus groups. An individual must receive ABO/Rh-matched blood. ABO incompatibilities are the most common cause of fatal transfusion reactions.

Crossmatching is performed after ABO/Rh typing. It is a process whereby serum from the recipient is mixed with the red blood cells from the donor. Antibodies to donor red cells present in the recipient serum will cause a positive crossmatch and preclude transfusion of those donor cells to this recipient.

Transfusion of Red Blood Cells

Red blood cell transfusions are available as (1) whole blood, (2) PRBCs, (3) washed red blood cells, (4) leukoreduced red blood cells, and (5) divided or pediatric unit red blood cells. There are no firm current indications for the transfusion of whole blood, with the exception of the need for massive transfusion or the need for lifesaving transfusion when component therapy is not available. Washed and leukoreduced red-cell preparations are used to transfuse red cells to patients who have had hypersensitivity or nonhemolytic febrile transfusion reactions to ordinary PRBCs, and for transplant patients. Transfusion of PRBCs is indicated when the red blood cell mass is decreased (as reflected in the hemoglobin concentration and/or hematocrit level) with a subsequent compromise of oxygen delivery to tissues and organs. The decision to transfuse, and the amount of blood to be transfused, is multifactorial and must be individualized on the basis of a number of factors, including (1) the reason for anemia; (2) the degree and acuity/chronicity of anemia; (3) underlying medical conditions, particularly cardiac, pulmonary, and renal disease; (4) anticipated future transfusion requirements; and (5) hemodynamic instability.

PRBCs are typically stored between 1 and 6 °C. The red blood cells have a shelf life of 42 days. One unit of PRBCs contains about 200 mL of red cells and 30 mL of plasma in a total volume of about 310 mL. The hematocrit of a typical unit of PRBCs is approximately 57%. Transfusion of one unit of PRBC into an average 70-kg person can be expected to raise the hemoglobin concentration by 1 g/dL and the hematocrit by 3%.

Transfusion Triggers

It is important to note that anemia alone is not an indication for transfusion in most populations; rather, the symptoms related to the anemia may trigger the decision to transfuse. Numerous retrospective studies in a variety of patient populations have found an association between blood transfusion and poor patient outcomes. At its core, blood product transfusions are tissue transplants, with all of the attendant immune problems. The decision to transfuse must be made on the basis of individual physiologic needs and clinical circumstances. Patients who are actively bleeding should receive balanced transfusion on the basis of their hemodynamic state and coagulation profile.

Transfusion of Fresh Frozen Plasma

Indications for transfusion of FFP include patients with laboratory evidence of multiple coagulation factor deficiency (eg, abnormally elevated PT or aPTT) with clinical bleeding or the need for an invasive procedure. Coagulation factor deficiencies can result from dilutional coagulopathy following massive transfusion or resuscitation, congenital synthesis defects, anticoagulant medications such as warfarin or heparin, liver disease, malnutrition, and other acquired disorders.

Transfusion of Platelets

Platelet transfusion is indicated for patients who have clinical bleeding, and either an absolute thrombocytopenia or a relative thrombocytopenia due to platelet dysfunction. Platelet dysfunction often occurs as a result of medical conditions, such as renal failure, or as a result of medications such as nonsteroidal anti-inflammatory drugs and clopidogrel (Plavix). Patients with normal platelet function typically do not experience clinical bleeding until the absolute platelet count drops to 30,000 to 50,000 platelets/µL and often even lower than this. In contrast, patients with dysfunctional platelets will often manifest clinical bleeding with platelet counts in the normal range. Additional information regarding the need for platelet transfusion can be obtained from a whole blood platelet function testing. Platelet suspensions contain some plasma and few red blood cells or leukocytes. The therapeutic effect of platelet transfusion depends upon the patient's pathologic state, existing platelet count, level of platelet function, weight of the patient, and the number of platelet concentrates transfused. The absolute rise in platelet count is also variable. A typical transfusion of six platelet concentrates can be expected to raise the platelet count by approximately 50,000 to 100,000 platelets/µL.

Complications of Blood Component Therapy

Transfusion of blood and blood components is safe and efficacious when used for the correct indications. However, transfusion is not without risk. There are multiple potential side effects associated with transfusion. These can be divided into (1) metabolic derangements, (2) immunologic reactions, (3) infectious complications, (4) volume overload, and (5) pulmonary complications. There are also special considerations for the transfusion of large amounts of blood products over a short period of time, such as in massive transfusion.

Metabolic Derangements

Metabolic complications of transfusion therapy are typically seen in the context of transfusion of large amounts of blood products, or transfusion of older blood products, or both. Most common are hypocalcemia, hyperkalemia, hypokalemia, and hypothermia.

The lethal triad (Figure 3-1) consists of the interrelation of acidosis, hypothermia, and coagulopathy and has been recognized as a significant cause of death for patients with trauma and/or massive blood loss. Successful resuscitation depends on breaking the cycle. Hypothermia, defined as core temperature of less than 35 °C, is a constant problem in trauma and may be present in a patient with otherwise normal vital signs. Hypothermia is seen in 50% of patients with trauma at initial presentation. Some populations are more susceptible to hypothermia, particularly older patients, frail patients, pediatric patients, burn patients, patients with diabetes, and those with thyroid dysfunction. Hypothermia results in impaired platelet function,

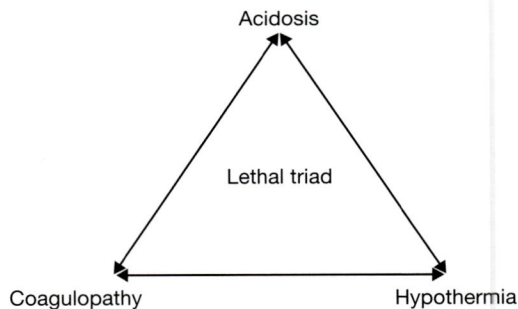

Figure 3-1. The lethal triad.

inhibition of clotting factors, and inappropriate activation of clot breakdown. Among other rewarming strategies, warmers for fluids and blood products being infused are important, because room temperature fluids contribute significantly to hypothermia.

Acidosis (pH <7.35) results in poor tissue perfusion because of decreased cardiac output. Decreased cardiac output is already present in patients with trauma who are bleeding, independent of acidosis, from decreased preload (due to blood loss) and peripheral vasoconstriction. Decreased cardiac output results in overall tissue hypoperfusion and anaerobic metabolism, resulting in more lactic acid production and a further decrease in the pH.

Multiple factors affect coagulopathy, including ongoing blood loss, cofactor consumption, dilutional coagulopathy due to intravenous (IV) fluid administration, and inadequate replacement of clotting factors. In addition, coagulation cofactors are progressively inhibited by decreasing pH and hypothermia. Coagulopathy results in continued bleeding in patients with trauma and is associated with a 4-fold increase in mortality.

The lethal triad begins and ends with bleeding, so the first step is to apply direct pressure to sites of bleeding. Take steps to maintain euthermia, and be aware that exposed patients are constantly losing heat. Resuscitate patients experiencing bleeding in a balanced fashion with blood products. Crystalloid solutions are low in pH (the pH of "normal saline" is 5.5), contribute to dilutional coagulopathy, and are often administered coldly. Thus, crystalloid use should be minimized and infused through a warmer whenever possible. By addressing all three factors in the lethal triad simultaneously, the cycle can be broken and the patient salvaged.

Immunologic Transfusion Reactions

Although ABO and Rh compatibility testing and crossmatching can obviate some of the more serious transfusion reactions, minor untested and unidentified antigens and antibodies can still precipitate immunologic reactions (Table 3-6). Immunologic transfusion reactions are (1) febrile reactions, (2) acute and delayed hemolytic transfusion reactions, (3) thrombocytopenia, (4) anaphylactic shock, (5) urticaria, (6) graft-versus-host disease, and (7) immune suppression.

Febrile reactions are the most common immunologic transfusion reactions. These reactions typically occur as a result of antileukocyte antibodies. Symptoms and signs

TABLE 3-6. Management of Transfusion Reactions		
	Reaction	**Management**
Minor transfusion reaction	Fever, rash, urticaria	Observation, antihistamines
Major transfusion reaction	Fever, chills, hypotension, bleeding in previously dry areas, hemoglobinuria, decreased urine output	Immediate cessation of transfusion; the unit of blood should be sent back to the blood bank for recrossmatch, volume expanders, pressors (mannitol, Lasix).

include fever, chills, and tachycardia. Hemodynamic instability can occur in severe cases. Patients with minor reactions can be managed expectantly, and the therapy is largely supportive. The transfusion should be stopped. Pretreatment with aspirin, antipyretics, and antihistamines can prevent future reactions. Alternatively, transfusion of leukocyte-reduced red cells can also be effective.

Acute hemolytic reactions can vary in severity from minor to catastrophic. Most hemolytic reactions occur as a result of a clerical error and transfusion of ABO-mismatched blood. They can begin quickly with administration of as little as 50 mL of donor blood. Symptoms include sensation of hot or cold, flushing, chest pain, and low back pain. Signs include fever, hypotension, tachycardia, hematuria, hemoglobinuria, bleeding, and possibly acute renal failure. Successful management of hemolytic transfusion reactions rests on early diagnosis and prompt intervention. The transfusion must be immediately stopped. The remaining transfusion blood and a sample of the patient's blood are returned to the laboratory for retyping and crossmatching. Transfused and patient blood is also sent for culture to differentiate from contamination. Care is primarily supportive. Hemodynamic instability is treated with volume expansion and pressors, if necessary. Some clinicians recommend the administration of mannitol and/or loop diuretics, such as furosemide, to maintain urine output. Severe renal failure may require hemodialysis.

Graft-versus-host disease occurs when patients who are immunosuppressed receive donor leukocytes in blood component therapy. These cells are unrecognized as foreign cells by the recipient, and they mount an immune response against recipient tissues. Onset of symptoms is often delayed for weeks and includes fever, rash, liver dysfunction, and diarrhea. This can be prevented by using leukocyte-reduced red cells and/or irradiated red cells.

Transmission of Infectious Agents

Transmission of infectious agents following transfusion is rare. Blood can transmit infections caused by bacteria, viruses, and parasites.

Transfusion-Related Acute Lung Injury

Transfusion-related acute lung injury (TRALI) occurs in about 1 out of every 5,000 transfusions. It can occur with transfusion of any blood component but is most common with transfusions that contain plasma, such as FFP or platelets. TRALI is characterized by noncardiogenic pulmonary edema following transfusion. The inciting event in TRALI is unknown but likely immunologic. Onset of pulmonary edema and respiratory insufficiency is generally within 1 to 2 hours of beginning the transfusion, but it can happen up to 6 hours after a transfusion. Recently, a delayed TRALI syndrome has been recognized, in which onset may be delayed up to 72 hours after transfusion. Treatment of TRALI is supportive.

SUGGESTED READINGS

Black JA, Pierce VS, Kerby JD, Holcomb JB. The evolution of blood transfusion in the trauma patient: whole blood has come full circle. *Semin Thromb Hemost*. 2020;46(2):215-220.

Bunch CM, Chang E, Moore EE, et al. SHock-INduced Endotheliopathy (SHINE): a mechanistic justification for viscoelastography-guided resuscitation of traumatic and nontraumatic shock. *Front Physiol*. 2023;14:1094845.

Cannon JW. Hemorrhagic shock. *New Engl J Med*. 2018;378: 370-379.

Carson JL, Stanworth SJ, Dennis JA, et al. Transfusion thresholds for guiding red blood cell transfusion. *Cochrane Database Syst Rev*. 2021;12(12):CD002042.

Delaney M, Wendel S, Bercovitz RS, et al. Transfusion reactions: prevention, diagnosis, and treatment. *Lancet*. 2016;388:2825-2836.

Dilday J, Lewis MR. Transfusion management in the trauma patient. *Review Curr Opin Crit Care*. 2022;28(6):725-731.

Orfanakis A, Deloughery T. Patients with disorders of thrombosis and hemostasis. *Med Clin North Am*. 2013;97:1161-1180.

Smith M, Wakam G, Wakefield T, Obi A. New trends in anticoagulation therapy. *Surg Clin North Am*. 2018;98:219-238.

Yu Y, Lian Z. Update on transfusion-related acute lung injury: an overview of its pathogenesis and management. *Front Immunol*. 2023;14:1175387.

SAMPLE QUESTIONS

QUESTIONS

Choose the best answer for each question.

1. A 21-year-old male patient arrives to the trauma bay with multiple gunshot wounds. After initial resuscitation, the patient is taken to the operating room for exploratory laparotomy. Within the next 4 hours, the patient receives more than 10 units of packed RBCs and 2 g of IV calcium. The patient continues to have diffuse oozing from surgical sites and venous access sites. Labs are remarkable for an aPTT of 100 second, INR of 5, and a platelet count of 20,000. What is the MOST likely cause of this patient's coagulopathy?

   A. Acute hemolytic transfusion reaction
   B. Dilutional coagulopathy
   C. Antiplatelet medication use at home
   D. Citrate-induced hypocalcemia
   E. von Willebrand disease

2. A 55-year-old woman is scheduled for a craniotomy to remove a brain tumor. She has a history of hypertension and hypercholesterolemia, and she underwent coronary artery angioplasty with a stent placed 6 months ago. Current medications include enalapril, pravastatin, and clopidogrel. Which one of the following tests would most likely be prolonged?

   A. aPTT
   B. Platelet function screening test
   C. PT
   D. Thrombin time
   E. Activated clotting time

3. A 50-year-old man is started on IV heparin for a peripheral arterial thrombosis. Three days later, it is noted that his platelet count has dropped from 200,000 to 35,000. What is the next best step in management?

   A. Discontinue heparin and administer argatroban.
   B. Continue heparin and administer argatroban.
   C. Discontinue heparin and administer aspirin.
   D. Discontinue heparin and administer warfarin (Coumadin).
   E. Continue heparin and administer a platelet transfusion.

4. A patient has ongoing bleeding after a damage-control surgery. DIC is suspected. Possible etiologies of DIC include all of the following except:

   A. The release of tissue debris into the bloodstream after trauma
   B. Several renal disease
   C. Extensive endothelial damage to vessels
   D. Hypotension
   E. Intravascular aggregations of platelets

5. A 65-year-old woman with severe symptomatic anemia secondary to chronic renal disease is being transfused with PRBCs. After 10 minutes of transfusion, she begins to complain of back pain, chest pain, and shortness of breath. The most likely diagnosis is which of the following?

   A. TRALI
   B. Delayed hemolytic transfusion reaction
   C. Acute hemolytic transfusion reaction
   D. Transfusion-related volume overload
   E. Transfusion-related hyperkalemia

ANSWERS AND EXPLANATIONS

1. **Answer: B**

   Massive transfusion of red blood cells may lead to bleeding because of dilution of clotting factors and platelets. Massive transfusion has been defined in various ways. The two most common definitions are: more than 10 units of PRBCs in 24 hours or replacement of whole blood volume in 24 hours. Proper MTPs consist of transfusing in a 1:1:1 ratio of RBC, plasma, and platelet units.

   The patient has no symptoms of an acute hemolytic transfusion reaction such as low back pain and flushing, and there is no reported hematuria, tachycardia, or hypotension. There is no history of antiplatelet drugs being taken at home. Citrate-induced hypocalcemia is not associated with bleeding but may be associated with cardiac arrhythmias. The patient's coagulation studies are not consistent with von Willebrand disease as the PT/INR is elevated and the platelet count is low; both of these parameters are normal in von Willebrand disease. For more information on this topic, see section "Complications of Blood Component Therapy."

2. **Answer: B**

   Clopidogrel is a platelet-inhibiting medication that is often used after the placement of intravascular stents to prevent thrombosis. Like aspirin (ASA [acetylsalicylic acid]), clopidogrel is nonreversible; therefore, it should be stopped 7 to 10 days before surgery if normal coagulation is required. Abnormal platelet function tests are often associated with platelet dysfunction. The aPTT (intrinsic and common pathways), PT (extrinsic and common pathway), and thrombin time (formation of fibrin from fibrinogen) evaluate specific aspects of the coagulation cascade. For more information on this topic, see section "Blood Component Therapy."

3. **Answer: A**

   HIT is a hypercoagulable state manifested by arterial and venous thromboses. HIT occurs as a result of antibody formation to heparin-platelet complexes and results in thrombocytopenia because of intravascular platelet activation and aggregation. There is no indication for platelet transfusion. HIT can occur because of administration of any type of heparin. Patients must be anticoagulated with an alternate agent such as argatroban or fondaparinux. In this setting, starting warfarin (Coumadin) without starting one of these alternate agents is contraindicated, because the initiation of warfarin therapy is associated with a transient hypercoagulable state. These patients may develop "coumadin-induced skin necrosis" if a long overlap period with heparin is not allowed. For more information on this topic, see section "Hypercoagulable States in the Surgical Patient."

4. **Answer: B**

DIC is characterized by intravascular coagulation and thrombosis that is diffuse rather than localized at the site of injury. This process results in the systemic deposition of platelet-fibrin microthrombi that cause diffuse tissue injury. The etiology of DIC may be any of the following: (1) the release of tissue debris into the bloodstream after trauma or an obstetrical catastrophe; (2) the introduction of intravascular aggregations of platelets as a result of activation by various materials, including ADP and thrombin (which may explain the occurrence of DIC in patients with severe septicemia or immune complex disease); (3) extensive endothelial damage, which denudes the vascular wall and stimulates coagulation and platelet adhesion (as seen in patients with widespread

burns or vasculitis); (4) hypotension that leads to stasis and prevents the normal circulating inhibitors of coagulation from reaching the sites of the microthrombi; (5) blockage of the reticuloendothelial system; (6) some types of operations that involve the prostate, lung, or malignant tumors; (7) severe liver disease; and (8) brain trauma or surgery because the brain is rich in thromboplastin, which activates clotting if released into the circulation. For more information on this topic, see section "Disseminated Intravascular Coagulation."

5. **Answer: C**

Acute hemolytic transfusion reactions are usually caused by clerical error resulting in the administration of ABO-mismatched blood. Host antibodies bind to antigens in donor red blood cells resulting in hemolysis. This may result in renal failure and shock. Patients complain of shortness of breath, chest pain, and back pain. The most appropriate course of action is to stop the transfusion, provide supportive therapy, and have the blood rechecked. TRALI usually occurs after completion of transfusions. Volume overload and hyperkalemia are unlikely to occur just minutes into a transfusion. For more information on this topic, see section "Immunologic Transfusion Reactions."

4

Surgical Shock

Bennett Berning and Charity Evans

In 1872, S.D. Gross described shock as "a rude unhinging of the machinery of life." The effects of the bodies malfunctioning cellular metabolism are initially reversible but can rapidly become irreversible, resulting in multiorgan failure (MOF) and death. Shock most commonly occurs from circulatory failure, resulting in systolic hypotension (<90 mm Hg). However, cellular and organ injury may develop without systolic hypotension, and not all etiologies of hypotension cause cellular or organ injury. Therefore, definitions of shock based on the circulatory measurement of systolic blood pressure (SBP) are potentially misleading and narrow in scope.

A broader definition of shock is a state of cellular and tissue hypoxia due to reduced oxygen delivery and increased oxygen consumption or inadequate oxygen utilization. Oxygen and blood volume delivery fails to meet the cellular metabolic and oxygen consumption needs. Recognizing shock and restoring circulation are the primary tenets for managing the patient with shock. This chapter describes the four main types of shock—hypovolemic, distributive, obstructive, and cardiogenic—and summarizes the pathophysiology, clinical guidelines, and various management strategies.

PATHOPHYSIOLOGY

The main function of circulation is to deliver oxygen to the cells. Reduced tissue perfusion or increased oxygen consumption results in cellular hypoxia, causing cell membrane ion pump dysfunction, intracellular edema, leakage of intracellular contents into the extracellular space, and inadequate regulation of intracellular pH. This ongoing process results in a further reduction in tissue perfusion from complex humoral and microcirculatory processes that impair regional blood flow, thereby exacerbating cellular hypoxia.

The major determinants of tissue perfusion are cardiac output (CO) and systematic vascular resistance (SVR), where blood pressure (BP) = CO × SVR. CO is the product of heart rate (HR) and stroke volume (SV): CO = HR × SV. SV is determined by preload, myocardial contractility, and afterload. SVR is regulated by vessel length, blood viscosity, and vessel diameter. Any biologic process that changes any of these physiologic parameters will alter BP and can result in shock. The measurement of the specific hemodynamic parameters will distinguish between the different classes of shock (Table 4-1). Most forms of shock will involve an alteration in CO and/or SVR.

Shock is a physiologic continuum that begins with an inciting event and progresses through several stages. Early shock, also known as preshock, is characterized by compensatory responses to diminished tissue perfusion, which are more amenable to therapy and likely to be reversible. In late shock, the compensatory mechanisms become overwhelmed with emerging signs and symptoms of end-organ

dysfunction. End-organ dysfunction refers to irreversible organ damage, MOF, and death.

INITIAL EVALUATION AND DIAGNOSTIC

History and Physical Examination

Diagnosing shock early (in any form) requires a high clinical suspicion for its presence and potential cause. Starting with a targeted history from the patient, their family members, and/or the medical record will provide potential etiology. Physical assessment of the patient should provide additional findings consistent with shock. Sentinel clinical exam findings include hypotension, oliguria, mental status changes, and cool and clammy skin. When present, sentinel findings of shock should prompt immediate therapeutic intervention and should not be delayed while awaiting additional laboratory and imaging studies.

Laboratory Studies

For patients with suspected shock, a broad set of laboratory studies should be obtained in a timely manner. Specific laboratory studies must include serum lactate, complete metabolic panel, cardiac enzymes, complete blood cell count, coagulation studies, and blood gas analysis. Results of these tests will help better differentiate the type and etiology of the shock state and help initiate early interventions.

Diagnostic Imaging

Various imaging modalities can be obtained rapidly and help diagnose potential causes of shock.

X-ray often is a first-line imaging modality. A simple chest radiography has the potential to detect the cause of shock in all forms (hypovolemic, distributive, cardiogenic, and obstructive). Some examples include hemothorax in the setting of trauma (hypovolemic shock), pneumonia or free air under diaphragm (distributive shock caused by sepsis), pulmonary edema or enlarged cardiac silhouette (cardiogenetic shock), tension pneumothorax (PTX; obstructive shock). In the setting of trauma, a pelvic x-ray may reveal significant pelvic fractures. If the patient is hemodynamically unstable, hypovolemic shock caused by significant hemorrhage would be high on the differential diagnosis.

Point-of-care ultrasonography (POCUS) has emerged as an important tool for the diagnosis and monitoring of various shock states. As ultrasound becomes more readily available and providers become more confident with its use, its role in the initial diagnosis of an undifferentiated shock state is invaluable. Various POCUS-related protocols have been created to help the clinician reveal the etiology of shock at the bedside. Examples include rapid ultrasound in shock

TABLE 4-1.   Hemodynamic Profiles of Shock in Adults

Physiologic Variable	Preload	Cardiac Function	Afterload	Tissue Perfusion
Clinical Measurement Used to Determine Physiologic Variable	Pulmonary Capillary Wedge Pressure	Cardiac Output	Systemic Vascular Resistance	Mixed Venous Oxyhemoglobin Saturation
Hypovolemic	↔ (early) or ↓ (late)	↔ (early) or ↓ (late)	↓	>65% (early) or <65% (late)
Cardiogenic	↓	↓	↓	<65%
Distributive	↔ (early) or ↓ (late)	↓ or ↓	↓	>65%
Obstructive				
Pulmonary embolism	↔ (early) or ↓ (late)	↔ (early) or ↓ (late)	↓	>65%
Pericardial tamponade	↓	↓	↓	<65%

(RUSH), focused cardiac ultrasound (FOCUS), abdominal and cardiac evaluation with sonography in shock (ACES), and focused assessment with sonography for trauma (FAST). There are many advantages that support the use of POCUS. Ultrasound is noninvasive, uses no ionizing radiation, is portable, and easily learned. In addition to its use as a tool for the diagnosis of various forms of shock, it can be used to help monitor a patient's responsiveness to fluid resuscitation. For these reasons, POCUS should be a first-line tool used in the evaluation of undifferentiated shock.

High-quality cross-sectional imaging, most commonly computed tomography (CT) scan, is a powerful diagnostic tool, especially when the etiology of shock is unclear. Hemorrhage, perforated hollow viscus, ischemic bowel, and PTX are only a few examples of various pathologies that could explain shock physiology during the initial assessment. Of note, it is imperative that the hemodynamics of a patient are stabilized before obtaining CT imaging.

Hemodynamic Monitoring

Several tools and maneuvers can be used to provide objective measures to assist in determining whether shock is present. In addition, once resuscitation is initiated one must assess progress and gain insight into whether or not a patient may or may not be responsive to additional fluid. These strategies include passive leg raise, analysis of SV variability, respiratory variation on arterial pressure tracing, and inferior vena cava distensibility/compressibility. The use of central venous pressure has been shown to be not a reliable tool and should not be used to make clinical decisions regarding fluid resuscitation. In addition, although the use of a pulmonary artery (PA) catheter may help differentiate between various states of shock, its use has not been proven to have a mortality benefit and its use should be reserved for only special patient populations. It is important to note that caution should be used when relying on a single tool to guide resuscitation, rather multiple objective measures should be used to help reveal the true clinical picture.

CATEGORIES OF SHOCK

Hypovolemic Shock

Hypovolemic shock results from reduced intravascular volume, causing a reduced preload and reduced CO.

Hypovolemic shock is divided into hemorrhagic and nonhemorrhagic, with hemorrhagic being the most common. Common etiologies of hypovolemia are listed in Table 4-2. The signs and symptoms of hemorrhagic shock are related to the amount of intravascular volume loss and subsequent decreased preload, as seen in Table 4-3.

Diagnosing hypovolemic shock starts with a thorough history and physical examination. Hemorrhagic shock may occur after trauma, following major surgical or invasive procedures, or present as a profound gastrointestinal (GI) bleed. Nonhemorrhagic hypovolemic shock may have an obvious source, such as GI loss due to significant emesis or diarrhea, but may be more overt, caused by loss of fluid into interstitial spaces (third spacing). On physical examination, patients will show signs of hypovolemia/anemia. Hypotension and tachycardia are expected but not required. Beware of medications that may alter the physiologic response to hypovolemia (eg, β-blockers). Additional physical examination findings may include, but are not limited to, pallor, lethargy, dry mucous membranes, skin tenting, and flat neck veins.

TABLE 4-2.   Common Etiologies of Hypovolemia

Hemorrhagic	Nonhemorrhagic
• Blunt or penetrating trauma • Upper gastrointestinal bleed • Lower gastrointestinal bleed • Intra- and postoperative bleeding • Ruptured abdominal aortic aneurysm • Aortoenteric fistula • Hemorrhagic pancreatitis • Iatrogenic • Tumor or abscess erosion into major vessel • Postpartum hemorrhage, uterine, or vaginal hemorrhage • Spontaneous retroperitoneal hemorrhage	• Gastrointestinal losses from diarrhea, vomiting, or external drainage • Skin losses • Renal losses • Third space losses into extravascular space or body cavities

TABLE 4-3. Classes of Hemorrhagic Shock

	I	II	III	IV
Blood loss (%)	<15 (<750 mL)	15-30 (750-1,500 mL)	30-40 (1,500-2,000 mL)	>40 (>2,000 mL)
Pulse	<100	>100	>120	>140
Blood pressure	Normal	Normal	↓	↓↓
Pulse pressure	Normal	Normal or ↓	↓↓	↓↓
Capillary refill (s)	<2	2-3	3-4	>5
Respiratory rate (breaths/min)	14-20	20-30	30-40	>40
Urine output (mL/h)	30 or more	20-30	5-10	Negligible
Mental status	Slightly anxious	Mildly anxious	Anxious and confused	Confused and lethargic

Hypovolemic shock causes significant laboratory derangements. Patients who are experiencing chronic or subacute bleeding may present with anemia (low hemoglobin [Hgb] or hematocrit [Hct]). Conversely, in the setting of profound acute blood loss, measurement of Hgb and Hct may not be reliable because Hgb and Hct are measures of concentration and will remain stable in a bleeding patient until compensatory mechanisms ensue. With dehydration, hemoconcentration may occur, resulting in an elevated Hgb and Hct. Nonhemorrhagic hypovolemia may lead to electrolyte abnormalities, depending on the fluid lost. GI losses from emesis or high-output nasogastric tube suctioning can lead to a hypokalemic, hyperchloremic metabolic alkalosis. GI losses from diarrhea, ileostomy output, or high-output pancreatic fistula may result in the loss of bicarbonate.

The management of hypovolemic shock is rapid volume repletion. Delaying volume resuscitation can lead to irreversible shock, MOF, and eventual death. Vasopressors generally should not be administered in the early stages of volume repletion, because they do not correct the primary problem and tend to further reduce tissue perfusion. The choice of replacement fluid depends upon the type of fluid that has been lost.

In hemorrhagic shock, isotonic crystalloid resuscitation should be avoided. Early blood product transfusion is required. If available, whole blood transfusion is ideal. The alternative is to transfuse packed red blood cells, fresh frozen plasma, and platelets in a 1:1:1 ratio. Early, balanced transfusion during hemorrhagic shock leads to less overall product transfused, improved coagulopathy, and decreased mortality. During the massive transfusion, the citrate in stored blood will lead to low free plasma calcium, so repletion is critical. Avoidance of hypothermia, acidosis, and coagulopathy, known as the "lethal triad," improves mortality for patients experiencing hemorrhagic shock. If the suspicion for active hemorrhage is high, permissive hypotension (limiting fluid resuscitation to allow for mild hypotension) can be considered until definitive hemorrhage control is achieved.

Isotonic solutions (Table 4-4) are the preferred fluid in hypovolemic shock that does not involve hemorrhage. Administered as a bolus of 20 to 30 mL/kg, and repeated every 5 to 10 minutes, fluid repletion should continue at the initial rate until clinical markers of resuscitation (BP, urine output, mental status, and peripheral perfusion) improve. Care must be taken to avoid fluid overload in certain patient populations. Examples include patients

TABLE 4-4. Components of Different Isotonic Intravenous Fluids

	Osmolarity (mOsm/L)	pH	Na+ (mmol)	Cl- (mmol)	K+ (mmol)	Ca2+ (mmol)	Glucose	Other
Lactated Ringer	273	6.5	130	109	4	3	–	Lactate: 28 mEq/L
Normal saline 0.9%	308	6.0	154	154	–	–	–	–
Albumin 5%	330	7.4	~145	–	≤2	–	–	Albumin: 50 g/L
Plasmalyte	294	7.4	140	98	5	3	–	Acetate: 27 mEq/L Gluconate: 23 mEq/L
Albumin 25%	330	7.4	~145	–	≤2	–	–	Albumin: 250 g/L
10% Dextran 40 in normal saline	310	4.9	154	154	–	–	–	Dextran: 100 g/L
Hetastarch 6% in normal saline	308	5.5	154	154	–	–	–	Hetastarch: 60 g/L

with heart failure, severe malnutrition, diabetic ketoacidosis, syndrome of inappropriate antidiuretic hormone, and extremes of age. Finally, one must address the source of volume loss and take measures to mitigate the amount of volume loss.

Distributive Shock

Distributive shock is the direct effect of excessive vasodilatation of the peripheral vasculature resulting in the impaired distribution of blood flow. Septic shock is the most common form of distributive shock encountered; however, anaphylactic, neurogenic shock, and adrenal crisis are also among this pathophysiology.

Septic Shock

The Surviving Sepsis Campaign, international guidelines for the management of sepsis and septic shock, published in 2021, defines sepsis as life-threatening organ dysfunction caused by a dysregulated host response to infection. Sepsis is identified through the use of the Sequential Organ Failure Assessment (SOFA) score (Table 4-5). The SOFA score assesses six major organ systems, applying a numeric value to the level of failure for each system. An acute increase of the SOFA score of 2 or more with suspected or documented infection is the clinical criteria for sepsis. A patient is in septic shock when circulatory and cellular/metabolic abnormalities are present. Clinically, this is defined as sepsis and vasopressor therapy is required to elevate mean arterial pressure (MAP) 65 mm Hg or more, with a lactate greater than 2 mmol/L after adequate fluid resuscitation. The development of septic shock significantly increases hospital mortality in excess of 40%.

The diagnosis of sepsis and septic shock starts with a thorough history and physical examination. Autonomic dysregulation will ensue resulting in hyperthermia or hypothermia, tachycardia, and tachypnea. Systemic hypoperfusion and microcirculatory dysfunction cause skin mottling and a cool sensation to touch. Additional symptoms and physical examination findings include poor mentation, low urine output, and GI dysmotility. Laboratory tests are often deranged, further assisting you in the diagnosis of sepsis/septic shock (Table 4-6).

The management of sepsis/septic shock is based on recommendations from the Surviving Sepsis Campaign, first presented in 2001, and updated and revised in 2021. The foundation for the treatment of sepsis/septic shock, first and foremost, is source control, which is often surgical in nature. In addition to aggressive source control, broad-spectrum antibiotics (including antifungals for high-risk patients) should be administered within the first hour after sepsis is suspected. Identification of the infectious source with cultures is recommended to assist in diagnosis and to inform antibiotic therapy. Attempts should be made to obtain cultures before antibiotic administration; however, obtaining cultures should not delay antibiotic administration. The risk of dying from septic shock increases by 10% per hour of delay to antibiotics, making timely administration a therapeutic priority.

It is not unexpected that many patients with sepsis or in septic shock may require critical care services. Multiorgan dysfunction is likely, and therapies should be tailored to support the patient through a dysregulated host response.

Aggressive, balanced isotonic crystalloid fluid resuscitation should be initiated early. Objective end points to resuscitation should help guide your therapy. As described earlier in the section describing hemodynamic monitoring, various tools and maneuvers can be used to provide objective measures to help guide your resuscitation. Frequent assessment and reassessment of the patient's response to volume is critical.

Intravenous (IV) vasopressor support is often needed to maintain MAP in patients with septic shock. Norepinephrine is the first-line agent with both α_1 (vasoconstrictive) and β_1 (inotropic) properties. The addition of vasopressin

TABLE 4-5. Sequential Organ Failure Assessment (SOFA) Score Criteria

SOFA Score	0	1	2	3	4
Respiratory: Pao_2/Fio_2 (mm Hg)	≥400	<400	<300	<200 and mechanically ventilated	<100 and mechanically ventilated
Coagulation: platelets $\times 10^3/\mu L$	≥150	<150	<100	<50	<20
Liver: bilirubin (mg/dL)	<1.2	1.2-1.9	2.0-5.9	6.0-11.9	>12.0
Cardiovascular: mean arterial pressure (MAP) or administration of vasopressors required	MAP ≥70 mm Hg	MAP ≥70 mm Hg	Dopamine ≤5 µg/kg/min or dobutamine (any dose)	Dopamine >5 µg/kg/min or epinephrine ≤0.1 µg/kg/min or norepinephrine ≤0.1 µg/kg/min	Dopamine >15 µg/kg/min or epinephrine >0.1 µg/kg/min or norepinephrine >0.1 µg/kg/min
Central nervous system: Glasgow coma scale	15	13-14	10-12	6-9	<6
Renal: creatinine (mg/dL) (or urine output)	<1.2	1.2-1.9	2.0-3.4	3.5-4.9 (or <500 mL/d)	>5.0 (or <200 mL/d)

TABLE 4-6. Common Laboratory Study Findings in Sepsis/Septic Shock

Laboratory Study	Common Finding in Sepsis/Septic Shock
CBC	• WBC >12,000/mm^3 or <4,000 mm^3 • >10% immature bands • Thrombocytopenia
BMP	• Decreased ionized calcium level • BUN: Cr ratio >20 can indicate under resuscitation. • Cl^- HCO_3, anion gap/base excess
LFTS	• Assess if liver or biliary tract are the source of infection. • Can reveal end-organ dysfunction of the liver
Coagulation studies (PT/INR, PTT, fibrinogen, TEG)	• Identify abnormalities to calculate SOFA score.
Lactate level	• Elevated due to hypoperfusion
Central venous oxygen saturation (Scvo$_2$)	• In early sepsis, metabolic demands will be higher, requiring more oxygen (Scvo$_2$ <75%). • Advanced end-organ failure and lack of ability of the organ systems to utilize oxygen for metabolic needs (Scvo$_2$ >75%)
Arterial blood gas	• Evaluates for acidosis • Guides adjustments when the patient is on a ventilator
Blood and urine cultures	• Identification of sepsis sources and guidance of antibiotic management
Procalcitonin	• Value >2 standard deviations above normal serve as a biomarker with greater specificity for infection than other cytokines.

BMP, basic metabolic panel; BUN, blood urea nitrogen; CBC, complete blood count; Cr, creatinine; INR, international normalized ratio; LFTS, liver function tests; PT, prothrombin time; PTT, partial thromboplastin time; SOFA, Sequential Organ Failure Assessment; TEG, thromboelastography; WBC, white blood cell count.

(a potent vasoconstrictor) can have a synergistic effect when used in combination with norepinephrine. Second- and third-line vasopressors include epinephrine and dopamine, respectively. Although dopamine provides vasoconstrictive properties in septic shock, it also has potent chronotropic properties, resulting in a significant risk for tachyarrhythmias. Phenylephrine should be avoided due to its pure α_1-agonist properties which do cause aggressive vasoconstriction, but result in a significant increase in afterload, causing strain on a heart in an already stressed state.

In addition to circulatory support, attention must be given to the other organ systems effected by the shock state. If mechanical support is required, lung protective strategies (tidal volume of 6 mL/kg) should be implemented per recommendations from the Acute Respiratory Distress Syndrome Network to prevent barotrauma or acute respiratory distress syndrome. Patients in septic shock can often develop adrenal insufficiency, and the addition of stress dose steroids (hydrocortisone) may allow these patients to be weaned from vasopressor support sooner. Finally, renal replacement therapy may be required in cases of severe acute kidney injury with hyperkalemia, severe acidosis, uremia, or volume overload.

Neurogenic Shock

Neurogenic shock is most commonly a result of traumatic injury to the spinal cord at the level of the sixth thoracic vertebra and higher and estimated to occur in up to 20% of cervical spine injuries. The damage results in complete dysregulation of the sympathetic nervous system, causing inappropriate vasodilation, resulting in hypotension, bradyarrhythmia, and temperature dysregulation. Neurogenic shock should not be confused with spinal shock characterized by transient state of depressed spinal cord function below the level of traumatic injury, with associated loss of reflexes and sensorimotor functions.

In the patient with traumatic injuries, the physical examination may suggest a high-level spinal cord injury. Patients will often present with hypotension and shock as well as bradycardia because of a loss of reflex sympathetic tachycardia. Other signs of spinal cord injury, such as diminished motor and sensory exam, priapism, and loss of rectal tone or reflexes, help confirm the diagnosis. It is vitally important that other forms of shock be ruled out first in the patient with trauma because hemorrhage is the number one cause of shock in this patient population.

Initial assessment should follow standard Advanced Trauma Life Support (ATLS) protocol, with a thorough primary and secondary survey. Standard laboratory studies should be obtained, but the core of the workup should be imaging. Isolated plain film imaging in the assessment for spine injury has fallen out of favor and replaced with high-quality cross-sectional imaging. Both CT and magnetic resonance imaging (MRI) should be used to fully assess the spine and spinal cord.

Initial treatment should be focused on the maintenance of adequate spinal cord perfusion. After ruling out other concomitant forms of shock, fluids and vasopressors may be required. As with all forms of shock, the first step in treatment is addressing fluid status with the goal of increasing the circulating volume. Infusion of isotonic crystalloid will help with hypotension from the vasodilation and further improve preload. Evidence supports that increasing MAP to a goal of greater than 85 mm Hg seems to correlate with improved neurologic recover. Adding vasopressor support if not obtained with fluid resuscitation may be required. Norepinephrine is the preferred first-line therapy as it provides action on both α- and β-receptors to counter both hypotension and bradycardia. Phenylephrine, a potent α-adrenergic receptor agonist, should be used with caution in patients with neurogenic shock as it may worsen bradycardia due to the unopposed α-stimulation.

Anaphylactic Shock

Anaphylactic shock is a form of distributive shock caused by a severe allergic reaction that largely effects the cardiovascular and respiratory systems. Immunoglobulin E (IgE) binds the source antigen, causing mast cells and basophils to have a massive release of inflammatory mediators (histamine). The massive release of these inflammatory mediators causes smooth muscle contraction within the bronchi, severe vasodilatation, leaking capillaries, and depressed cardiac contractility. Given this severe and rapid suppression of normal physiology, the recognition and diagnosis of anaphylactic shock in a timely manner is critical.

The majority of anaphylactic reactions are diagnosed clinically. Laboratory tests can help support the diagnosis. Obtaining plasma tryptase within the first 3 hours, plasma histamine within 15 to 20 minutes of presenting symptoms, and urine histamine metabolites within an hour may aid in the diagnosis of anaphylactic shock.

Treatment is supportive until the offending agent can be metabolized, and the source which caused anaphylaxis has been removed. Given the concern for significant angioedema associated with anaphylactic shock, there should be a low threshold for intubation. Airway edema should be treated with a course of steroids. If intubated, the presence of a cuff leak would suggest resolution of airway edema, making extubation safe. Epinephrine can be injected at a dose of 0.3 to 0.5 mg intramuscularly with repeat dosing every 5 to 15 minutes as needed. If possible, IV epinephrine should be administered, and a drip started to maintain an MAP of greater than 65 mm Hg. Albuterol nebulizers can help to relieve bronchospasms. Lastly, H_1 and H_2 antihistamines should be administered to effectively block histamine receptors.

Adrenal Crisis

The adrenal glands play a key role in the maintenance of BP through the production of cortisol and aldosterone. These hormones function to enhance the renin-angiotensin system as well as the production of endogenous epinephrine. Insufficient adrenal production can come in three forms:

- Primary adrenal insufficiency—inability of the adrenal glands to produce adequate levels of hormones, seen in Addison disease, or adrenal gland removal
- Secondary adrenal insufficiency—inability of the pituitary gland to provide adequate stimulation of the adrenal gland
- Tertiary adrenal crisis—insufficient exogenous steroid support

Diagnosis is made clinically as well as through various laboratory testing. The patient history and physical examination may include fatigue, lethargy, abdominal complaints, fever, psychiatric manifestations, and hypotension in all forms of adrenal crisis. Furthermore, electrolyte derangements such as hyponatremia and hyperkalemia may be present. Adrenal crisis may be the result of a lack of exogenous steroids as the patient may take them long term. Furthermore, adrenal crisis is usually the result of another pathologic influence, such as septic shock. Clinical hypotension that is refractory to volume replacement and vasopressor therapy is suggestive of adrenal crisis.

Treatment includes aggressive volume resuscitation with the addition of dextrose if hypoglycemia is present. If the patient has a history of steroid use chronically before admission, restarting should not be delayed. If there is concern for adrenal crisis secondary to septic shock, initiation for stress dose steroids should not be delayed. A cosyntropin stimulation test can be performed using 250 μg of cosyntropin, but the current recommendations from the Surviving Sepsis Campaign state that patients who remain on vasopressor medications or whose vasopressor medication dose is increasing should have a course of hydrocortisone 50 mg every 6 hours started, assuming adrenal crisis is playing a role in the patient deterioration. Furthermore, the infection or other offending pathology needs to be treated.

OBSTRUCTIVE SHOCK

Obstructive shock refers to impediment to flow of blood in the cardiopulmonary circuit, most commonly due to extracardiac causes, resulting in right ventricular dysfunction or collapse. The etiologies of obstructive shock are divided into two categories: pulmonary vascular and mechanical. Most causes of pulmonary vascular obstructive shock can be attributed to right ventricular failure from a hemodynamically significant pulmonary embolism (PE) or severe pulmonary hypertension (PH). Right ventricular failure occurs because the myocardium is unable to generate enough pressure to overcome the high pulmonary vascular resistance associated with PE or PH. This process can proceed to acute right heart syndrome, resulting in cardiogenic shock.

Mechanical causes of obstructive shock include tension PTX, pericardial tamponade, constrictive pericarditis, and restrictive cardiomyopathy. Mechanical obstructive shock presents clinically as hypovolemic shock, given the decreased preload from the reduced venous return to the right atrium or inadequate right ventricle filling.

Technically, PH, cardiomyopathies, and constrictive pericarditis cause impediment to the flow of blood in the cardiopulmonary circuit. However, these diseases are typically more progressive and diagnosed before the patient develops obstructive shock. PH presents with exertional dyspnea and fatigue, later progressing to overt right ventricular failure with exertional chest pain or syncope and congestion (peripheral edema, ascites, and pleural effusion). PH is diagnosed with imaging, including echocardiography to estimate PA pressure, and pulmonary function studies. PH is categorized into groups 1 to 5 on the basis of the etiology of the disease. Initial therapy is directed at the underlying cause of the PH, in addition to the administration of diuretics, oxygen, and anticoagulant therapies. Patients with persistent PH despite treatment of the underlying cause should be treated with advanced therapies according to the functional class of the World Health Organization.

Cardiomyopathies cause an impaired contraction of one or both ventricles, resulting in impaired systolic function, and may progress to overt heart failure. Patients present with atrial and/or ventricular arrhythmias, and sudden death can occur at any stage in the disease. Signs and symptoms are those consistent with heart failure (whether systolic or diastolic). Treatment is aimed at the underlying disease and the effects of heart failure.

Myocarditis refers to inflammation of the heart muscle. Patients present with varying symptoms ranging from no symptoms and changes on electrocardiogram to fulminant heart failure. Diagnosis is suspected on clinical examination and confirmed by histopathologic criteria on endomyocardial biopsy. Treatment depends on the etiology of the myocarditis and includes both specific therapies focused on the cause and nonspecific therapy aimed at the clinical manifestations, such as heart failure and arrhythmias.

Acute tamponade occurs most commonly secondary to trauma, insertion of a central venous catheter, or a thoracic procedure and can develop with relatively small volumes of pericardial fluid. Tamponade that develops less acutely is more likely to demonstrate distended neck veins, muffled heart sounds, and an increased paradoxical pulse (>15 mm Hg). It is important to distinguish this etiology of hypoperfusion from congestive heart failure (CHF) or cardiogenic shock because reducing fluid intake and administering a diuretic would reduce venous return further in tamponade. CHF usually results in normal or elevated BP, whereas tamponade results in hypotension. Therefore, tamponade simulates cardiogenic shock more closely than CHF. Because cardiogenic shock requires a major insult to myocardial function, hypotension with elevated central venous pressure (CVP) should increase a suspicion of tamponade or a tension PTX unless obvious evidence of severe myocardial malfunction is found.

Diagnosing tension PTX or pericardial tamponade is based primarily on clinical suspicion and physical findings. If life-threatening obstructive shock is present, further workup should not be pursued and the cause should be treated immediately, to avoid cardiopulmonary collapse and death. If the condition permits, imaging such as chest x-ray, CT chest, or echocardiogram can assist with the diagnosis of obstructive shock. Bedside POCUS (e-FAST) has utility in diagnosing both PTX and pericardial tamponade and should be used in cases where hemodynamic instability is present. Thoracic imaging in tension PTX may show a white visceral pleural line that is separated from the parietal pleura by a collection of gas, no pulmonary vessels visible beyond the visceral pleural line, with or without collapsed lung, shift of mediastinum to contralateral side, and depression of hemidiaphragm.

With symptomatic tension PTX, treatment consists of emergently releasing the tension (needle decompression or finger thoracostomy), followed by closed thoracostomy. Removal of the fluid surrounding the heart (pericardiocentesis/pericardial window/repair of a cardiac wound) is the most effective therapy, and it can result in a dramatic improvement in CO. However, venous return also improves as a result of increasing intravascular volume with IV fluid. Therefore, vigorous fluid administration should be provided despite an elevated CVP.

CARDIOGENIC SHOCK

Cardiogenic shock is defined as sudden failure directly involving the heart "pump" itself. This results in an inability of the heart to adequately supply blood to the end-organ systems of the body, creating a lack of oxygen delivery to tissues and, therefore, a shock state. Cardiac index (CI) is used to assess for cardiogenic shock, where CI = cardiac output/total body surface area (normal, 2.5-4 L/min/m^2; cardiogenic shock, ≤2.2 L/min/m^2).

Although the most common form of cardiogenic shock is caused by a myocardial infarction (MI), other cardiac pathology may also result in cardiogenic shock. These include cardiac arrhythmias, cardiomyopathy, heart valve problems, ventricular outflow obstruction such as with aortic valve stenosis or aortic dissection, and ventriculoseptal defects. Early recognition and diagnosis of cardiogenic shock is imperative because it can be rapidly fatal if not treated in a timely manner.

Diagnosis starts with a thorough history and physical examination. A high suspicion must be maintained in high-risk patients. Patients with a classic MI presentation will exhibit crushing substernal chest pain, which may radiate to the upper extremities, back, epigastric area, or jaw; however, patients with neuropathic changes to the innervation of the heart (ie, patients with diabetes or heart transplant patients) may present with atypical pain or nausea. A valvular cause may result in the auscultation of a new murmur. If the patient has developed left heart failure, it can result in pulmonary congestion, causing shortness of breath, hypoxemia, and tachypnea. In right heart failure, systemic congestion may cause jugular venous distention. Diagnostic modalities include the following:

- Laboratory studies: troponin, arterial blood gas, lactate, complete blood count, and basic metabolic panel
- Chest x-ray may be helpful in determining pulmonary congestion from heart failure.
- Electrocardiogram (ECG): New ST changes, new Q waves, or a new left bundle branch block suggest myocardial ischemic changes. Patients can also have an MI without changes in the ST segment.
- Transthoracic and/or transesophageal echocardiogram: depressed ejection fraction, valvular defects, cardiac wall motion abnormalities, and other potential mechanical cardiac defects

The treatment of cardiogenic shock begins with the establishment of good IV access. This may require a central line or PA catheter to provide continuous monitoring of heart function. Optimizing volume status will improve heart function. This is especially important in patients who are suffering from right heart failure related to a traumatic event. Oxygenation supplementation, intubation, and ventilator support may be needed. Medication administration includes the following:

- Aspirin 325 mg: given if the patient is experiencing an MI
- Nitroglycerin: should be given to help improve perfusion to the coronary arteries as long as BP can tolerate it
- Heparin infusion: given if the patient is experiencing an MI
- Norepinephrine or dopamine: to maintain an MAP of 65 mm Hg or more

- Dobutamine or milrinone: to help improve cardiac contractility. These inotropic agents can cause further hypotension, given their afterload reduction properties, so additional vasopressor medication may be required.

Percutaneous coronary intervention (PCI) is the mainstay of therapy for MI and should be completed within 120 minutes of the onset of symptoms for ST-segment elevation myocardial infarction (STEMI) and all patients with cardiogenic shock, regardless of the time of onset. If PCI cannot be completed within 120 minutes, fibrinolytic therapy should be initiated in the absence of contraindications. Strong consideration should be given to transferring the patient to a PCI center. Coronary artery bypass grafting is indicated in patients with STEMI and coronary anatomy not amenable to PCI who have ongoing or recurrent ischemia, cardiogenic shock, severe heart failure, or other high-risk features or mechanical defects.

Other forms of mechanical support include the insertion of an intra-aortic balloon pump. This device is used mainly for left ventricular failure and is placed in the proximal descending aorta usually through the femoral artery. When the heart is in systole, the pump is deflated to improve afterload reduction and offloading from the heart. When the heart is in diastole, the pump is inflated to better perfuse the coronary arteries.

Ventricular assist devices (VADs) are surgically inserted into one ventricle, or both, to help provide additional circulatory support to a failing heart. In worst-case scenarios, if cardiac function cannot recover enough to support circulation on its own, the VAD would be required as a surrogate before heart transplantation.

SUMMARY

Shock, or "a rude unhinging of the machinery of life," refers to a state of cellular and tissue hypoxia caused by reduced oxygen delivery and increased oxygen consumption or inadequate oxygen utilization. The effects of hypoxia on the body's cellular metabolism are initially reversible but can rapidly become irreversible, resulting in MOF and death. There are four main types of shock: hypovolemic, distributive, obstructive, and cardiogenic. Each presents with unique signs and symptoms with specific physiologic parameters. Laboratory studies and imaging exist to assist with diagnosis. Recognizing shock and restoring circulation are the primary tenets for managing the patient with shock. Without timely treatment, shock can lead to irreversible organ damage, MOF, and death.

SUGGESTED READINGS

Evans L, Rhodes A, Alhazzani W, et al. Surviving sepsis campaign: international guidelines for management of sepsis and septic shock 2021. *Intensive Care Med*. 2021;47(11):1181-1247.

Holcomb J, Tilley B, Baraniuk S, et al. Transfusion of plasma, platelets, and red blood cells in a 1:1:1 vs a 1:1:2 ratio and mortality in patients with severe trauma: the PROPPR randomized clinical trial. *JAMA*. 2015;313(5):471-482.

Welsford M, Nikolaou NI, Beygui F, et al. Part 5: acute coronary syndromes. 2015 international consensus on cardiopulmonary resuscitation and emergency cardiovascular care science with treatment recommendations. *Circulation*. 2015;132(16 suppl 1):S146-S176.

SAMPLE QUESTIONS

QUESTIONS

Choose the best answer for each question.

1. Shock is best described as

   A. a state of hypotension.
   B. a state of low CO.
   C. a state of low vascular resistance.
   D. a state of cellular and tissue hypoxia.
   E. a state of profound depression of the vital processes.

2. The major determinants of tissue perfusion are

   A. systemic vascular resistance and CO.
   B. preload, afterload, and contractility.
   C. wedge pressure, systemic vascular resistance, and pulmonary vascular resistance.
   D. CVP, MAP, and HR.
   E. wedge pressure, MAP, and pulmonary vascular resistance.

3. The first step in the management of hypovolemic shock is

   A. determining the cause.
   B. vasopressors to increase BP.
   C. inotropes to increase HR.
   D. rapid fluid replacement to restore preload.
   E. rapid intubation for respiratory support.

4. The most common cause of shock in surgical patients is decreased venous return. What clinical conditions cause decreased venous return?

   A. Intra-abdominal infection
   B. Tension PTX
   C. Pericardial tamponade
   D. Massive hemorrhage
   E. All the above

5. Which of the following is true?

   A. A 10% loss of blood volume results in tachycardia but not hypotension.
   B. A 20% loss of blood volume results in tachycardia and hypotension.
   C. A 35% loss of blood volume results in tachycardia but not hypotension.
   D. Vital signs and physical findings of a patient with hypovolemia show evidence of hypoperfusion roughly in proportion to the amount of volume deficit.
   E. Agitation, tachypnea, and peripheral vasoconstriction are seen only in patients with hypovolemic shock.

ANSWERS AND EXPLANATIONS

1. **Answer: D**

   Although all of these are true to some extent, the most accurate answer is D. For more information on this topic, please see the Introduction section at the beginning of this chapter.

2. **Answer: A**

   The major determinants of tissue perfusion are CO and SVR, where BP = CO × SVR. Any biologic process that changes any of these physiologic parameters will alter BP and can result in shock. For more information on this topic, please see section "Pathophysiology."

3. **Answer: D**

   Although determining the cause of hypovolemic shock is important for determining what needs to be done later, restoring volume should be started first. Vasopressors may reduce tissue perfusion, and inotropes are usually unnecessary and possibly harmful because patients are already tachycardic. For more information on this topic, please see section "Hypovolemic Shock."

4. **Answer: E**

   The most obvious answer is massive bleeding. However, increased pressure in the chest with tension PTX, pericardial tamponade, or decreased venous volume due to third spacing from intra-abdominal infection can also cause decreased venous return. For more information on this topic, please see section "Categories of Shock."

5. **Answer: D**

   A 10% blood volume loss does not produce changes in vital signs. A 20% loss will cause tachycardia but not hypotension. A 30% loss will cause tachycardia and hypotension. Agitation, tachypnea, and vasoconstriction are seen with any etiology of hypoperfusion. For more information on this topic, please see section "Hypovolemic Shock."

Wounds and Wound Healing

Jessica Beth O'Connell and Steven Farley

A wound is a disruption of the normal anatomic relations of tissues as a result of injury. The injury may be intentional (eg, an elective surgical incision) or unintentional (eg, trauma). A complex interaction of the biochemical, cellular, and physiologic processes leads to wound healing.

PHASES OF WOUND HEALING

Wound healing occurs in three phases: (1) inflammatory or substrate phase, (2) proliferative phase, and (3) maturation. Distinct biochemical and physiologic events characterize each phase and are correlated with gross morphologic changes in the wound.

Figure 5-1 shows an overview of the phases of normal wound healing, comparing cells and collagen concentrations with wound strength over time.

Primary Hemostasis

Primary hemostasis and recruitment of inflammatory cells occur in the first 1 to 2 hours after injury. The first cellular elements to enter the wound are platelets, which come into contact with damaged collagen at the site of injury. Platelets release α granules containing multiple growth factors such as platelet-derived growth factor and transforming

growth factor β. Inflammatory cells arrive and release a variety of cytokines and growth factors.

Substrate (Inflammatory) Phase

The substrate/inflammatory phase lasts approximately 3 days. The primary cells involved are polymorphonuclear leukocytes (PMNs) and macrophages. PMNs arrive first and remain the predominant cell type for approximately 48 hours. PMNs originate many inflammatory mediators, such as complement and kallikrein. Monocytes enter after the PMNs, reaching maximum numbers approximately 24 hours later. Monocytes evolve into macrophages, which phagocytize cellular debris in the wound. Small numbers of bacteria can be neutralized by the macrophages; however, a large number of bacteria can overwhelm the leukocytes resulting in a clinical infection.

Proliferative Phase

As debris and bacteria are being removed from the wound, substrates for collagen synthesis are assembled. The proliferative phase is the second stage of wound healing; it begins on day 3 and continues for approximately 6 weeks. This phase is characterized by additional cellular migration and proliferation, angiogenesis, and the production of collagen

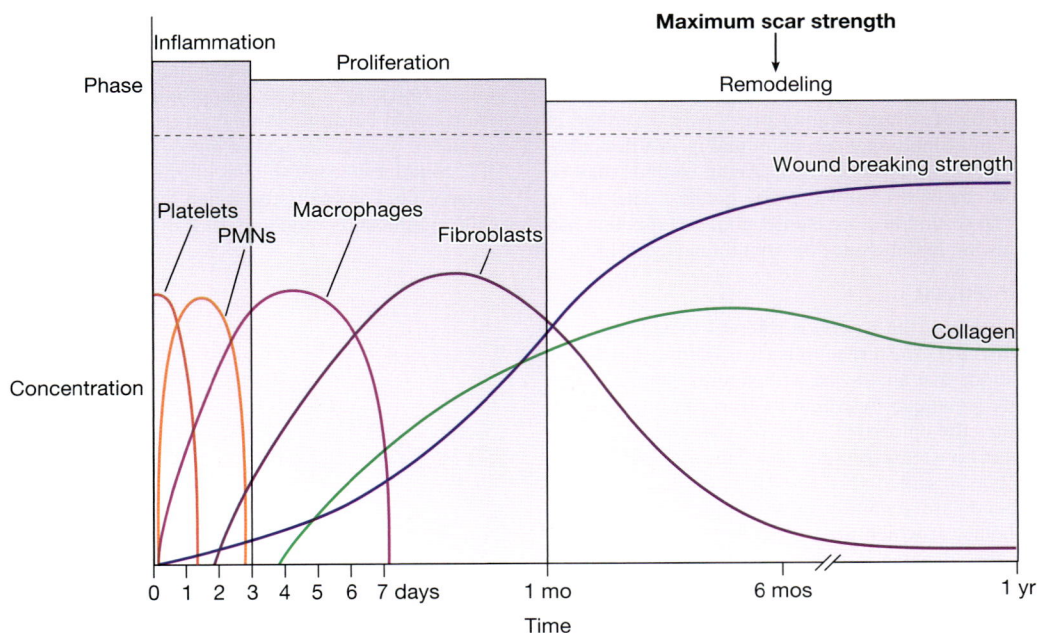

Figure 5-1. Phases of wound healing comparing cells and collagen concentrations with wound strength over time. PMNs, polymorphonuclear leukocytes.

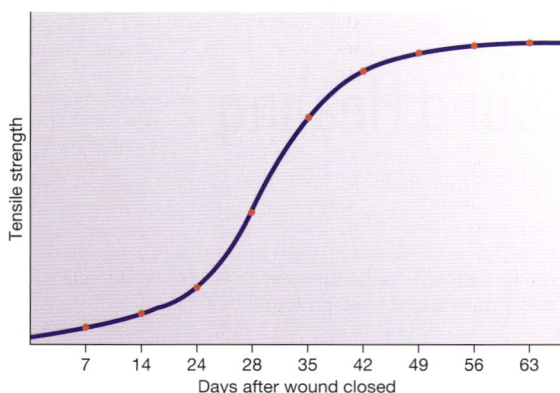

Figure 5-2. Wound tensile strength as a function of time.

in the wound, resulting in increased wound strength. The primary cell in this phase is the fibroblast. Collagen deposition begins between 3 and 5 days after the initial trauma and peaks around 4 to 6 weeks. At 1 week after injury, a wound possesses only 5% of its final tensile strength; at 1 month, it has 50%. A completely healed wound maintains 80% of the skin's original tensile strength (Figure 5-2).

Maturation Phase (Remodeling)

The third phase is the maturation phase, characterized by the remodeling and strengthening of collagen in the wound by intermolecular cross-linking. The wound scar gradually flattens and becomes less prominent and more pale and supple. Wound maturation in the adult takes at least 6 and sometimes up to 12 months.

APPROACHES TO WOUND MANAGEMENT

Acute wounds include all surgical incisions as well as acute trauma. Acute wounds are expected to pursue the normal phases of wound healing previously described in an orderly and timely manner, culminating in full epithelialization and formation of a scar. Acute wounds may be managed in one of several ways. The greatest deterrent to acute normal wound healing is infection, and it is this fact that informs the initial choice of wound management.

Primary Intention

Primary closure of the wound is referred to as *healing by primary intention*. The term applies to all surgical incisions and lacerations that are closed with sutures, staples, adhesive, or any technique by which the surgeon intentionally approximates the epidermal edges of a wound. It also includes tissue transfer techniques and flaps that may be employed by plastic surgeons to close larger defects. Primarily closed wounds are generally fully reepithelialized within 24 to 48 hours, at which time a surgical dressing may be removed. The advantages of this approach to wound management are that it is easy for the patient to manage, there is a rapid return of function of the wounded tissue, and the final cosmetic result is superior. The major disadvantage of primary closure of a wound, however, is the risk of wound infection that can occur in the closed space created.

Secondary Intention

An alternative to primary closure of a full-thickness wound is to leave it open or let it *heal by secondary intention*. These wounds are treated with a variety of wound dressings that may include silver or other antimicrobial agents, "wet-to-dry" dressings, or negative-pressure wound therapy, where a porous sponge is placed into the wound and connected to negative pressure. The negative pressure applied stimulates more rapid closure of the wound, while simultaneously promoting drainage and creating a moist wound environment favorable for the ingrowth of granulation tissue. The new healing tissues, termed "granulation tissue," is characterized by friable reddish moist "granules" of tiny capillary buds. Granulation tissue forms in the base of the open wound (Figure 5-3). Epithelial cells cannot migrate across granulation tissue, however, so healing by secondary intention occurs primarily by wound contraction. Myofibroblasts at the edges of the wound gradually draw the edges of the wound together. Wound contraction occurs to a greater extent in areas of the body where the surrounding tissues are redundant, such as the abdomen and buttock, and is not as pronounced in areas such as the scalp or pretibial area where the skin is taut. The disadvantages of leaving a wound open are that daily dressing changes are required until the wound is healed; costs are greater; and dressing changes are uncomfortable for the patient. The advantage of this method of wound management is that wound infection is much less common. Thus, secondary intention is appropriate for wounds that are highly contaminated, such as a subcutaneous abscess after incision and drainage, or where the likelihood of surgical site infection is deemed too great. Wounds that have not been closed primarily for more than 24 hours are usually considered too contaminated and left to heal by secondary intention.

Delayed Primary Closure

In delayed primary closure (DPC), sometimes called *healing by tertiary intention*, the wound is initially managed by secondary intention. After approximately 5 days, if the wound is clean and granulation tissue is abundant, the wound edges are actively reapproximated. This approach is successful because granulation tissue, while not sterile, is extremely vascular and is highly resistant to infection. DPC combines the advantages of primary wound closure in terms of final cosmetic result and rapid return to function, while significantly reducing the risk of wound infection.

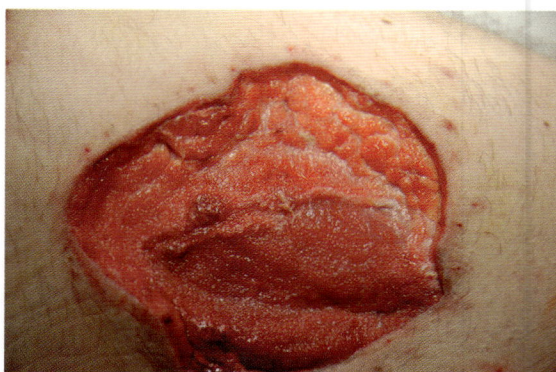

Figure 5-3. Granulation bed.

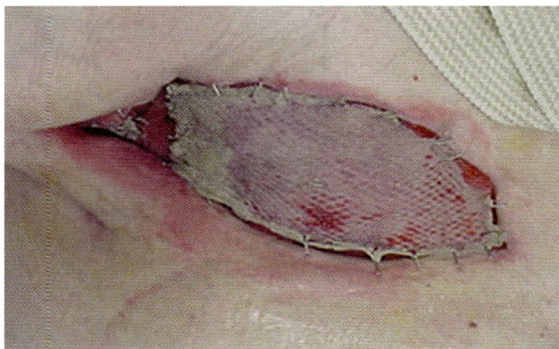

Figure 5-4. Initial placement of split-thickness skin graft.

Skin Grafting

For large surface area full-thickness wounds that cannot be closed primarily and healing by secondary intention would be lengthy, skin grafting is an option. Split-thickness skin grafts consist of epidermis and a portion of the underlying dermis, which are harvested (Figure 5-4). For the first 48 hours, the grafted skin derives its nutrients by passive absorption from the recipient bed, a process known as imbibition. Thereafter, the graft becomes revascularized and adherent to the bed, and the wound closes as a result of a combination of contraction and epithelialization.

FACTORS THAT AFFECT WOUND HEALING

Many local and systemic factors affect wound healing. The physician should be actively working to correct any abnormality that can prevent or slow wound healing (Table 5-1).

Local Factors

Meticulous care of the wound is important. Infection decreases the rate of wound healing and detrimentally affects proper granulation tissue formation, decreases oxygen delivery, and depletes the wound of needed nutrients. Wounds must be cleaned and debrided of all nonviable tissue. All wounds have some degree of contamination; if the body is able to control bacterial proliferation in a wound, that wound will heal. The use of cleansing agents helps reduce contamination. Grossly contaminated wounds should be cleaned as completely as possible to remove particulate matter (foreign bodies) and should be irrigated copiously with saline. Highly contaminated wounds should be left open to heal by secondary intention. Physicians should keep in mind the potential for *Clostridium tetani* in wounds with devitalized tissue and administer tetanus prophylaxis as indicated.

Bleeding must be controlled to prevent hematoma formation. Hematomas and seromas may become infected and can disrupt the wound, impairing wound healing.

Hypoxia and ischemia, from any cause, impede healing by reducing the amount of nutrients and oxygen that are available at the wound site. Radiation affects local wound healing in a peculiar way because of the decreased vascularity and increased fibrosis in irradiated tissues. Because adipose tissues are relatively poorly vascularized, obesity is a risk factor for poor wound healing.

Edema of any kind must be controlled. If there is too much fluid in the subdermal and subcutaneous tissues, movement of inflammatory chemokines and growth factors to the wound bed can be impeded.

Systemic Factors

In addition to controlling local factors, the physician must address systemic issues that can affect wound healing. Nutrition is an extremely important factor in wound healing. Patients need adequate protein, calories, and vitamins to support wound healing. Folic acid is critical to the proper formation of collagen. Vitamin C deficiency, the cause of scurvy, is characterized by impaired wound healing, as well as cutaneous sores and a hemorrhagic gingivitis. Vitamin E is an antioxidant, aids in immune function and fibroblast stimulation, and inhibits prostaglandin synthesis. Selenium is important for lymphocyte function and protects membranes from free radical damage. Zinc is possibly the most essential element for wound healing, because zinc deficiency leads to decreased fibroblast proliferation, decreased collagen synthesis, and likely decreased lymphocyte cellular immunity. Adequate fat intake is required for the absorption of vitamins A, D, E, and K. Vitamin K is essential for the synthesis of clotting factors II, VII, IX, and X; decreased clotting factors can lead to hematoma formation and altered wound healing. Vitamin A increases the inflammatory response, increases collagen synthesis, and increases the influx of macrophages into a wound. Magnesium is required for protein synthesis, and zinc is a cofactor for RNA and DNA polymerase. Deficiency of any one of these nutrients, vitamins, or trace elements will adversely affect wound healing. One should have a low threshold to check circulating albumin and prealbumin levels and for any vitamin deficiencies if any concern.

Poorly controlled diabetes mellitus results in hyperglycemia, which directly impairs wound healing and alters collagen formation. Hyperglycemia also inhibits neutrophil, fibroblast, and endothelial cell proliferation within the wound.

Certain medications will also impair wound healing. For example, corticosteroids blunt the inflammatory response, decrease the available vitamin A in the wound, and alter the deposition and remodeling of collagen. Cancer chemotherapy agents, including those that cause neutropenia as well as those that inhibit angiogenesis, negatively affect wound healing.

Chronic illnesses (including immune deficiency, cancer, uremia, liver disease, and jaundice) will predispose patients to infection, protein deficiency, and malnutrition, which, as noted previously, can affect wound healing.

TABLE 5-1. Factors That Affect Wound Healing	
Local Factors	**Systemic Factors**
• Infection	• Malnutrition
• Ischemia	• Diabetes mellitus
• Hematoma	• Corticosteroid use
• Seroma	• Chronic illness
• Foreign body	• Cancer
• Hypoxia	• Immune deficiency states
• Radiation	• Smoking
• Obesity	• Old age
• Tension	• Edema

Smoking has a systemic effect by decreasing the oxygen-carrying capacity of hemoglobin, causing vasoconstriction, and hypoxia results in a decrease in oxygen delivery to the wound, which impedes healing. Smoking may also decrease collagen formation within a wound. Every physician should encourage patients to stop smoking for general health reasons.

MANAGEMENT OF CHRONIC WOUNDS

A chronic wound is one in which the reparative processes of normal wound healing, as described earlier, fail to occur in an orderly and timely sequence. Most often, chronic wounds are stalled in the inflammatory phase of healing and have poor granulation tissue formation, altered cell cycles, and biochemical imbalances. Examples include a diabetic foot wound, venous stasis ulcers, fistula-in-ano, and chronic osteomyelitis. In general, wounds are considered stalled if significant wound healing has not occurred within 4 weeks.

Chronic wounds are clinically challenging to manage and require time and patience. Malnutrition, uremia, and the hyperglycemia of diabetes are examples of systemic factors that retard healing. Edema, infection, arterial insufficiency (ischemia), fecal soiling, and pressure on the wound are examples of local factors that can impair healing. Appreciation of the role of these factors and judicious intervention to counter them are key to successful management.

Advanced Care for Chronic Wounds

Management of chronic wounds requires a significant investment of resources, and many novel and technically sophisticated methods for stimulating wound healing have been devised in recent decades. Compared with medical interventions for other diseases, wound care therapy has not been as rigorously subjected to randomized prospective trials as it is difficult to create comparable cohorts when patients have varied comorbidities and various causes for their wounds. However, there are some studies that show modest improvement in healing chronic wounds with a variety of modalities, including the following:

1. Intermittent negative-pressure wound therapy
2. Topical broad-spectrum antimicrobial compounds
3. Topical growth factors and collagen preparations to promote healing
4. Topical enzymatic debridement preparations
5. Topical foams and occlusive dressings to promote a moist wound environment
6. Biologic (cell-based) dressings
7. Stem cell therapy
8. Hyperbaric oxygen therapy

Along with continued evaluation of these modalities, ongoing investigation of newer wound treatment technologies includes nanotherapeutics, advanced stem cell therapy, bioengineered skin grafts, and 3D bioprinting-based strategies.

SUGGESTED READINGS

Bainbridge P. Wound healing and the role of fibroblasts. *J Wound Care*. 2013;22(8):407-412.

Bryant R, Nix D, eds. *Acute & Chronic Wounds: Current Management Concepts*. 5th ed. Elsevier; 2016.

Greaves NS, Ashcroft KJ, Baguneid M, et al. Current understanding of molecular and cellular mechanisms in fibroplasia and angiogenesis during acute wound healing. *J Dermatol Sci*. 2013;72(3):206-217.

Huang C, Leavitt T, Bayler LR, et al. Effect of negative pressure wound therapy on wound healing. *Curr Probl Surg*. 2014;51(7):301-331.

Praveen K, Narala S, Nyavanandi D, et al. Innovative treatment strategies to accelerate wound healing: trajectory and recent advancements. *Cells*. 2022;11(15):2439.

Zielins E, Atashroo D, Zeshaan M, et al. Wound healing: an update. *Regen Med*. 2014;9(6):817-830.

SAMPLE QUESTIONS

QUESTIONS

Choose the best answer for each question.

1. The passive absorption of nutrients by a skin graft from the recipient wound bed is called
   A. epithelialization.
   B. revascularization.
   C. imbibition.
   D. granulation.
   E. healing by secondary intention.

2. A 45-year-old female presents to the emergency department with a 2-day history of nausea, anorexia, and right lower quadrant abdominal pain. Her computed tomography shows appendicitis with a localized abscess. Her intraoperative findings include perforation of the base of the appendix involving the cecum. You convert to an open procedure through a midline incision. After completing the procedure, you close the fascia but leave the skin and subcutaneous tissue layers open. The wound is packed with moist gauze and then covered with dry gauze and tape. This is an example of
   A. primary closure.
   B. healing by secondary intention.
   C. DPC.
   D. skin graft closure.
   E. None of the above

3. A 68-year-old female undergoes an emergency exploratory laparotomy for an incarcerated ventral incisional hernia. Her abdominal wall closure includes placement of a mesh underlay. On postoperative day 6, a wound hematoma is discovered. The wound is left open to heal via secondary intention. Her past medical history is

remarkable for obesity, lupus, type 2 diabetes, hypertension, and tobacco use. Smoking affects wound healing via

A. inhibition of prostaglandin synthesis.
B. inactivation of factors II, VII, IX, and X.
C. decreased oxygen-carrying capacity of hemoglobin.
D. decreased collagen formation.
E. C and D

4. You perform an uncomplicated open umbilical hernia repair on a 22-year-old triathlete. On postoperative day 5, they call to ask you if they can start swimming. You inform them the following:

A. They can resume swimming because the wound possesses 100% of its initial tensile strength.
B. Their wound possesses only about 5% of its final tensile strength.
C. They can resume swimming without a dressing, because the wound possesses 80% of its initial tensile strength by postoperative day 2.
D. At 1 month, the wound possesses 50% tensile strength.
E. B and D

5. A paraplegic nursing home resident presents for evaluation of a sacral ulcer. There is overlying eschar at the edges, along with necrotic fat. The wound is surgically debrided and a wound vac is placed. Negative-pressure therapy has the following effects:

A. Stimulates more rapid closure of the wound
B. Creates a moist environment favorable for ingrowth of granulation tissue
C. Combines the advantage of primary closure and rapid return to function
D. A and B
E. A, B, and C

ANSWERS AND EXPLANATIONS

1. **Answer: C**

For the first 48 hours following skin grafting, the grafted skin derives its nutrients by passive absorption from the recipient bed, a process known as imbibition. Thereafter, the graft becomes revascularized and adherent to the bed, and each interstice closes as a result of a combination of contraction and epithelialization, closing the wound. For more information on this topic, see section "Skin Grafting."

2. **Answer: B**

This wound involves a perforated viscus with an abscess and is, therefore, a dirty wound. Leaving the

wound open allows it to heal by secondary intention from the base upward through granulation tissue ingrowth. Wet-to-dry dressings provide debridement of infected and devitalized tissue, reducing the bacterial load. Wet-to-dry dressings also provide a moist environment favorable for granulation tissue ingrowth. Granulation tissue, characterized by friable reddish moist "granules" of tiny capillary buds, will form in the base of the open wound. Healing by secondary intention occurs primarily by wound contraction. Myofibroblasts at the edges of the wound gradually draw the edges of the wound together. For more information on this topic, see section "Secondary Intention."

3. **Answer: E**

Smoking has a systemic effect by decreasing the oxygen-carrying capacity of hemoglobin, and hypoxia results in a decrease in oxygen delivery to the wound, which impedes healing. Smoking may also decrease collagen formation within a wound. Every physician should encourage patients to stop smoking for general health reasons. For more information on this topic, see section "Factors That Affect Wound Healing."

4. **Answer: E**

At 1 week after injury, a wound possesses only 5% of its final tensile strength; at 1 month, it possesses 50%. The proliferative phase is the second stage of wound healing and lasts from day 3, continuing for approximately 4 to 5 weeks. The primary cell in this phase is the fibroblast. Collagen deposition begins between 3 and 5 days after wounding and peaks around 4 to 6 weeks. For more information on this topic, see section "Proliferative Phase."

5. **Answer: D**

The wound vac devices consist of a porous sponge placed into the wound connected to negative pressure. Negative-pressure therapy applied to the wound is a method of wound healing that promotes new tissue growth and assists in contraction of the wound. The negative pressure applied stimulates more rapid closure of the wound, while simultaneously promoting drainage and creating a moist wound environment favorable for the ingrowth of granulation tissue. Granulation tissue, characterized by friable reddish moist "granules" of tiny capillary buds, will form in the base of the open wound. For more information on this topic, see section "Secondary Intention."

6 Surgical Infection

Ho H. Phan

The term *surgical infection* refers to infections that occur postoperatively and that are associated with the surgical sites, as well as *de novo* infections that require urgent surgical evaluation and treatment. In addition, those who study surgical infection focus on proven ways to prevent surgical infection. This chapter reviews the basic principles associated with surgical infections, including the risks, sources, diagnosis, and treatment for many commonly seen diseases.

PATHOGENESIS OF INFECTION

Scheduled operations, traumatic injury, and nontraumatic local bacterial invasion can all lead to severe infections that may require surgical intervention. Following bacterial soilage of host tissues, the body initiates a well-defined process of host defense. There are several host factors that will affect bacterial virulence and the cellular host response, which in turn alter the pathogenesis of the infectious disease (Table 6-1). Retained wound hematomas provide an iron-rich environment that will potentiate bacterial growth, whereas the hemoglobin content will inhibit the effectiveness of the neutrophil response in eradicating the microorganisms. Blood is an excellent bacterial growth agar, and meticulous care must be given prior to wound closure in obtaining hemostasis. Likewise, dead tissue provides a means of bacterial growth unable to be penetrated by host defenses. Careful wound debridement and irrigation of all nonviable tissue is necessary for adequate healing. Foreign bodies, such as sutures, drains, urinary catheters, and intravenous catheters, provide potential portals of bacterial entry and must be evaluated for their risk of infection versus benefit and necessity for patient care.

Systemic factors (eg, shock, hypovolemia, hypoxia, comorbid disease) will also affect the host's response to infection. Shock leads to tissue hypoperfusion and metabolic acidosis that weakens host defense mechanisms. Hypoperfusion of end-organ tissue and subsequent cellular dysfunction increases septic complications in patients who have traumatic injury or who are postoperative from elective surgery. Oxygenation is an essential metabolic component for phagocytosis and intracellular killing. Inadequate oxygen delivery (related to both hypoperfusion and inadequate oxygenation) results in acidosis at the site of bacterial contamination and will significantly increase the likelihood of subsequent infection. Patient comorbid diseases must also be considered when assessing infection risk. Patients with diabetes have impaired neutrophil function and microcirculatory disease, whereas patients who are obese frequently have poor tissue perfusion secondary to poor blood supply in adipose tissue. Malnutrition will increase the vulnerability of the host to infection, and alcoholism impairs the host immune response. The use of systemic corticosteroids is common in many disease states. Steroid use, cancer chemotherapy, and transplant immunosuppression will all greatly increase the host risk for postoperative or surgical infection. A chronic disease that alters immune system function also poses infectious risk following injury or surgery.

PREVENTION OF SURGICAL INFECTIONS

Surgical Preparation and Perioperative Management

The prevention of surgical site infections (SSIs) begins with adequate wound preparation. Most surgical infections are due to contamination of the patient's own endogenous flora. Therefore, appropriate preparation of the surgical site is necessary to minimize the source of contamination. The patients should shower or bathe with soap or an antiseptic agent on the night before the day of the operation. Body hair should be clipped, not shaven, to prevent skin irritation and breakdown that can create a portal of bacterial entry into the wound bed. Hair removal should occur immediately before the planned procedure. Skin preparation should include the use of an alcohol-based antiseptic agent to reduce the number of endogenous flora. The sterile attire and aseptic techniques utilized are also designed to minimize the source of intraoperative contamination. Reducing operative time, maintaining normothermia, and controlling the glucose level during the procedure have also been shown to significantly reduce the rate of SSI.

Good surgical technique also plays a role in the reduction of postoperative infection. Devitalized tissue and foreign materials should be debrided to effectively remove any nidus for bacterial growth. Likewise, adequate

TABLE 6-1. Risk Factors That Increase the Incidence of Surgical Infection	
Local Wound	**Systemic**
Wound hematoma	Advanced age
Necrotic tissue	Shock (hypoxia, acidosis)
Foreign body	Diabetes mellitus
Obesity	Protein-calorie malnutrition
Contamination	Acute and chronic alcoholism
	Corticosteroid therapy
	Cancer chemotherapy
	Immunosuppression (acquired and induced)
	Remote site infection

hemostasis and the lavage of any large blood clots from the wound will reduce the risk for SSI. Maintenance of adequate tissue perfusion and oxygenation by intraoperative volume replacement and oxygen supplementation may also reduce SSIs.

Perioperative Antibiotics

The use of perioperative prophylactic antibiotics relates to the magnitude of surgical intervention and the presumptive microbes to be encountered in the elective surgical setting. Adequate dosing of the antibiotic to obtain maximal tissue and serum concentration at the time of making the incision is necessary for infection prevention. In general, antibiotics administered after the contaminating event are not effective in the prevention of surgical infections. The use of preoperative antibiotics has been shown to reduce the rate of SSIs, leading to a reduction in intensive care unit and hospital length of stay, hospital costs, risk of readmission, and mortality.

To ensure adequate serum and tissue levels, initial antibiotics are given within 1 hour prior to the incision. Some agents, such as fluoroquinolones and vancomycin, require administration over 1 to 2 hours; therefore, the administration of these agents should begin 120 minutes before surgical incision. Intraoperative redosing is needed if the duration of the procedure exceeds two half-lives of the antibiotic or if there is excessive blood loss during the procedure. The chosen agent should be well tolerated and safe, have a long half-life, and possess an antimicrobial spectrum appropriate for the planned procedure. Perioperative antibiotic use requires an understanding of the type of case to be performed and the level of contamination perceived (Table 6-2). Clean cases with little risk of contamination do not require antibiotic coverage. However, prophylaxis is utilized in clean cases where prosthetic material (ie, mesh, vascular graft orthopedic device) is used as a means to reduce the likelihood of device infection. For cases in which there is a risk of minimal endogenous contamination (clean contaminated), the source must be considered, because the SSI risk for these cases is 3 times higher than that of clean cases. Upper intestinal tract surgery requires gram-positive and gram-negative coverage, whereas lower intestinal tract surgery requires the addition of anaerobic coverage. Contaminated cases involve gross spillage from bowel perforation and polymicrobial bacterial involvement. The overall risk of site infection for contaminated cases increases 5- to 10-fold over clean cases. Dirty wounds involve existing contaminated or established infection and are at the highest risk for infection to develop, reaching approximately 50% in most series. Antibiotics are considered therapeutic in these cases with dirty wounds.

Perioperative antibiotic therapy is continued in the postoperative setting for less than 24 hours. For the majority of surgical cases, antibiotic infusion for more than 24 hours has been shown to increase bacterial resistance and have no further improvement on SSI rates. In certain surgical interventions, such as cardiac surgery, use may be extended to 48 hours. When antibiotics are used to treat existing infection, the empiric agent is usually continued until specific cultures dictate a more specific agent. Should the prophylactic agent need to be extended for the treatment of established infection, such as in the case of ruptured appendicitis, appropriate chart documentation should indicate the shift from prophylaxis to a treatment modality.

ESTABLISHED INFECTION

Early and appropriate diagnosis and treatment of surgical infections should be a major priority. If infection is suspected, early and appropriate empiric antibiotic therapy targeting the organisms commonly associated with the suspected diagnosis should be started. Choosing the correct empiric antibiotic for the right indication can have a significant impact on the outcome of patients with infections. The risk of mortality increases when empiric antibiotic therapy is delayed or inadequate. Identification of the offending organism(s) and antibiotic sensitivity should also be prioritized, and if necessary, the antibiotics should be narrowed or changed to the specific sensitivity profile. Source control to remove an ongoing source of infection by surgical drainage and/or debridement is also critical. Some minor and superficial infections only require bedside drainage, while more complex and invasive infections require surgical exploration, operative drainage, and radical debridement. It is also important to continue to assess the patient's response to treatment on a regular basis. If there is no sign of improvement after treatment, consideration should be given to changing antibiotic coverage or additional drainage and/or debridement for source control.

Surgical infections can be grouped as community acquired or hospital acquired. Community-acquired infections

TABLE 6-2. Classification of Surgical Wounds

Wound	Bacterial Contamination	Source of Contamination	Infection Frequency	Examples
Clean	Gram positive	Operating room environment, surgical team, patient's skin	3%	Inguinal hernia, thyroidectomy, mastectomy, aortic graft
Clean contaminated	Polymicrobial	Endogenous colonization of the patient	5%-15%	Elective colon resection, gastric resection, gastrostomy tube, common bile duct exploration
Contaminated	Polymicrobial	Gross contamination	15%-40%	"Spill" during elective GI surgery, perforated ulcer
Dirty	Polymicrobial	Established infection	40%-50%	Drainage of intra-abdominal abscess, resection of infracted bowel

are processes that were present before and, in many cases, are the reason the patient requires treatment. Hospital-acquired infections occur as a consequence of or during treatment and are termed *nosocomial*.

Nosocomial Infections

Nosocomial infection is by far the most common complication affecting hospitalized patients. It is estimated that 5% of hospitalized patients will acquire at least one nosocomial infection during their stay. Nosocomial infections are associated with a significant increase in morbidity and mortality and are often preventable.

Postoperative Fever

Fever that occurs in the postoperative period can be an early indication of developing infection. The traditional six "Ws" listed in Table 6-3 provide a systematic approach to help identify an etiology for the fever. Early temperature elevation is usually due to pulmonary atelectasis, which usually responds to deep breathing exercises and expectoration of secretions from the airway. Later in the postoperative course, fever points to the surgical wound, urinary tract, intravenous catheter site phlebitis, or deep vein thrombophlebitis as potential sources. The development of deep infections or abscess is usually identified as a late occurrence. Drug fever is an unusual event and should be considered only when all other obvious causes of fever have been ruled out. A postoperative fever should stimulate a careful patient examination and chart review to identify an etiology. Antibiotic treatment should be initiated only when a specific infectious source has been identified.

Surgical Site Infections

SSIs account for approximately 20% of all hospital-acquired infections, leading to increased cost and prolonged hospitalization, and are divided into categories on the basis of the level of tissue penetration. The diagnosis of superficial surgical infection is made in the majority of cases with an examination of the incision and surrounding skin demonstrating erythema and purulent drainage. For deep SSI and organ-space infection, fever and/or leukocytosis may also be present.

Superficial SSI involves the skin and subcutaneous tissues and is the most common type of SSI. Clinically, it ranges from simple cellulitis to overt infection of the wound bed above the fascia. Treatment includes oral antibiotics (gram-positive coverage) for cellulitis and reopening of the wound for those infections with purulent drainage.

Deep SSIs extend into the muscle and fascia. Treatment of deep SSIs requires reopening of the wounds and frequently sharp surgical debridement of the necrotic tissue. Deep SSI of abdominal wounds can lead to fascial necrosis and fascial dehiscence. In some of these cases, debridement of necrotic fascia and reapproximation is the best treatment course to prevent evisceration of abdominal contents. In more severe cases, the infections can spread along the fascial plane, causing fascial necrosis, systemic infection, and sepsis. Source control with radical debridement and intravenous broad-spectrum antibiotics is required for the successful treatment in these severe infections. Because of extensive tissue loss, reconstruction of the abdominal wall in these cases can be challenging.

Organ-space SSIs are infections that involve the body cavity where the operations were performed. These infections include secondary peritonitis, intra-abdominal abscess, and empyema. They are often related to inadequate source control from the original bacterial contamination event. Sometimes, a subfascial collection can manifest as wound drainage as the abscess attempts to extrude itself from the deeper space between fascial sutures. This can be difficult to differentiate from deep SSIs without the help of imaging studies. Intra-abdominal infections are usually polymicrobial, and broad-spectrum empiric antibiotic coverage should be started when the diagnosis is made. Anaerobic coverage should be considered on the basis of the most likely source and indigenous bacterial contaminants. Intrathoracic infections are less frequently polymicrobial, and antibiotic selection should be targeted at the most commonly occurring organisms for each patient's particular disease state. Patients with deep-space infections can become quite ill very quickly because of systemic extension of the infection and sepsis. Rapid diagnosis and treatment are necessary to prevent further morbidity and mortality. Computed tomography (CT) with contrast is a helpful diagnostic tool when this type of infection is suspected. Many isolated collections are amenable to percutaneous drainage utilizing radiographic guidance; however, those with ongoing contamination from infected implanted devices or anastomotic breakdown will require operative intervention.

Intra-Abdominal Infections

Intra-abdominal infections following abdominal surgery is a type of organ-space SSI. Postoperative intra-abdominal infection generally manifests in two clinical settings. The first and less common setting is diffuse peritonitis with florid sepsis. This is usually associated with major dehiscence of a bowel anastomosis or perforation with gross spillage of enteric or biliary contents. In these cases, reoperation is required for source control. Diffuse abdominal pain, peritonitis, fever, leukocytosis, and toxic septic state (rather than imaging studies) are the most important indicators of the need for reoperation in this setting. The second and more common setting is intra-abdominal abscess formation resulting from a small anastomotic leak or intraoperative contamination. Usually, persistent fever, leukocytosis, or ileus prompts the workup for intra-abdominal abscess. CT with enteric and intravenous contrast is the most useful diagnostic test to evaluate for intra-abdominal

TABLE 6-3. The "Ws" of Postoperative Fever

Site/Source	Postoperative Timing (d)
Wind	1-2
Water	2-3
Wound	3-5
Walking (deep vein thrombosis)	5-7
"**W**ound" abscess	7-10
Wonder drugs	Anytime, provided other etiologies have been ruled out.

abscess, demonstrating a well-organized fluid collection with peripheral contrast enhancement. Percutaneous drainage guided by ultrasound or CT is the initial intervention of choice for localized accessible abscesses. Operative source control is needed when there is (1) a source of ongoing contamination such as bowel perforation or an anastomotic leak or fistula, (2) devitalized tissue requiring debridement, (3) failure of percutaneous drainage, or (4) progression to generalized peritonitis.

In all cases of intra-abdominal infections, primary source control is an imperative step in the treatment plan. Systemic antibiotics alone will seldom be adequate therapy. Antibiotic therapy for intra-abdominal infections should appropriately cover the organisms that are inherent in the source of contamination. After adequate primary source control, the duration of antibiotics for intra-abdominal infections should not be longer than 2 days after resolution of fever and leukocytosis. A recent randomized controlled trial of short-course antimicrobial therapy for intraabdominal infection (STOP-IT) demonstrated similar outcome in patients with intra-abdominal infections treated with a 4-day course of antibiotics compared with those treated with a longer course.

Empyema

Pleural effusions are common in complicated surgical patients. Most often these are caused by volume overload, sympathetic effusions, or parapneumonic effusion. When a postoperative patient with systemic signs of infection (fever, systemic inflammatory response syndrome, and/or leukocytosis) develops a pleural effusion, the composition of the fluid should be determined by thoracentesis. A transudative effusion is caused by increased hydrostatic forces and has low protein content, whereas an exudative effusion is caused by increased permeability and has high protein content. Determining the fluid lactate dehydrogenase (LDH), glucose, pH, cell count, and Gram stain can help determine the type of effusion. Exudative effusions due to inflammation have a pH less than 7.2, a glucose less than 60 mg/dL, and/or an LDH greater than 3 times serum levels. They may be Gram stain or culture positive, although in up to one-third of patients with empyema, organisms are not identified in the fluid. The diagnosis can usually be confirmed by a CT scan and the identification of a loculated rim-enhancing pleural collection. In symptomatic patients or in patients with effusions associated with the characteristics of an exudate on thoracentesis sampling, adequate drainage of the pleural space should be accomplished. Although repeat therapeutic thoracentesis may be sufficient in some cases, surgical drainage is usually required either with video-assisted thoracic surgery or, for more advanced cases, thoracotomy and decortication. In select cases, fibrinolytic therapy by the instillation of a fibrinolytic agent in combination with DNAse through the existing chest tube can be used as a treatment modality.

Hospital- and Ventilator-Associated Pneumonia

Hospital-associated pneumonia and ventilator-associated pneumonia (VAP) together account for 22% of all hospital-acquired infections, making them the most common hospital-acquired infections. Approximately 10% of patients who require mechanical ventilation are diagnosed with VAP, and this rate has not declined over the past decade. The duration of mechanical ventilation, hospitalization, mortality, and treatment costs in patients who are on mechanical ventilation diagnosed with VAP are substantially higher when compared with those without VAP.

The diagnosis of VAP is suspected when the patient has an infiltrate/consolidation on chest x-ray that is new or progressive, along with clinical signs of fever, leukocytosis or leukopenia, new onset or increased purulent sputum production, and worsening gas exchange. Patients with suspected VAP should be further evaluated by bronchoscope-guided bronchial sampling (bronchoalveolar lavage or protected bronchial brushing) or blind bronchial sampling (mini-bronchoalveolar lavage) for quantitative cultures. Alternatively, noninvasive sampling with endotracheal aspiration for semiquantitative cultures can be done to guide antibiotic therapy. A positive quantitative culture is defined as greater than or equal to 10^4 colony-forming units (CFU)/mL for bronchoalveolar lavage and greater than or equal to 10^3 CFU/mL for protective bronchial brushing. The threshold for a positive endotracheal aspirate is 10^5 CPU/mL.

Once VAP is suspected, empiric antibiotic(s) must be chosen. This will largely be based on the patient's risk of having resistant organisms. In all patients with VAP, antibiotic coverage should include *Staphylococcus aureus, Pseudomonas aeruginosa,* and gram-negative bacteria. Examples of empiric agents are piperacillin-tazobactam, cefepime, levofloxacin, imipenem, and meropenem. Patients who are in shock, are immunocompromised, have been in the hospital for 5 days or more, or have acute respiratory distress syndrome at the time of diagnosis are at high risk for infections with multidrug-resistant organisms. In this setting, empiric antibiotic coverage should also include methicillin-resistant *Staphylococcus aureus* (MRSA) coverage. Once the causative organism is identified by culture, empiric antibiotics should then be tailored to the narrowest possible spectrum to cover the organism(s). Patients with semiquantitative or quantitative cultures below the diagnostic threshold should have their empiric antibiotics discontinued. Specific antibiotic treatment for 7 days is sufficient for most patients with VAP.

Attempts at VAP prevention have led to the development of a group of interventions that when bundled together seems to have a great impact when compared with any individual effort. The basic principles for VAP prevention are to (1) minimize sedation and sedation interruption daily, (2) assess readiness for extubation daily with spontaneous breathing trials, (3) maintain and improve physical conditioning by early mobility, (4) minimize pooling of secretions above the endotracheal tube cuff by using an endotracheal tube with a subglottic suction device, (5) elevate the head of the bed 30° to 45°, and (6) maintain the ventilator circuit (change only when visibly soiled or malfunctional). Adherence to these recommendations has demonstrated a significant reduction in the length of time patients require ventilator assistance, which leads to a reduction in VAP rates.

Urinary Tract Infections

The greatest risk factor for developing a urinary tract infection (UTI) is the presence of an indwelling bladder catheter. The rate of catheter-related UTI is directly related to the duration of catheter placement. Therefore, the need for a urinary catheter in every patient should be evaluated daily, and catheters should be removed as soon as they are no longer indicated. Other prevention strategies include aseptic placement, maintenance of the closed drainage system, and daily urethral hygiene.

The diagnosis of postoperative UTI is traditionally made with a quantitative bacterial culture of more than 100,000 organisms/mL of urine. However, bacteriuria does not mean invasive urinary sepsis and is usually not the source of fever in postsurgical patients. In most cases, positive urinary cultures with an indwelling catheter are usually clear after removal of the catheter. In the absence of a functional or anatomic obstruction to urine flow, systemic bacteremia from the urinary tract is uncommon, and a postoperative fever should not be attributed to the urinary tract even with positive urinary cultures. Surveillance for other sources of fever should be undertaken in these clinical scenarios.

Catheter-Related Bloodstream Infections

Catheter-related bloodstream infection (CRBSI) is defined as the presence of bacteremia that originated from an intravenous catheter. CRBSI accounts for 11% of hospital-acquired infections and is associated with increased intensive care unit (ICU) stay, hospital stay, and mortality. The risk for CRBSI is substantially greater for central venous catheters compared to peripheral venous catheters. CRBSI can arise from organisms invading at the catheter entry site or from organisms being introduced through the lumen of the catheter. Organisms associated with CRBSI come from the normal flora of the skin, and *S. aureus* is the most common, followed by *P. aeruginosa*, *Candida* species, and other gram-negative bacilli.

CRBSI is suspected when fever and other signs of sepsis are present in a patient with a central venous catheter. Examination of the entry site may reveal local signs of infection, such as erythema, swelling, tenderness, and purulent drainage. However, most cases do not manifest local signs of infection, so the absence of these signs does not rule out CRBSI. The diagnosis of CRBSI is made based on positive blood culture in the setting of fever or sepsis, and the source of infection is attributed to the intravenous catheter. There are several ways to demonstrate that the positive blood culture is attributed to the catheter. One method is the removal of the catheter under sterile condition, and the catheter tip is sent for semiquantitative or quantitative cultures. Greater than 15 CFU/catheter tip for semiquantitative culture or greater than 10^3 CFU/catheter tip for quantitative culture is considered positive. Another method is quantitative paired blood culture. In this method, the blood culture drawn from the central catheter must have 5 times the colony count as blood culture drawn simultaneously from a peripheral vein. The third method is differential time positivity. In this method, blood from the central catheter demonstrates microbial growth at least 2 hours earlier than growth detected in blood taken from the peripheral vein. For all of these methods, the species growing from the catheter tip or blood from the central catheter must be the same as the species growing from blood taken from the peripheral vein.

Management of CRBSI should include the removal of the infected catheter. Empiric antibiotics should be started as soon as blood cultures have been sent. Empiric antibiotics should include vancomycin to cover for MRSA and fourth-generation cephalosporin, β-lactam/β-lactamase

inhibitor combination, or carbapenem to cover for *Pseudomonas* and gram-negative organisms. For patients with femoral line or patients on total peripheral nutrition, coverage for *Candida* species should be considered. Once identification and sensitivity data are obtained, antibiotic coverage should be narrowed. Duration of antibiotic therapy depends on the severity of illness, patients' immunologic status, and the species involved, and can range from 7 to 14 days for gram-negative bacilli, 14 days for *Enterococcus* and *Candida*, and up to 4 to 6 weeks for *S. aureus*. Since the risk of associated endocarditis is high in patients with *S. aureus* bloodstream infection, a transesophageal echocardiogram (TEE) should be considered to rule out endocarditis. A negative TEE can help the decision of a shorter antibiotic course.

Clostridioides difficile Infections

Clostridioides difficile (formerly known as *Clostridium difficile,* commonly known as *C. difficile* or *C. diff*) is the organism causing antibiotic-associated diarrhea and colitis. *C. difficile* is highly transmissible via the fecal to oral route by the ingestion of spores, and hospitalized patients harboring *C. difficile* can serve as a source for transmission through contacts. Not all patients with *C. difficile* cultured from their stool have diarrhea or colitis. Up to 10% of hospitalized or long-term facility care patients can be asymptomatic carriers of *C. difficile*. Exotoxins, toxin A and toxin B (coded by *tcdA* and *tcdB* genes, respectively) produced by *C. difficile* are responsible for the death of colonocytes, disruption of intercellular tight junctions, loss of intestinal barrier function, and inflammation. Local tissue injury and inflammation then result in diarrhea.

Antibiotic use is the most widely known risk factor for *C. difficile* infection (CDI). The antibiotics most frequently associated with CDI are fluoroquinolones, clindamycin, and broad-spectrum β-lactams, although any antibiotics can be implicated. Other risk factors include advanced age, hospitalization, immunosuppression, severe comorbid illness, and gastric acid suppression with proton pump inhibitors.

The most common symptom of CDI is diarrhea (more than three episodes per day), usually watery and rarely bloody. In patients on or were recently on antibiotics therapy who develop diarrhea that is unexplained, a suspicion for CDI should be raised. Other associated symptoms include fever, abdominal cramping, nausea, anorexia, and vomiting. Patients with more severe infections may have diffuse abdominal tenderness and distension, signs of hypovolemia, evidence of worsening renal function, and markedly elevated white blood cell (WBC) count. In fulminant infections, shock, hypotension, or toxic megacolon is present.

The diagnosis of CDI requires the detection of *C. difficile* toxin or *C. difficile* organism in stool sample. Three tests are commonly used: polymerase chain reaction (PCR) for the *tcdB* gene, enzyme immunoassay (EIA) for glutamate dehydrogenase (GDH, an enzyme produced by *C. difficile*), and enzyme immunoassay for toxins A and B. PCR for *tcdB* and EIA for GDH and are often used as the initial screening tests. Enzyme immunoassay for toxins A and B is less sensitive but is highly specific. It is often used as a confirmatory test following *tcdB* PCR or GDH assay. Cell culture for *C. difficile* and cytotoxicity assay are not routinely used in clinical settings.

The first step in the treatment of patients with CDI is discontinuation of the inciting antibiotics as soon as possible.

Although either oral fidaxomicin or oral vancomycin can be used for the treatment of patients with an initial CDI episode, fidaxomicin is preferred over oral vancomycin because it is shown to have a lower recurrence rate. Both medications when given orally have very little systemic absorption and therefore have low side effects. Intravenous vancomycin is not secreted into the colon and therefore it is not effective against CDI. Metronidazole administered either orally or intravenously is less effective for CDI, but it can be used if oral fidaxomicin or oral vancomycin is not available. In patients who have associated ileus, orally administered antibiotics may not progress into the colon. In these situations, rectally administered vancomycin should be used in conjunction with an oral regimen to ensure that there are effective antibiotics in the colonic lumen. The standard duration for treatment of initial CDI is 10 days.

Surgery is generally only considered in patients with fulminant CDI. Some patients with fulminant disease may still respond to antibiotics and support therapy. In patients whose disease continues to progress, especially if they are already on maximal medical therapy, surgical intervention may be required. Some of the indications for surgical intervention are shock with escalating pressor support, perforation, colonic necrosis, and abdominal compartment syndrome. Surgical intervention usually involves total abdominal colectomy and ileostomy creation. Mortality rate for this patient population is very high, ranging from 20% to 50% depending on the series.

Recurrent CDI can occur in up to 20% of patients. Recurrence is defined by the resolution of symptoms, followed by reappearance of symptoms within 2 months after discontinuation of treatment. In patients with recurrent episodes of CDI, a fidaxomicin standard regimen or extended-pulsed regimen is recommended. Vancomycin taper regimen over 6 to 8 weeks can also be used as an alternative. Bezlotoxumab, a monoclonal antibody to toxin B given intravenously as a one-time infusion used in conjunction with antibiotics treatment, has been shown to reduce recurrent episodes and should be considered. Fecal microbial transplant (FMT) is a treatment modality in which stool from a healthy donor pool is instilled in the colon of a patient with recurrent CDI by way of colonoscopy. The cure rate for recurrent CDIs using FMT in conjunction with antibiotics has been shown to be up to 90%. FMT is not widely available and should be avoided in patients who are immunosuppressed and patients with inflammatory bowel disease.

The primary prevention strategies against CDI are minimization of antibiotic use, environmental cleaning, isolation of patients with CDI, and rigorous hand hygiene. It is important to note that alcohol gels do not inactivate spores, thus hand washing with soap and water is necessary to prevent the spread of CDI.

Community-Acquired Infections
Skin and Soft Tissue Infections
Common soft tissue infections are outlined in Table 6-4. Cellulitis as manifested by blanching erythema is caused by *Streptococci*, which respond to penicillin therapy.

TABLE 6-4. Common Soft Tissue Infections

Infection	Etiology	Typical Organism(s)	Physical Findings	Treatment
Cellulitis	Break in skin barrier	*Streptococcus*	Warm to touch, diffuse erythema, tenderness	Systemic antibiotics and local wound care
Furuncle, carbuncle	Bacterial growth within skin glands and crypts	*Staphylococcus*	Localized induration, erythema, tenderness, swelling with purulent drainage	Incision and drainage, systemic antibiotics
Hidradenitis suppurativa	Bacterial growth within apocrine sweat glands	*Staphylococcus*	Multiple small localized subcutaneous abscesses, drainage, commonly from axilla and groin	Incision and drainage of small lesions, systemic antibiotics; large areas will require wide local excision and skin grafting.
Lymphangitis	Infection within lymphatics	*Streptococcus*	Diffuse swelling and erythema of distal extremity with areas of inflamed streaks along lymphatic channels	Local wound care, systemic antibiotics, removal of any foreign body, elevation of extremity
Gangrene, NSTIs	Destruction of healthy tissue by virulent microbial enzymes	Synergistic: *Streptococcus/ Staphylococcus* Mixed aerobic/ anaerobic Clostridium	Necrotic skin/fascia, swelling and induration, foul-smelling discharge, crepitus with subcutaneous emphysema, frequently with toxic systemic signs and symptoms of sepsis	Radical debridement/amputation of involved tissues, aggressive local wound care with frequent debridement as necessary, parenteral broad-spectrum antibiotics

NSTIs, necrotizing soft tissue infections.

Staphylococci may also be the cause of cellulitis, particularly if gross suppuration (pus) is present at the affected site. Suppurative lesions require local incision and drainage in addition to antibiotic therapy. Increasingly, the offending organism is community-acquired MRSA, which is particularly virulent and can cause local tissue necrosis.

Soft tissue infections characterized by pathogen invasion, tissue necrosis, and systemic signs of sepsis are collectively termed necrotizing soft tissue infections (NSTIs). Necrotizing infection can be classified on the basis of the depth of invasion (eg, necrotizing adipositis, fasciitis, or myositis). All are surgical emergencies requiring aggressive fluid resuscitation, intravenous broad-spectrum antimicrobials, and wide surgical debridement of the necrotic tissue. Delay in recognition and treatment will lead to extensive tissue loss, limb loss, and mortality. The most characteristic finding is pain out of proportion to physical appearance. Other early clinical manifestations include edema beyond the area of erythema, skin anesthesia, epidermolysis, and skin discoloration. Bullae, crepitus, foul-smelling drainage, and dermal gangrene are late manifestations and are usually associated with systemic sepsis. Leukocytosis and hyponatremia, if present, can support clinical suspicion. Radiographic imaging (x-ray and CT) may reveal asymmetric tissue inflammation and occult soft tissue gas. However, soft tissue emphysema is detected only in 39% of patients, and its absence does not rule out NSTIs. Surgical exploration of the affected area is often necessary to definitively rule in or rule out NSTIs. Fournier gangrene is an eponym that specifically applies to NSTI of the genitalia and perineum. The vast majority of these infections are polymicrobial. Antibiotic coverage for these patients should include MRSA, gram-negative organisms, and anaerobic organisms. A protein synthesis inhibitor such as clindamycin or linezolid is commonly used because it theoretically reduces toxin production.

Two monomicrobial NSTIs deserve specific attention: group A streptococcus (GAS) infection and clostridial myonecrosis. Necrotizing streptococcal gangrene rarely occurs in surgical patients. These infections are characterized by nonblanching erythema, with blisters and frank necrosis of the skin. Nonblanching erythema indicates subdermal thrombosis of the nutrient blood supply of the skin. Extensive surgical debridement of the affected area and a combination of high-dose penicillin and clindamycin are the appropriate treatment. A Gram stain of blister fluid or tissue obtained during the debridement is useful in differentiating this infection from other necrotizing infections of the skin and skin structures.

Clostridial myonecrosis and clostridial cellulitis are fulminant life-threatening infections characterized by tissue necrosis and rapidly advancing crepitus (gas gangrene). Either may occur as early as 1 day postoperatively or after tissue injury, most commonly from puncture wounds, and carries a high mortality rate. When *Clostridium* gas gangrene is diagnosed, immediate radical surgical debridement is necessary. Antibiotic therapy should include high-dose penicillin. Clindamycin is a reasonable alternative in patients with penicillin allergy, as is tigecycline, a glycylcycline related to tetracycline. Hyperbaric oxygen therapy to vastly increase local O_2 concentration, directly kill bacteria, and support WBC oxidative burst has also been successfully utilized as an adjunct for NSTI in general, and clostridial myonecrosis and GAS in particular, but it is not a substitute for aggressive surgical debridement. Adequate surgical debridement without primary wound closure prevents clostridial myonecrosis or cellulitis in most patients with high-risk wounds.

Tetanus

Tetanus (lockjaw) is caused by the neurotoxin produced by *Clostridium tetani* that affects the brain, spinal cord, and peripheral nerves. After an incubation period of 3 to 21 days, prodromal symptoms of restlessness and headache are followed by descending muscular spasms, beginning with masseter muscle stiffness, neck stiffness, and difficulty swallowing, and spreading to the rest of the body. Violent generalized tonic muscle spasms usually follow within 24 hours of symptom onset, culminating in acute respiratory arrest, which may require ventilator support. Autonomic nerve involvement may lead to episodic tachycardia and hypertension. The diagnosis is made clinically rather than by microbiology because the organism is isolated in only 30% of the cases. The keystone of management is the prevention of exotoxin production by debridement and cleansing of all wounds in which devitalized, contaminated tissue is present, coupled with an immunization program. Tetanus immunoglobulin (TIG) is recommended for patients with tetanus. TIG can only help remove unbound toxin and cannot affect toxin already bound to nerve endings. It is usually given intramuscularly and infiltrated around the wound. All patients who sustain tetanus-prone wounds, as described in Table 6-5, should receive tetanus prophylaxis in accordance with the recommendations of the Centers for Disease Control and Prevention, as outlined in Table 6-6. Patients with high-risk wounds who have not completed the primary three-shot series of tetanus immunization should be given TIG in addition to tetanus immunization. Tetanus in persons with a documented primary series of tetanus toxoid is exceedingly rare.

Breast Abscess

Breast abscess, characterized by localized severe tenderness, swelling, and redness associated with a mass, is a common staphylococcal soft tissue infection. Risk factors for breast abscess include breast feeding, maternal age greater than 30, first pregnancy, gestational age more than 41 weeks, smoking, and obesity. Development of breast abscess in a nonlactating woman should alert the physician to the possibility of an underlying malignancy. The diagnosis is made on the basis of clinical examination with confirmation by ultrasound and aspiration of purulent fluid. Antistaphylococcal antibiotics and serial ultrasound–guided

TABLE 6-5. Tetanus Risk by Wound Type		
	Tetanus Prone	**Nontetanus Prone**
Type	Crush Avulsion Puncture Extensive abrasion Burns or frostbite	Sharp/clean Minor wound
Contaminants (soil, dirt, saliva, feces)	Present	Absent

TABLE 6-6. Guide to Tetanus Prophylaxis in Routine Wound Management

Characteristics	Nontetanus-Prone Wounds		Tetanus-Prone Wounds	
	DTaP, Tdap, or Td[a]	TIG	Tdap or Td[a]	TIG
History of absorbed tetanus toxoid (doses)				
Unknown or <3 doses	Yes	No	Yes	Yes
≥3 doses	No[b]	No	No[c]	No

DTaP, diphtheria-tetanus-pertussis; Td, tetanus and diphtheria; Tdap, tetanus-diphtheria-pertussis; TIG, tetanus immunoglobulin.
[a]DTaP is recommended for children below 7 years of age. Tdap is preferred to Td for persons aged 11 years or older who have not previously received Tdap. Persons aged 7 years or older who are not fully vaccinated against pertussis, tetanus, or diphtheria should receive one dose of Tdap (preferably the first) for wound management and as part of the catch-up series; if additional tetanus toxoid–containing doses are required, either Td or Tdap vaccine can be used.
[b]Yes, if above 10 years since the last tetanus toxoid–containing vaccine dose.
[c]Yes, if above 5 years since the last tetanus toxoid–containing vaccine dose.
Tiwari TSP, Moro PL, Acosta AM. Chapter 21: Tetanus. In: Epidemiology and Prevention of Vaccine-Preventable Diseases. Public Health Foundation.
https://www.cdc.gov/pinkbook/hcp/table-of-contents/chapter-21-tetanus.html

aspiration should be the initial treatment option. Usually, two to three serial aspirations separated by 2 to 3 days are required for complete resolution. In cases when the overlying skin is compromised or when serial aspiration fails, surgical drainage is required. Surgical drainage as the initial treatment is acceptable; however, it is associated with worse cosmetic outcome and a higher rate of mammary duct/milk fistula. Mothers who are breastfeeding should be encouraged to continue feeding or pumping even in the setting of breast infection. In patients at risk for malignancy, a biopsy should be performed.

Perirectal Abscess

Perirectal abscesses result from infection within the crypts of the anorectal canal and present as a tender mass in the perianal area. Perirectal abscess can extend into the pelvis above the pelvic floor and can be fatal, especially in patients with diabetes or who are immunocompromised. Perirectal abscesses are exquisitely tender and usually require general anesthesia to be examined and to establish adequate drainage. Antibiotic coverage is usually broad spectrum, targeting both anaerobes and aerobes, and is necessary in patients with bacteremia and patients with associated cellulitis. Invasive infection may result in subcutaneous tissue necrosis, which requires wide debridement for salvage.

Biliary Tract Infections

Biliary tract infections are usually a consequence of obstruction within the biliary tree, involving either the cystic or the common bile duct. The bacteria most commonly involved include *Escherichia coli*, *Klebsiella* spp., and *Enterococcus* spp., whereas anaerobes are not commonly encountered. In patients with previous biliary-enteric anastomosis, the likelihood of anaerobic organism involvement is increased. Antibiotics are utilized as an adjunct to surgical and/or endoscopic intervention for effective drainage and infection resolution.

Acute cholecystitis is the most common inflammatory condition in the biliary tract. It begins as an obstruction of the cystic duct by gallstone. Entrapped bacteria convert inflammation into an invasive infectious process. Increased endoluminal pressure, combined with invasive bacterial infection into the wall, may also compromise the blood supply of the gallbladder walls, resulting in ischemia, necrosis, and perforation. The most effective treatment for acute cholecystitis is cholecystectomy.

Infection proximal to a common duct obstruction causes ascending cholangitis. Patients present with fulminant fever, right upper quadrant abdominal pain, and jaundice (Charcot triad); the addition of hypotension and altered mental status is known as *Reynold pentad*. These patients usually manifest with severe sepsis or septic shock, accompanied by hemodynamic instability, which requires aggressive intravenous fluid resuscitation to maintain mean arterial pressure. Prompt common bile duct drainage, together with the administration of empiric systemic antibiotics, is imperative. The common duct can be drained by endoscopic means (endoscopic retrograde cholangiopancreatography with stone extraction and sphincterotomy of the sphincter of Oddi), percutaneous transhepatic cholangio-catheter placement, or surgical exploration of the common bile duct. Cholecystectomy should be undertaken once the patient's septic pathology has been corrected.

Acute Peritonitis

Acute peritonitis occurs when bacteria are present within the normally sterile peritoneal cavity. Primary peritonitis is spontaneous bacterial peritonitis that occurs without a breach of the gastrointestinal (GI) tract or peritoneal cavity. It is usually monomicrobial and is more commonly seen in patients with ascites associated with liver disease and in those who are immunocompromised. Secondary peritonitis occurs as a result of spillage of gut organisms from the GI tract or contamination from indwelling catheters (peritoneal dialysis catheters). It is usually polymicrobial.

Peritonitis causes acute abdominal pain, usually accompanied by fever and leukocytosis. Examination of the abdomen typically demonstrates marked tenderness with voluntary guarding and percussion tenderness. Involuntary guarding with board-like rigidity is characteristic of generalized peritonitis. An upright chest x-ray commonly shows pneumoperitoneum beneath a hemidiaphragm. CT is more sensitive for pneumoperitoneum, and a small amount of free air can be readily demonstrated by CT that may not be initially apparent on plain radiography (Figure 6-1).

Perforated gastroduodenal ulcers usually present with acute onset abdominal pain with little or no antecedent history of abdominal discomfort. Approximately 80% of patients have pneumoperitoneum on an upright chest film. The perforation allows gastric acid, bile, as well as oral microflora to gain access to the peritoneal space. Operative

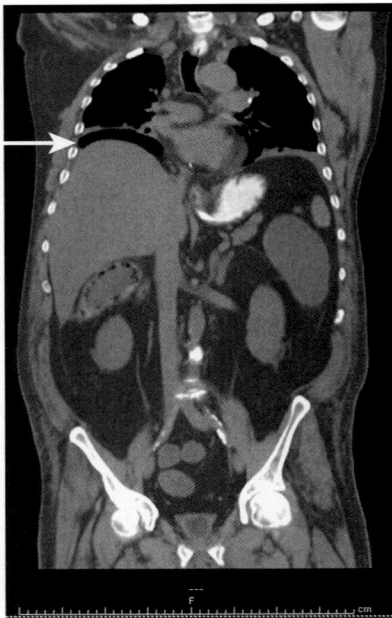

Figure 6-1. Coronal imaging of the abdomen with free intraperitoneal air under the right hemidiaphragm (indicated by arrow).

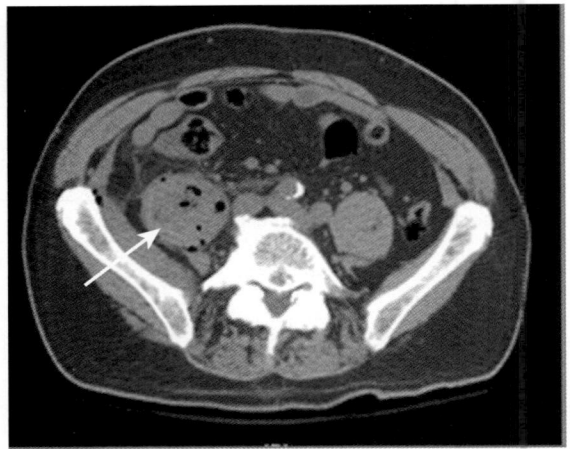

Figure 6-2. Localized psoas abscess (indicated by arrow) following appendectomy for perforated, gangrenous appendicitis.

repair of the perforation is usually necessary for source control. All patients with ulcer-associated perforation should be assessed for the presence of *Helicobacter pylori* infection. Perioperative antibiotic therapy to address oral aerobes and anaerobes is generally indicated for acute perforations for less than 24 hours. Established infection with peritonitis and abscess indicates a need for longer therapeutic antibiotics whose duration exceeds 24 hours. Importantly, perforation in patients with achlorhydria (endogenous or medication induced) should prompt empiric antifungal therapy as well.

Acute appendicitis causes localized peritoneal irritation, and appendiceal perforation commonly causes generalized peritonitis. In the absence of an appropriate operation, perforation may occur within 24 hours of symptom onset. Patients typically demonstrate the characteristic findings of acute, diffuse peritoneal irritation when the perforation is not contained, whereas a contained perforation with periappendiceal abscess formation (Figure 6-2) may induce only right lower quadrant pain and tenderness. Antibiotic therapy is directed against both aerobic (*E. coli*) and anaerobic (*Bacteroides fragilis*) enteric organisms. Treatment depends on the hemodynamic status of the patient and the presence or absence of a localized collection that is amenable to percutaneous drainage. Patients without a localized collection should undergo an emergent operation for source control.

Colonic perforation with diffuse peritonitis creates the most virulent type of peritonitis, because the colonic aerobic and anaerobic floral densities are high. Patients generally demonstrate peritonitis, hemodynamic instability, and septic shock. After volume resuscitation and initiation of broad-spectrum antibiotics, surgical intervention is generally required to manage the perforation, drain purulent collections, debride nonviable tissue, and decontaminate the

fecal materials. The etiology of colonic perforation may vary (ischemia, diverticulitis, perforated colon cancer, etc). CT findings may include a thickened bowel wall, mesenteric stranding, pneumatosis intestinalis, pericolonic fluid collections, and pneumoperitoneum. Colon perforations usually require resection of the perforated segment and diversion of the fecal stream as part of their management. Selected patients who present with a localized perforation (including mesocolonic perforation) may be initially managed without immediate operation, provided the leak is adequately drained.

Hand Infections

Although generally not life threatening, hand infections may lead to severe morbidity from loss of function as a result of tissue loss, scar, and contracture. Paronychia is a staphylococcal infection of the proximal fingernail that erupts at the sulcus of the nail border. Simple drainage and hot soaks usually provide adequate therapy. Felons are deep infections of the terminal phalanx pulp space. These infections usually occur after distal phalanx–penetrating injuries and are treated by drainage. A subungual abscess is the extension of a deep paronychia and is diagnosed by fluctuance beneath the nail. Removal of the nail is usually necessary to permit adequate drainage. Neglected infections of the fingers may result in tenosynovitis, an infection that extends along the tendon sheath of the digit. Drainage requires opening the sheath along its entire length to prevent necrosis of the tendon.

Penetrating injury or spread from a contiguous fascial compartment may lead to infection in one of three deep-space compartments in the hand. A thenar space infection causes swelling and pain directly over the thenar eminence. The thumb is held in abduction to reduce pain and tendon stretch. Loss of the normal concavity as a result of tense, painful swelling of the palm is characteristic of a midpalmar space abscess. Rarely, infection of the hypothenar space presents in a similar fashion, with swelling and painful movement. Urgent incision and drainage are required for these infections, and empiric broad-spectrum antibiotics, later based on culture data, are generally continued for 10 days depending on the response to therapy.

Human bites of the hand are common, and the potential infectious nature should not be underestimated. Contamination of these wounds with polymicrobial aerobic and anaerobic oral flora contributes to invasive deep-space infections, including tenosynovitis. Copious irrigation, debridement of devitalized tissue, hand elevation, and broad-spectrum antibiotics are required to reduce the potential for infectious complications. Human bites are the only penetrating injury of the hand in which primary closure is not done. Human oral flora includes the invasive pathogen *Eikenella corrodens*, an organism that is known to suppurate along tendon sheaths, leading to extensive tissue destruction. The hand and upper extremity are often injured by animal bites as well. Debridement and irrigation are required (as for human bites), but the pathogens involved are likely to be aerobic *Pasteurella* species from both dogs and cats.

Foot Infections

Foot infections result from direct injury or, more commonly, from mechanical and metabolic derangements that occur in patients with diabetes. Trauma-related infections are best prevented by adequate wound cleansing at the time of injury. Established infections should raise concern that a retained foreign body or underlying osteomyelitis is present. All foreign bodies associated with infection require localization and removal for healing to occur. Osteomyelitis requires operative debridement and long-term antibiotics.

Foot infections in patients with diabetes are a common problem because of neuropathy, the resultant bone deformities, and the vascular compromise that occurs in this population, which leads to ischemic and pressure-related ulceration. Ulcers on the plantar aspect of the forefoot underneath a metatarsal head are typical for such pressure ulcers. A thorough examination of the infected foot should determine the extent of vascular and neurologic impairment. Plantar space infections may present with dorsal cellulitis, and all cases of dorsal cellulitis should trigger a search for a plantar source. Osteomyelitis in a diabetic foot wound can be present even when the wound itself does not show evidence of active infection. Wounds with exposed bone or those that probe to bone are highly suspicious of underlying osteomyelitis, and they should be evaluated further. Diabetic foot infections are usually polymicrobial in nature, including *Pseudomonas*,

which is highly prevalent in this patient population. Cultures of involved tissue (not just surface swabs) should be obtained, followed by initial empiric broad-spectrum antibiotic therapy, debridement, and drainage. Efforts should focus on limb salvage in these patients because amputation is a frequent morbid consequence of these complex infections. Such efforts may require the management of concomitant vascular disease by revascularization procedures. Antibiotics alone may be insufficient to clear the infection and allow tissue healing without specific wound dressings, correction of pressure points by orthotic footwear, and/or surgical debridement and arterial inflow improvement.

SUMMARY

The term *surgical infections* has now been expanded to encompass an entire host of disease states for which evaluation by a surgeon and potential surgical intervention are necessary. Surgical infections require a myriad of treatment techniques ranging from antibiotics to incision and drainage to radical debridement to organ removal. A prompt diagnosis with rapid surgical treatment will limit morbidity and mortality in many of these diseases.

SUGGESTED READINGS

Berrios-Torres SI, Umscheid CA, Bratzler DW, et al. Centers for Disease Control and Prevention guideline for the prevention of surgical site infection, 2017. *JAMA Surgery*. 2017;152(8):784-791.

Johnson S, Lavergne V, Skinner AM, et al. Clinical practice guideline by the Infectious Diseases Society of America (ISDA) and Society for Healthcare Epidemiology of America (SHEA): 2021 focused update guidelines on management of *Clostridioides difficile* infection in adults. *Clin Infect Dis*. 2021;73(5):e1029-e1044.

Kalil AC, Metersky ML, Klompas M, et al. Management of adults with hospital-acquired and ventilator-associated pneumonia: 2016 clinical practice guidelines by the Infectious Diseases Society of America and the American Thoracic Society. *Clin Infect Dis*. 2016;63(5):e61-e111.

O'Grady NP, Alexander M, Burns LA, et al. Summary of recommendations: guidelines for the prevention of intravascular catheter-related infections. *Clini Infect Dis*. 2011;52(9):1087-1099.

Phan HH, Cocanour CS. Necrotizing soft tissue infections in the intensive care unit. *Crit Care Med*. 2010;38(9 suppl):S460-S468.

SAMPLE QUESTIONS

QUESTIONS

Choose the best answer for each question.

1. A 32-year-old man is seen in the emergency department 45 minutes after a motor vehicle collision. His only injury is a long linear laceration beginning on the left temporal forehead at the hairline and extending posteriorly for 10 cm. The edges are still bleeding briskly, and the emergency medical technicians described a large amount of blood at the scene. He did not lose consciousness. His last tetanus booster was 4 years ago. Which of the following is required for tetanus prophylaxis in this patient?

A. TIG only
B. Nothing further at this time
C. Tetanus toxoid only
D. TIG followed by a single tetanus toxoid booster
E. TIG followed by three tetanus boosters

2. A 48-year-old man is being evaluated in the emergency department with fevers, chills, and abdominal pain for the past 24 hours. He has a history of hepatitis C infection following a blood transfusion 14 years ago for a large scalp laceration and orthopedic injuries sustained in a motor vehicle collision. He has not been to a physician for 5 years.

He does not smoke or drink alcohol. He takes no medications. His temperature is 39 °C, and his vital signs are as follows: blood pressure (BP) of 90/50 mm Hg, pulse of 110/min, and respirations of 26/min. A CT scan shows a single stone in the gallbladder that does not appear to be obstructing. The bile ducts are of normal caliber, and the gallbladder wall is not thickened. There is a moderate amount of fluid, mild small bowel distension, and stranding around the sigmoid colon as well as a small amount of free intraperitoneal gas around the liver. An aspirate of the peritoneal fluid shows leukocytes and mixed gram-positive and gram-negative bacteria on Gram stain. Laboratory values show a white blood cell count of 19,000/mm^3, a total bilirubin of 1.2 mg/dL, and an alkaline phosphatase of 40 U/L. In addition to fluid resuscitation and broad-spectrum antibiotics, what is the best step in management?

A. Laparoscopic cholecystectomy
B. Long-term antibiotics only
C. Laparotomy
D. Magnetic resonance cholangiopancreatography
E. Endoscopic retrograde cholangiopancreatography

3. A 72-year-old woman underwent an operative fixation of an intertrochanteric femur fracture 7 days ago. Her urinary catheter was removed on postoperative day 5. Now, she is complaining of burning with urination and urinary urgency. Her urinalysis is positive for leukocytes and bacteria. Which of the following statements is NOT correct about this condition?

A. The diagnosis is made with quantitative bacterial culture.
B. The rate of infection is unrelated to the duration of the indwelling urinary catheter.
C. This condition is rarely the cause of postoperative fever.
D. This complication adds to the cost of hospital care.
E. Prevention of this condition involves maintenance of the close drainage of the urinary catheter and aseptic placement.

4. A 30-year-old man is in the hospital recovering from splenectomy for a ruptured spleen sustained in a motor vehicle collision. He has otherwise been healthy and was not taking medications prior to the injury. A temperature of 102 °F is noted on the second postoperative day. Vital signs are as follows: a BP of 130/80 mm Hg, a pulse of 100/min, and a respiration rate of 18/min. His pain is moderately controlled with morphine using patient-controlled analgesia. Breath sounds are diminished at both bases, more so on the left. His abdomen is mildly distended, soft, and tender near the incision. The incision appears to be healing without a problem. What is the most likely cause for his fever?

A. Atelectasis and pulmonary infection
B. Peritonitis
C. UTI
D. Suppurative thrombophlebitis
E. Cardiac contusion

5. A 25-year-old man is seen in the emergency department because of a painful swollen forearm. Two days ago, he sustained a small laceration to his left forearm while clearing brush. It caused only minor discomfort until about 12 hours ago when the area around the laceration became redder and more swollen. He has otherwise been healthy. He takes no medications. His temperature is 38 °C. There is a 2-cm superficial laceration on the dorsum of his left forearm with a 15-cm diameter–surrounding erythema that is quite tender. The edges of the erythema were marked, and 20 minutes later, the erythema extended 1 cm further beyond the mark. The most likely causative organism is

A. MRSA.
B. group-A β-hemolytic streptococcus.
C. *E. coli.*
D. *Streptococcus faecalis.*
E. *Candida albicans.*

ANSWERS AND EXPLANATIONS

1. **Answer: B**

   Wounds prone to the development of tetanus include those with extensive contamination with soil, deep puncture wounds from metal objects, exposure injury complicated with frostbite, and wounds greater than 6 hours from the time of injury (see Table 6-6). Linear lacerations in general are not prone to tetanus. The extent of blood loss does not affect the need for tetanus booster administration. The patient last received tetanus toxoid less than 5 years ago, so nothing further is required. For more information on this topic, see section "Tetanus."

2. **Answer: C**

   This patient has secondary peritonitis. This usually involves perforation of a hollow viscus and thus involves contamination of the peritoneal cavity with multiple organisms. Gram stain and culture of the peritoneal fluid usually shows a single organism in patients with primary peritonitis, and this can be treated with antibiotics without surgical intervention. In this scenario, the CT scan shows stranding around the sigmoid and fluid and evidence of free air suggestive of diverticulitis with fecal peritonitis. Laparotomy with washout and correction of underlying cause is indicated. Patients with underlying liver disease are prone to gallstones, which is a common finding. There is no evidence of common bile duct obstruction that warrants further investigation because the alkaline phosphatase is normal. For more information on this topic, see section "Acute Peritonitis."

3. **Answer: B**

   The rate of catheter-related infection is directly related to the duration of the urinary catheter being in place. The diagnosis of UTI is usually made with a quantitative bacteria culture of more than 100,000 organisms/mL urine. UTI is rarely the cause of postoperative fever. UTI adds to the cost of care for hospitalized patients, and prevention requires aseptic placement and maintenance of a closed drainage system. For more information on this topic, see section "Urinary Tract Infections."

4. **Answer: A**

Early postoperative fever is usually the result of atelectasis and subsequent pulmonary infection (see Table 6-4). In this scenario, because of the close proximity of the left hemidiaphragm to the spleen, an infiltrate in the left lower lobe of the lung is highly probable. An adequately drained urinary tract in a young person seldom gives a high fever this early in the postoperative period. Although peritonitis from injury to a surrounding structure during the splenectomy (ie, pancreas, stomach, or bowel) is a

possibility, it is much less likely than a pulmonary source. Cardiac contusion does not elicit a febrile response. For more information on this topic, see section "Postoperative Fever."

5. **Answer: B**

Although cellulitis may be caused by any organism, the most likely early organism would be group-A β-hemolytic streptococcus. MRSA more commonly causes local inflammation and pus formation. The other three species are rarely isolated from skin infections but are more commonly seen in infections involving the GI tract. For more information on this topic, see sections "Urinary Tract Infections" and "Skin and Soft Tissue Infections."

7 Trauma

Jared M. Huston and Felix Y. Lui

OVERVIEW AND EPIDEMIOLOGY

Unintentional injury remains the leading cause of death in the United States for individuals aged 1 to 44 years and is the fourth most common cause of mortality after the first year of life. In 2021, 45,404 people died following motor vehicle collision, and the total deaths from firearms were 47,286. There are over 30 million nonfatal injuries annually in the United States. Patient care advances have decreased trauma fatality rates over time, including improved computed tomography (CT) and magnetic resonance imaging (MRI), minimally invasive surgical and interventional techniques, abbreviated (damage control) operations, advancements in resuscitation, and regionalization of trauma care.

INITIAL ASSESSMENT

Advanced Trauma Life Support (ATLS) remains the gold standard approach for providing care to injured patients. It offers an invaluable framework for prioritizing patient management, focusing on the (1) primary survey, (2) resuscitation, (3) secondary survey, and (4) definitive care.

Primary Survey

The primary survey is focused on the identification and immediate treatment of life-threatening injuries while initiating resuscitation. It is described by the acronym ABCDE. The **A**irway is assessed for patency and stability. Next, **B**reathing and **C**irculation are evaluated. **D**isability is determined by the overall assessment of the neurologic status. Finally, **E**xposure is a complete examination of the entire external anatomy for additional injuries and/or hemorrhage. Injuries identified at each step are treated before moving on to the next.

Airway

If a patient lacks a patent airway, respiratory gas exchange cannot occur and death becomes imminent. Airway patency is assessed by asking the patient to speak. Normal voice and speech indicate patent airway and intact cognition. Stridor, hoarseness, or pain when speaking, as well as cyanosis, agitation, or tachypnea are concerning signs for possible airway injury. Complex facial fractures, massive tissue disruption of the chest, oropharyngeal swelling, and blood in the oropharynx can quickly obstruct the airway and should prompt immediate intervention to stabilize and protect the airway.

An upward chin tip (chin lift) and pulling the mandible anteriorly (jaw thrust) while maintaining c-spine immobilization are two simple maneuvers that may reopen the airway and assure oxygenation and ventilation. In an obtunded patient, the tongue may partially or completely obstruct the glottis, and so insertion of a nasal or oral airway can promptly reestablish a patent airway. Nasopharyngeal devices are better tolerated in the conscious patient but should not be used in the presence of midface injuries. The most definitive approach to secure the airway is endotracheal intubation. This procedure requires skill and experience and involves passing an endotracheal tube with an inflatable cuff through the mouth and vocal cords into the trachea. Rapid sequence intubation with a sedative (etomidate) and paralytic (succinylcholine) agent is utilized to reduce the risk of pulmonary aspiration in patients with depressed consciousness or a prominent gag reflex.

If the glottis cannot be intubated orally, a surgical airway must be performed. This can be achieved by performing a cricothyroidotomy or placement of a large-bore needle. Figure 7-1 illustrates the incision used for an open cricothyroidotomy. Once the cricothyroid membrane is opened, a 6F or smaller endotracheal tube is placed directly into the trachea. The needle cricothyroidotomy is quicker to perform than the open approach but is less stable and provides limited airflow. A large-bore (16-18 gauge) intravenous (IV) catheter is passed directly through the cricothyroid membrane.

Breathing

Breathing is assessed by inspecting and palpating the chest for symmetric movement and auscultating for breath sounds with a stethoscope, along with pulse oximetry monitoring. Cyanosis and poor oxygen saturation may indicate inadequate ventilation. A tension pneumothorax can result from lung injury. Air from the lung enters the pleural space, and intrapleural pressure increases with each respiration. As the pressure rises, the mediastinum (heart) shifts to the contralateral side and impedes venous return. This decreases preload and cardiac output, resulting in obstructive shock. On physical examination, the combination of absent breath sounds and shock indicates tension pneumothorax until proven otherwise. Late findings may include jugular venous distension or tracheal deviation. Immediate treatment is directed at decompressing the intrapleural hypertension with a needle thoracostomy. This is accomplished by placing a large-bore angiocatheter into the second intercostal space at the midclavicular line and then inserting a chest tube at the anterior or mid-axillary line in the fourth or fifth intercostal space.

Circulation

The evaluation of the circulation focuses on prompt recognition and reversal of shock through intervention and resuscitation. Shock is defined as inadequate tissue perfusion resulting in anaerobic metabolism, and prolonged tissue hypoxia causes organ dysfunction, irreversible tissue damage, and, eventually, death. Tachycardia, tachypnea, hypotension, mental status change, agitation, anxiety, and oliguria are common signs and symptoms of shock.

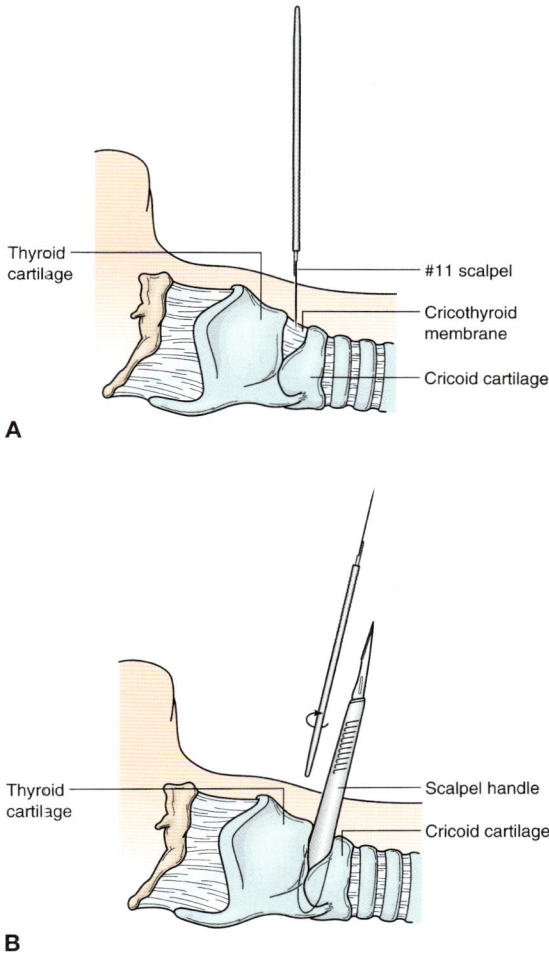

A

B

Figure 7-1. Open cricothyroidotomy. A. A 2-cm transverse incision is made through the skin, subcutaneous tissues, and cricothyroid membrane. B. After the cricothyroid membrane is incised, the handle of the scalpel is inserted and rotated 90° to facilitate insertion of a size 6 cuffed endotracheal tube.

Additional signs include cool, clammy, or cyanotic skin and diminished peripheral pulses.

The most common cause of shock after injury is hemorrhage. Treatment involves restoration of circulating blood volume, initially with boluses of an isotonic crystalloid solution such as lactated Ringer solution or normal saline. In severe shock, transfusion of blood products in a 1:1:1 ratio including packed red blood cells, plasma, and platelets (balanced resuscitation) should be initiated. The severity of hemorrhagic shock is classified according to the percentage of circulating blood volume loss (Table 7-1). While external bleeding from traumatic extremity wounds may be controlled temporarily with direct pressure or a tourniquet, intrathoracic or intra-abdominal hemorrhage may require more invasive measures, such as tube thoracostomy, surgical intervention, or angiography with embolization. Other less common causes of shock include cardiogenic, obstructive (tension pneumothorax and cardiac tamponade), and neurogenic (spinal cord injury).

Disability

A quick assessment of neurologic function provides a measure of disability. The Glasgow Coma Scale (GCS) score, based on the patient's best verbal, motor, and eye-opening responses, is calculated and guides subsequent evaluation and treatment (Table 7-2).

Exposure

The last step in the primary survey is removal of all clothing to allow a complete head-to-toe examination for injury or bleeding. Removing wet and contaminated clothing is important to prevent hypothermia and toxicity. Once completed, the patient should be covered with warm linens and/or heating devices to prevent hypothermia, which exacerbates coagulopathy and worsens acidosis.

Adjunctive Studies and Resuscitation

The results of the primary survey determine the need for further diagnostic studies. Radiographs of the chest, cervical spine, and pelvis assist with the identification of potentially life-threatening injuries. Ultrasonography (FAST [focused assessment with sonography for trauma]) of the abdomen is performed in patients who are hemodynamically unstable sustaining blunt injury to detect intraperitoneal hemorrhage. A nasogastric (NG) tube should be placed to relieve gastric distension. The tube should not be placed nasally when there is a basilar skull fracture or extensive facial fractures. A urinary catheter is a useful adjunct to monitor urine output and may help diagnose bladder injury. Blood at the penile meatus and/or a disruption of the pubic symphysis, which is seen with some pelvic fractures, are signs of urethral transection. If present, retrograde urethrography (RUG) should be performed to assess the integrity of the urethra. In the event of a urethral disruption, suprapubic catheterization should be performed.

Secondary Survey

The purpose of the secondary survey is to identify and treat additional injuries not recognized during the primary survey; it includes a comprehensive physical examination and, where possible, a medical history, including allergies, last meal, tetanus immunization status, and medications.

HEAD INJURY

Traumatic brain injuries (TBIs) are the leading cause of trauma-related mortality and long-term disability. Although primary injury to the brain (incurred at the moment of impact) is difficult to treat, propagation of the injury (secondary injury) can be prevented or limited with proper treatment. Hypotension is the most common cause of secondary brain injury.

Anatomy and Physiology

Anatomic features contribute to certain patterns of injury to the head. Lacerations are common injuries that may involve the skin, subcutaneous fat, and galea aponeurotica. Blunt force may result in a contusion and/or hematoma of the scalp without violation of the skin. Blood vessels held securely by the subcutaneous connective tissue cannot retract when severed and result in significant hemorrhage. In

TABLE 7-1. Classification of Hemorrhage

	Class I	Class II	Class III	Class IV
Blood loss (mL) 70-kg person	<750	750-1,500	1,500-2,000	>2,000
Blood volume loss (%)	<15	15-30	30-40	>40
Heart rate (beats/min)	<100	>100	>120	>140
Blood pressure	Normal	Normal	Decreased	Decreased
Pulse pressure	Normal	Decreased	Decreased	Decreased
Respiratory rate (breaths/min)	14-20	20-30	30-40	>35
Urine output (mL/h)	>30	20-30	5-15	Negligible
Capillary refill (s)	Normal	>2	>2	>2
Mental status	Slight anxiety	Mild anxiety	Anxious/confused	Confused/lethargic
Fluid management	Crystalloid	Crystalloid	Crystalloid and blood	Crystalloid and blood

addition, muscles attached to the galea aponeurotica contract in opposite directions, which may hold the wound and vessel lumen open and increase bleeding.

Within the cranium, the dura mater is a thick, dense fibrous layer that encloses the brain and spinal cord. It

TABLE 7-2. Glasgow Coma Scale

Assessment Area	Score
Eye opening (E)	
Spontaneous	4
To speech	3
To pain	2
None	1
Motor response (M)	
Obeys commands	6
Localizes pain	5
Withdraws to pain	4
Decorticate posturing (abnormal flexion)	3
Decerebrate posturing (abnormal extension)	2
None (flaccid)	1
Verbal response (V)	
Oriented	5
Confused conversation	4
Inappropriate words	3
Incomprehensible sounds	2
None	1

Glasgow Coma Scale (GCS) score = $E + M + V$; best = 15, worst = 3.

forms the dural venous sinuses, diaphragma sellae, falx cerebri, falx cerebelli, and tentorium cerebelli. Cerebral venous blood flows into the dural sinuses through bridging veins, which can be torn when blunt force is applied to the head, resulting in a subdural hemorrhage. The meningeal artery lies between the skull and the dura. Fractures of the temporal and parietal bones of the cranial vault can lacerate these arteries and cause an epidural hematoma. The vascular pia directly covers the brain. Injuries to the blood vessels of the pia as well as the underlying brain can cause subarachnoid hemorrhage or intraparenchymal contusion.

The skull and vertebral bodies of the spine function as a rigid, bony case, which contains the spinal cord, cerebrospinal fluid (CSF), and blood. Increased intracranial pressure (ICP) due to bleeding or edema can alter the cerebral blood flow (CBF) or compress the brain and adjacent structures. Because the volume within the skull is fixed, an increase in volume of one of the three tissues may elevate ICP. When the ICP exceeds 20 mm Hg, decreased CBF may result in ischemia.

Besides ICP, CBF is affected by cerebral vascular resistance (CVR) and cerebral perfusion pressure (CPP). CPP is the difference between the mean arterial pressure (MAP) and ICP. As flow equals the change in pressure divided by resistance ($Q = \Delta P/r$), CBF equals perfusion divided by resistance (CBF = CPP/CVR). Under normal circumstances, CBF remains constant over a wide range of CPP by alterations in vascular resistance known as *autoregulation*. This autoregulation can be impaired or lost after brain injury. As ICP rises, the cardiovascular system maintains CPP by increasing the MAP. This early response to increased ICP is associated with bradycardia and a decreased respiratory rate, known as the *Cushing reflex*. Continued elevation of the ICP may eventually result in herniation and brain death.

The tentorium cerebelli is a stiff and unyielding membrane dividing the hemispheres from the cerebellum. The brainstem passes through this tentorium. Any increased pressure within the cranium pushes the brain past the tentcrium and compresses adjacent structures, such as the oculomotor nerve, resulting in dilated and immobile (fixed) ipsilateral pupil. As the ICP continues to increase, herniation progresses, resulting in the corticospinal (pyramidal) tract in the cerebral peduncle being compressed. This results in contralateral spastic weakness and a positive Babinski sign. With further increase in the ICP, the brainstem is compressed against the tentorium, causing dysfunction of the cardiorespiratory centers in the medulla. The associated hypertension and bradycardia that follow usually signal impending brain herniation.

Clinical Evaluation

Assessment of the neurologic system begins during the primary survey and includes pertinent injury details such as loss of consciousness, seizure activity, postinjury alertness, and extremity motor function. A complete neurologic examination focuses on the level of consciousness, pupillary function, sensation, and presence of lateralizing extremity weakness. The assessment is frequently repeated to detect and document changes. It should be noted that hypotension in patients with head injury indicates blood loss until proven otherwise and should not be attributed to the brain injury.

The GCS score is a widely accepted and reproducible method to quantify a patient's neurologic examination (see Table 7-1). It assigns scores between 3 (worst possible) and 15 (normal) for eye-opening response (E), verbal response (V), and motor response (M). The score quantitates the severity of the head injury and is used as a prognostic indicator of outcome. Score of 3 or 4 is associated with combined mortality or vegetative state nearing 97%. Mortality rates approach 65% with a score of 5 or 6 and 28% with a score of 7 or 8. Multiple factors unrelated to the head injury may affect the GCS score, such as sedatives, shock, alcohol consumption, and recreational drug use.

Other signs of head injury are identified during the secondary survey. Some scalp lacerations are obvious, but others may be hidden by hair. Bony step-offs, indicative of a skull fracture, may be palpated. Periorbital ecchymoses (raccoon eyes), perimastoid ecchymosis (Battle sign), hemotympanum, and leakage of CSF from the nose (rhinorrhea) or ear (otorrhea) are all signs of a basilar skull fracture.

Intracranial injury is diagnosed by obtaining a noncontrast head CT (Figures 7-2 to 7-4). This imaging modality allows localization of extra-axial hemorrhage, brain swelling, midline shift, hydrocephalus, and skull fractures. Although recognizing a skull fracture is important, diagnosing the underlying brain injury is more consequential. Brain injuries can occur with or without skull fractures and vice versa. Concomitant cervical spine injury occurs in up to 15% of patients with head injury. Thus, radiologic evaluation of the cervical spine should occur at the time of brain imaging.

Management of Head Injuries

TBI management should focus on minimizing increases in ICP, which may worsen the initial insult.

A ventricular catheter placed into the lateral ventricle of the brain through a burr hole allows continuous ICP monitoring as well as drainage of CSF to reduce ICP. A pressure monitor can be placed within the subarachnoid

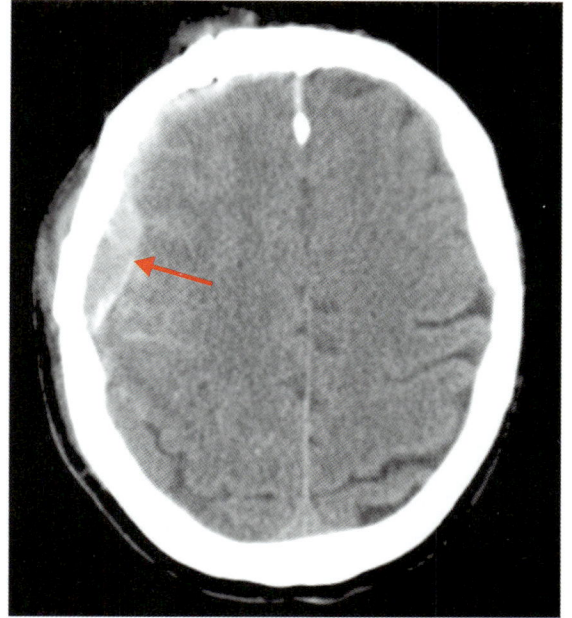

Figure 7-2. Epidural hematoma. A convex or lens-shaped (arrow) collection of blood is typical.

space when drainage is not desired or when the ventricles cannot be cannulated. Other monitoring techniques involve placement of a fiberoptic transducer into the epidural space, subdural space, or lateral ventricle as well as the use of probes that detect brain tissue oxygen levels, often in combination with ICP monitoring.

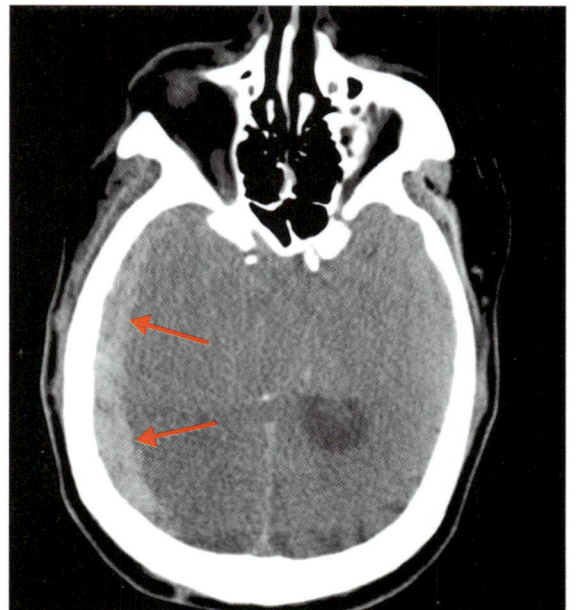

Figure 7-3. Acute subdural hemorrhage. High-density blood is present in a crescentic or concave shape (arrows) along the right cerebral hemisphere.

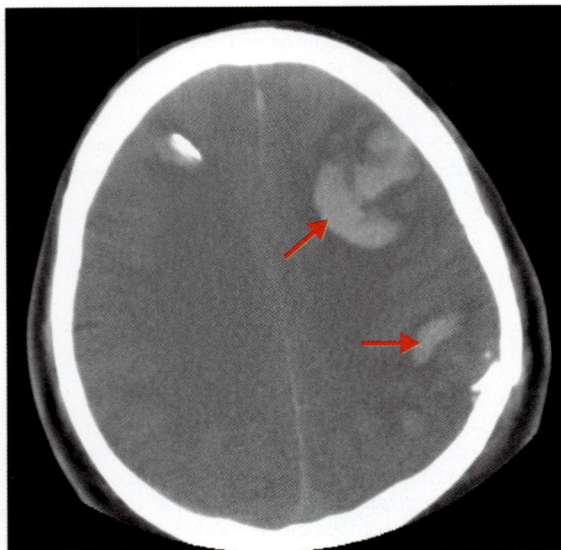

Figure 7-4. Traumatic subarachnoid hemorrhage with intra-parenchymal cerebral contusions. Multiple foci of acute hemorrhage (arrows) are noted within the left cerebral hemisphere.

Additional interventions to regulate ICP include maintaining the neck in a neutral position, head elevation, sedation, hypertonic saline, IV fluid limitation, and mannitol. Sedation reduces posturing and combative behavior as well as the metabolic demand of brain tissue. Moderate hyperventilation to a $PaCO_2$ of 32 to 35 mm Hg transiently lowers ICP but may worsen cerebral ischemia and is only used when there is an acute increase in ICP.

IV fluids are administered judiciously to ensure adequate cardiac output. Mannitol is a free-radical scavenger and osmotic diuretic that effectively reduces brain swelling and lowers ICP. However, it may cause hypotension in patients with hemorrhage. Hypertonic saline solutions may be administered IV to decrease brain swelling and maintain euvolemia. Patients with TBI should be closely observed for seizures and receive prophylaxis and/or treatment with anticonvulsants and antiepileptic medications.

Operative management of TBI continues to evolve. Epidural hematomas generally require surgical evacuation when large or associated with decreasing mental status. Prognosis is very good with prompt treatment. Subdural hematomas causing significant mass effects require emergent evacuation, but prognosis is more guarded and outcome is based on the degree of injury to the underlying brain parenchyma. Subarachnoid hemorrhage and diffuse axonal injury (DAI) are mostly managed nonoperatively. Prognosis is variable and is dependent on the severity of injury. Full recovery may take months or years.

Finally, even with isolated TBI, the body as a whole must be supported. Early enteral nutrition is an important adjunct once the initial resuscitation of a patient with brain injury has concluded. The best possible TBI outcome is achieved with attention to ICP control while meeting the body's underlying metabolic demands.

INJURIES OF THE SPINE AND SPINAL CORD

Blunt force trauma to the torso frequently results in injury to the vertebral column and may occur with or without overt neurologic compromise at the time of initial presentation. Since the cervical spine is the most frequent site of spinal injury, immobilization with a hard collar is warranted to protect against further injury until the spine is evaluated clinically and with radiologic imaging. The use of long backboards for thoracic and lumbar spinal "protection" is no longer recommended because of the high incidence of pressure injury (decubitus ulcer) as a result of prolonged immobilization.

The internal spinal canal space is wide in the higher spine but has more soft tissue elements packed in its confines. The canal narrows as it traverses down but the volume of nerve occupying that space decreases as nerve roots exit, making the lower cervical and highest upper thoracic canal the most likely to have spinal cord injury even without bony fracture present. The thoracic spinal column is stabilized and buttressed by the ribs, making it far less mobile and reducing the probability of injury. Approximately 15% of injuries occur at the thoracolumbar junction because of the transition from stabilized, inflexible thoracic spine to the more flexible lumbar spinal elements. In adults, the spinal cord ends at the level of the first lumbar vertebral body becoming the cauda equina. The cauda equina is more mobile and has a larger space to occupy in the lumbar vertebral ring. Thus, it is less likely to be injured with fractures involving the distal lumbar vertebral bodies.

Fracture of a vertebral body may not initially present with neurologic deficits because of intoxication, altered mental status, or coma with paralysis. A patient may sustain a bony fracture, dislocation, ligamentous injury, or even spinal cord injury without any radiographic abnormality (SCIWORA). These patients should initially be maintained in spine precautions until it is determined that the injury is stable or unstable. Any life-threatening injuries should be addressed first while the spine is protected from movement. This includes the use of a cervical collar. Moderate or severe head injury eliminates clinical examination of the cervical spine. Thus, a cervical collar should be maintained until the spine surgeon has determined that it can be removed.

The flexible and relatively exposed cervical spine is usually the most frequent site of injury to the spinal column after blunt trauma. Fractures of a cervical vertebral body account for approximately 50% of all spinal injuries. In adults, the most common level of injury is the fifth cervical vertebra. In contrast, the pediatric (under 8 years) spine is most commonly injured at the second or third cervical vertebral level. Since the phrenic nerve is composed of fibers originating from the C3 to C5 spinal nerves, it is more common to see impaired diaphragmatic function in children with a cervical spine injury when compared with adults. Blunt injury to the spinal column and spinal cord may occur with flexion, extension, rotation, or axial loading. Shallow water diving injuries frequently result in permanent paralysis in young adults because of fractures from axial loading on the cervical spine. In adults, the proximal spinal cord (C1-C4) only occupies 50% of the spinal canal space. It is important to remember that a patient with an unstable injury involving the proximal cervical spine may not have a cord injury initially until interventions such as intubation without spinal stabilization, allowing displacement of the unstable injury. Symptoms and clinical findings after a penetrating injury to the bony spine or spinal cord will typically have obvious signs of injury. Delayed presentation of neurologic findings is rare after penetrating injury and may result from a contusive force without direct injury to the cord. Patients involved with high energy blunt force that results in a cervical fracture may have another noncontiguous fracture of the spinal column. The reported incidence ranges from 5% to 30%.

Like head injury, spinal nerve injury consists of primary and secondary injury. Primary injury occurs at the time of traumatic event, while secondary injury is delayed as a result of ischemia due to hypotension and hypoxia. The incidence of primary injury has decreased with improvements in the design of seatbelts and airbags as well as injury prevention programs. Secondary injury is determined by the level of care provided at the accident scene, during transport, and on presentation at the hospital. The incidence of secondary injury is reduced by timely and appropriate early care provided by emergency medical services (EMS), nurses, and physicians. Reduction of unnecessary motion and maintaining adequate perfusion pressure and oxygenation are important first steps to reduce secondary injury during the prehospital and early phases of care.

Initial injury to the spinal cord is classified as partial or complete. A partial injury may deteriorate into a complete injury over time. In contrast, a complete injury presenting with no motor or sensory function below the injury site rarely improves unless proper care protocols are initiated early and maintained. During the secondary survey, the physical examination includes palpation of the entire spine looking for swelling, masses, crepitus, tenderness, or deformity. Gross motor and sensory function should be assessed using light touch or pin prick. In the awake patient, it is recommended that the examination start by evaluating the nerve roots distal to the obvious level of injury and then move cephalad. Beginning the examination at the insensate level and moving to the level of sensation allows for a precise diagnosis of the level of injury. Key sensory dermatome levels include C5 (deltoid), T4 (nipple), and T10 (umbilicus). Reflexes and motor function should be assessed for strength and symmetry. Extremity muscle groups are innervated by identifiable spinal segments, making it possible to pinpoint the precise level of cord injury (Table 7-3).

Injuries at the C5 level and above may result in phrenic nerve dysfunction characterized by abdominal breathing, inability to inhale deeply, and progressive respiratory insufficiency. As noted previously, the phrenic nerve originates in the C3, C4, and C5 nerve roots. Patients exhibiting these symptoms should be considered for endotracheal intubation during the primary survey.

Injuries to the cervical spine, and occasionally the upper thoracic spine, can disrupt the sympathetic chain, resulting in neurogenic shock due to loss of precapillary sphincter tone. Impaired peripheral sympathetic tone coupled with an intact parasympathetic tone may result in vasodilation causing hypotension. The blood volume of a 70-kg adult is 5 L, but with neurogenic shock, it can increase to 15 L and result in hypotension, ischemia, and peripheral organ damage. Initial supportive treatment consists of aggressive fluid resuscitation to increase the effective circulating volume. If hypotension persists, addition of vasopressors and/or inotropes should be considered. While hypotension in patients with trauma is considered blood loss until proven otherwise, proximal spinal cord injuries can cause hypotension in the absence of hemorrhage. Hypotension with associated bradyarrhythmia is often the best sign to differentiate neurogenic from hemorrhagic shock. Other signs of neurogenic shock may include tetraplegia and warm extremities. In contrast, hemorrhagic shock manifests with tachycardia and pale, cool extremities.

When the initial and subsequent treatment are optimized, an incomplete cord injury has a better prognosis for recovery. Incomplete cord injuries include central cord syndrome, anterior cord syndrome, and Brown-Séquard syndrome (hemi-transection). Central cord syndrome is

TABLE 7-3. Segmental Motor Innervation by the Spinal Cord

Motor Function	Muscle Groups	Spinal Cord Segments
Shoulder extension	Deltoid	C5
Elbow flexion	Biceps brachii, brachialis	C5, C6
Wrist extension	Extensor carpi radialis longus and brevis	C6, C7
Elbow extension	Triceps brachii	C7, C8
Finger flexion	Flexor digitorum profundus and superficialis	C8
Finger abduction/adduction	Interossei	C8, T1
Thigh adduction	Adductor longus and brevis	L2, L3
Knee extension	Quadriceps	L3, L4
Ankle dorsiflexion	Tibialis anterior	L4, L5
First toe extension	Extensor hallucis longus	L5, S1
Ankle plantar flexion	Gastrocnemius, soleus	S1, S2

the most common, presenting with weakness in the upper versus lower extremities as a result of injury due to cervical hyperextension in the presence of preexisting canal stenosis. It is more common in older adults with osteoarthritis.

Nerve injury without cervical or thoracic bony fracture may occur but is more often seen in children or older patients and is termed *spinal cord injury without any radiographic abnormality*. This is usually a result of ligamentous injury or hyperextension injury, resulting in cord contusion or stretch. Central cord syndrome is an adult variant of SCIWORA. The concept of SCIWORA was developed before the widespread availability of CT or MRI when plain radiographs of the spinal column were standard. Plain films of the spinal column can miss up to 20% of bony injuries, especially in the lower cervical and upper thoracic regions. Many patients thought to have SCIWORA will have evidence of injury on CT or MRI. CT of the cervical spine is considered the "gold standard" for spine imaging. Three-dimensional CT reconstruction of the spinal column increases the diagnostic yield and can be done without increasing the original radiation dose.

Assessment of ligamentous injury, spinal cord contusion, epidural hematoma, and herniated discs is usually performed with MRI. This imaging requires a hemodynamically stable and cooperative patient. The additional information provided by MRI aids in treatment and management, thus improving overall outcomes.

Clinical clearance of the cervical spine may be performed during the secondary survey but should be delayed in unstable patients. Established protocols (Nexus, Canadian C-spine Rule) may allow for reliable evaluation of the cervical spine and safe removal of the cervical collar without the need for imaging. These protocols require an awake patient free of drugs, alcohol, or pain medications who can follow commands, has no cervical pain or limitation of motion, and has no distracting injuries. Any patient not fulfilling these criteria must have the neck immobilized until further evaluation can be completed. Any noncompliant patient who demands removal of a protective collar must be warned of the risks of paralysis as a potential result of removing the collar.

THORACIC INJURY

Thoracic trauma accounts for approximately 25% of trauma-related deaths and follows TBI as the second most common cause of death after injury. Life-threatening chest injuries may be fatal if not promptly diagnosed and treated, including tension pneumothorax, open pneumothorax, cardiac tamponade, massive hemothorax, and flail chest. The majority of thoracic injuries can be treated nonoperatively by maneuvers, such as establishing a definitive airway or tube thoracostomy. Only 10% to 15% of thoracic injuries require formal operative intervention via median sternotomy or thoracotomy. The principles of ATLS provide a stepwise framework for diagnosing life-threatening injuries and those that may cause morbidity and mortality if diagnosis is significantly delayed.

Life-Threatening Injuries Detected During Primary Survey

Tension pneumothorax results from gas accumulation under pressure within the pleural cavity. It may occur after blunt or penetrating thoracic trauma. Open pneumothorax occurs in the setting of a penetrating injury to the thorax when the chest wall wound remains patent. This allows air to preferentially enter through the chest wall defect rather than the trachea, resulting in collapse of the underlying lung. Clinically, the passage of air through the chest wound results in an audible "sucking" sound. Respiratory failure may occur as the work of breathing increases because airflow via the wound prevents the generation of adequate negative inspiratory force to entrain air via the tracheobronchial tree. In the prehospital setting, open pneumothorax may be treated by placing a partially occlusive dressing over the thoracic wound and securing it to the skin with tape on three sides. This creates a one-way valve that allows egress of accumulated pleural gas during exhalation but prevents inflow from the atmosphere during inhalation. The result is partial reexpansion of the lung and an improvement in gas exchange. In effect, this maneuver converts an open pneumothorax into a simple pneumothorax. Upon arrival to a hospital, a chest tube must be inserted through a separate incision to allow for complete reexpansion of the lung. Operative debridement and closure of the wound may be required.

Cardiac tamponade is an immediately life-threatening event that may occur after penetrating or blunt precordial injury. The most common scenario is a stab wound along the left sternal border with laceration of the right ventricle. Blood escaping from the heart accumulates within the nondistensible pericardial space, resulting in compromise of right ventricular relaxation during diastole and tamponade. The triad of muffled heart sounds, jugular venous distension, and hypotension (Beck triad) in a patient with a penetrating wound to the precordium is the classic presentation for cardiac tamponade. Other physical findings may include Kussmaul sign (increasing jugular vein distension [JVD] with inspiration) and pulsus paradoxus (drop in systolic blood pressure [BP] ≥ 10 mm Hg during inspiration). However, these findings are quite variable, and their absence does not preclude the presence of tamponade. Diagnosis is confirmed by ultrasound, usually FAST, which is the diagnostic test for hemopericardium and tamponade (Figure 7-5). Treatment of tamponade includes volume resuscitation to increase

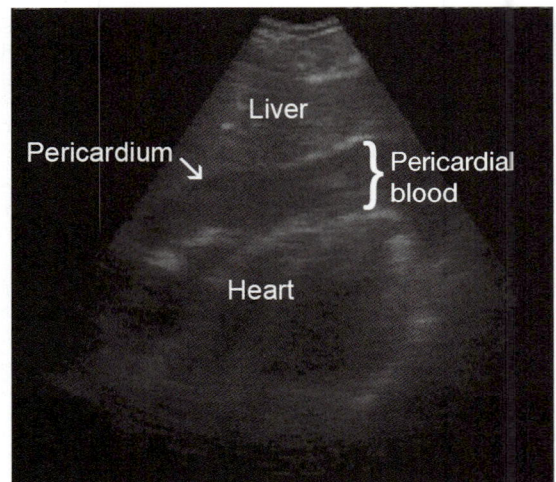

Figure 7-5. Penetrating cardiac injury with hemopericardium visualized on bedside ultrasound. Note the large amount of blood outside the heart within the pericardial sac.

cardiac output and immediate surgical decompression to release the tamponade and repair the underlying cardiac injury. In patients with cardiac tamponade who experience cardiac arrest in the resuscitation area, prompt emergency department (ED) resuscitative thoracotomy should be performed. Pericardiocentesis may be considered in situations where resuscitative thoracotomy and pericardial window in the operating room are not options due to surgeon inexperience or lack of necessary equipment, though salvage rates are extremely low with this approach.

Massive hemothorax is defined as loss of 1,500 mL or more of blood into the pleural space during the first hour after injury, or ongoing blood loss of 200 mL/h of blood over 4 hours. The source of bleeding is most frequently intercostal vessels, but lacerated lung parenchyma, intercostal muscles, great vessels, or atrial injuries may contribute to ongoing bleeding. Clinical diagnosis may reveal diminished breath sounds and dullness to percussion. These physical findings may be difficult to determine in a noisy ED. Chest x-ray or ultrasound may confirm the presence of hemothorax. Initial treatment involves tube thoracostomy (Figure 7-6) and volume resuscitation to restore euvolemia. Operative control of hemorrhage is indicated for hemodynamically stable patients with the abovementioned criteria. Emergent thoracotomy is also indicated when intrathoracic hemorrhage is the cause of hemodynamically instability, regardless of the amount of chest tube drainage. Autotransfusion of shed blood may be a useful adjunct to decrease utilization of banked blood products. Postprocedural x-rays should be obtained to confirm satisfactory evacuation of the hemothorax and tube location. Retained hemothorax should be treated by early thoracoscopic evacuation, usually within 5 days, as the risk of infection (empyema) or entrapped lung increases significantly after this time frame, particularly in older patients.

Flail chest occurs when two or more contiguous ribs are fractured in two or more places. This creates an unstable segment of the chest wall that moves out of phase during spontaneous (negative pressure) respiration. It can be recognized on inspection by the paradoxical movement of the flail segment. Treatment may require positive pressure ventilation, including mechanical ventilation. Operative stabilization of the flail segment with rib plating reduces morbidity in select patients. Pulmonary contusion is commonly associated with flail chest. The underlying contusion results in ventilation-perfusion mismatch and is the primary cause of hypoxia and hypercarbia seen with flail chest. Pulmonary contusion, coupled with pain from fractured ribs, impairs respiratory function. Treatment involves aggressive pain control measures, as well as tube thoracostomy for an associated pneumothorax or hemothorax. Patients who develop respiratory failure require intubation with mechanical ventilation. IV fluids should be administered judiciously because aggressive hydration is associated with sequestering of fluid in the contused lung, which may increase ventilation-perfusion mismatch and exacerbate hypoxia and hypercarbia.

Potentially Severe Injuries Detected During Secondary Survey

Simple pneumothorax occurs when gas enters the pleural space, causing partial or complete collapse of the ipsilateral lung. Gas may be introduced from the atmosphere in a

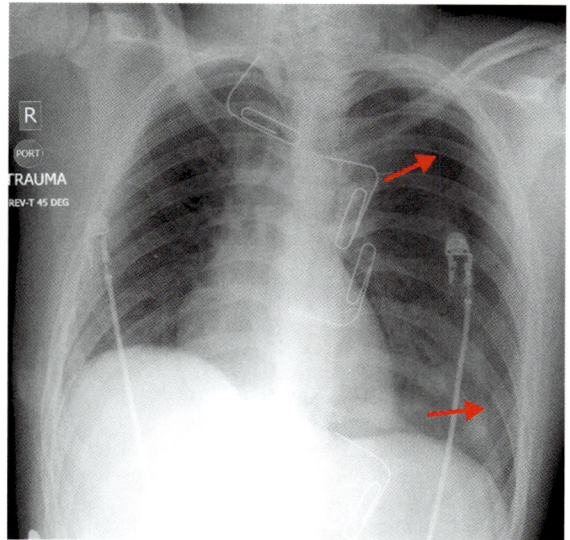

A

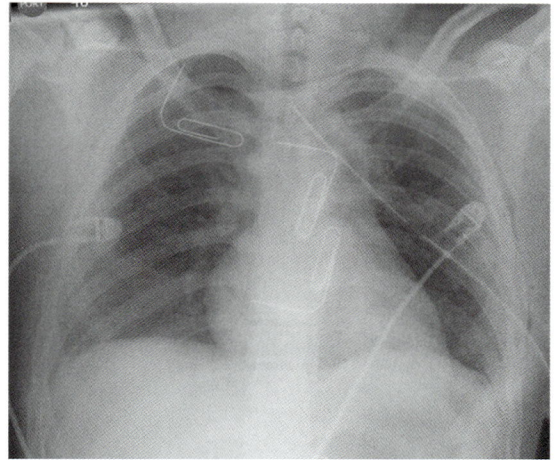

B

Figure 7-6. Left pneumothorax after penetrating chest injury. A. Lung markings are absent along the periphery of the left hemithorax, lateral to border of collapsed lung (red arrows). B. After insertion of a left chest tube, the lung has reexpanded.

penetrating injury, or it may emanate from an injury to the lung parenchyma or tracheobronchial tree. Physical examination typically reveals diminished breath sounds on the affected side, though this finding is variable in the noisy environment of the trauma resuscitation area. Hyperresonance to percussion may be present. Diagnosis is made by plain radiography of the chest or bedside ultrasound. Posttraumatic pneumothorax visible on plain radiography of the chest requires tube thoracostomy for reexpansion of the lung. Narrow-bore (pigtail) chest catheters may be considered as well. Pneumothorax seen on CT, but not on plain film, requires close observation but often does not necessitate chest tube placement. Positive pressure ventilation may result in tension pneumothorax in patients with small CT-diagnosed pneumothoraces, so chest tube placement should be considered before mechanical ventilation.

Blunt aortic injury (BAI) is a relatively uncommon but potentially lethal injury associated with rapid deceleration mechanisms, including motor vehicle collisions and falls from heights. BAI most often results from a shearing force that occurs at the junction of the mobile aortic arch with the immobile descending aorta in the posterior mediastinum. Direct compression of the aorta may play a role as well. Full-thickness aortic rupture results in rapid exsanguination and death at the scene. In survivors, the rupture is typically contained by the adventitial layers of the aorta. Intimal flaps or pseudoaneurysms may develop as well. BAI is suggested by mediastinal widening (>8 cm) seen on chest x-ray. Additional radiographic signs associated with BAI include apical capping, loss of normal aortic contour, depression of the left mainstem bronchus, loss of the paratracheal stripe, obliteration of the aortopulmonary window, NG tube deviation, left hemothorax, and fractures of the first or second ribs (Figure 7-7). However, the absence of these findings does not rule out aortic injury, and patients with a concerning mechanism of injury should undergo contrast-enhanced CT angiography (Figure 7-8). Left untreated, a significant number of aortic injuries can progress to free rupture and death. Endovascular techniques (transcatheter aortic valve replacement or TVAR) have replaced open repair via a left posterolateral thoracotomy. Paraplegia may result when the stent graft occludes the intercostal vessels, resulting in spinal cord ischemia. Occasionally, aortic repair must be delayed because of other life-threatening injuries or comorbidities. In such cases, aggressive BP control is necessary to decrease the risk of free aortic rupture.

Rib fractures are the most common thoracic injury after blunt trauma. Fractured ribs are diagnosed on physical examination by noting point tenderness along a rib. They may or may not be seen on chest x-ray. CT of the thorax is more sensitive for diagnosing rib fractures but is not required to make the diagnosis. The location of fractured ribs also helps identify associated injuries. Fractures of the first three ribs are associated with aortic or great vessel injury. Fractures of the mid-thoracic ribs are frequently associated with pulmonary contusion and/or hemopneumothorax. Lower rib fractures are associated with diaphragmatic,

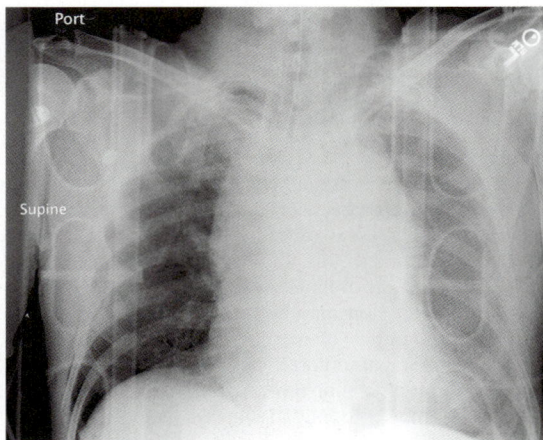

Figure 7-8. Chest computed tomography in a patient with blunt aortic injury. Blood is present within the mediastinum (white arrow), and a pseudoaneurysm of the descending aorta is depicted by the red arrow.

liver, and spleen injuries. Rib fracture management consists of providing adequate (multimodal) analgesia to allow for oxygenation, ventilation, and clearance of secretions. Young healthy patients with one or two rib fractures and adequate tidal volumes may be safely managed with oral analgesics and discharged from the ED. Older patients, or those with multiple rib fractures, generally require inpatient admission for pain control. IV patient-controlled analgesia and thoracic epidural catheterization are options that provide effective analgesia and avoid intubation. The goal of treatment is to avoid splinting from pain, which impairs secretion clearance and which may result in atelectasis and subsequent pneumonia. Older patients with multiple rib fractures have worse outcomes and often require admission to a critical care setting.

Emergency Department Thoracotomy

Patients presenting to the ED in profound shock or in pulseless electrical activity may not respond to cardiopulmonary resuscitation (CPR) and volume resuscitation. In select cases, resuscitative left anterolateral thoracotomy may be beneficial and is considered a lifesaving maneuver. Resuscitative thoracotomy allows several goals to be accomplished quickly, including pericardiotomy for release of cardiac tamponade, open cardiac massage (which is superior to closed chest compression to restore perfusion, particularly in hypovolemia), cross-clamping of the descending aorta at the diaphragm, intracardiac administration of resuscitative drugs, direct control of intrathoracic hemorrhage, and potential relief of air embolism. This procedure should be considered in penetrating trauma survivors who lose vital signs less than 15 minutes before arrival or in the ED. Patients with pericardial tamponade and cardiac arrest are candidates for ED thoracotomy as well. In contrast, patients with prolonged cardiac arrest after penetrating injury, massive blunt trauma with prehospital cardiac arrest and pulseless electrical activity do not benefit from ED thoracotomy. Resuscitative thoracotomy should not be performed unless a surgeon capable of managing complex truncal injuries is immediately available. The survival rate for ED thoracotomy is highest with knife injuries to the right heart or atrium, but still only ranges from 1% to 10% in most studies. Resuscitative endovascular balloon occlusion of the aorta (REBOA) is a novel alternative to resuscitative

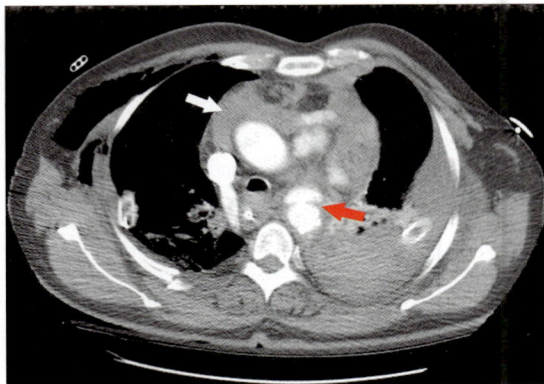

Figure 7-7. Chest x-ray in a patient with blunt aortic injury. The mediastinum is markedly widened, the aortic contour is abnormal, a left apical cap is present, the trachea is deviated toward the right, upper rib fractures are present, and a left hemothorax is noted.

thoracotomy in patients with exsanguinating hemorrhage below the diaphragm, but it is a temporizing measure that eventually requires definitive surgical control.

ABDOMINAL INJURY

Background

Abdominal trauma results from penetrating wounds or blunt force. Penetrating injuries can occur with low energy stab wounds and high energy gunshot wounds. Blunt traumatic injury occurs after falls, assaults, crush injuries, and motor vehicle collisions.

Unexplained hypotension in an injured patient requires immediate consideration of intra-abdominal injury. Life-threatening intra-abdominal hemorrhage is a common source of shock that must be considered during the primary survey. Rapid diagnosis and treatment of intra-abdominal hemorrhage is critical.

Anatomic Considerations

The torso is divided into several regions (Figure 7-9). The *flank* is defined as the region between the anterior and posterior axillary lines, the lower ribs, and the iliac crest. The back is bounded by the spinous processes, the posterior axillary line, the lower ribs, and the iliac bone. Injuries to any of these areas can involve the peritoneal cavity and/or retroperitoneum. The abdominal contents are partially protected by the rib cage, the pelvis, and the lumbar spine as well as the abdominal wall musculature. The pancreas, kidneys, bladder, aorta, inferior vena cava (IVC), duodenum, ascending and descending colon, and rectum reside in the retroperitoneum.

The location, volume, and size of these organs affect the injury patterns observed with both blunt and penetrating traumas. For example, penetrating wounds in the third trimester of pregnancy more commonly involve the uterus and/or fetus. The small intestine and mesentery are most frequently injured with penetrating wounds. During rapid deceleration that occurs with motor vehicle collision, the liver and spleen are more mobile relative to hollow viscus organs, resulting in a higher frequency of injury.

Initial Evaluation

The history and mechanism of traumatic injury are important to determine the relative risk and location of injuries. This is frequently provided by prehospital personnel and can be quickly obtained while the patient is being transferred to the gurney. The examination starts with complete exposure and thorough examination of the entire body, including the abdomen, flanks, and back. Identification of old scars, bruising, puncture wounds, lacerations, asymmetry, and distension provide clues for determining underlying organ injury.

Palpation of the abdomen in patients with trauma is essential but may be unreliable due to altered mental status from alcohol, drug use, head injury, or shock. Palpation may reveal focal or diffuse tenderness, signs of peritoneal irritation, distension due to intra-abdominal hemorrhage, and fascial and muscular defects in the abdominal wall. The sensitivity of abdominal palpation to detect intra-abdominal hemorrhage is low. Examination of the pelvis should be performed to identify pelvic bony tenderness or instability. Serial abdominal examinations should be performed to minimize the risk of missed injury. Digital rectal examination should be performed in cases of suspected intra-abdominal trauma or pelvic fracture.

Adjunctive Diagnostic Tools

If there is no evidence of urethral injury or a high-riding prostate on rectal examination, insertion of a urinary catheter can help guide fluid resuscitation and reveal hematuria from renal or bladder injuries. A supine abdominal x-ray of the abdomen and pelvis may be useful to determine the presence and location of bullets or other foreign bodies (Figure 7-10) or to identify unstable pelvic fractures. The

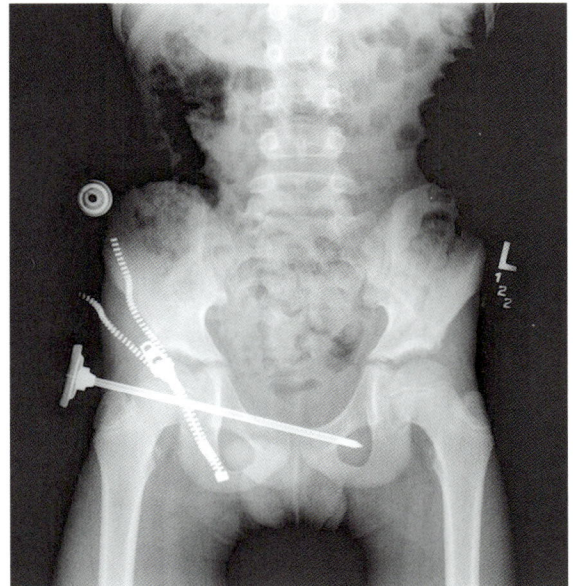

Figure 7-10. Penetrating trauma with impaled foreign body. Plain x-ray revealed trajectory concerning for peritoneal penetration and pelvic organ injury.

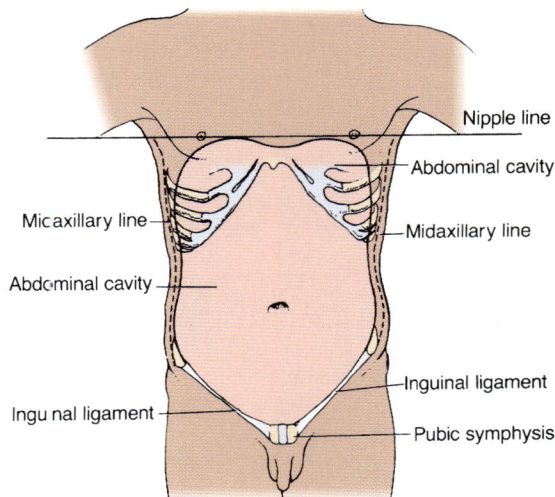

Figure 7-9. Surface landmarks of the abdominal cavity.

Nipple line
Abdominal cavity
Midaxillary line
Midaxillary line
Abdominal cavity
Inguinal ligament
Inguinal ligament
Pubic symphysis

FAST ultrasound examination is quick and easy to perform and has supplanted diagnostic peritoneal lavage to assess for intraperitoneal bleeding. FAST evaluates for free fluid in the abdomen or pericardium using ultrasonographic views of the right and left upper quadrants, pericardium, and pelvis (Figure 7-11). It is accurate under many conditions and may be reliably performed by surgeons, emergency physicians, and radiologists.

Contrast-enhanced CT scanning has transformed the evaluation of abdominal injury and is the gold standard for identifying injuries to intraperitoneal and retroperitoneal organs in hemodynamically stable patients.

Operative Care

A hypotensive victim of blunt abdominal trauma who does not respond to volume resuscitation is considered to have an intra-abdominal source of bleeding until proven otherwise. Spinal cord or neurologic injury can cause hypotension, but uncontrolled intra-abdominal hemorrhage occurs far more frequently. The most common source of hemorrhage is the spleen and/or liver. Rapid surgical management to secure hemostasis is required.

Penetrating wounds with peritonitis require prompt laparotomy, as the incidence of visceral injury is extremely high. Bullets may ricochet and fragment, and one should never assume that skin wounds from penetrating injury connect in a straight line. Hemodynamically stable patients with a penetrating wound in the right upper quadrant or right thoracoabdominal region may be managed nonoperatively with isolated liver injury. In addition, stable patients without peritonitis may have wounds that are limited to the abdominal wall. CT scans can help avoid a nontherapeutic laparotomy. Low-velocity injury to the abdomen from sharp objects should undergo diagnostic laparoscopy or local wound exploration to determine whether the peritoneum or fascia is violated. When present, laparotomy is indicated to manage injuries.

Penetrating flank and back wounds from firearms are managed like other penetrating wounds but may have more extensive injuries due to blast effect. Triple-phase contrast-enhanced CT with oral, IV, and rectal contrast allows for accurate identification of injuries in stable patients. Penetrating

trauma to these regions causes retroperitoneal organ injury more frequently. Any patient with hypotension with a penetrating abdominal, flank, or back wound should undergo emergent exploratory laparotomy to control bleeding.

INJURY TO SPECIFIC ORGANS

Liver

Blunt liver injuries are graded from I to VI in severity. Grade I injuries include small capsular hematomas or parenchymal lacerations less than 1 cm in depth, while grade VI injuries result from avulsion of the liver from its vascular pedicles (Table 7-4). Most low-grade liver injuries are self-limited. CT scan is the diagnostic modality of choice, providing anatomic detail and accurate grading of the injury (Figure 7-12) in the hemodynamically stable patient. Ongoing bleeding with active contrast extravasation seen on CT may require angioembolization. Higher grade liver injuries, including those involving the hepatic veins or retrohepatic IVC, may result in massive hemorrhage requiring emergent operative intervention and damage control surgical techniques, as outlined in a subsequent section.

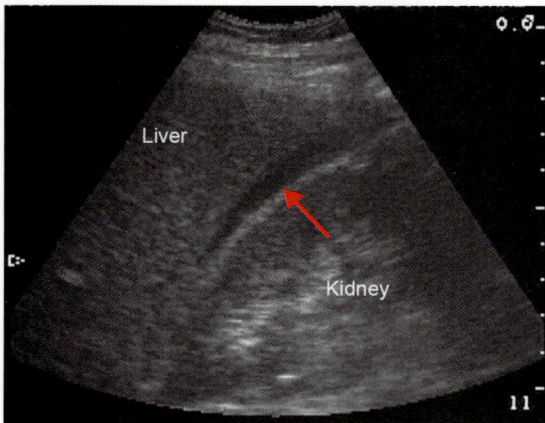

Figure 7-11. Positive FAST examination. Hypoechoic (red arrow) blood is noted in Morison pouch between the liver and the right kidney.

TABLE 7-4. Liver Injury Scale

Grade[a]		Injury Description
I	Hematoma	Subcapsular, nonexpanding, <10% surface area
	Laceration	Capsular tear, nonbleeding, <1 cm in depth
II	Hematoma	Subcapsular, nonexpanding, 10%-50% surface area
		Intraparenchymal, nonexpanding, <10 cm in diameter
	Laceration	Capsular tear, active bleeding; 1-3 cm parenchymal depth, <10 cm in length
III	Hematoma	Subcapsular, >50% surface area or expanding; ruptured subcapsular hematoma with active bleeding; intraparenchymal hematoma >10 cm or expanding
	Laceration	>3 cm parenchymal depth
IV	Hematoma	Ruptured intraparenchymal hematoma with active bleeding
	Laceration	Parenchymal disruption involving 25%-75% of hepatic lobe or 1-3 segments within a single lobe
V	Laceration	Parenchymal disruption involving >75% of hepatic lobe or >3 segments within a single lobe
	Vascular	Juxtahepatic venous injuries (ie, retrohepatic vena cava/central major hepatic veins)
VI	Vascular	Hepatic avulsion

[a]Advance one grade for multiple injuries up to grade III.

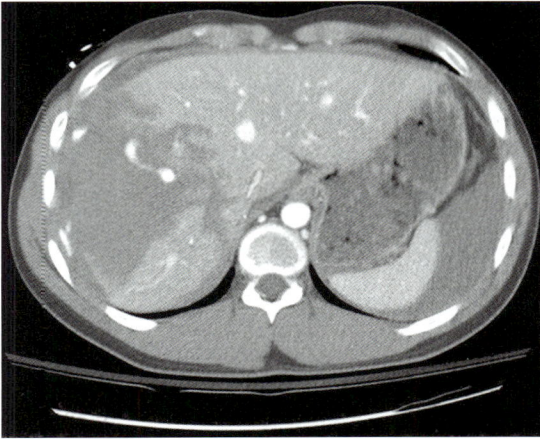

Figure 7-12. Computed tomography scan of the abdomen in a patient with blunt abdominal trauma and extensive hepatic injury.

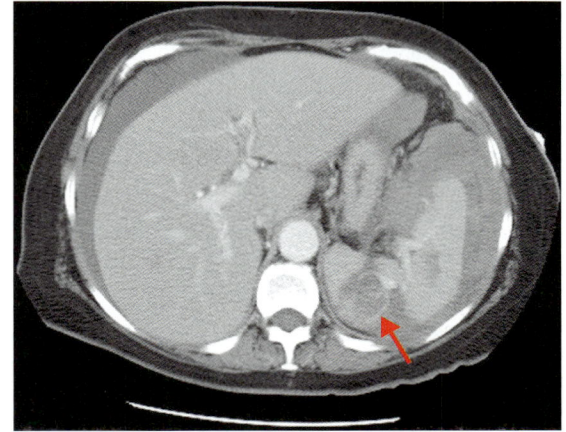

Figure 7-13. Splenic injury, as demonstrated by computed tomography of the abdomen. Diffuse hemoperitoneum is present, along with active extravasation of IV contrast (red arrow).

Spleen

The spleen is frequently injured in blunt abdominal trauma. As with the liver, higher grade injuries (Table 7-5) are more likely to require intervention. Splenic salvage is preferred but must be balanced with the risk of bleeding and death. CT scan allows for accurate assessment of the degree of

splenic injury and also assesses for concomitant injuries. Nonoperative management is used for hemodynamically stable patients, particularly with low-grade injuries (Figure 7-13). Recurrent hemorrhage or development of peritonitis signals failure of nonoperative management and requires expeditious laparotomy or embolization. Splenic injury with active bleeding and hypotension requires total splenectomy or, less commonly, splenorrhaphy. Hemodynamically stable patients with IV contrast extravasation on dynamic CT scan require angioembolization with possible splenic salvage (Figure 7-14). Splenectomized patients should undergo postoperative vaccination for encapsulated bacterial organisms (*Streptococcus pneumoniae*, *Neisseria meningitidis*, *Haemophilus influenzae*) to reduce the risk of overwhelming postsplenectomy sepsis (OPSS), which is rare but potentially fatal.

TABLE 7-5. Splenic Injury Scale

Grade[a]		Injury Description
I	Hematoma	Subcapsular, nonexpanding, <10% surface area
	Laceration	Capsular tear, nonbleeding, <1 cm in depth
II	Hematoma	Subcapsular, nonexpanding, 10%-50% surface area
		Intraparenchymal, nonexpanding, <5 cm in diameter
	Laceration	Capsular tear, active bleeding; 1-3 cm parenchymal depth that does not involve a trabecular vessel
III	Hematoma	Subcapsular, >50% surface area or expanding; ruptured subcapsular hematoma with active bleeding; intraparenchymal hematoma >5 cm or expanding
	Laceration	>3 cm parenchymal depth or involving trabecular vessels
IV	Hematoma	Ruptured intraparenchymal hematoma with active bleeding
	Laceration	Laceration involving segmental or hilar vessels producing major devascularization (>25% of spleen)
V	Laceration	Completely shattered spleen
	Vascular	Hilar vascular injury, which devascularizes spleen

[a]Advance one grade for multiple injuries up to grade III.

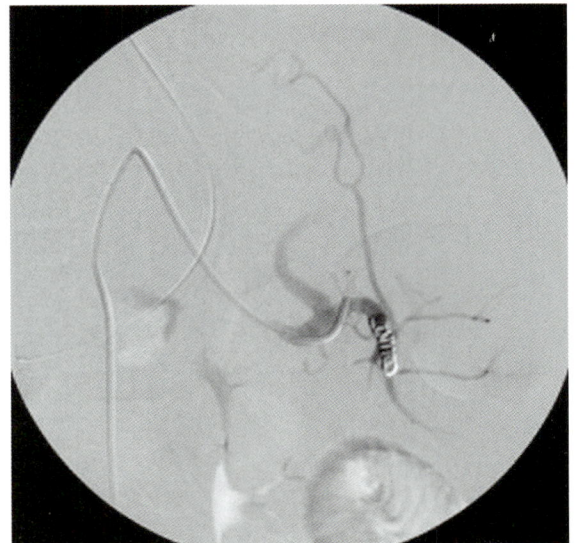

Figure 7-14. Angiographic embolization of splenic hemorrhage after blunt abdominal trauma. Metallic coils have been placed within the splenic artery.

Pancreas

Injury to the pancreas is uncommon due to its retroperitoneal location. This protected location also makes diagnosis by physical examination difficult. Any patient presenting with significant blunt force to the lower chest and upper abdomen should undergo CT imaging for early diagnosis of potential pancreatic injury. Transection of the body of the pancreas may occur by compression against the vertebral column, such as with a handlebar or high-riding seatbelt. When the fractured parenchyma is to the left of the superior mesenteric artery, distal pancreatectomy with or without splenic salvage is the optimal management. Injuries of the pancreatic head are especially challenging. Initial management includes hemorrhage control and drainage of the disrupted pancreatic tissue. Small injuries of the pancreas not involving the main pancreatic duct may be managed with drainage alone. Stab wounds to the back can injure the pancreatic parenchyma and ducts. Evaluation may include CT scanning, magnetic resonance cholangiopancreatography (MRCP), and endoscopic retrograde cholangiopancreatography (ERCP).

Diaphragm

Blunt rupture of the diaphragm usually extends from the gastroesophageal (GE) junction into the tendinous portion of the central diaphragm. Rarely, blunt injury may result in complete avulsion of the posterior muscular insertion from the ribs (Figure 7-15). Repair is done with interrupted or running permanent suture to minimize the risk of recurrence. Care should be taken to avoid injury to the branches of the phrenic nerve.

Low-velocity penetrating injury to the diaphragm can occur without pneumothorax or evidence of peritoneal injury. Left-sided diaphragmatic injuries are particularly concerning because of the subsequent risk of diaphragmatic hernia and visceral incarceration. In addition, left-sided diaphragmatic wounds are commonly associated with injuries of the stomach, colon, spleen, and small intestine. Unfortunately, small penetrating injuries of the diaphragm are not readily diagnosed by CT. For these reasons, there

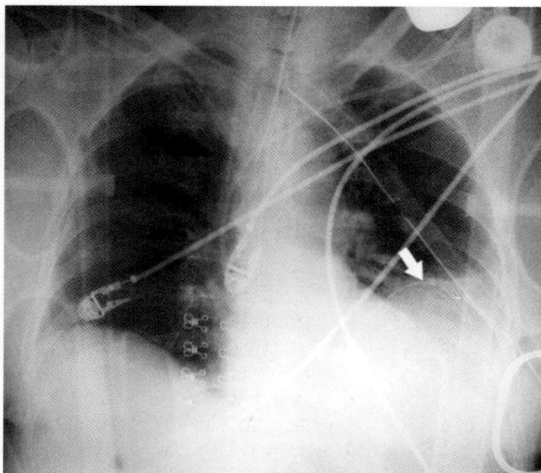

Figure 7-15. Blunt rupture of the left diaphragm. The nasogastric tube is visualized in the left hemithorax (arrow).

should be a low threshold for diagnostic laparoscopy or thoracoscopic evaluation of the left hemidiaphragm after penetrating injury to the thoracoabdominal region. Small injuries of the right diaphragm may be managed without surgical repair because the liver protects against herniation.

Kidneys

The kidneys are relatively protected from injury because of their retroperitoneal location, as well as encasement within Gerota fascia. Blunt renal trauma rarely requires operative intervention unless there is ureteral injury or disruption of the renal pelvis. Nephrectomy may be necessary for massive parenchymal destruction (grade IV or higher) or hilar injury. Under most circumstances, penetrating injuries are self-limiting unless major vessels are involved. Foley catheter drainage should be maintained for 7 to 10 days, or until hematuria resolves.

Small Intestine and Mesentery

Perforation of the small intestine may occur following blunt force compression, or by avulsion of the mesenteric blood supply. Small bowel contusion may result in delayed perforation. An abdominal "seatbelt sign" increases the risk for bowel injury. Mesenteric tears with hemorrhage from the arcade vessels can occur after deceleration injury and should be suspected when peritoneal fluid is seen on CT without accompanying solid organ injury. The small bowel and mesentery are frequently injured by knife and gunshot wounds. Repair is generally straightforward and involves closure with absorbable or nonabsorbable suture. Stapled repair or resection with anastomosis is appropriate for severe injuries or those involving the mesentery.

Colon

Injury to the large intestine from low- and high-velocity projectiles can often be repaired primarily. More extensive wounds that involve the mesentery may require resection with primary anastomosis. Colostomy is seldom required in colonic trauma. Injuries to the extraperitoneal rectum should be considered for fecal diversion to avoid perineal sepsis. Patients with colonic trauma and multiple other injuries or profound shock may require temporary diverting colostomy because of the increased risk for anastomotic dehiscence.

Damage Control

Patients presenting with shock and ongoing hypotension benefit from abbreviated laparotomy to control hemorrhage and/or enteric contamination. This is referred to as *damage control laparotomy*. The "lethal triad" of hypothermia, acidosis, and coagulopathy is worsened by prolonged operation and is almost universally fatal if not avoided. Control of immediate life-threatening hemorrhage is achieved by suturing of bleeding vessels and packing solid organ injuries with laparotomy pads. Injured segments of the intestine are resected and left in discontinuity to minimize operative time. Damage control surgery usually takes 60 to 90 minutes, with expedient transfer of the patient to the intensive care unit for ongoing resuscitation, rewarming, and correction of coagulopathy. Once stabilized, usually 12 to 48 hours after initial presentation, the patient is returned to the operating room for staged removal of hemostatic packing, reconstruction of the gastrointestinal tract, and definitive repair of other injuries.

Abdominal Compartment Syndrome

Aggressive crystalloid or blood product resuscitation may result in sequestering of fluids in the retroperitoneum and peritoneal cavity (third spacing) raising intra-abdominal pressure. This compromises blood flow to the abdominal and retroperitoneal viscera. Diaphragmatic excursion is reduced and evident by increased airway pressure, reduced tidal volumes, hypoxia, and eventual hypercapnia. The clinical triad of decreased urine output, increased airway pressures, and a tense distended abdomen should prompt concern for the development of abdominal compartment syndrome (ACS). When left untreated or when there is a delay in diagnosis, ACS results in multiple organ dysfunction syndrome (MODS) and is commonly fatal. Diagnosis is facilitated by measuring bladder pressure, which indirectly reflects intraperitoneal pressure. An intraperitoneal pressure greater than 25 mm Hg with associated organ dysfunction constitutes ACS. Treatment requires prompt decompression via midline laparotomy. This restores pulmonary function and renal perfusion, and urinary output increases. The abdominal fascia can be closed after several days when swelling subsides, but occasionally prolonged wound care, skin grafting, or complex closure techniques are required.

PELVIC FRACTURES

Significant force is required to fracture the large bones of the pelvis, such as after motor vehicle collisions, pedestrian-vehicle collisions, and falls from great heights. The fracture patterns are classified by the mechanism of injury: anteroposterior (AP) compression, lateral compression (LC), or vertical shear. Of the three forces of transmitted energy, the LC mechanism is most common and most stable because it is less likely to lead to ligamentous disruption of the sacroiliac joint. The AP compression fracture pattern (Figure 7-16) may result in an open book pelvic fracture. The symphysis pubis is disrupted and the iliac wings open, leading to variable amounts of sacroiliac ligamentous disruption. The appearance of the pelvis on radiologic imaging does not necessarily indicate the full extent of pelvic

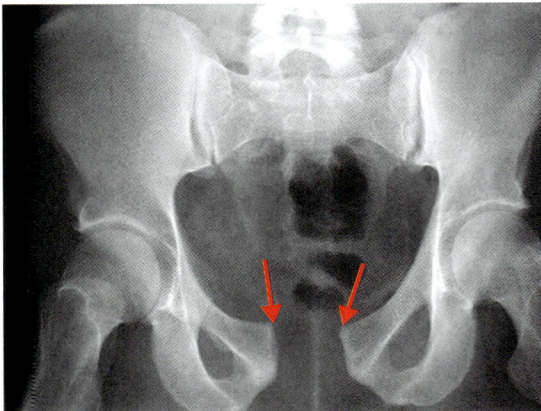

Figure 7-16. **Open book pelvic fracture from anteroposterior compression injury with widening of pubic symphysis (red arrows).**

bone distraction that occurred on initial impact. The least common but most unstable pelvic ring disruption results from vertical shear injury, which is caused by a severe vertical force that may disrupt the hemipelvis from the spine, or create a fracture through the iliac wing. This fracture pattern is frequently associated with underlying abdominal, pelvic, or vascular injuries.

Pelvic fractures may be suspected on the basis of history and physical findings. If the patient is conscious, tenderness to palpation is usually present. There may be bruising to the lower abdomen, hips, buttocks, or lower back. The bony pelvis should be palpated gently to elicit tenderness, deformity (such as a widened symphysis pubis), or movement with compression. Examination should include inspection of the perineum for open wounds, which signifies open pelvic fracture. The lower extremities should be examined for alignment, length discrepancy, and pelvic pain with movement. In symptomatic patients, a plain x-ray of the pelvis is indicated to evaluate for pelvic fracture. Dynamic helical CT scan of the pelvis offers a means of evaluating integrity of the bony pelvis, as well as internal pelvic structures. Hemorrhage associated with pelvic fracture is related to the fracture edges, presacral venous plexus, or, in approximately 10% of patients, an arterial source. Extravasation of IV contrast is a sign of ongoing arterial hemorrhage and should prompt consideration for early angioembolization.

Because of the high kinetic energy necessary to disrupt the pelvic ring, rapid assessment for other sources of blood loss should be performed. Bleeding from the fracture edges or small veins can be minimized by bony stabilization to maintain pelvic volume. There are several simple methods to achieve this, ranging from wrapping a sheet tightly around the pelvis to applying a pelvic binder. These methods work best for AP compression injuries to restore the alignment of the pelvic bones. Ongoing bleeding from an arterial source requires intervention. As a general rule, surgical exploration is not the best option to control pelvic hemorrhage as opening the retroperitoneum risks releasing the tamponade. If the patient is taken to surgery for other injuries, such as a ruptured spleen, the pelvic hematoma can be packed separately with laparotomy pads. A bony external fixator may be placed by orthopedic surgery. The preferred method to control arterial hemorrhage is catheter-directed angioembolization.

Lower genitourinary injuries can occur with pelvic fractures because of the close proximity of the bladder and prostate to the pubic bones; they are usually suspected because of hematuria. Blunt mechanisms produce two types of bladder injury—intraperitoneal and extraperitoneal lacerations. Extraperitoneal injury results from the ligamentous attachments, which secure the bladder to the pelvic bones, tearing the bladder wall. The diagnosis is made by a cystogram demonstrating extravasation into the retroperitoneum. Treatment is decompression of the bladder with a Foley catheter until the laceration heals, typically 7 to 10 days. Blunt force to the lower abdominal wall when the bladder is distended results in a disruption of the dome of the bladder, which is intraperitoneal. This injury may or may not be associated with pelvic fractures. The diagnosis is made by abdominopelvic CT or dedicated CT cystogram, revealing contrast extravasation into the peritoneal cavity. Intraperitoneal bladder injury requires surgical exploration and repair. Typical signs associated with urethral injury are scrotal hematoma, blood at the urethral meatus, and a high-riding or nonpalpable prostate gland on rectal examination. A retrograde urethrogram should be done to evaluate for injury before attempting Foley insertion. Blind passage of a catheter in a patient with a partial urethral tear can lead to worsening of the injury or complete transection. Inability to pass a catheter or identification of a urethral injury requires urologic consultation for definitive management. The urethra can also be injured directly with penetrating trauma or blunt force mechanisms, such as straddle injuries.

PENETRATING NECK TRAUMA

The neck is a highly complex anatomic region with critical vascular, neurologic, and aerodigestive structures concentrated within a very small area. Any wound that violates the platysma muscle carries a risk of injury to the great vessels, trachea, esophagus, and spinal cord and, therefore, requires further assessment. For purposes of clinical evaluation and management of penetrating wounds, the anterior neck (from the midline to the anterior border of the sternocleidomastoid muscle) is divided into three zones as illustrated in Figure 7-17.

Initial evaluation of patients with penetrating neck wounds is determined by the physical examination and physiologic status. Shock or hard signs of injury to any of the vital structures in zones I and II mandate treatment by an immediate endovascular or operative exploration

to control hemorrhage. In the hemodynamically stable patient, a more selective approach is taken for zone I and zone III injuries because of the difficulties in operative exposure in these areas. Controversy remains around the optimal approach for hemodynamically stable patients with an isolated zone II wound and no signs or symptoms of major injury. Traditional evaluation includes angiography, bronchoscopy, and esophagoscopy in conjunction with esophagography.

There is a growing body of literature to support contrast-enhanced CT for evaluation of penetrating neck injury. Several prospective studies evaluating CT angiography in penetrating neck trauma have demonstrated a sensitivity approaching 100% and a negative predictive value over 90%. One of the recognized limitations of the use of CT in the evaluation of penetrating neck trauma is the difficulty in detecting the trajectory of knife wounds. Specifically, small pharyngoesophageal wounds are difficult to detect with CT scan. Despite these limitations, the literature supports an increasing role for the use of CT in evaluating stable patients with a penetrating wound to any zone of the anterior neck.

Aerodigestive Tract Injury

Aerodigestive tract injuries are seen in 10% of penetrating trauma to the neck. Airway management is paramount. The need for a surgical airway (cricothyroidotomy) should always be considered in any patient who might have a tenuous or compromised airway.

The preferred method of evaluating for an injury to the larynx and trachea involves a combination of direct

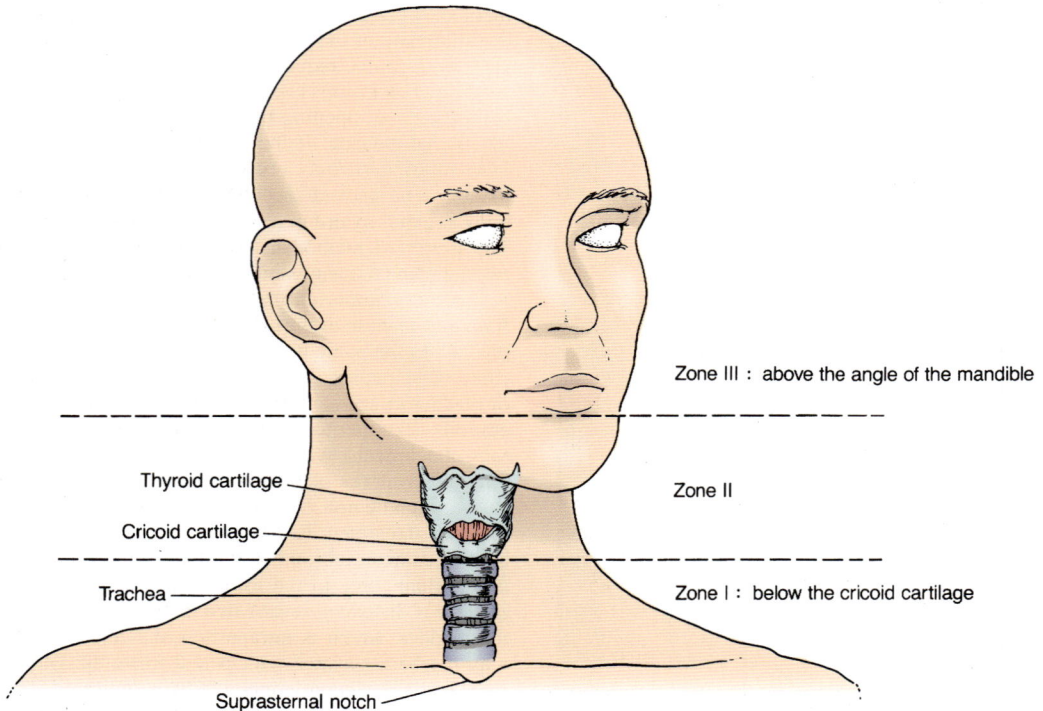

Zone III : above the angle of the mandible

Zone II

Zone I : below the cricoid cartilage

Thyroid cartilage

Cricoid cartilage

Trachea

Suprasternal notch

Figure 7-17. Zones of the neck.

laryngoscopy and bronchoscopy. Laryngeal injuries are classified as supraglottic, glottic, and subglottic. Supraglottic injuries typically result in a depression of the superior notch of the thyroid cartilage and are associated with a vertical fracture of the thyroid cartilage. Disruption of the thyroid cartilage results in a glottic injury. An injury to the subglottic region usually involves the lower thyroid and cricoid cartilage. Early definitive repair for any laryngeal injury should be the goal because of the higher incidence of stricture formation with delayed repair. Subglottic injury to the trachea should be repaired in one layer with absorbable suture. When there is an associated esophageal or arterial injury, the risk of fistulization between the two repairs is reduced by interposing a vascularized pedicle of omohyoid or sternocleidomastoid muscle. Operative management of cervical esophageal injuries requires meticulous debridement, a two-layer closure of the wound, and closed suction drainage. Injuries limited to the hypopharyngeal region can be safely managed conservatively with an NG tube for feeding and an empiric course of parenteral antibiotics.

Vascular Injury

The approach to evaluation of a vascular injury in the neck is dictated by the patient's hemodynamic status and neurologic assessment. Observation or expectant management is advocated for patients who are comatose. Simple ligation of an artery is an option for those patients presenting with exsanguination or when a temporary shunt cannot be placed. The carotid artery should be repaired when the patient has an intact or alternating neurologic examination. Repair may be performed by a direct operative approach or using endovascular techniques in the stable patient. Angiographic intervention is particularly applicable in zone III injuries to the internal carotid artery located at the base of the skull because of the difficulty in accessing this area surgically.

The most common vascular injury with penetrating wounds is the internal jugular vein. In the patient who is hemodynamically unstable, any venous injury should be managed by simple ligation. Otherwise, an injury to the internal jugular vein should be repaired by lateral venorrhaphy or patch venoplasty. Despite the method of repair, subsequent thrombosis is common.

Associated Spinal Cord Injury

Approximately 10% of penetrating neck wounds are associated with a spinal cord or brachial plexus injury. Injuries to the spinal cord above the fourth cervical vertebrae are associated with a high mortality. The utility of steroids in the management of spinal cord injury remains controversial.

EXTREMITY TRAUMA

Extremity injuries are common in both blunt and penetrating traumas and may range in severity from trivial to limb and even life threatening. During the primary survey, potentially lethal injuries such as major vascular injuries, open fractures, crush injuries, and near amputations should be stabilized by application of a splint. The history obtained from prehospital personnel may indicate significant blood loss at the scene or during transport. Exsanguinating hemorrhage from a major vascular injury should be treated initially with direct pressure or by application of a tourniquet proximal to the wound. During the secondary survey, a detailed neurovascular examination of each extremity should be performed and include evaluation of peripheral pulses, sensation, motor function, and range of motion. Palpation may elicit tenderness suggestive of fracture or soft tissue injury. Deformity of the extremity is typically associated with fractures and/or dislocations.

Vascular injuries can be obvious or occult. The "hard signs" of acute injury include pulsatile bleeding, expanding hematoma, bruit, and a pale, cool, pulseless extremity with or without paresthesia or paralysis. Hard signs of a vascular injury are an indication for immediate operative exploration. Physical findings that may be suggestive, but not diagnostic for vascular injury, are termed "soft signs." These are nonexpanding hematoma or diminished pulses. Doppler ultrasound provides a useful adjunct to examination of the vascular system and allows calculation of the ankle-brachial index (ABI). The ABI is calculated by measuring the systolic BP (by Doppler probe) divided by the systolic pressure in the brachial artery. Normally, this ratio is 1 or higher; values less than 0.9 are suggestive of arterial injury or occlusion. In this setting, further diagnostic evaluation with CT angiography is indicated. (See the Vascular chapter for a more detailed discussion of the diagnosis and management of extremity vascular injuries and their sequelae.)

Radiographic imaging is indicated for any extremity deformity, bony tenderness, or joint swelling as part of the secondary survey. If a fracture is identified, imaging should also include the bones above and below the fracture. Fractures are characterized by bony location, comminution, angulation, and whether they are closed or open with communication to the skin. Open fractures lead to bacterial contamination and risk of complications, such as wound infection, osteomyelitis, poor bone healing, and, ultimately, poor functional outcome.

While a detailed discussion of extremity fractures falls outside the scope of this chapter, certain basic principles may be universally applied. Splinting a fracture improves pain control, minimizes secondary soft tissue damage, and diminishes bleeding from the soft tissues and bone edges. Femoral shaft fractures may be associated with significant blood loss into the soft tissues and should be addressed with appropriate resuscitative measures, including transfusion of blood as necessary. Patients with bilateral femur fractures may present with shock, even in the absence of other injuries. Neurovascular status should also be reassessed and the findings documented before and after manipulation of the injured extremity. Open fractures are potentially limb-threatening injuries. Treatment involves prompt operative debridement of devitalized tissue, copious irrigation to remove dirt and other contaminants, fracture reduction, and early administration of IV antibiotics mainly targeting gram-positive organisms.

Dislocations should be splinted in place for transport. Reduction of the dislocation should be done as soon as possible. Imaging is indicated before reduction to rule out an associated fracture that might impede reduction. Prolonged dislocation can cause traction injury to nearby nerves and vessels and thus significant morbidity.

Compartment syndrome may occur after blunt or penetrating trauma in any extremity and results from soft tissue edema and hemorrhage. When this swelling occurs in an unyielding fascial compartment, interstitial pressure rises. In the initial phases, this increase in pressure may diminish venous capillary outflow and worsen cellular injury, resulting in further swelling and interstitial fluid accumulation. If left uncorrected, compartment syndrome may result in permanent nerve injury or muscle necrosis that may necessitate amputation. The muscular damage associated with compartment syndrome may lead to rhabdomyolysis and result in myoglobinuria. Early signs of compartment syndrome include pain, paresthesia, and diminished sensation. The affected compartment is typically swollen and tense. Diminished or absent pulses are late findings and are associated with irreversible ischemia. The diagnosis is typically made by history and physical examination findings. Direct measurement of compartmental pressures may be accomplished with commercially available devices when the diagnosis is equivocal. In patients with brain injury or those who are comatose, direct measurement of compartmental pressures should be performed. Treatment is prompt fasciotomy of all the involved compartments. Fasciotomy allows the injured muscle to swell without concomitant increases in pressure. Perfusion is maintained, and secondary damage is minimized. Compartment syndrome may occur in any extremity but is most commonly associated with crush injuries of the calf, with or without bony fractures.

Rhabdomyolysis and subsequent myoglobinuria may develop after significant muscular injury or in the setting of compartment syndrome. Myoglobin is nephrotoxic and precipitates in the acidic milieu of the renal tubules. Treatment involves aggressive hydration with isotonic IV fluids. Alkalinization of the urine with IV sodium bicarbonate and osmotic diuresis with mannitol are adjunctive measures. Debridement of all necrotic tissue is mandatory to eliminate rhabdomyolysis causing myoglobinuria.

TRAUMA IN PREGNANCY

The leading causes of injury among pregnant women are transportation-related trauma, falls, and assault. Motor vehicle collision is the most common mechanism, resulting in fetal death, followed by firearms, and then falls. Pregnant women between 15 and 19 years of age are at greatest risk for trauma-related fetal demise.

Assault is a frequent cause of injuries in pregnant patients. It is estimated that 10% to 30% of women are physically abused during pregnancy, and of these, 5% are severe enough to result in fetal death. Thus, it is mandatory for all members of the health care team to be versed in recognizing the signs and symptoms of physical abuse.

The priorities for the treatment of the pregnant patient are the same as those for the nonpregnant patient. Prevention of hypotension when the patient is supine is accomplished by repositioning to displace the uterus off the vena cava and aorta while maintaining alignment of the spine. This can be accomplished by three simple maneuvers: placing the patient in the left lateral decubitus position, placing the patient in the right lateral decubitus position, or placing the patient in the knee-chest position when supine. Alternatively, the uterus can be manually displaced to the patient's left side. Since the physiologic hypervolemia of pregnancy

may mask the early signs of shock, early crystalloid resuscitation should be initiated, even in the normotensive patient. The secondary survey should include a prenatal history and associated comorbid factors. A urine pregnancy test should be obtained in all injured women of childbearing age, and, when positive, early obstetrical consultation is recommended.

Abdominal examination may reveal evidence of uterine rupture when fetal parts can be palpable through the abdominal wall. A speculum examination should be performed followed by the bimanual examination only if there is no evidence of vaginal bleeding. The examination focuses vaginal blood, ruptured amniotic membranes, active contractions, a bulging perineum, and an abnormal fetal heart rate or rhythm. Drainage of cloudy white or green fluid from the cervical *os* is indicative of ruptured membranes. This is an obstetrical emergency requiring urgent cesarean section. Bloody amniotic fluid is indicative of either placental abruption or placenta previa. When this occurs during the first trimester, there is a high risk of spontaneous abortion.

Rh typing is essential in the pregnant patient with trauma. The Rh antigen is well developed by 6 weeks of gestation, and as little as 0.001 mL of fetal blood can cause sensitization of the Rh-negative mother. Therefore, all Rh-negative women should receive Rho (D) immune globulin, unless the injury is minor and remote from the uterus.

In cases of severe trauma in late-term pregnancy, perimortem cesarean section may be necessary. This maneuver may be considered in cases of impending or actual maternal cardiac arrest; fetal survival has been reported when performed within 4 minutes after loss of maternal vital signs.

PEDIATRIC TRAUMA

Pediatric trauma is the number one cause of death of children, as well as the number one cause of permanent disability in those under 14 years of age. In children over 1 year and under 14 years of age, firearms recently surpassed motor vehicle collisions as the number one cause of death related to injury. Other common causes include drowning and thermal injury.

Although the resuscitation priorities (ABCDE algorithm) are the same for children as for adults, anatomic and physiologic differences require modifications to the approach. Assessment of the child's airway is the first step. Most children do not have preexisting pulmonary disease; thus, a room air oxygen saturation less than 90% generally indicates ineffective gas exchange. If oxygenation is difficult, then a pneumothorax or aspiration should be considered. In the injured child, hyperventilation is common after TBI or shock. With either condition, intubation and mechanical ventilation are appropriate. The injured child who is combative because of hypoxia or emotional distress may also need to be intubated to facilitate further diagnostic testing. A chest x-ray should be obtained to confirm the correct position of the endotracheal tube since a right mainstem intubation is a common complication. The Broselow Pediatric Resuscitation Measuring Tape has become the standard for assisting in the management of trauma in children. This device is placed on the bed next to the child, and the height measurement allows estimation of weight for determining appropriate sizing of resuscitative equipment and dosing of medications and other therapeutic maneuvers.

Age-specific hypotension is an indication for volume resuscitation of the injured child. Cardiovascular compensation by tachycardia and vasoconstriction will maintain BP in the child who has had significant blood loss. Therefore, a normal BP does not connote a normal circulating blood volume. A child's blood volume is approximately 8% of body weight or 80 mL/kg. Clinical signs of decreased organ perfusion in conjunction with altered mentation are the classic findings of hemorrhagic shock. Initial resuscitation is begun with 20 mL/kg of an isotonic crystalloid solution, such as 0.9% normal saline, or lactated Ringer solution. If there is no improvement in perfusion after a second bolus of crystalloid, then a 10 mL/kg bolus of either cross-matched or O-negative packed red blood cells should be administered.

Hypothermia is common in the injured child and may occur at any time of the year. The response to hypothermia includes catecholamine release, with an increase in oxygen consumption and metabolic acidosis. Hypothermia and acidosis may then contribute to posttraumatic coagulopathy. The rate of cooling and subsequent hypothermia can be reduced by warming the room (>37 °C), using warmed IV fluids and blood (39 °C), heated air-warming blankets, and external warmed blankets during the initial resuscitation.

In a child, the comparatively thin abdominal wall musculature and flexible rib cage provide relatively little protection for the abdomen from blunt injury, and thus abdominal injuries are common in children. In addition to physical examination, adjunctive tests include FAST and CT scan. CT imaging of the head, chest, abdomen, and pelvis are the accepted diagnostic radiologic studies of choice in the hemodynamically stable children. In the hemodynamically normal children, the vast majority of solid organ injuries can be managed without surgical intervention. As in adults, hollow viscus perforation should be managed by prompt surgical repair.

TRAUMA IN THE OLDER INDIVIDUAL

The older population (age ≥65 years) is the fastest growing age group in the United States. Injury is the fifth leading cause of death in the older individual. Within this group, 42% reported some type of long-lasting condition or a disability. Of those aged 65 to 74 years, one-third reported at least one disability; that number climbs to 72% in people aged 85 years and above.

Common injury mechanisms in the geriatric population include falls, motor vehicle collisions, automobile versus pedestrian collisions, assaults, and burns. Motor vehicle collision victims over the age of 85 have a fatality rate that is 7 to 9 times higher than that of younger adults. Adult pedestrian injuries are more common in lower socioeconomic groups who are more likely to travel by walking. The slower pace and restricted mobility associated with aging result in the older pedestrian requiring longer times to cross a street, which places them at higher risk for being struck by oncoming vehicles.

Interpersonal violence is increasing as a cause of injury in the older individual. In the United States, 5% of all homicides involve survivors aged 65 years and above. The overall incidence of abuse in older patients is estimated to be 2% to 10% and should always be considered when caring for the geriatric patient. Substance misuse also should be considered in older patients. Consideration of causes of altered mental status should include brain injury, stroke, delirium, dementia, or intoxication.

Older patients with trauma have higher injury-related mortality when compared with younger patients. Much of this is due to reduced function in all organs that occurs with aging and also the increased incidence of comorbid conditions. The prevalence of preexisting conditions increases with age and can be as high as 80% in those over 95 years.

The most frequent comorbidities in the older patients involve the cardiovascular system. These diseases compromise the ability of older patient with trauma to respond to hypovolemia. Rather than mounting a tachycardia and increase in cardiac output, there is an increase in systemic vascular resistance, resulting in a falsely reassuring BP. In fact, a normal BP in an older trauma survivor frequently corresponds to profound shock when perfusion is assessed using systemic markers, such as serum lactate and base deficit. Cardiac physiology is also affected by medications prescribed for hypertension and arrhythmias.

Aging also affects pulmonary function. There is a decrease in the alveolar surface area that reduces the surface tension and thus gas exchange and forced expiratory flow. Gross anatomic changes in the thorax of the older patients include the development of kyphosis, which results in a reduction of the transverse thoracic diameter. The loss of bone density is associated with an increased rigidity of the chest wall. Chest wall compliance decreases with age, resulting in increased work of breathing. In older women, osteoporosis increases the risk for rib fractures and pulmonary contusion. Age has been shown to be the strongest predictor of outcome and is directly proportional to mortality in patients with multiple rib fractures.

In the geriatric patient, the initial GCS score may be less reliable and more reflective of chronic disease of the central nervous system or systemic disease. A significant TBI can result from apparently minor trauma because of the changes with aging of the meninges and a reduction in brain volume. Thus, any older patient with a change in mental status should prompt a thorough evaluation for TBI, including a noncontrast CT scan of the head. In addition, many older patients are prescribed anticoagulants. Otherwise minor head injuries may become devastating intracranial hemorrhages in the patient who is on anticoagulation. Morbidity and mortality are reduced by prompt correction of coagulopathy.

Renal function begins to deteriorate at the age of 30. The number of functioning nephrons decreases by 10% per decade, whereas the remaining functional units hypertrophy. Glomerular filtration rate begins to decrease at 50, declining by 0.75 to 1 mL/min/y.

Traumatic injury in the older patients is more likely to produce bowel and mesenteric infarction. The diagnosis of an intraperitoneal injury by physical examination is less reliable. Gastrointestinal tract wounds are associated with a 3- to 4-fold increase in mortality when compared with younger cohorts.

Cell-mediated immunity is diminished with a decrease in peripheral T-cell count and function. The antibody response to stimuli is depressed, and this places the older patients at increased risk for infection. With severe trauma, they may be more prone to the development of MODS.

Normal thermoregulatory mechanisms become less responsive with aging. Cutaneous vasoconstriction and shivering are less effective, placing the older patients at increased risk for the development of hypothermia in cold environments, and after significant volume loss. Efforts to prevent hypothermia must be initiated in the prehospital setting.

SUGGESTED READINGS

Centers for Disease Control and Prevention. Web-based Injury Statistics Query and Reporting System. Accessed October 21, 2024. https://wisqars.cdc.gov.

Centers for Disease Control and Prevention. Mortality in the United States, 2016. National Center for Health Statistics. Accessed August 6, 2018. https://www.cdc.gov/nchs/products/databriefs/db293.htm

Chang R, Holcomb JB. Optimal fluid therapy for traumatic hemorrhagic shock. *Crit Care Clin.* 2017;33(1):15-36.

Holcomb JB, Tilley BC, Baraniuk S, et al. Transfusion of plasma, platelets, and red blood cells in a 1:1:1 vs a 1:1:2 ratio and mortality in patients with severe trauma: the PROPPR randomized clinical trial. *JAMA.* 2015;313(5):471-482.

Stocchetti N, Taccone FS, Citerio G, et al. Neuroprotection in acute brain injury: an up-to-date review. *Crit Care.* 2015;19(1):186.

SAMPLE QUESTIONS

QUESTIONS

Choose the best answer for each question.

1. A 43-year-old woman was an unrestrained driver involved in a high-speed motor vehicle collision into a tree. She is noted to have extensive facial injuries, including fractures to the midface and mandible with bleeding in the airway. Her oxygen saturation is 88%. She does not open her eyes, moans to deep stimulation, and has extensor flexion of her extremities on noxious stimulation. The optimal management of her airway is

   A. nasopharyngeal airway.
   B. oropharyngeal airway.
   C. fiberoptic nasal intubation.
   D. endotracheal intubation.
   E. surgical cricothyroidotomy.

2. A 65-year-old man is struck by a car while riding a moped. On arrival, his respiratory rate is 18/min, his heart rate is 95 beats/min, and his BP is 78/54 mm Hg. His oxygen saturation is 93%. He complains of chest pain and shortness of breath and has right chest wall tenderness and decreased breath sounds. He moves all extremities to command. The most likely cause of his hemodynamic instability is

   A. neurogenic shock.
   B. cardiogenic shock.
   C. hemorrhagic shock.
   D. distributive shock.
   E. obstructive shock.

3. A 23-year-old man is brought in by EMS after a fall off his second story roof. He presents unresponsive, with a heart rate of 40 beats/min and a BP of 165/90 mm Hg. His GCS is 3. His physical examination shows a laceration to his right scalp; bruising of his chest wall; a nontender, nondistended abdomen; and deformity of his right forearm. His FAST examination is positive. The next step of his management should be

   A. endotracheal intubation.
   B. administration of an antihypertensive agent.

   C. resuscitative thoracotomy.
   D. CT scan of his head.
   E. exploratory laparotomy.

4. A 70-year-old woman is brought in after a fall down a flight of stairs. She is disoriented to time and place, is somnolent, and complains of neck and back pain. She cannot feel or move her lower extremities. She localizes pain in her upper extremities. Her heart rate is 46 beats/min, and her BP is 75/34 mm Hg. This patient most likely has

   A. high cervical spine injury.
   B. low cervical spine injury.
   C. high thoracic spine injury.
   D. low thoracic spine injury.
   E. lumbar spine injury.

5. A 38-year-old unbelted male driver is involved in a head-on motor vehicle collision and is brought to the ED with a heart rate of 115 beats/min and BP of 65/28 mm Hg. He is awake and anxious, complaining of shortness of breath and chest wall tenderness. He has decreased breath sounds on the right, bruising across his chest, and chest wall tenderness. The next step should be

   A. orotracheal intubation.
   B. nasotracheal intubation.
   C. ED thoracotomy.
   D. chest tube placement.
   E. needle thoracostomy.

ANSWERS AND EXPLANATIONS

1. **Answer: D**

   Establishment of an airway can be challenging in patients with complex facial injuries. Owing to her injuries, this patient requires immediate placement of a secure airway. Nasal instrumentation and intubation should be avoided because of the concern for a skull base fracture. Endotracheal intubation should be the initial modality for establishing an airway. Emergent surgical cricothyroidotomy may be required if orotracheal intubation is unsuccessful. For more information on this topic, see section "Airway."

2. **Answer: C**

After traumatic injuries, hemorrhage accounts for the majority of cases of persistent hypotension. The patient in this scenario does not present with signs or symptoms of neurologic injury that would suggest neurogenic shock. While cardiogenic or obstructive shock is possible, hemorrhagic shock from a hemothorax is the more likely diagnosis. For more information on this topic, see section "Circulation."

3. **Answer: A**

The constellation of hypertension and bradycardia with a slow respiratory rate is suggestive of a Cushing reflex because of increased ICPs. Immediate establishment of an airway with eventual head CT is essential. Management of hyperventilation, elevation of the head, administration of mannitol, and surgical decompression may be required. For more information on this topic, see section "Head Injury."

4. **Answer: C**

The combination of bradycardia and hypotension in a patient with suspected spinal injury is concerning for neurogenic shock due to loss of sympathetic vasomotor tone. Cervical and high thoracic spinal injuries can cause neurogenic shock. This patient shows no deficits consistent with cervical spine injury; therefore, a high thoracic injury is the most likely etiology. For more information on this topic, see section "Injuries of the Spine and Spinal Cord."

5. **Answer: E**

This patient presents with hypotension with a probable tension pneumothorax. Immediate decompression with needle thoracostomy is required. Chest tube placement will be needed after decompression but requires more time to perform in a patient in extremis. Establishment of an airway is not required, and in the setting of tension pneumothorax, administration of sedation and paralytics can worsen hypotension. In the presence of vital signs, ED thoracotomy is not indicated. For more information on this topic, see section "Breathing."

8

Burns

Jong Lee and Tina Palmieri

Major burn injury is considered by many to be one of the most devastating of all injuries, a perception that is all too often correct. To patients, acute burns are the "ultimate agony," and the short- and long-term consequences of burn injury present enormous psychological, social, and physical challenges to meaningful recovery. Burn treatment is labor-intensive, both physically and psychologically challenging. Burn injury encompasses virtually every facet of medical and surgical care. As such, major burn injury is often used as a paradigm for the most severe physiologic derangements that can accompany trauma.

Burns are also a major public health problem. In the United States, more than 450,000 patients seek medical attention for burns every year. Over 3,700 people die every year of burn-related injuries, primarily from house fires, and about 40,000 patients are hospitalized. In addition, several recent disasters, both nationally and internationally, have involved major fires with subsequent burn injuries. This chapter presents basic burn pathophysiology and practical guidelines for the treatment of acute burns.

A *note on illustrations*: Burns are uniquely *visual* injuries, and the ability to assess burns by sight is an essential skill both for planning initial burn care and for making decisions about things such as the need for surgery, the presence of infection, and the extent of scarring. Clinicians who cannot assess burn extent and depth accurately often make significant errors in burn evaluation and treatment. For that reason, familiarity with the appearance of burn injuries is an important objective of this chapter.

PATHOPHYSIOLOGY OF BURN INJURY

The skin can be injured by a variety of agents, including direct heat from flames or scalding liquids, contact with hot objects or corrosive chemicals, and electrical current. Burns are classified according to the depth of injury. Figure 8-1 shows these injuries in relation to the structures of the skin, knowledge of which will help the reader understand the physiologic effects of burns of various depths, and the findings seen on examination.

Epidermal burns ("first-degree burns") involve only the epidermis. Within minutes of injury, dermal capillaries dilate so that these burns present as red, moderately painful areas that blanch with direct pressure, indicating the continued presence of dermal perfusion. Blistering is absent from true epidermal injuries, and the initial erythema usually resolves within a few hours. Epidermal burn injuries are limited in their physiologic effects, and even extensive burns usually require only supportive care, which consists of pain control (oral analgesics), adequate oral fluids, and application of a soothing topical compound. Healing

occurs within a few days because the injured epidermis peels off, revealing new skin beneath. Because scarring occurs in the dermis, epidermal burns do not form the scar tissue. Sunburns are often limited to the epidermis, although deeper injuries can result.

Partial-thickness burns ("second-degree burns") extend into, but not through, the dermis. These injuries vary greatly in both appearance and significance, depending on their exact depth. Superficial partial-thickness burns (Figure 8-2) typically present with reddened skin that forms blisters composed of epidermis and filled with proteinaceous fluid that escapes from the damaged capillaries. The underlying dermis is pink, moist, blanches on direct pressure, and is usually very painful, because cutaneous nerves, which reside in the deeper dermis, are intact.

Deep partial-thickness injuries look very different from more superficial burns. Coagulation necrosis of the upper dermis often gives these wounds a dry, thickened texture. Erythema is often absent, and these wounds may be a variety of colors but are most often waxy white. Because epidermal appendages penetrate far into—sometimes through—the dermis, even a very deep dermal burn can heal if followed long enough. These wounds also vary in

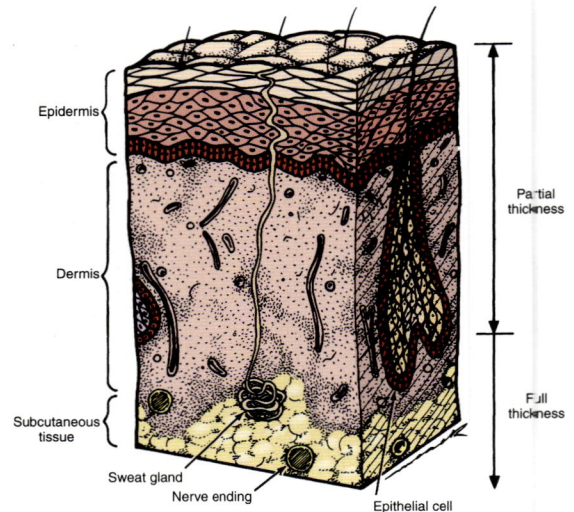

Figure 8-1. Anatomy of the skin showing major skin structures and their relation to partial- and full-thickness burns. Epithelial cells make up the lining of hair follicles and sweat glands, and these structures penetrate deeply into—sometimes through—the dermis. Even very deep partial-thickness burns can heal if these "epidermal appendages" survive. Dermal capillaries and nerve endings also reside in the deep dermis and survive most partial-thickness burns.

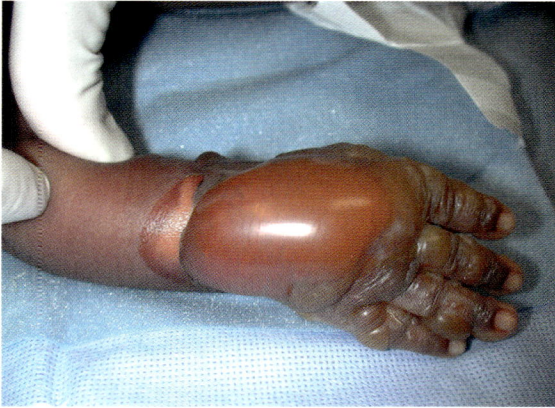
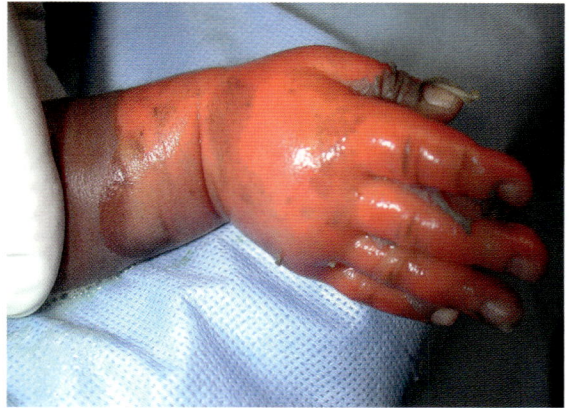

A   **B**

Figure 8-2. Superficial partial-thickness burns that occurred when this child reached into a pot of hot water. A. Distended, fluid-filled blisters that are characteristic of superficial injuries (deeper burns will form blisters, but usually they do not contain much fluid). B. After debridement of blisters, the underlying dermis is bright red, moist, and painful, and blanches readily with direct pressure. Removing blisters from these wounds is uncomfortable but facilitates wound care. In addition, the removal of blistered skin permits a more accurate assessment of burn extent and depth.

the amount of pain they produce; very deep wounds cause the destruction of many dermal nerve endings and are less painful than more superficial injuries. Such wounds heal with scars, however, because the damaged dermis does not regenerate; instead, it is replaced by the scar tissue, which is often rigid, tender, and friable. For this reason, many deep dermal burns are best treated with an excision of the burned tissue and skin grafting. An example of a deep partial-thickness burn is illustrated in Figure 8-3.

During the first 24 to 48 hours after injury, burn wounds develop a coating of dead tissue, coagulated serum, and debris called *eschar*. The exact depth of partial-thickness burns is often difficult to judge, particularly after eschar forms. The appearance of the wound changes dramatically as eschar develops and again as it separates during

wound healing. Partial-thickness burns should demonstrate eschar separation within 10 to 14 days, revealing punctate areas of new epidermal growth called skin "*buds*," which develop from the epidermal linings of hair follicles and sweat glands (Figure 8-4). Burns of "indeterminate" depth—those that have some features of both partial- and full-thickness injuries—can often be treated conservatively for 10 to 14 days; wounds that remain unhealed should undergo grafting.

Full-thickness burns ("third-degree burns") occur when all layers of the skin are destroyed. These wounds are usually covered with dry, avascular coagulum, which is relatively insensate due to the destruction of nerve endings. The wound surface may be almost any color, from waxy white in the case of chemical burns, to a completely black,

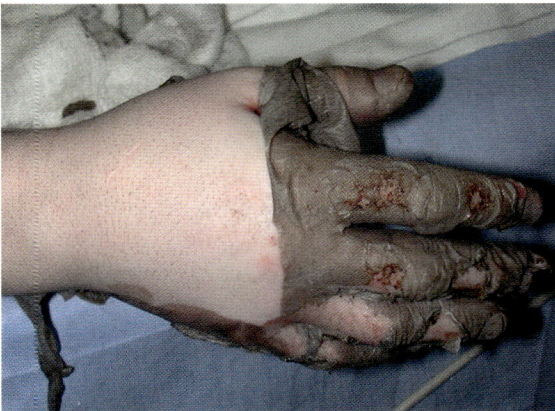

Figure 8-3. Partial-thickness injuries can vary greatly in appearance depending on the etiology and duration of exposure. This photograph shows a deep burn of the dorsal hand from an electrical flash injury. The epidermis is loose and slides off almost like a glove, revealing a waxy white dermis, which has relatively little remaining sensation. Note that there is no fluid beneath the blistered epidermis.

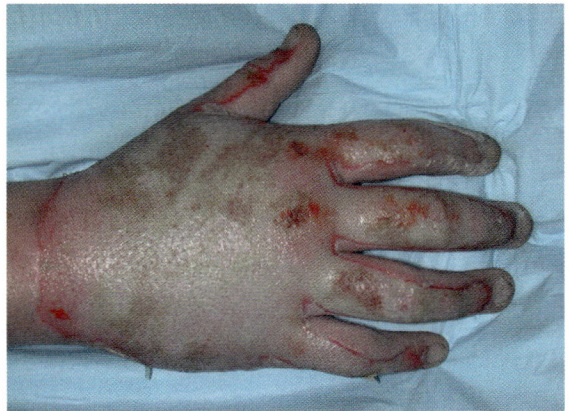

Figure 8-4. This burn of the dorsal hand is about 10 days old. Areas of different burn depth are apparent. There is still some fairly solid eschar over the dorsal hand and fingers, but eschar has separated over the proximal (wrist) edge, revealing pink healing tissue. Regularly spaced, small, darker red spots are epidermal appendages ("skin buds"), where the epidermis is growing upward from hair follicles. The appearance of uniform skin buds indicates that the wound will heal reliably within about 14 days.

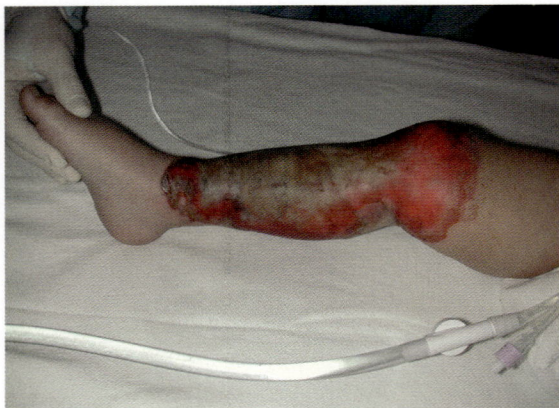

Figure 8-5. Full-thickness burn of the leg. This little boy was playing with matches and gasoline and ignited his pant leg. The wound is a variety of colors, from dull white to black, but almost the entire wound is dry, leathery, and insensate. The contraction of dermal proteins, causing a tourniquet-like effect, is apparent.

charred surface from flame injury. Full-thickness scald burns are often a dark cherry red color, but the surface is dry and does not blanch with pressure. In addition, as dermal proteins are coagulated, they contract, often forming a tight, tourniquet-like constriction, which can cause circulatory compromise in the extremities. Very small, full-thickness burns can heal by contraction, but larger injuries require skin grafting because even the deepest epidermal appendages are destroyed. Figure 8-5 illustrates the appearance of full-thickness burns, which can be very dramatic. An additional category of burn injury, termed "fourth-degree" burns, is sometimes used to describe injuries that extend to the bone.

PATHOPHYSIOLOGY OF INHALATION INJURY

Inhalation injury is a unique complication of injury from flames and smoke that is an important facet of burn treatment. Although inhalation injury is often less apparent than other manifestations of burn injury on initial presentation, it can cause severe morbidity and mortality that may overshadow those of cutaneous burns. These injuries most commonly occur during a fire in an enclosed space; therefore, detailed information regarding the location of the patient during the fire is a critical point in the history. The treatment of inhalation injury is largely supportive. Endotracheal intubation to secure the edematous airway is mandatory. Ventilator support with positive end-expiratory pressure (PEEP) is most helpful in combating the airway collapse.

Inhalation injury can present in three different ways in burn patients. First, patients exposed to large amounts of toxic smoke frequently present with *carbon monoxide (CO) poisoning*. CO poisoning is a common cause of immediate death in patients injured in building fires and often accounts for the majority of deaths in mass casualty incidents. CO is produced from an *incomplete* combustion of normal household items, such as wood and cotton. CO competitively binds to oxygen receptors on the hemoglobin molecule to produce carboxyhemoglobin (COHb),

which cannot transport oxygen. The tissue delivery of oxygen consequently decreases and severe hypoxia ensues. Oxygen-enriched tissues, such as the heart and brain, are the most vulnerable. At low levels, CO poisoning is initially asymptomatic, but as the COHb level rises, symptoms increase. CO poisoning is particularly deadly because of its tendency to impair mental function. The patient will initially experience headache, progressing to dizziness, weakness, and syncope. In the later stages, coma, seizures, and death result (see Table 8-1). CO poisoning should be strongly suspected in any patient who presents with altered mental status following exposure to smoke. Remember that pulse oximetry is not accurate in detecting CO poisoning; an arterial blood gas with direct measurement of hemoglobin saturation must be obtained to detect CO toxicity.

The treatment of CO poisoning should consist of 100% oxygen and must begin as soon as possible, ideally before the patient reaches the hospital. Endotracheal intubation may be needed both to protect the impaired airway and to adequately deliver such high levels of oxygen. If a more rapid decrease in COHb concentration is deemed necessary

TABLE 8-1. Signs and Symptoms at Various Concentrations of Carboxyhemoglobin	
COHb Concentration (%)	**Symptoms**
0-10	None (normal value may range up to 10% in smokers)
10-20	Tightness over forehead, mild headache, dilation of cutaneous blood vessels
20-30	Headache and throbbing in the temples
30-40	Severe headache, weakness, dizziness, dimness of vision, nausea, vomiting, and collapse
40-50	As above; syncope, increased pulse, and respiratory rate
50-60	Syncope, tachycardia, tachypnea, coma, intermittent seizures, Cheyne-Stokes respirations
60-70	Coma, intermittent seizures, depressed cardiac and respiratory function, possible death
70-80	Bradycardia, slow respirations, death within hours
80-90	Death within an hour
90-100	Death within minutes

COHb, carboxyhemoglobin.
Reprinted from Einhorn IN. Physiological and toxicological aspects of smoke produced during the combustion of polymeric materials. *Environ Health Perspect.* 1975;11:163-189; Schulte JH. Effects of mild carbon monoxide intoxication. *Arch Environ Health.* 1963;7:524-530; and Traber DL, Herndon DN, Enkhbaatar P, Maybauer MO, Maybauer DM. The pathophysiology of inhalation injury. In: Herndon, DN, ed. *Total Burn Care.* 3rd ed. Saunders Elsevier; 2007:248-261. Schulte JH. Heldref Publications; and Herndon DN. *Total Burn Care.* 3rd ed. Saunders Elsevier; 2007:250. Copyright © 2007 Elsevier. With permission.

(usually because of acute neurologic symptoms), hyperbaric oxygen (HBO) therapy may be used. HBO works by providing higher concentrations of oxygen to compete with CO for hemoglobin binding. Oxygen administered at three atmospheres of pressure produces a Pao$_2$ as high as 1,500 mm Hg. This provides a significant amount of dissolved oxygen for immediate use and reduces the half-life of COHb from about 80 minutes at one atmosphere of pressure down to about 20 minutes. Appropriate equipment and personnel are required to perform HBO, and its use must be prioritized with other important aspects of care for acutely burned patients, including fluid resuscitation.

Burn patients may also present with *upper airway injury*. Unlike other forms of inhalation injury, which are chemical injuries, upper airway injury is produced by heat. Flash burns and explosions may produce instantaneous deep burns of the face and oropharynx, which lead to rapid, life-threatening airway edema. Swelling occurs progressively over the 24 hours following injury, and facial/airway edema can arise very precipitously. Massive facial swelling can accompany scald or chemical burns, even in the absence of flames or smoke. Figure 8-6 illustrates this process. The assessment of airway patency and swelling is an important component of the initial evaluation of every burn patient (see Figure 8-6). Early endotracheal intubation is essential to support the airway during acute care of these patients.

Patients who inhale significant quantities of smoke can suffer *lower airway injuries*, the so-called "*true*" *inhalation injury*. Cotton, wood, and paper are the most abundant fuels burned during a house/building fire. Large amounts of CO, formaldehyde, formic acid, cyanide, and hydrochloric acid are produced from the incomplete combustion of these materials. The inhalation of toxic compounds causes severe damage to the mucosal cells of the airway. Cyanide, generated as a byproduct of burning plastics, has been reported as a cause of death following smoke inhalation. The hallmark of cyanide toxicity is a persistent metabolic acidosis that is not responsive to fluid resuscitation. The treatment is the administration of hydroxocobalamin, which turns urine a dark purple color. In smoke inhalation injury, the dead/damaged lung parenchyma cells slough, producing plugging, segmental collapse, and bronchiectasis. Pneumonia can occur in multiple lung segments in these patients. However, this cascade of events often takes several days to develop; symptoms may be completely absent for the first 24 to 48 hours of care, so a high index of suspicion is critical for the detection and timely treatment of these injuries. The performance of fiberoptic bronchoscopy is an important part of the initial evaluation of patients trapped in enclosed spaces.

INITIAL CARE OF THE BURN PATIENT

Burn patients should be considered victims of multiple trauma, and many of the same treatment priorities and algorithms apply to their care as to other patients with trauma. It will be assumed that the reader is familiar with the principles of Advanced Trauma Life Support outlined in Chapter 7; this chapter on burns focuses on the aspects of care that are unique to burn injuries.

Stop the Burning Process

A unique problem of burn trauma is the tendency for burns to continue producing tissue damage for minutes to hours after the initial burn has occurred. This process can further injure the patient. For example, placing an oxygen mask on a victim of flame injury runs the risk of reigniting smoldering clothing. Stopping the burning process before proceeding with any other measures is critical. Flame burns should be extinguished completely by dousing with water, smothering, or rolling patients on the ground. Hot liquids—especially viscous liquids like tar or plastics—can remain hot enough to burn for some time; they should be

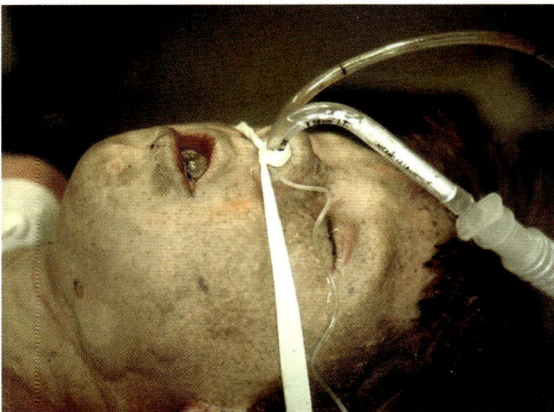
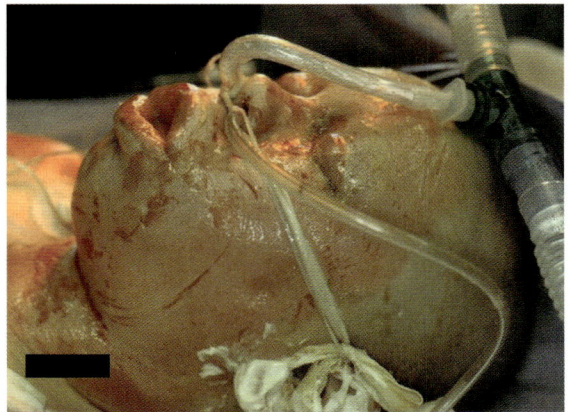

A   **B**

Figure 8-6. This young man suffered an extensive burn injury from a glass explosion. A. About 45 minutes after injury. He has extensive deep burns on the face, which are indicated by the grayish, dry skin and charring about the lips. Although he was breathing normally, prophylactic intubation was performed. B. A few hours after the first photo. He has massive facial edema affecting his lips, eyelids, and neck. Without an endotracheal tube, it is likely that his airway would occlude. In treating extensive burns of this nature, it is important to consider intubation early, before evidence of airway compromise develops. Also note that this patient has been nasally intubated. These are old photos; nasal intubation is rarely used today.

cooled immediately with cool water or moist compresses. Once cooled, such compounds can then be left in place on the patient if necessary. Caustic chemicals must be diluted immediately and completely with copious amounts of water. In recent years, widespread concern over possible acts of terrorism and mass casualty incidents involving toxic chemicals has heightened awareness of the need to decontaminate patients thoroughly both to protect the care team and to spare victims further harm.

Victims of electrocution can themselves conduct current to rescue workers. Such patients cannot be approached until the source of current is shut off.

Primary Survey

The primary survey is a quick examination designed to detect and treat immediately life-threatening conditions, beginning with the evaluation of *airway, breathing, and circulation* (the ABCs). In performing the primary survey in burn patients, special attention should be paid to the possible existence of *inhalation injury*, which is a major source of both immediate- and long-term morbidity and mortality. As discussed previously, inhalation injury should be suspected whenever the patient has been exposed to smoke. All three types of inhalation injury—CO poisoning, upper airway edema, and lower airway obstruction and hypoxemia—may be present simultaneously, or any of the three may occur alone. Even in the absence of smoke exposure, patients with severe facial burns can develop massive swelling that can lead to an obstruction of the supraglottic airway. Remember again that edema is progressive, and the signs of airway compromise may be absent until several hours following injury; patients should be followed and reexamined regularly for this. Also during the primary survey, the examiner should note the evidence of circulatory compromise in extremities caused by severe edema and constricting burn wounds. See Chapter 7 for a more detailed review of the signs and symptoms of vascular compromise accompanying trauma to the extremities.

Resuscitation

Initial resuscitation of burn patients is similar to that of other patients. If injuries appear to be major, two large-bore lines placed intravenously should be secured. A Foley catheter should be placed to aid in resuscitation. Formal calculation of fluid requirements should not be performed until after the secondary survey is completed. The performance of fluid resuscitation is an important ongoing part of the definitive treatment of burn injuries and is discussed in detail in the following paragraphs.

Secondary Survey

All too often, the presence of a dramatic burn wound distracts the examiner from detecting other, more urgent injuries. In addition, the swelling, discoloration, and pain that accompany burns can obscure underlying abdominal tenderness, extremity fractures, or cyanosis. For these reasons, it is imperative that a comprehensive, head-to-toe examination of every burn patient be conducted. Only after completing the secondary survey should burns be debrided by removing blistered skin and washing the burn wound thoroughly. The location, extent, and depth of burn wounds should be documented. There are two common ways of estimating the burn size. One, the "Rule of Nines"

is performed by dividing the body into its component parts and assigning 9% of the total body surface area (TBSA) to each part. As an alternative, the Lund and Browder chart can be used (Figure 8-7). These charts are used to calculate the total burn size, expressed as *percent total body surface area* (%TBSA). Only partial-thickness (second-degree) and full-thickness (third-degree) burn wounds should be included in this estimate of total burn size. An easy way to estimate small burns is to remember that the palm of the patient's hand (with fingers) is approximately 1% of the patient's body surface area (BSA). This estimate of burn size is used to guide fluid resuscitation, nutrition, and other aspects of care. Wounds should not be dressed with antibiotic creams or ointments, or wrapped with dressings, until a secondary assessment has been completed and the burn has been evaluated.

Burn Center Referral

Over the past 50 years, specialized burn facilities have been developed to care for patients with serious burns. The American Burn Association and the American College of Surgeons have defined criteria for burn centers, similar to those developed for trauma centers. These criteria require that institutions maintain significant multidisciplinary expertise in all phases of burn treatment, and commit space, resources, and personnel to the care of patients with burns. In addition, specific guidelines for referral of patients to burn centers have been developed; these are contained in Table 8-2. The guidelines are widely used as standards for treatment. As a more general rule, surgeons who do not work in burn centers should treat only patients with burns they are experienced in treating and should consider consultation with a burn center for *any* questions regarding patient management.

DEFINITIVE CARE OF BURN INJURIES

Following the initial assessment, burn patients require treatment for a number of physiologic consequences of injury. Support for several different problems may be required simultaneously, although the importance and magnitude of these problems change at different times after burn. To help in organizing treatment priorities and protocols, many physicians divide burn care into three periods: *resuscitation, wound closure,* and *rehabilitation*. It should be emphasized, however, that these distinctions are somewhat artificial, that many aspects of care overlap, and that careful attention to the individual patient's needs is essential at all stages of treatment.

Resuscitation Period

This period lasts for the first 24 to 48 hours following injury. Once an acutely burned patient has been evaluated and stabilized, as described previously, fluid resuscitation is the most important goal of initial treatment. Burn injury produces a loss of capillary integrity, which results in edema formation. With large ($\geq$15%-20% TBSA) burns, capillary leakage becomes systemic, producing total body edema, and severely depleting circulating volume, a phenomenon known as *burn shock*. In general, patients with burns of 10% to 15% TBSA or greater require formal fluid

BURN ESTIMATE AND DIAGRAM
AGE vs AREA

Area	Birth 1 y	1-4 y	5-9 y	10-14 y	15 y	Adult	2º	3º	Total	Donor Areas
Head	19	17	13	11	9	7				
Neck	2	2	2	2	2	2				
Ant. Trunk	13	13	13	13	13	13				
Post. Trunk	13	13	13	13	13	13				
R. Buttock	2½	2½	2½	2½	2½	2½				
L. Buttock	2½	2½	2½	2½	2½	2½				
Genitalia	1	1	1	1	1	1				
R. U. Arm	4	4	4	4	4	4				
L. U. Arm	4	4	4	4	4	4				
R. L. Arm	3	3	3	3	3	3				
L. L. Arm	3	3	3	3	3	3				
R. Hand	2½	2½	2½	2½	2½	2½				
L. Hand	2½	2½	2½	2½	2½	2½				
R. Thigh	5½	6½	8	8½	9	9½				
L. Thigh	5½	6½	8	8½	9	9½				
R. Leg	5	5	5½	6	6½	7				
L. Leg	5	5	5½	6	6½	7				
R. Foot	3½	3½	3½	3½	3½	3½				
L. Foot	3½	3½	3½	3½	3½	3½				
						TOTAL				

Cause of Burn_____

Date of Burn_____

Time of Burn_____

Age_____

Sex_____

Weight_____

BURN DIAGRAM

LUND AND BROWDER CHART

COLOR CODE

Red—3º

Blue—2º

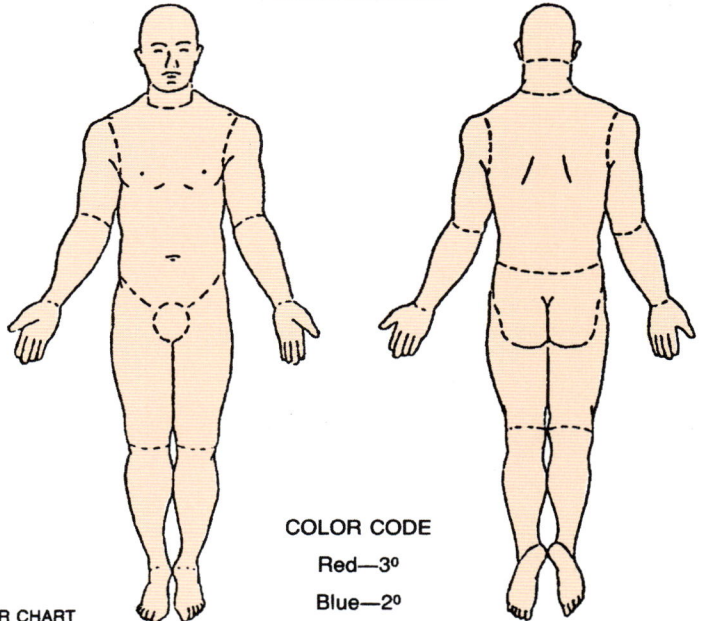

Figure 8-7. Lund and Browder chart. This diagram was developed during World War II to help document and estimate the extent of burn injuries. Following initial debridement, the examiner should draw the burn injuries on the figure, calculate how much of each body area is burned, and then add all areas to produce a total burn size. Inexperienced providers tend to overestimate burn size and underestimate depth. We hope that the figures included in this chapter will help readers evaluate burn wounds more accurately.

TABLE 8-2. Criteria for Referral to a Burn Center

1. Partial-thickness burns >10% TBSA

2. Burns that involve the face, hand, feet, genitalia, perineum, or major joints

3. Third-degree burns in any age group

4. Electrical burns, including lightning injury

5. Chemical burns

6. Inhalation injury

7. Burn injury in patients with preexisting medical disorders that could complicate management, prolong recovery, or affect mortality

8. Any patient with burns and concomitant trauma (such as fractures) in which the burn injury poses the greatest risk of morbidity or mortality. In such cases, if the trauma poses a greater immediate risk, the patient's condition may be stabilized initially in a trauma center before transfer to a burn center. Physician judgment will be necessary in such situations and should be in concert with the regional medical control plan and triage protocols.

9. Burned children in hospitals without qualified personnel or equipment for the care of children

10. Burn injury in patients who will require special social, emotional, or rehabilitative intervention

TBSA, total body surface area.

resuscitation. These fluid losses can exceed those of any other injury or disease; truly remarkable amounts of fluid may be required for the successful resuscitation of patients with very large burns.

A host of algorithms have been developed for burn resuscitation, but most successful regimens share several basic concepts. These are illustrated in Table 8-3. The American Burn Association's Advanced Burn Life Support (ABLS) course recommends fluid resuscitation of 2 mL/kg/% TBSA burn in adult patients, 3 mL/kg/% TBSA burn in pediatric patients, and 4 mL/kg/% TBSA burn in patients with electrical injury.

This formula calls for isotonic crystalloid fluid (lactated Ringer solution) to be given at an initial rate determined from burn size and body weight. Edema formation occurs throughout the first 24 hours after burn but is most pronounced during the first 8 hours; therefore, half the total fluid is given during that period. However, because inhalation injury, multiple trauma, and other factors can influence an individual's fluid requirements, regimens like the Consensus formula really only tell you where to *begin* resuscitation. Fluid administration should thereafter be guided by frequent and repeated evaluation of the patient. The maintenance of adequate urine output (≥30 mL/h in adults; 1-1.5 mL/kg/h in children) is used as an indicator of appropriate fluid intake and an important goal of treatment. The infusion rate is adjusted according to urine output and gradually decreased until a maintenance rate is reached. Vital signs, hematocrit, and other laboratory tests should be carefully monitored as well.

Fluid resuscitation does not stop fluid leakage into the interstitium; it is intended only to keep up with

TABLE 8-3. Principles of Fluid Resuscitation for Burns: The American Burn Association's ABLS Course Recommendation

Principles

A. Resuscitation should consist primarily of isotonic crystalloid solution because it is inexpensive, readily available, and can be given in large quantities without harmful side effects.

B. Because injured capillaries are porous to proteins for the first several hours after injury, colloid-containing fluids are not used initially.

C. Resuscitation requirements are proportional to burn size and the patient's body weight.

D. Edema formation is most rapid during the first hours after injury but continues for at least 24 h. Therefore, half the calculated fluid is given in the first 8 h following the burn.

E. Formulas only tell you where to BEGIN resuscitation, which must then be guided by patient response: urine output, vital signs, and mental status.

Practice: The American Burn Association's ABLS Course Recommendation

A. The formula: 2 mL lactated Ringer × body weight (kg) × %TBSA burns = total fluid for the first 24 h.

B. For the first 8 h after injury, give half the total calculation.

C. For the second and third 8 h after injury, give one-fourth of the total calculation.

Example

A. A 220-lb (100 kg) man is burned while filling the gas tank on his boat. He is wearing a swimming suit and is burned over all of both legs, his chest, and both arms. The calculated burn size is 65% TBSA.

B. Calculated fluid requirements using 2 mL/kg/%TBSA burn:

2 mL × 100 kg × 65% TBSA burn = 13,000 mL in 24 h

TABLE 8-3. Principles of Fluid Resuscitation for Burns: The American Burn Association's ABLS Course Recommendation (*continued*)

	= 6,500 in first 8 h = 812 mL/h
	= 3,250 mL in each of the second and third 8 h = 406 mL/h

C. Adjust according to patient response.

1. You select an initial rate of 812 mL/h on the basis of a calculation of 2 mL/kg/%TBSA. After 6 h, the patient received 4,872 mL of lactated Ringer. Urine output, which was initially good, has fallen to 20 mL in the past hour. Heart rate is 132 beats/min, and BP is 106/50 mm Hg.

2. At this point, you should increase the fluid rate, typically by about 10%-20%. All indications point to inadequate resuscitation.

3. You increase fluids by 20%, to 974 mL/h. Two hours later, urine output again drops, to 15 mL/h. Heart rate is 128 beats/min, and BP is 98/52 mm Hg.

4. You should again increase fluids. Most experts would NOT consider the use of a diuretic at this point in time. Individual fluid requirements vary significantly, and this man appears to need more than the minimum requirements. Your response to decreasing urine output should be to increase fluids.

5. Three hours later, urine output has increased to 95 mL/h. Heart rate has dropped to 90 beats/min, and BP is 135/85 mm Hg.

6. You should now begin to decrease fluids by 10%-15% per hour, with continued attention to urine output and vital signs. Fluid resuscitation is a dynamic process and requires continuous attention to detail.

ABLS, American Burn Association's Advanced Burn Life Support; BP, blood pressure; TBSA, total body surface area.

ongoing losses, which decrease over time. As resuscitation proceeds, therefore, so does tissue edema. Fluid accumulating beneath the constricted eschar of a deep burn increases tissue hydrostatic pressure, sometimes to the point that circulation is compromised. Frequent evaluation of extremity pulses, sensory and motor function, and pain is essential to diagnose the progressive ischemia of a compartment syndrome. The treatment of compromised circulation in a circumferential burn is escharotomy. An escharotomy is an incision made through the rigid, leathery eschar to relieve the compression produced by ongoing edema and, thus, restore distal circulation. Figure 8-8 illustrates an escharotomy of the upper extremity. Compression by edema can also affect the chest and abdomen, resulting in respiratory compromise. Escharotomies can be performed on the torso and should provide immediate relief. Because escharotomies are always made through burn wounds, they are repaired during burn wound excision and skin grafting and usually leave no additional scars.

However, escharotomies do not always provide adequate relief of edema-related pressure. When burns of the extremity are particularly deep, incisions through the underlying muscle fascia ("fasciotomies") may be required to produce adequate decompression. This is more commonly required for high-voltage electrical injuries (Figure 8-9). In addition, massive fluid accumulation within the tissues of the abdomen can produce an abdominal compartment syndrome and require decompressive laparotomy to relieve this compression.

RESPIRATORY SUPPORT

Resuscitation of the patient with moderate-to-severe inhalation injury usually requires modifications. An inhalation injury is essentially a burn to the inside of the lungs, and the Consensus formula must be adjusted appropriately. The amount of fluid given should still be adjusted according to patient response, but it is common for the patient

with inhalation injury to have higher fluid requirements from unseen fluid loss caused by lung injury. Ventilatory support and close monitoring of systemic arterial pressure, lactic acid, and urine output must be used to help titrate the amount of fluids the patient is receiving. The development of acute respiratory distress syndrome (ARDS) is very common with a severe inhalation injury. Overresuscitation with intravenous fluids can worsen the ARDS and should be avoided if at all possible. ARDS is diagnosed by a "ground-glass" appearance on chest radiograph coupled with the clinical syndrome of worsening respiratory failure. Aggressive modes of ventilator support are necessary to combat hypoxemia in patients with ARDS. Conventional ventilator settings must have adequate PEEP and

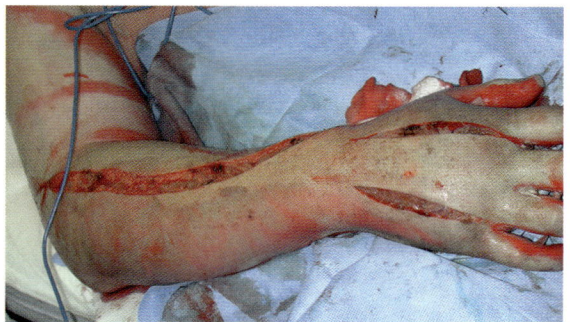

Figure 8-8. Escharotomy of the upper extremity. This extensively burned arm and hand developed progressive tense edema, numbness and tingling, and deep throbbing pain. Intramuscular pressures were measured using a sterile needle connected to a pressure transducer and were in excess of 30 cm H_2O. Escharotomies were performed at the bedside using deep sedation and electrocautery. The wound edges have separated markedly because of the underlying edema. It should be remembered that escharotomy does not reduce the *swelling* associated with the burn injury, but it is done to relieve the *compression* produced by edema accumulation beneath the unyielding surface of a deep burn injury.

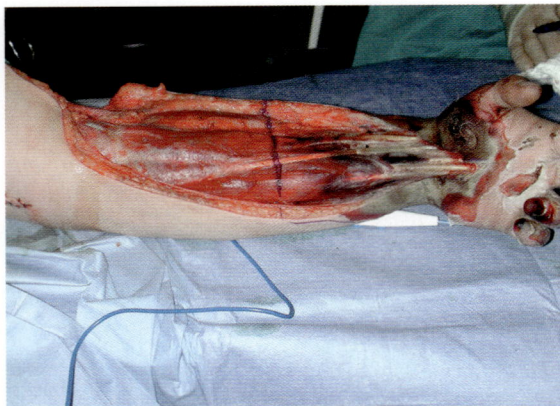

Figure 8-9. High-voltage electrical injury of the hand. Charring and full-thickness injury of the base of the palm is apparent. The fingers and wrist are "fixed" in flexion because of coagulation necrosis of the flexor muscles of the forearm. Brownish necrosis of the flexor tendons and distal muscles is apparent. Note the dramatic separation of the skin edges following fasciotomy. The hand is unsalvageable; the blue line indicates the approximate level of amputation to be performed.

low tidal volumes to minimize barotrauma. Newer ventilator modes, such as airway pressure release ventilation and pressure-regulated volume control, may be useful in ARDS, as they reduce barotrauma. The treatment team must remain vigilant with respiratory care and patient positioning to reduce the risk of pneumonia from inhalation injuries. ARDS secondary to inhalation injury can progress to chronic respiratory failure; these patients may require tracheostomy and long-term ventilator support.

Wound Coverage Period

This phase of treatment begins following fluid resuscitation and lasts for days to weeks until the burn wound either heals primarily or is successfully replaced with skin grafts. This period comprises most of the patient's hospital care and is the period of most intensive treatment. Patients who attain successful wound closure usually survive, although they may face prolonged rehabilitation following this period of care.

EXCISION AND SKIN GRAFTING

Deeply burned skin is a great liability to the patient. Not only does burn eschar serve as a source of infection, but the loss of skin integrity causes increased evaporative fluid losses and an intense inflammatory response that can escalate, leading to multiple organ failure and death. If followed conservatively, deep eschar will eventually separate spontaneously, but this can take weeks, during which the patient is exposed to ongoing stress and the risk of infection. For these reasons, most burn centers now employ early excision, in which burned skin is excised off the underlying tissue. Two techniques are available: fascial and tangential excision. In fascial excision, the scalpel or cautery is used to excise the entire skin and subcutaneous tissue, usually to the level of the underlying fascia. Although this procedure is easy to perform and permits good skin graft "take," it is disfiguring and leads to joint stiffness and poor mobility (Figure 8-10). In tangential excision, sequential thin slices of skin are removed with a dermatome or a blade until viable tissue is encountered. This technique requires skill and produces significant bleeding. However, the cosmetic and

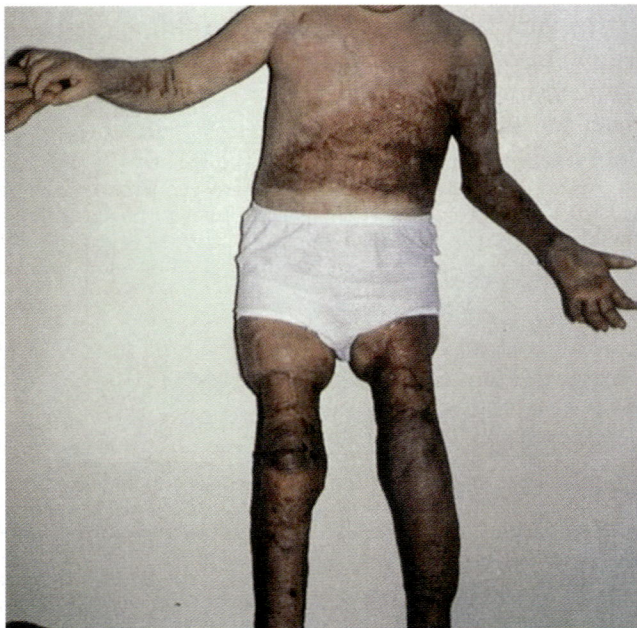

Figure 8-10. The long-term result of fascial excision and skin grafting. Fascia is well vascularized and will "take" skin grafts well. However, the resulting wound is stiff, and the lack of subcutaneous padding results in chronic discomfort and poor joint mobility, as well as the obvious problems with appearance.

functional results of grafting this type of wound are often superior to those of fascial excision. Tangential excision of deep partial-thickness burns permits salvaging intact dermal elements, which improves the results of skin grafting. Most surgeons wait until fluid resuscitation has been completed before beginning excisional therapy in order to permit the stabilization of cardiovascular function and intravascular volume, which can be further compromised by surgical blood loss. Limited burns of mixed or indeterminate depth can be followed for 10 to 14 days before the decision to proceed to surgery must be made.

Skin grafting is usually performed at the same time as excision. At present, permanent coverage of an excised wound can be achieved only with the patient's own skin, called an *autograft*. Autografting can be performed using full-thickness or split-thickness skin grafts. Full-thickness grafts are obtained by excising an ellipse of skin from the groin or flank, which is closed with sutures. Split-thickness grafts are obtained by using a dermatome to procure intact skin at the level of the superficial dermis, typically 0.004 to 0.015 inches in depth. This yields a graft with sufficient dermis for secure coverage of the excised burn, while leaving a wound superficial enough to heal spontaneously in 7 to 14 days. In treating very large burns, the urgency to remove eschar often requires that excision be performed, even if no donor sites are available for grafting. Although the best functional and cosmetic results are obtained when sheet grafts are placed, when insufficient autograft is available, several techniques can be used to obtain wound coverage. First, skin can be expanded by meshing or cutting multiple small slits in the skin. Many skin grafts are meshed to facilitate application and graft "take." These grafts leave a permanent mesh pattern in the skin but produce durable coverage. Widely meshed autografts will cover larger areas, although the interstices of the mesh are prone to desiccation. The most widely used skin substitute is cadaver allograft, skin obtained from tissue banks. Other skin substitutes include human amniotic membrane and various synthetic materials. In recent years, considerable research has been devoted to the development of a man-made "artificial dermis," which could be taken off the shelf and used to cover large burn wounds. Some of these products are used routinely, particularly in reconstructive surgery, but they still require coverage with thin autografts. Finally, it is possible to grow a patient's own epidermal cells in culture. These cultured epidermal autografts are expensive, fragile, and easily lost because of infection. Nonetheless, they have proved lifesaving in some patients with massive burns.

INFECTION CONTROL

Although the skin surface after burning is virtually sterile for 24 to 48 hours, it is gradually repopulated with bacteria. Burn eschar—especially the thick, avascular eschar of deep burns—is an ideal culture medium for bacteria, which will rapidly multiply on such a surface. These bacteria may colonize burn eschar harmlessly, or, by penetrating through the burn wound, invade intact tissues and overwhelm local defenses, producing invasive infection, termed *burn wound sepsis*. Infection is also exacerbated by the immunosuppression that accompanies severe burn injury. Burn wound

sepsis is often fatal and, until recently, has been the most common cause of death in hospitalized burn patients. With modern methods of wound management, however, it is now an infrequent occurrence in burn centers.

Much of the increased survival from burns achieved in the past 50 years is due to improved understanding and the treatment of burn wound infections. Beginning in the 1940s, systemic antibiotics like penicillin, as well as some topical agents, were used to control microbial contamination of burn wounds. The first widely used topical antimicrobial, silver nitrate solution, proved particularly effective in controlling infections caused by *Staphylococcus* and *Streptococcus* species. A variety of gram-negative infections then began to predominate as causes of burn wound infection. The development in the 1960s of two powerful topical agents, mafenide acetate and silver sulfadiazine, helped control many gram-negative bacteria, which were then replaced by resistant *Pseudomonas* as a leading cause of infection. More recently, a host of powerful systemic antibiotics, and numerous other topical agents, have helped control *Pseudomonas* infections. This success has been followed by—and to some extent, caused—the emergence of multidrug-resistant bacteria (such as methicillin-resistant *Staphylococcus aureus*, *Acinetobacter baumannii*, and vancomycin-resistant *Enterococcus*), as well as fungi and other exotic organisms, as important clinical pathogens in burn patients. This problem is magnified by the development in many burn centers of entrenched, endemic microbial populations, which have proven very difficult to eradicate. Thus, because the medical community has developed evermore powerful antimicrobials for burn care, we have seen the microbial fauna adapt and continue to present new and unforeseen problems.

The most effective technique in the battle against burn wound infection is early burn excision and skin grafting, as discussed previously. Meticulous wound care is an essential part of burn treatment during the repair phase. Beginning immediately after burn, wounds must be washed regularly and carefully debrided of old topical creams and ointments, dried serum, and bits of loose eschar. Topical antimicrobials are effective only for a few hours, and most experts agree that their replacement, as well as regular and thorough debridement, should be performed at least twice daily. There are some products that adhere to wounds and release antibiotics (usually silver) slowly; their use should be supervised by an experienced clinician because infection developing beneath these products can be particularly difficult to diagnose and treat. This is also true for freshly grafted burn wounds and skin graft donor sites.

As the prevention and treatment of burn wound infection have become more successful, other problems have gained prominence as causes of morbidity and mortality in burn patients. Pneumonia has emerged as the most common, and often the most troublesome, infection seen in burn patients. The bronchiectasis and mucous plugging that accompany inhalation injury create an environment rife for the development of infections and render them difficult to clear. Pneumonia, in turn, often serves as a stimulus for systemic inflammation and infection, leading to the development of multiple organ failure. Other infectious complications can occur as well, including wound, urinary tract, and bloodstream infections. Septic thrombophlebitis can even occur in veins cannulated for vascular access.

NUTRITIONAL SUPPORT

As part of the hormonal response to burn trauma, metabolic rate rises dramatically and can exceed twice normal for prolonged periods, with a corresponding increase in nitrogen excretion. The massive catabolism after burn can result in a fatal degree of inanition within a few weeks if left untreated. In response to the increased metabolic demands of a major burn, skeletal muscle is broken down to provide an available energy substrate. This results in increased nitrogen excretion and a loss of lean body mass, which can exceed a half pound per day. Cardiac muscle and respiratory muscles are not immune from these effects, and as muscle wasting continues, both heart failure and respiratory failure can occur with wasting of respiratory muscles and immune compromise, resulting in pulmonary infection and death. A loss of as little as 15% lean body mass can be fatal within a few weeks of injury. For this reason, burn patients require aggressive nutritional support and close nutritional monitoring throughout the wound closure phase of treatment. Enteral feeding is superior to intravenous nutrition in burn patients; patients with large burns should have the placement of enteral feeding tubes as soon as possible and the infusion of a high-protein diet until they can demonstrate adequate oral intake. A variety of formulas have been used to predict the caloric requirements of burn patients. None is entirely satisfactory, due in large part to the wide variation seen among individuals and the fluctuations in energy expenditure that occur during the postburn course. Many experts recommend the routine measurement of energy expenditure using indirect calorimetry and of protein utilization by determining nitrogen balance at least weekly. The technique of indirect calorimetry calculates the energy requirements of an individual by measuring the oxygen consumed during normal breathing. The provision of a basic high-protein diet (1.5-2.0 g protein/kg body weight daily), in quantities sufficient to satisfy caloric requirements, remains the most important principle in the nutritional management of such patients.

The Rehabilitation Phase

Once burns are closed, major emphasis is shifted to rehabilitation. Providers should remember the adage that *rehabilitation begins at the time of injury*; do not wait for wound closure. As burn wounds heal, they contract because of the presence of myofibroblasts that begin to accumulate within wounds shortly after injury and continue to proliferate within the scar. If unopposed, burn scar contractures can immobilize extremities and produce significant disfigurement. Much of the therapy provided during burn rehabilitation is aimed at preventing and correcting contractures. This therapy is more effective if begun soon after injury, while the scar tissue is still pliable, and before it can "set" into significant contractures. The scar tissue remains inflamed and continues to remodel and reshape itself for at least a year following injury. In addition to motion and stretching exercises, compression garments are frequently used to reduce the growth of hypertrophic scars. These custom-made garments are worn until the scar tissue softens and erythema fades. Figure 8-11 shows a custom-made clear facemask used for the same purpose. The process of recovering completely from a major burn is long and labor-intensive, but the vast majority of burn patients can

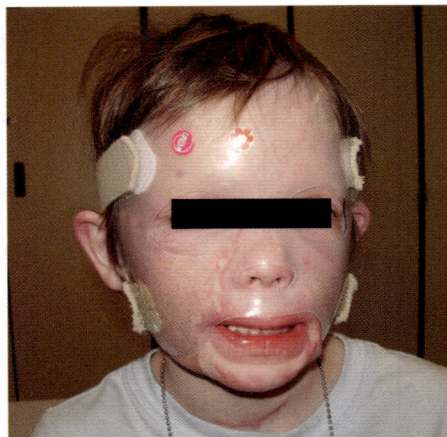

Figure 8-11. Compressive face mask. The child was burned in an automobile fire and required extensive skin grafting to her face. Long-term use of elastic face masks tends to produce deformities of the mandible in children; these masks are unattractive and socially stigmatizing. Instead, a rigid mask of clear plastic, which the patient wears for most of every day, was custom-made. This compresses the skin grafts as they remodel, resulting in a smoother result with fewer hypertrophic scars and contractures. Such masks are typically worn for at least a year following injury.

return to active and useful lives with appropriate therapy. The vast majority of patients return to work or school, even following burns of 70% TBSA or greater.

Reconstructive surgery may be needed to correct particularly difficult contractures, resurface areas of unstable wound coverage, or improve cosmesis. This surgery is usually postponed until burn scars mature and soften. However, many reconstructive procedures can be avoided by early and continued application of physical therapy and other rehabilitative techniques.

SPECIAL PROBLEMS IN BURN CARE

Comprehensive care of burn patients often involves a number of issues that either are not regularly encountered in other surgical practices or present themselves in unique ways. These include the unique features of electrical and chemical injuries, the care of patients with minor burns, problems with pain control and itching, and the increasing trend for burn centers to treat other nonburn conditions. These are reviewed here.

Chemical and Electrical Burns

Both chemical and electrical injuries can present unique challenges in diagnosis and treatment. The degree of tissue damage produced by chemicals is determined by the nature of the agent, its concentration, and the duration of skin contact. Three classes of chemicals commonly produce skin injuries. Alkalis dissolve and combine with the proteins of the tissues to form alkaline proteinates, which contain hydroxide ions. These ions induce further chemical reactions, penetrating deeper into the tissue. Acids induce protein breakdown by hydrolysis, which results in an eschar that does not penetrate as deeply as the alkalis. These agents also induce thermal injury by heat generation with contact of the skin, further causing tissue damage. Organic compounds such as petroleum products, phenols, and others injure tissue by their fat-solvent action, which dissolves cell membranes. All three types of agents also pose the risk of systemic absorption and toxicity.

A careful history should be obtained to identify the responsible chemical. Prompt treatment is imperative in minimizing tissue damage. Providers should wear protective gear and detoxify the patient completely before other care is delivered. It is critical that the chemical be neutralized by decontamination before a primary survey can be conducted safely. All patient clothing should be removed, any dry powders should be brushed off the skin, and all chemicals should then be thoroughly irrigated with copious volumes of water. Hot chemicals such as tar can be left in place once cooled completely. If the chemical composition is known, monitoring of the pH of the irrigated solution will give a good indication of irrigation effectiveness and completion. The local poison control center may provide important information on specific chemical injuries, their severity, and possible adjunctive treatment, but initial detoxification should always be instituted as quickly as possible.

Patients may have metabolic disturbances from pH abnormalities or from specific chemical toxicities (such as organophosphates). An arterial blood gas, electrolytes, and hepatic enzymes should be obtained. If the patient's condition deteriorates—such as obvious progression of the wound and/or progressive metabolic deterioration—urgent surgery may be needed to remove the wound entirely. Resuscitation should be guided by BSA involved. The depth of injury can be difficult to determine with chemical injuries: Some may be more superficial than they appear, particularly in the case of acids, whereas alkaline injuries may penetrate beyond that which is apparent on examination and will require more fluid for effective resuscitation volume. Once initial care and resuscitation are completed, chemical wounds are managed in the same way as other burn injuries.

Electrical injuries occur when current enters a part of the body, such as the hand, and proceeds through tissues with the lowest resistance, generally nerves, blood vessels, and muscles, to exit through ground. Electrical injuries are classified as low voltage (<1,000 V) and high voltage (>1,000 V). Low-voltage injury, which typically results from household (120 V) current, is generally limited to the area surrounding the injury. The skin has high resistance to electrical current, and many low-voltage injuries produce only small cutaneous burns. However, with high-voltage injuries, typically from industrial current contact, the skin involvement may be limited, but associated underlying soft tissue damage may be extensive. Current travels preferentially beneath the skin, because deeper tissues have less resistance; tissues having the highest resistance generate the most heat. Deep tissues appear to retain heat so that the tissues next to the bones, especially between two bones, often sustain more severe injury than more superficial tissue does. In fact, the superficial muscle may appear uninjured, while the deeper muscle near the bones may be damaged. Thus, the true extent of tissue damage with high-voltage injury may be impossible to determine on initial inspection. See Figure 8-9 for an example of a high-voltage electrical injury.

Electrical injuries can cause a variety of wounds. Current flow through tissues, as described earlier, can result in deep tissue damage. In addition, current passing from its source to ground can generate an electrical arc or "flash" injury. Flame injuries can also result from an ignition of clothing without actual current flow through the patient. Electrical injury may also be associated with falls and can produce blunt trauma from tetanic muscle contractions. Lightning injuries are a type of very high-voltage direct current injuries. The blast associated with lightning strikes can produce significant trauma, including ruptured eardrums. Late complications include the development of cataracts and peripheral neuropathy.

In assessing a victim of electrical injury, the first step is to be sure that no potential for continued electrical damage exists. Current sources must be disconnected before the patient can be approached. Electrical injury can result in dysrhythmia, and many patients die from electrically induced ventricular fibrillation or cardiac standstill; therefore, immediate attention to resuscitation is essential. All victims of electric shock should have an electrocardiogram (ECG) obtained; victims of high-voltage injury (and low-voltage injuries associated with abnormal ECG findings) should be monitored on telemetry for at least 24 hours. Because of the potential for multiple trauma from falls and muscle tetany, patients should be immobilized and treated as patients with multiple trauma. Victims of high-voltage injury should be referred to a burn center and will require formal resuscitation. These injuries often result in muscle damage and rhabdomyolysis; if untreated, this will lead to compartment syndromes and acute kidney injury. Pigmented urine with myoglobin will appear tea colored. Intravenous fluid should be given to maintain adequate urine output, which should be 100 mL/h or greater until the urine is clear or myoglobinuria is resolved. The use of bicarbonate to alkalinize urine and mannitol as an osmotic diuresis to enhance renal clearance of myoglobin has not been proven in prospective studies. Therefore, the use of these adjunct treatments should be individualized according to practitioners' experience.

When compartment syndrome is suspected or myoglobinuria does not improve with resuscitation, emergent fasciotomy or exploration of muscles and debridement of the necrotic muscle may be needed. Early amputation of an affected limb may be required in severe cases. Figure 8-9 illustrates such a case.

Care of Outpatient and Minor Burns

Although burn centers concentrate on the care of patients with major injuries, many burn patients have small burns and can be managed on an outpatient basis. More than a half million emergency department visits annually are related to burns, and over 75% are limited injuries (<10% TBSA). Even such small burns, however, can be serious injuries, with significant associated pain, potential for infection, and disability. The overarching goals of treatment are to relieve pain, prevent infection, and encourage optimal healing with the least amount of scar formation.

Burns that involve small areas of injury can often be treated in a primary care or emergency department setting. Any burn patient with the evidence of inhalation injury, circumferential burns, burns to the face, hands, or perineum, or significant comorbidities is best referred to a burn center. Minor burns in children or older individuals are less than 5% TBSA. The size of burns is often overestimated, and the use of standardized tools such as the Lund and Browder chart (see Figure 8-7) is helpful in deciding on the most appropriate location and method of treatment.

As with major burns, treatment begins with removal of the offending agent and cooling the injury. It has been shown that ice water or ice cubes increase necrosis in experimental burns but that tap water at 12 to 25 °C is effective at reducing damage and providing initial pain relief. However, cooling should be applied only for a short time, because complications such as frostbite and hypothermia can result from prolonged cooling. After patient assessment and calculation of the burn depth and size, a decision is made regarding treatment in the outpatient setting, hospital admission, or burn unit transfer. Criteria for referral of burn injuries to specialized centers for care are listed in Table 8-2.

Epidermal burns without blistering do not require topical care. The treatment of superficial partial-thickness injuries should begin by thoroughly washing the wound. Although controversy exists regarding the treatment of blisters, they can often be left intact. However, once they rupture, blisters should be debrided to facilitate cleansing of the wound. Once washed and debrided, burns can be covered with a variety of topical agents, including antibiotic creams (silver sulfadiazine, mafenide acetate) or ointments (neomycin sulfate, bacitracin). Historically, silver nitrate and silver sulfadiazine have been used to inhibit bacterial growth in burns. Because these substances are inactivated in a burn wound environment, they require frequent reapplication. Although the evidence for the direct benefits of such topical care for minor burns is lacking, it is unquestionably true that dressing these wounds relieves discomfort and provides psychological benefit to the patient. Encouraging frequent washing and reapplying topical compounds may provide their most important benefit. More recently, a variety of other silver-containing dressings (silver imbedded in hydrofibers or on polyethylene mesh, and nanocrystalline silver) have been developed for burn care. These dressings can be left on wounds for longer periods, lengthening the time between dressing changes, which reduces pain compared with traditional silver preparations. They are also cost-effective, considering the need for fewer dressing changes.

Oral antibiotics are not required for uninfected burns. Topical antibiotics and absorptive dressings are useful for most contaminated burns. Burns should be inspected daily to assess for infection and changes that become evident rapidly when infection occurs.

Deep partial-thickness burns or third-degree burns are covered initially with an antibiotic ointment and dressed. Depending on local expertise and size of the burn, they should be considered for local excision and grafting. Because these wounds heal by contraction and generate considerable scar formation, all but the smallest burns should be excised. The depth of the burn may be difficult to determine initially, so frequent examination is required. Burns can deepen during the first few days because of infection or desiccation. As described previously, small burns should heal within a few weeks; burns taking longer than 3 weeks will likely form hypertrophic scars and provide an unstable epithelium. For this reason, early excision is optimal.

Treatment of Itching and Pain

Morbidity from burns extends beyond the acute phase of treatment. The pain and anxiety associated with burn injury is a significant problem. Control of pain is essential to quality patient care. Pain should be assessed whenever other vital signs are taken and treated promptly and effectively. A variety of standard scales are available to quantify pain by both patients and providers.

Analgesics are most effective for acute burn pain when given on a scheduled basis, before pain can escalate. The intravenous route is preferred during the resuscitation phase; intramuscular injections should be avoided because of highly unpredictable absorption and plasma levels and the pain of the injections themselves. Once resuscitation is completed, oral or enteral medications can be used to supplement injections as needed. The dose, route, and type of medication should be evaluated frequently to make sure pain is satisfactorily controlled.

The most commonly used analgesics for controlling acute burn pain are opioids. Morphine is most widely used. Fentanyl is shorter acting and avoids oversedation following a procedure. In addition to opioid analgesics, anesthetic agents such as ketamine and nitrous oxide can be used to provide short-term relief of pain and anxiety during procedures. For outpatient treatment, combinations of hydrocodone or oxycodone with acetaminophen are often sufficient. Nonsteroidal anti-inflammatory drugs can be used for the relief of mild-to-moderate pain or as adjuncts to hydrocodone/oxycodone.

Anxiety is prevalent in burn patients and can exacerbate pain. Lorazepam, diazepam, and midazolam are the main anxiolytics used in the treatment of burn-related anxiety and are often used in combination with opiate analgesics; α_2-adrenergic agonists such as clonidine and dexmedetomidine can also have excellent sedative, analgesic, and anxiolytic effects and have been used in burn patients with good results. Table 8-4 lists a number of medications commonly used for analgesia and sedation in burn centers. It should be noted that many of these agents should be used only in an inpatient, monitored setting.

Medications by themselves often do not control pain and anxiety completely. A variety of nonpharmacologic therapies have been tried to alleviate pain associated with burn injury, including cognitive techniques (breathing exercises, reinforcement of positive behavior, use of age-appropriate imagery, and behavioral rehearsal). Another approach to pain control is distraction. Distracting patients' attention using music therapy, movies, and games can help them better tolerate pain. Virtual reality systems can immerse patients' attention in a computer-generated world and engage them in multisensory interactions with that world, including touch, sight, and sound, providing profound relief of pain and anxiety. Studies have shown a significant reduction in pain in burn patients during dressing changes and rehabilitative therapies using virtual reality systems. Augmented virtual reality involves a virtual image being overlaid onto the physical world instead of immersion into an artificial virtual world to focus patient perception away from a noxious stimulus. Hypnosis can reduce pain and can be used as an effective nonpharmacologic approach to burn pain. Hypnosis uses a combination of relaxation, imagery, and cognitive-based approach.

TABLE 8-4. List of Analgesia and Sedatives Typically Used in Adult Burn Treatment

Agent	Recommended Dosages	Comment
Opiates		
Morphine sulfate	0.03-0.1 mg/kg IV	Morphine, fentanyl, and hydromorphone (Dilaudid) are the most widely used acute analgesics. All three agents can be used with patient-controlled analgesia devices for effective pain control. Oral preparations of these and other narcotics are preferred for long term and outpatient use, but remember to use equianalgesic doses when transitioning from IV to oral agents.
Fentanyl	50-100 µg IV, 0.5-1 µg/kg IV	
Hydromorphone	1-2 mg IV, 0.02 mg/kg IV	
Oxycodone	5-10 mg PO q4-6h	These two widely used oral analgesics are less powerful than morphine and fentanyl but share the same risks of respiratory depression and dependency. They are often used in the rehabilitative phase of burn care and for outpatients. A long-acting form of oxycodone is available.
Hydrocodone	5-10 mg PO q4-6h	
Benzodiazepines		
Midazolam	0.03-0.1 mg/kg IV	These are widely used benzodiazepines for sedation and relief of anxiety. They are not good analgesics, however, so other medications should be used to provide adequate pain control.
Lorazepam	1-4 mg IV, 0.04-0.08 mg/kg IV	
Diazepam	2-10 mg IV, 0.04-0.3 mg/kg IV	
Other agents		
Propofol	0.5-1 mg/kg IV	Frequently used for short-term sedation for procedures and for sedation of patients on mechanical ventilation. Airway support is required for use.
Ketamine	0.5-1 mg/kg IV	Can be given intramuscularly for short procedures in the outpatient setting. Associated with emergence problems, including delirium and nightmares. Can be used at a very low-dose continuous infusion (0.1 mg/kg/h).
Dexmedetomidine	0.3-0.7 µg/kg/h IV	Increasingly popular both for short-term sedation and for a more prolonged sedation of patients on mechanical ventilation.
Clonidine	0.1-0.3 mg q6-12h PO	Also available as a sustained-release patch. Should not be used as a single agent for pain control.

IV, intravenous; PO, by mouth.

In addition to pain, itching can be a severe, prolonged problem in burn patients. In a study from one outpatient burn clinic, 50% of the patients recalled moderate-to-severe pruritus. This often interfered with sleep and with the quality of life in general. At times, it causes wound breakdown because of scratching. Pruritus occurred in 32% of the cases with burns smaller than 2% TBSA, almost as frequent as pruritus in major burns. Although pruritus recedes with time, it can last for up to 12 years after the burn. Treatment is often not effective, with only 36% of patients in that study reporting benefit. Topical drugs (tricyclic histamine receptor blockers, doxepin) as well as gabapentin, dapsone, ondansetron, and H_1-/H_2-blocker combination therapy have been employed. Simple cooling, transcutaneous electrical nerve stimulation, and massage have also been useful.

Burn Unit Treatment of Other Injuries

As burn units have evolved into centers for multidisciplinary expertise, they have often been used to treat other conditions that require critical care, specialized wound management, physical therapy, and rehabilitation. Among the conditions often referred to burn centers are the major exfoliative skin disorders and necrotizing soft tissue infections.

SKIN DISORDERS

Toxic epidermal necrolysis (TEN) and Stevens-Johnson syndrome (SJS) are rare, life-threatening exfoliative disorders involving the skin. They are caused by cell-mediated immune reactions, resulting in the destruction of basal epithelial cells by CD8-positive T cells and macrophages in the superficial dermis. T cells then migrate into the epidermis, causing keratinocyte injury and epidermal necrolysis, analogous to the graft-versus-host disease that occurs in bone marrow transplant recipients. The disorders are distinguished primarily by the extent of cutaneous involvement: TEN is defined as greater than 30% BSA desquamation, whereas SJS has less than 10% BSA involvement. Patients with 10% to 30% BSA involvement have an SJS/TEN "overlap." Because TEN is the most severe form of this disorder, it is most frequently referred to burn centers for care.

Drug exposure causes 80% of all TEN cases. Dilantin and sulfonamide antibiotics are involved in 40% of all cases; however, other agents, such as nonsteroidal anti-inflammatory agents, other antibiotics, other anticonvulsants, upper respiratory tract infections, and viral illness have also been implicated. High-risk groups include patients with seizure disorders, metastatic cancer (particularly brain metastases), urinary tract infections, allogenic bone marrow transplants, and human immunodeficiency virus (HIV) infections.

A viral-like prodromal phase consisting of fever and malaise is frequently reported shortly after exposure to the inciting agent. Following this, a macular rash develops that spreads, often becoming confluent. The syndrome may involve any mucosal surface, including the oropharynx, eyes, gastrointestinal tract, genitourinary tract, and tracheobronchial tree. Patients have evidence of epidermal necrosis with large areas of epidermal detachment on physical examination. Nikolsky sign, the separation of the epidermis with digital pressure, is a common physical finding. This is illustrated in Figure 8-12.

TEN and SJS treatment begins with immediate discontinuation of the inciting agent. Skin biopsy at the edge of the blistered area and adjacent uninvolved skin should be performed to distinguish TEN/SJS from infectious (staphylococcal scalded skin syndrome, viral exanthem) or immunologic disorders. Once diagnosis is confirmed, wound management is a critical component of treatment, as secondary skin infections are the major cause of death. Because TEN involves separation of the dermal-epidermal junction, it is similar to a partial-thickness burn wound, which can heal without operative intervention, provided that appropriate supportive therapy is given. Debridement of devitalized tissue and the use of appropriate temporary wound coverage are vital. A wide range of regimens for temporary wound coverage have been proposed, including biosynthetic wound dressings, xenograft, allograft, Xeroform gauze, 0.5% silver nitrate soaks, and antimicrobial

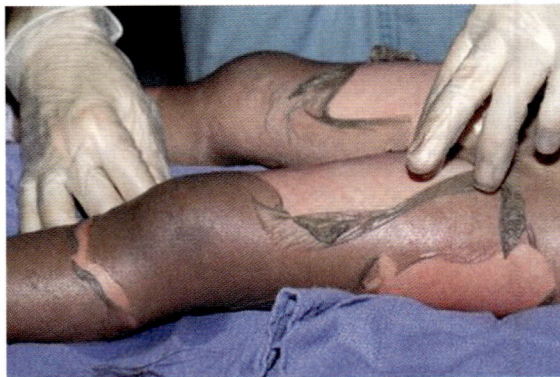

Figure 8-12. Severe toxic epidermal necrolysis. This child demonstrates confluent epidermal sloughing, which is readily removed with gentle pressure (Nikolsky sign).

wound dressings. Sulfa-containing topical agents are generally avoided because of their involvement in the etiology of TEN. To date, there are no clinical trials that prove the superiority of any given regimen. What does appear to make a difference is protocol-driven care by an experienced burn center. This includes fluid therapy, wound care, ventilator support when needed, aggressive nutrition, and physical therapy. Ocular involvement is frequent, and as many as half of the survivors have severe long-term sequelae. Ophthalmologic consultation should be obtained early in the course of the disease in order to diagnose and treat pseudomembranous or membranous conjunctivitis.

A number of systemic therapies for TEN and SJS have been proposed as well. Although systemic steroids reduce the inflammatory response, they have not improved survival in TEN or SJS after the development of desquamation. The use of immunoglobulin was recommended because of its inhibition of CD95 in an experimental model. However, clinical studies have not demonstrated the benefit of immunoglobulin administration.

Mortality from TEN ranges from 20% to 75%. A multicenter review of 199 patients treated in U.S. burn centers reported a mortality of 32%. Mortality risk from TEN has been associated with multiple factors, including age more than 40 years, the presence of malignancy, more than 10% TBSA of sloughed epidermis, elevations in blood urea nitrogen level and serum glucose, acidosis (serum bicarbonate <20 mEq/L), and heart rate greater than 120 beats/min. Mortality is due primarily to sepsis, multisystem organ failure, and cardiopulmonary complications. Long-term sequelae include abnormal pigmentation, a loss of nail plates, phimosis in men, vaginal synechiae in women, dysphagia, conjunctival scarring, lacrimal duct damage with decreased tear production, ectropion, and symblepharon. Close follow-up and referral to appropriate specialists is needed to optimize long-term outcomes.

NECROTIZING SOFT TISSUE INFECTIONS

The term *necrotizing soft tissue infections* encompasses a variety of severe infections of the skin, subcutaneous tissue, and muscle that require immediate surgical excision and debridement. The continued use of other terms such as *necrotizing fasciitis*, *Fournier gangrene*, and *Meleney gangrene* has led to substantial confusion in the literature. Regardless of terminology, these infections share several characteristics: Most are rapidly progressive, produce severe toxicity, and lead to a necrosis of involved tissues, which may spread rapidly. These infections are discussed in more detail in Chapter 6, but are mentioned here because their appropriate treatment often results in large wounds that burn centers are well equipped to treat. Like burn patients, such patients often require aggressive fluid resuscitation, meticulous wound care and surgery, critical care support, and prolonged rehabilitation.

SUGGESTED READINGS

Cancio LC. Initial assessment and fluid resuscitation of burn patients. *Surg Clin North Am*. 2014;94(4):741-754.

Deutsch CJ, Tan A, Smailes S, Dziewulski P. The diagnosis and management of inhalation injury: an evidence based approach. *Burns*. 2018;44(5):1040-1051.

Guilabert P, Usúa G, Martín N, Abarca L, Barret JP, Colomina MJ. Fluid resuscitation management in patients with burns: update. *Br J Anaesth*. 2016;117(3):284-296.

Rae L, Fidler P, Gibran N. The physiologic basis of burn shock and the need for aggressive fluid resuscitation. *Crit Care Clin*. 2016;32(4):491-505.

SAMPLE QUESTIONS

QUESTIONS

Choose the best answer for each question.

1. A 63-year-old man with chronic obstructive pulmonary disease caught his home on fire while smoking in bed. He was trapped in the house for an unknown time period before firefighters extricated him. He presents to the emergency department with severe facial blistering, singed nasal hairs, black intraoral mucosa, a swollen tongue, and carbonaceous sputum. His pulse oximetry reads 85% on room air, and he is obtunded. What is the next best step in management?

   A. Administer racemic epinephrine and steroids.
   B. Draw an arterial blood gas for COHb levels.
   C. Secure his airway by endotracheal intubation.
   D. Place him on 10 L oxygen by humidified facemask.
   E. Transfer him to the HBO chamber.

2. A 25-year-old man suffers burns to 40% of his TBSA in an explosion at a natural gas drilling site. He requires emergent intubation and fluid resuscitation. During his first week of hospitalization, he undergoes a major operative procedure for excision and skin grafting. By the end of the third week in the hospital, his weight (which originally increased with resuscitation) has come back down, and he weighs 12 lb less than before the injury. What is the most likely cause for his weight loss?

   A. Decreased nitrogen excretion and resulting catabolism
   B. Increased nitrogen excretion and resulting catabolism
   C. Protein malnutrition with respiratory muscle wasting
   D. Use of enteral feeding does not meet the caloric requirement.
   E. Underfeeding from frequent NPO (nil per os) for procedures

3. A 27-year-old man is sprayed with concentrated sulfuric acid while working in an oil refinery, sustaining burns to his face, hands, and forearms. He is brought immediately to the emergency department. On initial examination, he is awake and in pain. His clothes are soaked with acid. In addition to providing appropriate protection for all health care workers, the first step in management should be to

   A. debride his burns and complete a Lund and Browder chart.
   B. immediately place the patient in a decontamination shower.
   C. perform a secondary survey.
   D. begin fluid resuscitation.
   E. contact the local burn center for referral.

4. A 6-year-old girl was burned in a house fire from which she was unable to escape. She was found unconscious by firefighters, who intubated her at the scene. On arrival in the burn center, she is found to have carbonaceous sputum, elevated COHb levels, and burns to 30% TBSA. You should inform her parents that inhalation injury significantly increases the mortality rate of patients with major burns *mostly* due to

   A. increased metabolic rate and protein-calorie malnutrition.
   B. persistent pulmonary infection and eventual development of multiple organ dysfunction.
   C. hypoxia.
   D. airway obstruction.
   E. increased fluid requirements for resuscitation.

5. A 19-year-old man is seen in the emergency department 20 minutes after a high-speed head-on collision with a tree, in which his car caught fire. In the emergency department, he is alert, but he does not remember what happened. He admits to drinking a few beers earlier. His blood pressure is

75/40 mm Hg, and his heart rate is 140. His airway is patent. Breath sounds are equal bilaterally. Arterial blood gases reveal a Pao_2 of 140, a Sao_2 of 98%, a $Paco_2$ of 34, and a pH of 7.33. He has burns to 15% TBSA, involving his anterior trunk and legs. His abdomen is covered with burns but appears distended; tenderness is hard to determine because of painful burn wounds. What is the most likely cause of his hypotension?

A. Smoke inhalation injury
B. Burn shock
C. Intra-abdominal hemorrhage
D. Ethanol intoxication
E. Closed head injury

ANSWERS AND EXPLANATIONS

1. **Answer: C**

   This man presents with every manifestation of inhalation injury, which is the most frequent cause of death in victims of structural fires. Oxygen therapy is essential, but he likely does not have an adequate airway. Securing his airway is the first principle of treatment. For more information on this topic, see section "Primary Survey."

2. **Answer: B**

   In response to the increased metabolic demands of a major burn, skeletal muscle is broken down to provide an available energy substrate. This results in increased nitrogen excretion and a loss of lean body mass, which can exceed a half pound per day. Cardiac muscle and respiratory muscles are not immune from these effects, and as muscle wasting continues, both heart failure and respiratory failure can occur. A loss of as little as 15% lean body mass can lead to a fatal degree of inanition within a few weeks of injury. For more information on this topic, see section "Nutritional Support."

3. **Answer: B**

   The patient illustrates the danger that health care workers face when dealing with hazardous material spills. Unwary physicians and nurses who attempt to help this man could suffer serious burns from the acid on his clothing, which is continuing to burn the patient as well. This chemical must be neutralized by decontamination before a primary survey can be conducted safely. All of the other answers are appropriate steps in treatment but should not be performed until after the patient is decontaminated. For more information on this topic, see section "Chemical and Electrical Burns."

4. **Answer: B**

   Although inhalation injury can produce immediate death from CO poisoning and hypoxia, patients who survive the initial event should survive this problem. Similarly, airway obstruction is usually a treatable problem with a limited time course. Pneumonia is the most worrisome complication of smoke inhalation because it is often persistent/recurrent and difficult to treat. Persistent infection—including pneumonia—often leads to the development of the multiple organ dysfunction syndrome, which can be fatal. For more information on this topic, see sections "Pathophysiology of Inhalation Injury" and "Infection Control."

5. **Answer: C**

   This patient illustrates the importance of the secondary survey in victims of burn injury. This man's burns are too limited in extent to cause severe shock, especially so soon after injury. Smoke inhalation is doubtful, especially with good blood gases. There is no evidence for ethanol intoxication or closed head injury. Unless a second injury (ie, abdominal trauma) is *considered*, it will not be diagnosed. For more information on this topic, see section "Secondary Survey."

9

Surgical Critical Care

Brian J. Daley and Nicole A. Stassen

Surgical critical care involves treating patients who have developed or may develop complex physiologic derangements of one or more of the body's organ systems, with the goal of maximizing outcomes. Hypovolemia, or most directly, hypoperfusion, from either blood loss or maldistribution, is the hallmark of a surgical critical illness. The surgical intensive care unit (SICU) of the 21st century integrates sophisticated technologies along with management by a multidisciplinary team including nurses, respiratory therapists; pharmacists; physical, occupational, and speech therapists; dietitians; and social workers. Systematic programs for care, or protocols, are developed for ventilator weaning, resuscitation, transfusion, burn care, and so on. These protocols are based on both published research evidence and expert consensus guidelines that link care delivered to outcome.

RESPIRATORY FAILURE

Prevention and Respiratory Monitoring

Tachypnea is one of the best predictors of critical illness. Preventing respiratory failure must begin in the preoperative phase in elective cases and immediately in emergent cases. Inadequate postoperative or posttrauma pain control can result in poor respiratory effort leading to secretions that are not cleared adequately, and pneumonia may result. Multimodal pain control regimens include regional pain management with epidurals and nerve blocks as well as nonnarcotic analgesics. Narcotics (either intravenous or oral) are often inappropriate as they may produce respiratory depression, especially in the older adults.

Monitoring of respiration uses continuous pulse oximetry of oxygen saturation, treated with titration of supplemental oxygen. Carbon dioxide levels are also monitored by sensors in the breathing circuit or by arterial blood gases.

Interventions

Respiratory failure occurs from hypoxia (low partial pressure of oxygen [PaO_2]), hypoventilation (high partial pressure of carbon dioxide [PCO_2]), or both. It is important to determine the cause of respiratory failure and initiate treatment. Treatment for hypoxia involves increasing the oxygen available for transport into the pulmonary circulation (increased oxygen concentrations and mean airway pressures), while treatment for hypercarbia involves increasing minute ventilation. For hypoxia, the first intervention is to administer high-flow oxygen. If oxygen alone is ineffective, then positive pressure ventilation often helps. Noninvasive positive pressure ventilation can be provided via a tightly fitting face mask as continuous positive airway pressure (CPAP) or bilevel positive airway pressure

(BiPAP), which provides separate pressures for inspiration and expiration. These modalities are most effective with rapidly reversible causes of respiratory failure (eg, fluid overload).

If these methods are not effective, invasive positive pressure ventilation is required. Tracheal intubation with a cuffed tube allows the delivery of high concentrations of oxygen and positive pressure ventilation. Indications for intubation include inadequate oxygenation, inadequate ventilation, increased work of breathing, and inability to protect the airway from aspiration.

Mechanical Ventilation

Ventilation modes are categorized as volume controlled (VC) or pressure controlled (PC). In VC, the ventilator inflates the lungs to a preset tidal volume, regardless of the airway pressure generated. VC modes are further categorized as assist control (AC) and intermittent mandatory ventilation (IMV). In AC, all breaths, whether initiated by the ventilator or by the patient, provide the set tidal volume. In IMV, machine tidal volumes are given at a set rate. Additional pressure support is given for spontaneous breaths and can be used either as a stand-alone or as a supplement to IMV. Additional pressure in the ventilator circuit at the end of expiration, called *positive end-expiratory pressure* (PEEP), helps to prevent alveolar collapse and maintains them as functional parts of the lung in oxygenation and ventilation.

Barotrauma is a repetitive injury to the lungs that can result in continued inflammation, pneumothorax, and impaired ventilation and tends to occur more frequently with VC modes. PC modes deliver flow to a set inspiratory pressure allowing for a decreased incidence of barotrauma with these modes. Pressure support ventilation (PSV) is one type of PC ventilation that is based on inspiratory demand and flow decreasing to a certain level. Since the patient controls the respiratory rate and receives support rapidly, patients may find this mode more comfortable than VC ventilation. Airway pressure is set by the clinician. The tidal volume provided to the patient is variable and is determined by the resistance of the alveoli or lung compliance.

In severe hypoxemia, inversing the inspiratory:expiratory (I:E) ratio can help recruit alveoli and improve oxygenation. In normal spontaneous breathing, the expiratory time is about twice as long as the inspiratory time (an I:E ratio of 1:2). An I:E ratio of 1:1.5 to 1:4 is normal for an adult on mechanical ventilation. A ratio is termed *inverse* when the I:E ratio is 2:1 or higher. The extension of the inspiratory/expiratory time leads to an increased mean airway pressure and potentially to improved oxygenation.

Adult respiratory distress syndrome (ARDS) is a result of global inflammation from infection, trauma, or other insults, resulting in changes in the alveoli, which impair oxygenation and ventilation. A lung-protective ventilatory strategy limits tidal volumes to 6 to 8 mL/kg to prevent barotrauma. Combinations of PEEP and the fraction of inspired oxygen (Fio_2) are adjusted to maintain adequate Pao_2.

Weaning

The initial issue in determining whether to wean a patient from the ventilator is to determine whether all acute issues have been resolved. Fio_2 must be titrated down, and PEEP must be low. A daily trial of spontaneous breathing on minimal support (pressure support of 5 cm H_2O) is effective in determining weaning readiness. If the patient tolerates the trial with an adequate respiratory rate, tidal volume, and oxygen saturation, the patient can be extubated. The rapid shallow breathing index (frequency/tidal volume in liters) is a vetted method of predicting successful extubation.

CARDIOVASCULAR FAILURE

Hemodynamic Monitoring

Arterial Catheterization

Arterial catheterization allows for the continuous measurement of blood pressure (BP) and arterial blood collection for laboratory studies. Complications of arterial catheterization are rare but include infection, bleeding, vascular injury (pseudoaneurysm and arteriovenous fistula), distal ischemia, and thromboembolism. BP readings must be carefully assessed because malpositioning of the transducer or dampening of the waveform by air bubbles or excessive length gives incorrect values. BP can be overestimated if the system is incorrectly calibrated.

Central Venous Catheterization

Central venous catheters (CVCs) are common in critically ill patients (Figure 9-1). Indications for central venous catheterization include the need for monitoring of central venous pressure (CVP) readings, administration of medications that may be irritating to peripheral vessels, and inability to obtain peripheral access. Special CVCs, often called "*introducers*," are used for large-volume resuscitation. Complications of CVCs include pneumothorax, malpositioning, infection, thrombosis, vascular injury, air embolism, and arrhythmia. Confirmation of placement in the desired location is necessary before infusing potent agents. A CVC should be removed when the need for central access is finished.

Other Methods of Hemodynamic Monitoring

Less invasive methods of hemodynamic monitoring can often be used. Increased pulse pressure (pulse contour wave analysis) variability during mechanical ventilation can be a simple method for identifying hypovolemia. Very narrow pulse pressures suggest poor stroke volume, as in profound hypovolemia or cardiac dysfunction.

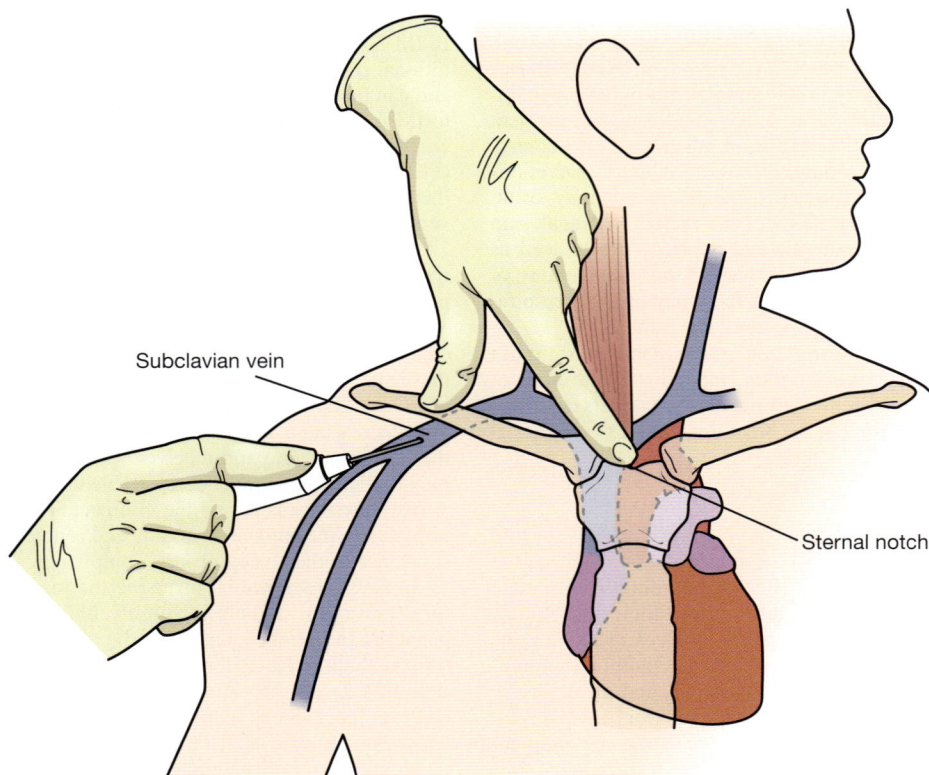

Subclavian vein

Sternal notch

Figure 9-1. Central venous catheterization is often accomplished via the subclavian vein. Understanding the anatomic relationships between the clavicle, subclavian vein, and the underlying pleura is important for safe cannulation.

Echocardiography can provide evidence of cardiac dysfunction or pericardial fluid, as well as an estimation of volume status. Esophageal Doppler monitoring uses flow to estimate stroke volume. Many practitioners follow base deficit or lactate levels to gauge both adequate volume resuscitation and cardiac function.

Hemodynamic Support

Inotropes

In cardiac failure, sepsis-induced myocardial dysfunction, or cardiogenic shock, the contractile function of the myocardium is depressed. Inotropic support with agents such as norepinephrine, dobutamine, epinephrine, and phosphodiesterase inhibitors enhances cardiac function and oxygen delivery. Vasopressors, which increase vascular tone, may also be needed.

Epinephrine is a potent naturally secreted adrenal hormone that has marked effects on contractility and increasing vascular tone. A precursor of epinephrine, norepinephrine is the agent of choice in sepsis. Both agents increase myocardial oxygen consumption and decrease visceral blood flow. Dobutamine increases myocardial contractility and heart rate; however, myocardial oxygen consumption is increased and may worsen cardiac function. Because peripheral vasodilation can occur, dobutamine may not be the best inotrope in a patient with hypotension. Dobutamine may lead to tachyarrhythmias, which also affect cardiac output. Phosphodiesterase inhibitors increase myocardial contractility coupled with myocardial and vascular smooth muscle relaxation. These agents may exacerbate hypotension and tachyarrhythmias, but less so than dobutamine.

Vasopressors

Norepinephrine is a potent vasoconstrictor, making it a first-line agent for distributive shock, such as sepsis. Phenylephrine can be effective in patients with vasodilatory shock, but it can decrease stroke volume by increased afterload. Vasopressin, a pituitary hormone regulating volume status, has positive effects in refractory septic shock by stimulating vasopressin receptors, bypassing catecholamine receptors, and increasing sensitivity to catecholamines.

Cardiogenic Shock

Cardiogenic shock is caused by decreased cardiac function from myocardial infarction, sepsis, trauma, or medications. Dysrhythmias may also contribute to poor cardiac function and shock. For example, tachycardia affects cardiac output by reducing filling time and stroke volume, and bradycardia reduces cardiac output directly. Valvular dysfunction may also lead to cardiogenic shock. Echocardiography is helpful in defining the cause of shock and directing therapy. First-line treatment involves optimization of volume status and inotropes. Mechanical circulatory support, such as the intra-aortic balloon pump (Figure 9-2), may also be beneficial, and newer ventricular assist devices such as the left ventricular assist device (LVAD) and Impella may be needed. A general approach to the patient in shock is presented in Figure 9-3.

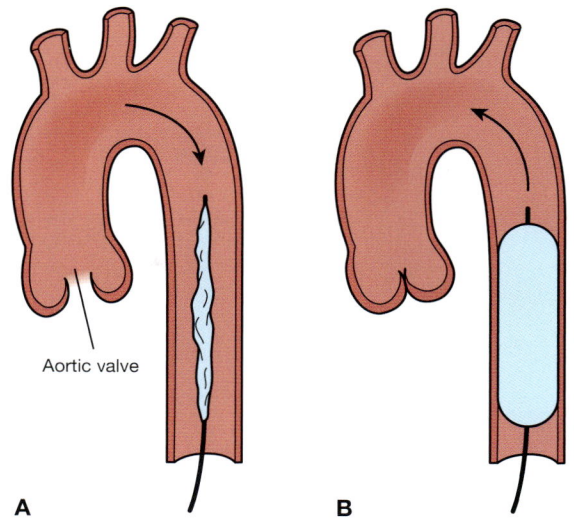

Figure 9-2. A. The intra-aortic balloon pump is placed via the femoral artery into the proximal, descending aorta. B. The balloon is inflated during diastole to increase coronary and cerebral perfusion; it is then deflated just before systole to decrease afterload.

Extracorporeal Membrane Oxygenation

Extracorporeal membrane oxygenation (ECMO) is an invasive modality to replace the respiratory system, the cardiac system, or both as a bridge to recovery or transplant of those organ systems when other therapies have failed. ECMO uses a pump to take blood from the body and allows respiration to occur. The pump can replace or assist the pumping ability of the heart, and the membrane can allow oxygen transfer into the blood and carbon dioxide removal from the blood. In venovenous ECMO, blood drawn from a CVC is returned to the venous system after oxygenation and CO_2 gas exchange to bypass the lungs. In venoarterial ECMO, blood is drawn from a central vein and returned to the arterial system, bypassing the heart and lungs, and effectively replacing the heart and lungs. ECMO poses high risks and frequent complications and is associated with high mortality.

Cardiac Arrest

With sudden cardiac arrest in the ICU, acute myocardial infarction, pulmonary embolism (PE), acute respiratory decompensation (aspiration or mucous plugging), tension pneumothorax, or massive hemorrhage must be considered. First-line treatment for any cardiac arrest not caused by blood loss is the initiation of cardiopulmonary resuscitation (CPR; the 2015 Advanced Cardiovascular Life Support [ACLS] Guidelines). Asystole and pulseless electrical activity (PEA) are frequently caused by reversible factors: hypovolemia, hypoxia, hydrogen ions (acidosis), hypo- or hyperkalemia, hypoglycemia, hypothermia, toxins, tamponade (cardiac), tension pneumothorax, and thrombosis (coronary or pulmonary).

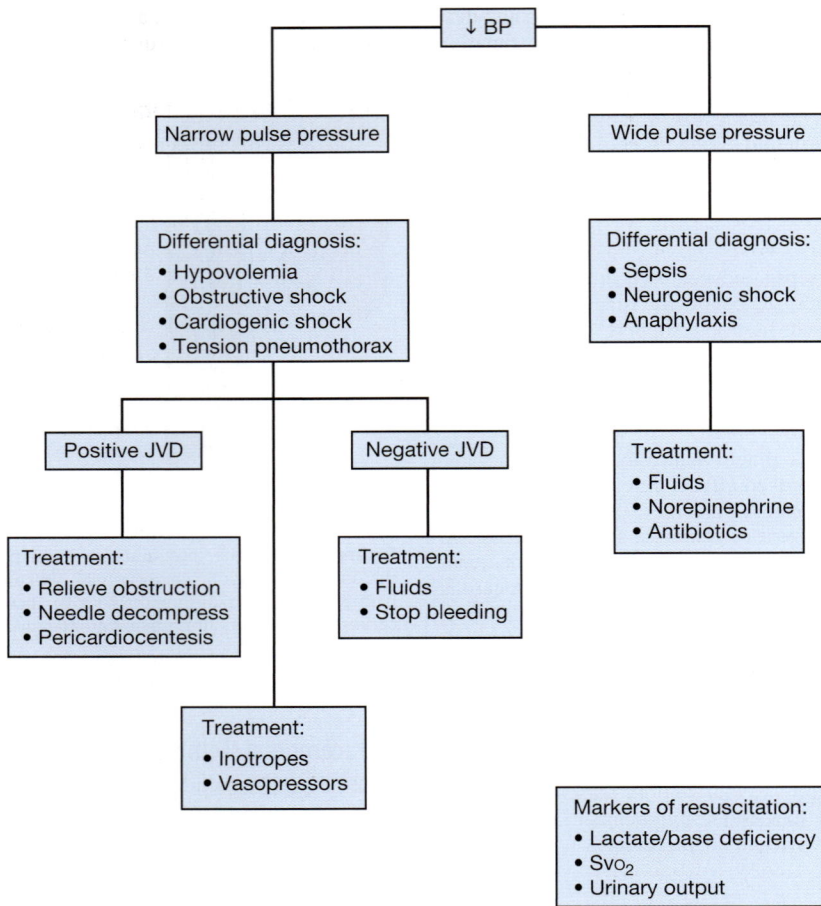

Figure 9-3. Bedside shock diagnosis and treatment. BP, blood pressure; JVD, jugular venous distension; Svo$_2$, mixed venous oxygen saturation.

ACUTE KIDNEY INJURY

Acute kidney injury (AKI) occurs in 5% to 10% of hospitalized patients. The criteria for the diagnosis have been defined by global consensus (Kidney Disease Improving Global Outcomes [KDIGO]) based on serum creatinine levels (Table 9-1). AKI results in the retention of nitrogenous waste; fluid, electrolyte, and acid-base imbalance; and alters the effects of the many medications excreted through the kidneys. AKI is associated with a significant increase in morbidity and a mortality increase of 150% to 300%, depending on severity. Although the kidney is unique in its ability to regulate its own blood flow, the critically ill patient is at risk for hypoperfusion resulting from hemorrhage, hypovolemia, cardiac pump failure, and use of medications that cause vasoconstriction. Nephrotoxic agents such as intravenous contrast, antibiotics, and antifungal agents are common in the ICU.

Renal Monitoring

Primary preventive strategies include ensuring adequate volume status, maintaining perfusion pressure by keeping the mean arterial pressure (MAP) greater than 60 mm Hg and limiting exposure to potentially nephrotoxic agents.

Early identification of renal dysfunction allows earlier treatment and results in an improved outcome. Urine output is an indicator of systemic perfusion and is easy to monitor. An adult should make at least 0.25 to 0.5 mL/kg/h and

TABLE 9-1. Staging of Acute Kidney Injury

Stage	Serum Creatinine	Urine Output
1	1.5-1.9 × baseline or >0.3 mg/dL increase	<0.5 mL/kg/h for 6-12 h
2	2.0-2.9 × baseline	<0.5 mL/kg/h for >12 h
3	3 × baseline or >4 mg/dL or RRT or GFR <35 mL/min in patients <18 y	Anuria <12 h

GFR, glomerular filtration rate; RRT, renal replacement therapy.
From Kidney International. KDIGO clinical practice guidelines 2012. Accessed July 7, 2018. http://www.kidney-international.org Reprinted from Woo KT, Chan CM. KDIGO clinical practice guidelines for bisphosphonate treatment in chronic kidney disease. *Kidney Int.* 2011;80(5):553-554. Copyright © 2011 International Society of Nephrology. With permission.

children 0.5 to 1 mL/kg/h. Production of urine in amounts less than this should prompt immediate investigation. There are limitations to using urine output as a monitor of systemic perfusion and a measure of renal function. It is possible to have high-output renal failure, in which the kidney produces large volumes of urine but is not reabsorbing electrolytes or excreting nitrogenous waste products. The other markers for inadequate perfusion, lactate and base deficit, remain the best measures. Serum creatinine levels measure renal function serially in the critical care setting.

$$\text{Creatine clearance (mL/min)} = \frac{[\text{urine Cr (mg/dL)} \times \text{volume (mL/24 h)}]}{\text{serum Cr (mg/dL)} \times 1,440 \text{ (min/24 h)}}$$

Measuring the renal concentrating ability distinguishes oliguria caused by prerenal factors, such as hypovolemia, from that caused by impaired tubular function. Sodium and water reabsorption is compromised in cases of intrinsic renal failure but not in prerenal azotemia. The fractional excretion of sodium (Fe_{Na}) distinguishes prerenal from renal causes of azotemia. Fe_{Na} is calculated as

$$Fe_{Na} = [\text{Urine Na} \times \text{Serum Cr}] / [\text{Urine Cr} \times \text{Serum Na}] \times 100$$

In normal individuals, the Fe_{Na} is less than 1% to 2%. In a patient experiencing oliguria, a value of less than 1% suggests a prerenal cause. A value of greater than 2% to 3% suggests compromised tubular function.

In the SICU, blood urea nitrogen (BUN) is of limited value, because it is affected by the production of nitrogenous wastes, from high-protein diets, reabsorption of hematomas, and blood from the gastrointestinal (GI) tract.

Management of Acute Kidney Injury

The first step for managing any patient with AKI is to acquire a relevant history, including baseline state of health, baseline laboratory values, hypotension status, and recent exposure to known *nephrotoxins*. The clinician should then calculate the Fe_{Na}. Postrenal failure is determined by the placement or flushing of a urinary catheter. Ultrasound imaging can rule out bilateral obstruction of the ureters. The most common type of AKI in the SICU is acute tubular necrosis secondary to ischemia. Once the cause of AKI is determined, renal perfusion is optimized with appropriate volume and cautious use of vasoactive agents. An all too common mistake in surgical patients is to assume that the prerenal etiology is solely a lack of volume. Although this is a very common cause, decreased cardiac output is also frequent and may require inotropic or vasopressor support. Dopamine at low doses increases sodium excretion, thus increasing urine output, but large clinical trials have demonstrated no improvement in AKI. Ensuring adequate oxygenation is also important when resuscitating the injured kidney.

Because of the kidney's role in eliminating many medications, the doses of many medications need to be adjusted ("renal dosing"), and some medications need to be discontinued. Medications known for their nephrotoxicity should be avoided. Renal dysfunction can also lead to platelet dysfunction and an increased risk of bleeding.

Renal Replacement Therapy

Indications for renal replacement therapy (RRT) or dialysis are volume overload, electrolyte disturbances (often hyperkalemia), metabolic acidosis, and severe azotemia. All forms of RRT rely on the p; a subset of RRT, ultrafiltration, achieves volume removal by using a pressure gradient to drive water across the membrane. RRT is classified as intermittent or continuous. An example of intermittent RRT is hemodialysis, which allows rapid removal of solute and volume and rapid correction of electrolytes and acidosis. Its disadvantage is hypotension due to rapid shifts in volume. Continuous RRT is gradual; therefore, volume removal, azotemia, electrolyte balance, and acid-base status may be better managed.

RRT requires large-bore venous access (Figure 9-4). In acute situations, nontunneled and noncuffed CVCs are usually used. Typically, these are placed in the internal jugular or femoral veins, sparing the subclavian veins from stenoses or thrombosis that could complicate long-term access. In addition, the risk of creating a pneumothorax is lower with an internal jugular catheter. For long-term access, tunneled and cuffed dialysis catheters can be placed in the central veins to decrease the risk of infection. Alternatively, an arteriovenous graft can be surgically created directly between an artery and vein, using a prosthetic graft material such as polytetrafluoroethylene.

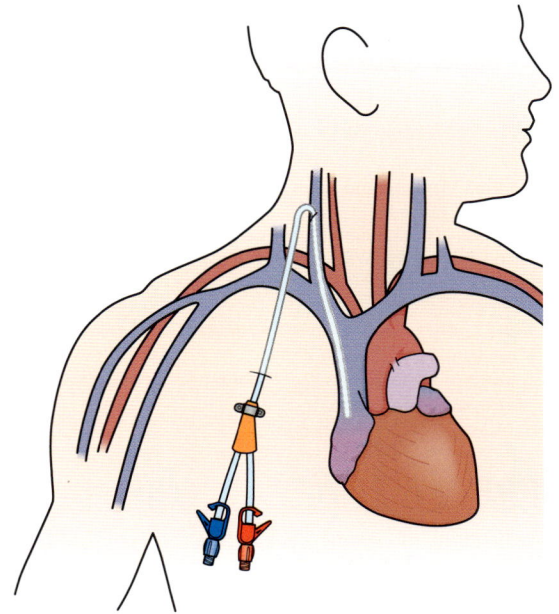

Figure 9-4. Patients with chronic renal failure require long-term venous access for dialysis. A dialysis catheter with an adherent antibiotic- or silver-impregnated cuff can be tunneled under the skin.

Oliguria

Rule out urinary obstruction → Bladder catheter Ultrasound

Blood volume / Cardiac output / Inotropes → Ensure good renal blood flow

Dx: renal parenchymal disease → Confirm by urine electrolytes and clearance

Diuretic trial (Furosemide, 100-500 mg)

Polyuria

Dx: some nephrons functional

- Expect azotemia
- Full nutrition
- Intermittent hemodialysis as needed for solute clearance

Oliguria

Dx: no nephrons functional

Isolate renal failure
- Full nutrition
- Intermittent hemodialysis as needed for volume and solute control

Multiple-organ failure
- Full nutrition
- CAVH or CVVH for volume
- CAVHD or CVVHD for solute control

Chronic renal failure

Renal recovery

Dx: some or all nephrons recovered

DX: no nephrons recovered

Chronic dialysis

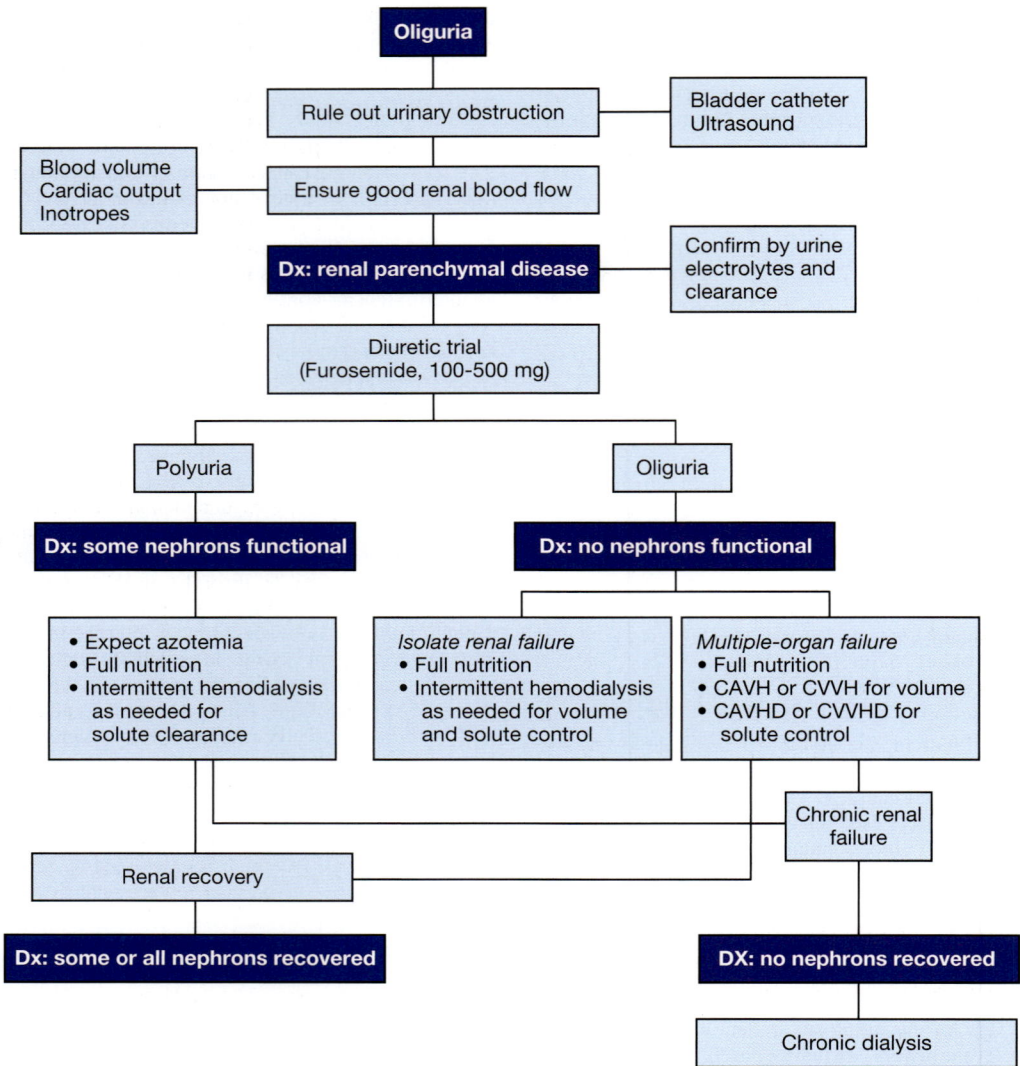

Figure 9-5. Workup and management of acute renal failure. CAVH, continuous arteriovenous hemofiltration; CAVHD, continuous arteriovenous hemodiafiltration; CVVH, continuous venovenous hemofiltration; CVVHD, continuous venovenous hemodiafiltration; Dx, diagnosis. (Reprinted with permission from Mulholland MW, Lillemoe KD, Doherty GM, et al, eds. *Greenfield's Surgery*. 4th ed. Lippincott Williams & Wilkins; 2006:208.)

A general approach to the patient with acute renal failure is illustrated in Figure 9-5.

LIVER FAILURE

Complications of chronic liver failure that may result in ICU admission include variceal hemorrhage, encephalopathy, spontaneous bacterial peritonitis, and hepatorenal syndrome. In addition, liver disease may be a comorbidity of patients presenting with another disease process. Global hypoperfusion can also create liver dysfunction. See Chapters 19 and 20 for diagnosis and treatment options.

GASTROINTESTINAL FUNCTION

Normal GI tract function is expected in the SICU; however, vomiting, diarrhea, and constipation are common and may be the result of illness, injury, drugs, immobility, or a combination of factors. Simple measures, including elevating the head of the bed and assuring frequent laxation, prevent intolerance.

Gastrointestinal Integrity

Changes in the gut anatomy fall into two major areas: loss of mucosal integrity or ischemia. Gastric erosion, often called *stress-related mucosal disease* (SRMD), thought to be due to reduced mucosal perfusion, can lead to gastritis or ulceration. Improved hemodynamic resuscitation has reduced gastric ulceration, but there are subsets of SICU patients (upper GI bleeding, prolonged ventilation [>48 hours], and coagulopathy) who require acid prophylaxis. Prophylaxis for SRMD involves H_2 antagonists, proton pump inhibitors, or cytoprotective agents. Enteral feeding promotes increased blood flow and reduces intraluminal pH. The colon can also ulcerate or blister from the toxin produced by *Clostridium difficile*.

Ischemia to the gut can occur from obstruction of splanchnic blood flow to the vessels from embolism or from hypotension or vasoactive agents. Ischemia is marked by abdominal pain and lactic acidosis, but early signs of abdominal tenderness and peritoneal rebound may be absent. Ischemia may also result from nonocclusive mesenteric ischemia (NOMI) with global inadequate perfusion. Treatment requires improved hemodynamics.

Abdominal Compartment Syndrome

Abdominal compartment syndrome is a result of elevated intraperitoneal pressures that affect extraperitoneal organ systems. Intraperitoneal pressures, measured via the bladder, greater than 25 cm H_2O indicate abdominal hypertension. Abdominal compartment syndrome manifests as impaired pulmonary function, urinary output/renal function, and venous return, leading to hypotension. Early recognition is critical; treatment is decompression of the peritoneal cavity by paracentesis, intraluminal decompression, muscle paralysis, or opening the fascia surgically.

ENDOCRINE DYSFUNCTION

Critical illness can cause profound alterations in the endocrine system. A normal endocrine system is needed for the appropriate physiologic responses to trauma and stress. As a result, patients with preexisting endocrine disease or those with unrecognized endocrine abnormalities are difficult to manage and have an increased rate of complications and mortality.

Adrenal

In the general population, the incidence of adrenal insufficiency is less than 0.1%, but it may be as high as 28% in critically ill patients. Adrenal insufficiency potentiates the vasoconstrictor actions of both endogenous and exogenous catecholamines. Critically ill patients are at risk for the development of adrenal insufficiency in critical illness (AICI). These patients have hypotension, unresponsiveness to catecholamine infusions, and/or ventilator dependence. Electrolyte abnormalities (hyponatremia, hyperkalemia) and hypoglycemia may also be present and not recognized as adrenal insufficiency. Random serum cortisol levels that are less than 20 μg/dL may be sufficient to diagnose AICI. If the patient is in refractory shock, the Surviving Sepsis Guidelines of 2016 support empiric treatment with steroids.

Glucose Disorders

Hyperglycemia occurs in many critically ill and injured patients and is due to increased sympathetic and adrenal activity and activation of the cytokine cascade. Certain medications such as β-blockers, catecholamines, total parenteral nutrition, and glucocorticoids promote hyperglycemia. Hyperglycemia also stems from decreased insulin release and peripheral insulin resistance.

Hyperglycemia is associated with an increased risk of in-hospital mortality. Tight control of blood glucose improves outcomes in critically ill and injured patients; however, glucose control that is too strict may be more dangerous because of hypoglycemia, so the proper range of appropriate blood glucose levels for specific subgroups of intensive care patients is required.

Thyroid Disorders

Critical illness may alter the production of thyroid hormone, through regulatory changes in thyroid-stimulating hormone (TSH), peripheral metabolism, or alteration in binding proteins. Thyroid storm is severe hyperthyroidism precipitated by surgery, trauma, childbirth, and critical illness. The symptoms are high fever (105-106 °F), high-output cardiac failure, and mental status changes. The diagnosis is based on a nondetectable TSH and elevation of T3 (triiodothyronine) and T4 (thyroxine) levels. Decreasing production and release of T3 and T4, blocking their peripheral actions, and addressing the primary cause are the mainstays of treatment.

Hypothyroidism is also common in the SICU. Although rare, myxedema coma is the most severe, with mortality rates of more than 60%. Clinical features include reduced metabolic rate, hypothermia, ileus, bradycardia, decreased cardiac contractility, hypotension, and hypoventilation. An elevated TSH, low T4, hyponatremia, and low glucose are typically present. Treatment is external warming, infusion of glucose, and thyroxine replacement. An isolated decrease in T3 with normal TSH is called *euthyroid sick syndrome*. Currently, replacement therapy is not recommended.

NEUROLOGIC DYSFUNCTION

Sedation/Analgesia

SICU patients frequently require analgesia and/or sedation, particularly during mechanical ventilation. Guidelines from the Society of Critical Care Medicine outline tools for assessing a patient's level of pain and delirium. Excessive dosing of medications for analgesia and sedation can cause prolonged time on the ventilator or in the SICU. For pain, a narcotic infusion is usually used. Adjuvants, such as nonsteroidal anti-inflammatory drugs (NSAIDs) or regional anesthesia, can decrease the need for narcotics.

Sedation with short-acting medications is preferred. The goal is to have a calm but responsive patient. Deeper levels of sedation may be required in some circumstances, such as high airway pressures or intracranial hypertension, or during a procedure. To decrease the danger of sedative medications, which can lead to delayed awakening, longer days of mechanical ventilation, and prolonged SICU stay, a daily interruption of sedation has become a standard practice.

Delirium

Delirium is acute or fluctuating mental status and inattention, plus disordered thinking or altered level of consciousness. Initial management includes the reversal of any immediately life-threatening issues. A rapid evaluation for reversible causes can be divided into the patient (eg, alcoholism, endocrine disorders), acute illness (eg, sepsis, head trauma), complications (eg, hypoxemia, hypovolemia, and electrolyte abnormalities), and iatrogenic factors (eg, medications). Sepsis is a frequent cause of delirium. When organic causes of delirium have been excluded, further management is multimodal and includes altering environmental factors such as light and sound, restoration of the sleep-wake cycle, minimization of deliriogenic medications like narcotics and benzodiazepines, and initiation of antipsychotic medications.

Alcohol Withdrawal Syndrome

When patients who regularly misuse alcohol or benzodiazepines cease or reduce their intake, they risk withdrawal. Initial signs are hypertension, tachycardia, tachypnea, fever, and diaphoresis. These symptoms can occur within hours. Delirium usually occurs 2 to 3 days later, as well as the most feared complication, seizures.

Traumatic Brain Injury

SICU care for traumatic brain injury (TBI) involves reducing secondary injury from hypotension or hypoxemia. Any episodes of hypotension or hypoxemia can significantly impact the outcome of TBI.

The Glasgow Coma Scale (see Chapter 7) is useful for categorizing the severity of TBI and following the patient's course. The Brain Injury Foundation and the Trauma Quality Improvement Program have published guidelines. Management of patients with severe TBI is focused on adequate tissue perfusion by control of intracranial pressure (ICP). Other interventions are discussed in Chapter 7.

Brain Death

Brain death is defined as the cessation of all functions of the brain. It can occur while other systems function normally. Diagnosis is set by state laws and hospital protocols. Before brain death is considered, any confounding issues must be ruled out. The examination for brain death includes the testing of all cranial nerves, no response to central painful stimuli, and apnea demonstrated with P_{CO_2} greater than 60 Torr.

SYSTEMIC INFLAMMATORY RESPONSE SYNDROME

Certain physiologic and laboratory parameters change due to injury, infection, or inflammation; together, these are called *systemic inflammatory response syndrome* (SIRS). It is usually the first sign of an ongoing process, and it serves as a warning sign. The criteria for SIRS are listed in Table 9-2. If SIRS is associated with infection or suspected infection, it is considered sepsis. If sepsis has progressed to impair an organ or body system, it is severe sepsis. Sepsis with hypotension is septic shock. A newer assessment tool, the Sequential Organ Function Assessment (SOFA), can also be calculated to assess the severity of sepsis.

Organ dysfunction is common in the SICU as a result of hypoperfusion or SIRS (Figure 9-6). If more

TABLE 9-2. Systemic Inflammatory Response Syndrome

Temperature	<36 °C or >38 °C
Heart rate	>90 beats/min
Respiratory rate	>20 breaths/min (or P_{aCO_2} <32 mm Hg)
Leukocyte count	<4,000 or >12,000 cells/mm^3 (or >10% bands)

than one system is affected, multiple-organ dysfunction syndrome (MODS) is present. Individual organ failure can be tabulated and scored (Table 9-3). The sum of the scores correlates with mortality. Mortality increases linearly to greater than 80% when four organs fail. The most common organ system that fails and requires support is the respiratory system, followed by the cardiac and renal systems.

INFECTIOUS DISEASES

Sepsis remains a leading cause of death. Virtually, any surgical intervention and the intravenous access and monitoring devices utilized in the ICU place patients at additional risk for infections and sepsis. The Society of Critical Care Medicine has repeatedly revised guidelines for the treatment of sepsis as part of its Surviving Sepsis Campaign. Critical components include rapid identification of sepsis with a rapid SOFA score of altered mentation, systolic blood pressure (SBP) less than 100 mm Hg and respirations greater than 22 breaths/min, aggressive goal-directed resuscitation with fluids and vasopressors for MAP greater than 65 mm Hg, source control of the septic focus, and early administration of appropriate antibiotic therapy. Serum lactate and procalcitonin determine the duration of resuscitation and antimicrobial treatment, respectively.

In the SICU, secondary and tertiary peritonitis are frequently associated with appendicitis, diverticulitis, anastomotic dehiscence, and perforated ulcers. Another common source of sepsis in the SICU is ventilator-associated pneumonia (VAP). VAP occurs in 9% to 24% of patients with respiratory failure. Patients on the ventilator have a 3% per day risk of developing VAP. Development of pneumonia increases ICU stay and mortality. Simple things to prevent VAP include good oral hygiene, keeping the head of the bed elevated, and mobilizing patients. Good hand washing by health care workers prevents patient-to-patient cross-contamination and contamination of the ventilator circuit. Further, malnutrition weakens the immune system, emphasizing the need for nutritional support. These interventions are pooled into a ventilator bundle or protocol to help reduce VAP.

The optimal method of diagnosis of VAP in the ICU includes quantitative culture obtained by bronchoalveolar lavage (BAL) or protected specimen brush. Treatment with early, broad-spectrum coverage avoids inadequate or inappropriate coverage and reduces morbidity and mortality. Antibiotics should ultimately be narrowed, based on final culture results.

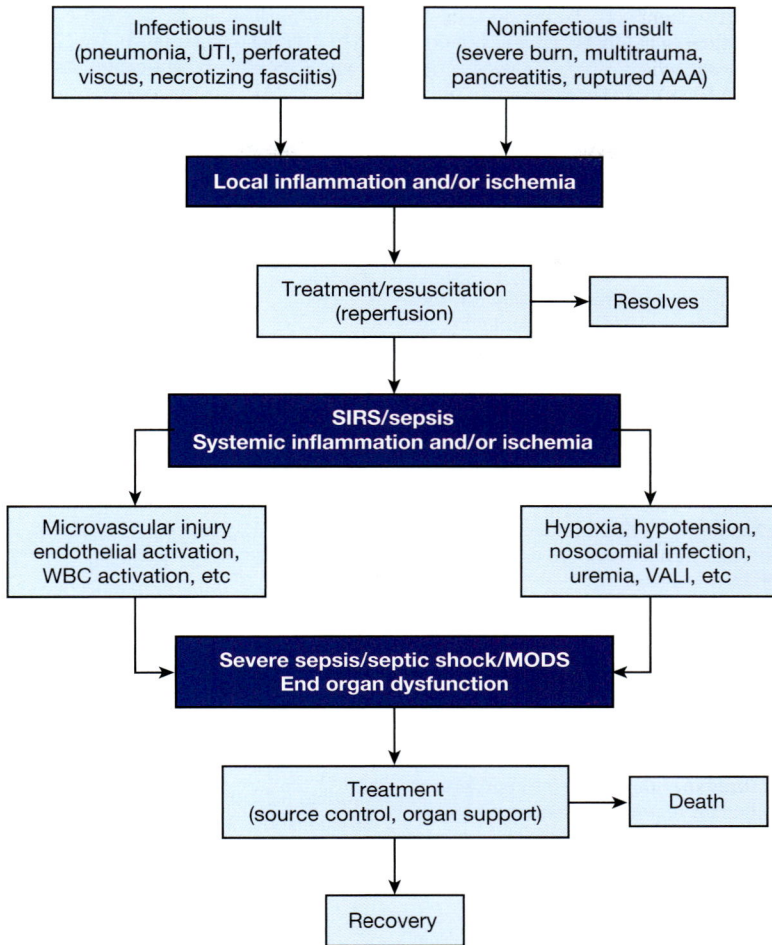

Figure 9-6. Pathophysiology of multiple-organ dysfunction. AAA, abdominal aortic aneurysm; MODS, multiple-organ dysfunction syndrome; SIRS, systemic inflammatory response syndrome; UTI, urinary tract infection; VALI, ventilator-associated lung injury; WBC, white blood count. (Reprinted with permission from Fischer JE, Bland KI, eds. *Mastery of Surgery*. 5th ed. Lippincott Williams & Wilkins; 2006:114.)

TABLE 9-3. Multiple-Organ Dysfunction Score

	Score				
Organ System	0	1	2	3	4
Respiratory (PO_2/FIO_2)	>300	226-300	151-225	76-150	≤75
Renal (serum creatinine, mg/dL)	≤1.1	1.2-2.3	2.4-3.9	4.0-5.6	>5.7
Hepatic (serum bilirubin, mg/dL)	≤1.1	1.2-3.5	3.6-7.1	7.2-14.1	>14.2
Cardiovascular (PAR)	≤10	10.1-15	15.1-20	20.1-30	>30
Hematologic (platelet count, $\times 10^3$)	>120	81-120	51-80	21-50	≤20
Neurologic (GCS)	15	13-14	10-12	7-9	≤6

PAR = heart rate × (CVP/mean arterial pressure).
CVP, central venous pressure; GCS, Glasgow Coma Scale score; PAR, pressure-adjusted heart rate.
Adapted with permission from Marshall JC, Cook DJ, Christou NV, Bernard GR, Sprung CL, Sibbald WJ. Multiple organ dysfunction score: a reliable descriptor of a complex clinical outcome. *Crit Care Med*. 1995;23(10):1638-1652.

Urinary catheters are also a source of infection. Each day, the necessity of a catheter should be assessed to ensure removal as early as possible.

Antibiotics, although necessary in the SICU, can alter the flora in the colon, allowing *C. difficile* to flourish. Diagnosis is made by demonstrating the presence of the *C. difficile* toxin in a stool sample. Treatment is by administration of oral or intravenous metronidazole or oral vancomycin.

Critically ill patients, particularly those with hypotension, diabetes mellitus, mechanical ventilation, and parenteral nutrition, are at risk of acalculous cholecystitis, which is caused by biliary stasis and ischemia of the gallbladder wall. Diagnostic criteria include wall thickening and pericholecystic fluid on ultrasound and right upper quadrant tenderness (Murphy sign). Treatment includes broad-spectrum antibiotic coverage and placement of a cholecystostomy tube or cholecystectomy.

Another cause of sepsis is catheter-related blood stream infection (CRBSI). Any type of intravascular catheter poses a risk of CRBSI. Risk of sepsis increases with the location (femoral being the highest), the number of lumens, and the frequency of use, as well as with the use of parenteral nutrition. The need for intravascular catheters should be assessed on a daily basis.

END POINTS OF RESUSCITATION

For patients with shock, therapy needs to be early and aggressive (for further discussion of shock, see Chapter 4), but treatment must be titrated with the use of appropriate monitoring, including hemodynamic parameters and evidence of adequate end-organ perfusion. Once the patient is adequately volume loaded, the next consideration is adequacy of cardiac output. Echocardiography can estimate cardiac output and volume status.

Measurement of either base deficit or lactate levels can reflect anaerobic metabolism. Base deficit is confounded by other causes of metabolic acidosis, such as alcohol intoxication, hyperchloremia, or preexisting acid-base disorders. Lactate can be increased in sepsis, even when global oxygen delivery is normal, because of inhibition of pyruvate dehydrogenase, cytopathic hypoxia, increased release of alanine from muscle, and decreased hepatic clearance.

PREVENTING COMPLICATIONS IN THE SURGICAL INTENSIVE CARE UNIT

Other complications may arise that may increase morbidity and mortality. Deep vein thrombosis (DVT), with or without the associated PE, and SRMD are the most common. Prophylactic measures are employed in an effort to reduce the incidence of these complications.

Deep Vein Thrombosis

DVT, often within the large veins of the lower extremities and pelvis, may occur in 20% to 70% of hospitalized patients, depending on the patient population studied and surveillance strategy. Prophylaxis for DVT includes early ambulation, pneumatic compression devices, and the administration of low-dose heparin (unfractionated or low-molecular weight). The initial treatment of DVT requires therapeutic anticoagulation.

Stress-Related Mucosal Disease

SRMD has been seen historically in burn patients (Curling ulcer) and patients with TBI (Cushing ulcer) and may be significant in 3% to 6% of patients. Other patients at risk include those on mechanical ventilation, as well as those with major trauma or sepsis or those being treated with steroids.

ETHICS

Ethical issues frequently arise in the SICU, especially those focused on quality and end-of-life care. It is best to establish the person responsible for making decisions and have discussions before life-threatening events occur. As patients develop multiple-organ system dysfunction or irreversible neurologic dysfunction, prognosis and the goals of care should be discussed. The ethical principles of beneficence and nonmaleficence should direct the goals of care. Involvement by nursing staff, social services, palliative care services, and clergy is often helpful with these discussions.

CONCLUSIONS

Surgical patients frequently require critical care. The surgical intensivist-led multidisciplinary critical care team must be able to manage the complexities involved in these patients in order to optimize patient outcomes. The challenge for the surgical intensivist is to simultaneously diagnose the patients' conditions, while initiating appropriate therapy, focusing on the whole patient and their treatment goals.

SUGGESTED READINGS

Barr J, Fraser GL, Puntillo K, et al. Clinical practice guidelines for the management of pain, agitation, and delirium in adult patients in the intensive care unit. *Crit Care Med.* 2013;41(1):263-306. doi:10.1097/CCM.0b013e3182783b72

Fan E, Brodie D, Slutsky AS. Acute respiratory distress syndrome. Advances in diagnosis and treatment. *JAMA.* 2018;319(7): 698-710. doi:10.1001/jama.2017.21907

Plurad DS, Chiu W, Raja AS, et al. Monitoring modalities and assessment of fluid status: a practice management guideline from the Eastern Association for the Surgery of Trauma. *J Trauma Acute Care Surg.* 2018;84(1):37-49. doi:10.1097/TA.0000000000001719

Rhodes A, Evans LE, Alhazzani W, et al. Surviving sepsis campaign: International Guidelines for Management of Sepsis and Septic Shock: 2016. *Crit Care Med.* 2017;45(3):486-552. doi:10.1097/CCM.0000000000002255

Singer M, Deutschman CS, Seymour CW, et al. The third international consensus definitions for sepsis and septic shock (sepsis-3). *JAMA.* 2016;315(8):801-810. doi:10.1001/jama.2016.0287

SAMPLE QUESTIONS

QUESTIONS

Choose the best answer for each question.

1. A 68-year-old woman in the SICU is comatose 10 days after a motor vehicle crash during which she sustained a fractured right femur treated with an intramedullary rod within 24 hours of the injury. There were no other injuries noted on admission. She remains intubated because of hypoventilation. Vital signs are BP of 100/60 mm Hg and pulse of 52 beats/min. Her temperature is 35.4 °C. Her physical exam is otherwise normal. The surgical site is healing, with no signs of infection. An electrocardiogram (ECG) shows sinus rhythm with low-voltage QRS. Computed tomographic scan of her head is normal for her age. Laboratory studies show the following:

   Hemoglobin: 8.2 g/dL
   Sodium: 138 mEq/L
   Potassium: 3.7 mEq/L
   TSH: 16.4 µU/mL (ref: 0.5-5.0 µU/mL)
   T4: 0.5 µg/dL (ref: 5-12 µg/dL)

   What is the most likely diagnosis for her condition?

   A. Sick euthyroid syndrome
   B. Thyroid storm
   C. Myxedema coma
   D. AICI
   E. Graves disease

2. A 70-year-old woman is hypotensive 2 days after undergoing an open low anterior resection for sigmoid cancer. The surgery went well, with minimal blood loss. She was quite healthy and active prior to surgery. Since surgery, she has been receiving maintenance intravenous fluids and was stable until a few hours ago. Despite receiving boluses of normal saline and starting norepinephrine and vasopressin, she remains hypotensive. She is intubated because of lethargy and tachypnea. Her temperature is 37.4 °C. Her abdomen is soft and tender only near the lower midline incision. There is minimal urine output from a Foley catheter. Laboratory studies show the following:

   Hematocrit: 33% (36% the day before)
   Sodium: 129 mEq/L
   Potassium: 5.1 mEq/L
   Glucose: 108 mg/dL
   Arterial blood gases (ABGs) on 40% F_{IO_2}—pH: 7.39
   P_{CO_2}: 38 mm Hg
   P_{O_2}: 130 mm Hg
   U/A: no bacteria, negative leukocyte esterase

   What is the most likely diagnosis?

   A. Hemorrhage
   B. Anastomotic leak
   C. PE
   D. Acute adrenal insufficiency
   E. Urosepsis

3. A 71-year-old man is in the ICU with septic shock secondary to pneumonia. His BP is 85/40 mm Hg, and his heart rate is 95 beats/min. Which of the following medications would be the most appropriate to use to treat his hypotension?

   A. Epinephrine
   B. Dobutamine
   C. Milrinone
   D. Dopamine
   E. Norepinephrine

4. A 90-year-old man becomes lethargic after repair of an incarcerated ventral hernia. He has not been eating well and is maintained on intravenous fluids. He has been receiving his usual dose of oral hypoglycemic medication, and his glucose is 600 mg/dL. Which of the following is associated with worsening hyperglycemia in a postoperative patient?

   A. Oliguria
   B. Paralytic ileus
   C. Reduced cardiac output
   D. Hepatic encephalopathy
   E. Central nervous system dysfunction

5. The nurse in the unit calls because the 60-year-old man postoperative day 2 from his pancreaticoduodenectomy develops a temperature of 38.4 °C. His heart rate is 90 beats/min, and his BP is 130/80 mm Hg with 18 respirations a minute. What is the most common cause of fever for a postoperative patient in the first 48 hours following surgery?

   A. Wound infection
   B. Atelectasis
   C. SIRS
   D. Bacteremia
   E. Anesthetic reaction

ANSWERS AND EXPLANATIONS

1. **Answer: C**

   Although rare, myxedema coma is the most severe form of hypothyroidism. Typical features of this condition include mental status changes ranging from lethargy to coma, hypothermia, sinus bradycardia, low-voltage QRS complex on ECG, hypoventilation, and ileus. An elevated TSH and severely depressed T4 levels confirm the diagnosis. Sick euthyroid syndrome may be an adaptation to critical illness and is noteworthy for a depressed T3 level. Thyroid storm is severe hyperthyroidism and has features opposite of myxedema coma, including fever, high-output cardiac failure, and nearly nondetectable TSH, with elevated T3 and T4 levels. The hallmark of AICI is hypotension refractory to fluids and vasoactive medications. For more information on this topic, please see section "Endocrine Dysfunction."

2. **Answer: D**

   Adrenal insufficiency (AICI) typically presents with hypotension refractory to fluid resuscitation and vasoactive medications. Ventilator dependence, hyponatremia, hyperkalemia, and hypoglycemia can occur but are less commonly attributed to adrenal dysfunction. Although frequently seen with chronic adrenal insufficiency, hyperpigmentation, abdominal pain, nausea, weight loss, and fatigue are not typical symptoms in the critical care setting. For more information about this topic, please see section "Adrenal" under "Endocrine Dysfunction."

3. **Answer: E**

   Dobutamine is a β-agonist. Milrinone is a phosphodiesterase inhibitor. Both are commonly used for the management of cardiogenic shock. Epinephrine and dopamine have mixed α- and β-receptor activity. Dopamine also stimulates dopaminergic receptors. Tachycardia is a frequent side effect. Norepinephrine stimulates mainly α receptors, with some β-receptor activity. Thus, it is the drug of choice for patients with distributive shock, for example, sepsis. For more information, see section "Inotropes."

4. **Answer: E**

   Hyperglycemia occurs in many critically ill and injured patients. Although diabetes may be the etiology in a few patients, hyperglycemia caused by increased sympathetic and adrenal activity and activation of the cytokine cascade are the most common causes in critically ill patients. Hyperglycemia causes organ dysfunction in the cardiovascular, cerebrovascular, neuromuscular, and immunologic systems. Hyperglycemia induces cardiac arrhythmias, depletes intravascular volume because of osmotic diuresis, and increases urine output. The hyperglycemia leads to osmotic loads that dehydrate the brain and cause lethargy. For more information on this topic, please see section "Glucose Disorders."

5. **Answer: B**

   The criteria for SIRS are somewhat, but purposefully vague to trigger evaluation (see Table 9-3). Two criteria must be present, and there must be a plausible situation present (eg, the normal physiology seen with exercise meets the criteria for SIRS). If SIRS is present from infection or suspected infection, this is called *sepsis*. If sepsis has progressed to impair the normal function of an organ or body system, it is called *severe sepsis*. Sepsis with hypotension is septic shock. When SIRS criteria are not fully met, one then follows the usual physiologic causes, and atelectasis is a very common cause of fever particularly within the first 48 hours postoperatively. For more information on this topic, please see section "Systemic Inflammatory Response Syndrome."

10 Abdominal Wall, Including Hernia

Tess C. Huy, David C. Chen, and Ian T. MacQueen

A hernia of the abdominal wall is a clear, defined defect in the muscles and fascia through which abdominal contents can protrude. This can potentially cause trapping of the contents (incarceration), bowel obstruction, and ischemia (strangulation), depending on what structures are involved and how tightly and long they have been entrapped. Hernias can occur in various regions of the abdominal wall (Figure 10-1) and may present as first-time hernias or recurrences from previous repairs. For the purposes of this discussion, hernias will be grouped into two primary categories: ventral hernias of the anterior abdominal wall and groin hernias of the myopectineal orifice (MPO).

Other less common hernias will be briefly discussed separately. These rare hernias include flank, lumbar, obturator, sciatic, and perineal hernias. Compared to the first two categories of hernias, these hernias pose increased diagnostic challenges, and thus primary care physicians, radiologists, and surgeons must be familiar with their presentation and diagnostic workup.

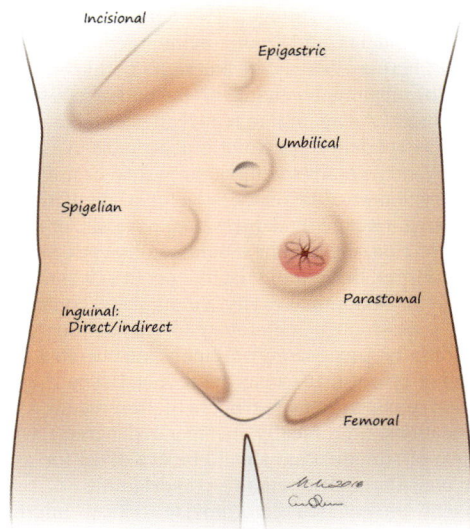

Figure 10-1. Possible sites of abdominal wall and groin hernias. Myopectineal orifice hernias include inguinal and femoral hernias. (Illustrated by Charlotte R. Spear and Marco A. Marchionni.)

ABDOMINAL WALL HERNIAS

Anatomy

Abdominal Wall Layers

The anatomy of the abdominal wall can be divided into lateral and central areas, separated by the linea semilunaris, also called the *semilunar line*. Each region is comprised of several layers (Figure 10-2).

The lateral abdominal wall is composed of three muscle layers with somewhat less prominent fascial layers. The external oblique muscle forms the most superficial layer, followed by the internal oblique muscle and then the transversus abdominis muscle. The transversalis fascia is the innermost layer, underlying the transversus abdominis muscle, and is closely associated with the peritoneum.

The central abdominal wall consists of the rectus muscle that is encased by the anterior and posterior rectus sheaths. The anterior rectus sheath runs from the xiphoid to the pubis. It is formed by the external oblique aponeurosis and half the internal oblique aponeurosis superiorly and the external oblique, internal oblique, and transversus abdominis aponeuroses inferiorly. The posterior rectus sheath is formed from half the internal oblique aponeurosis and the transversus abdominus aponeurosis superiorly until inferior to the umbilicus when all the aponeuroses move anteriorly to join the anterior rectus sheath. This demarcation is called the *arcuate line*. Above the arcuate line, the central abdominal wall consists of the anterior and posterior rectus sheath and rectus muscle while below the arcuate line, it consists of the transversalis fascia, rectus muscle, and anterior rectus sheath. The anterior and posterior rectus sheath fuse in the midline to form the linea alba.

Blood Supply and Innervation

The blood supply to the central abdominal wall is derived from the superior and inferior epigastric vessels, which run in a craniocaudal direction on the deep surface of the rectus muscle. Perforator vessels supplying the overlying muscle, skin, and subcutaneous tissue branch off the epigastric vessels and exit anteriorly along the length of the rectus abdominis. Blood supply and innervation for the lateral aspect of the abdominal wall come primarily from segmental branches, which run from lateral to medial.

Main Hernia Types

Hernias of the anterior abdominal wall can be divided into several types. Primary ventral hernias are hernias with no associated prior incision and are located anywhere along the midline. Umbilical hernias are a subset of ventral hernias occurring specifically at or adjacent to the umbilicus, usually producing a protrusion of the umbilical skin.

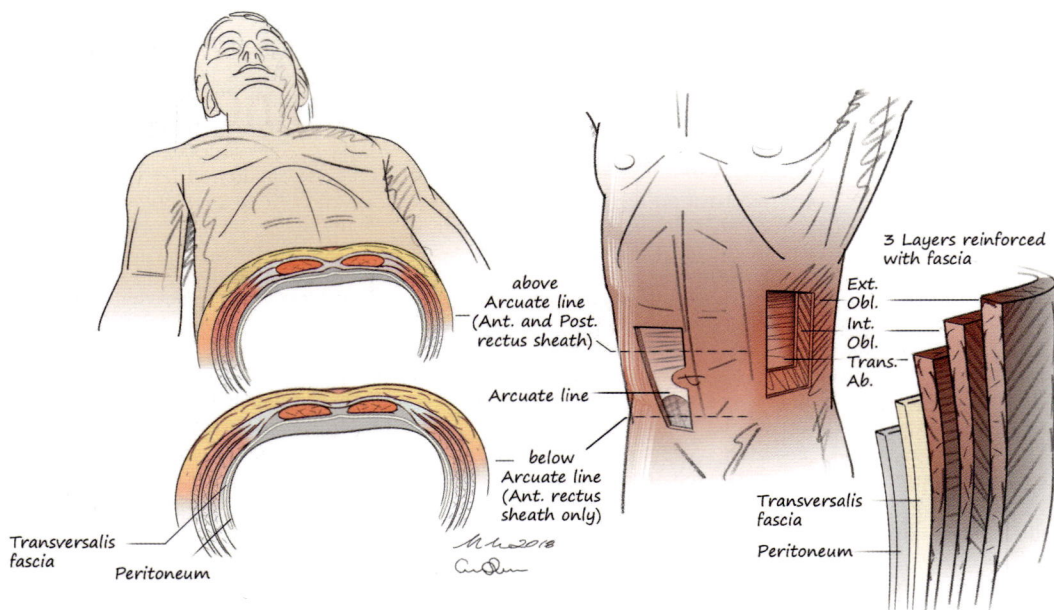

Figure 10-2. Layers of the main abdominal wall, including the changes above and below the arcuate line. Ant, anterior; ext, external; int, internal; obl, oblique; post, posterior; trans. ab, transversus abdominis. (Illustrated by Charlotte R. Spear and Marco A. Marchionni.)

Incisional hernias develop along prior surgical incisions and may be located anywhere on the abdominal wall.

Clinical Considerations

The overall goal in hernia management is to address symptoms, minimize the patient's risk of incarceration or strangulation, and minimize complications of repair, including hernia recurrence. Clinical presentation, surgical history, hernia-specific factors, and patient factors all play significant roles.

Clinical Presentation

Hernias have two typical presentation patterns: asymptomatic and symptomatic. Asymptomatic hernias are typically found during evaluation by a health care provider but may be noticed by the patient. These hernias may not require repair, as discussed in the following paragraphs. Asymptomatic hernias are most often reducible, meaning the hernia contents can be returned to the true abdominal cavity. This may occur either spontaneously, such as when a patient lies in the supine position, or manually, where the patient or health care provider pushes the contents back into the abdomen. Among reducible hernias, those with smaller fascial defects or those requiring difficult manual reduction may pose a greater risk of complications.

Symptomatic hernias may present in a variety of ways, both with subacute and acute symptoms. The most common subacute presentation is pain at the hernia site or abdominal cramping. This may occur continuously or intermittently and is often exacerbated by heavy lifting or physical activity. Symptomatic hernias should be fixed if the risk-benefit analysis favors repair. Of note, reducible hernias may still be symptomatic.

Acute presentation of hernias includes incarceration and strangulation. Incarceration of a hernia is defined by trapping of the contents within the hernia, such that the hernia contents are no longer reducible. Incarceration alone, especially without pain, is not necessarily an indication for emergent management. However, incarcerated hernias are at increased risk for strangulation, defined as ischemia of the hernia contents, and require more urgent attention than reducible hernias. Newly incarcerated hernias should be reduced or repaired depending on the patient's history and clinical status. An attempt to reduce the hernia under sedation by an experienced provider is acceptable in a hemodynamically stable patient without a physical examination or laboratory abnormalities suggestive of strangulation, such as erythema, marked tenderness, leukocytosis, or acidosis. After reduction, the patient should be observed to rule out the possibility that strangulated contents were reduced back into the abdominal cavity. Strangulated contents may infarct, necessitating exploratory abdominal surgery (eg, laparotomy or laparoscopy). Acutely incarcerated hernias containing bowel that cannot be reduced should undergo emergent repair within 4 to 6 hours of presentation to avoid complications. Chronically incarcerated hernias with no evidence of strangulation should be evaluated for surgical repair, considering the patient's comorbidities.

Patient presentation can provide critical information regarding the need for urgent or emergent hernia repair. Intractable nausea and vomiting, severe pain, tachycardia, fever, focal peritonitis, leukocytosis, acidosis, or obstruction on imaging indicate likely strangulation and point to the need for emergent surgery. Strangulation is also identified by the presence of focal peritonitis, acidosis, leukocytosis, or change of color in the overlying skin, suggesting necrosis of underlying tissues. If the hernia contents are suspected to be strangulated, emergent surgical intervention is required and the hernia should be reduced intraoperatively rather than at bedside. If there are infarcted organs in the hernia contents, resection is lifesaving and is the operative priority, with hernia repair becoming a secondary consideration.

Surgical History

Patient history can provide useful information regarding the nature of prior abdominal pathology and the likelihood of intra-abdominal adhesions. Both are factors that may affect hernia repair. Prior abdominal incisions, prior fascial dehiscence, or postoperative abdominal wound infection all increase the risk for incisional hernia. A history of prior abdominal tubes or ostomies may create disruptions in the abdominal wall, which will affect how hernia repair should be conducted. Prior operative notes and discharge summaries can be very helpful in this regard.

Hernia-Specific Factors

Adequate characterization of the hernia defect and determination of the exact location are useful in operative planning. If hernia size and location cannot be established by physical examination alone, computed tomography (CT) is useful to confirm the defect location and size, in addition to providing information about visceral involvement, the surrounding abdominal wall, and the position of any stoma, previously placed mesh, or other implantable devices. Imaging can also assist the surgeon in determining the patient's odds of emergent repair and hernia-related complications with models using the hernia size, hernia-to-abdominal wall angle, and hernia-to-neck ratio. Generally speaking, a greater hernia sac size in comparison to the hernia neck size is associated with a higher risk of an incarceration event or emergency repair.

Patient Factors

Modifiable Risk Factors

The decision for hernia repair should focus on modifiable risk factors, such as functional status, smoking, obesity, and medical comorbidities to reduce perioperative morbidity. Nutritional optimization for the undernourished patient is critical to ensure adequate wound healing, especially with the large incisions used for open repair of hernias of the anterior abdominal wall. Weight management for obesity reduces overall perioperative morbidity, wound issues, and the risk of hernia recurrence after repair. Smoking cessation is helpful from both a pulmonary complication and wound healing standpoint and should be mandated for elective repair. Diabetes is associated with perioperative morbidity and mortality, poorer wound healing, and increased risk of infection. For patients with diabetes, hemoglobin A_{1c} should be normalized to less than 8 if possible, prior to elective surgery. Perioperative venous thromboembolism prophylaxis may also need to be considered. Routine mechanical prophylaxis with compression devices is appropriate for most patients, but high-risk patients may benefit from chemoprophylaxis (anticoagulation) as well. Patients already on anticoagulation will require a plan to manage anticoagulation.

Perioperative Planning

In addition to the reduction of modifiable risk factors, prehabilitation improves preoperative strength, mobility, and overall recovery for patients with poor functional status. Plans may need to be in place for alternative, nonnarcotic pain control options—lidocaine drip, regional blocks of the transversus abdominis plane (TAP), and spinal or epidural blocks—which may reduce respiratory depression and aid in improving postoperative pain control, ambulation, and early return of bowel function. Often, such interventions are incorporated into perioperative prehabilitation and enhanced recovery protocols.

Patient Counseling

Preoperative patient counseling typically includes evaluating the patient's risk of hernia-related complications and surgical risks. By balancing the two risk profiles, the surgeon can decide to proceed with operative or nonoperative management. Clinical obstructive symptoms, previous incarceration, and emergency department visits for a symptomatic hernia are useful in determining the patient's risk for future incarceration or strangulation. Ultrasound, CT, and other imaging also enable the physician to determine the risk of hernia complications, according to risk model calculations and hernia-to-neck ratio. Recurrence risk after repair should focus on individual patient factors such as prior abdominal surgery, obesity, age, smoking status, overall activity level, and hernia size. Specific risks of hernia repair should be reviewed, including the risks of recurrence, seroma, mesh infection, and visceral injury, all of which are discussed in the following paragraphs. Available online risk assessment tools, including the American College of Surgeons risk calculator, can be very useful for patient education, especially in patients at higher risk for perioperative morbidity and mortality.

Surgical Approaches

The technique chosen must minimize the risk of recurrence while also limiting the potential for morbidity. Options for repair of hernias of the abdominal wall include primary, mesh, and component separation repairs, performed by an open or minimally invasive approach.

Primary Repair

Primary repair involves closure of the hernia defect with suture alone. This approach is reserved for primary hernias that are at low risk for recurrence, such as hernia defects less than 1 to 2 cm without surrounding rectus diastasis. This technique is not appropriate for incisional or recurrent hernias. Perceived benefits of primary repair of a ventral abdominal wall hernia must be carefully considered, as mesh repairs have lower recurrence rates.

Mesh Repair

Mesh repair involves the placement of mesh to strengthen the repair and distribute tissue tension to minimize recurrence risk. Hernia mesh types include permanent (ie, nonabsorbable) synthetic mesh, absorbable synthetic mesh (including slowly absorbable meshes sometimes termed "*biosynthetic*"), and biologic meshes. Most commonly, permanent synthetic mesh is used to reinforce the closure of hernia defects. After implantation, abdominal wall tissue grows into the mesh, incorporating it into the abdominal wall to strengthen the repair.

The use of mesh reduces the risk of recurrence but can also be associated with certain complications. Mesh can be associated with seroma formation, infection, and erosion into surrounding tissue. Erosion can be especially problematic when the mesh is located within the peritoneal space, in direct contact with visceral structures. Some meshes are intended for intraperitoneal implantation and manufactured with biochemical properties to mitigate this risk. Mesh is a foreign body, and as such, infection involving mesh can be difficult to eradicate. Infected permanent mesh often requires removal. The problem of refractory mesh infection is self-limited in the case of biologic and absorbable meshes, as any synthetic foreign material in these meshes is eventually dissolved. For this reason, biologic and absorbable synthetics are often used in damage control situations of intra-abdominal contamination or urgent repair in the setting of uncontrolled risk factors, where the risk of mesh infection is high. When the risk of mesh infection is very high, primary repair may be used even for large defects, accepting the risk of recurrence while minimizing the risk of mesh-related problems.

Mesh can be implanted in a variety of locations and by a range of techniques (Figure 10-3). It can be placed superficial to the anterior fascia of the abdominal wall (onlay), in the preperitoneal space, or in an intraperitoneal position. By dividing the medial border of the posterior rectus sheath, the mesh may also be placed between the rectus muscle and the posterior rectus sheaths, known as the *retrorectus* or *retromuscular position*. It is ideal to close the midline abdominal wall fascia in addition to using mesh, though this is not always anatomically possible. When native tissues cannot be brought together, the mesh may be used to bridge across a hernia defect.

Component Separation Repair

This is a specific type of mesh repair that is generally reserved for larger, more complex midline abdominal wall hernias, including recurrent hernias. This type of hernia repair involves the separation of the individual layers of the abdominal wall to gain length for tissue approximation to close the hernia defect while relieving tension on the fascial closure. There are multiple techniques including anterior component separation, retrorectus repair, and posterior component separation with a transversus abdominis release (TAR). All these techniques require specialized training to perform.

Anterior component separation is performed by dividing the external oblique aponeurosis lateral to the semilunar line along the length of the abdominal wall (Figure 10-4). Incision of this aponeurosis allows the remaining muscle layers to be pulled across a large hernia defect, approximating healthy tissue at the midline. These maneuvers can produce up to 10 to 12 cm of advancement toward the midline for defect closure and are most commonly used with an onlay mesh.

Retrorectus repair involves dividing the medial border of the posterior rectus sheath and developing a plane between the rectus muscle and the posterior rectus sheath bilaterally. This plane can be extended from the costal margin to the pubic symphysis, extending to the preperitoneal space inferior to the arcuate line. A posterior layer of the posterior rectus sheath and peritoneum is then closed to cover and protect the viscera, and mesh is placed into the retrorectus space. The anterior rectus sheaths are closed over this in the midline. This repair can be technically challenging but allows for adequate-size mesh placement for medium-sized hernias while protecting against mesh erosion into the viscera or through the subcutaneous tissues.

For large hernias, a posterior component separation via TAR may be added to a retrorectus repair to allow for more laxity for abdominal wall closure and to allow for the placement of a larger mesh. After the retrorectus dissection is completed, the posterior lamella of the posterior rectus sheath and transversus abdominis muscle are divided just medial to the neurovascular bundles innervating the rectus muscle. This allows dissection in a preperitoneal or pre-transversalis plane into the far lateral abdomen. This may be extended to the retropubic space inferiorly and to the central tendon of the diaphragm superiorly, allowing wide mesh reinforcement of the entire anterior abdominal wall.

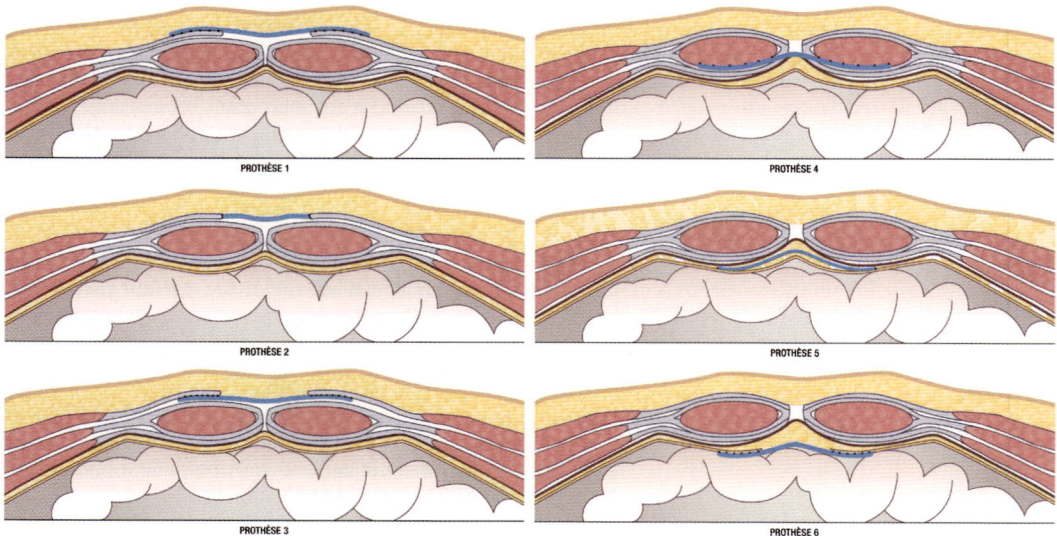

PROTHÈSE 1

PROTHÈSE 4

PROTHÈSE 2

PROTHÈSE 5

PROTHÈSE 3

PROTHÈSE 6

Figure 10-3. Positions in which mesh can be implanted during hernia repair. Note that sublay and retrorectus mesh fall under section "Component Separation Repair." (Illustration by Nancy Beauregard, CHU de Québec—Université Laval, Quebec, Canada.)

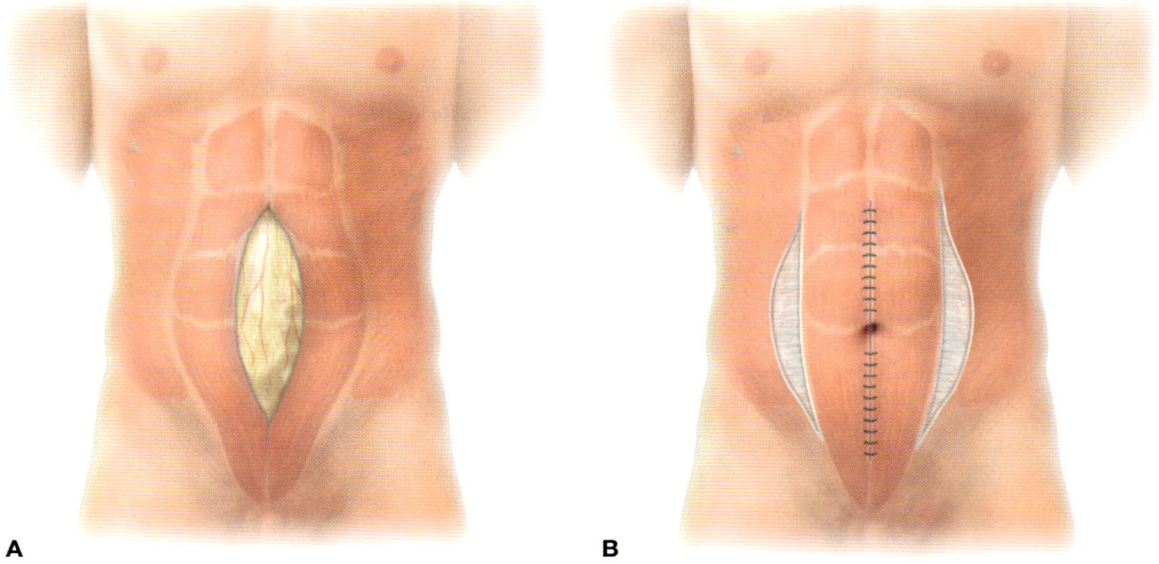

A **B**

Figure 10-4. A. A midline ventral hernia. B. A postoperative view after hernia repair with anterior component separation. Note the relaxing incision of the external oblique aponeurosis laterally to the rectus muscles. The deeper abdominal wall layers are still present, keeping the abdominal wall intact. (Images from Wexner SD, Fleshman JW, Fischer JE. *Master Techniques in General Surgery Colon and Rectal Surgery Abdominal Operations*. Lippincott Williams & Wilkins; 2019. Copyright © 2019 Wolters Kluwer.)

Component separation techniques require specialized training to perform safely and effectively. Importantly, anterior and posterior component separation cannot be used together as the abdominal wall will become destabilized.

Minimally Invasive Versus Open Approach

Abdominal wall hernias can be repaired as described previously through an open incision or through a minimally invasive (laparoscopic or robotic) approach. The advantages to minimally invasive approaches are decreased potential incisional morbidity, shorter length of stay, and quicker recovery when compared with open approaches, though these outcomes have not been extensively studied, and heterogeneity in surgical technique, mesh location, and so on, makes it difficult to draw clear conclusions comparing these approaches. The best-studied benefit of minimally invasive repair is a significant reduction in surgical site infections. It is generally accepted that minimally invasive repair can be more difficult and often requires specialized training, especially if the mesh is to be placed in an extraperitoneal location. Patients who undergo these approaches must also be able to tolerate general anesthesia to allow for intraoperative paralysis.

The open approach generally has the advantage of potentially being more straightforward and having a shorter operative time. The open approach may also avoid the need for paralysis, general anesthesia, or extensive adhesiolysis. Finally, an open approach is appropriate when concomitant skin removal or scar revision is required.

Common Postoperative Issues

Seroma

Seroma can develop in the space previously occupied by the hernia contents or in other potential spaces that may have been created during dissection (Figure 10-5). Often, the peritoneal hernia sac is excised to reduce the risk of seroma formation, but sac excision does not completely eliminate the risk of seroma, especially among large hernias. Seromas can often be palpated, and the bulging raises concerns for possible hernia recurrence. On examination, the seroma will not increase in size with Valsalva, whereas hernia recurrence will, and seromas typically are not painful. If physical examination is insufficient to confirm the diagnosis, ultrasound or CT can be used to clarify. In general, seromas will resorb over time and do not require any intervention. Drainage of an otherwise uncomplicated seroma is not recommended because it can lead to infection.

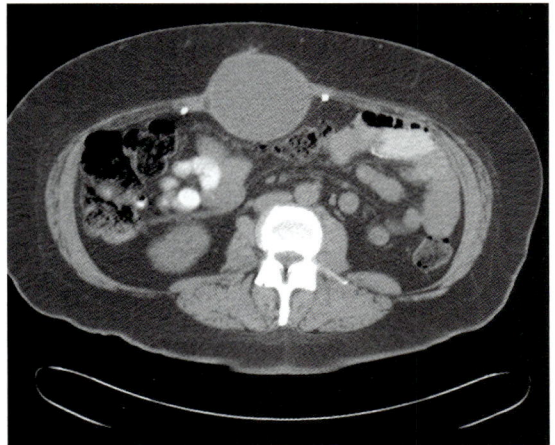

Figure 10-5. A postoperative seroma after incisional hernia repair as seen on computed tomography (axial view). Note the radiodensity on either side of the fluid collection representing tacks placed to fixate the edges of the mesh.

Infection

Surgical site infection is problematic in hernia repair because it can lead to poor fascial healing or mesh infection requiring explantation, both of which increase the risk of hernia recurrence. Prevention is critical through the use of preoperative antibiotics, avoidance of mesh implantation in contaminated fields, optimization of patient comorbidities, and using a minimally invasive approach when appropriate. Early recognition and management of superficial infection is critical in limiting the spread of infection from superficial tissues to the underlying mesh.

Neuropathic Symptoms

Periodically, patients undergoing abdominal wall hernia repair develop neuropathic symptoms related to intraoperative nerve damage presenting as numbness, tingling, and hyperesthesia. Typically, minor issues are self-limited, although some patients require local injection, steroids, and medications for neuropathic symptoms. This is a more significant issue with the hernias of the MPO.

Recurrence

All hernias have the potential to recur following repair. Prior abdominal surgery, particularly with prior incisional wound infections, obesity, age, smoking, patient level of activity, and the presence of chronic coughing or straining are factors that increase recurrence risk. Patients who have undergone hernia repair should be evaluated when new or recurrent symptoms arise to rule out the development of recurrent hernia. If physical examination is insufficient, further imaging with ultrasound or CT is appropriate.

Special Situations

Several special abdominal hernias exist outside of these broad categories; these are generally beyond the scope of this chapter. There are two exceptions worth mentioning. First, the Spigelian hernia occurs at the junction of the inferior edge of the posterior rectus sheath and the lateral border of the rectus abdominis, at the arcuate line (Figure 10-6). It has a characteristic location in the right or left lower quadrant and usually involves only the posterior elements.

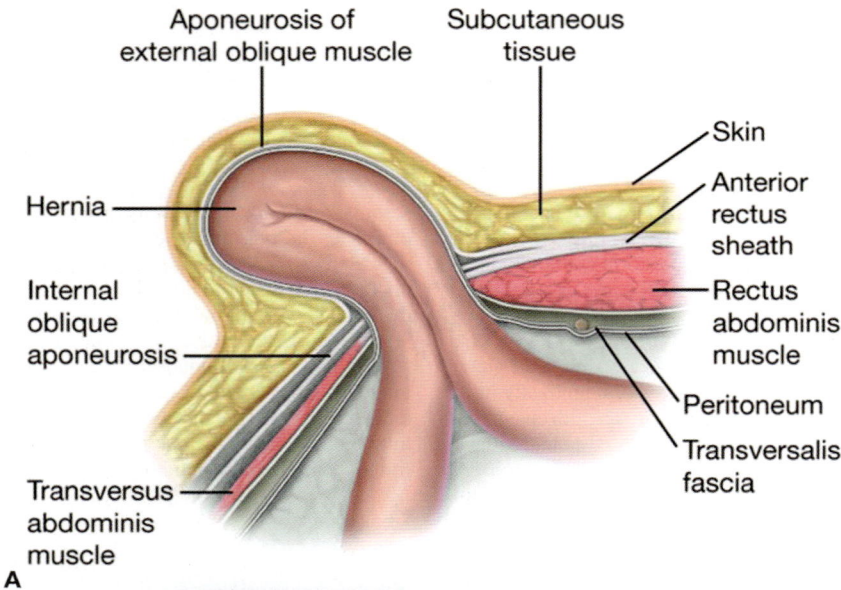

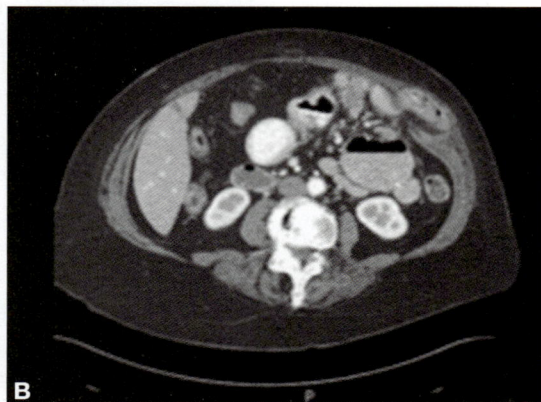

Figure 10-6. Spigelian hernia. A. Schematic axial view. B. Spigelian hernia as seen on computed tomography (axial view). Note that the external oblique remains intact overlying this hernia. (A. From Jones DB, Fischer JE. *Master Techniques in Surgery: Hernia.* Lippincott Williams & Wilkins, A Wolters Kluwer business; 2013.)

Separated
rectus abdominus
muscle bellies

A

B

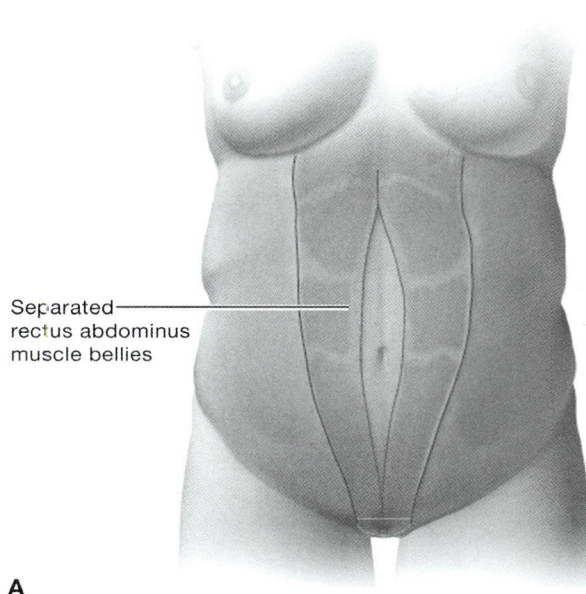

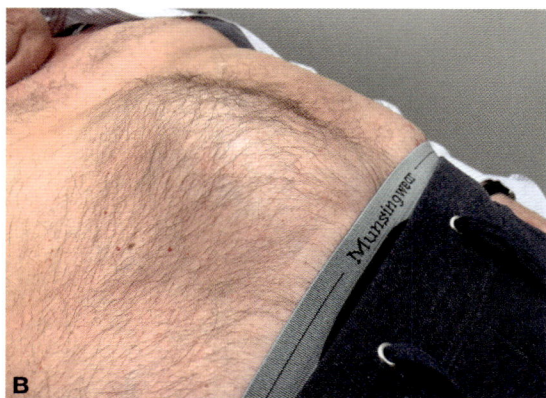

Figure 10-7. A. A schematic of rectus diastasis. B. A patient with rectus diastasis. Note the bulging of the upper midline abdomen when the patient does a "sit-up" maneuver. (A. Reprinted with permission from Irion JM, Irion GL. *Women's Health in Physical Therapy*. 1st ed. Lippincott Williams & Wilkins. Copyright © 2010 Lippincott Williams & Wilkins, A Wolters Kluwer business.)

Because it does not typically penetrate the anterior portion of the abdominal wall, it may not be a visible or palpable bulge on the surface.

Second, parastomal hernias develop within the fascial opening of an ostomy, with herniation of additional viscera alongside the stoma. Parastomal hernias can affect stomal function. Many options are available to repair parastomal hernias, including minimally invasive or open procedures, as well as relocation of the stoma to an area of intact abdominal wall.

Finally, it is important to note that the term *hernia* implies at least a partial defect in the abdominal wall. On the contrary, rectus diastasis is a thinning of the upper midline abdominal wall without a defect. This is caused by stretching and attenuation of the linea alba from increased intra-abdominal pressure and pregnancy, causing the rectus muscles to deviate laterally (Figure 10-7). Rectus diastasis often presents as a bulge on Valsalva and can be confused with a ventral midline hernia. Because only attenuation is present without a true abdominal wall defect, rectus diastasis does not carry any risks of incarceration or strangulation and does not require intervention.

MYOPECTINEAL ORIFICE (GROIN) HERNIAS

Anatomy

The groin hernia is notable for its complex anatomy. Groin hernias are caused by a defect of the MPO of Fruchaud. The MPO is an area of inherent weakness in the pelvis caused by the embryologic egress of the testicle or round ligament and the iliac neurovascular bundle from the intra-abdominal compartment.

Myopectineal Orifice Boundaries

There are clear boundaries of the MPO. The inferior boundary is a ridge on the superior pubic ramus known as the *pectineal line* or *Cooper ligament*. The lateral boundary is the medial edge of the iliopsoas muscle. The superior boundary is made of muscle fibers from the transversus abdominis and internal oblique, the aponeurosis of which is the conjoint tendon. These fibers curve to intersect the medial boundary, the lateral edge of the anterior rectus sheath. Of note, in 3% to 6% of cases, the conjoint tendon continues parallel to the rectus, inserting upon the pubic tubercle itself.

The irregular three-dimensional shape of the MPO differs in appearance when viewed from the anterior perspective (as seen in an open inguinal hernia repair) or the posterior perspective (as in a minimally invasive approach) (see Figure 10-8).

Myopectineal Orifice Spaces

There are three types of MPO hernias: femoral, indirect inguinal, and direct inguinal hernias, differentiated by the area of the MPO in which they occur (see Figure 10-8). The MPO is subdivided into two spaces by the ilioinguinal ligament (Poupart ligament), which runs obliquely from the anterior superior iliac crest to the pubic tubercle. The area inferior to the ilioinguinal ligament is called the "*femoral canal.*" This inferior space of the MPO is where the femoral nerve, artery, vein, and lymphatics run. The potential space between the common femoral vein and lymphatics is commonly called the "*femoral space*" and is where femoral hernias occur. Superior to the ilioinguinal ligament is the inguinal space and is where the spermatic cord or round ligament exits the abdominal cavity and traverses medially. This is the space where the two most common types of MPO hernia, indirect and direct inguinal hernias, can be found.

Inguinal Canal Anatomy

Understanding the similarities and differences between direct and indirect inguinal hernias requires knowledge of the anatomy of the superior space of the MPO and the inguinal canal. In contrast to the main abdominal wall, the MPO does not contain any muscular layers. The superior space of the MPO is bounded by the diagonal line of the ilioinguinal

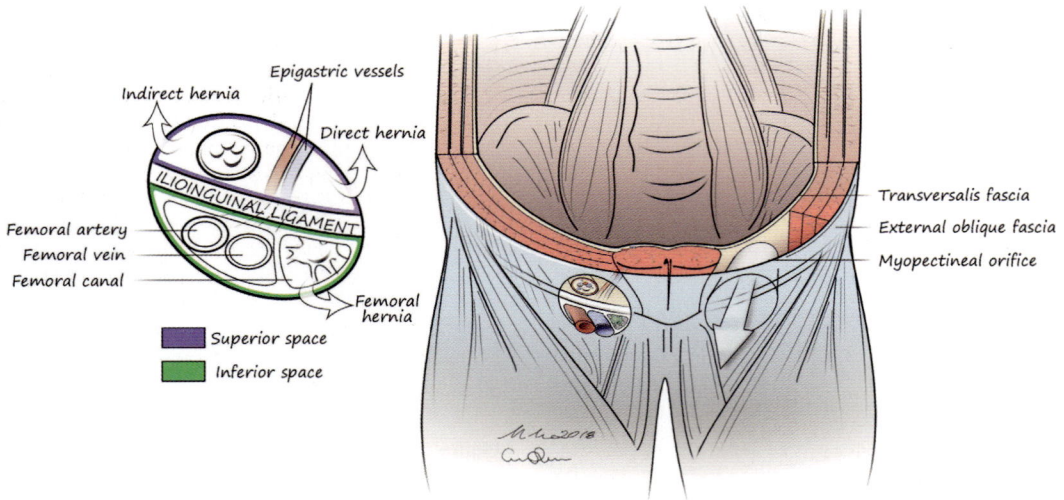

Figure 10-8. A schematic of the myopectineal orifice (MPO). Note the cylindrical shape that tunnels through the lower abdominal wall on the left groin. The right groin shows the anatomic structures passing through the space, with the relevant labels and locations of MPO hernias shown in the inset, left. (Illustrated by Charlotte R. Spear and Marco A. Marchionni.)

ligament inferiorly and laterally, the rectus muscle medially, the transversalis fascia posteriorly, the aponeurosis of the external oblique anteriorly, and the conjoint tendon superiorly. The entrance of the spermatic cord or round ligament to the inguinal canal is through a cephalad, a posterior opening in the transversalis fascia. This is termed the *deep* or *internal inguinal ring* and is covered anteriorly by the aponeurosis of the external oblique. The exit of the canal is a caudal anterior opening through the external oblique aponeurosis, called the *superficial* or *external inguinal ring*, which is covered posteriorly by the transversalis fascia. This angled penetration through the abdominal wall layers at two different points maximizes the closure of the inguinal canal after the descent of the testicle. The male inguinal canal contains the spermatic cord, while the female inguinal canal contains the round ligament. Given the greater complexity of the spermatic cord and the increased prevalence of inguinal hernias in males, inguinal hernia anatomy is commonly described using a male example, which will be continued here.

Inguinal Canal Spaces

Both direct and indirect hernias are caused by protrusion of abdominal contents through the MPO superior to the inguinal ligament. The difference between the indirect and direct hernias is the exact location of the transversalis defect. Just as the MPO is divided into superior (inguinal canal) and inferior spaces (femoral canal) by the ilioinguinal ligament, the superior space is subdivided vertically into two spaces by the inferior epigastric artery and vein (see Figure 10-8).

An indirect inguinal hernia occurs when abdominal contents herniate lateral to the epigastric vessels through a weakened internal inguinal ring. The sac will follow the spermatic cord within the abdominal wall. This is the same course taken by a pediatric inguinal hernia or hydrocele, and most hydroceles found later in life do have an associated indirect hernia and are congenital. A direct inguinal hernia occurs medial to the inferior epigastric vessels. The direct space is historically named Hesselbach triangle, covering a large part of the floor

of the inguinal canal. When there is a defect in the Hesselbach triangle, the hernia sac goes directly into the inguinal canal, and the distal aspect will abut the spermatic cord but does not travel through the internal ring along with it.

Myopectineal Orifice Hernia Types

In summary, there are three spaces where hernias can occur within the MPO. The space below the ilioinguinal ligament, the inferior space of the MPO, is where femoral hernias occur. The two spaces above the ilioinguinal ligament are the lateral indirect space and the medial direct space, which can each develop hernias of the same name. A patient may have a hernia in one, two, or all three of these spaces. A hernia in both the direct and indirect space is called a "*pantaloon hernia*" describing a "leg" of the peritoneum in both spaces, split by the fixed epigastric vessels.

The most common of the three MPO hernias in women is the indirect hernia. It is important to note that women have a much higher incidence of femoral hernias than men, as a wider pelvis means a wider potential opening into the femoral space.

Special Situations

Other presentations of MPO hernias include Richter hernia, where only a portion of the circumference of the bowel is incarcerated or strangulated through the hernia defect. This may pose diagnostic challenges because patients may not have symptoms of bowel obstruction despite the presence of incarcerated and strangulated bowel. A sliding hernia occurs when an intra-abdominal organ constitutes a portion of the hernia sac. In these cases, attempts to open the hernia sac may cause visceral injury. A Littre hernia occurs when a symptomatic Meckel diverticulum is found in the hernia sac, and an Amyand hernia contains the appendix.

Clinical Considerations

Patient Presentation

The management of patients with groin hernias depends on the severity of symptoms. It has been shown that an asymptomatic hernia or a minimally symptomatic inguinal hernia rarely causes complications, and watchful waiting is safe. Despite this, most inguinal hernias will progress to requiring repair in the future, typically for the development of symptoms. Asymptomatic femoral hernias should be repaired because they are more likely to incarcerate or strangulate.

Patients with symptomatic MPO hernias have a bulge in the groin. The bulge may enlarge with increases in intra-abdominal pressure, such as lifting or coughing. MPO hernias are typically associated with discomfort, frank pain, burning, or a dull ache that is worse after a long day of standing. On physical examination, the bulge of a direct or indirect inguinal hernia will initiate above the ilioinguinal ligament but may extend all the way into the scrotum or labia majora. A femoral hernia will be felt entirely below the ilioinguinal ligament. If physical examination is not confirmatory, further imaging with ultrasound or CT is helpful.

The issues of incarceration and strangulation apply to MPO hernias in much the same way as main abdominal wall hernias. Reduction of newly incarcerated hernias may be attempted in a hemodynamically stable patient without lab abnormalities, with postreduction monitoring. Clinical signs concerning strangulation will warrant operative exploration, sometimes requiring a separate laparotomy incision if the extent of ischemia cannot be fully evaluated via a groin incision.

Surgical History

Operative strategy will be different for recurrent groin hernias as compared to primary hernias. A history of prior abdominal surgery may signify the need for distant lysis of adhesions in a planned minimally invasive repair.

Hernia-Specific Factors

The primary assessment in the evaluation of a groin hernia is to determine whether it is an inguinal or femoral hernia. This can often but not always be determined by physical examination. Physical examination cannot typically differentiate direct from indirect hernias, but this is readily determined by imaging. Surgical techniques for the repair of direct and indirect inguinal hernias are identical, whereas femoral hernias, lying in the inferior space of the MPO, require different repair techniques because the closure of a different MPO space is required.

Surgical Approaches

Surgical options for MPO hernias are based on surgeon preference and experience, as well as the presentation of the patient. All surgical approaches adhere to the same overriding principles: hernia repairs should be performed in a tension-free manner, and mesh should not be used in contaminated wounds.

There are a variety of surgical approaches to hernias of the MPO, but these can be broadly divided into two categories: the anterior (open) approach and the posterior (minimally invasive) approach.

Anterior Approach

The anterior, open approach for inguinal hernias requires an incision over the inguinal canal. The roof of the canal (aponeurosis of the external oblique) is opened, the hernia is reduced, and the direct and/or indirect defects in the floor of the inguinal canal are repaired. This can be done with or without mesh, but a mesh repair is standard for the MPO today due to its lower recurrence rates and decreased tension.

Lichtenstein Mesh Repair

The Lichtenstein repair, named for the surgeon who popularized the technique, is an anterior repair performed with mesh overlying the anterior surface of the floor of the inguinal canal. In a typical Lichtenstein repair, the mesh is affixed to the floor of the inguinal canal and covers both the direct and indirect spaces of the MPO. The edges of the mesh are fitted to the boundaries of the superior space of the MPO. The inferior portion of the mesh is sutured to the inferior inguinal ligament (Figure 10-9). A keyhole is fashioned in the mesh superiorly to allow the spermatic cord to enter the inguinal canal, thus creating a new internal inguinal ring. The aponeurosis of the external oblique is closed over the mesh but left open inferiorly, creating a new external inguinal ring.

Tissue Repairs

Despite the prevalence and benefits of mesh repair, it is important to understand the use of tissue repairs. These repairs are useful in contaminated fields because they eliminate the need for placement of mesh, thus limiting the risk of infection, and are, therefore, still used today, albeit rarely. Tissue repairs are summarized in Table 10-1.

Posterior Approach

The posterior approach for inguinal and femoral hernias is usually performed either laparoscopically or robotically. The two primary minimally invasive techniques are the total extraperitoneal (TEP) approach and the transabdominal preperitoneal (TAPP) approach. Both posterior approaches use minimally invasive incisions and always use mesh. The posterior mesh approach is the only mainstream approach in which a single piece of mesh will cover all three spaces of the MPO (direct, indirect, and femoral). It is for this reason that femoral hernias should be repaired with a posterior approach when patient factors and surgeon technical expertise allow.

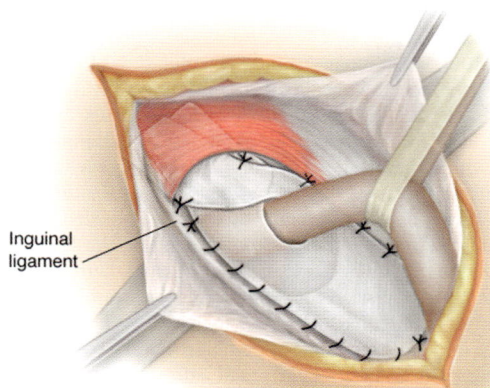

Inguinal ligament

Figure 10-9. In a Lichtenstein repair, the mesh is used to bridge the aponeurotic arch superiorly and the inguinal ligament inferiorly. (From Hawn MT, Mulholland MW. *Operative Techniques in Foregut Surgery.* Wolters Kluwer Health; 2015. Copyright © 2015 Wolters Kluwer Health.)

TABLE 10-1. Myopectineal Hernia Tissue Repairs

	Tissue Closed	Myopectineal Orifice Hernia Types	Notes
McVay	Conjoint tendon to Cooper ligament medially, conjoint tendon to ilioinguinal ligament laterally	Femoral Direct Indirect	• Relaxing incision is needed to reduce tension.[a]
Bassini	Conjoint tendon to ilioinguinal ligament	Direct Indirect	• Relaxing incision is needed to reduce tension.[a] • Will NOT repair femoral hernia
Shouldice	Complex, multilayered repair	Direct Indirect	• Reportedly tension-free • Will NOT repair femoral hernia • May have lowest recurrence rate of tissue repairs

[a]Similar to the process described for hernias of the main abdominal wall, under section "Component Separation Repair."

The primary difference between the two posterior techniques is the placement of the camera and instruments relative to the peritoneum. The TEP procedure does not involve entering the peritoneal cavity. A space is made between the rectus muscle and the peritoneum through which the entire operation is performed using laparoscopic equipment only. With the TAPP procedure, the abdomen is entered in the same fashion as any other minimally invasive procedure. A peritoneal flap is then created over the MPO, the mesh is placed, and the peritoneum is sutured close. This can be done laparoscopically or robotically. Both procedures place a piece of mesh between the peritoneum and the MPO and are equally useful for direct, indirect, and femoral hernias (Figure 10-10). Options for mesh fixation include self-fixating mesh, sutures, and tacks.

Choosing a Technique

Surgical repair of MPO hernias has evolved. Large, open, mesh-free repairs such as the McVay and Bassini repairs have been supplanted with less morbid, open, mesh repairs such as the Lichtenstein repair. Meanwhile, minimally invasive technologies have advanced. The optimal surgical approach to groin hernia repair must consider the specific needs of the patient and the technical capabilities of the surgeon.

As a rule, mesh repairs should be offered to all patients regardless of whether an open or minimally invasive approach is chosen. Exceptions to this are in cases of contamination of the surgical field, as in cases of strangulated hernias with ischemia, necrosis, or inadvertent bowel injury.

Minimally invasive surgery has benefit in evaluating and treating bilateral MPO hernias. A posteriorly placed mesh covers all three MPO hernia spaces including the femoral space. Due to the ability to repair occult femoral hernias, this is the preferred approach for groin hernias in women.

Finally, minimally invasive techniques have been shown to improve the speed of patient recovery because of less acute pain and allow early and safe return to normal activities. Minimally invasive repair is recommended for unilateral, first-time, and femoral hernia repairs when expertise in these techniques is available.

Common Postoperative Issues

Repair of MPO hernias, whether by an anterior or posterior approach, is performed in the outpatient setting. As patients leave the medical setting immediately after completion of the repair, it is critical to counsel them regarding expected postoperative conditions. It is common for the patient to experience postoperative swelling or ecchymoses in the scrotum, labia, or penis. The use of a scrotal support may help with these symptoms in male patients.

Neuropathic Symptoms

Neuropathic symptoms are much more common following MPO hernia repair compared with the main abdominal wall hernia repair. If an open approach is used, a zone of hypoesthesia may be observed at the skin incision. With regrowth of superficial innervation, the patient may notice symptoms of paresthesia such as burning or tingling.

Unfortunately, 5% to 10% of patients will experience chronic pain following MPO hernia repair. Chronic pain is defined as pain at the repair site that persists longer than 12 weeks. In these patients, it is important to distinguish neuropathic pain from nociceptive pain to ensure appropriate management. Unlike neuropathic pain, which results from nerve injury, nociceptive pain results from injury to tissues.

There are several nerves that can be entrapped or damaged in the zone of groin hernia repair. During anterior repair, these include the ilioinguinal nerve, the iliohypogastric nerve, and the genital branch of the genitofemoral nerve. The ilioinguinal nerve runs within the inguinal canal and along the course of the spermatic cord or round ligament. Patients with injury to this nerve may present with pain along the groin crease, radiating to the medial thigh, scrotum, or labia. On examination, there may be numbness or hyperesthesia over this distribution. The iliohypogastric nerve lies between the external and internal oblique muscles. If the iliohypogastric nerve is injured, patients may report numbness or pain over the lower abdomen and groin. The genitofemoral nerve passes through the internal inguinal ring and courses within the spermatic cord, innervating the skin of the scrotum. This may be damaged during open or minimally invasive repair. Finally, damage to the femoral branch of the genitofemoral nerve or the lateral femoral cutaneous nerve causes numbness to the anterior and lateral thigh. These are typically only susceptible to injury during posterior repair.

Nociceptive pain is often related to bulky or folded mesh. Post-herniorrhaphy orchialgia, or testicular pain, is neuropathic pain that may be caused by injury to the paravasal nerves. It must be distinguished from scrotal and groin pain.

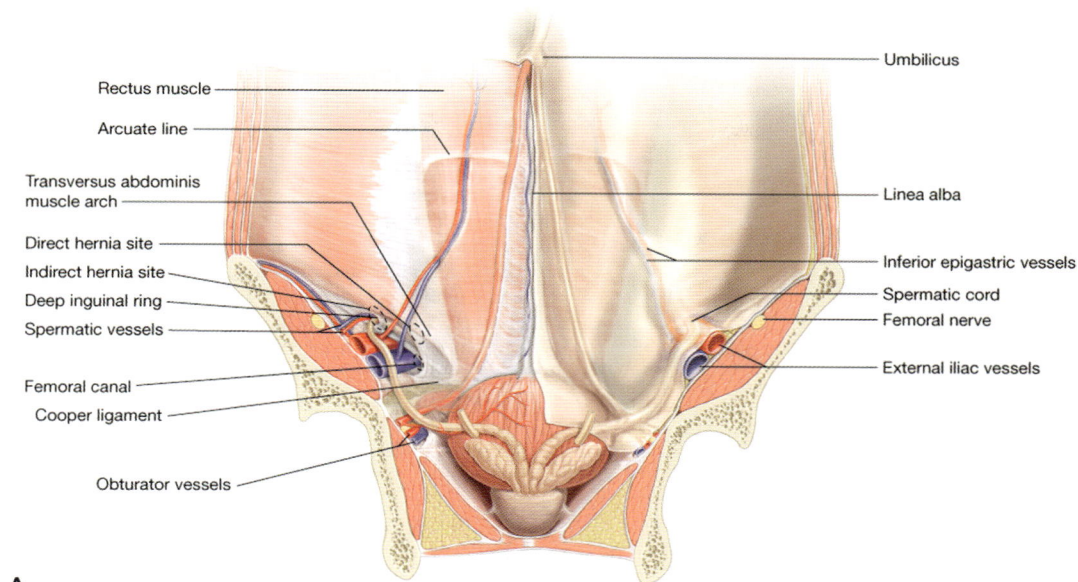

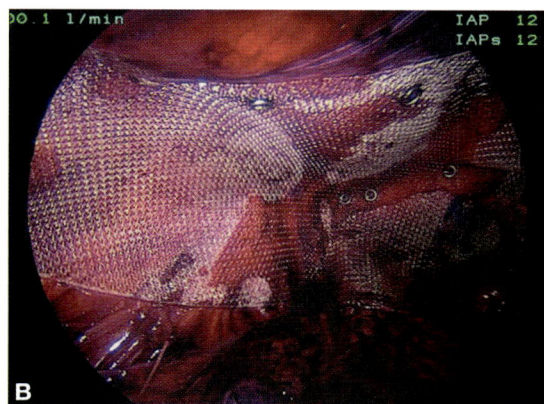

Figure 10-10. A. Anatomy of the inguinal canal, intra-abdominal view. B. Laparoscopic repair using total extra-peritoneal approach. The mesh covers the entire inguinal floor, including the posterior rectus sheath and its insertion on the pubis. (A. Reprinted with permission from Hawn MT, Mulholland MW, eds. *Operative Techniques in Foregut Surgery*. 1st ed. Wolters Kluwer Health; 2015; Figure 34-1; B. From Jones DB, Fischer JE. *Master Techniques in Surgery: Hernia*. Lippincott Williams & Wilkins; 2013.)

Initial pain management strategies include watchful waiting followed by pharmacologic analgesics including nonsteroidal anti-inflammatory drugs (NSAIDs), gabapentinoids, tricyclic antidepressants, and others. If pain continues, local injections are used for diagnostic and therapeutic purposes. Surgery is reserved for refractory cases and includes triple neurectomy and removal of mesh and fixation devices. In cases of post-herniorrhaphy orchialgia, resection of the lamina propria of the vas deferens is additionally required.

Orchitis

Restriction of blood flow to or from the testicle may cause orchitis. This is more common in recurrent hernia repair because the pampiniform venous plexus will have been compromised in these patients because of scarring from prior repair. The patient may present with a swollen and tender testicle; this must be differentiated from the swelling alone that commonly follows MPO hernia repair. Orchitis is generally self-limiting, and NSAIDs should be sufficient treatment. It is uncommon to fully devascularize the testicle because there is collateral circulation from other

arteries. In the long term, however, testicular atrophy can be expected in any testicle with compromised circulation.

Meshoma

A rarer complication of hernia repair includes meshoma formed by shrinkage or folding of the mesh to form a bulky mass. Folded mesh and incorrectly secured mesh may contribute to this complication. Patients may report pain and are at higher risk of hernia recurrence and erosion into adjacent organs due to mesh displacement. Management depends on patient symptomatology and the presence of hernia recurrence or erosion into nearby organs.

Pubic Inguinal Pain Syndrome

There are times when a patient will present with groin pain and no clear hernia on examination. This presentation was first recognized in athletes, causing it to historically be called "*sports hernia*." This term is imprecise and is used to refer to a spectrum of actual pathologic processes including athletic pubalgia, occult true hernias, urologic problems, and more (Table 10-2). Of these, athletic pubalgia is typically

TABLE 10-2. Differential Diagnosis of Inguinodynia

Type	Examples
Sports/work injuries	Adductor muscle strain Inguinal canal disruption Osteitis pubis
Hip joint injuries	Stress fracture Avulsion fracture Degenerative joint disease Labral tear Femoro-acetabular impingement Osteonecrosis
Genitourinary	Round ligament pain Varicocele Prostatitis Orchialgia Urinary tract infection Endometriosis
Gastrointestinal	Intra-abdominal adhesions Inflammatory bowel disease Diverticulitis Irritable bowel syndrome

the most common, representing injury to the muscles or tendons of the muscles and ligaments that insert onto the pubis.

A detailed history will often demonstrate that the patient acutely felt a tear or a strain when lifting, coughing, or participating in sports that require rapid acceleration. Exacerbating factors need to be elicited, such as the complaint of an ongoing pulling or tearing sensation in the groin with activity. In addition, sudden movements such as forceful rotation may exacerbate the pain, whereas rest will mitigate the symptoms, although the pain will return with the resumption of activities. In cases of chronic groin pain, there will often be an evolution of symptoms, typically worsening with ongoing activity. Most importantly, it must be determined whether the patient has ever felt a groin bulge. All patients should be asked about changes in their bowel or bladder habits because associated pelvic floor weakness could cause constipation or urinary frequency.

The examination should begin with the patient in an upright position. If an inguinal hernia is present, it should be easily palpated, especially with a Valsalva maneuver. If no hernia is demonstrated, an examination of the groin is repeated in the supine position. The purpose of this is to isolate and demonstrate the injured muscular or tendon insertion points. To evaluate the adductor longus, the hip should be rotated, flexed, and extended with and without resistance. The patient may have pain with digital pressure on the adductor longus insertion with this maneuver. The insertions of the rectus muscle, transversalis fascia, and aponeurosis of the external oblique onto the pubis should be assessed as well. Palpation of these insertion points during a "sit-up" maneuver may be helpful in identifying the injured structure. On examination of the pubic tubercle, pain upon palpation suggests osteitis pubis as the source.

As discussed previously, radiologic studies rarely play a role in diagnosing a patient with a demonstrable inguinal hernia. An ultrasound may be used in the difficult-to-examine groin to rule out a hernia or testicular pathology. A CT can evaluate other

pathologies of the groin and is less operator dependent than an ultrasound. Magnetic resonance imaging (MRI), however, is the examination of choice when tendon and muscle injuries are suspected in pubic inguinal pain syndrome. MRI can reveal asymmetric development of the muscles or inflammation of the pubic fascia. If osteitis pubis is suspected, a bone scan may be ordered.

When pain in the inguinal region is the major complaint and a symptomatic hernia is not the primary cause, nonsurgical treatment is the best approach. Numerous studies have demonstrated that pain prior to surgery is the greatest predictor of developing chronic, debilitating pain after surgery. The significance of this cannot be overstated. Nonsurgical management is the next best step and includes NSAIDs, limitation of activity, and physical therapy/rehabilitation. Eventual surgical management of a concurrent inguinal hernia in unresolved groin strain is a decision that requires substantial thought by the surgeon, as well as candid discussion with the patient regarding the likelihood of a positive outcome.

OTHER HERNIAS

There are several types of abdominal hernias that do not fit into the broad categories of ventral abdominal wall hernias and hernias of the MPO. Several of these are briefly discussed later, though the management of these hernias is not within the scope of this chapter.

Obturator Hernia

An obturator hernia is the result of a defect in the pelvic floor at the obturator canal, an area inferior to the MPO (Figure 10-11). There is commonly small bowel herniating through the defect, which causes symptoms of impingement of the obturator nerve. Classic presentation is of a thin or emaciated, multiparous woman with crampy abdominal pain and medial thigh pain; thus, this hernia is often nicknamed "the little old lady hernia."

The diagnosis of an obturator hernia is difficult and requires a very high level of suspicion because the hernia is rare and its presentation is intermittent. In the acute setting, the patient may have a severe, concurrent small bowel obstruction. On examination, the patient may have paresthesias or shooting pain on the anteromedial thigh. The pinching of the nerve by the hernia contents is exacerbated by medial rotation of the thigh, a clinical maneuver called the "*Howship-Romberg sign.*" Rarely, the hernia itself can be felt as a tender mass on a rectal examination. Typically, the diagnosis is made by a CT or during surgery for the management of a small bowel obstruction.

With the increasing popularity of minimally invasive hernia repair for MPO hernias, asymptomatic, early obturator hernias are being identified more frequently. However, these are not generally repaired independently, but rather at the time of surgical management of a small bowel obstruction.

Sciatic Hernia

A sciatic hernia is one of the rarest hernias and occurs when visceral contents protrude through the greater or lesser sciatic foramen of the pelvis. They can occur in three different locations: supra-piriformis, infra-piriformis, or spino-tuberous. Symptomatic patients report dull pelvic

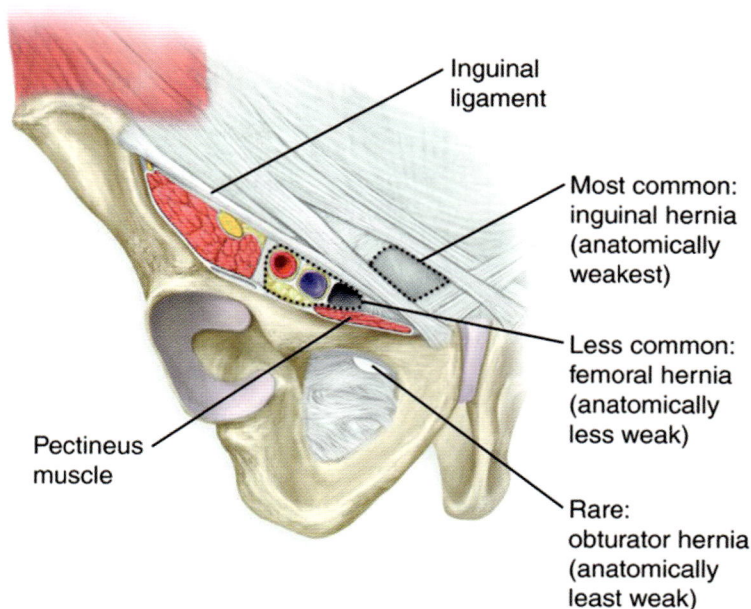

Figure 10-11. Schematic depiction of the relationship of the obturator hernia compared with hernias of the myopectineal orifice. (From Jones DB, Fischer JE. *Master Techniques in Surgery: Hernia*. Lippincott Williams & Wilkins. Copyright © 2013 Lippincott Williams & Wilkins, A Wolters Kluwer business.)

pressure radiating to the gluteal muscles or posterior thigh. If the sciatic nerve is compressed, they may also report sharp shooting pain down the posterior thigh and leg. Sciatic hernias can be palpated as a reducible mass deep to the gluteus muscle, which protrudes with cough. Rectal and vaginal examination can aid in diagnosis. However, CT with rectal contrast and excretory urography can diagnose hernias containing colon or ureters, respectively.

Flank Hernia

Flank hernias occur when intra-abdominal contents protrude through a defect in the flank muscles lateral to the semilunar line. They can be congenital, incisional, or traumatic. Congenital flank hernias include lumbar hernias, in which contents herniate through the superior or inferior lumbar triangles. Given their location near bony prominences and major neurovascular structures, management and mesh placement for the repair of flank hernias can be challenging.

Perineal Hernia

Perineal hernias occur from a pelvic floor defect anterior or posterior to the superficial transverse perineal muscles. Primary and secondary hernias can occur. Primary perineal hernias often occur due to increased intra-abdominal pressure from constipation or pregnancy. Postoperative complications after pelvic surgery (abdominoperineal resection, pelvic exenteration, and coccyx or distal sacrum resection) may result in secondary perineal hernias. Symptoms typically present as pain exacerbated by standing up. Patients may report difficulty urinating or defecating. Perineal hernias may be palpated on bimanual rectovaginal examination, however, are typically diagnosed with pelvic ultrasound or CT. Difficulty with urination and defecation and skin erosion typically require repair.

CONCLUSION

Hernia anatomy, no matter the site, is complex and can be confusing. The most important principles in this chapter relate to the identification of hernias that require surgical attention for elective or emergent repair, the understanding of how to improve patient risk factors prior to surgery, and the complications that can occur postoperatively. These concepts will be clearest with a good understanding of the anatomy and the principles guiding best practices for repair.

SUGGESTED READINGS

American College of Surgeons. ACS surgical risk calculator. Accessed May, 2018. http://riskcalculator.facs.org/RiskCalculator/.

Augenstein VA, Colavita PD, Wormer BA, et al. CeDAR: Carolinas equation for determining associated risks. *J Am Coll Surg*. 2015;221(4):S65-S66.

Daes J, Felix E. Critical view of the myopectineal orifice. *Ann Surg*. 2017;266(1):e1-e2. doi:10.1097/SLA.0000000000002104

Ellatar O, Choi HR, Dills VD, et al. Groin injuries (athletic pubalgia) and return to play. *Sports Health*. 2016;8(4):313-323.

Fitzgibbons RJ, Giobbie-Harder A, Gibbs JO, et al. Watchful waiting vs repair of inguinal hernia in minimally symptomatic men: a randomized clinical trial. *JAMA*. 2006;295(3):285-292. doi:10.1001/jama.295.3.285

Guidelines. EHS: European Hernia Society. Accessed March 8, 2024. https://europeanherniasociety.eu/category/guidelines/

HerniaSurge Group. International guidelines for groin hernia management. *Hernia*. 2018;22(1):1-165.

Novitsky YW, Elliott HL, Orenstein SB, Rosen MJ. Transversus abdominis muscle release: a novel approach to posterior component separation during complex abdominal wall reconstruction. *Am J Surg*. 2012;204(5):709-716. doi:10.1016/j.amjsurg.2012.02.008

SAMPLE QUESTIONS

QUESTIONS

Choose the best answer for each question.

1. A 57-year-old male construction worker presents to the office with a complaint of a bulge in his midline abdominal wall. He first noticed it about 2 years after he underwent an uncomplicated open splenectomy following a fall at work. He reports that the bulge has been getting larger, and he will have occasional slight pain at the site with heavy lifting. He was diagnosed with diabetes mellitus 2 weeks ago and started to take an oral hypoglycemic agent last week. He is a current smoker and obese. Physical examination confirms an easily reducible incisional hernia with a palpable defect of 6 cm. What is the next best step in his care?

   A. CT of the abdomen and pelvis for operative planning
   B. Optimizing modifiable risk factors to reduce postoperative complications
   C. Elective open hernia repair with biologic mesh
   D. Emergent open hernia repair due to the risk of strangulation
   E. TAP block to alleviate the patient's discomfort

2. A 42-year-old female presents to the office with a complaint of a bulge in her upper midline abdominal wall. Her medical history consists of spontaneous vaginal delivery of full-term triplets. She reports that the bulge has become more prominent since recovering from the birth of her children, but she otherwise has no complaints. Physical examination reveals an otherwise thin woman with a midline abdominal bulge on Valsalva and laterally displaced rectus muscles, but there is no visible or palpable mass or hernia defect. In addition to ordering a CT of the abdomen and pelvis for confirmation, how should this patient best be counseled?

   A. Reassure her that as you cannot feel the defect, it must be small, and watchful waiting is appropriate.
   B. Inform her that you are concerned about the presence of Spigelian hernia.
   C. Reassure her that her condition is not a true abdominal wall defect and requires no intervention.
   D. Inform her that you will need to optimize her risk factors prior to hernia repair.
   E. Ask her to take time off from work to minimize her chances of incarceration.

3. A 27-year-old man presents to the emergency department for severe abdominal pain located at his umbilicus over the last 4 hours. He reports having a bulge at his umbilicus for 3 years, which would "come and go," but is now "stuck." His temperature is 101.7 °F, his heart rate is 115 beats/min, and his blood pressure is 143/92 mm Hg. His physical examination reveals a softly distended abdomen with severe tenderness to palpation at a 5-cm bulge

effacing the umbilicus. The skin overlying the bulge has a purple discoloration. His white blood cell (WBC) count and lactate are elevated. What is the next best step in his management?

   A. Admit the patient to the hospital for observation.
   B. Administer narcotics for pain control and acetaminophen for fever.
   C. Plan for elective hernia repair with biologic mesh.
   D. Administer sedation for manual hernia reduction.
   E. Transfer the patient to the operating room for emergent exploration.

4. A 65-year-old woman presents to the clinic with a complaint of a bulge in her left lower quadrant. She reports that she has some mild, persistent discomfort at the site. She has a history of end colostomy for perforated diverticulitis, which was reversed 5 years ago. Physical examination reveals an incarcerated hernia underlying her stoma site scar with a palpable defect of 2 cm. The patient reports she would prefer to not have another surgery. What is important for her to understand regarding a nonoperative approach in her case?

   A. She is at a higher risk for infection because this is the site of a prior stoma.
   B. She is at a higher risk for complications because the hernia is incarcerated.
   C. She is at a higher risk for complications because the hernia is not on the midline.
   D. She is at a higher risk for the hernia enlarging because it is not on the midline.
   E. She is at a higher risk for strangulation because of her age.

5. A 39-year-old man presents to the office for consultation regarding the repair of his incisional hernia. The hernia occurred after an exploratory laparotomy following a motor vehicle collision and is increasingly painful with activity. His past medical history consists of well-controlled asthma requiring a rescue inhaler once a month and diabetes mellitus with a recent hemoglobin A_{1c} of 6.5%. He is sedentary and enjoys playing video games. Physical examination reveals a body mass index of 44.2 kg/m^2 and a periumbilical midline bulge that is reducible. Which of this patient's factors predict a higher risk of hernia recurrence after repair?

   A. Prior surgery due to trauma
   B. Increased coughing due to asthma
   C. Presence of diabetes mellitus
   D. Low activity level
   E. Morbid obesity

ANSWERS AND EXPLANATIONS

1. **Answer: B**

   Prehabilitation and reduction of modifiable risk factors are critical in planning for the repair of asymptomatic or minimally symptomatic hernias. For this patient, weight management will reduce morbidity and the risk of recurrence, smoking cessation will assist wound healing, and his hemoglobin A_{1c} must be less than 8 prior to elective repair of his hernia. CT is not necessary in this first-time hernia. There are no issues of contamination to suggest that biologic mesh should be used. Emergent repair is not necessary for a reducible hernia. TAP block is used for pain control in the postoperative setting. For more information on this topic, please see section "Patient Factors."

2. **Answer: C**

This woman has rectus diastasis, as shown by the physical examination finding of a midline bulge with lateral displacement of the rectus muscles and the absence of a hernia defect. She was at risk for this condition because of her prior pregnancy. Rectus diastasis is not a condition requiring surgical repair, and therefore, she can be reassured and does not require optimization of risk factors. Also, because diastasis has no true defect of the abdominal wall, there is no chance of incarceration. Small hernia defects are at a higher risk of complications, and watchful waiting may not be appropriate. Although a Spigelian hernia would not have a palpable defect, it is located off the midline. For more information on this topic, please see section "Main Hernia Types."

3. **Answer: E**

This patient has an acutely incarcerated hernia. However, his fever, tachycardia, skin discoloration, elevated WBC count, and lactate are extremely concerning for strangulation of hernia contents. Therefore, he requires emergent operative intervention, and the hernia should not be reduced for fear of reducing ischemic or necrotic tissue back into the abdomen. Observation is appropriate after the manual reduction of an acutely incarcerated hernia in a non-ill-appearing patient. Symptomatic control with acetaminophen and narcotics will not resolve the primary issue, and strangulation of the contents prevents the consideration of elective hernia repair. For more information on this topic, please see section "Clinical Presentation."

4. **Answer: B**

This woman has an incisional hernia, which has all the same risk factors as any other hernia of the main abdominal wall. The patient's age and the hernia location off the midline do not impart any increased risks. The increased risk of infection is present only with active (current) contamination, not a history of bowel spillage from the stoma at the site. The fact that the hernia is incarcerated means it is at higher risk for bowel obstruction or strangulation than a reducible hernia. The patient must understand her increased risk in order to proceed with observation. For more information on this topic, please see section "Clinical Considerations" under the heading "Abdominal Wall Hernias."

5. **Answer: E**

Modifiable risk factors must be minimized prior to elective hernia repair. However, both this patient's asthma and diabetes are very well controlled, and improvement is unlikely to be made. Low activity level will reduce, not increase, his risk of recurrence. The reason for his prior surgery, a traumatic injury, does not affect recurrence risk. Morbid obesity, on the contrary, is the largest risk factor affecting the recurrence rate after hernia repair. For more information on this topic, please see section "Patient Factors."

11

Esophagus

Emily Speer, James N. Lau, and James A. McCoy

The esophagus connects the oropharynx to the stomach. The complex anatomy and physiology of the esophagus belie its simple function as a conduit for passage of oral contents into the stomach. Regardless of the medical specialty chosen, the future physician will likely encounter a clinical situation where knowledge of esophageal diseases will prove useful. Although this chapter covers various topics on esophageal disease, the medical student should focus on the workup and management of three commonly encountered esophageal diseases: gastroesophageal reflux disease (GERD), esophageal carcinoma, and esophageal perforation.

ANATOMY

General Anatomy

The esophagus, a muscular alimentary tube of approximately 25 cm length, connects the pharynx to the stomach. The esophagus starts at the level of the cricoid cartilage (level of the 6th cervical vertebra) and ends just below the diaphragm (level of the 11th thoracic vertebra). It can be subdivided into four segments, the cervical esophagus (3-5 cm long), the proximal and middle thoracic esophagus (18-22 cm long), and the distal abdominal esophagus (3-6 cm long). For endoscopic mapping purposes, the esophagus starts at around 15 cm from the incisors and ends at about 40 cm from the incisors. It traverses the thorax in the posterior mediastinum. Structures closely associated with the esophagus include the trachea and left atrium (both anterior to the esophagus) and the descending thoracic aorta. The aorta travels along the left of the esophagus and then swings posterior to the esophagus as it passes through the diaphragm (Figure 11-1). Because the aorta runs along the left side of the esophagus, most surgical approaches to the esophagus are performed through a right thoracotomy (Figure 11-2).

Three anatomic areas of esophageal narrowing are of clinical significance, because ingested foreign bodies often lodge there and food impaction can occur there. They include the proximal esophagus at the level of the cricopharyngeus muscle, the midesophagus at the level of the aortic arch, and a distal narrowing at the level of the diaphragm (Figure 11-3). There are two functional sphincters in the esophagus: an upper esophageal sphincter (UES), at the level of the cricopharyngeus muscle, and a lower esophageal sphincter (LES), between the esophagus and the stomach.

Arterial Supply

The cervical esophagus is supplied by the inferior thyroid artery from the thyrocervical trunk artery. The thoracic esophagus is supplied by the bronchial arteries and smaller esophageal arteries from the thoracic aorta. The distal esophagus is supplied by branches of the left gastric artery (Figure 11-4).

Venous Drainage

The cervical esophagus drains mainly through the inferior thyroid vein. The thoracic esophagus drains mainly through the azygos vein and hemiazygos vein. The distal esophagus is drained through the coronary and left gastric vein, which drain into the portal venous system (Figure 11-5). In liver cirrhosis with portal vein hypertension, the lower esophageal venous plexus provides collateral drainage from the portal venous system to the azygos veins, leading to esophageal varices.

Lymphatic Drainage

Lymphatics from the cervical esophagus drain into the deep cervical (jugular) lymph nodes. The thoracic esophagus drains into lymph nodes found in the posterior mediastinum, such as the paratracheal and pulmonary hilar lymph nodes. The distal esophagus drains into the celiac, left gastric, and parahiatal lymph nodes (Figure 11-6). In esophageal carcinoma, initial lymph node spread is determined by the location of the tumor.

Innervation

Innervation of the esophagus is based on the autonomic nervous system with sympathetic and parasympathetic fibers exerting opposing effects. The proximal esophagus receives its nerve fibers through the recurrent laryngeal nerves of the vagus nerve and cervical sympathetic chain. Damage to the recurrent nerve disrupts not only the vocal cords but also the swallowing mechanism of the upper esophagus, increasing the risk of aspiration. The mid- and distal esophagus receives autonomic innervations from the vagus and thoracic sympathetic chain. An intramural nerve plexus of sympathetic and parasympathetic fibers is located in the muscularis propria, between the circular and longitudinal muscle layers (myenteric plexus). The myenteric plexus controls peristaltic activity of the esophagus and, when damaged, can lead to achalasia (failure of the LES muscle to relax along with esophageal body aperistalsis). Afferent visceral pain fibers of the esophagus travel via sympathetic fibers to the upper thoracic spinal cord, sharing a similar pathway with cardiac sensory fibers. As a result, pain from the heart (angina) can resemble esophageal pain (spasm, acid reflux). The motor innervation of the esophagus is supplied through the vagus.

Histology

The esophageal wall consists of four main layers: (1) mucosa (containing a layer of superficial and deep mucosa), (2) submucosa, (3) muscularis propria (made up of two layers, an inner circular layer and an outer longitudinal layer), and (4) adventitia (paraesophageal tissue). The esophagus does not have a serosal layer, unlike most of the gastrointestinal (GI) tract. On endoscopic ultrasound (EUS) imaging, the esophagus is seen as five discrete boundaries, correlating to the two layers of the mucosa: (1) superficial mucosa and

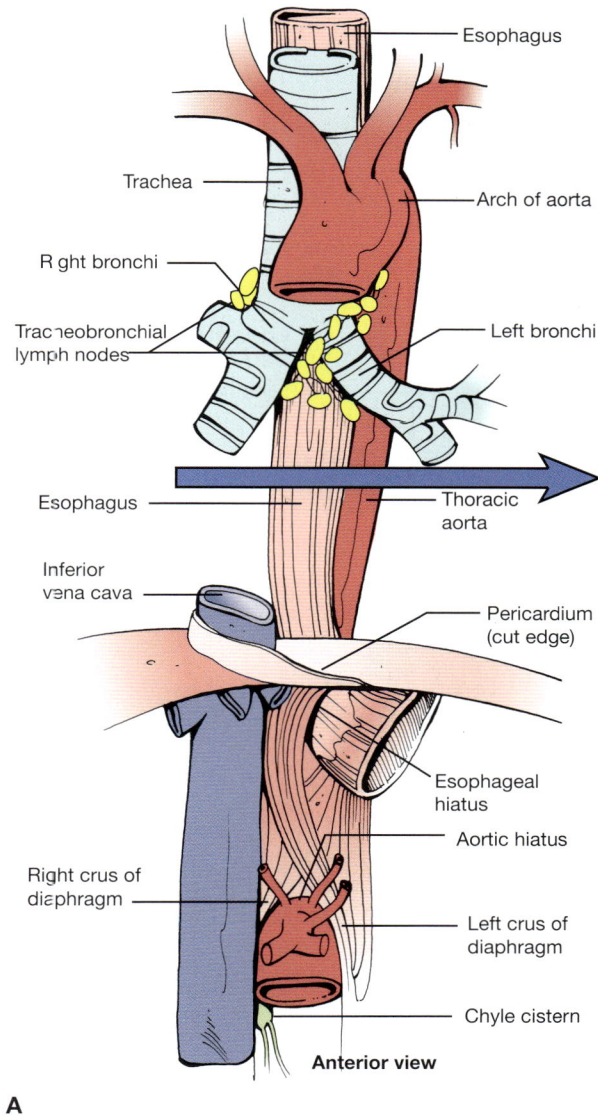

CT Scan Cross-Section

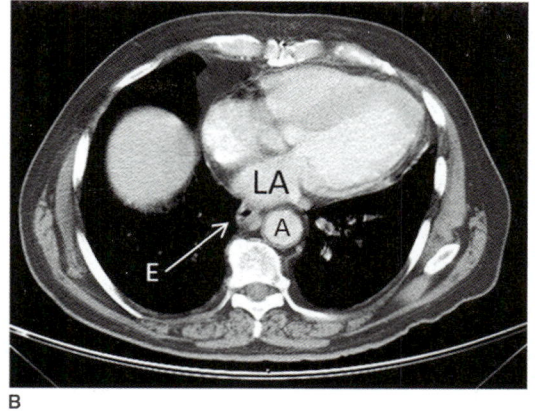

B

Figure 11-1. A. Anterior view with the lung and the heart removed to expose the posterior mediastinum where the esophagus and the aorta run (arrow indicates cross-section imaging in B). B. Computed tomography (CT) scan shows a cross-sectional cut at the shown level with the aorta (A) on the left and the arrow indicates the heart anterior of the esophagus (E). LA, left atrium. (A. Reprinted with permission from Fischer JE, Jones DB, Pomposelli FB, et al. *Fischer's Mastery of Surgery.* 6th ed. Lippincott Williams & Wilkins; 2012:793.)

(2) deep mucosa, (3) submucosa, (4) muscularis propria, and (5) adventitia (Figure 11-7). The muscularis propria layer of the esophagus transitions from striated muscle fibers (proximal 1/3) to smooth muscle fibers (distal 2/3). The entire length of the esophagus is normally lined with nonkeratinizing stratified squamous epithelium, whereas the immediately downstream proximal stomach is lined with gastric oxyntic mucosa. In GERD, there is abnormal reflux of gastric contents into the distal esophagus, which can lead to abnormal transformation of normal squamous epithelial cells into metaplastic intestinal columnar cells (Barrett esophagus) (Figure 11-8).

PHYSIOLOGY

At rest, most of the esophagus is in a relaxed state, except for the UES and LES where resting pressures are high (30-120 mm Hg for the UES and 15-30 mm Hg for the

LES). The resting high pressure of the LES helps prevent reflux and regurgitation of digestive material backup into the stomach. The swallowing mechanism is voluntarily initiated from the nucleus ambiguous (located in the medulla). When the swallowing mechanism is initiated, there is temporary relaxation of the UES, allowing the food to enter the upper esophagus. The bolus is propelled down the esophagus by a primary peristaltic wave. The LES relaxes in anticipation of the food bolus, allowing the food to enter the stomach. After passage of the bolus, the LES returns to its normal high resting pressure, preventing reflux of stomach contents.

Normally, swallowing a bolus of food causes a primary peristaltic wave. Secondary peristaltic waves are not part of the normal swallowing mechanism but occur with esophageal dilatation or irritation, or if there is obstruction that prevents bolus progression. It is believed to represent a "backup" clearing process of residual material in the

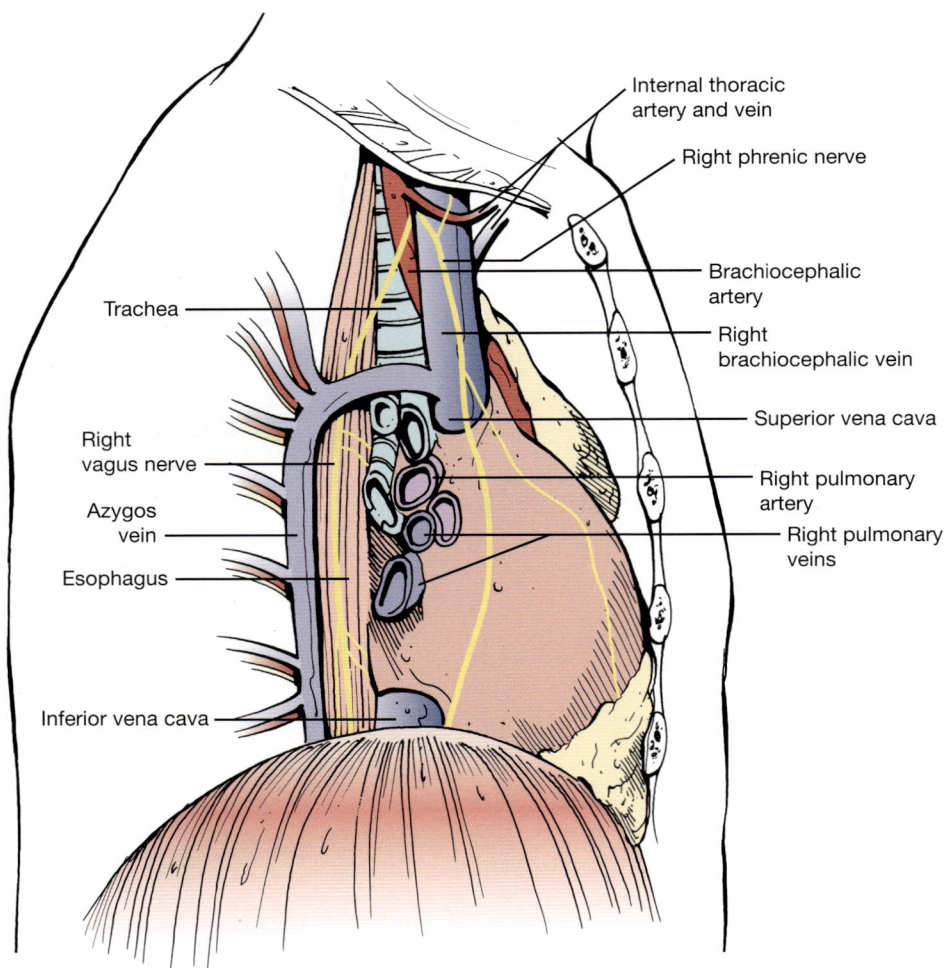

Figure 11-2. Esophageal anatomy from a surgeon's perspective. Through a right thoracotomy, most of the thoracic esophagus is accessible. As a result, proximal and mid-thoracic esophageal lesions are best approached through the right chest. (Reprinted with permission from Fischer JE, Jones DB, Pomposelli FB, et al. *Fischer's Mastery of Surgery.* 6th ed. Lippincott Williams & Wilkins; 2012:793.)

esophagus after the swallowing process. Tertiary waves are abnormal, nonpropulsive "fibrillation" of the esophagus. Figure 11-9 shows the typical peristaltic activity initiated by the swallow mechanism and the method of intraluminal manometry to record this process.

ESOPHAGEAL DISORDERS: CLINICAL PRESENTATION AND SIGNS

Detecting esophageal disorders requires meticulous attention to the symptoms described by the patient because they may be manifestations of disease in other organ systems (eg, angina pectoris or asthma) or signs of a systemic problem (eg, collagen vascular or neurologic disorders). To better assess the patient, the student should become familiar with several terms.

Difficulty with the transition of ingested substances from the mouth to the stomach is called "*dysphagia*." The patient usually complains that food becomes "stuck" and is often able to define the point of obstruction. Dysphagia

can occur with both liquids and solids, and pain is usually not a component of the process. Odynophagia is painful swallowing. It can be caused by esophageal infection (eg, *Candida* esophagitis, cytomegalovirus, or herpesvirus infection), a foreign body in the esophagus, or injury to the esophagus. Globus hystericus is a "lump in the throat"; these patients must be evaluated carefully because the sensation may represent a mass lesion and not a psychological symptom.

Heartburn is a burning sensation that rises up into the chest or throat. Reflux or regurgitation is a sensation of fluid or liquid form the stomach coming up into the throat. Both are symptoms of GERD, but they do not necessarily secure the diagnosis of true GERD, because they can also be associated with achalasia, functional heartburn (hypersensitive esophagus), and esophageal strictures. In exploring the diagnosis of GERD, it is best to allow patients to describe their symptom complex in their own words. Heartburn that spontaneously disappears over a period of months without therapy may be a sign of a severe disease process (eg, esophageal stricture or carcinoma).

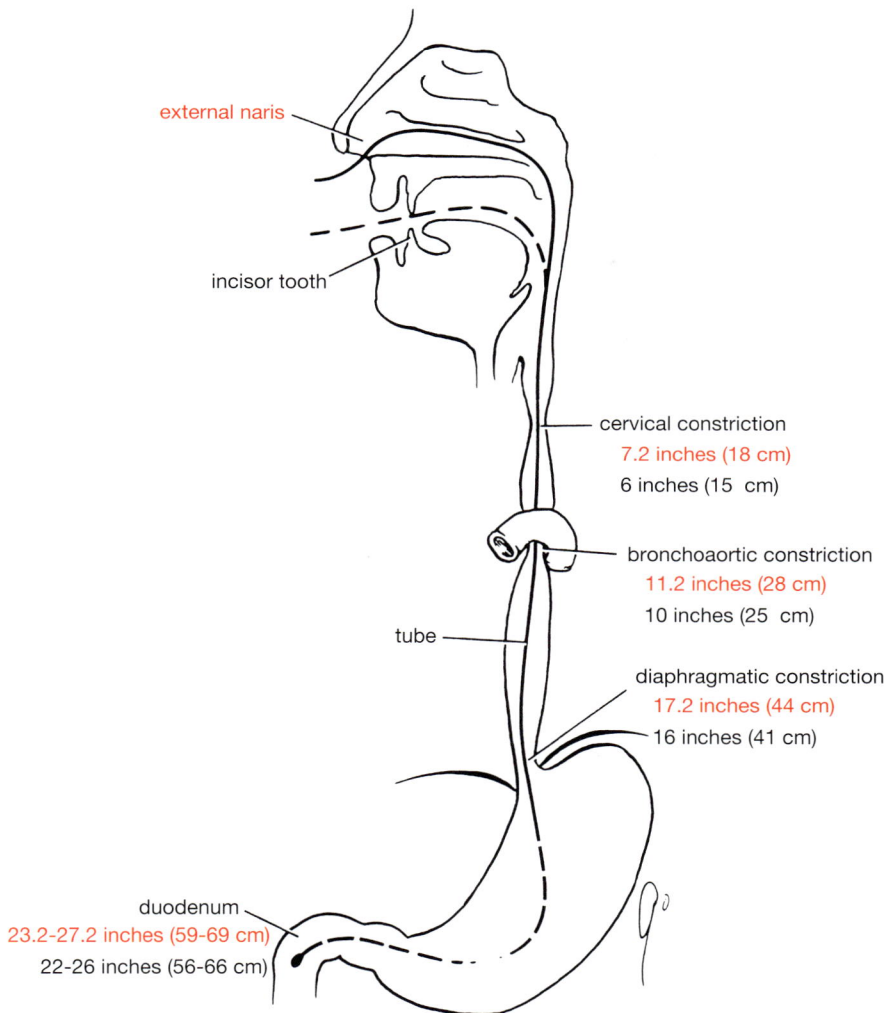

Figure 11-3. **Three areas of normally occurring esophageal constriction where foreign bodies and food impaction have a tendency to become lodged.** (Reprinted with permission from Snell R. *Clinical Anatomy*. 10th ed. Lippincott Williams & Wilkins; 2019.)

Recurrent episodes of bronchitis or pneumonia, particularly in the very young and the older patients, may be signs of recurrent aspiration of esophageal or gastric contents because of esophageal obstruction, congenital malformation, diverticula, large hiatal hernias, or esophageal motility disorders. Esophageal disease must also be considered in the differential diagnosis of anemia and bleeding. Ulcerative esophagitis is the most common cause of esophageal bleeding and usually causes occult blood in the stool.

Hiccup, or singultus, is a sign of diaphragmatic irritation and may indicate a diaphragmatic hernia, acute gastric dilation, or subendocardial myocardial infarction.

Esophageal disease may cause signs and symptoms that are often indistinguishable from those of angina pectoris because of the common sensory pathway of the esophageal and cardiac sympathetic nerves. Some historical features may help differentiate between the two disease processes. Symptoms related to the esophagus are typically aggravated by changes in body position, particularly bending over. The symptoms are relieved by belching and only marginally relieved by nitroglycerin (although it can significantly relieve symptoms of spastic esophageal disorders such as distal esophageal spasm). In any case, cardiac and esophageal evaluation must proceed simultaneously because myocardial ischemia and esophagitis are both common diseases.

DIAGNOSTIC EVALUATION OF THE ESOPHAGUS

Barium Esophagography

In most cases, a contrast esophagram is the first study obtained for the workup of esophageal dysphagia, regurgitation, or heartburn. The patient swallows barium plus or minus a 13-mm barium tablet, while monitored with real-time video, to grossly assess esophageal motility and to look for hiatal hernias, diverticula, or obstruction. When

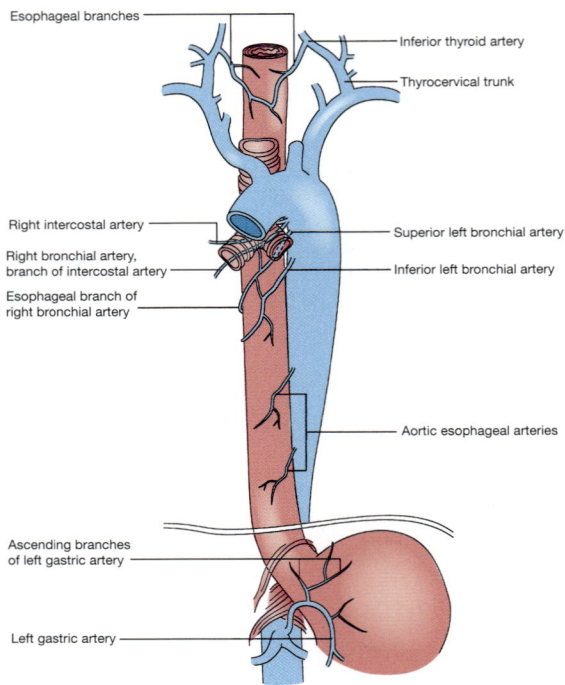

Figure 11-4. Arterial supply to the esophagus. The thoracic esophagus is supplied by multiple small branches arising from the descending thoracic aorta. Because of the small size of these arterial vessels, blunt and "blind" dissection of the esophagus is possible without the risk for severe bleeding. (Reprinted with permission from Mulholland MW. *Greenfield's Surgery*. 6th ed. Lippincott Williams & Wilkins; 2016.)

a hiatal hernia is suspected, video recording is performed in various positions to increase intra-abdominal pressures, maximizing the yield for identifying the presence of the hernia. Barium study also provides a good visualization of any esophageal structural disease. Because of its general availability and usefulness in identifying motility and structural disorders, the esophagram is the preferred initial study.

Esophageal Manometry

Esophageal manometry allows for direct, simultaneous measurement of intraluminal pressures at multiple levels. Manometry study is used to assess the function of both the UES and the LES, and it also identifies esophageal body contraction abnormalities seen in esophageal motility disorders. Esophageal manometry is performed by nasally inserting a tube containing multiple levels of solid state pressure transducers into the esophageal lumen. Peristaltic wave activity and sphincter function are studied by measuring intraluminal pressure along the esophagus during "wet" swallows with water and "viscous" swallows with a thicker solution (see Figure 11-9). Manometry is indicated in the workup of achalasia, esophageal spasm, and GERD.

Esophageal pH Monitoring

The monitoring of distal esophageal pH is the gold standard for securing the diagnosis of GERD. This is

performed in a 24-hour outpatient study, where a pH probe sensor is inserted via a nasal catheter to the level just above the LES. The patient is then encouraged to go through a "normal day," with routine meals and activities, while both proximal and distal esophageal pH are monitored continuously (Figure 11-10). Using these nasal catheter probes (called *pH/impedance probes*), both acid and nonacid reflux can be measured. Wireless technology has made pH probe transducers (inserted endoscopically) more tolerable for patients. Because of the greater comfort, these wireless pH probes can be left in longer (allowing for studies of up to 48-96 hours), increasing the yield for detecting acid reflux. However, nonacid reflux cannot currently be measured using these devices. In addition, acid exposure can be measured only in the location of the esophagus in which the device is implanted (whereas the nasal catheter probes can measure reflux exposure in the proximal and distal esophagus simultaneously). Proton pump inhibitors (PPIs) and H_2-blockers are discontinued for approximately 7 days before a pH study for GERD is performed.

The 24-hour pH study is used to collect six measures of abnormal pH (<4) exposure in the distal esophagus: (1) percentage of total time with pH less than 4, (2) percentage of upright time with pH less than 4, (3) percentage of supine time with pH less than 4.0, (4) number of episodes with pH less than 4, (5) number of episodes more than 5 minutes with pH less than 4, and (6) longest episode (in minutes) with pH less than 4. The patient's results are compared with those of normal subjects, and a composite score is calculated on the basis of "normal" mean and the standard deviation values of these measures. This composite score is commonly known as the *DeMeester score*. A DeMeester score greater than 14.72 is believed to be very specific in identifying the patient who would benefit from antireflux surgery.

Imaging Studies

Compared with other available studies, computed tomography (CT) and magnetic resonance imaging (MRI) provide limited additional information when assessing for esophageal disease. Esophagram, endoscopy, and EUS provide superior local structural evaluation of the esophagus. However, CT and MRI can provide a useful assessment of distant metastasis in esophageal carcinoma, especially when combined with positron emission tomography (PET) scanning (an important step in the staging of esophageal cancer). CT and MRI can provide some information regarding disease involvement of surrounding structures, such as the aorta, trachea, and lymph nodes. It should be emphasized that apparent involvement of these structures on CT scan does not alone exclude surgical resectability, because it is difficult to differentiate between inflammatory changes and direct carcinomatous invasion. The CT scan with on-table contrast swallow is useful in the workup of suspected esophageal perforation, as is a standard chest x-ray showing a left-sided pleural effusion.

Upper Endoscopy

Direct endoscopic examination of the esophagus is mandatory for all esophageal diseases. It has a role in the diagnosis and treatment of various esophageal diseases. Endoscopy allows for direct visualization of any pathology, and it provides access for biopsies. Through endoscopy, the physician

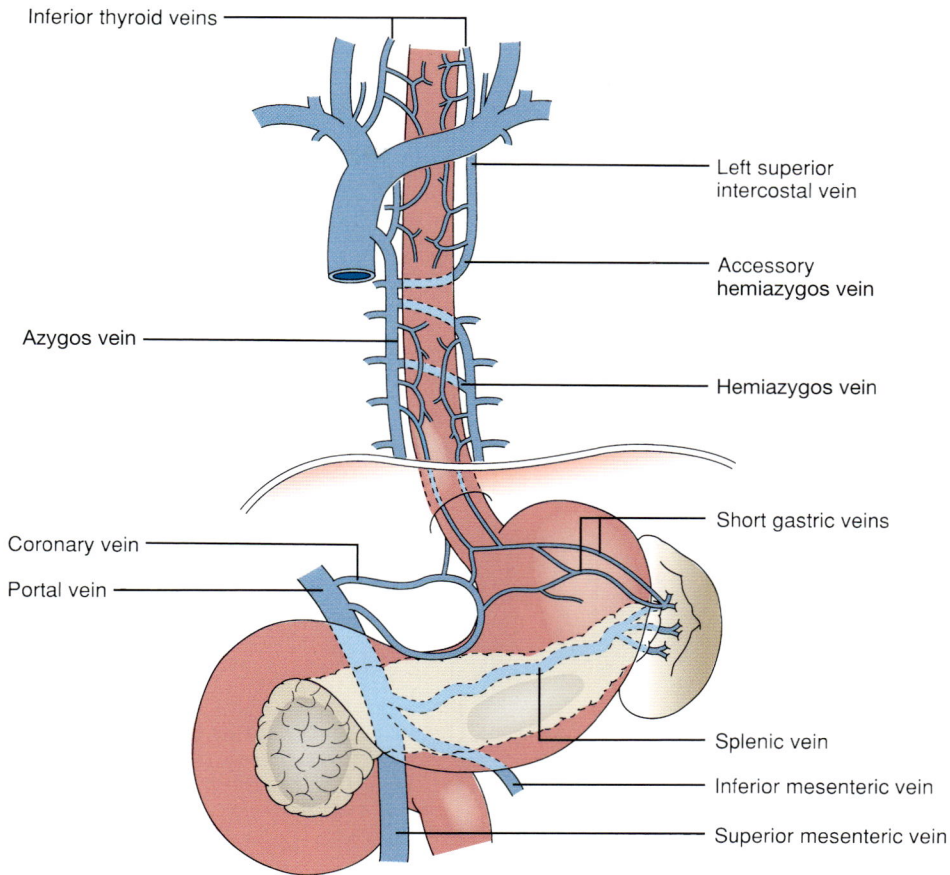

Figure 11-5. Venous drainage of the esophagus. Most of the drainage occurs through the azygos vein system, which communicates with the portal venous system via the coronary and short gastric veins. In portal vein hypertension, these collaterals enlarge and can lead to esophageal varices. (Reprinted with permission from Mulholland MW. *Greenfield's Surgery*. 6th ed. Lippincott Williams & Wilkins; 2016.)

can perform dilatations of strictures and inject pharmacologic agents to treat varices and LES disorders. When esophageal diverticular disease is suspected, or in severe caustic esophageal injury, endoscopy is performed with caution, because there is increased risk for perforation. In GERD, endoscopic examination is used to evaluate the extent of reflux esophagitis, look for the presence of Barrett esophagus and/or dysplasia, delineate the anatomy of hernias, and much more. Advanced endoscopy techniques can now also be used to perform incisionless surgeries, such as endoscopic cricopharyngeal myotomy for Zenker diverticuli and per oral endoscopic myotomy (POEM) for achalasia.

Endoscopic Ultrasound

EUS of the esophagus is used to obtain detailed imaging of esophageal wall and adjacent lymph node pathology. To perform EUS, an ultrasound probe is introduced endoscopically to the area of interest. Detailed imaging of the esophageal wall is seen as five discrete layers, and any adjacent lymph nodes can also be visualized for guided biopsy. EUS is used in the staging workup of esophageal cancer. With EUS, tumor depth and invasion can be evaluated for

T staging, and abnormal lymph nodes can be located for fine-needle aspiration N staging (Figure 11-11). EUS is also useful in identifying other intramural lesions, such as leiomyomas.

ESOPHAGEAL DISEASES

GERD and esophageal carcinoma are the most frequently encountered esophageal diseases. A thorough fund of knowledge in these two esophageal entities forms the essential basis for this chapter. In addition, esophageal perforation is commonly referred to the surgeon as an emergency consultation, and a thorough understanding on the workup and management of it will complete the basic foundation for managing esophageal disease. Because of their significance, these three esophageal disorders are presented first, whereas other less commonly encountered diseases are added at the end for completeness. The common surgical procedures of the esophagus are described within each of these clinical scenarios, but the surgical approach and techniques can be applied to almost any esophageal pathology.

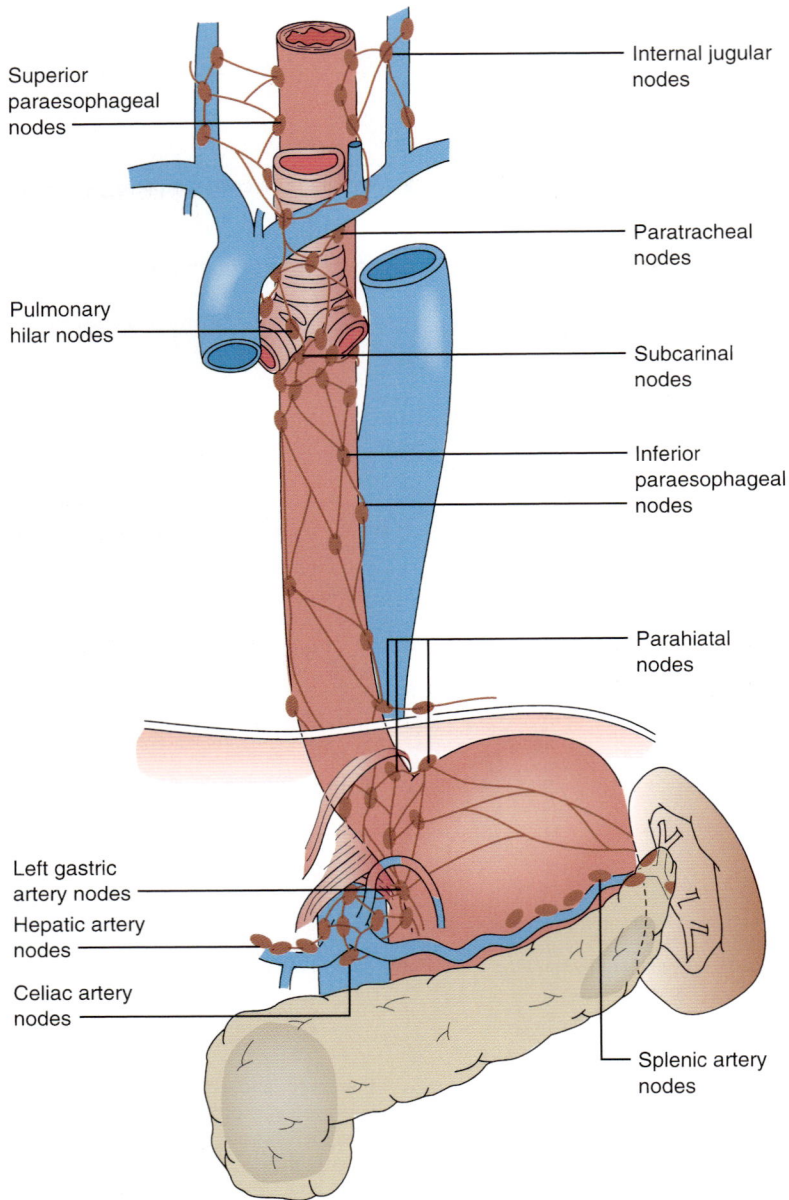

Figure 11-6. Lymphatic drainage of the esophagus. Lymphatic drainage and tumor spread from distal esophageal cancer occur to the inferior paraesophageal and celiac lymph nodes, whereas the proximal/midesophageal cancers spread to superior paraesophageal, paratracheal, and internal jugular lymph nodes. (Reprinted with permission from Mulholland MW. *Greenfield's Surgery*. 6th ed. Lippincott Williams & Wilkins; 2016.)

Gastroesophageal Reflux Disease

Gastroesophageal reflux is the backward flow of gastric contents into the distal esophagus, past the LES. Occasional reflux of gastric contents into the distal esophagus is seen as a "physiologically normal" process, which makes the distinction between "normal" and "pathologic" GERD difficult to define. GERD is caused primarily by an incompetent LES. LES competence depends on total sphincter length, resting pressure, and intra-abdominal length. Poor LES function is commonly caused by prolapse into the chest, as in a hiatal hernia, increased intragastric pressures, food- or drug-induced LES relaxation, or esophageal motility disorders. Although GERD is frequently associated with a hiatal hernia, not all patients with GERD have a hiatal hernia (numbers vary between 50% and 90%), and not all patients with hiatal hernia have GERD (numbers vary between 13% and 84%).

GERD symptoms can be classified into two subtypes: typical and atypical. The typical symptoms of GERD are heartburn and regurgitation. These symptoms (along with a positive response to antireflux medications) are the

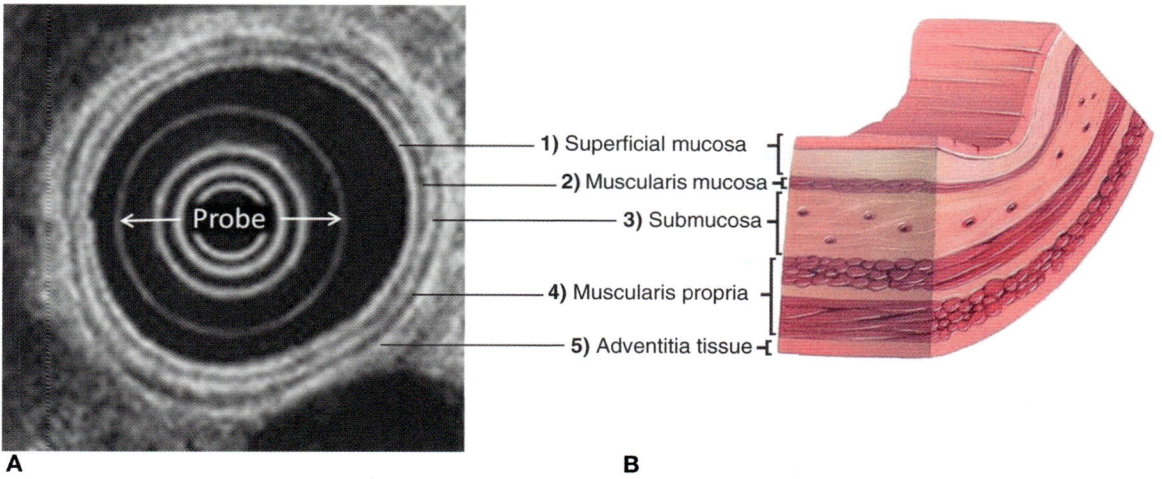

Figure 11-7. A. Endoscopic ultrasound (EUS) of the esophagus. B. The five histologic layers of the esophagus correlating with those seen on the ultrasound. EUS provides an accurate picture of the depth of tumor wall invasion, an important step in staging esophageal cancers.

Gastroesophageal junction   Endoscopy

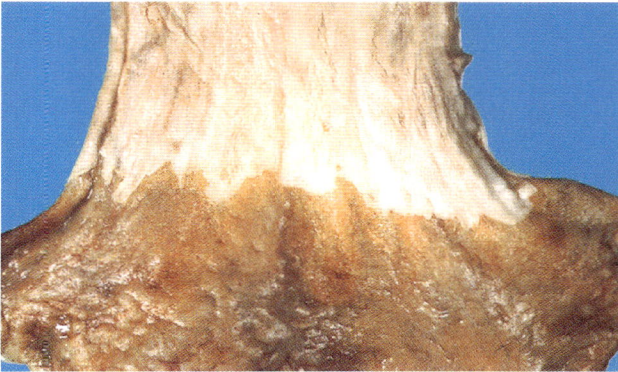

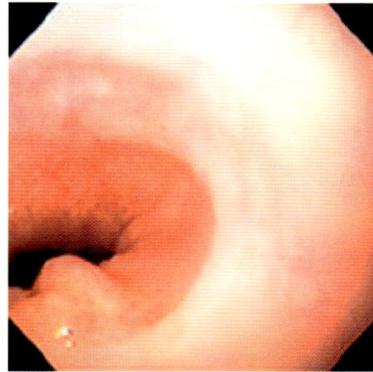

Normal

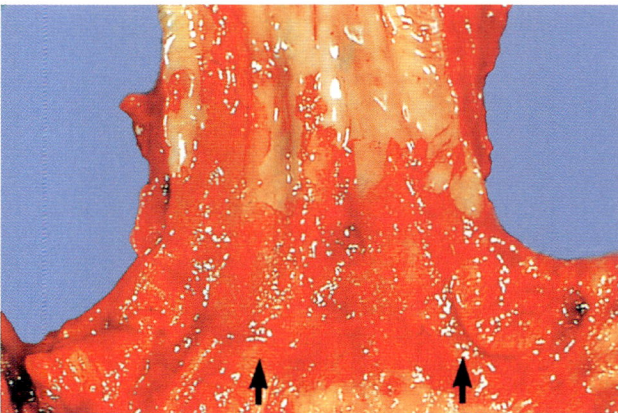

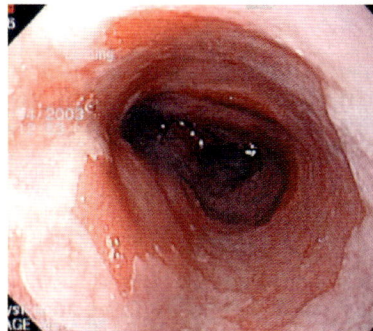

Barrett

Figure 11-8. Photographs showing the normal demarcated squamocolumnar junction of the gastroesophageal junction when compared with the abnormal Barrett columnar cell esophagitis (seen in gastroesophageal reflux disease). A and B. The anatomic and endoscopic appearance of a normal demarcated squamocolumnar junction. C and D. Barrett esophagus, where "tongues" of abnormal pink columnar cells are seen invading into the whitish normal squamous tissue zone. Arrows show the "Barrett esophagus" findings. (A-D. Reprinted with permission from Mulholland MW. *Greenfield's Surgery*. 6th ed. Lippincott Williams & Wilkins; 2016.)

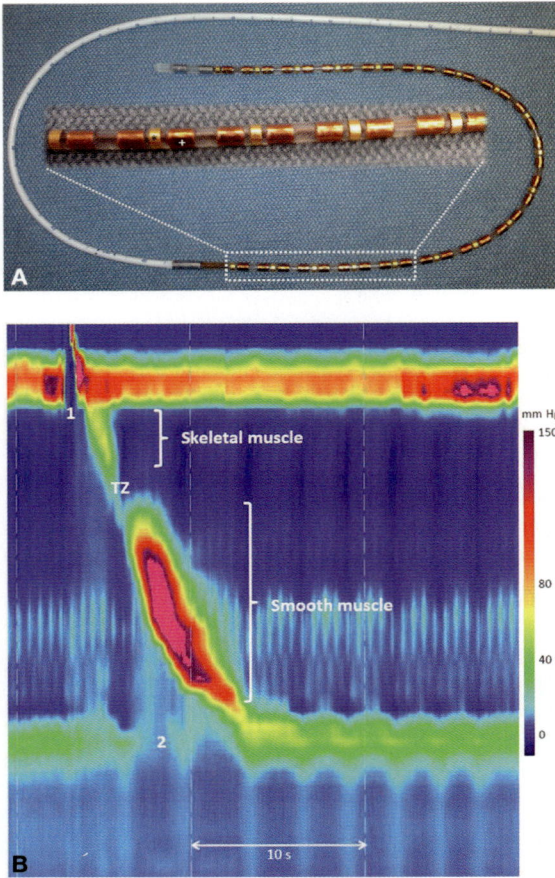

Figure 11-9. The technique for recording esophageal peristaltic activity. A. A catheter with multilevel pressure transducers is inserted into the esophagus to temporally measure intraluminal pressures during swallows. B. Actual recordings of esophageal activity at different levels during dry swallow. (Reprinted with permission from Swanstrom LL, Soper NJ. *Mastery of Endoscopic and Laparoscopic Surgery.* 4th ed. Lippincott Williams & Wilkins; 2013; Figures 7-6 and 7-8.)

strongest predictors of good response to antireflux surgery in patients with abnormal pH/impedance results. Atypical symptoms of GERD (such as cough, hoarseness, chest pain, and asthma) respond less reliably to antireflux surgery. Regardless, it is important to note that the diagnosis of GERD cannot be secured with symptoms alone, because patients with typical symptoms do not always have true GERD. Late complications of GERD include stricture of the distal esophagus (peptic stricture) and intestinal metaplasia of the distal esophageal mucosa (Barrett esophagus). The concern with Barrett esophagus is its predisposition to the development of dysplasia, which can lead to malignant transformation of the distal esophagus. Dysplasia can be either low grade or high grade, based on histologic analysis. Current recommendations for managing patients with Barrett esophagus associated with low-grade dysplasia include routine follow-up endoscopy every 6 to 12 months with four-quadrant biopsies every 1 to 2 cm of involved esophagus. Management of high-grade dysplasia is evolving and can involve anything from endoscopic therapy to esophagectomy. Barrett esophagus with high-grade dysplasia should be managed by an esophageal specialist.

Diagnosis

Aggressive workup of GERD is usually reserved for when surgical intervention is being considered, or if late complications are present, such as stricture or Barrett esophagus. The workup for GERD should include (1) esophageal pH study, (2) barium swallow, and (3) upper endoscopy. Esophageal manometry is often done to exclude esophageal motility disorders and to tailor the choice of antireflux surgery. Gastric emptying studies can also be obtained in patients with bloating, nausea, or vomiting symptoms to rule out gastric emptying disorders. Appropriate preoperative workup is essential to ensure the best chances for surgical success.

Medical Treatment

Currently, the initial therapies for GERD should include behavioral modifications and the use of PPIs. Behavioral modifications include avoiding eating late at night, sleeping at an incline, and avoiding agents that relax the LES (such as alcohol or peppermint) (Table 11-1). PPIs have been found to successfully control symptoms in the majority of patients with GERD (>90% success) For patients who fail nonoperative management or desire to avoid the potentially negative side effects of PPIs (decreased bone mineral density, *Clostridium difficile* colitis, kidney issues), surgical intervention is a good option. The development of "less invasive" laparoscopic procedures for GERD has reduced the threshold for surgical intervention.

Surgical Treatment

Unlike medications, antireflux surgery addresses the underlying anatomic cause of GERD by augmenting a weak LES and mitigating the reflux of gastric contents up into the esophagus. Predictors of successful response to surgery include (1) a positive pH test, (2) the presence of typical reflux symptoms, and (3) symptomatic relief with PPIs. Although fundoplication may reverse or prevent dysplastic progression of small areas of Barrett esophagus in many patients, there is currently no evidence that it prevents the development of esophageal adenocarcinoma. The principles of antireflux surgery include (1) restoration of a 2- to 3-cm intra-abdominal segment of esophagus, (2) closure of the diaphragm, and (3) reinforcement of the LES, usually with a fundoplication. The purpose of the fundoplication wrap is to accentuate or recreate the gastroesophageal flap mechanism (where distension of the stomach fundus leads to external compression of the LES, reinforcing its closure, mimicking the esophageal clasp fibers). Numerous antireflux procedures have been described: the Nissen, Belsey, Hill, Dor, and Toupet procedures. These procedures can be categorized into complete or partial stomach wraps and transabdominal versus thoracic surgical approaches (Table 11-2).

Currently, the Nissen fundoplication is the most commonly performed antireflux procedure. It is usually performed through a transabdominal approach and consists of a complete (360°) fundoplication wrap, whereas other fundoplications are considered partial wraps (Figure 11-12).

Some surgeons believe there is less postoperative dysphagia and gas bloat after a partial wrap, whereas other surgeons believe there is a lower recurrence rate of GERD after a complete wrap. In the end, if the principles of antireflux surgery are followed (restoration of the intra-abdominal esophageal length, closure of the diaphragmatic

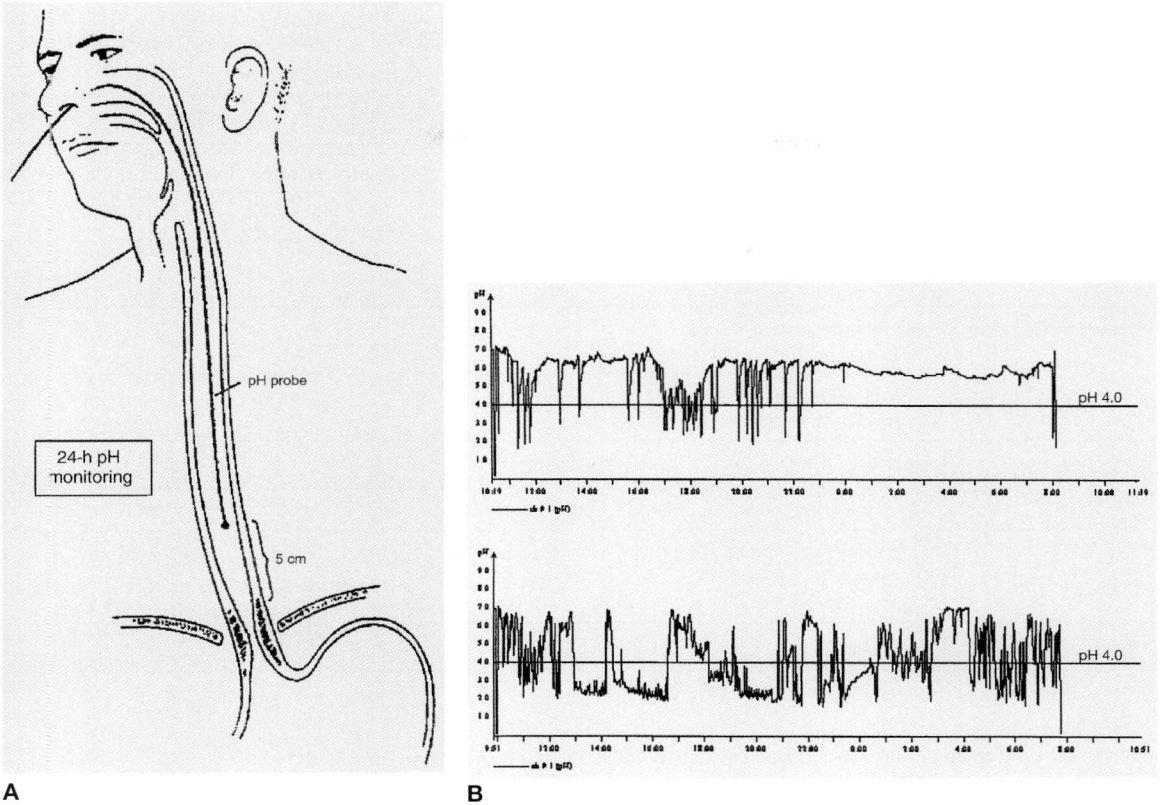

Figure 11-10. A 24-hour pH monitoring study. A. A pH electrode is inserted nasally and positioned 5 cm above the lower esophageal sphincter. B. pH tracings in patients with abnormal acid reflux. In the upper tracing, short episodes of pH less than 4.0 (line) suggest defective lower esophageal function. In the lower tracing, the episodes of pH less than 4.0 (line) are prolonged, suggesting poor esophageal clearance of acid reflux. (Reprinted from Shields TW, Lociciero J, Reed CE, Feins RH. *General Thoracic Surgery*. 7th ed. Lippincott Williams & Wilkins; 2009:1713, 1709. With permission.)

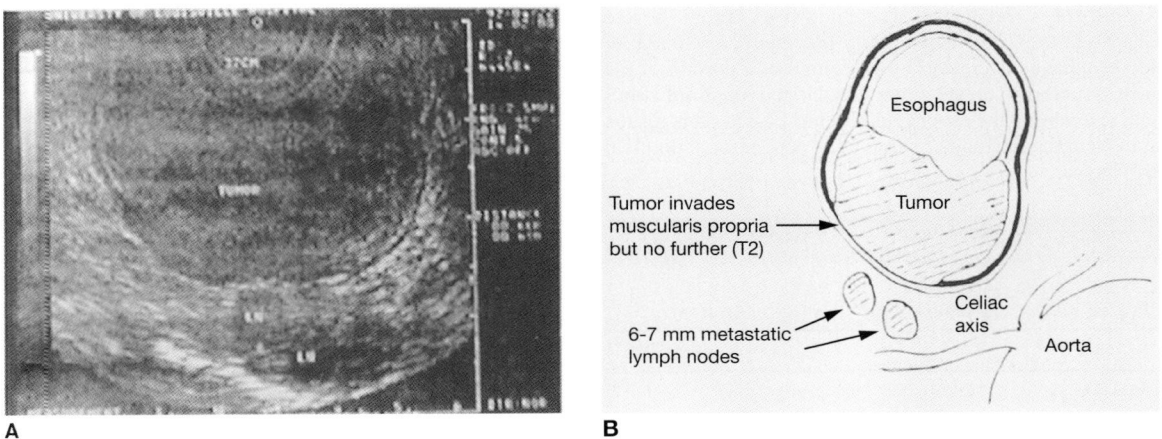

Figure 11-11. Endoscopic ultrasound (EUS) is the most accurate means to determine the depth of tumor invasion in the esophageal wall. A. Example of an actual ultrasound image of esophageal tumor. B. Correlating schematic drawing. Tumor depth invasion (T staging) has strong prognostic implications in the treatment and outcome of esophageal cancer (see Table 11-3 for staging details). EUS is also valuable in identifying and guiding fine-needle aspiration of suspicious paraesophageal lymph nodes. (Reprinted with permission from Shields TW, Lociciero J, Reed CE, Feins RH. *General Thoracic Surgery*. 7th ed. Lippincott Williams & Wilkins; 2009:1713-1999.)

TABLE 11-1. Behavioral Modifications for Treating GERD

	Modification	LES Competency	Gastric Pressure and Emptying	Mucosal Irritant
Dietary behavior	Eat small meals.		+	
Dietary content	Avoid acidic foods.			+
	Avoid fatty meals.	+	+	
	Avoid caffeine, chocolate.	+		
Postural modification	Elevate the head of the bed.		+	
	Avoid lying down after meals.		+	
Social habits	Avoid smoking.	+		+
	Avoid alcohol.	+	+	+
Medications	Avoid anticholinergics, calcium, β-blockers, xanthines, and aspirin.	+	+	+
Obesity	Lose weight.		+	

GERD, gastroesophageal reflux disease; LES, lower esophageal sphincter.

defect, and reinforcement of the LES), excellent results have been reported for the various antireflux procedures (success rates of >90%). Mortality should be less than 1%. Newer antireflux procedures are based on these same principles and differ mainly on the surgical approach (laparoscopic vs robotic vs endoscopic) and the type of LES reinforcement employed (magnetic sphincter augmentation devices, radiofrequency ablation, bulking agents, etc). The Collis gastroplasty procedure (also known as a "*wedge fundectomy*") is used in combination with a fundoplication when there is esophageal shortening from chronic severe GERD. In the Collis gastroplasty procedure, a segment of neo-esophagus is created by wedging out a portion of the gastric fundus to create a new tubularized length of stomach, resembling the esophagus (Figure 11-13). This results in the lengthening and creation of a "neo" intra-abdominal esophagus.

TABLE 11-2. Antireflux Procedures

Procedure	Degree of Stomach Wrap	Surgical Approach
Nissen	360	Abdominal or thoracic
Belsey-Mark	240	Thoracic
Toupet	Posterior 270	Abdominal
Dor	Anterior 180	Abdominal
Hill	0[a]	Abdominal

[a]Although the Hill procedure does not attempt to wrap the stomach around the distal esophagus, it still follows the key principle of reinforcing the lower esophageal sphincter by accentuating the gastroesophageal flap valve.

Esophageal Carcinoma

Between 1987 and 2007, the incidence and mortality rate for esophageal cancer have remained constant despite significant shifts in histologic type in the United States. Incidence per year has remained around 4 to 5 per 100,000, with mortality rate being similar at 4 to 5 per 100,000. Overall survival for patients diagnosed with esophageal cancer remains dismal at around 20% for 5 years, mainly because of advanced disease at the time of diagnosis. There are two histologic types of esophageal cancer, squamous cell carcinoma (SCC) and adenocarcinoma. Although both types of esophageal carcinoma carry a poor prognosis and are managed similarly, their etiology, epidemiology, and anatomic characteristics are different enough to warrant distinction between the two.

Until recently, SCC was the most common type of esophageal cancer seen in North America and Europe (recently, adenocarcinoma has surpassed SCC in prevalence). There is a higher incidence of SCC seen in African Americans and males (near 4:1 ratio). SCC is seen mainly in the mid- to proximal segment of the esophagus but can also involve the distal segment. There has been a strong association between alcohol and tobacco consumption with SCC. Other factors believed to increase risk for SCC include a high dietary intake of nitrosamine, dietary deficiencies in vitamins and minerals (including Plummer-Vinson syndrome), genetic predisposition (tylosis), achalasia, and a history of caustic injury to the esophagus.

Adenocarcinoma has surpassed SCC as the most common esophageal cancer type encountered in North America and Europe. Its incidence in the Western world has increased 4-fold over the past two decades. The prevalence

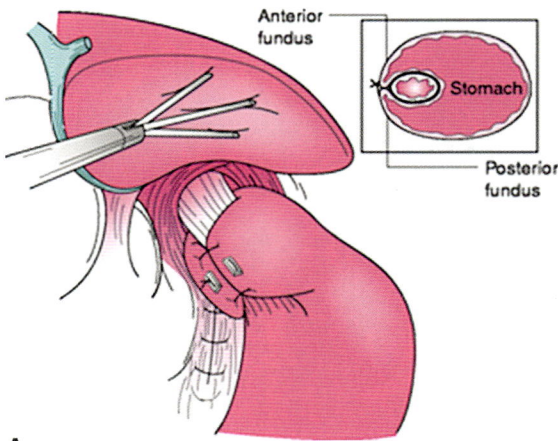

A

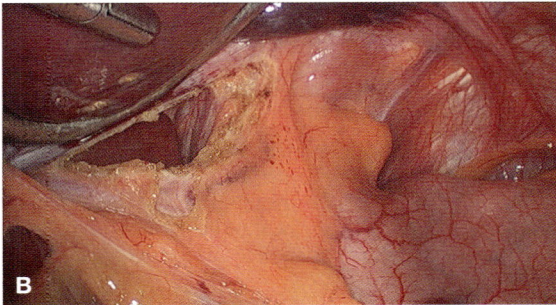

B

Figure 11-12. A. The Nissen fundoplication procedure is a full 360° wrap. The gastroesophageal flap is recreated where a portion of the fundus overlaps the distal esophagus to provide external compression support of competency for the distal esophagus. B. Endoscopic picture of fundoplication. (A. Reprinted with permission from Mulholland MW, Lillemoe KD, Doherty GM, et al. *Greenfield's Surgery*. 4th ed. Lippincott Williams & Wilkins; 2006. B. Reprinted with permission from Luketich JD. *Master Techniques in Surgery: Esophageal Surgery*. 1st ed. Wolters Kluwer Health; 2014.)

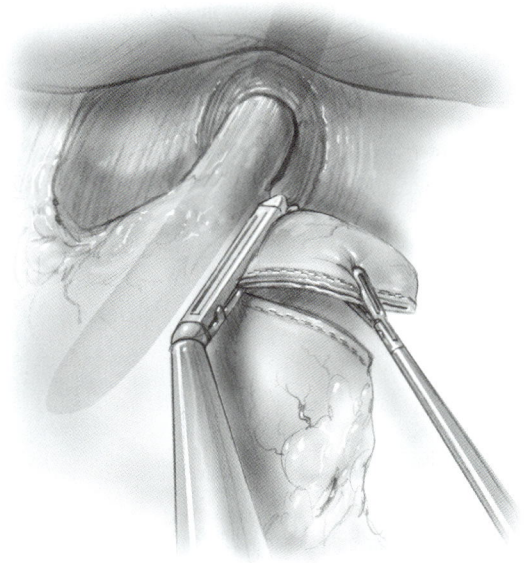

Figure 11-13. **When the esophagus is shortened and retracted into the chest from chronic gastroesophageal reflux disease, the Collis gastroplasty procedure is used to recreate a distal "esophageal" tube from the stomach.** The shortened esophagus is lengthened 5 cm by stapling the fundus into a tube of "neo" esophagus. (Reprinted with permission from Swanstrom LL, Soper NJ. *Mastery of Endoscopic and Laparoscopic Surgery*. 4th ed. Wolters Kluwer; 2013.)

of adenocarcinoma is higher in Whites than in African Americans. It involves the distal esophagus and is associated with Barrett esophagus from GERD. Although the association between adenocarcinoma and Barrett disease is not disputed, the role for PPI and antireflux procedures as a means to slow or reverse Barrett disease (thereby reducing the risk for developing adenocarcinoma) remains controversial.

Diagnosis

Because of the increased prevalence of adenocarcinoma in the West, the clinical presentation and history for esophageal carcinoma have changed. Both types of esophageal cancer usually present with dysphagia to solid food and weight loss, but with adenocarcinoma, a history of reflux disease is frequently associated. On presentation, the patients with adenocarcinoma are usually healthier, with less advanced disease, especially if they have been undergoing surveillance endoscopy of Barrett disease. Patients with

SCC usually present with more advanced disease, greater weight loss, and a history of smoking and alcohol misuse.

Workup for esophageal cancer is mainly intended to confirm the diagnosis and stage the cancer. Initial diagnostic study is frequently the barium swallow to evaluate the cause of dysphagia. Barium swallow is the first study performed and will typically demonstrate stricture with irregular filling defect (Figure 11-14).

CT scan can be useful in defining the extent of the tumor and abnormal-appearing lymph nodes. However, CT scan alone is not enough to prove tumor invasion of adjacent structures, because distinction between local inflammatory reaction and tumor invasion is not possible. Endoscopic evaluation is mandatory for histologic confirmation of esophageal cancer. In patients with Barrett dysplasia, endoscopic surveillance with routine biopsies helps identify early malignant changes. EUS is performed to define the depth of tumor invasion and in assisting with localizing adjacent suspicious lymph nodes for fine-needle aspiration. In tumors involving the proximal and midesophagus, bronchoscopy is performed to rule out tracheobronchial involvement. The combination of CT scan and PET scan is helpful in identifying distant metastasis. Other than lymph nodes, the distant organs most commonly involved with metastatic disease are the liver and the lungs.

Staging

Once diagnostic studies are completed, the esophageal cancer can be staged using the current 2017 TNM (tumor, node, metastasis) staging definitions from the American Joint Committee on Cancer. In the most recent update on

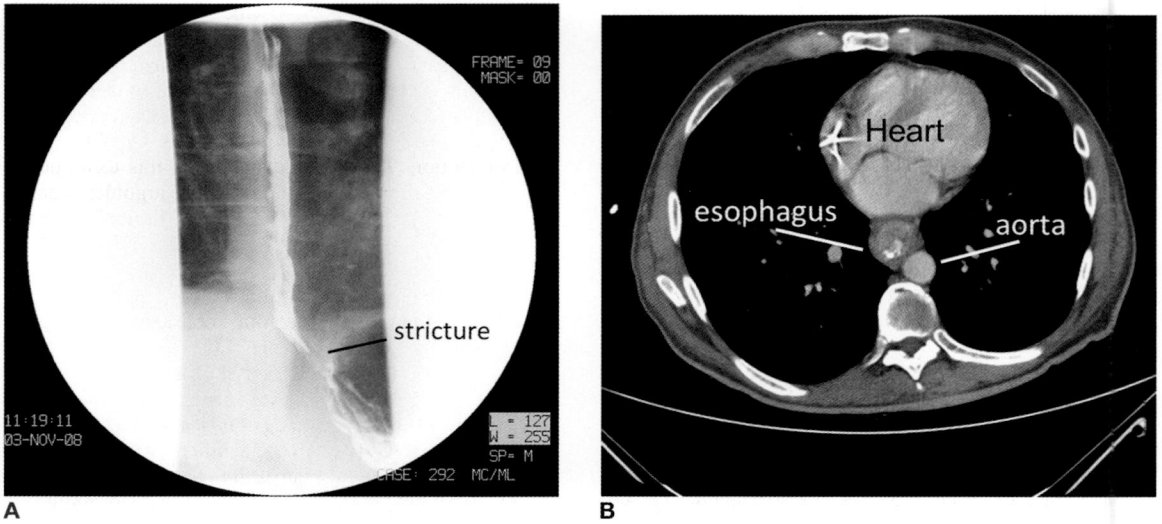

Figure 11-14. Barium swallow (A) and corresponding computed tomography scan cut demonstrating a distal esophageal cancer (B).

esophageal cancer staging, squamous cell and adenocarcinoma are graded differently, with tumor location used only for the staging of SCC. Remembering the TNM criteria for each stage is difficult, but a useful guideline to remember is the distinction between early (≤stage IIa) from more advanced stages of esophageal cancer. For stages IIa or earlier, there is limited local tumor invasion and no lymph node involvement, with no metastasis. A more detailed description of early-stage esophageal cancer is shown in Table 11-3.

The distinction between early stages (I and IIa) and more advanced stages (IIb and IV) is useful, because current 5-year survival is 50% or greater for the early stages when compared with less than 30% for advanced stages.

Surgical Treatment

Surgical resection remains the best chance for the cure of esophageal cancer. Despite significant improvements in surgical morbidity and mortality, long-term outcome after attempted curative resection remains poor, with most series reporting an overall 5-year survival rate of 20%. Only in the early stages (contained tumor with no lymph node involvement, or tumors that show complete regression after preoperative chemoradiation) has there been a significant long-term survival of more than 50%.

Surgical treatment of esophageal carcinoma is based upon the principle of complete local resection of the tumor with reconstruction of the alimentary tract by using another segment of the GI tract. Variations on the procedure depend upon what segment of the GI tract is used for esophageal reconstruction and the surgical approach used for resecting the tumor.

Esophageal Substitutes

Esophageal substitutes that have been used for reconstruction include the stomach, colon, and jejunum. Which of these is used depends upon availability, location of the resected esophageal segment, and surgeon preference. Surgeons who have an interest in performing esophagectomies should be familiar with more than one technique, because options may be limited by the clinical history (prior gastrectomy, vascular disease, etc).

The stomach is the most frequently used conduit in esophagectomies. The advantage of using the stomach includes its rich vascular supply, ease of surgical mobilization as a vascularized pedicle, and the need to create fewer GI anastomoses. When used as a conduit, the left gastric and the short gastric arteries are divided, allowing the fundus to be mobilized into the chest or neck. The stomach is then left with blood flow coming from the right

TABLE 11-3. Criteria for Early Stage (≤IIa) of Esophageal Cancer					
	T	**N**	**M**	**G**	**Location**
Adenocarcinoma stage ≤IIa	≤T2	N0	M0	Any	Not applicable
Squamous cell carcinoma stage ≤IIa	T1	N0	M0	Any	Any
	T2-T3	N0	M0	G1	Any
	T2-T3	N0	M0	G2-G3	Lower

G, grade; M, metastasis; N, node; T, tumor.

gastric and gastroduodenal arteries. Because the vagus is divided during esophageal resection, a pyloromyotomy is often performed to facilitate gastric emptying. The drawbacks of using the stomach as a conduit include the risk of ischemia in the fundus because of dependent collateral flow and postoperative gastroesophageal reflux symptoms after destruction of the LES mechanisms. Reflux appears to be more common when an intrathoracic gastroesophageal anastomosis is used, when compared with a cervical anastomosis.

The left colon can also be used as an esophageal substitute, and it is the next most frequently used after the stomach. Some surgeons prefer using the left colon to the stomach because of its longer available length, favorable vascular anatomy, and close size match with the esophagus. The left colon is used in an isoperistaltic manner, with a vascular pedicle dependent upon the left colic artery branch of the inferior mesenteric artery. When compared with the stomach, the colon has the advantage of a longer and more relaxed reach to the cervical esophagus. The colon is also more resistant to acid reflux. The disadvantages of using the colon include the need to perform two additional anastomoses and the greater technical experience needed in assessing and mobilizing the colon vasculature. Preoperative colonoscopy and visceral angiography is required to verify the absence of pathology and adequate blood supply to the colon.

There are two ways of routing the colon interposition graft. The preferred route is through the resected esophageal space in the posterior mediastinum. An alternate route is through the retrosternum, which is used if the posterior mediastinal space is not available because of extensive disease or scarring, or if the diseased esophagus cannot be safely removed. The retrosternal route is not optimal because of a more circuitous route, increasing the risk of obstruction because of kinking of the conduit, especially at the thoracic inlet.

The jejunum is rarely used as an esophageal substitute. It is occasionally used as a free graft, especially when a short segment of the cervical esophagus is resected. The jejunal free graft is placed as an interposition graft between the esophageal ends, with its vascular supply reconstructed through microvascular anastomosis of the jejunal vessels to the neck vessels. A pedicled jejunal graft for extensive esophageal reconstruction is difficult to create because of its unfavorable vascular anatomy. Jejunal reconstruction via a Roux-en-Y connection (see Chapter 12 for description) can be used when total gastrectomy is combined with distal esophagectomy.

Surgical Procedures

Surgical resection of the esophagus can be performed by either a thoracotomy or a transhiatal approach. Both frequently require a concomitant incision through either an abdominal incision or a cervical incision, or both. Each technique has its proponents, claiming advantages in operative mortality, postoperative morbidity, and cancer survival. The thoracotomy approach for esophageal resection has been the historical standard, with proponents claiming a cleaner and visually direct resection of the tumor. However, because a thoracotomy is often associated with a higher morbidity than an abdominal incision, the transhiatal approach was introduced. This approach, which

avoids a thoracotomy, may provide significant advantages in certain clinical scenarios, such as in some patients with poor pulmonary function, or those who have had previous major thoracic procedures. A transhiatal esophagectomy is performed via a cervical and abdominal incision, with the esophagus and the tumor removed partly by blunt, blind hand dissection. The main advantage of this technique is avoidance of a thoracotomy incision. The argument against transhiatal esophagectomy is the risk of limited access to uncontrolled bleeding and the limited resection of large tumors involving the surrounding esophageal tissue. Although there have been multiple retrospective studies supporting either the thoracotomy or transhiatal surgical approach (with respect to cancer survival and perioperative complications), the surgeon should be familiar with both surgical techniques. Tumor location, clinical history, or patient functional status may enhance the theoretical advantages of one approach over the other.

Three main surgical approaches have been described in performing a thoracotomy. The most common approach is via the right thorax combined with an abdominal incision (Ivor Lewis). In an Ivor Lewis approach, the gastroesophageal anastomosis is located in the right chest (Figure 11-15). For tumors involving the proximal and midesophagus, a three-incision (abdominal, right thoracotomy, and cervical) approach has been described (McKeown). The McKeown procedure is similar to the Ivor Lewis approach, other than the addition of the third cervical incision and a cervical gastroesophageal anastomosis. The potential advantages of the McKeown procedure include wider surgical margins due to more extensive proximal resection of the esophagus and construction of a cervical anastomosis, where the consequences of a possible anastomotic leak are less severe than an intrathoracic anastomotic leak. For a distal esophageal tumor extending into the stomach with extensive local disease, a left thoracoabdominal incision has been advocated by some, through which an extensive "en bloc" resection can be performed with the theoretical benefit of a cleaner oncologic resection.

To avoid the morbidity of performing a thoracotomy, a transhiatal approach for esophageal resection has been proposed. The operation consists of two incisions: an abdominal incision and a cervical incision. The stomach and lower esophagus are mobilized via the abdomen, and a cervical incision is used to mobilize the upper esophagus. Part of the removal of the midesophagus is performed by a blunt, blind hand dissection (Figure 11-16). The fundus of the stomach is mobilized to the neck for a cervical anastomosis. Arguments for a transhiatal approach include avoidance of a painful thoracotomy incision, reduced lung trauma from mechanical retraction, and avoidance of an intrathoracic anastomosis. Concerns with using the transhiatal approach include a limited resection of large tumors (especially those involving the midesophagus), greater potential for local tumor spillage from blunt dissection, and the greater stretch of the stomach to reach the neck. The extra distance required for the stomach to reach the neck can contribute to an increased risk for anastomotic failure because of tension and ischemia. The transhiatal approach seems to be ideally suited for local limited disease involving the distal esophagus, as commonly seen with malignant transformation of Barrett disease.

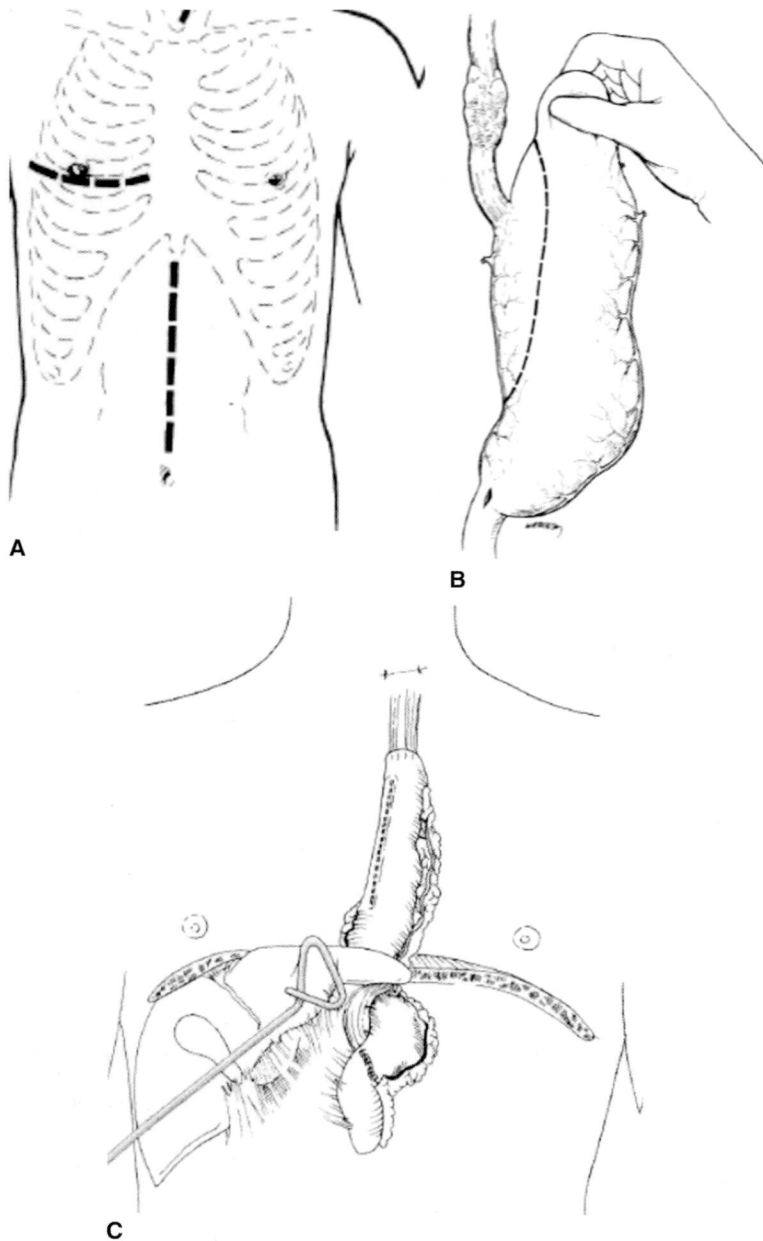

Figure 11-15. A. In the Ivor Lewis approach for esophageal resection, two separate incisions are made. B. The initial abdominal incision is used to mobilize the esophageal replacement conduit (usually the stomach) into the right chest. C. A second incision is made into the right chest, to complete the resection of the distal esophagus and to reestablish gastrointestinal continuity by anastomosing the stomach to the proximal esophagus. (Reprinted with permission from Kaiser LR, Kron IL, Spray TL. *Mastery of Cardiothoracic Surgery.* 2nd ed. Lippincott Williams & Wilkins; 2007:145, 143, 161. With permission.)

Again, it should be emphasized that despite strong proponents for each of the abovementioned approaches, there is no definitive study demonstrating a clear advantage of one technique over the other. Understanding of the theoretical benefit and drawbacks of each technique, and the familiarity of using more than one surgical approach, would allow the surgeon to map a treatment course best serving the individual patient.

More recently, the advent of laparoscopic techniques for esophageal resection has started to provide an alternate approach to patients with resectable esophageal cancer. The laparoscopic equivalent of the thoracotomy and transhiatal esophagectomies has been described with similar long-term cancer survival outcomes, but with reduced surgical morbidity due to less invasive incisions. There

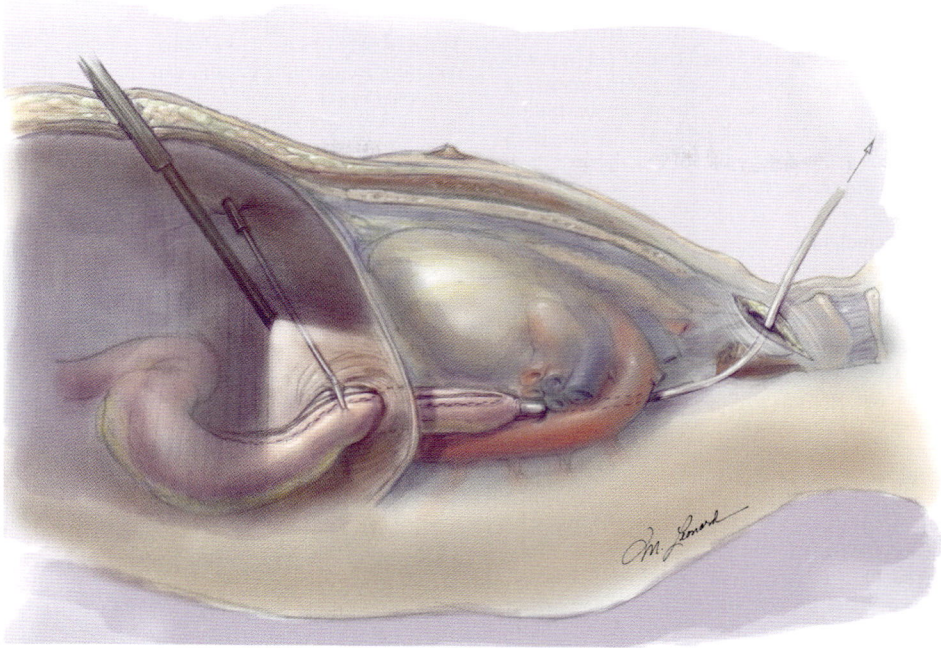

Figure 11-16. As the chest tube is withdrawn through the cervicotomy, the attached gastric conduit is carefully followed laparoscopically to make sure it does not twist, tear, or suffer undue tension. (Reprinted with permission from Swanström LL, Soper NJS. *Mastery of Endoscopic and Laparoscopic Surgery.* 4th ed. Lippincott Williams & Wilkins, A Wolters Kluwer business; 2014.)

is a long learning curve, and currently, only limited centers have the expertise to perform successful laparoscopic esophagectomy. As more surgeons gain expertise in minimally invasive techniques, especially robotics, the operative morbidity for esophageal cancer will decline.

Neoadjuvant Therapy

Because of the dismal prognosis in advanced esophageal cancer, the role for neoadjuvant (preoperative) therapy has been intensively pursued. Because most esophageal cancer presents at an advanced stage, the goal of neoadjuvant therapy is to "downstage" the tumor and improve cancer survival after surgical resection. Multiple prospective randomized trials have been conducted, with many studies showing improved cancer survival with neoadjuvant chemoradiation and surgery, as opposed to surgery alone. Most neoadjuvant chemoradiation therapy protocols include a course of 5-fluorouracil and cisplatinum with 45 Gy radiation over 6 to 7 weeks, followed by surgical resection a month after completion of treatment. Not all studies demonstrated improved survival, and the cost of increased perioperative mortality and morbidity must be weighed in. The greatest survival benefit occurs in the patient who demonstrates a complete response to neoadjuvant therapy (with no residual tumor found in the resected specimen).

In summary, the use of neoadjuvant chemotherapy remains controversial, and its use is dependent on the institution or physician. The benefit of some survival improvement with neoadjuvant therapy must be balanced against the treatment cost, the increased perioperative morbidity, and the delay in surgical intervention to complete chemoradiation therapy.

Palliative Management

Palliative interventions for patients with terminal esophageal carcinoma are directed toward the relief of severe dysphagia and obstruction. With advances in endoscopic approaches such as stents, laser coring, and phototherapy, surgical intervention is rarely indicated for palliation. Chemoradiation remains an effective means of palliation, and its effect is more durable. However, the benefit of palliative chemoradiation does not occur immediately and takes several weeks before the patient sees any improvement. Most endoscopic palliative interventions can provide immediate relief, but there is a higher risk of complications because of perforation, and their effects may not be long-lasting.

Dilatation

Immediate improvement of dysphagia can be obtained using dilators or balloon expansion. These techniques of dilatation are relatively simple and readily available in most hospitals, but their effect is usually of short duration. The main risk is that of perforation.

Stents

Endoscopically placed expandable metal stents have replaced plastic, rigid tubes for treating obstructing lesions. They can provide immediate relief but require expertise in sizing and placement. Recurrence of obstructive symptoms can occur within a few months, requiring reintervention. Complications include stent migration, food impaction, and perforation. Stents are used for mid- and distal esophageal tumors and can be associated with significant reflux when placed in the distal esophagus.

Laser and Photodynamic Therapy

Endoscopically guided laser "coring" of obstructing tumors can be effective but carries a high risk of perforation. Photodynamic therapy consists of using photosensitizing agents followed by local light therapy to ablate the tumor. Because of the limited depth of penetration by the laser light, the risk of perforation is reduced, but the extent of tumor debulking is, therefore, limited.

Radiation and Chemoradiation

Chemoradiation therapy can be very effective and durable in reducing tumor mass and improving dysphagia. Compared with the other palliative modalities, there is less limitation from tumor location and size or the availability of endoscopic expertise. The limiting factor of chemoradiation is the lag period of weeks to achieve effect and systemic debilitation from chemotherapy.

Ideally, centers treating patients with advanced esophageal cancer should have expertise in multiple options of palliation, because it is likely that the patients will need more than one approach for their disease. Ultimately, the goal of palliation is to provide a "comfortable" quality of life in the limited time available for the patient. Any aggressive palliative intervention must be weighed against potential for major complications and the need for acute hospitalization.

ESOPHAGEAL PERFORATION

Traumatic injury to the esophagus is a frequently encountered surgical emergency seen in thoracic surgery. It is useful to separate injury occurring at the cervical esophagus from that occurring at the thoracic esophagus. The etiology, prognosis, and management differ, depending on the location of the perforation.

Cervical Esophageal Injury

The majority of cervical esophagus injuries are caused by endoscopic instrumentation, especially at the level of the cricopharyngeal sphincter. Penetrating trauma to the neck is another common cause of cervical esophageal injury, because it is more vulnerable because of its location when compared with the thoracic esophagus. The immediate concern of cervical esophageal injury is sepsis. The ability for infection from a cervical esophageal injury to rapidly extend into the posterior mediastinum (posterior descending mediastinitis) is a classically described entity. The retrovisceral space is located posterior to the esophagus and anterior to the prevertebral fascia. This space connects the paracervical esophageal space to the posterior mediastinum, providing a route for infection to rapidly descend from the neck into the mediastinum (Figure 11-17).

Initial symptoms of cervical esophageal injury include pain with swallowing and neck flexion. Tenderness and crepitus may be present. On plain x-ray films, air may be seen in the retrovisceral space, possibly extending down to create pneumomediastinum. Indication for surgical intervention in suspected cervical esophageal injury can be based on history, clinical examination, and simple x-rays. A positive barium esophagram study is not mandatory, because up to 20% of these studies may be negative.

The treatment of cervical esophageal injury consists of intravenous antibiotics, surgical debridement, and drainage. Surgical approach is through a cervical incision on the side of injury. Drainage and debridement of the retrovisceral space is performed, extending down to the superior posterior mediastinum if infection extends downward. A gastrostomy tube is placed if a prolonged period of limited oral intake is anticipated. Primary repair of the esophageal injury is attempted, but not required because most cervical

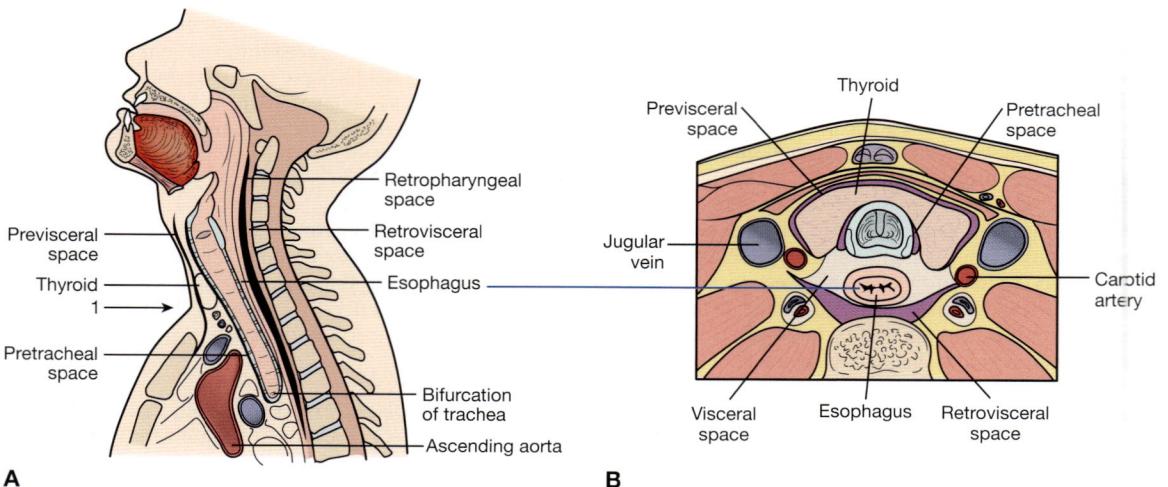

Figure 11-17. **The retropharyngeal space and the retrovisceral space are a plane of loose connective tissue running behind the pharynx and esophagus, anterior to the vertebral bodies.** This tissue plane is a potential space connecting the posterior pharynx and esophagus down into the posterior mediastinum (A). Because it consists of loose connective tissue, infections arising from the pharynx or cervical esophagus can travel quickly down into the posterior mediastinum (posterior descending mediastinitis). The numeral (1) represents the level of cross-sectional view illustrated in (B).

esophageal injuries will heal with adequate drainage, restricted oral intake, and the absence of distal esophageal obstruction. If there is an associated tracheal injury, a pedicled muscle flap is incorporated into the procedure to prevent tracheoesophageal fistula formation.

Thoracic Esophageal Injury

Thoracic esophageal perforation is most commonly caused by the instrumentation of a diseased esophagus, usually after attempted dilatation of a distal esophageal obstruction such as a peptic stricture. Spontaneous rupture of the distal esophagus can occur, though, after violent retching and emesis (Boerhaave syndrome). Major perforation of the thoracic esophagus usually presents with acute signs of sepsis, and it is commonly associated with chest pain, respiratory distress, and pleural effusion. A recent history of esophageal instrumentation or violent emesis, associated with an acute onset of clinical distress, should lead to a suspicion of esophageal perforation. Historically, patients with a Boerhaave tear present in a more clinically dramatic manner and have a worse prognosis because of greater contamination from spillage of esophageal and gastric contents into the chest cavity. It should be noted that, similar to Boerhaave syndrome, a Mallory-Weiss tear is a gastroesophageal junction tear that also occurs after forceful vomiting. However, Mallory-Weiss tears are nontransmural and primarily cause upper GI bleeding.

Workup of suspected thoracic esophageal perforation starts with plain x-rays, which may demonstrate pneumomediastinum and pleural effusion. An upper GI swallow or CT scan with an on-table swallow of contrast is helpful in determining the extent of injury and infection. Assessment for the presence of concomitant esophageal disease is needed to help determine optimal surgical management.

Treatment options include expectant medical management or surgical intervention. There has been much debate about nonoperative management with antibiotics, nasogastric drainage, and distal tube feeds or parental nutrition. However, nonoperative management should be the exception, and not the rule, as specific criteria need to be met for the medical management of esophageal perforation. They include a limited perforation contained within the neck or mediastinum and a clinically stable patient. Surgical principles for managing esophageal perforation include good debridement of infected tissues, two-layer repair of the mucosa and muscularis layers, and reinforcement (often using a pedicled intercostal muscle flap). Any concomitant esophageal disease needs to be identified and addressed, because a residual obstruction or pathology can place tension on the surgical repair. This includes concomitant myotomy for achalasia, dilatation of fibrotic strictures, and, in some cases, esophagectomy for obstructing esophageal carcinoma. In the presence of terminal esophageal cancer, T-tube drainage via the perforation or intraluminal stenting may be alternatives to consider. Surgical esophageal exclusion has been used in managing significant esophageal injury when the patient is too ill to tolerate an extended surgical procedure for repair. Esophageal exclusion is achieved by stapling off the injured segment, cervical drainage by a spit fistula (cervical esophagostomy), feeding jejunostomy tube, wide drainage, and local debridement. Spontaneous recanalization across the staple line can occur, or reconstruction with a gastric, colonic, or jejunal conduit can be offered after recovery.

HIATAL HERNIAS

There are four types of hiatal hernias described. The most common type is the sliding hiatal hernia (type I), which is frequently associated with GERD. In type I, the gastroesophageal junction slides in and out of the chest through the esophageal hiatus. In the other three types of hiatal hernias, there is a component of prolapse of the stomach or other abdominal organs into the chest.

In a type II (true paraesophageal) hernia, there is isolated stomach prolapsed through a weakened phrenoesophageal ligament, but with preservation of the gastroesophageal junction in the abdomen. A type III hernia is a combination of sliding and paraesophageal hernia, and type IV involves herniation of other organs, such as the colon or spleen (Figure 11-18).

Plain chest radiography can demonstrate the presence of an air-fluid level in the mediastinum or left chest consistent with herniation of the stomach. Contrast upper GI is considered the gold standard for identifying the presence of hiatal hernias. CT scan can provide further details on the anatomy of the hernia but is usually unnecessary.

Asymptomatic type I hiatal hernias can be observed, because there is no risk for incarceration. Surgical intervention for the type I hernia is usually done for symptoms of gastroesophageal reflex, and operative approaches are similar to the ones described in section "Gastroesophageal Reflux Disease."

Management of asymptomatic type II hernias is controversial. Because of the potential for acute strangulation and ischemia, some physicians believe that elective repair should be recommended for asymptomatic paraesophageal hernias. However, the incidence of acute incarceration and infarction is considered rare, and close observation with patient education seems a reasonable alternative to prophylactic surgery.

Surgical repair of any type of hiatal hernia is typically indicated when symptoms (postprandial pain, dysphagia, GERD, dyspnea, etc) are present. Key operative steps include complete reduction of the hernia sac, mobilization of the thoracic esophagus to achieve 2 to 3 cm of intra-abdominal esophageal length, tension-free closure of the diaphragmatic defect (with or without an absorbable mesh), and fundoplication (Figure 11-19).

In chronically debilitated older patients who are not candidates for a lengthy surgery, simple laparoscopic hernia reduction with gastropexy (either with sutures or with a percutaneous gastrostomy tube) is often satisfactory to alleviate symptoms associated with large paraesophageal hernias.

ESOPHAGEAL MOTILITY DISORDERS

Achalasia

One of the most notorious motility disorders affecting the esophagus is achalasia, which translates as "failure to relax." The primary abnormality is believed to be a degenerative disease of the myenteric (Auerbach) neural plexus.

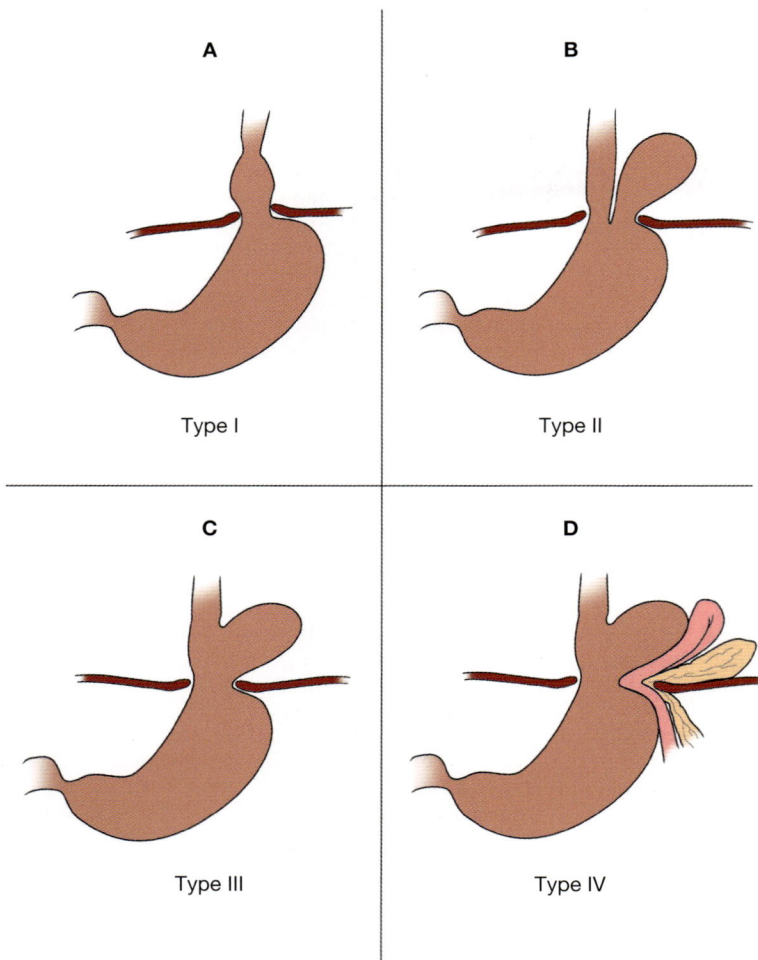

Figure 11-18. Type I and type II hiatal hernias. A. In type I (often associated with gastroesophageal reflux disease), the gastroesophageal junction and proximal stomach slide into the chest because of weakening of the esophageal hiatus. B. In type II, the gastroesophageal junction remains anchored in the abdomen, and a weakening in the phrenoesophageal ligament allows the stomach to prolapse into the mediastinum. C. In type III, the gastroesophageal junction and the stomach migrate into the chest. This is the most common paraesophageal hernia (not counting type I). D. Type IV is type III with other intra-abdominal viscera in the chest. (Reprinted with permission from Luketich JD. *Master Techniques in Surgery: Esophageal Surgery*. 1st ed. Wolters Kluwer Health; 2014.)

This leads to denervation of the esophagus with resultant failure of relaxation of the LES upon swallowing and absent esophageal peristalsis. The primary complaint in patients with achalasia is progressive dysphagia to solids and then liquids. Because patients commonly complain of regurgitation symptoms, they are often initially misdiagnosed as having GERD.

Achalasia is often diagnosed on a barium swallow study, which shows a classic "bird's-beak sign" where contrast meets a gradually tapering obstruction at the LES, resembling a bird's beak (Figure 11-20). On manometric studies, there is failure of the LES to relax with swallowing, combined with the absence of normal peristaltic contractions of the esophagus. Endoscopy is always performed to rule out other possible causes of chronic distal obstruction, which can also lead to proximal esophageal dilatation, such as carcinoma (pseudoachalasia).

Treatment of achalasia is limited to palliative interventions, because the disease cannot be cured. Interventions are directed toward relieving LES spasm through medical management, endoscopic intervention, or surgical myotomy. Initial approach sometimes includes the use of oral/sublingual nitrates and calcium channel blockers to promote LES relaxation prior to meals, but unfortunately, medications almost never give patients any durable relief

of symptoms. Therefore, the current mainstays of treatment for achalasia are endoscopic balloon dilatation of the LES and surgical myotomy. Endoscopic pneumatic balloon dilation is the most effective nonsurgical intervention available to patients with achalasia. Dilations can last anywhere from a few months to a few years, but repeated dilations are often necessary. Because of the cumulative risk of perforation with repeated dilations, surgical myotomy is often preferentially performed in younger patients. Endoscopic injection of the LES with botulinum toxin has also been used but with limited success.

Surgical myotomy (called *Heller* myotomy) can be performed through a transthoracic or transabdominal incision (Figure 11-21). Studies have been done to demonstrate the advantage of one approach over the other, but ultimately, surgeon preference and clinical history are major determinants of surgical technique. Currently, a laparoscopic approach for the myotomy provides better patient comfort and the advantage of better visualization of the myotomy, possibly improving long-term outcomes (Figure 11-22). Many surgeons emphasize the importance of extending the myotomy toward the stomach for at least 2 to 3 cm. Fundoplication is performed concomitantly to prevent gastroesophageal reflux after making the LES incompetent.

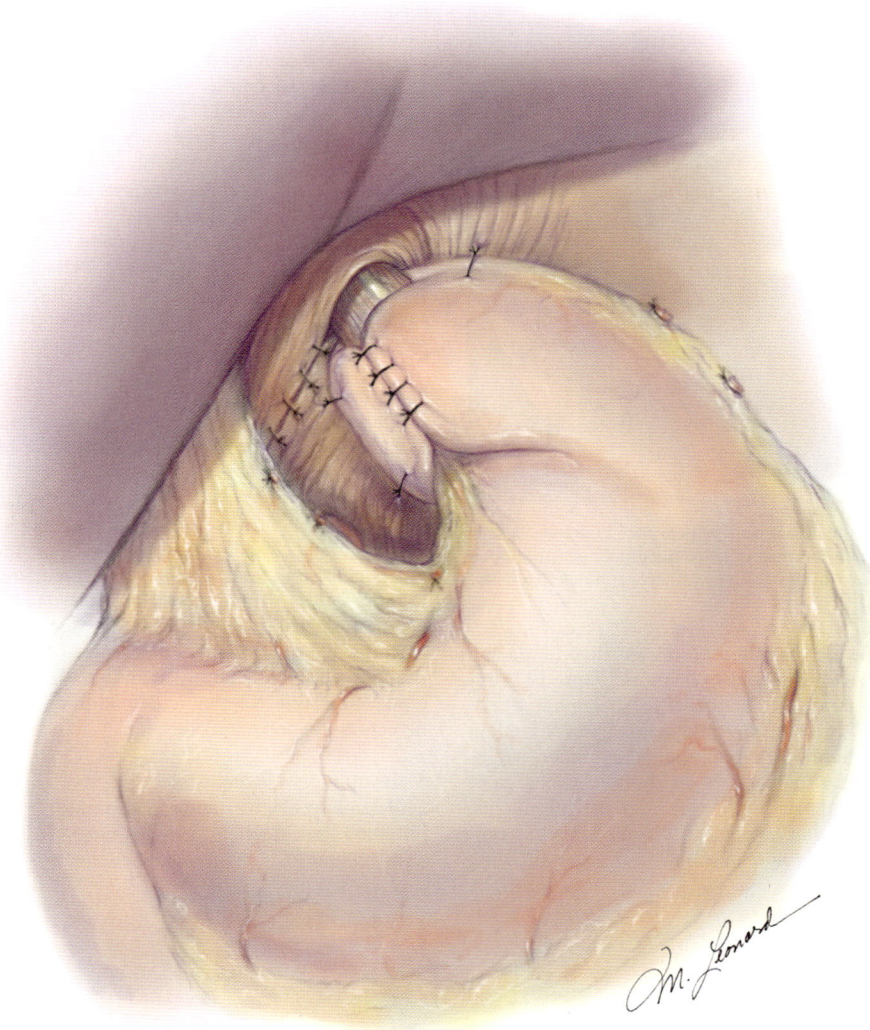

Figure 11-19. A fundoplication anchored to the diaphragm and crura. (Reprinted with permission from Swanstrom LL, Soper NJ. *Mastery of Endoscopic and Laparoscopic Surgery.* 4th ed. Wolters Kluwer; 2013.)

Endoscopic surgical therapy is increasingly available for achalasia. POEM involves endoscopically creating a submucosal tunnel and then performing a myotomy of the LES. Reflux rates after this procedure can be high, as a fundoplication is not performed concomitantly.

Major and Minor Disorders of Peristalsis

Major and minor disorders of esophageal peristalsis include such disorders as ineffective esophageal motility (IEM), distal esophageal spasm, and hypercontractile (jackhammer) esophagus. IEM is often asymptomatic but can manifest as dysphagia. There is no known treatment for this disorder, but esophageal prokinetic medications have been tried with some success. Spastic esophageal disorders (such as distal esophageal spasm and jackhammer esophagus) usually present as dysphagia and noncardiac chest pain. Management is typically limited to medical treatment with nitrates

and calcium channel blockers, but long myotomy has also been described to have good symptomatic improvement.

Esophageal Diverticula

An esophageal diverticulum is an outpouching from the wall and is classified as either a pulsion or a traction diverticulum. Pulsion diverticula are more common and are almost always associated with esophageal motility dysfunction. They are usually located in the proximal or distal esophagus. Because they lack a full muscle layer, pulsion diverticula are considered to be false diverticula. Traction diverticula are usually located in the midesophagus and often develop from a local lymph node inflammatory reaction, causing traction on the esophageal wall. Interestingly, they are almost always associated with esophageal dysmotility as well. Traction diverticula are true diverticula in that all layers of the esophageal wall are involved.

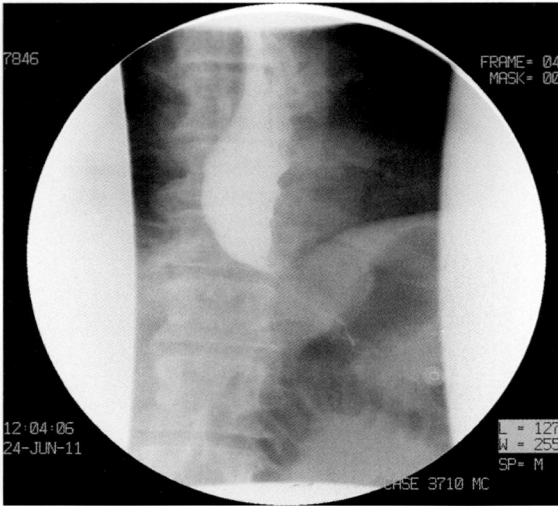

Figure 11-20. Classic bird's-beak appearance of achalasia seen during barium swallow because of proximal esophageal dilatation associated with failure of the distal esophageal sphincter to relax.

Zenker Diverticula

Zenker diverticula are classified as pulsion diverticula and occur in the cervical esophagus. They are caused by uncoordinated or impaired relaxation of the cricopharyngeus muscle on swallowing, causing obstruction and subsequent proximal outpouching of the mucosa and submucosa. Anatomically, they occur posteriorly, in the transition area of weakness between the hypopharynx and the esophagus, just above the cricopharyngeus muscle. Patients are typically older individuals and may have some swallowing disorders associated with previous transient ischemic attacks or strokes. Patients with symptomatic Zenker have regurgitation of recently swallowed food or pills, dysphagia, choking, or halitosis. Diagnosis is confirmed by barium swallow (Figure 11-23).

Endoscopy is not necessary for diagnosis but, if performed, should be done with caution, because perforation can occur. Patients with symptoms are treated with cricopharyngeal myotomy and diverticulectomy or diverticulopexy (inversion and fixation of the diverticulum to promote drainage by gravity). Newer endoscopic approaches have been described where the cricopharyngeus muscle is divided with an endoscopic stapler or electrocautery, creating an esophagodiverticulostomy.

Epiphrenic Diverticula

Epiphrenic diverticula occur in the distal third of the esophagus and are generally pulsion diverticula associated with dysfunction of the LES. Epiphrenic diverticula can be caused from complications of GERD, such as stricture. Symptoms of these diverticula are similar to other esophageal diverticula, including dysphagia, regurgitation of undigested food, and occult aspiration. When symptomatic, they are referred for surgical intervention. Workup includes barium swallow and manometric studies to identify esophageal dysmotility. A surgical approach for epiphrenic diverticula is usually through a left thoracotomy, with diverticulum resection and repair, followed by stricture dilatation or an extensive distal myectomy to prevent recurrence.

Midesophageal Diverticula

Midesophageal diverticula are commonly associated with inflamed paratracheal lymph node disease associated with tuberculosis, histoplasmosis, or lung cancer and are

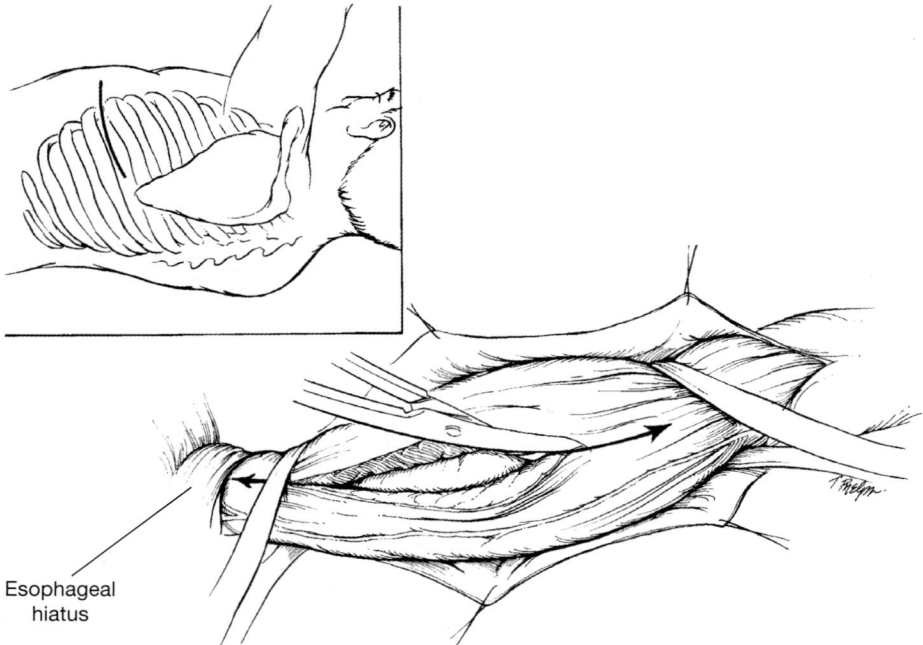

Esophageal hiatus

Figure 11-21. Heller myotomy for the treatment of achalasia, in which the distal esophageal sphincter is divided down to the mucosa. Some surgeons combine a fundoplication procedure to minimize reflux, although there is some controversy with a risk for causing residual distal obstruction Arrows indicate the direction in which the myotomy can go, longitudinally caudally toward GE junction and cranially. (Reprinted with permission from Kaiser LR, Kron IL, Spray TL. *Mastery of Cardiothoracic Surgery*. 2nd ed. Lippincott Williams & Wilkins; 2007:166.)

A　　　　　　　　　　　　　　　　　　　　　**B**

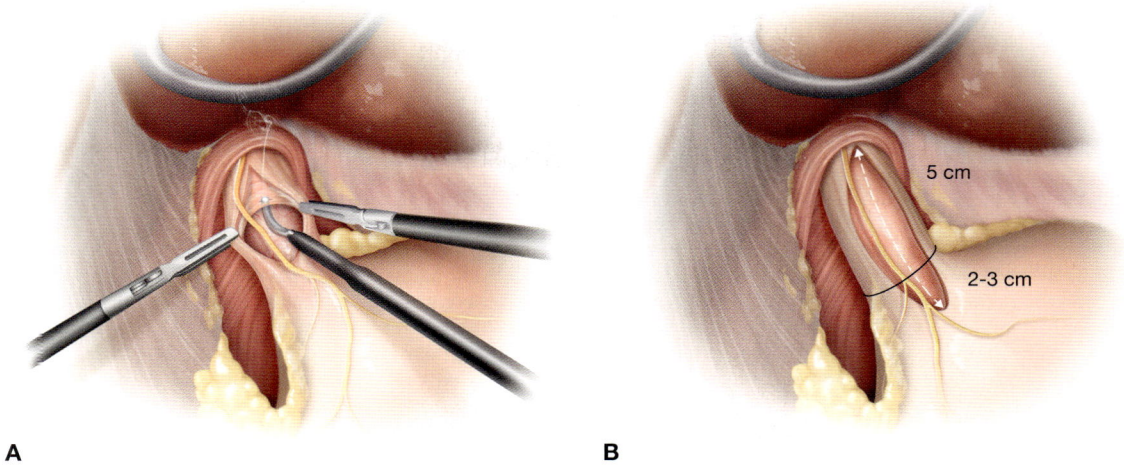

Figure 11-22. Heller myotomy. A. Circular fibers incised with cautery after splitting the longitudinal fibers laparoscopically. Mucosal preservation is key. B. Emphasis on a 5-cm myotomy with 2 to 3 cm on the stomach side to prevent inadequate myotomy. (Reprinted with permission from Luketich JD. *Master Techniques in Surgery: Esophageal Surgery.* 1st ed. Wolters Kluwer Health; 2014.)

usually true diverticula. Pulsion diverticula can also occur in the midesophagus and are associated with esophageal dysmotility, such as distal esophageal spasm or achalasia. Usually, they are asymptomatic and are left alone. Fistula formation to the trachea or adjacent blood vessels can occur, which will lead to respiratory and bleeding symptoms. Surgical treatment consists of excision of the diverticula and repair of the adjacent structure. Frequently, an interposition flap of tissue is used to prevent recurrence and promote healing.

BENIGN ESOPHAGEAL LESIONS

Benign esophageal lesions are uncommon and are categorized by location in the esophageal wall. They are usually asymptomatic and discovered incidentally, although some can present with dysphagia. The most common benign neoplasm is the leiomyoma, which is located in the muscularis layer. Overlying mucosa is almost always uninvolved. The second most common benign mass is an esophageal cyst, which is located in the outermost adventitial layer, partially involving

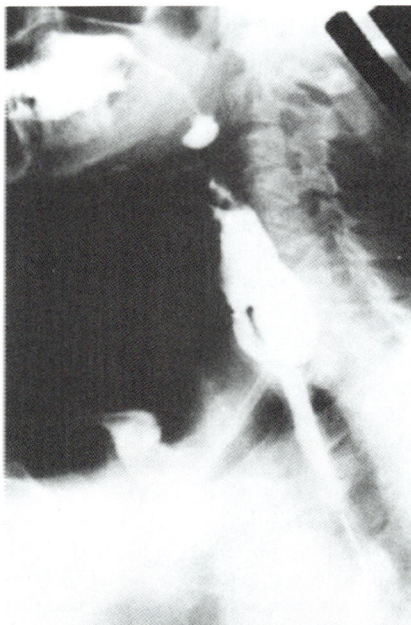

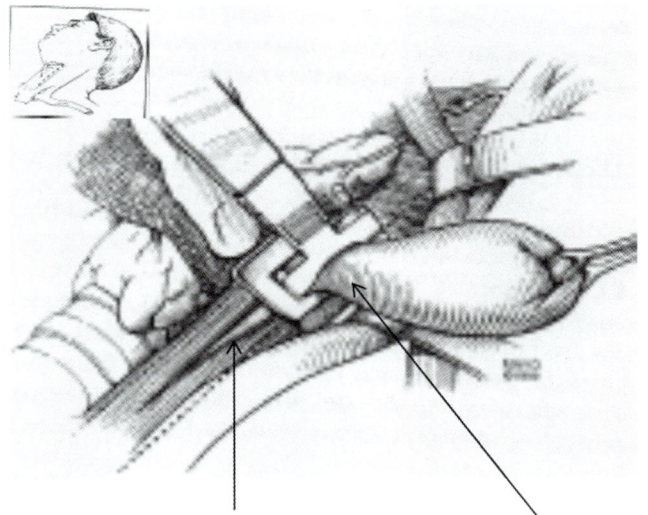

A　　　　　　　　　　　　　　　　　　　　　**B**

Figure 11-23. A. Barium swallow shows a Zenker diverticulum. B. Surgical treatment consists of a cricopharyngeal myotomy to relieve obstruction and usually a diverticulectomy. (Reprinted with permission from Shields TW, Lociciero J, Reed CE, Feins RH. *General Thoracic Surgery.* 7th ed. Lippincott Williams & Wilkins; 2009:1963-1965.)

the muscularis layer. The granular cell tumor and fibrovascular polyp are the most common mucosal/submucosal lesions. Most of these lesions occur in the mid- to distal esophagus and commonly present with dysphagia. Barium swallow demonstrates a smooth well-defined mass occupying the lumen of the esophagus. Diagnostic workup includes direct endoscopic visualization and EUS (Figure 11-24).

In general, small asymptomatic masses can be observed, because there is minimal risk for malignant transformation of these lesions. These lesions can be serially monitored using EUS. Fine-needle aspiration or biopsies should be avoided, because these rarely provide adequate differentiation between a benign leiomyoma and a malignant leiomyosarcoma. In addition, invasive manipulation of a cyst can result in iatrogenic infection requiring immediate surgical resection. When symptomatic, leiomyomas can be surgically removed by enucleation of the lesion with reapproximation of the muscle layer. Resection can be approached via standard thoracotomy, video-assisted thoracoscopic approach, or endoscopic approach (for smaller lesions). As expected, prognosis is excellent with good results and almost no recurrence.

FOREIGN BODY INGESTION

Foreign body ingestion is most common in toddlers and mentally ill adults. In this patient population, the history must be confirmed with appropriate imaging studies. In adults, most foreign body ingestion is caused by food impaction (poorly chewed meat or bones). The majority of impaction occurs at the level of the cricopharyngeus

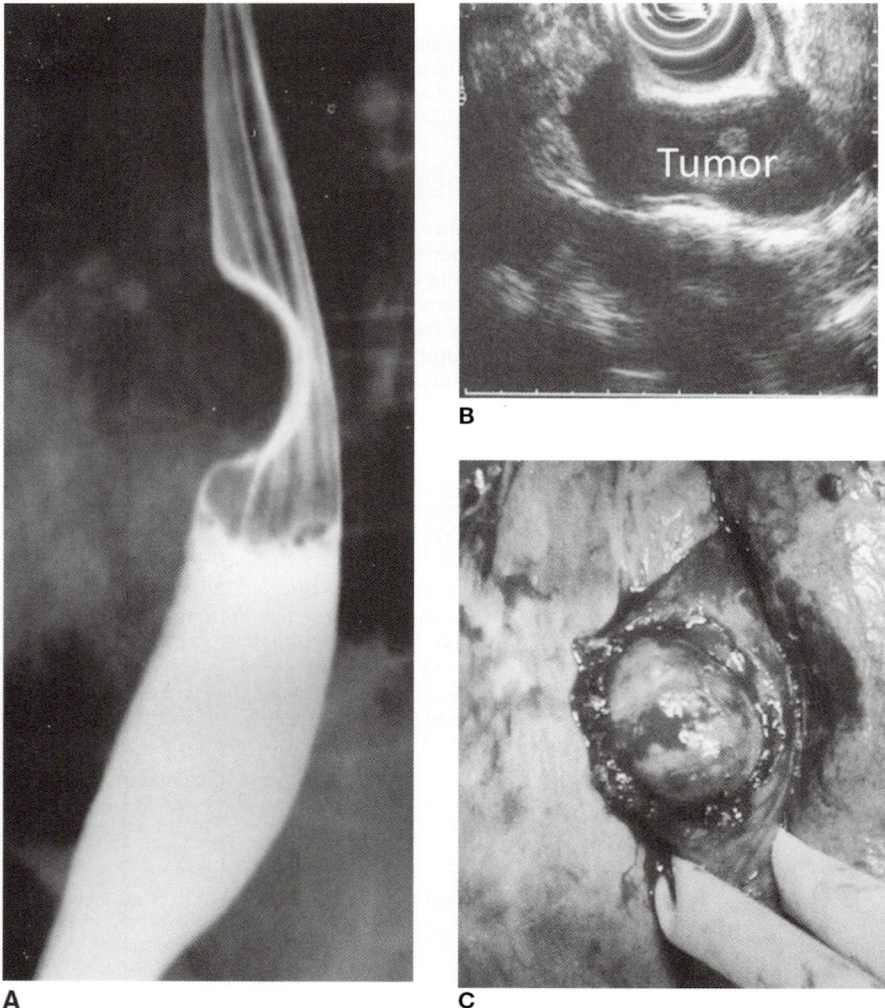

Figure 11-24. Typical appearance of an intramural leiomyoma on (A) barium swallow and (B) endoscopic ultrasound. If surgery is pursued, the leiomyoma is removed by (C) enucleation. (A. Reprinted from Orringer MB. Tumors of the esophagus. In: Sabiston DC Jr, ed. *Textbook of Surgery*. 13th ed. WB Saunders, 1986:736. With permission. Copyright © 1989 Elsevier. With permission. B and C. Reprinted from Shields TW, Lociciero J, Reed CE, Feins RH. *General Thoracic Surgery*. 7th ed. Lippincott Williams & Wilkins; 2009:1978, 1980. With permission.)

muscle or at the level of a peptic stricture in the distal esophagus. Symptoms typically include the inability to swallow secretions, drooling, and chest pain. Available imaging modalities include plain x-rays of the neck and chest, including lateral views of the neck to rule out cervical or mediastinal emphysema. Barium study is contraindicated because there is a high risk for aspiration, and contrast delineation does not add to the management of these patients. CT scan of the neck and chest can provide useful additional information. Underlying esophageal disease should be considered (eg, foreign body lodged on an acid-induced stricture), especially if impaction occurs in the distal esophagus.

Once the diagnosis is confirmed, the patient is best treated with gentle extraction using an esophagoscope under general anesthesia. In rare instances where endoscopic removal is not possible, or there is associated perforation, open surgical removal may be necessary. Perforation of the esophagus is the most serious complication to rule out in a patient after extraction of the foreign body. A contrast study to exclude esophageal perforation can be performed before the patient is discharged. If perforation of the esophagus is identified, management is as described in section "Esophageal Perforation."

INGESTION OF CAUSTIC MATERIALS

Ingestion of caustic materials, either accidentally (as by children) or intentionally (as by an adult in a suicide attempt), is a medical emergency. Compared with ingestion of acid products, ingestion of alkaline products (eg, Drano, Liquid Plumr) results in greater full-thickness esophageal injury. Ingestion of acidic material often leads to more superficial injury, and the ability to ingest large volumes of acid is limited by the extreme burning sensation they create in the mouth. The long-term complication from ingestion of caustic material is stricture formation.

Evaluation

The most important aspect of treatment is the early identification of the etiologic agent (eg, acid, alkaline, specific toxin), because each agent requires a different approach. Second, careful physical examination of the oropharyngeal cavity is required to estimate the severity of injury, and the physician should be prepared for emergent fiberoptic endotracheal intubation, because these patients may develop rapid upper airway edema. Flexible endoscopy is urgently performed to assess the extent of injury and should be performed early (within 24 hours) to minimize the risk of perforation. Injury severity is graded by the degree of depth, from superficial first-degree burns to transmural third-degree burns. The risk of perforation and stricture formation increases with the depth of injury.

Treatment

Induced vomiting and neutralization of caustic substances are not suggested because they are potentially harmful

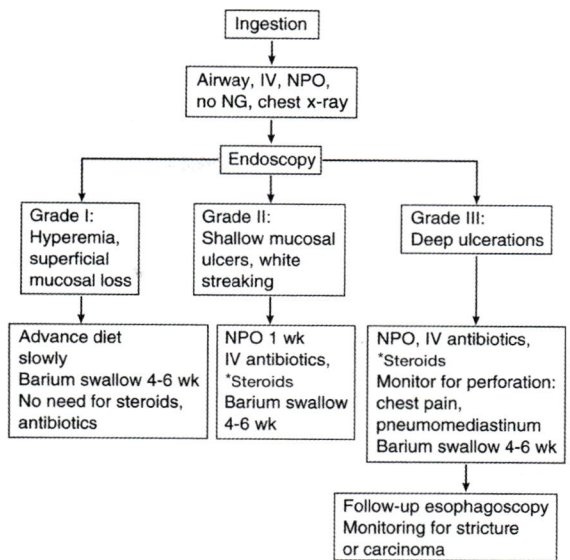

Figure 11-25. Algorithm for caustic ingestion. IV, intravenous; NG, nasogastric tube; NPO, nothing by mouth. *Steroids have not proven to be effective in preventing stricture formation.

and ineffective. In addition, induced vomiting exposes the esophagus to the caustic substance a second time. Airway maintenance is the first priority, followed by the maintenance of esophageal patency. During initial endoscopic evaluation, if second- or third-degree burns are identified but the stomach is relatively spared, percutaneous gastrostomy may be performed for nutritional intake and future access for string-guided retrograde dilatation to prevent stricture formation. The use of antibiotics as adjuvant therapy is controversial. Steroids have not been proven effective in preventing stricture formation. Other than stricture formation, long-term complications include the increased risk for developing SCC of the esophagus. Surgical resection, if indicated because of perforation or refractory stricture formation, is challenging because of extensive scarring in the tissues surrounding the esophagus. Surgical resection frequently requires the use of colon interposition, because the stomach is frequently damaged. If scarring is deemed too intense to preclude safe esophageal resection, a substernal route for colonic interposition is performed. Figure 11-25 shows an algorithm for caustic ingestion.

SUGGESTED READINGS

Jobe BA, Richter JE, Hoppo T, et al. Preoperative diagnostic workup before antireflux surgery: an evidence and experience-based consensus of the Esophageal Diagnostic Advisory Panel. *J Am Coll Surg.* 2013;217(4):586-597.

Kahrilas PJ, Bredenoord AJ, Fox M, et al. The Chicago Classification of esophageal motility disorders, v3.0. *Neurogastroenterol Motil.* 2015;27:160-174.

Okusanya OT, Hess NR, Luketich JD, Sarkaria IS. This video demonstrates the key steps in performing a successful robotic assisted minimally invasive esophagectomy. *Asvide.* 2017;4:363.

SAMPLE QUESTIONS

QUESTIONS

Choose the best answer for each question.

1. A 50-year-old man has the onset of chest pain shortly after he undergoes pneumatic dilatation of the LES to treat achalasia. An upper GI water-soluble contrast study shows free extravasation of the contrast material at the level of the distal esophagus. The decision is made to take the patient to the operating room for immediate repair. The best surgical incision to use is a(n)

   A. median sternotomy.
   B. right thoracotomy.
   C. left thoracotomy.
   D. abdominal incision.
   E. left thoracoabdominal incision.

2. A 50-year-old woman comes to the clinic because of severe heartburn and regurgitation after meals and on lying down. She has been on long-term PPIs with good relief of symptoms but now wants to have antireflux surgery. Her body mass index is 32.4. The preoperative study most useful in predicting symptomatic relief from antireflux surgery is a(n)

   A. contrast barium swallow.
   B. CT scan of the chest and abdomen.
   C. upper endoscopy.
   D. esophageal manometry study.
   E. 24-hour pH monitoring study.

3. A 43-year-old woman is being considered for antireflux surgery. She has a long history of reflux symptoms that are now only partially controlled with lifestyle changes and a PPI. Upper endoscopy showed a small hiatal hernia and a short segment of intestinal metaplasia, but no evidence of dysplasia. She wants to know the possible advantage of the Toupet (partial) fundoplication when compared with the Nissen (full) fundoplication. The theoretical advantage for the Toupet fundoplication procedure is

   A. reduced morbidity and mortality when compared with the Nissen procedure.
   B. better long-term relief from GERD.
   C. reduced postoperative symptoms of dysphagia and gas bloat.
   D. prevention of malignant progression of Barrett disease.
   E. avoidance of a thoracotomy incision.

4. A 74-year-old man has a recent diagnosis of adenocarcinoma of the distal esophagus. He has a long history of reflux and Barrett esophagus, and a recent upper endoscopy and biopsies confirmed the diagnosis. A staging workup is planned. What is the best study for assessing T (tumor invasion depth)?

   A. Barium swallow
   B. CT scan with oral and intravenous contrast
   C. Upper endoscopy with rebiopsy
   D. PET scan
   E. EUS

5. A frail 85-year-old man underwent upper endoscopy with dilation and biopsy of a distal esophageal stricture. Concerned about a perforation, the endoscopist obtained a water-soluble contrast upper GI study that confirmed a perforation. Nonsurgical management is acceptable if

   A. the patient has a new left pleural effusion.
   B. the patient has an obstructing carcinoma.
   C. the patient develops pain.
   D. the perforation is over 24 hours old.
   E. the upper GI study shows leak of contrast, which drains back into the esophagus.

ANSWERS AND EXPLANATIONS

1. **Answer: C**

   The best exposure of the distal thoracic esophagus is through a left thoracotomy. Anatomically, the upper and middle thoracic esophagus runs along the right side of the aorta, but the distal esophagus swings anteriorly and then to the left of the aorta to exit into the abdomen. The esophagus is not accessible through a median sternotomy because it lies in the posterior mediastinum with the heart lying anterior to it. A right thoracotomy is used to expose the proximal and middle thoracic esophagus. A left thoracoabdominal incision is a large morbid incision and is not necessary for the repair of the perforation and to perform a myotomy. For more information on this topic, see section "General Anatomy."

2. **Answer: E**

   Evidence of abnormal acid reflux obtained from a positive 24-hour pH study is the best indicator for the likely benefit of an antireflux procedure in GERD. The other studies offered earlier can provide additional information on GERD but are not as sensitive in identifying potential surgical candidates for antireflux procedure. A barium swallow can identify a hiatal hernia, associated strictures, or shortened esophagus. A CT scan provides very little additional information but may demonstrate the presence of a hiatal hernia. Upper endoscopy is useful in identifying and monitoring the progression of Barrett disease. Manometric study, when abnormal, is useful in identifying motility dysfunction, which may affect surgical outcome. For more information on this topic, see section "Diagnosis" under the heading "Gastroesophageal Reflux Disease."

3. **Answer: C**

   Because the Toupet procedure is a partial fundoplication, there is less risk for developing dysphagia or from having difficulty burping when compared with a full encircling fundoplication. Both the Toupet and Nissen procedures can be performed laparoscopically with minimal morbidity and mortality. Because the Nissen is a full fundoplication, many proponents argue that it provides better protection from recurrent reflux. No antireflux procedure has been conclusively shown to prevent or reverse Barrett disease, and continued periodic endoscopic monitoring is recommended. Both the Toupet and Nissen procedures are usually performed through an abdominal incision. For more information on this topic, see section "Surgical Treatment" under the heading "Gastroesophageal Reflux Disease."

4. **Answer: E**

   The EUS is the best way to assess the depth of tumor invasion (T stage) and is also useful in identifying adjacent abnormal lymph nodes for fine-needle aspiration (N stage). A barium swallow is a good initial study in the workup of dysphagia and helps locate the level of the lesion. A CT scan may show gross invasion of adjacent structures but cannot differentiate tumor depth. Upper endoscopy is used to obtain biopsies to confirm carcinoma, but the depth of invasion cannot be determined from the biopsy specimen. A PET scan is used to identify distant metastasis but does not have the resolution to determine tumor depth. For more information on this topic, see section "Diagnosis" under the heading "Esophageal Carcinoma."

5. **Answer: E**

   Conservative management is acceptable if contrast study shows a contained leak that drains back into the esophageal lumen. A new left pleural effusion is indicative of a more severe leak, which should not be managed conservatively. Obstructing lesions cannot be ignored, because any obstructions will exacerbate the leak. Pain is indicative of excessive leak of GI contents into the mediastinum and pleura, which cannot be managed conservatively. Duration of perforation should not dictate whether surgical intervention is pursued. For more information on this topic, see section "Thoracic Esophageal Injury."

12 Stomach and Duodenum

John T. Paige and Sajani N. Shah

ANATOMY

Stomach

The stomach is a gastrointestinal (GI) capacitance organ usually located in the left hypochondrium and epigastrium, interposed between the esophagus and duodenum. There are anatomic relationships with the diaphragm superiorly, the spleen and liver laterally, the pancreas posteriorly, and the greater omentum inferiorly. Normally, the stomach can expand to accommodate a liter or more of ingested food, which it prepares for digestion and absorption.

The gastroesophageal (GE) junction forms histologically by a mucosal change from squamous to columnar epithelium and functionally by a high-pressure zone known as the lower esophageal sphincter (LES). In healthy individuals, the LES is intraperitoneal, more than 2 cm long, and has a resting pressure above 6 mm Hg. A hypotonic LES or hiatal hernia may contribute to gastroesophageal reflux disease (GERD). With swallowing, a coordinated relaxation of the LES occurs to facilitate the entry of food into the stomach. Impaired LES relaxation and esophageal aperistalsis define the condition called achalasia.

The gastroduodenal junction is marked histologically by a definite mucosal change from gastric epithelium to intestinal epithelium (striated columnar cells with interspersed goblet cells) and functionally by a discreet 1- to 3-cm long smooth muscle valve known as the pylorus. The pylorus prevents reflux of duodenal contents into the stomach and, in association with the antral pump, controls gastric emptying. After ingestion of a meal, particles larger than 3 to 5 mm remain in the stomach until the final "cleansing" wave of peristalsis occurs several hours later.

The stomach has three distinct regions based on histologic and physiologic differences. The most proximal portion, the *fundus*, plays a crucial role in capacitance by undergoing receptive relaxation. As food traverses the pharynx and esophagus, vagal stimulation causes relaxation of the fundus, limiting intragastric pressure increases as food is stored. The fundus is the site of the autonomic pacemaker that is responsible for initiating gastric motor activity. The middle portion of the stomach, the *corpus*, contains most of the acid-producing parietal cells, as well as pepsinogen-producing chief cells and enterochromaffin-like (ECL) cells. The corpus is important for hydrochloric acid (HCl) secretion, storage of gastric contents, and peristaltic grinding against the pylorus. The most distal region, the *antrum*, contains G cells, which produce gastrin, but not the parietal cells. For this reason, a surgeon performing an antrectomy for ulcer disease must be certain to extend the resection to the proximal duodenum, since *retained antrum* in this now isolated, non–acid containing segment will hypersecrete gastrin causing recurrent ulcers in the remaining proximal stomach or at the anastomosis to small bowel (marginal ulcer). Finally, mucus-secreting goblet cells are throughout the entire stomach.

The wall of the stomach has four layers: the mucosa, submucosa, muscularis, and serosa. The mucosa has a coarse rugal pattern and a complex glandular structure. The muscularis mucosa separates the mucosa from the submucosa. Its abundant blood supply arises from the rich vascular network of the submucosa. The muscularis surrounds the submucosa in three layers of smooth muscle: the outermost longitudinal, the middle circular, and the innermost oblique. The gastric pacemaker in the fundus is located in the circular muscle layer. The serosa overlies the muscularis and is the outermost covering.

The arterial blood supply to the stomach includes the right and left gastric arteries, the right and left gastroepiploic arteries, the short gastric arteries, and the gastroduodenal artery (Figure 12-1). Because of this abundant blood supply, unintended surgical devascularization of the stomach rarely occurs. Sympathetic innervation parallels arterial flow.

Parasympathetic innervation via the vagus nerves contributes to HCl production by the parietal cell mass and motor activity of the stomach. As the vagus nerves traverse the mediastinum, the left trunk rotates so that it enters the abdomen anterior to the esophagus (Figure 12-2), whereas the right trunk rotates so that it enters posterior to the esophagus. The right vagus gives off a posterior branch to the celiac plexus, from which nerves pass to the midgut (pancreas, small intestine, and proximal colon), and, sometimes, a small branch that travels behind the esophagus to innervate the stomach, known as the criminal nerve of Grassi. When not properly identified and divided during a parietal cell or truncal vagotomy, this nerve will continue to stimulate acid secretion in the stomach, leading to recurrent peptic ulcer disease (PUD). The left vagus gives off a hepatic branch that passes through the gastrohepatic ligament and innervates the gallbladder, biliary tract, and liver. Below these branches, both vagus nerves continue down the lesser curvature and give off side branches that innervate the stomach and terminal branches that innervate the pylorus (crow's foot).

Duodenum

The duodenum is a "C-shaped," mostly retroperitoneal, 25- to 30-cm tube connecting the stomach to the jejunum. Anatomically, it is divided into four regions: the duodenal bulb (first part), the descending duodenum (second part), the transverse duodenum (third part), and the ascending duodenum (fourth part). The *duodenal bulb* receives chyme from the stomach via the pylorus. The *descending duodenum* receives enzymes from the pancreas and bile from the liver via the ampulla of Vater at the posteromedial

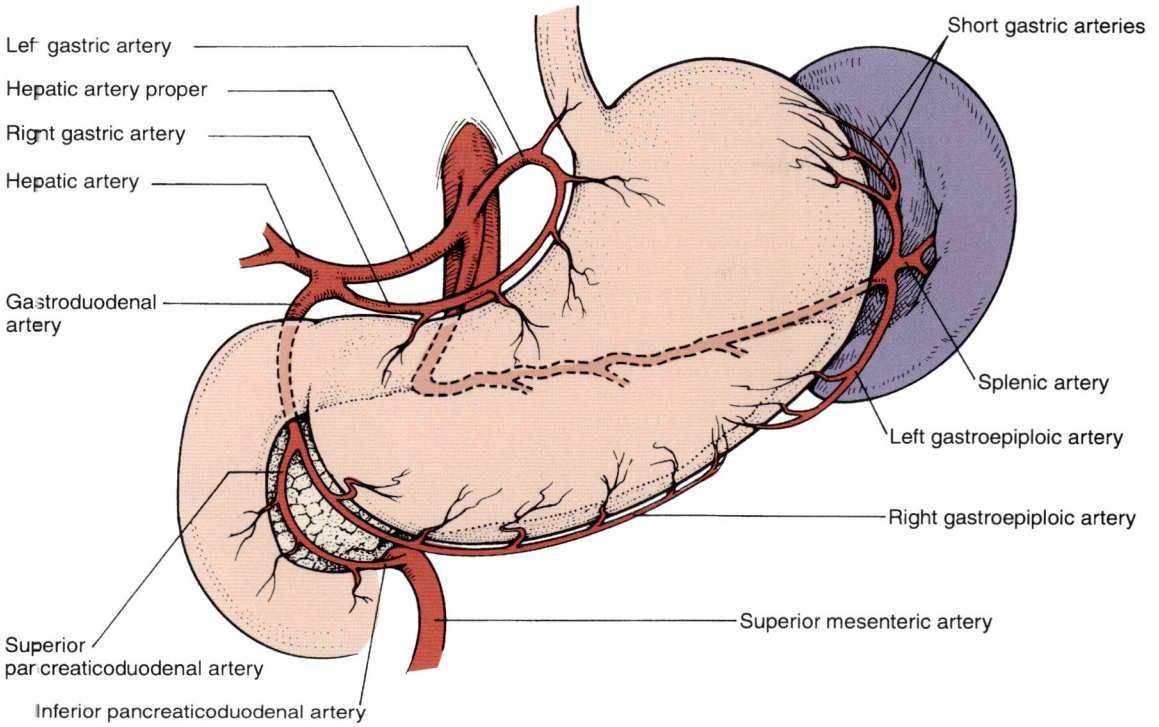

Figure 12-1. The major arteries that supply the stomach. The gastroduodenal artery is located behind the duodenum. Posterior penetrating duodenal ulcers may erode into this artery and cause hemorrhage.

aspect. In addition, the accessory pancreatic duct empties through the nearby lesser duodenal papilla. The *transverse duodenum* crosses the midline from right to left, and the *ascending duodenum* becomes the jejunum at the ligament of Treitz, where the small bowel becomes an intraperitoneal organ. The descending duodenum contains the intestinal pacemaker. Brunner glands throughout the duodenum

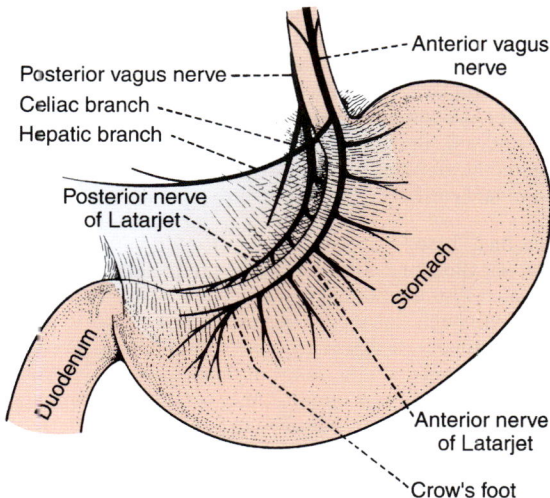

Figure 12-2. Branches of the vagus nerve innervate the stomach, pylorus, and duodenum. If the distal nerve of Latarjet is denervated, the pylorus does not relax in response to normal stimuli.

are the sites of mucus secretion, protecting the duodenal mucosa from gastric acid injury.

The duodenum is also an endocrine organ, with the secretion of secretin and cholecystokinin (CCK) in response to the arrival of gastric acid and ingested fats. These hormones signal the hepatobiliary system to deliver bile and the pancreas to deliver bicarbonate and digestive enzymes such as trypsin, lipase, and amylase.

The blood supply to the duodenum comes primarily from the gastroduodenal artery and the superior mesenteric artery, although other smaller vessels are contributors (Figure 12-1). The gastroduodenal artery is the first branch of the hepatic artery proper. It courses immediately posterior to the duodenal bulb and divides into the superior pancreaticoduodenal arcades. A duodenal ulcer that penetrates through the posterior wall of the duodenal bulb does so in the vicinity of the gastroduodenal artery. Exposure of the vessel wall to the digestive enzymes and acid can result in erosion and massive bleeding. The superior mesenteric artery arises from the descending aorta and supplies the inferior pancreaticoduodenal arcades.

PHYSIOLOGY

Hydrochloric Acid Secretion

Gastric acid secretion is a complex, highly regulated process in which multiple specialized gastric and duodenal cells play an essential role. A well-developed mucosal defensive mechanism is also present in the stomach to protect it from caustic injury. The parietal cell rests at the heart of this elaborate system.

Gastric acid secretion occurs under basal and stimulated conditions. The basal acid secretion occurs in a circadian rhythm, with the highest levels occurring during the night and lower levels during the morning hours. When stimulated, the parietal cell undergoes morphologic and functional changes. The former includes a fusion of many cytoplasmic tubulovesicles, on which proton pumps rest, with the canalicular membrane moving the proton pumps to a position in which they can actively exchange H^+ for K^+. The H^+, K^+-ATPase is responsible for creating the concentrated acid environment within the lumen of the stomach. It accomplishes this task by actively secreting hydrogen ion against a 1,000,000:1 concentration gradient. Gastric acid secretion is an active process that requires a high amount of energy provided by adenosine triphosphate (ATP). Chloride ion transport into the lumen occurs in conjunction with this process. Water and bicarbonate are by-products of this reaction, and they passively diffuse into the plasma and extracellular space. When stimulated, 60% to 70% of proton pumps in the parietal cell become active. The proton pumps are recycled back to the inactive state in cytoplasmic vesicles once parietal cell activation ceases. Direct blockage of this fundamental step inhibits gastric acid production. Proton pump inhibitors (PPIs), developed by the pharmaceutical industry, work in this manner. They have dramatically altered the therapy of duodenal ulcer and gastric reflux disease.

The parietal cell membrane has three important receptors involved in HCl secretion: a cholecystokinin B (CCK_B) gastrin receptor, a muscarinic 3 (M_3) acetylcholine (Ach) receptor, and a histamine 2 (H_2) receptor. Activation of gastrin and M3 receptors leads to activation of the protein kinase C/phosphoinositide pathway, while activation of H_2 receptors by histamine leads to activation of the adenylate cyclase pathway with an increase in cyclic adenosine monophosphate (cAMP). Each pathway regulates a series of kinase cascades that control the pump mechanism. These receptors engage in a synergism in which simultaneous activation of two or more of them by the appropriate ligand augments acid secretion. Conversely, when any one of these sites is blocked, the other sites become less responsive to stimulation. Thus, interruption of vagal innervation blunts the parietal cell response to gastrin.

Mechanisms of Acid Stimulation

The capacity of the stomach to secrete HCl is almost linearly proportional to parietal cell mass. Gastric acid secretion by the parietal cell mass occurs in a sequential order divided into three general phases: cephalic, gastric, and intestinal. Each phase has distinct mechanisms of activation.

Cephalic Phase

This initial phase is mediated by the central nervous system (CNS) and stimulated by the sight, smell, or thought of food that activates afferent neural pathways to the CNS. Efferent activity proceeds from the hypothalamus to the stomach via the vagus nerve. Ach release by the vagus has three actions:

1. Directly: Ach stimulates the parietal cell directly by binding to its M_3 receptor. Activation of this receptor leads to an intracellular cascade resulting in the release of HCl.

2. Indirectly: Ach stimulates acid secretion by activating antral cells that produce gastrin-releasing protein (GRP). GRP then promotes gastrin secretion from antral G cells.

3. Ach can stimulate the ECL cells to release histamine, which subsequently stimulates gastric acid secretion through H_2-receptor stimulation.

In addition to food's visual and olfactory stimulation of acid release, its actual physical presence in the mouth activates the vagal pathway. Surgical division of the vagal nerves supplying the parietal cell mass blunts this parasympathetic response, decreasing acid secretion. In addition, anticholinergic blockade of the M_3 receptor can inhibit the response. Such anticholinergic agents produce multiple side effects and are ineffective compared to other clinically available acid inhibitors, precluding their use.

Gastric Phase

The gastric phase starts once the food enters the stomach. Stretch receptors within the stomach activate intragastric parasympathetic reflex pathways that promote further Ach release. In addition, chemical and stretch receptors within the antrum detect alkalinization, antral distension, and the presence of amino acids. In response, the G cells release gastrin. The gastrin enters the venous circulation and exerts both a direct and indirect effect:

1. Directly: Some gastrin binds the CCK_B receptors on the parietal cells, promoting HCl secretion. This direct mechanism of action is the weaker of the two.

2. Indirectly: Gastrin promotes acid secretion mainly via the ECL cells. Here, gastrin activates receptors, causing histamine release from the ECL cells. The histamine then binds the H_2 receptors on the parietal cells, stimulating acid release.

Gastrin is the most potent stimulus for acid secretion in humans. It exhibits marked heterogeneity, breaking into multiple fragments from the initial preprogastrin produced by the G cells. Three main forms include 14-, 17-, and 34-amino acid species. Of these, the 17-amino acid gastrin is the most biologically active in stimulating acid secretion. It has a short half-life of only 2 to 3 minutes, and, like all fragments, undergoes neutralization in the small intestine and kidney.

Certain foods can also stimulate acid secretion. Both alcohol and caffeine act directly on the mucosa to increase HCl release. Proteins also seem to promote acid secretion indirectly via their breakdown products (amino acids) as described earlier.

Intestinal Phase

The intestinal phase of gastric acid production occurs with the arrival of the products of digestion in the small intestine. Although knowledge regarding this phase is somewhat limited, it is associated with substantial elevations in various serum peptides. Some of them, like enterooxyntin, stimulate gastric acid output. Other peptides are inhibitory (see section "Mechanisms of Acid Suppression and Mucosal Protection"). The parietal cell H_2 receptor may play an important role in this phase of acid secretion.

Mechanisms of Acid Suppression and Mucosal Protection

When stimulated, the parietal cell mass in the stomach can drop the pH to as low as 1.0. In this acidic environment, pepsinogen activates to pepsin and begins to hydrolyze proteins into peptones and amino acids. Unchecked, this process would lead to severe caustic injury and autodigestion of the stomach. Fortunately, several mechanisms exist to suppress acid secretion and protect the gastric mucosal lining.

Endocrine-Mediated Acid Suppression

The release of acidic chyme into the duodenum stimulates the secretion of numerous gut-inhibiting hormones (the so-called enterogastrones: secretin, somatostatin, vasoactive intestinal peptide [VIP], glucose-dependent insulinotropic polypeptide [GIP], neurotensin) that help suppress gastric acid production. Secretin, a 27-amino acid peptide released by duodenal S cells, plays an important role in this suppression. Luminal acidity, biliary salts, and fatty acids stimulate its secretion. In turn, secretin inhibits gastrin release, gastric acid secretion, and gastric motility. Somatostatin, a tetradecapeptide, is another important mediator. Its secretion is stimulated by a drop in gastric pH, after which it acts directly on the parietal cells to inhibit acid secretion. In addition, it inhibits gastrin release when gastric luminal pH drops to less than 1.5. Finally, somatostatin reduces histamine release from ECL cells. CCK and GIP, both released by cells in the duodenum, also act to suppress gastric acid production. Thus, an enterogastric feedback mechanism exists in which duodenal peptides help suppress acid production in the stomach once food enters the intestines.

Gastric Mucosal Protection

Within the stomach is a sophisticated, highly efficient barrier system that protects the gastric mucosal lining from caustic injury and digestion. The first barrier is a mucus-bicarbonate layer produced by the gastric epithelial cells. The mucus is a mucopolysaccharide that attaches to the luminal surface of the gastric mucosa, creating a protective mucous gel barrier that impedes diffusion of ions and molecules such as pepsin into the cells. The bicarbonate secretion occurs in exchange for chloride ions. The amount of bicarbonate produced by the stomach can only neutralize a small portion of the maximum acid output. The gastric lining preservation occurs due to the gel-like mucosal barrier trapping the secreted bicarbonate. Any back diffusion of hydrogen ions into it, therefore, leads to their rapid neutralization and clearance. As a result, even though the pH in the stomach may drop to as low as 1.0, the pH at the luminal surface of the mucosal cells rarely falls below 7.0. When this mechanism is not functioning adequately, as seen in *Helicobacter pylori* infection, damage to the mucosa can occur, and gastritis or gastric ulcers can result. Calcium, prostaglandins, cholinergic input, and luminal acidification stimulate bicarbonate secretion.

The second barrier is prostaglandins that play an important role in gastric epithelial defense/repair by stimulating mucus-bicarbonate secretion by epithelial cells, inhibiting HCl secretion by parietal cells, and improving gastric mucosal blood flow.

Vitamin B₁₂ (Cobalamin) Absorption

Vitamin B_{12} is a water-soluble vitamin with a key role in the normal functioning of the nervous system and in the formation of blood cells. The stomach and duodenum play an important role in vitamin B_{12} (cobalamin) absorption. To be properly absorbed in the terminal ileum, vitamin B_{12} must be complexed to intrinsic factor (IF). The parietal cells in the stomach produce this glycoprotein, and it then binds to vitamin B_{12} after pancreatic proteases have isolated it in the proximal small bowel. Failure of any step in this sequence can result in vitamin B_{12} deficiency with the subsequent development of megaloblastic anemia, irreversible sensory neuropathy, and dementia.

The Schilling test is an effective means of determining the cause of vitamin B_{12} deficiency, which could be either pernicious anemia or small intestinal bacterial overgrowth. In the first part of the test, a patient takes an oral dose of radiolabeled cobalamin followed by an intramuscular injection of unlabeled vitamin. The excretion of cobalamin in the urine is then determined by collecting a 24-hour urine sample. An abnormal value corresponds to less than 10% excretion of vitamin. Abnormal results trigger a repeat Schilling test using radiolabeled cobalamin bound to IF. Urinary excretion in this case will be normal if IF deficiency, as seen in pernicious anemia, is responsible for the poor vitamin B_{12} absorption. It will remain abnormal in cases of bacterial overgrowth or ileal disease causing the vitamin deficiency. Finally, the Schilling test can also be administered using radiolabeled cobalamin bound to proteins in scrambled eggs. An abnormal result in this situation would suggest a failure of the vitamin to dissociate from the ingested food, as occurs in patients with achlorhydria.

Duodenal Bicarbonate Secretion

Like the stomach, the duodenum has several mechanisms of mucosal protection. Brunner glands produce mucus, helping to create a protective barrier over the mucosa. In addition, the duodenal cells secrete sodium bicarbonate via a transmucosal electrical gradient. This production is up to 6 times greater than that of the stomach. As a result, the sodium bicarbonate can neutralize all of the hydrogen ions entering the duodenal bulb. Additional bicarbonate comes from the pancreas. It, however, neutralizes only a small amount of the total acid load.

Duodenal bicarbonate is stimulated locally by mucosal irritation. Pancreatic bicarbonate release occurs in response to secretin stimulation. It increases the volume of pancreatic secretions of bicarbonate and water. The cells of origin of these secretions are the centroacinar cells.

BENIGN GASTRIC DISEASE

Gastric Ulcer Disease

PUD includes benign ulcers of the stomach and duodenum. In most cases, gastric and duodenal ulcers have similar pathophysiology, clinical presentation, medical therapies, and surgical indications. Certain factors with respect to gastric ulcers, such as their risk of underlying malignancy, must be considered during evaluation and management. This chapter, therefore, discusses each entity in separate sections to emphasize such differences. Because of overlap, however, the sections on duodenal ulcer disease will discuss similarities between duodenal and gastric ulcers.

Improved understanding of the role of *H. pylori* and nonsteroidal anti-inflammatory drugs (NSAIDs) in the formation of PUD has led to a dramatic shift in treatment algorithms away from surgery. Both of these etiologies promote the development of ulcers by altering the balance between the protective and potentially harmful components of the gastric environment. *H. pylori* infection causes chronic active gastritis, with dysregulation of gastrin and acid secretion. NSAIDs inhibit cyclooxygenase 1 (cox-1), an essential component of prostaglandin synthesis, thereby altering local blood flow, mucus production, and bicarbonate secretion in the stomach. In such cases, acid and pepsin activity overcome gastric mucosal defensive mechanisms, exposing the lining of the stomach to damage. Taken together worldwide, *H. pylori* infection and NSAID use, either alone or in combination, remain the cause of most benign gastric ulcers. Tobacco use is an important associated risk factor. Although alcohol is a strong promoter of acid secretion and can cause mucosal damage, evidence for its direct role in ulcerogenesis is lacking.

Classification

Developed before the current understanding of PUD etiology, the classification scheme for gastric ulcers takes into consideration the anatomic location and associated pathophysiology to better direct therapy. They occur along the lesser curvature of the stomach between the junction of the fundus and the antrum. Type II gastric ulcers arise in combination with duodenal ulcers. Type III gastric ulcers develop in the prepyloric region. Type IV gastric ulcers are the least frequent. They occur high on the lesser curve near the GE junction. Type I and IV ulcers are associated with normal or low acid output; type II and III ulcers, like those found in the duodenum, are associated with gastric acid hypersecretion.

The characteristics and behavior of *H. pylori* likely explain the patterns behind the above-noted classification scheme for gastric ulcers. These small, curved, microaerophilic, gram-negative rods spread from person to person via gastro-oral or fecal-oral transmission, and they can colonize the antrum of the stomach, causing local mucosal inflammation. In patients with a high gastric acid output, this colonization can extend distally into the duodenal bulb if the duodenal mucosa undergoes gastric metaplasia. In patients with a low gastric acid output, the colonization spreads more proximally into the cardia, with particularly dense activity at the transition zone between the antrum and the cardia. Such observations help explain why type I and IV gastric ulcers are associated with low acid output, why type II ulcers are associated with duodenal ulcers, and why type II and III ulcers are associated with acid hypersecretion.

Type V gastric ulcers are NSAID-induced ulcers. These ulcerations can occur anywhere in the stomach. They respond differently to treatment than the other classifications.

Clinical Presentation and Evaluation

The clinical presentation of benign gastric ulcers depends on the severity of the disease process. In uncomplicated gastric ulcers, patients typically complain of a characteristic gnawing epigastric pain that can radiate to the back. Often, since this pain is associated with the ingestion of food, patients develop anorexia and weight loss. In cases of complicated gastric ulcers, patients may or may not have these antecedent symptoms prior to perforation or bleeding. Up to 10% of NSAID-induced ulcers present as a complicated disease without warning. The presentation, evaluation, and initial treatment of complicated gastric ulcers follow the algorithm presented for complicated duodenal ulcers later in this chapter.

Evaluation of a patient suspected of having an uncomplicated gastric ulcer begins with a thorough history and physical examination. In addition to determining the duration and character of symptoms, identification of risk factors is essential. In particular, inquiries regarding current tobacco or NSAID use, prior PUD, or history of *H. pylori* infection are key. Physical examination should focus on searching for signs of a malignant process.

Esophagogastroduodenoscopy (EGD) confirms the presence of an ulcer. This study involves the passage of a fiberoptic scope from the mouth into the esophagus, stomach, and duodenum with a detailed examination of the mucosa. Photographs taken at the time of such a study provide documentation and can serve as a comparison in subsequent evaluations of healing. Approximately 2% to 4% of gastric ulcers harbor an underlying malignancy. Consequently, all gastric ulcers require multiple biopsies at the time of endoscopy to establish the presence or absence of carcinoma. Endoscopic features suggestive of malignancy include a bunched-up ulcer border or large (>3 cm) ulcer size. Biopsy specimens should include samples incorporating the margin of the ulcer. Cytology and brushings are also helpful as an adjunct to biopsy. Despite such guidelines, false-negative results are still possible due to the small sample size of the biopsy specimens. The presence of achlorhydria in a patient with gastric ulceration is also suggestive of a malignant process. Finally, all patients with gastric ulcers, like those with duodenal ulcers, require testing to determine the presence or absence of *H. pylori* infection. Samples obtained at the time of endoscopy can serve such a purpose.

On occasion, ulceration is discernable on computed tomography (CT) obtained to work up unknown abdominal pain. CT, however, is not a recommended diagnostic study due to its poor sensitivity and specificity for ulcer disease. Historically, a barium upper GI contrast study was the diagnostic test of choice, revealing a small crater extending outward from the stomach (Figure 12-3). It is not used currently.

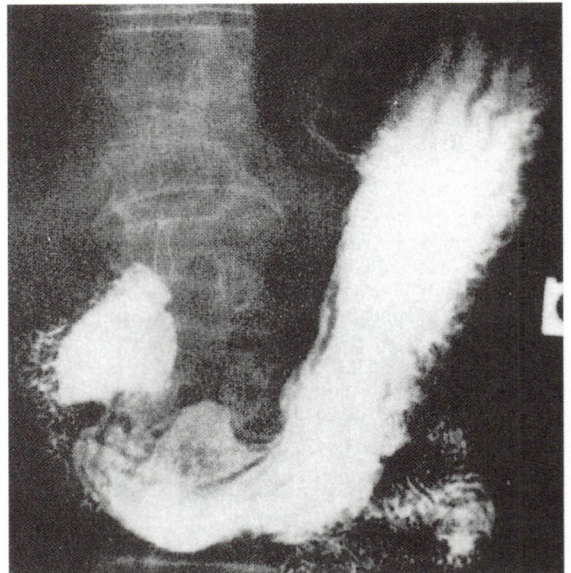

Figure 12-3. Moderate-sized ulcer seen on the lesser curve of the distal stomach in this barium upper gastrointestinal (GI) study.

Medical Treatment

First-line therapy for uncomplicated gastric ulcer disease is medical and follows guidelines similar to those for uncomplicated duodenal ulcer disease. In brief, this regimen includes cessation of all potential ulcerogenic agents (tobacco, NSAIDs, aspirin, steroids, alcohol), treatment of *H. pylori* infection with appropriate antibiotics, and acid suppression therapy using PPIs (Table 12-1).

Additional options for gastric ulcer treatment include the administration of cytoprotective agents such as sucralfate and misoprostol. Sucralfate is an aluminum salt containing sulfated sucrose. On ingestion, the sucrose polymerizes, coating the gastric ulcer with a protective barrier that prevents further injury. Misoprostol is a prostaglandin E1 analogue that promotes gastric mucosal protection by enhancing the defensive mechanisms of the gastric lining. Even with the best medical therapy, refractory and recurrent gastric ulcer disease often may occur.

Repeat endoscopy is mandatory after initiating medical treatment of a gastric ulcer. After 6 weeks, the ulcer should show substantial (>50%) healing. While another course of medical therapy followed by endoscopy may be applied, failure of a gastric ulcer to heal completely with adequate medical therapy and follow-up is highly suggestive of an underlying malignant process. As such, each EGD should include multiple biopsy specimens taken at the margin of the ulcer. Careful histologic review of these specimens is important. Even so, despite the best efforts of pathologists, false-negative results do occur. Other tests such as cross-sectional imaging and endoscopic ultrasound can further characterize a lesion. Still, even in the absence of a definitive diagnosis, failure of ulcer healing is an indication for elective operation unless a compelling reason exists to preclude a given patient as an operative candidate.

Surgical Treatment

Standard operative therapy for nonhealing, obstructing, or refractory gastric ulcers includes excision because of the possibility of malignancy. For ulcer types I, II, and III, a generous antrectomy (50% gastrectomy) is most commonly performed, and GI continuity is restored to the proximal duodenum (Billroth I reconstruction, Figure 12-4), a loop of proximal jejunum (Billroth II reconstruction, Figure 12-5),

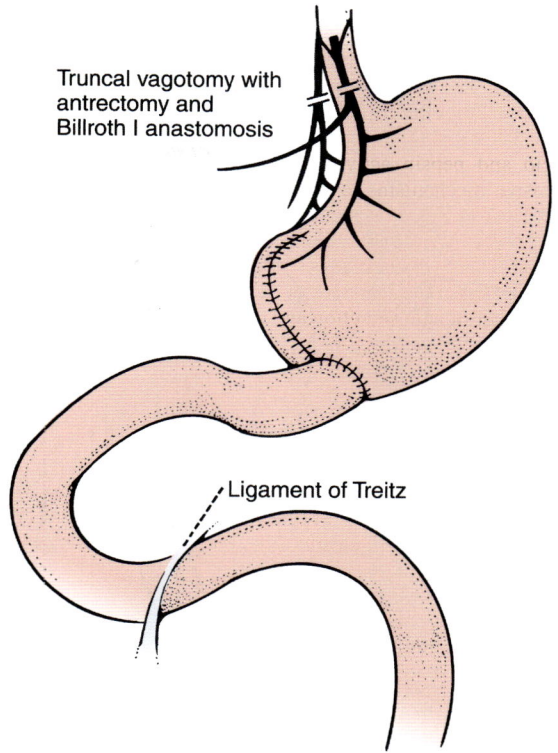

Figure 12-4. An antrectomy removes the distal portion of the stomach, where gastrin is produced. In addition, it removes the pylorus, thus allowing gastric emptying after vagotomy. In a Billroth I reconstruction, the duodenum is anastomosed to the stomach in continuity.

or a transposed limb of jejunum isolated from biliopancreatic secretions (Roux-en-Y reconstruction). All of these reconstructions carry the risk of marginal ulcer formation on the intestinal side of the gastroenteric anastomosis. Roux-en-Y reconstruction, in particular, may be associated with impaired gastric emptying and intestinal transit. Patients with type II and III ulcers often receive truncal vagotomies

TABLE 12-1. Useful Medications Related to PUD			
Medication	**Action/Class**	**Indication**	**Dosage**
Clarithromycin	Antibiotic	*Helicobacter pylori* infection	500 mg po bid (triple therapy)
Amoxicillin	Antibiotic	*H. pylori infection*	1 g po bid (triple therapy)
Metronidazole	Antibiotic	*H. pylori infection*	400 mg po bid (triple therapy) 400 mg po tid (quadruple therapy)
Tetracycline	Antibiotic	*H. pylori infection*	500 mg po daily (quadruple therapy)
Bismuth	Antacid	*H. pylori infection*	120 mg po daily (quadruple therapy)
Omeprazole	Proton pump inhibitor	*H. pylori infection/ulcer healing*	20 mg po bid (triple and quadruple therapy) 80 mg IV bolus then 8 mg/h × 72 h (bleeding ulcer) 20 mg po/IV daily prophylaxis

bid, twice a day; IV, intravenous; po, orally; PUD, peptic ulcer disease; tid, 3 times a day.

Truncal vagotomy with
antrectomy and
Billroth II anastomosis

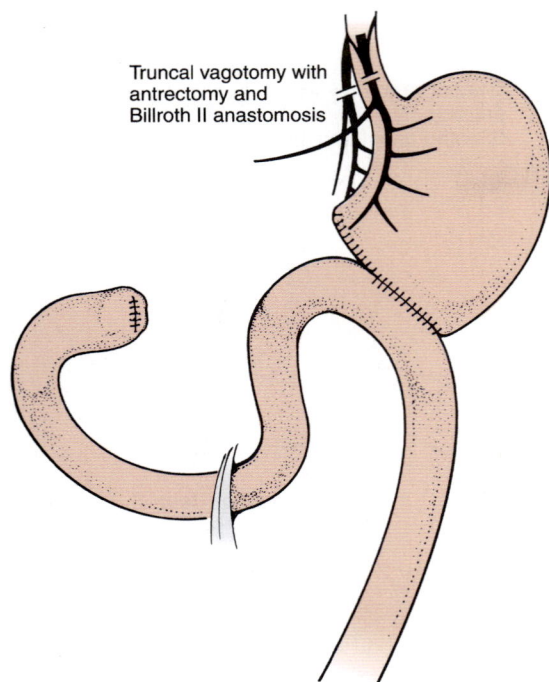

Figure 12-5. In a Billroth II reconstruction, the duodenum is not attached to the stomach; the stomach is anastomosed to a proximal loop of the jejunum. This procedure is particularly useful when the duodenum is extensively scarred.

in addition to antrectomy to further decrease gastric acid secretion. Type IV ulcers, given their proximal location, may require near-total gastrectomy with Roux-en-Y reconstruction, though local excision is also an option. Every resected gastric ulcer must undergo a careful histologic review to verify that a gastric carcinoma is not in the depths of the crater. For this reason, complete excision of the ulcer is always required. If a gastric carcinoma is present, appropriate evaluation and adjunctive treatment are necessary. The recurrence rate after surgical treatment of a gastric ulcer is very low.

In the case of an emergent operation for a perforated pyloric channel ulcer that was previously unrecognized, many surgeons will choose to treat it by oversewing the perforation and/or placing an omental patch without resection. In these situations, the patient is often acutely ill, has not yet undergone evaluation and treatment for *H. pylori* infection or NSAID injury, and the risk of malignancy is low. In this strategy, a follow-up endoscopy is required to confirm complete healing.

Acute Gastritis

Acute gastritis produces an inflammation of the stomach mucosa that may be associated with erosions and hemorrhage. Presenting symptoms vary and may include nausea, vomiting, hematemesis, melena, or hematochezia. *H. pylori* infection, NSAID or aspirin use, bile reflux, alcohol ingestion, irradiation, and local trauma can all contribute to this inflammatory response. Treatment involves acid suppression, removal of the noxious agent, occasional gastric decompression, and nutritional support.

Stress Gastritis

Stress gastritis is another important cause of acute inflammation. It typically occurs in patients suffering from severe physiologic stress, and, if not properly recognized and treated, can lead to significant morbidity and mortality. Patients develop mucosal erosions beginning in the proximal stomach and progressing rapidly throughout the rest of the organ. Classic presentations include ulcer formation in major burn victims (Curling ulcer) and patients with CNS injury (Cushing ulcer). Positive pressure ventilation for greater than 48 hours and the presence of a coagulopathy are also major risk factors. Stress gastritis also occurs in other critically ill patients, such as those with severe trauma, organ failure, or sepsis. Early application of medical prophylaxis for critically ill patients in the intensive care unit using PPIs, H_2-receptor blockers, sucralfate, or misoprostol is necessary since stress gastritis typically develops within 48 hours of the onset of physiologic stress. Without ulcer prophylaxis, about three-quarters of critically ill patients will develop stress ulceration.

Once stress gastritis is present, aggressive acid suppression is essential. Intraluminal pH should not decrease below 4.0 since platelet aggregation and clot stabilization are less effective below this threshold. Primary treatment includes administration of PPIs or H_2 blockers. Sucralfate serves as a secondary therapy in situations in which PPIs or H_2 blockers cannot be used.

Hemorrhage is the most common complication of stress gastritis. It can be occult, overt, or life threatening. Patients may present with blood per rectum or in nasogastric aspirate, or with a drop in blood count or unexplained hemodynamic instability. Immediate treatment should focus on initial fluid resuscitation and stabilization. Upper endoscopy confirms the diagnosis. Gastric lavage to clear the stomach of clots before endoscopy is useful. Electrocautery, heater probe, injection of vasoconstrictive agents, or laser therapy can treat isolated sites of bleeding. Acid suppression is necessary, and the blood bank should be ready for immediate or subsequent transfusion as clinical parameters mandate. Serial blood counts aid in confirming the resolution of the bleed.

In cases of persistent bleeding, more invasive interventions are required. Selective visceral angiography (typically of the left gastric artery) with embolization is one such option. Operative therapy is another. Of the several possible surgical interventions, selective suturing of the bleeding erosions, with possible vagotomy and pyloroplasty (see section "Intractibility under Complicated Peptic Ulcer Disease"), is an expeditious, conservative procedure that controls hemorrhage in approximately 50% of patients. Total gastrectomy is a preferred option in cases of recurrent bleeding.

Hypertrophic Gastritis (Ménétrier Disease)

Hypertrophic gastritis, also known as Ménétrier disease, is a rare disorder of the lining of the stomach characterized by massive hypertrophy of the gastric rugae. It is autoimmune in character, and overexpression of tumor necrosis factor (TNF)-β may play a role. Hyperplasia of the mucus-secreting cells in the corpus and fundus leads to thickening of the mucosal folds. Patients may present with epigastric pain, nausea, vomiting, occult hemorrhage, anorexia, weight loss, and diarrhea. Progression of the disease can result in a protein-losing gastropathy causing hypoproteinemia and peripheral edema. Upper endoscopy with mucosal biopsy is usually sufficient for diagnosis, although a full-thickness surgical biopsy is sometimes required.

Treatment is typically nonoperative and includes acid suppression therapy with PPIs and H_2-receptor antagonists A high-protein diet and careful monitoring of nutritional status are essential. Anticholinergic medications are sometimes useful in decreasing protein loss from gastropathy. In rare instances, total gastrectomy may be required. Ménétrier disease is a risk factor for the development of adenocarcinoma of the stomach.

Mallory-Weiss Syndrome

An upper GI hemorrhage secondary to linear tearing of the mucosa at the GE junction is a well-described phenomenon known as Mallory-Weiss syndrome. Typically, these tears form after episodes in which a strong Valsalva maneuver causes mechanical stress on the mucosa in this region. Retching (often from acute alcohol intoxication), heavy lifting, childbirth, vomiting, blunt abdominal trauma, and seizures can all result in this syndrome. Patients typically present with hematemesis, melena, or hematochezia after such an antecedent history. Evaluation focuses on hemodynamic assessment and verification of a tear as the bleeding source. Nasogastric intubation and gastric lavage are the first steps in management. The presence of blood should prompt endoscopic evaluation. Retroflexion of the flexible endoscope allows for the identification of the tears. Nuclear scintigraphy or selective angiography can also provide a diagnosis if endoscopy is unavailable. Laboratory investigations should include the determination of coagulation parameters and serial blood counts. Blood draw should include a type and crossmatch.

Initial therapy involves fluid resuscitation and stabilization. PPIs or H_2-receptor blockers provide acid suppression. Most bleeding will stop without further intervention; however, if bleeding persists, repeat endoscopy may be required with electrocautery, heater probe, or injection therapy of the tear. Selective angiography with embolization may also be therapeutic. Surgery is a last resort. The presence of subserosal staining along the lesser curve at the time of exploration is pathognomonic. Gastrotomy with oversewing of all tears is undertaken. Rebleeding after any of the above interventions typically occurs within 24 hours.

Gastric Polyps

The increased utilization of diagnostic upper GI endoscopy has led to an increase in the identification of gastric polyps. Hyperplastic polyps are more common and are typically benign, although cancerous transformation rarely occurs. Adenomatous polyps have a higher risk of malignant degeneration, especially those greater than 1.5 cm. In the presence of a gastric polyp, the physician should consider the possibility of polyposis syndromes with additional polyps within the GI tract.

Peutz-Jeghers syndrome is one such example. This condition involves the presence of multiple benign polyps in the small intestine and melanin spots on the lips and buccal mucosa. Polyps can also occur in other portions of the GI tract It is an autosomal dominant trait with a high degree of penetrance. In these patients, the tumors are hamartomas and infrequently malignant, making conservative therapy the preferred option.

Bezoar

A bezoar is an accumulation of a large mass of indigestible fiber within the stomach. A phytobezoar consists exclusively of vegetable fiber, whereas a trichobezoar is made up of hair. Trichobezoars are more common in children and among inmates of mental institutions. Patients with large bezoars can sometimes present with gastric outlet obstruction. Although most bezoars may be broken up using the endoscope, some require surgical gastrotomy for removal.

MALIGNANT GASTRIC DISEASE

Adenocarcinoma of the Stomach

Almost 95% of stomach cancers are adenocarcinomas. Worldwide, adenocarcinoma remains a leading cause of cancer-related death. Its overall incidence, however, has been steadily declining over the last 50 years. In addition, marked regional variability exists. While the frequency of adenocarcinoma in the United States and Europe remains relatively low, it is considerably higher in Asia, particularly Japan and China. High rates of disease also exist in Russia, Chile, and Finland. Environmental factors, especially diet, seem to account for this discrepancy since émigrés from these high-risk areas who settle in the United States have a lower incidence of the disease.

Important risk factors for gastric adenocarcinoma include *H. pylori* infection, pernicious anemia, achlorhydria, and chronic gastritis. A history of caustic injury from lye ingestion also increases the risk of malignant degeneration. Finally, the presence of adenomatous polyps in the stomach is a risk factor for carcinogenesis.

Classification of Gastric Adenocarcinoma

Various histologic and clinical classification schemes exist for adenocarcinoma of the stomach. In the United States, a cancer's endoscopic appearance can be divided into one of four subtypes: ulcerative, polypoid, scirrhous, or superficial spreading Of these, ulcerative carcinomas are by far the most frequent. Even though some differences in prognosis do exist between certain subtypes, the usefulness of this classification system is somewhat limited.

Two distinct histologic types of gastric adenocarcinoma exist: intestinal and diffuse. The intestinal type is more common in regions having a high incidence of disease. Typically, it occurs in older patients and spreads hematogenously. Histologically, cells are well differentiated with glandular elements. The diffuse type occurs in younger patients and has an association with blood type A. It spreads via the lymphatics and local extension. On histology, cells are poorly differentiated with characteristic signet ring cells. *Linitis plastica* is the term used to describe the complete infiltration of the stomach with carcinoma. In this situation, the stomach can look like a leather bottle. Patients with this variant of gastric cancer have a particularly poor prognosis.

Clinical Presentation and Evaluation

The clinical presentation of gastric adenocarcinoma depends on its stage. Early cancers are usually asymptomatic. As a result, in the United States, they often go unrecognized until later in their progression. In Japan, an aggressive endoscopic screening protocol has resulted in more frequently diagnosed early-stage cancer. The low incidence of gastric carcinoma in the United States, however, makes the cost of such a screening prohibitive.

More advanced disease leads to the development of symptoms. Patients can complain of vague epigastric pain similar to that produced by gastric ulceration. Often, it can be present for an extended period. Unexplained weight loss is another early complaint. As the disease progresses, patients begin to have more specific symptoms. Dysphagia, hematemesis, melena, nausea, or vomiting develops. Patients may also present with new onset iron deficiency anemia or guaiac-positive stools.

The initial evaluation for a patient suspected of having gastric carcinoma begins with a thorough history and physical examination. History should include the determination of risk factors and the presence of decreased energy or unintentional weight loss. Physical examination should focus on signs of advanced disease. An enlarged left supraclavicular lymph node (Virchow node) or a palpable umbilical node (Sister Mary Joseph node) indicates distant lymphatic spread. In addition, a palpable rectal ridge (Blumer shelf) or the presence of ascites suggests peritoneal dissemination. All these findings are ominous signs and worrisome for extensive disease. On abdominal examination, the presence of an epigastric mass may indicate a locally advanced tumor.

Diagnostic workup and clinical staging should follow the National Comprehensive Cancer Network (NCCN) consensus guidelines. Upper endoscopy is essential to characterize the location and extent of the disease. In addition, multiple biopsies of the lesion are required to obtain a histologic diagnosis. Often, endoscopic ultrasound can aid in determining the depth of tumor invasion, an important aspect of staging. Metastatic spread to the lungs, liver, and ovaries (Krukenberg tumor) does occur. Imaging studies to rule out such involvement are therefore necessary. CT of the chest, abdomen, and pelvis are adequate screening modalities. Positron emission tomography (PET) is useful for clinical staging, especially in detecting advanced disease. Its accuracy is low, however, in the setting of poorly differentiated or mucinous adenocarcinoma. Laboratory investigations include a complete blood cell count, electrolytes, creatinine level, and liver function tests.

Peritoneal dissemination is present in 20% to 30% of patients with gastric carcinoma. These lesions are difficult to identify using conventional CT. As a result, laparoscopy has become a key component of staging. Patients who do not have any evidence of metastatic disease on initial workup now undergo laparoscopic staging. During this procedure, careful inspection of the abdomen for evidence of peritoneal, hepatic, or omental disease occurs with a biopsy of any suspicious lesions. Abdominal washings are sent for cytology, and the local extent of the tumor is determined. The presence of metastatic disease precludes curative resection and can help avoid an unnecessary laparotomy.

Treatment

In the presence of localized disease, curative resection is possible. Considerable debate exists regarding the extent of such a resection. For most distal lesions, many surgeons favor a radical subtotal gastrectomy involving the removal of approximately 85% of the stomach and the entire omentum. The proximal portion of the resected specimen requires immediate frozen section analysis by the pathologist to verify that it is free of tumor involvement. Only after verification of a clear proximal margin is GI continuity restored by means of a Roux-en-Y gastrojejunostomy. Large distal lesions or proximal tumors will typically require total gastrectomy. Splenectomy or pancreatectomy may also be part of the operative procedure. They should only occur, however, when they are unavoidable.

The extent of lymph node dissection at the time of resection remains a topic of discussion. The Japanese favor a radical lymphadenectomy. In the United States, a less extensive dissection is undertaken. Comparisons between the two approaches in Japan point toward improved survival in those patients having radical lymph node removal. In Western countries, results are less definitive. In fact, the more extensive dissections seem to cause higher morbidity without an overall survival benefit. Nonetheless, long-term results do point to a reduction in locoregional recurrence and cancer-specific survival. Regardless of the extent of the dissection, the surgeon must harvest at least 15 lymph nodes as part of the lymphadenectomy for adequate staging of lymph node disease. Key lymph node basins to include in a lymphadenectomy are the infrapyloric, left gastric, and right paracardiac regions. Currently, patients should undergo perioperative (pre- and postoperative) chemotherapy in resectable lesions that clinically appear to invade beyond the lamina propria or have positive nodes. The most effective regimen includes 5-fluorouracil, leucovorin, oxaliplatin, and docetaxel. In patients undergoing resection without preoperative chemotherapy, postoperative chemotherapy has utility in large-size tumors (ie, T3 and T4) and node-positive disease, typically with capecitabine and oxaliplatin. The addition of chemoradiotherapy with chemotherapy may also have utility in such settings. Similarly, it decreases local recurrence rates in patients who do not undergo a radical lymphadenectomy or who have positive margins after resection. Less invasive lesions (ie, those only invading the submucosa) typically do not require preoperative chemoradiotherapy. Several studies investigating preoperative chemoradiotherapy with perioperative chemotherapy are currently accruing patients. The best cure rates occur in Japan, where a high percentage of the superficial spreading type disease is present. Even with this type of tumor, the 5-year survival rate can be less than 50%. In most studies from English-speaking countries, curative resection is associated with a 5-year survival rate of less than 10%. Pathologic staging of the resected specimen is the best predictor of survival. In patients who had an incidental carcinoma found during stomach surgery for a supposed benign disease, the 5-year survival rate approaches 75%.

Although the majority of patients with metastatic disease are incurable, recent data suggest that aggressive surgical resection of residual disease can lead to long-term survival in select patients whose disease appears resectable after initial chemotherapy. In patients with isolated gross peritoneal disease, cytoreductive surgery with or without hyperthermic intraperitoneal chemotherapy (HIPEC) is an option at specialized centers. Its efficacy, however, remains controversial. Patients with occult peritoneal disease (eg, positive cytology) have very poor prognoses. Studies are currently underway to investigate HIPEC in these situations.

Palliative therapy should focus on quality of life. Because the morbidity and mortality associated with palliative surgery can be high, its judicious use is paramount. In selected patients with good preoperative status, it may be beneficial. The resection should include the lesion, with an adequate cephalic margin, and the entire stomach distal to the tumor. Clear indications for palliative surgical intervention include proximal or distal tumor obstruction and bleeding. Endoscopic stent placement, especially in patients with short life expectancy, and laser therapy are also palliative options.

Gastric Lymphoma

The stomach is the primary source of almost two-thirds of all GI lymphomas. Patients with gastric lymphoma tend to be older and male. The non-Hodgkin variant predominates. The two major subtypes include the low-grade marginal zone B-cell lymphoma of the mucosa-associated lymphoid tissue (MALT) and the high-grade diffuse large B-cell lymphoma (DLBCL). MALT arises in the setting of chronic gastritis due to *H. pylori* infection. Patients typically present with symptoms similar to those seen in gastric adenocarcinoma. Upper abdominal pain, unexplained weight loss, fatigue, and bleeding can occur. Diffuse involvement of the stomach wall in MALT can present with perforation. Upper endoscopy with tissue biopsies remains the primary means of diagnosis of primary gastric lymphomas. Sometimes, however, the presence of lymphoma is only determined at the time of surgical exploration. Once one has established the diagnosis of primary gastric lymphoma, its staging should follow that undertaken for other lymphomas. It typically includes chest, abdomen, and pelvic CT; bone may also play a role. Finally, PET/CT can be useful in patients with the DLBCL subtype.

The treatment of primary gastric lymphoma has traditionally included a wide range of interventions, ranging from chemotherapy, radiation, and surgery, alone or in combination. More recently, immunochemotherapy involving rituximab, cyclophosphamide, doxorubicin, vincristine, and prednisone (R-CHOP), has resulted in high 5-year survival rates in patients with DLBCL. In patients with early-stage MALT, *H. pylori* eradication alone can lead to cure rates approaching 75%. Surgical intervention is currently an intervention reserved only for major complications including hemorrhage and perforation.

Gastrointestinal Stromal Tumor

Gastrointestinal stromal tumors (GISTs) constitute the most common form of GI tract sarcomas. They are submucosal growths arising from a variety of cell types. Over half of these masses are located in the stomach. GISTs can be either benign or malignant, but, unless direct invasion is present, differentiation between the two is often difficult. Large tumor size (>6 cm) and tumor necrosis suggest malignancy. Typically, the finding of more than 10 mitotic figures per 50 high-powered fields on histologic examination is indicative of malignancy.

The clinical presentation of GISTs is similar to other gastric tumors. Many patients are asymptomatic. Nonspecific abdominal pain can occur. Bleeding and obstruction can be manifestations. Finally, some patients present with an abdominal mass. Evaluation typically involves upper endoscopy, which reveals a submucosal mass. Central ulceration may be present. Biopsy is usually nondiagnostic. Endoscopic ultrasound is a useful adjunct. Chest, abdominal, and pelvic CT aids in determining the tumor size,

presence of invasion, and evidence of metastasis. The liver is the most common site for disseminated disease. PET/CT is useful in cases of ambiguous results on imaging. Genetic next-generation sequencing (NGS) helps tailor chemotherapy by identifying mutations most susceptible to certain drugs.

Treatment of suitable stomach GISTs involves local excision with negative histologic margins. Because of the risk of malignancy in the tumor, enucleation is not an option. Disruption of the tumor capsule with consequent tumor spillage increases the risk of recurrence. The extent of the tumor influences the gastric resection pursued. Patient survival following resection depends on the presence of malignancy. The prognosis for a benign lesion is excellent. Malignant GIST, however, can be quite aggressive.

Gastric GISTs less than 2 cm require fine needle aspiration or core needle biopsy under endoscopic ultrasound guidance. Tumors without high-risk features can undergo endoscopic observation. Those GISTs with high-risk features such as a large number of mitoses or tumor necrosis require resection. In situations where resection might lead to high morbidity, NGS-guided neoadjuvant therapy using imatinib mesylate or its derivatives can shrink the tumor to minimize potential morbidity and allow for resection. In successfully resected disease, the use of adjuvant chemotherapy with these substrates depends on the presence of high-risk features (tumor spillage, large size, high mitotic index). In the setting of metastatic disease, debulking surgery in combination with chemotherapy has a role in treatment.

BENIGN DUODENAL DISEASE

Uncomplicated Duodenal Ulcer Disease

Globally, PUD affects approximately 4 million people each year. In the United States, it accounts for billions of dollars in health care expenditures. Duodenal ulcers constitute the majority of this disease burden. They typically form in the duodenal bulb. *H. pylori* and NSAIDs are important ulcerogenic agents. An association with tobacco also exists. In contrast to gastric ulcers, duodenal ulcers rarely harbor any underlying malignancy. Their workup and treatment, therefore, differ somewhat from the evaluation and therapy of gastric ulcers.

Most duodenal ulcer disease is uncomplicated. The identification of *H. pylori* as a potential ulcerogenic agent and the development of effective acid suppression medications were seminal events in the evolution of care, shifting its treatment from the domain of the surgeon to that of the internist.

Clinical Presentation and Evaluation

The clinical presentation of uncomplicated duodenal ulceration has features similar to that of uncomplicated gastric ulcer disease. Patients often complain of a burning epigastric abdominal pain that is gnawing in character. It may radiate to the back, especially if the ulcer is located in the posterior aspect of the duodenal bulb. Certain aspects of presentation, however, are different from uncomplicated gastric ulceration. The pain typically occurs 1 to 3 hours after food ingestion and is worse with fasting. It may awaken patients from sleep. Relief from pain typically occurs after the use of over-the-counter acid suppressants. Food intake can also improve pain, leading to weight gain in some patients.

A thorough history and physical examination remain important components of the initial evaluation of the patient suspected of having uncomplicated duodenal ulceration. In addition to characterizing the nature of the pain, risk factors are determined. They include a history of PUD, prior *H. pylori* infection, NSAID ingestion, or tobacco use. Physical examination focuses on the abdomen. Mild epigastric tenderness on palpation may be present. Signs of occult blood loss may be present. Pallor, orthostasis, and guaiac-positive stools are significant findings.

Diagnostic Testing
The diagnosis of uncomplicated duodenal ulceration is often empiric. In the patient with typical signs and symptoms, noninvasive testing for the presence of *H. pylori* infection is undertaken. Both quantitative and qualitative serologic antibody testing exist. These studies have the advantage of low cost and wide availability. Their accuracy, however, depends on the probability of infection. In developed countries, they are particularly useful at identifying active *H. pylori* infection among younger patients because of its low incidence. The presence of antibody in older individuals, however, is a less reliable indicator of active disease.

Urease testing and fecal antigen testing are both effective in diagnosing active disease and documenting successful eradication. The urease tests detect increased carbon dioxide in blood or breath due to *H. pylori*'s hydrolyzing urea with its urease. The antigen test identifies *H. pylori*–specific antigen in the stool. PPIs and bismuth compounds can lead to false-negative results.

In patients with characteristic symptoms, upper endoscopy is the diagnostic modality of choice. In such cases, it leads to direct visualization and characterization of the ulceration. It can also identify concomitant disease or suggest an alternative diagnosis. Finally, it provides a means of obtaining biopsies. Typically, antral tissue biopsy allows for the detection of *H. pylori* via rapid urease testing, culture growth, or histologic analysis.

Treatment
First-line therapy of uncomplicated duodenal ulcer disease focuses on promoting ulcer healing and preventing its recurrence. Patients should stop all ulcerogenic agents, especially tobacco and NSAID/aspirin use. They should start on acid suppression therapy. Finally, if *H. pylori* infection is present, its eradication is mandatory. Due to the tenacity of the organism and growing antibiotic resistance, two or more antibiotics are required to treat adequately any infection, typically in combination with PPIs or H_2-receptor antagonists.

The preferred method of eradication is clarithromycin-based triple therapy of at least 7-day duration. This regimen includes clarithromycin paired with amoxicillin or metronidazole and acid suppression. In situations in which clarithromycin resistance is high, traditional quadruple therapy using an acid suppression drug, bismuth, metronidazole, and tetracycline for 7 to 14 days is the alternative treatment. Successful eradication requires confirmation with urease or fecal antigen testing. With eradication of *H. pylori*, rapid healing of duodenal ulcers and resolution of gastritis occur. In addition, recurrence rates for both duodenal and gastric ulcers are lower.

Acid suppression therapy is necessary until complete healing of the ulcer occurs. If the etiology of the ulcer is apparent, discontinuation of PPIs or H_2-receptor antagonists occurs over a relatively short time interval. If the etiology of the ulcer is unclear, their administration continues until its cause is determined and treated.

Complicated Peptic Ulcer Disease
Complicated PUD has four main manifestations: perforation, hemorrhage, gastric outlet obstruction, and intractability. As a result, the presentation, evaluation, and initial treatment of complicated duodenal ulcer disease and complicated gastric ulcer disease are the same. Differences in care can arise at the time of surgical intervention.

Clinical Presentation and Evaluation
The type of complication determines the clinical presentation and evaluation. Patients with perforated ulcers present with acute onset of severe epigastric pain. Often, they are able to report the exact time of day that the symptoms began. Physical examination usually reveals tachycardia and evidence of a rigid (surgical) abdomen resulting from diffuse chemical peritonitis. Occasionally, however, a more localized peritonitis may develop as gastric acid drains into the right paracolic gutter. In such cases, the patient presents with right lower quadrant rebound tenderness very similar to that seen in acute appendicitis. Evaluation should include an upright chest radiograph. Evidence of free intraperitoneal air (pneumoperitoneum) outlining the diaphragm or liver is diagnostic of a perforated intra-abdominal viscus (Figure 12-6). Patients should also have a complete blood count and a basic metabolic panel drawn.

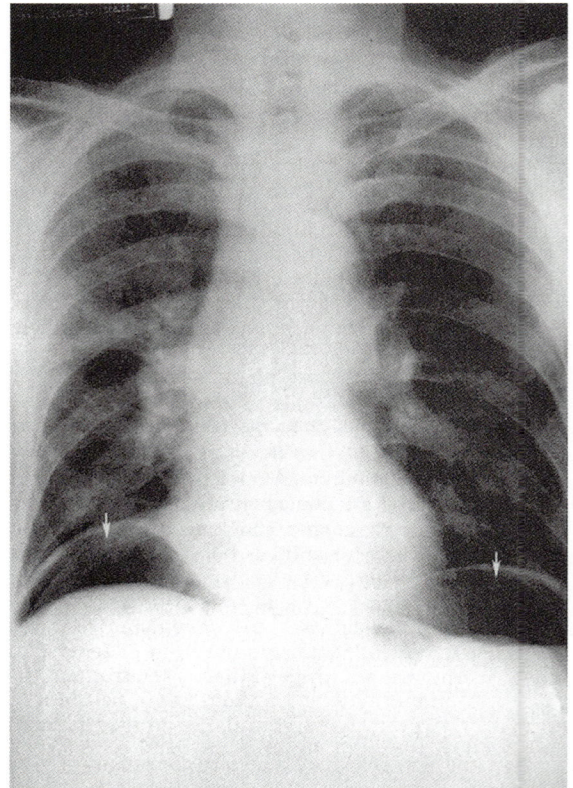

Figure 12-6. An upright posteroanterior chest radiograph often shows subdiaphragmatic air (white arrows) in patients with a perforated ulcer.

A patient presenting with a bleeding ulcer will report hematemesis, melena, or blood per rectum. Massive bleeding can occur, and some patients may exhibit signs of early or late shock. Physical examination may reveal hypotension, tachycardia, pallor, mental status changes, and active bleeding. In such cases, volume resuscitation with crystalloid or whole blood is required. Evaluation of any GI hemorrhage should focus on determining the site of bleeding. The first step involves the placement of a nasogastric tube followed by gastric lavage. The presence of blood suggests an upper GI source. Endoscopy is confirmatory, and it allows characterization of the ulcer and determination of *H. pylori* status. Patients with bleeding ulcers should have serial hematocrits followed and coagulation parameters determined. Finally, blood type and crossmatch should be ready at all times.

Patients with gastric outlet obstruction resulting from chronic ulcer scarring will complain of inability to tolerate oral intake. In particular, they may report projectile vomiting of food shortly after eating, much like infants with pyloric stenosis. A history of weight loss is common. These patients often delay seeking medical attention. As a result, they suffer from varying degrees of dehydration. Physical examination may reveal upper abdominal fullness, decreased skin turgor, dry mucus membranes, or epigastric peristaltic waves. Evaluation should focus on assessing the extent of metabolic derangement. Electrolyte and creatinine levels are informative. Often, these patients develop a hypokalemic, hypochloremic metabolic alkalosis. In severe cases, they will have evidence of paradoxical aciduria as the distal renal tubules sacrifice hydrogen ions for potassium (see Chapter 2).

Finally, patients with intractable ulcers will have symptoms of persistent disease after adequate nonoperative therapy. Often, these individuals will have undergone multiple treatments for ulceration without relief or healing. In addition, they may develop a recurrence of the disease after an apparently successful initial therapy. Fortunately, such patients are becoming less frequent. Physical examination in these patients mirrors findings seen in uncomplicated PUD. Intractability should alert the clinician to the possibility of rarer causes of ulceration (see the section "Zollinger-Ellison Syndrome").

Treatment

The treatment of complicated PUD typically involves an initial stabilization phase. During this period, the patient undergoes resuscitation and receives nonoperative therapies. Depending on a patient's complication and response to treatment, this phase can be definitive. Otherwise, the patient will require operative intervention. Surgical intervention should pursue two objectives: (1) proper treatment of the complication and (2) performance of a definitive antisecretory procedure to minimize recurrence. A full discussion of antisecretory procedures is present in section "Intractability."

Perforation

A perforated ulcer is a surgical emergency. Preparation for the operating room includes fluid resuscitation and nasogastric decompression. At the time of surgical exploration, identification of the site of perforation is essential. Typically, the perforation occurs on the anterior aspect of the duodenal bulb. Due to the effectiveness of medical therapy, the performance of a definitive acid-reducing surgery during acute surgical treatment of a perforation is no longer mandatory. Typically, the surgeon oversews the ulcer and buttresses it with a tag of omentum (Graham patch). In the postoperative period, the patient then undergoes intensive treatment with PPIs and antibiotics to eradicate *H. pylori*. Both open and laparoscopic repair of simple perforated duodenal ulcers is possible.

Complex perforated duodenal ulcers can be therapeutic challenges. Large, friable ulcers are difficult to close. In such circumstances, extensive procedures are required. They focus on patching the opening or excluding it from the flow of GI contents. Adequate drainage of the duodenal region is essential.

In rare cases, patients with a perforated ulcer undergo nonoperative therapy. Typically, the patient is a clinically stable older individual with multiple medical problems who presents relatively late (12 or more hours) after the onset of symptoms. Because of the high operative risk, these patients have therapy consisting of nasogastric decompression, volume resuscitation, nothing by mouth, and serial abdominal examinations with blood laboratories. If the perforation has sealed off, they will improve and avoid operation. Any clinical deterioration, however, requires surgical intervention.

Hemorrhage

In patients who have upper GI hemorrhage, initial stabilization is necessary with placement of at least two large-bore intravenous lines and volume resuscitation following Advanced Trauma Life Support (ATLS) guidelines. Stabilization also includes nasogastric decompression, high-dose PPI therapy, and correction of coagulation abnormalities.

Upper endoscopy constitutes the first-line therapy for ulcer hemorrhage. Options include electrocautery, heater probe, or injection therapy. Using such techniques, most cases of bleeding stop without surgical intervention. Endoscopic signs worrisome for risk of rebleeding include active hemorrhage at the time of endoscopy, a visible vessel in the ulcer crater, and fresh clot on the ulcer. Repeat endoscopy can occur with rebleeding. In patients with high operative risk, angiography with selective embolization is an option.

Refractory bleeding requires surgical intervention. In general, a transfusion requirement of six or more units of blood over the first 12 hours is an indication of surgery. Older patients or those who are hemodynamically unstable may require earlier operative therapy. Younger, more stable patients may undergo a longer period of resuscitation. At the time of laparotomy, the surgeon ligates the bleeding artery. In the case of a posterior duodenal ulcer, duodenotomy with three-point U-stitch fixation of the ulcer bed is necessary. In a type IV gastric ulcer, left gastric artery ligation may be necessary.

Gastric Outlet Obstruction

In patients with gastric outlet obstruction, the stomach is decompressed with a nasogastric tube for 5 or 6 days or until it returns to near-normal size. During this time, the patient has nothing by mouth and receives intravenous nutrition and fluids. Because the patient is hypochloremic and alkalotic, initial resuscitation should be with a normal saline crystalloid solution with careful monitoring of electrolytes.

Most cases of gastric outlet obstruction require operative intervention because of the cicatricial scarring around the site of the ulcer. Such procedures require either the removal of the obstruction or its bypass. Typical treatment involves antrectomy with appropriate reconstruction. If antrectomy is not possible, drainage of the stomach via a gastroenterostomy is necessary. In either case, the surgeon should perform an acid-reducing procedure as well.

In some cases, the gastric outlet obstruction develops due to mucosal edema rather than scarring. The prolonged nasogastric decompression helps decrease the swelling and provides resolution of the obstruction. Endoscopy, however, is still required to characterize the extent of scarring, biopsy any suspicious lesions, and screen for *H. pylori*.

Intractability

Patients with ulcers unresponsive to conventional medical management have intractable disease. They may require surgical intervention to decrease acid secretion. The surgeon can alter such secretion through interruption of the vagal neural pathway with or without removal of the gastrin-producing cells in the antrum.

The most straightforward approach to vagal interruption is by means of a truncal vagotomy. In this procedure, all vagal trunks at or above the esophageal hiatus of the diaphragm are completely transected. This intervention denervates the entire parietal cell mass. Unfortunately, truncal vagotomy also denervates the antral pump, the pyloric sphincter mechanism, and most of the abdominal viscera, disrupting gastric motility. A gastric drainage procedure to facilitate gastric emptying is therefore necessary. Otherwise, gastric antral dilation occurs, stimulating gastrin release. The most common complementary drainage procedure is pyloroplasty, which involves incising the pylorus horizontally and closing it vertically (Figure 12-7). Various eponymous modifications of pyloroplasty have been proposed. If pyloroplasty is not possible, gastroenterostomy is an alternative. Many surgeons add distal gastrectomy (antrectomy) to the truncal vagotomy (Figure 12-4). Antrectomy augments the effect of vagotomy by removing the bulk of the gastrin-producing cells (G cells). This combination interrupts both the cephalic phase and the gastric phase of acid stimulation. Truncal vagotomy with antrectomy has a lower ulcer recurrence rate than truncal vagotomy with pyloroplasty.

Selective vagotomy and highly selective vagotomy were attempts in the past to limit complications associated with truncal vagotomy while keeping recurrence rates low. Due to their technical difficulty and higher recurrence rates, they have fallen out of use with the advent of successful medical therapy for ulcer disease.

Duodenal Polyps

Duodenal polyps typically arise as part of an inherited familial disorder. Familial adenomatous polyposis (FAP) is a well-known one. This autosomal dominant syndrome involving mutations in the adenomatous polyposis coli (APC) gene results in the development of multiple adenomatous polyps in the colon and gastroduodenal region. Because of the possibility of malignant degeneration of these polyps, these patients require close monitoring. They typically require early prophylactic removal of the colon. Starting around 25 years of age, all patients need routine endoscopic surveillance of the stomach and duodenum with the removal of any polyps. Interval follow-up or the need for surgery depends on the number of polyps present, their size, histology, and the presence of dysplasia. Evidence of cancer or villous adenoma in a duodenal polyp requires surgical excision. Depending on the location of the polyps, segmental duodenectomy, pylorus-sparing pancreaticoduodenectomy, and pancreaticoduodenectomy are surgical options. Another important condition is Peutz-Jeghers syndrome (see section "Gastric Polyps").

MALIGNANT DUODENAL DISEASE

Zollinger-Ellison Syndrome

Although very rare, Zollinger-Ellison syndrome (ZES) is the most common functioning neuroendocrine tumor (NET) disorder of the duodenum. It is the direct result of a gastrin-producing neoplasm (gastrinoma). The resultant hypergastrinemia causes near-maximal stimulation of the parietal cell mass and constant HCl secretion. Over two-thirds of these tumors are located in an anatomic triangle whose apices include the junction of the cystic duct with the common bile duct, the junction of the second and third portions of the duodenum, and the neck of the pancreas.

Gastrinomas can occur sporadically or as part of an inherited familial disorder. A strong association exists with the multiple endocrine neoplasia type 1 (MEN-1) syndrome. Patients with this disorder develop a clinical constellation of pituitary adenomas, hyperparathyroidism, and pancreatic islet cell tumors (of which gastrinomas are the most common). Approximately 60% of all gastrinomas are malignant. Five-year survival in the setting of metastatic disease is poor, improving some with locoregional disease. In the setting of localized disease, long-term survival is possible.

Clinical Presentation and Evaluation

A high degree of suspicion is necessary to identify patients with ZES. Often, unusual clinical presentations

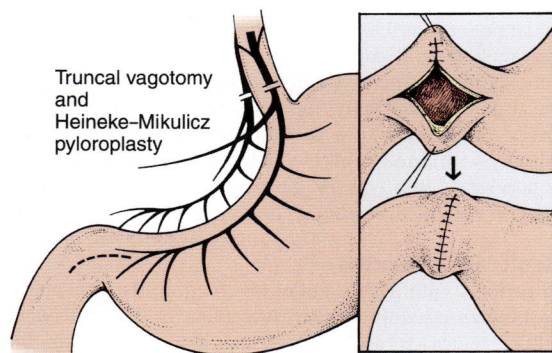

Figure 12-7. When the trunk of the vagus nerve is divided, a pyloroplasty is also performed to allow gastric emptying. This pyloroplasty is the most common type performed.

Truncal vagotomy and Heineke–Mikulicz pyloroplasty

suggest the diagnosis. Symptoms of ulcer disease with concomitant chronic or severe diathesis with can result from multiple duodenal ulcers or ulceration in atypical locations (jejunum or ileum). Patients may also report a personal or family history of refractory PUD or neuroendocrine disease.

Evaluation begins with a thorough history and physical examination focused on establishing the presence of any of the above-mentioned associations. In particular, a personal or family history of MEN-1 and its associated disorders may be present. Diagnosis rests on establishing the presence of hypergastrinemia with hypersecretion of acid. A fasting serum gastrin level and gastric pH testing are necessary. The surgeon must make sure that the patient has discontinued any PPIs for at least 1 week prior to testing because they tend to increase gastrin levels and decrease gastric pH. The presence of elevated gastrin levels above 1,000 pg/mL in the setting of a gastric pH less than 2 is diagnostic. Abnormal values less than 1,000 pg/mL with gastric pH less than 2 should prompt further confirmatory testing. The investigation of choice is the secretin stimulation test. In addition to being safe, it has high specificity and sensitivity. After the intravenous infusion of secretin, blood draws at 2, 5, 10, 15, 30, 45, and 60 minutes occur with calculation of fasting serum gastrin levels. In patients with ZES, an elevation in the baseline gastrin value occurs, typically greater than or equal to 200 pg/mL. With the diagnosis of ZES, further evaluation should focus on tumor localization and clinical staging. Commonly used imaging modalities include CT, magnetic resonance imaging, and ultrasonography. Somatostatin receptor scintigraphy and, more recently, somatostatin PET/CT are effective in identifying disease. Endoscopic ultrasound is also useful in tumor localization. These neoplasms are often quite small and, as a result, their preoperative localization can be difficult. A thorough search is useful, however, because knowing the site of the primary tumor helps with operative planning. The liver is the most common site for metastatic disease.

Finally, all patients with newly diagnosed ZES should undergo some form of screening for MEN-1 syndrome. Although genetic testing is available, it requires thorough pretest counseling. A more straightforward screen is to obtain a serum calcium level. If it is elevated, a parathyroid hormone level should be determined. The presence of hyperparathyroidism is highly suggestive of concomitant MEN-1 (see Chapter 18).

Treatment

Traditional therapy for ZES involved total gastrectomy with esophageal anastomosis, a procedure associated with high mortality, pernicious anemia, malnutrition, and weight loss. Advances in care, however, have drastically changed the approach to ZES. Patients start high-dose PPIs to lower the production of HCl, prevent ulcer diathesis, and improve hypersecretory diarrhea. Patients having sporadic gastrinoma without metastasis should undergo surgical exploration and, with successful localization, removal of the tumor by enucleation. Successful removal of the neoplasm can result in cure. Lymphadenectomy should accompany enucleation.

The role of surgery in patients having gastrinoma in association with MEN-1 is more complex. If hyperparathyroidism is present, the patient should first undergo a parathyroidectomy because it attenuates gastrin release. Because cure is rarer in patients with MEN-1, some experts do not recommend surgical exploration in patients without metastasis. Others recommend resection in tumors greater than 2 cm in size. Since enucleation seldom results in cure in this group of patients, pancreaticoduodenectomy is the preferred choice of operation.

The presence of metastatic disease decreases survival. Some experts recommend surgical debulking in combination with medical therapy if 80% of disease removal is feasible. Other options include chemotherapy and hepatic embolization. Hormonal manipulation using long-acting synthetic analogues of somatostatin (octreotide) can also be effective. Octreotide suppresses the elevated gastrin concentrations and may help in slowing tumor growth. All patients with metastatic disease, as well as those whose tumors are not located at surgical exploration, require continued PPI therapy. Recently, combined capecitabine and temozolomide therapy and peptide receptor radionuclide therapy have shown promise in treating patients with metastatic disease.

Adenocarcinoma of the Duodenum

The duodenum is the most common site for adenocarcinoma in the small bowel. Approximately two-thirds of these lesions are located in the second part of the duodenum, usually in the periampullary region. Fortunately, it is a rare disease because patients typically present late in its course. Symptoms can range from nonspecific abdominal pain with weight loss to those of intestinal or gastric outlet obstruction. Some patients will present with melena or hematochezia due to ulceration of the lesion. Physical examination often is unremarkable. Upper endoscopy with tissue biopsy makes the diagnosis. CT is helpful in determining evidence of local invasion or metastatic spread.

In resectable disease, surgical excision is possible. Pancreaticoduodenectomy is typically the preferred intervention for tumors in the first or second portion of the duodenum. An extended small bowel resection with duodenojejunostomy is effective when the tumor is limited to the third or fourth portion of the duodenum. Patients with unresectable disease or evidence of metastasis at the time of exploration should have a diverting gastroenterostomy. Postoperative radiation therapy may be helpful. In patients with positive lymph nodes, prognosis is very poor, with 5-year survivals below 15%.

Duodenal Lymphoma

Lymphoma of the duodenum is also relatively rare; most small bowel primaries occur in the ileum. The clinical presentation is similar to that for duodenal adenocarcinoma. Abdominal pain, weight loss, and fatigue are common. Complications include perforation, bleeding, or obstruction. Endoscopy may be helpful in diagnosing duodenal lymphomas. CT assists in determining disease extent. In the setting of a diagnosis made prior to surgical exploration, the patient should undergo complete clinical staging, following guidelines similar to those for gastric lymphoma. In resectable disease, the surgeon should perform wide surgical excision with staging. Adjuvant chemotherapy is an option in the postoperative period. Patients with disseminated disease receive chemotherapy and local radiation.

POSTGASTRECTOMY COMPLICATIONS

Postgastrectomy Syndromes

Changes in anatomy, physiology, and reconstruction combine to produce the postgastrectomy syndromes commonly encountered after resection. Workup of patients presenting with symptoms associated with them includes an upper GI series to assess the extent of gastric resection, type of reconstruction, gastric motility, and gastric emptying. CT is also useful in diagnosis and ruling out other differentials. Endoscopy allows for direct visualization of the anatomy and biopsy of suspicious lesions. When necessary, a radionuclide-labeled gastric emptying study can lend insight into gastric physiology.

A useful way to approach postgastrectomy syndromes is to categorize them according to their predominant etiology. This sort of classification aids in understanding the pathophysiology involved. Groupings include syndromes related to gastric reservoir dysfunction, vagal denervation, and reconstruction anatomy as well as those disorders due to long-term complications.

Disorders Related to Gastric Reservoir Dysfunction
Early Dumping Syndrome
Early dumping syndrome arises with the ingestion of high osmolarity foods. The typical inciting meal contains a large quantity of simple and complex sugars (eg, milk products). Approximately 15 minutes after its ingestion, the patient develops vasomotor symptoms including anxiety, weakness, tachycardia, diaphoresis, and palpitations. Weakness may be so severe that the patient desires to lie down. Other associated symptoms include crampy abdominal pain, borborygmi, and diarrhea. Gradually, the symptoms clear.

This early dumping syndrome results from uncontrolled emptying of hypertonic fluid into the small intestine. Fluid moves rapidly from the intravascular space into the intraluminal space, producing acute intravascular volume depletion. As the simple sugars are absorbed and as dilution of the hypertonic solution occurs, symptoms gradually abate. Fluid shifts from the intracellular space and absorption from the intestinal lumen restore intravascular volume. The release of several hormonal substances, including serotonin, neurotensin, histamine, glucagon, VIP, and kinins, also contributes to the symptom complex.

Initial therapy for early dumping syndrome includes slowly eating frequent, small meals at least 6 times a day, avoiding complex sugar foods, consuming liquids at least 30 minutes before or after eating solid foods, and eating a diet high in protein and fiber. In refractory cases, somatostatin analogues are useful. Its use may follow a trial of acarbose (see section "Late Dumping Syndrome"). In some patients with Billroth I or II anastomoses and recalcitrant symptoms, surgical revision of these reconstructions to a Roux-en-Y gastrojejunostomy may be necessary.

Late Dumping Syndrome
As in early dumping, the patient suddenly has anxiety, diaphoresis, tachycardia, palpitations, weakness, fatigue, and a desire to lie down. In late dumping, the symptoms usually begin within 3 hours after the meal. This variant of dumping is not associated with borborygmi or diarrhea. The physiologic explanation for late dumping involves rapid changes in serum glucose and insulin levels. After the meal, a large bolus of glucose-containing chyme is present in the small intestine. In this setting, glucose absorption occurs much more rapidly than when an intact pylorus aids in metering gastric emptying. Extremely high serum glucose levels may occur shortly after the meal and may elicit a profound release of insulin. The insulin response exceeds what is necessary to clear the glucose from the blood, and subsequently, hypoglycemia results. Thus, the symptoms of late dumping are the direct result of rapid fluctuations in serum glucose levels.

As in early dumping syndrome, initial therapy involves diet modification. In addition, a small snack (eg, crackers and peanut butter) 2 hours after meals is helpful in ameliorating symptoms. If diet modification fails, acarbose, an α-glycosidase hydrolase inhibitor, can prevent symptoms of late dumping syndrome. Refractory cases require revisional surgery to a Billroth I or Roux-en-Y gastrojejunostomy. Table 12-2 summarizes the differences between early and late dumping syndromes.

Metabolic Disturbances
Although a variety of metabolic abnormalities can occur after gastric resection, anemias are the most common. Vitamin B_{12} or folate deficiency from decreased absorption can lead to megaloblastic anemia in patients not receiving appropriate supplementation. Iron deficiency secondary to altered absorption or chronic blood loss can produce microcytic anemia requiring iron replacement therapy and treatment of any chronic bleeding.

Altered bowel function is common following gastric reconstructions. Patients can develop frequent, loose stools postoperatively (see Table 12-3 for medications to treat postgastrectomy syndromes). The increased intestinal transit, if rapid enough, can lead to steatorrhea. Calcium

TABLE 12-2. Comparison of Early Versus Late Dumping Pathophysiology		
	Early Dumping	**Late Dumping**
Presentation	15-30 min after a hyperosmolar meal	1-3 h following a hyperosmolar meal
Symptoms	Abdominal: nausea, vomiting, diarrhea, abdominal cramps Vasomotor: sweating, weakness, palpitations, dizziness	Vasomotor: sweating, weakness, palpitations, difficulty concentrating, hunger
Etiology	Rapid emptying of hyperosmolar contents into the small bowel causing osmotic shifts and release of vasoactive substances	Rapid change in serum glucose and insulin levels resulting in rapid decline in blood glucose levels (hypoglycemia)

TABLE 12-3. Useful Medications Related to Postgastrectomy Syndromes

Medication	Action	Indication	Dosage
Acarbose	α-Glucosidase hydrolase inhibitor	Late dumping syndrome	50-100 mg po tid
Cholestyramine	Bile salt binding agent	Postvagotomy diarrhea, alkaline reflux gastritis	1 packet daily to start
Somatostatin	Secretory inhibitor	Postvagotomy diarrhea, dumping syndrome	Long-acting form—20 mg IM monthly
Metoclopramide	Promotility agent	Gastric atony	10 mg po 30 min before each meal and at bedtime
Sucralfate	GI protectant	Marginal ulcer, alkaline reflux gastritis	1 g po qid
Diphenoxylate hydrochloride	Antidiarrheal agent	Postvagotomy diarrhea	5 mg po qid
Loperamide	Antidiarrheal agent	Postvagotomy diarrhea	4 mg followed by 2 mg po after each unformed stool; not to exceed 16 mg/d

GI, gastrointestinal; IM, intramuscularly; po, orally; qid, 4 times a day; tid, 3 times a day.

and magnesium can chelate to intestinal fats, leading to decreased absorption with resultant osteomalacia. Supplemental calcium as well as bisphosphonates can prevent such bone loss.

Disorders Related to Vagal Denervation
Postvagotomy Diarrhea
Almost half the patients who undergo truncal vagotomy experience a change in bowel habits (ie, increased frequency, more liquid consistency). In most cases, the symptoms improve or disappear with time. In a small percentage of patients (<1%), severe diarrhea persists and does not relent with time. The diarrhea can be explosive, have no relation to meals, and occur without warning. Vagal denervation leads to enhanced intestinal motility. Rapid gastric emptying, bile malabsorption, and bacterial overgrowth can also play a role.

Treatment includes fluid restriction, including ingesting solids that are low in fluid content. Antidiarrheal agents such as loperamide may be of benefit. Cholestyramine, which binds bile salts, or somatostatin analogues may also be used. Antibiotics are a consideration for bacterial overgrowth. If the postvagotomy diarrhea is severe or is refractory to medical management, a reversed 10-cm segment of jejunum is inserted 100 cm distal to the ligament of Treitz. This procedure delays small bowel transit time, but it has many inherent problems, making its use infrequent.

Gastric Atony
Many gastric reconstructions result in the denervation of the stomach and ablation of the pylorus, altering gastric motility. Rapid emptying of liquids occurs, resulting in early and late dumping syndromes (see section "Disorders Related to Gastric Reservoir Dysfunction"). Gastric atony leads to delayed emptying of solids. It typically occurs more frequently in patients with Billroth I reconstructions. Symptoms can include abdominal fullness after oral intake and relief after explosive vomiting. Treatment is conservative; such symptoms will improve with time and not require intervention. This includes ingestion of small meals throughout the course of the day and avoidance of tobacco and alcohol. Promotility agents such as metoclopramide or erythromycin may be beneficial. Frequently, symptoms will improve over time, and they may not require any intervention.

Cholelithiasis
Vagal denervation of the gallbladder can lead to bile stasis with subsequent development of cholelithiasis. Another contributing factor is a decrease in the release of CCK from the duodenum due to its bypass leading to bile stasis. The more extensive the gastrectomy, the sooner the interval to the development of cholelithiasis. Some surgeons advocate cholecystectomy at the time of radical gastrectomy due to this fact.

Disorders Related to Reconstruction Anatomy
Afferent Loop Obstruction
Afferent loop obstruction occurs only after gastrectomy with a Billroth II reconstruction. It is usually associated with a kink in the afferent limb adjacent to the anastomosis. Pancreatic and biliary secretions build up in the afferent limb, causing its distension. Patients develop severe, crushing, crampy abdominal pain immediately after the ingestion of a meal. Within 45 minutes, the patient then feels an abdominal rush that is associated with increased pain, followed by nausea and vomiting of a dark brown, bitter-tasting material that has the consistency of motor oil with subsequent resolution of symptoms due to the spontaneous, forceful decompression of the obstructed afferent limb. Patients with afferent limb obstruction often develop profound weight loss because of food fear. Treatment involves exploratory laparotomy with the conversion of the Billroth II anastomosis to either a Roux-en-Y gastrojejunostomy or a Billroth I gastroduodenostomy.

Efferent Loop Obstruction

Efferent loop obstruction results from mechanical obstruction of the small bowel at the site of a Billroth II gastrojejunostomy or beyond. Symptoms include abdominal distension, nausea, and emesis. Obstruction is typically secondary to adhesions or herniation. Exploratory laparotomy with lysis of adhesions, reduction and repair of hernias, or anastomotic revision constitutes treatment.

Roux Stasis Syndrome

Roux stasis syndrome develops due to transection of the proximal small bowel leading to disruption of motility. Combined with vagal denervation, small bowel transit time decreases, leading to stasis. Patients develop abdominal discomfort and distension with nonbilious vomiting. In severe cases, patients restrict their intake to liquids only with subsequent malnutrition and weight loss. Initial therapy includes diet modification with augmented caloric intake as necessary. Promotility agents are adjuncts. Surgical therapy involves resection of the gastric remnant with Roux-en-Y revision.

Alkaline Reflux Gastritis

Alkaline reflux gastritis results from the reflux of duodenal, pancreatic, and biliary contents into the denervated stomach, typically occurring after Billroth I and II reconstructions. These patients have weakness, weight loss, persistent nausea, and epigastric abdominal pain that often radiates to the back. In addition, they are often anemic. Upper endoscopy will reveal an edematous, bile-stained gastric epithelium that is atrophic and erythematous. Mucosal biopsies taken away from the anastomosis demonstrate inflammatory changes with a characteristic corkscrew appearance of submucosal blood vessels. Nuclear scintigraphy will often demonstrate delayed gastric emptying.

Although clinicians have advocated a variety of medical regimens to treat alkaline reflux gastritis (eg, oral ingestion of cholestyramine, antacids, H_2 blockers, or metoclopramide), none is uniformly satisfactory. Surgical correction consists of diverting the duodenal contents away from the stomach with a long-limb Roux-en-Y gastrojejunostomy. A minimum distance of between 40 and 60 cm of the Roux limb and the entry point of the biliopancreatic limb draining the digestive juices into the intestine is typically effective at preventing future reflux gastritis. Another surgical option is the Braun enteroenterostomy. It involves the creation of a jejunojejunostomy between the afferent and efferent limbs of a Billroth II reconstruction between 40 and 60 cm from the gastrojejunostomy.

Long-Term Complications
Marginal Ulcer Disease

Marginal ulcers develop on the jejunal side of a gastrojejunostomy anastomosis. They occur secondary to ischemia. Smoking is a contributing factor. Patients may present with abdominal pain during eating, as well as nausea and vomiting. Upper endoscopy reveals an ulcer no more than 2 cm from the anastomosis located on the jejunal limb. Initial therapy includes discontinuing tobacco use and initiation of a PPI. In severe cases, patients may need to stop oral intake and begin total parental nutrition in order to promote healing through bowel rest and nutritional supplementation.

If the ulcer is recalcitrant to medical management, surgical revision of the anastomosis is required.

Recurrent Ulcer Disease

Recurrent ulcer disease following surgical intervention in benign PUD is most commonly due to incomplete vagotomy. Often, the posterior vagal trunk or a branch of the right posterior nerve (criminal nerve of Grassi) remains intact. After truncal vagotomy and antrectomy, the recurrent ulcer rate is around 2%. Upper endoscopy confirms the diagnosis of persistent vagal innervation. Congo red demonstrates areas of pH drop in the gastric mucosa after the administration of an acid secretagogue (pentagastrin). Such regions have intact vagal innervation. Treatment options include long-term PPIs or reoperative vagotomy.

For patients with recurrent ulceration and verified complete vagotomy, a more thorough evaluation is required. In particular, a search for a neuroendocrine etiology is necessary. Patient history should include an inquiry into a family history of MEN-1. Blood calcium, parathyroid hormone, and gastrin level determinations can help rule out hyperparathyroidism or gastrinoma.

SURGICAL TREATMENT OF OBESITY

Obesity

Obesity is a complex and chronic illness associated with weight-related mortality, cardiovascular disease, diabetes, liver disease, obstructive sleep apnea (OSA), malignancy, functional impairment, as well as many other disorders. The medical costs of obesity exceed $100 billion per year. Over one-third of American adults are obese, and obesity rates continue to increase. Weight loss surgery (WLS) is the most effective intervention to reduce body weight and obesity-associated diseases among patients who are obese and has become a widely accepted approach to treating these disorders. Obesity is the result of an imbalance in energy homeostasis. A positive caloric accumulation leads to the storage of excess energy as fat. This positive balance can be due to either increased energy intake or decreased energy expenditure. A mere 10 kcal/d (one saltine cracker) of extra energy can result in a 1-lb weight gain over the course of a year. Both genetic and environmental influences are responsible for the development of obesity. For example, energy intake may increase secondary to altered appetite regulation, a genetic influence, or as a result of greater food availability, an environmental cause. Likewise, energy expenditure can be decreased due to a genetically determined low body metabolism or from an environmentally related sedentary lifestyle. Such a plethora of potential sources for weight gain emphasizes the multifactorial nature of obesity. An understanding of the classification, evaluation, and treatment of patients who are obese is essential for providing quality care to this often-marginalized group of people.

Physiology of Appetite Regulation

Appetite regulation has become an area of intense research over the last decade, increasing our understanding of energy homeostasis. The body's energy metabolism, adiposity, and weight are carefully held in balance by central neural networks using dynamic feedback loops involving multiple, coordinated central and peripheral biohormonal circuits, each linked to the gut, pancreas, and adipose tissue. Factors impacting weight include energy intake-expenditure balance, lipid storage, and glucose usage, which are under the control of different neuroendocrine systems, such as the gut-brain axis and metabolic hormones.

The hypothalamus, stomach, and adipocyte all play important roles in this complex process (Figure 12-8). Food intake is triggered by the release of the hormone ghrelin from gastric oxyntic cells. This compound stimulates the release of neuropeptides in the "hunger center" of the hypothalamus, increasing caloric consumption. To signal adequate caloric load, the adipocyte releases the hormone leptin, which activates the "satiety center" of the hypothalamus. In this manner, food intake is decreased.

The stomach, adipocyte, and hypothalamus, therefore, constitute an intricate hormonal axis that helps to control energy homeostasis via regulation of appetite. Defects within this axis can lead to energy imbalance with important metabolic consequences. For example, leptin-receptor deficiency results in loss of the satiety signal and the development of obesity. It is one of the few disorders for which exogenous leptin administration is potentially curative. Likewise, ghrelin overproduction is thought to contribute to the hyperphagia and obesity seen in patients with Prader-Willi syndrome.

Incretins are hormones secreted from enteroendocrine cells after nutrient intake that stimulate insulin secretion from β cells in a glucose-dependent manner. GIP and glucagon-like peptide-1 (GLP-1) are two known incretins. GLP-1 is secreted from L cells in the ileum and colon by direct contact with nutrients (fat, protein, and glucose) and neuronal input from the upper intestine. GLP-1 has a variety of peripheral and central effects. It has a satiety effect manifested by its blood-borne transfer to the hypothalamus and paracrine fashion action on vagal afferents. It stimulates glucose-dependent insulin release from the pancreas, slows gastric emptying, and inhibits inappropriate glucagon release.

Classification of Obesity

Obesity is defined by the World Health Organization (WHO) as an "abnormal or excessive fat accumulation that presents a risk to health," commonly classified by the body mass index (BMI). BMI is simple to calculate, but it does have its limitations where factors such as age, muscle mass, and ethnicity can influence its relationship with body fat. Anthropometric measures such as skinfold thickness, waist circumference, and waist-to-hip ratio are increasingly used to assess an individual's risk of obesity-related conditions such as type 2 diabetes mellitus (T2DM) and cardiovascular disease.

Despite the limitations of BMI to accurately risk stratify patients with obesity for their future health risk, it is the most feasible and widely used criteria to identify and classify patients with overweight or obesity. It is calculated by dividing an individual's weight in kilograms by the square of their height in meters:

$$BMI = weight\ (kg)/[height\ (m)]^2.$$

Using the BMI, a person can be classified into various weight categories reflecting total body fat (Table 12-4). Even though helpful, the BMI can occasionally overestimate (as in bodybuilders) or underestimate (as in the older people) total body fat. The classification system based on BMI provides the basis by which individuals are treated for overweight and obesity.

Clinical Presentation and Evaluation

Patients with severe obesity (Class III obesity) may come to medical attention because of poor quality of life, problems with self-image, or to prevent or reduce medical conditions associated with obesity. These *comorbidities* may stem from the metabolic changes related to excess

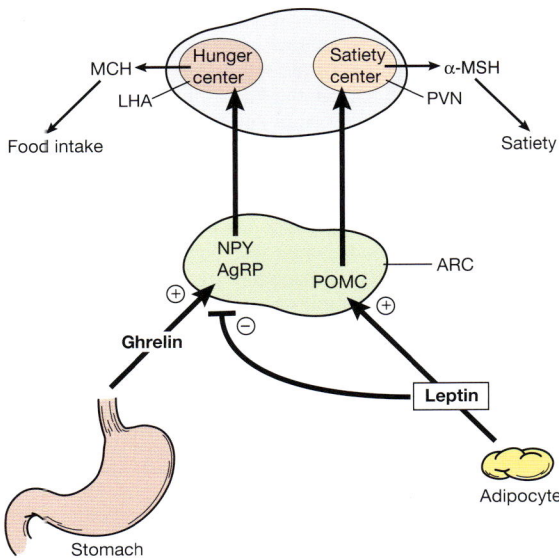

Figure 12-8. Hormonal axis controlling energy homeostasis. Ghrelin and leptin activate first-order neurons in the ARC of the hypothalamus, leading to stimulation of the hunger and satiety centers. AgRP, agouti-related protein; ARC, arcuate nucleus; LHA, lateral hypothalamic area; MCH, melanin-concentrating hormone; NPY, neuropeptide Y; POMC, proopiomelanocortin; PVN, paraventricular nucleus; α-MSH, α-melanocyte-stimulating hormone.

TABLE 12-4. Weight Classification and Risk of Illness Based on Body Mass Index (BMI)		
BMI Range	**Weight Classification**	**Risk of Illness**
<18.5	Underweight	Increased
18.5-24.9	Ideal weight	Normal
25.0-29.9	Overweight	Increased
30.0-39.9	Obese	High/very high
40.0 or greater	Severely obese	Extremely high

Adapted with permission from Bessesen DH, Kushner R. *Evaluation and Management of Obesity.* Hanley and Belfus; 2002.

fat, namely insulin resistance, atherosclerosis, dyslip-idemia, vein thrombosis, and cholelithiasis, or from the physical strains that obesity places on the body, namely sleep apnea, degenerative joint disease (DJD), GERD, and urinary stress incontinence. In addition, some disorders have a combined metabolic and physical etiology, such as hypertension, infertility, psychosocial illnesses, and heart failure.

According to a 1991 National Institutes of Health (NIH) consensus conference on GI surgery for severe obesity, adult patients are candidates for surgery if they meet BMI criteria for clinically severe obesity, have failed attempts at diet and exercise, and are motivated and well informed. In addition, they recommend that patients who are candidates for bariatric surgery should be evaluated by a "multidisciplinary team with access to medical, surgical, psychiatric, and nutritional exper-tise." The value of assessments is based on the recogni-tion of the complexity of the disease of obesity and the ability to provide a comprehensive risk/benefit analysis when considering surgery. This may also facilitate the patient's ability to comprehend the lifelong changes that can be expected after surgery, benefiting from the exper-tise of different health care providers. Studies have sug-gested that the addition of a multidisciplinary team to the perioperative care of the patient may decrease rates of complications.

There are no absolute contraindications to bariatric surgery. Relative contraindications include severe heart failure, unstable coronary artery disease, end-stage lung disease, active cancer diagnosis or treatment, cirrhosis with portal hypertension, uncontrolled drug or alcohol de-pendency, and severely impaired intellectual capacity.

Preoperative preparation is similar for all bariatric procedures. The components include determining a pa-tient's indications for surgery, identifying issues that may interfere with the success of the surgery, and assessing and treating comorbid diseases. The typical assessment includes psychological testing, nutrition evaluation, and medical assessment.

Patients referred for bariatric surgery are more likely than the overall population to have psychopathologies such as somatization, social phobia, obsessive-compulsive disorder, substance misuse, binge-eating disorder, post-traumatic stress disorder, generalized anxiety disorder, and depression. Most bariatric programs therefore require

psychological evaluation before allowing a bariatric pro-cedure. An extensive assessment performed by a mental health professional will allow appropriate therapy for poorly controlled psychological conditions and will iden-tify any history of physical or mental abuse that might in-terfere with postsurgical recovery and success.

Preoperative nutritional counseling should include an assessment of actual and required caloric intake, screen-ing for detrimental eating habits, and education regarding required postoperative dietary changes. Sometimes, a pre-operative very-low-calorie diet (VLCD) is implemented to reduce liver volume to improve access for a minimally invasive bariatric approach. In association, a fitness evalu-ation is useful to determine the baseline level of function and to provide education and resources about a postopera-tive exercise program.

Medical assessment includes a thorough history and a physical examination with a systematic review to rule out treatable endocrine causes of obesity and to identify comorbidities that may complicate the surgery. Routine studies include baseline nutritional measures, as well as cardiovascular assessment by electrocardiogram and pos-sible stress test to identify occult coronary artery disease. Respiratory evaluation may include chest x-ray, blood gas, and pulmonary function tests, with specific attention to the possibility of obesity hypoventilatory syndrome (day-time hypercapnia). Medical conditions need to be opti-mized using a multidisciplinary approach prior to surgical intervention.

Treatment

Managing patients who are overweight and who are obese requires a variety of skills of various health care practitioners (physicians, nutritionists, registered dieti-tians, psychologists, and exercise physiologists) work-ing as a team to help patients learn to make the changes they need to make over the long term. In 1998, the NIH developed guidelines on the Identification, Evaluation, and Treatment of Overweight and Obesity based on BMI for appropriate weight loss interventions (Table 12-5). These criteria help health care workers in determining the best weight loss approach for a person of any given size. Treatment for people who are overweight and obese falls into three broad categories: behavior modification (diet and exercise), pharmacotherapy, and surgical inter-vention. All three therapies are able to induce a degree

TABLE 12-5. National Institutes of Health Guidelines for Treatment of Overweight and Obesity

BMI Range	Behavior Modification	Pharmacotherapy	Surgery
25.0-26.9	Yes[a]	No	No
27.0-29.9	Yes[a]	Yes[a]	No
30.0-34.9	Yes	Yes	No
35.0-39.9	Yes	Yes	Yes[a]
40 or more	Yes	Yes	Yes

BMI, body mass index.
[a]Comorbidities present.
From Executive summary. *Obes Res.* 1998;6:51S-179S. https://onlinelibrary.wiley.com/doi/abs/10.1002/j.1550-8528.1998.tb00690.x?sid=nlm%3Apubmed

of weight loss. Only bariatric surgery, however, has been successful in helping people lose a significant amount of weight and keeping it off.

Behavior Modification

The 1998 NIH guidelines recommend behavior modification for any patient who is obese and for those individuals who are overweight with comorbid conditions. Two main forms of modification exist: reduction in energy intake (diet) and augmentation in energy expenditure (exercise). Dietary modification is an effective means of inducing weight loss. There are two forms; the most common one is the low-calorie diet (LCD), which aims for an energy deficit ranging from 500 to 1,000 kcal/d. For women, this negative energy balance is reached at 1,000 to 1,200 kcal/d. For men, it requires an intake of 1,200 to 1,500 kcal/d. Following such guidelines, patients will lose about 0.45 to 0.90 kg/wk. The goal of such therapy is a 10% weight loss over 6 months. The second form is a VLCD, which limits energy intake to less than 800 kcal/d. It often consists of high-protein liquid meals supplemented with essential vitamins, minerals, fatty acids, and electrolytes. Short-term weight loss can be dramatic, with some individuals losing up to 20 kg in as little as 3 months. The long-term weight loss from VLCDs, however, is not different from that produced by LCDs. VLCDs should not be used routinely for weight loss therapy because they require special monitoring due to the increased risk of complications (hyperuricemia, gout, cardiac complications, and cholelithiasis). As a result, they are not recommended as therapies in the 1998 NIH guidelines.

LCDs fall into two categories: those that primarily restrict fat intake and those that primarily restrict carbohydrate intake. Both diets produce weight loss that is insufficient to affect any major change in health status. A description of each type of diet follows.

Reduced-carbohydrate diets: These diets are based on the belief that increased carbohydrate consumption is responsible for weight gain. They therefore focus on severely limiting carbohydrate intake in an attempt to lose weight. Even though these diets can cause a decrease in weight, it is often due to diuresis from depletion of glycogen stores. Furthermore, ketogenesis resulting from the low availability of carbohydrates leads to appetite suppression. Weight, therefore, is often regained when the diet is abandoned and carbohydrates are reintroduced. Finally, to keep carbohydrate intake low, protein and fat content are increased. The high fat exposes the individual to the risk of atherosclerotic changes and their sequelae. The high protein is potentially detrimental to renal function, especially in borderline cases. Care should be taken, therefore, in pursuing these reduced-carbohydrate programs.

Reduced-fat diets: Since fat is the most energy-dense macronutrient (having 9 kcal/g), its reduction is useful in decreasing total energy consumption. In fact, both reduced-carbohydrate and reduced-fat diets are really only effective in the setting of decreased caloric intake. A reduced-fat diet provides the additional benefit of decreasing atherosclerotic risk. It is therefore the recommended approach in promoting weight loss.

Physical activity: Unlike decreasing energy intake, increasing energy expenditure is much less effective in causing weight loss. It results in minimal reductions, both alone and in combination with dietary restriction. Typical recommendations suggest increasing activity to reach an energy expenditure of 1,000 kcal/wk. Such an energy deficit can be obtained in a single day of dietary restriction, showing why increased activity does not lead to significant weight loss. It is, however, very effective in preventing weight regain after successful loss because of its role in long-term weight maintenance.

Energy expenditure comes from three main sources. The basal metabolic rate (BMR) produces the most energy. It is defined as the amount of energy required to keep sodium and potassium where they belong, to keep the body warm, to pump blood, to breathe, and to perform other basic functions. A small contribution comes from the thermic effect (TEF) of the digestion of food. Physical activity produces the rest. Of the three, physical activity is modifiable. It can be increased by adjusting lifestyle habits, such as taking stairs instead of an elevator or engaging in structured exercise. The latter is the most useful in reaching recommended energy expenditure goals. For example, walking two miles a day for 5 days a week will produce an expenditure of 1,000 kcal/wk.

Although often effective over the short term, behavior modification fails to result in many long-term successes. Maintaining a dietary restriction or structured exercise protocol can be difficult, and people often lapse. The lost weight is regained with additional pounds. Unfortunately, only a small fraction of individuals who lose weight by behavior modification are able to keep it off.

Pharmacotherapy

Pharmacotherapy can enhance weight loss in selected patients who are obese and should be used only as a part of a comprehensive weight management program that includes behavior therapy, diet, and physical activity. However, effective use of weight loss medications requires long-term therapy and monitoring. Trials showed that initial responders tend to continue to respond, whereas initial nonresponders are less likely to respond even with increased dosages. The 1998 NIH guidelines recommend pharmacotherapy for individuals who are obese for long-term weight management in adults with a BMI of at least 30 or BMI of at least 27 and comorbid conditions.

There are a large number of anti-obesity drugs in different stages of development. The medications currently approved in the United States for the treatment of obesity are short-term phentermine, a combination of phentermine/topiramate, orlistat, a combination of naltrexone and bupropion, liraglutide, and semaglutide.

Phentermine HCl is a centrally acting sympathomimetic, which enhances the release of serotonin, norepinephrine, and dopamine and leads to weight loss through appetite suppression. It is approved in the United States for short-term use (15-37.5 mg/d in one to two divided doses) and used to be one of the more prescribed anti-obesity drugs because of its low cost. The longest randomized controlled trial (RCT) involving phentermine (36 weeks) led to a maximum mean placebo-subtracted weight loss of 8.2 kg. Its most common side effects include dry mouth, insomnia, dizziness, palpitations, flushing, fatigue, and constipation.

Topiramate, a γ-aminobutyric acid (GABA) receptor agonist, decreases appetite and increases satiety. It also increases energy expenditure. Phentermine is a sympathomimetic that suppresses appetite by increasing norepinephrine and to a lesser extent, dopamine. The phentermine/topiramate (PHEN/TPM) combination was approved in 2012 for obesity management by the U.S. Food and Drug Administration (FDA). The combination results in more weight loss compared with its monotherapy components. A 5% weight loss was reported in 75% of those receiving phentermine-topiramate versus 23% of those receiving placebo. The dosage affected the efficacy, and a limiting factor was the association of phentermine-topiramate with nervous system side effects. Adverse effects include dry mouth, psychiatric side effects including depression, anxiety, and loss of concentration. Studies also reported increased heart rate with PHEN/TPM.

Orlistat is a potent pancreatic lipase inhibitor. It promotes weight loss by reducing intestinal fat absorption by roughly 30%. The higher the fat content of the ingested food, the more effective is the drug. Side effects include steatorrhea, fecal leakage, bloating, and increased flatulence. Long-term use results in about 10% weight loss. Initial dosing is 120 mg tid. Weight regain is common after its cessation.

GLP-1 agonists (liraglutide and semaglutide) have shown promising results in the reduction of body weight in patients who are obese with and without diabetes. They are also successful at improving glycemic control by stimulating insulin secretion and inhibiting glucagon secretion without the onset of hypoglycemia. Although their weight loss effects are well known, the mechanism underlying these effects is still debatable. Most investigations into the underlying mechanisms of GLP-1 on appetite and weight loss have focused on liraglutide. The most notable known mechanisms are linked with the central and peripheral nervous systems through direct activation of the hypothalamus and hindbrain or indirect activation via the vagus nerve, resulting in reduced appetite and food intake. GLP-1s are also known to delay gastric emptying, but the effect on patients' total weight loss seems to be minimal. These medications are meant to be used long term and have weight loss results from 7% to 20% in 1 year. Contraindications to utilizing GLP-1 agonists include hypersensitivity and pregnancy as prohibitions to prescribing this class of medications. In addition, patients with severe GI diseases such as gastroparesis, pancreatitis, and inflammatory bowel disease should avoid GLP-1 analogues. Lastly, GLP-1 agonists are not recommended in patient populations with a personal or family history significant for MEN-2A, MEN-2B, or medullary thyroid cancer.

Developments in the basic sciences suggest targeting the regulatory signals and pathways with different new drugs that have different mechanisms of action. Most of this work is still undergoing investigation. Included in the list are recombinant leptin, drugs acting on neuropeptide Y receptor subtypes responsible for feeding effects, CCK agonists, β3-adrenergic receptor agonists, and drugs targeting uncoupling protein 3 in human skeletal muscles. Also on the list are endocannabinoid system blockers, which have a weight loss effect. They are used in many countries but not in the United States.

TABLE 12-6. Indication for Bariatric Surgery for Morbid Obesity
Individuals with a BMI of 40 kg/m² or greater
Individuals with a BMI of 35-40 kg/m² with significant obesity-related comorbidity

BMI, body mass index.

Surgical Intervention

Surgery remains the only proven modality effective in inducing and maintaining weight loss and in reducing lifetime obesity-related morbidities and mortality. In 1991, an NIH Consensus Development Conference established criteria by which patients should be considered for operative treatment of obesity (Table 12-6). These guidelines have served as the basis for subsequent societal and organizational recommendations related to WLS.

In 2022, joint guidelines from the American Association of Clinical Endocrinologists, the Obesity Society, and the American Society for Metabolic and Bariatric Surgery advise that WLS should be considered for patients whose BMI is over 40 regardless of comorbidities, for patients with a BMI of 35 to 40 in the presence of a severe obesity-related comorbidity, and for patients with BMI 30 to 35 in the presence of a severe obesity-related comorbidity such as diabetes. They advise consideration of WLS for those with poorly controlled diabetes in patients with a BMI between 30 and 35. These guidelines also suggest lowering the BMI thresholds by 2.5 points for Asian populations.

Bariatric procedures induce weight loss by decreasing energy intake. Three mechanisms are responsible for this decrease (Table 12-7). Restrictive operations limit food intake by forcing the patient to eat smaller portions. Adjustable gastric banding (AGB) and sleeve gastrectomy (SG) are the most common examples of such interventions. Malabsorptive operations alter food processing by limiting its absorption in the intestines. Biliopancreatic diversion (BPD) with or without duodenal switch (BPD/DS) is the most popular of these procedures. Among combined restrictive and malabsorptive operations, the Roux-en-Y gastric bypass (RYGB) is the most common procedure. In

TABLE 12-7. Types of Weight Reduction Surgery
Restrictive procedures
Adjustable gastric banding (AGB)
Sleeve gastrectomy (SG)
Malabsorptive procedures
Biliopancreatic diversion (BPD)
Biliopancreatic diversion with duodenal switch (BPD/DS)
Combination of malabsorption and restriction
Roux-en-Y gastric bypass (RYGB)

general, restrictive procedures are less extensive than malabsorptive ones, but they sometimes result in less overall weight loss and cure of comorbid conditions. Malabsorptive procedures, on the other hand, have better weight loss but an increased risk of problems with malnutrition. Both types of operations can be performed by an open, laparoscopic, or robotic approach.

In the United States, procedures have shifted in the last several years, such that 61% of the estimated 252,000 primary bariatric procedures performed are SG followed by RYGB, which accounts for 17%. The AGB and BPD procedures each account for less than 2%. Revisional surgeries make up about 15% of the procedures. The jejunoileal bypass, vertical banded gastroplasty, and laparoscopic AGB procedures have been largely abandoned due to intolerable adverse effects, high rates of reoperation, or poor long-term efficacy. Intragastric balloons (IGBs) and endoscopic interventions are slowly gaining traction.

SG is currently the most common operative intervention for severe obesity in the United States. Surgeons remove approximately 85% of the stomach so that the stomach takes the shape of a tube or "sleeve" (see stomach in Figure 12-9). Initially used to bridge high-risk patients to BPD, SG was ultimately accepted as a stand-alone alternative. This procedure is not reversible. Unlike many other forms of bariatric surgery, the pylorus and stomach innervation remain intact. SG results in excellent weight loss and comorbidity reduction that exceeds, or is comparable to, that of other accepted bariatric procedures. Long-term data are limited, but the 3- and 5-year follow-up data have demonstrated the durability of the SG procedure.

RYGB was traditionally regarded as the standard of care and until 2013 was the most popular bariatric operation. RYGB involves dividing the stomach to create a small pouch composed of cardia and fundus known as the "gastric pouch." The jejunum is divided distal to the ligament of Treitz. The distal "roux limb" is anastomosed to the gastric pouch such that food bypasses the proximal "biliopancreatic limb," composed of the remnant stomach, duodenum, and associated pancreaticobiliary structures. Meanwhile, the biliopancreatic limb is anastomosed to the roux limb at about 100 cm along its length such that the two limbs converge and empty into a "common channel" (Figure 12-10). Weight loss averages from 75% to 85% excess body weight (EBW) within a couple of years. Nutritional problems tend to be less severe than BPD or BPD/DS. Long-term weight loss of 60% EBW at up to 15 years is documented.

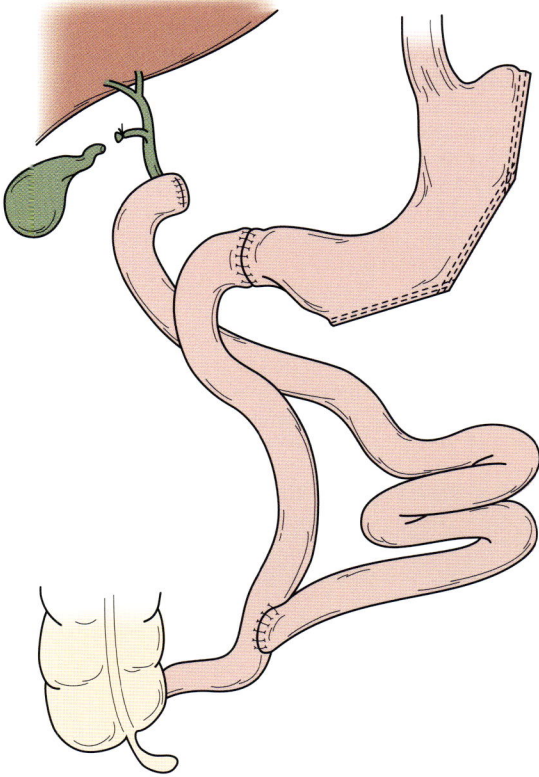

Figure 12-9. Biliopancreatic diversion with or without duodenal switch (BPD/DS). In a BPD/DS, the stomach is reduced in size, the gallbladder is removed, the proximal duodenum is divided and reanastomosed to the more distal small bowel, and a short common channel is created via a jejunoileostomy. Weight loss is predominantly secondary to malabsorption, and complications related to malnutrition are more frequent in this procedure.

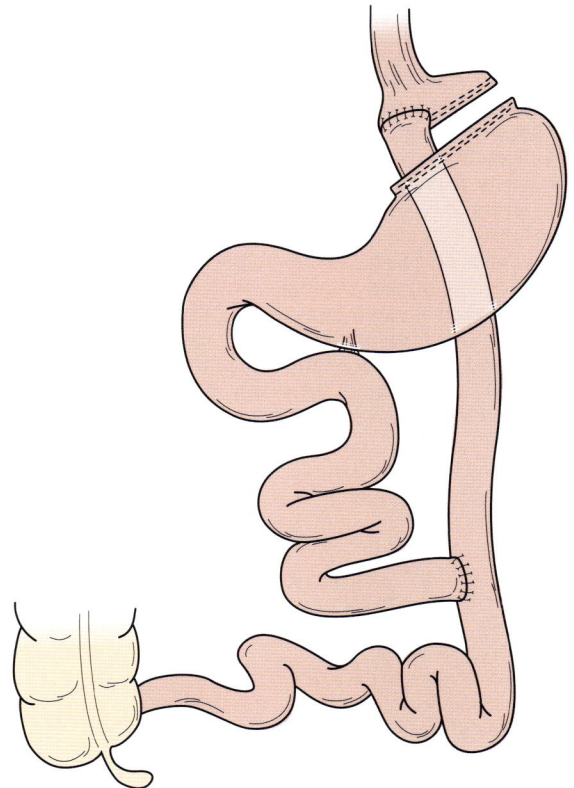

Figure 12-10. Roux-en-Y gastric bypass (RYGB). In a gastric bypass, the stomach is transected unevenly, creating a small proximal pouch. A Roux-en-Y gastrojejunostomy is then created. Weight loss occurs due to decreased food intake as well as some malabsorption. Gastric bypass is currently the most common bariatric procedure performed in the United States.

BPD and BPD/DS are more complex procedures. BPD is a subtotal gastrectomy with a very distal Roux-en-Y reconstruction. BPD/DS involves SG, duodenal transection with duodenojejunostomy creation, and very distal jejunoileostomy (Figure 12-9). Both operations can result in 70% to 90% EBW loss within the first few years, but nutritional problems can be severe. Given their complexity and issues with malnutrition, BPD and BPD/DS have not enjoyed the same popularity as other bariatric procedures in the United States.

AGB has significantly decreased in popularity in recent years. Key aspects of this procedure include the creation of a proximal gastric pouch using an inflatable band and the placement of an access port (Figure 12-11). A pars flaccida technique is used to create a posterior gastric tunnel from the lesser curve to the angle of His. The band is then positioned and secured by imbricating its anterior aspect. The distal fundus is sutured to the proximal gastric pouch. The port is placed on the abdominal muscle fascia. Adjustments of the band are made by instilling a sterile solution percutaneously via the access port. However, AGB is associated with an unacceptably high rate of 10%. Although some authors advocate for its continued utility in selected patients, its use has declined precipitously over the last decade and has been nearly abandoned in favor of RYGB and SG.

Intragastric Balloons

The IGB has been a useful anti-obesity intervention since 1985 and commonly consists of an endoscopically deployed silicone balloon that is filled with saline and inflated in the stomach for a duration of 6 months. IGBs provide an alternative option for weight loss in those patients who decline or are not fit for bariatric surgery. Currently, there are several balloon models, filled with liquid or air. The most widely used is the nonadjustable liquid-filled balloon due to its lower rate of complications. It is made of a transparent silicone elastomer, with a self-sealing valve through which the balloon is filled, with volumes from 400 to 700 mL. It floats freely inside the stomach, increasing satiety and decreasing gastric reservoir capacity and food intake. It can be kept in the stomach for up to 6 months, with a new generation of balloons allowing 12 months

of stay. The mechanism of action of IGBs appears to be multifactorial, involving physiologic and neurohormonal changes. The device functions as an artificial bezoar, filling the stomach and leading to early satiety. Also, alterations in gut hormones and gastric motility have been shown. A recent review of IGBs meta-analyzed four controlled trials and found the devices led to a mean total body weight loss of 9.7%, which is significant but small in relation to standard weight loss surgical interventions.

Endoscopic Interventions

In recent years, we have seen the rapid development of endoscopic therapeutic devices for the treatment of obesity, either as adjuncts to bariatric surgery or as an alternative for individuals who may not be suitable surgical candidates, who decline surgery because of its associated risks, or who would prefer to choose a less invasive therapeutic strategy. Current devices work on a variety of mechanisms including the reduction in gastric capacity or gastric contents or by excluding the proximal small intestine, thus mimicking the effects of surgery.

Complications of Bariatric Operations

Given the dramatic increase in bariatric surgical procedures, patients with a history of bariatric surgery are increasingly being seen by surgical and nonsurgical practitioners alike. Knowledge of the common complications of bariatric surgery is essential in the evaluation and treatment of such patients. Such complications can be classified as early, occurring perioperatively or before the patient is discharged from the hospital, or late, occurring after the patient has been discharged (Table 12-8). Late complications may occur within weeks of surgery or may take years to develop. Furthermore, each type of bariatric procedure has its own unique complications, in addition to the complications common to all surgical procedures, such as bleeding and infection.

Early Complications

Staple Line Leak

Leaks are the most dreaded complication of any bariatric procedure because they increase overall morbidity and mortality. A leak should be suspected and investigated in

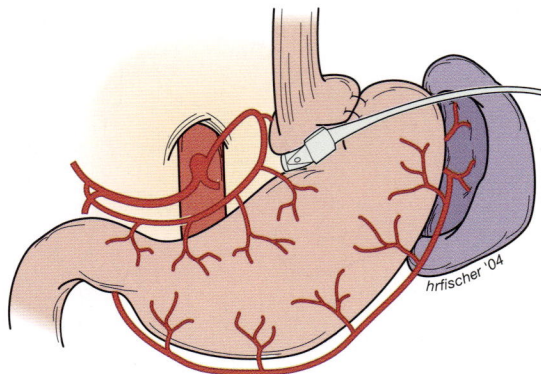

Figure 12-11. Adjustable gastric banding (AGB). An inflatable band is placed around the proximal portion of the stomach, creating a small pouch and restricting food intake. The stoma size into the distal stomach can be adjusted by inflating or deflating the band.

TABLE 12-8. Comparison of Early Versus Late Complications for Common Bariatric Procedures

Early Complications	Late Complications
Staple line leak[a,b,c]	Nutritional disturbances[a,b,c]
Deep venous thrombosis and pulmonary emboli[a,b,c]	Marginal ulcers and anastomotic strictures[a,b]
Bleeding[a,b,c]	Internal hernia[a,b]
Infection[a,b,c]	Afferent limb syndrome[a,b]
Splenic or visceral injury[a,b,c] Small bowel obstruction[a,c]	Cholelithiasis[a,b,c] Esophageal dilatation[a,b]

[a]Roux-en-Y gastric bypass.
[b]Biliopancreatic diversion +/− duodenal switch.
[c]Sleeve gastrectomy.

any patient with persistent tachycardia (>120 beats/min [bpm]), dyspnea, fever, and abdominal pain. The average time for symptoms of a leak to present is approximately 3 to 14 days after the operation, and sleeve leaks usually present 10 to 14 days after the index operation. Often the patient has been discharged home and may present to the emergency department. Sustained heart rates over 120 bpm are a particularly worrisome sign and should be addressed quickly.

Gastric bypass or BPD/DS leaks occur anywhere from 0.5% to 5%. The gastrojejunostomy is most likely to be the site of leakage. Classic signs and symptoms of peritonitis may not be present or may be difficult to recognize in the patient who is obese. Abdominal pain, unexplained tachycardia, tachypnea, and hypoxia should raise suspicion of a leak. Abnormal output from a drain placed at the anastomosis at the time of surgery is also highly suggestive. Imaging with an upper GI series or abdominal CT with oral contrast should be performed promptly. Conservative management with percutaneous drainage and parenteral nutrition may be attempted in the hemodynamically stable patient. If this is unsuccessful or if the patient is clinically unstable, immediate operative exploration, drainage, and repair (if possible) are performed.

Sleeve leaks, on the other hand, occurring in a high pressure system, are thought to be more common; they range in incidence from 1% to 3%. Most SG leaks occur at the uppermost extent of the sleeve, where the blood supply is tenuous. The high pressure comes from the pyloric sphincter and LES, or possibly due to a stenosis, twist in the SG, or kink. These anatomic narrowings must be addressed if the leak is to be treated successfully. Stable patients with leaks after an SG can undergo image-guided drainage procedures. Endoluminal intervention with covered stenting may be placed earlier in the treatment course to help control the leak. The stent should cover the LES through the pyloric sphincter to allow the leak to heal.

Bleeding

Postoperative bleeding that requires intervention occurs in up to 5% to 6% of cases in both the RYGB and SG. Fortunately, most patients are likely to stop without surgical intervention. Usual supportive treatment should be instituted promptly and includes establishing adequate venous access, crystalloid resuscitation, blood product transfusions, serial hematocrits, hemodynamic monitoring, correction of any coagulopathies, and stoppage of venous thromboembolism (VTE) chemoprophylaxis if it is being used. An experienced endoscopist can safely evaluate an anastomosis in the early postoperative period and perform therapeutic endoluminal interventions like clip application or epinephrine injections as first-line treatment.

Hemodynamic instability or failure of nonoperative management mandates emergency surgical management. The staple line is the most common site of bleeding after an SG, but splenic injury is also possible. After RYGB, the anastomoses are probable sites of bleeding, but intra-abdominal hemorrhage from the omentum, mesentery, and spleen are also potential areas. It is also important to determine if the bleeding is occurring intraluminally or intra-abdominally. If no obvious site is found, the surgeon must evaluate inside the gastric remnant, the biliopancreatic limb, and the Roux limb for bleeding sources.

Obstruction

Small bowel obstruction (SBO) can occur from misconstruction during RYGB or BPD/DS operations, internal herniation, adhesion formation (in both open and laparoscopic procedures), or port site hernia. Early SBO is usually caused by a technical error such as the failure to reapproximate the fascia from a port site or potential internal hernia sites. After an RYGB, an internal hernia can occur through the mesentery of the jejunojejunal anastomosis and posterior to the gastrojejunal anastomosis. If a retrocolic approach is used, an internal herniation can occur through the transverse mesocolon defect or through a Petersen defect, which is the space between the transverse mesocolon and the Roux limb as it passes through the mesocolon.

Deep Vein Thrombosis and Pulmonary Embolus

Bariatric patients are at increased risk for deep vein thrombosis (DVT) and pulmonary embolus (PE) for several reasons.

Adipose tissue itself causes metabolic changes that increase thrombogenesis. Patients who are obese are often less mobile, especially after surgery. Increased adipose tissue in the lower extremities compresses the veins and impairs venous outflow. Finally, venous stasis from general anesthesia and the prothrombotic, proinflammatory postsurgical state combine to render bariatric patients particularly susceptible to developing venous thrombosis. Aggressive prophylaxis is important to help minimize risk. Combination therapy including low-molecular-weight heparin, sequential compression devices, and early ambulation is recommended.

DVT typically presents as painful, unilateral swelling of a lower extremity. Diagnosis is made using duplex ultrasound of the affected extremity. However, given the limited sensitivity of ultrasound in patients who are obese, treatment is often instituted in the absence of a clearly positive study, if the clinical presentation is sufficiently suggestive. Either enoxaparin or unfractionated heparin may be used for initial treatment, followed by oral anticoagulation for 6 months.

PE can manifest as hypoxia, tachypnea, tachycardia, dyspnea, or chest pain. The severity of the presentation can range from mild symptoms to cardiovascular collapse. Diagnosis is usually made by helical CT. As with DVT, therapy consists of immediate institution of anticoagulation using enoxaparin or unfractionated heparin, followed by long-term anticoagulation. Therapy should be started presumptively if CT scanning cannot be obtained immediately. Patients deemed to be at unusually high risk of PE due to a history of DVT/PE, extreme obesity (BMI >60), or chronic venous stasis should be considered for postoperative extended thromboprophylaxis.

Late Complications
Nutritional Disturbances

Not surprisingly, the therapeutic nutrient restriction imposed by bariatric surgery may also lead to significant nutritional deficiencies. Such disturbances are more likely to occur in patients undergoing malabsorptive procedures, such as RYGB, than in restrictive procedures, such as gastric banding. Bariatric surgical patients are instructed to consume extra protein (60-80 g) on a daily basis to ensure that the metabolic demands of the body are met, but patients who do not adhere to the regimen may develop protein energy malnutrition. In addition, various vitamin and mineral deficiencies can occur. Of these, iron, vitamin B_{12}, folic acid, thiamine, calcium, and vitamin D deficiency are the most important. Iron deficiency is the most common and develops in up to 50% of gastric bypass patients. The gastric pouch produces only a very small amount of acid and therefore absorbs less iron. Also, the duodenum, a major location for iron and calcium absorption, is bypassed. Patients with preexisting iron deficiency and menstruating women should take 65 mg of elemental iron daily, plus vitamin C, which improves absorption. Vitamin B_{12} deficiency is the next most common and can produce neurologic symptoms and megaloblastic anemia. In gastric bypass, the distal stomach is isolated from the food stream, preventing IF from combining with vitamin B_{12} to permit absorption in the ileum. For this reason, gastric bypass patients are routinely administered intramuscular or sublingual vitamin B_{12}. Thiamine deficiency often presents with neuropathic symptoms, and daily thiamine supplementation, usually in the form of a multivitamin, is recommended. Calcium absorption is also decreased in bypass patients, and routine calcium and vitamin D supplementation is necessary to avoid osteoporosis and osteomalacia.

Because of the potential to develop serious nutritional disturbances, bariatric patients require lifelong follow-up. Such care usually involves yearly office visits to review adherence to dietary recommendations and measurement of vitamins B_{12}, A, D, and E, thiamine, folate, calcium, and prealbumin.

Marginal Ulcer

An ulcer occurring on the jejunal side of the gastrojejunostomy is termed a marginal ulcer. Such ulcers are thought to be caused by impaired perfusion of the jejunal mucosa due to interruption of the blood supply by the staple line at the anastomosis. Smoking and the use of NSAIDs or steroids such as prednisone may also contribute. Marginal ulcers may occur as early as several weeks or as late as 1 year postoperatively. Patients present with abdominal pain, upper GI bleeding, nausea, and vomiting. Patients may lose weight due to fear of eating, as food may worsen the symptoms. Diagnosis is made with upper endoscopy, and treatment consists of protection of the GI mucosa with PPIs and sucralfate. Total bowel rest with parenteral nutrition is sometimes necessary. If the ulcer is recalcitrant to conservative management, revision of the gastrojejunostomy may be necessary.

Stricture

Healing of the gastrojejunostomy may be complicated by the development of a stricture. This complication usually occurs within 6 months of the surgery. Patients typically complain of progressive intolerance of solids and liquids, with postprandial abdominal pain and vomiting. Upper endoscopy is the diagnostic procedure of choice. If a stricture is present, pneumatic balloon dilation can be performed to open the anastomosis. The endoscope should be able to enter into the Roux limb after dilation. Multiple dilatations are sometimes necessary.

Internal Hernia

Reconfiguration of the small intestine in gastric bypass necessitates the creation of openings in the mesentery. These defects may permit herniation of the colon or small bowel, with resultant partial or complete obstruction. The

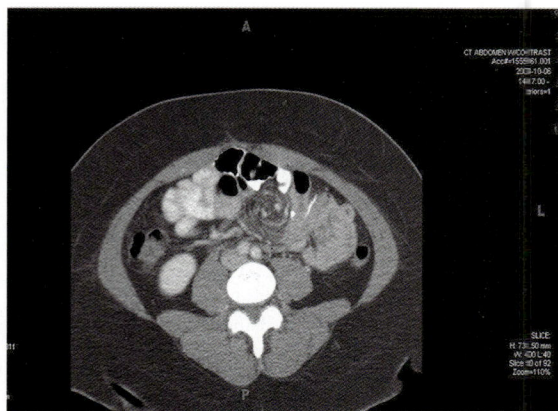

Figure 12-12. Computed tomography (CT) scan demonstrating an internal hernia following gastric bypass. Note the swirling of the mesenteric fat.

presenting symptoms are those of intestinal obstruction, namely, postprandial abdominal pain, nausea, and vomiting. Because the herniation may occur intermittently, symptoms may come and go. Furthermore, upper GI series and abdominal CT may be normal in a large percentage of cases, and diagnostic laparoscopy may be necessary to diagnose and repair the defect (Figure 12-12).

Biliopancreatic Limb Obstruction

Obstruction of the biliopancreatic limb, that is, the blind gastric pouch, duodenum, and proximal jejunum, may occur due to inflammation at the jejunojejunostomy. This complication, which typically occurs within 1 month postoperatively, results in the accumulation of bile and pancreatic secretions in the afferent limb and gastric remnant. Patients complain of abdominal pain, nausea, and nonbilious vomiting. Decompression can be accomplished through the placement of a percutaneous gastrostomy tube, which is then removed after the inflammation subsides and the jejunojejunostomy reopens (Figures 12-13 and 12-14).

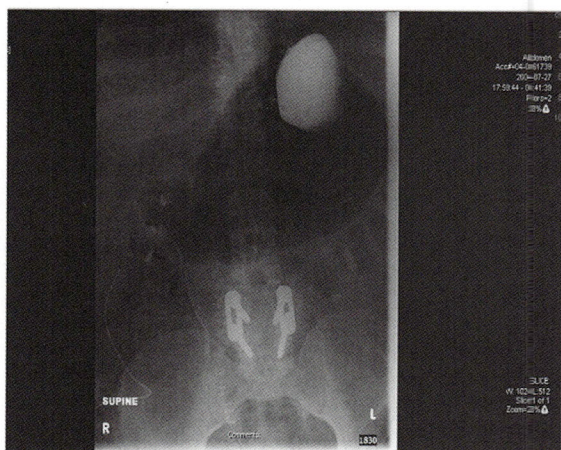

Figure 12-13. Abdominal x-ray of biliopancreatic limb obstruction following gastric bypass. Note the distended stomach remnant.

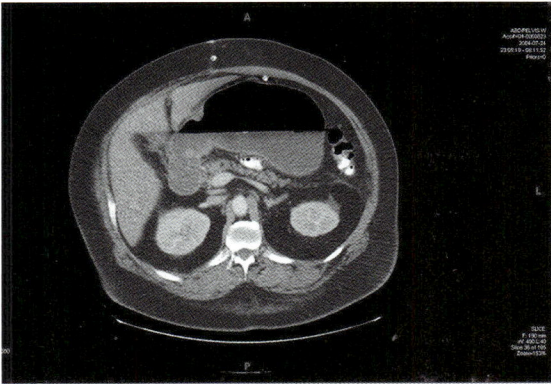

Figure 12-14. Abdominal computed tomography (CT) of biliopancreatic limb obstruction after gastric bypass. Note the distended gastric remnant filled with air and fluid.

Cholelithiasis

About a third of patients who are obese will develop cholelithiasis during the rapid weight loss following gastric bypass surgery. The risk is lower with restrictive procedures. This statistic has led to the routine administration of ursodeoxycholic acid, 300 mg twice daily, for 6 months postoperatively. This medication decreases the risk of developing cholelithiasis to around 2%. Side effects include diarrhea, dyspepsia, and abdominal pain. Although screening for gallstones with ultrasound is not routinely suggested for all patients, most surgeons will perform cholecystectomy at the time of initial operation if patients have known symptoms of biliary colic.

For a list of useful medications related to bariatric surgery complications, see Table 12-9.

Adjustable Gastric Band Complications

Gastric band complications include band slippage and erosion. Slippage of the band, which usually occurs as a late complication, results in movement of the distal stomach through the band with the formation of an enlarged proximal pouch. Food can become lodged in this region, causing nausea and vomiting. In addition, patients may develop reflux symptoms. In severe cases, gastric outlet obstruction occurs and the stomach can become strangulated. Overtightening of the gastric band can lead to dilation of the distal esophagus. Diagnosis of these complications is obtained with upper GI radiographs, which can show

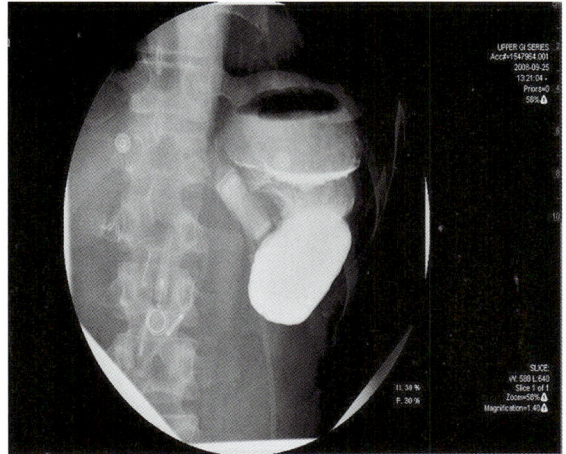

Figure 12-15. Upper gastrointestinal (GI) series demonstrating slippage of the adjustable gastric band. Note the dilated proximal pouch, failure of contrast passage into the distal stomach, and downward orientation of the band.

proximal dilation, poor movement of contrast, and improper orientation of the band (Figures 12-15 and 12-16). Initial treatment includes complete deflation of the band with a future plan to remove the band.

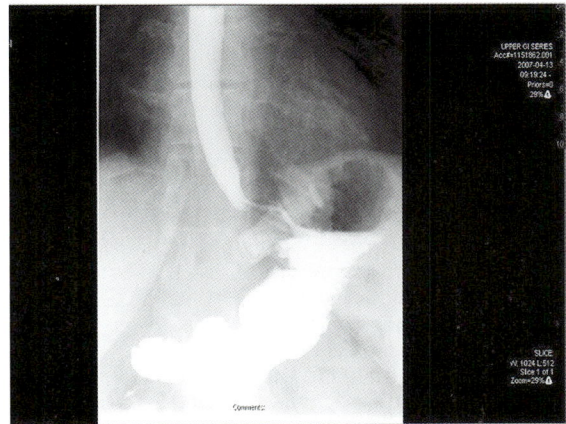

Figure 12-16. Upper gastrointestinal (GI) series demonstrating normal orientation of adjustable gastric band. Note the difference compared to Figure 12-15.

TABLE 12-9. Useful Medications Related to Bariatric Surgery Complications

Medication	Action	Indication	Dosage
Heparin	Antithrombin III inhibitor	DVT/PE	Heparin nomogram used in most hospitals for therapy 5,000 units subQ tid for prophylaxis
Low-molecular-weight heparin/enoxaparin	Antithrombin III inhibitor	DVT/PE	1 mg/kg subQ bid for therapy 40 mg subQ daily or bid for prophylaxis
Warfarin	Vitamin K–dependent protein inhibitor	DVT/PE	Dosage varies depending on patient factors. International normalized ratio (INR) goal of 2-3
Ursodeoxycholic acid	Gallstone formation inhibitor	Gallstones	300 mg po bid for prophylaxis

bid, twice a day; DVT, deep vein thrombosis; PE, pulmonary embolus; subQ, subcutaneous; tid, 3 times a day.

Benefits of Bariatric Operations

Surgical treatment of obesity ameliorates comorbid conditions, reduces mortality, and ultimately decreases health care costs. In a meta-analysis of 22,094 patients, WLS resolved diabetes in 76% of patients; hypertension was eliminated in 61.7%; OSA in 85.7%; and high cholesterol levels decreased in more than 70% of patients. A study from Canada reported an absolute mortality reduction of 5% when comparing 1,035 patients who underwent WLS with 5,746 matched controls in a 5-year follow-up. As little as 10% weight loss reduced hypertension, hypercholesterolemia, and type 2 diabetes; decreased the expected lifetime incidence of heart disease and stroke; and increased life expectancy. Most recently, the Swedish Obese Subjects (SOS) study found a 28% reduction in the adjusted overall mortality rate in the surgical group compared with conventionally treated controls.

Cost-effectiveness analyses (CEAs) have shown that gastric bypass provides net savings. In the United States, gastric bypass costs $35,000 per quality-adjusted life year (QALY) and appears to be more cost effective for women than for men, for individuals with a BMI greater than 40, and for younger individuals. Dialysis, for example, costs more at $50,000 QALY.

Surgical management is an effective treatment option for severe obesity, improves quality of life, decreases morbidity and mortality, and restores overall health.

SAMPLE QUESTIONS

QUESTIONS

Choose the best answer for each question.

1. A 60-year-old man comes to the emergency department because of hematemesis and bright red blood per rectum. He reports a history of gnawing epigastric pain radiating to the back, which improved with eating. His past medical history is significant only for frequent headaches and back pain, for which he takes NSAIDs and over-the-counter medications. On physical examination, he is pale, hypotensive, and tachycardic. After resuscitation, initial upper endoscopy reveals evidence of an upper GI hemorrhage and an ulcer in the posterior duodenal bulb. Which blood vessel is the most likely source of bleeding?

   A. Left gastric artery
   B. Right gastric artery
   C. Common hepatic artery
   D. Gastroduodenal artery
   E. Superior mesenteric artery

2. A 63-year-old man came to the office because of epigastric pain of 2 months' duration not relieved with antacids. He has a history of an adenomatous gastric polyp removed 3 years ago. At upper endoscopy, he was found to have another gastric polyp in his antrum that, on endoscopic ultrasound, appeared to be superficial and not associated with any enlarged lymph nodes. Pathologic analysis of the polyp reveals evidence of adenocarcinoma invading the submucosa. On clinical staging, there is no evidence of distant metastasis. The next step in therapy for this patient is

   A. a repeat endoscopy in 1 year.
   B. chemotherapy.
   C. chemoradiotherapy.
   D. gastric wedge resection.
   E. subtotal gastrectomy.

3. A 34-year-old woman is being evaluated for epigastric pain and is found to have an ulcer in the anterior duodenal bulb on upper endoscopy. Rapid urease testing of a mucosal biopsy of the antrum of the stomach is positive. Appropriate therapy at this time would include a 2-week course of omeprazole,

   A. amoxicillin, and metronidazole.
   B. tetracycline, and cephalexin.
   C. clarithromycin, and amoxicillin.
   D. cephalexin, and metronidazole.
   E. bismuth, and cephalexin.

4. A 53-year-old woman comes to the clinic for evaluation for weight loss. She has recently been diagnosed with diabetes, asthma, sleep apnea, and hypertension. Her BMI is 38 kg/m². Which of the following weight loss options is most appropriate for this patient?

   A. VLCD
   B. LCD
   C. Sibutramine
   D. Orlistat
   E. Gastric bypass

5. A 42-year-old woman comes to the emergency department with epigastric pain radiating to the right upper quadrant. She underwent a laparoscopic gastric bypass 6 months ago. She has lost approximately 80 lbs. over the 6 months. She is afebrile with stable vital signs. A right upper quadrant ultrasound is shown below. Which of the following medications would have been most effective in preventing this complication?

   A. Sucralfate
   B. Ursodeoxycholic acid
   C. Cholestyramine
   D. Calcium citrate
   E. Omeprazole

ANSWERS AND EXPLANATIONS

1. Answer: D

The patient presents to the emergency department with evidence of a massive upper GI hemorrhage (hematemesis with bright red blood with hypotension and tachycardia). His symptoms of gnawing epigastric pain radiating to the back, which improved with eating suggest a posterior bulb duodenal ulcer. Ulcers in this location can erode into the gastroduodenal artery as it passes behind the first portion of the duodenum, causing massive GI hemorrhage. The left gastric artery arises from the celiac axis. The common hepatic artery divides into the gastroduodenal and proper hepatic arteries. The right gastric artery arises from the proper hepatic artery. The superior mesenteric artery is a branch off the aorta. For more information on this topic, please see sections "Uncomplicated Duodenal Ulcer Disease" and "Complicated Peptic Ulcer Disease."

2. Answer: E

This patient has early-stage gastric cancer (ie, no evidence of metastasis or perigastric lymph nodes) on clinical staging and is a candidate for potentially curative resection. Patients with minimal evidence of gastric wall invasion (ie, mucosal or submucosal invasion) do not require any preoperative therapy and should proceed straight to surgical resection. In this patient with an antral lesion, a subtotal gastrectomy is indicated with frozen section analysis of surgical margins to ensure adequate resection. Wedge resection is not recommended. In patients with evidence of greater gastric wall invasion (ie, invasion to and beyond the lamina propria), perioperative chemotherapy with epirubicin, cisplatin, and 5-fluorouracil has been demonstrated to provide a survival benefit. For more information on this topic, please see section "Malignant Gastric Disease."

3. Answer: C

All patients presenting with duodenal ulceration should undergo testing for the presence of *H. pylori* infection. The rapid urease test can be performed on antral stomach biopsies and is indicative of infection if positive. If *H. pylori* infection is present, it should be eradicated. First-line therapy includes acid suppression in addition to clarithromycin and amoxicillin or clarithromycin and metronidazole for a minimum of 7 days. Traditional quadruple therapy is a second-line treatment and consists of acid suppression in addition to bismuth, metronidazole, and tetracycline for a minimum of 7 days. For more information on this topic, please see section "Uncomplicated Duodenal Ulcer Disease."

4. Answer: E

This patient has type II obesity with the life-threatening comorbidity of sleep apnea. As such, she qualifies for surgical intervention according to 1998 NIH guidelines. WLS is the only treatment option to demonstrate sustained, substantial weight loss. Gastric bypass, therefore, is indicated. VLCDs are not recommended for weight loss by the NIH guidelines. Although LCDs, sibutramine, and orlistat are all options for treating patients who are obese, those individuals who qualify for surgery should undergo it if they are deemed appropriate candidates. For more information on this topic, please see section "Surgical Treatment of Obesity."

5. Answer: B

This patient has developed symptomatic cholelithiasis following rapid weight loss after a bariatric procedure. The ultrasound shows several echogenic stones within the gallbladder. Without pharmacotherapy, the risk of gallstone formation during this period approaches 30%. The prophylactic use of ursodeoxycholic acid decreases the risk of gallstone formation to approximately 2%. Sucralfate is used to promote the healing of anastomotic ulcers. Cholestyramine is used in the treatment of alkaline reflux gastritis to bind bile salts. Calcium citrate is given to bariatric patients to prevent calcium deficiency and subsequent osteoporosis. Omeprazole is a PPI used in the treatment of anastomotic ulcers. For more information on this topic, please see section "Complications of Bariatric Operations."

Small Intestine and Appendix

Veronica F. Sullins and Justin P. Wagner

Diseases of the small intestine and appendix constitute some of the most common surgical emergencies. Acute appendicitis, mechanical small bowel obstruction (SBO), paralytic ileus, and inflammatory bowel disease (IBD) are particularly frequent problems encountered in the care of a patient with abdominal complaints. The small bowel and the mesentery are amazingly productive organs with complex physiology that includes digestive, nutritional, vascular, neurologic, immunologic, and endocrine functions. Alteration of these functions by disease, medication, and surgical intervention can have profound health implications.

DISEASES OF THE SMALL INTESTINE

Small Bowel Obstruction

The most frequent indication for surgery on the small intestine is SBO. With obstruction, the small intestine is blocked, causing fluid and gas to back up inside the lumen. This may result in abdominal distension, nausea, and vomiting. SBOs are classified as complete or partial. In a complete obstruction, no content can pass through the point of obstruction, while in a partial obstruction, there is some passage of content. Bowel ischemia can be caused by either direct compromise of the mesenteric blood supply (such as in acute volvulus) or increased intraluminal pressure that prevents perfusion of the bowel wall. A *closed-loop obstruction* refers to an alarming condition in which two sites of obstruction isolate a segment of the small bowel, which is then at great risk of acute ischemia, necrosis, and perforation. This condition requires emergent surgical correction.

Etiology of Small Bowel Obstruction
Extrinsic Causes

The most common causes of SBO are extrinsic to the small bowel itself. In industrialized nations, postsurgical adhesions, or scar tissue, are the most frequent cause of SBO. Adhesions are thought to be caused by disruption of the serosa, followed by fibrinocoagulative and inflammatory processes, resulting in adhesions between adjacent surfaces. Adhesions are present in at least two-thirds of patients who have undergone prior intraperitoneal surgery and in more than 90% of patients who have had two or more prior intra-abdominal operations. It is estimated that laparoscopic operations are associated with 80% fewer adhesions than open procedures. These adhesions can cause kinking or constriction of the small intestine, resulting in an obstruction of the bowel lumen. Approximately 3% to 9% of all patients who have had a prior abdominal

operation will subsequently develop SBO. Accordingly, postsurgical adhesive SBO is a substantial public health problem in industrialized countries. Adhesions may also be the cause of SBO during or following acute inflammatory conditions that involve intraperitoneal organs, even when managed without an operation. Some examples include acute diverticulitis, cholecystitis, appendicitis, IBD, pelvic inflammatory disease, or endometriosis. The initial presenting symptoms in any of these acute infectious or inflammatory conditions may include features of an SBO.

In areas of the world where abdominal surgery is less commonly performed, hernia is the most common cause of SBO. The most common sites of hernias include the umbilicus, inguinal regions, and at sites of prior incisions. Under these circumstances, a loop of small bowel protrudes through a defect in the abdominal wall. The kinking of the intestine at the neck of the hernia often creates a closed-loop SBO. If it is identified early, the bowel can be reduced back through the defect, alleviating the obstruction. Otherwise, edema of the bowel wall and distension of the bowel lumen will occur, leading to incarceration (the bowel cannot be reduced). This will eventually cause strangulation (the blood supply to the trapped bowel segment is completely blocked). Strangulation leads to intestinal ischemia, necrosis, and perforation. This predictable progression is why an SBO caused by an incarcerated hernia is a surgical emergency, requiring immediate operation.

A hernia in which only the antimesenteric wall of the small bowel is entrapped is called a "Richter" hernia. In this case, patients may present with an incarcerated palpable tissue mass, but without an SBO, as the lumen remains patent. Rarely, SBO can be caused by herniation of the small bowel through other defects, such as surgically created defects in the mesentery (called "internal hernias"), recesses in an area where the bowel normally transitions from a retroperitoneal to an intraperitoneal location ("paraduodenal hernia"), or defects in the diaphragm ("diaphragmatic hernia") that may include congenital, traumatic, iatrogenic, or hiatal hernias. Because the obstructed small bowel within any hernia is at high risk for strangulation, emergent operative correction is usually indicated.

Cancer that has metastasized to the peritoneum, or carcinomatosis, is another common cause of extrinsic SBO. Metastatic peritoneal implants, commonly from ovarian or colon cancer, may compress the small bowel lumen, causing an intestinal obstruction. Unfortunately, this process is often multifocal and may be incurable; however, in appropriate-risk cases, palliative operations to release or bypass points of obstruction may offer patients relief from severe pain, vomiting, and abdominal distension.

Less common causes of extrinsic SBOs include volvulus and superior mesenteric artery syndrome (SMAS). Volvulus, which is the twisting of the bowel on its mesentery, may occur because of intra-abdominal fibrous bands, congenital intestinal malrotation, or chronic massive bowel dilation. The twisting causes a closed-loop obstruction of the bowel itself, while twisting at the level of the mesentery causes obstruction of blood flow to the affected bowel (Figure 13-1). This situation requires emergent operative correction. SMAS may cause duodenal obstruction. In this setting, patients have rapid and significant weight loss due to compression of the third portion of the duodenum between the aorta and the SMA at its origin. Diagnosis is often made with computed tomographic angiography (CTA) or magnetic resonance arteriography (MRA), which identifies the point of obstruction in the duodenum and demonstrates the narrow aortomesenteric angle and decreased distance relative to normal. In some cases of SMAS, surgery is necessary either to liberate the point of obstruction or to bypass it by connecting a portion of the jejunum to the proximal duodenum.

Intrinsic Causes

Diseases intrinsic to the small bowel may include congenital anatomic anomalies or progressive thickening of the bowel wall due to inflammation, tumor, or metastasis. Congenital anomalies include duodenal atresia, annular pancreas, intraluminal webs, and jejunoileal atresia. In IBD, the lumen slowly becomes compromised by chronic inflammation and scarring, forming a stricture within the small bowel. Although liquid may pass, any solid or undigested particles may not be able to pass through the narrowed lumen, causing crampy abdominal pain. Strictures are classified as benign or malignant. The most common cause for a benign stricture is Crohn disease (see section "Crohn Disease of the Small Intestine"). Less common causes of benign stricture include radiation enteritis, ulcers associated with chronic nonsteroidal anti-inflammatory drug (NSAID) use, and anastomotic strictures following a previous small bowel resection. Malignant strictures can be caused by any primary small bowel malignancy, such as adenocarcinoma, gastrointestinal stromal tumors (GISTs), lymphoma, or by tumor metastases to the small intestine, such as malignant melanoma. Bowel obstructions from

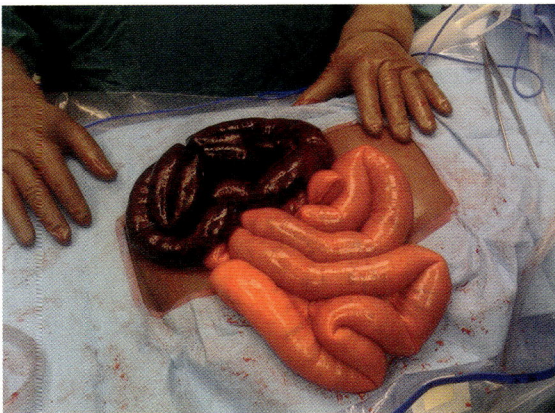

Figure 13-1. Operative photograph of the strangulated portion of the small intestine and the adjacent normal small intestine. The strangulation was caused by an adhesive band, leading to volvulus of the strangulated segment, which appears ischemic in this picture.

strictures are often incomplete and more commonly have an insidious onset. Many patients will describe weeks of crampy abdominal pain with associated weight loss. Because the mesentery is not compromised, strangulation is rare in these circumstances. Operative strategies for any of these conditions reflect a complex analysis of risks, benefits, and alternatives specific to each pathologic process.

Intraluminal Causes

Less commonly, an SBO results from the intraluminal impaction of a foreign body. In general, most foreign bodies that can move across the pylorus will also pass through the small bowel. In some cases, the ileocecal valve (ICV) may obstruct passage of larger foreign bodies. Phytobezoars are concretions of poorly digested fruit and vegetable fiber that act as a foreign body and can be the cause of an intraluminal obstruction. Gallstone ileus is a rare condition that most commonly affects older patients. In it, a large gallstone erodes through the gallbladder into an adjacent loop of adherent small bowel in the setting of acute cholecystitis, and when it becomes impacted at the ICV, it causes an SBO.

Intussusception is a condition in which a segment of the bowel "telescopes" within its own lumen, leading to obstruction. Some small children develop ileocolic intussusception, which involves spontaneous prolapse of the terminal ileum into the colon. First-line therapy for this condition is air or water-soluble contrast enema; however, failure of the enema to reduce the intussusception is an indication for surgical reduction. Small bowel intussusception may also occur as a sequela of acute viral syndromes. This condition is most commonly self-limited, but in rare cases, it persists on serial imaging studies, and an operative exploration may be indicated. In adults and some children, intussusception of the small bowel may be caused by peristalsis acting on a "lead point" such as an intraluminal polyp or tumor. If a lead point is suspected, operative exploration is warranted, and the surgeon may resect the intussuscepted small bowel for histologic evaluation.

Pathophysiology

Patients with SBO develop hypovolemia primarily from emesis, malabsorption, and hormone-mediated paradoxical fluid secretion triggered by distension of the bowel lumen. "Third space" fluid losses due to interstitial edema and transudation of fluid into the peritoneal cavity may also occur, especially in acute infectious and inflammatory conditions. The combination of all these types of fluid loss may lead to severe hypovolemia.

Electrolyte abnormalities vary with the location of the obstruction and duration of illness. In extremely proximal SBO, repeated bouts of vomiting gastric acid result in metabolic alkalosis. In distal partial SBO, succus is alkaline, and metabolic acidosis may result from malabsorptive diarrhea and/or bilious emesis. The severity of electrolyte derangements increases with the duration of illness. Initial phases of dehydration may result in hypokalemia and acidosis as sodium is reabsorbed by the renal system, while more advanced hypovolemia and ischemia may result in lactic acidosis and renal insufficiency.

The end-stage complication of SBO is strangulation of the involved bowel. In this setting, the bowel becomes ischemic and progresses to infarction and necrosis. Sepsis and perforation of the bowel may occur. Several clinical signs and laboratory values have been used to predict bowel compromise. Fever, tachycardia, leukocytosis, and localized abdominal tenderness have most commonly been cited as indicators of impending strangulation. In some series, the risk of strangulation increased from 7% when one of these signs is present to 67% when all four are noted. It is critical to recognize that bowel necrosis may evolve in the absence of these indicators, and all four may be present without necrosis. In sum, these indicators are associated with an increased likelihood of tissue loss and catastrophic complications. Thus, when they are abnormal in a patient with a clinical history suggesting SBO, surgeons must have a low threshold to operate urgently.

Clinical Presentation and Evaluation
History
Common presenting symptoms of SBO are shown in Table 13-1. It is critically important to obtain a detailed past medical history, including prior abdominal surgeries or illnesses. Patients should be asked about bulges or focal regions of reproducible pain or tenderness that may suggest a hernia. Reports of vague or chronic symptoms prior to obstructive symptoms may indicate inflammatory or neoplastic disease that warrants further investigation. Patients typically experience colicky abdominal pain in the periumbilical region that is poorly localized, as autonomic nerves convey this noxious signal. Pain may become steadier as peristaltic activity lessens and generalized bowel distension progresses. Localized pain and tenderness signify parietal peritoneal irritation (focal peritonitis), while tenderness of the entire abdomen (generalized peritonitis) develops as a result of bowel ischemia, necrosis, and perforation. Nausea and vomiting are common complaints in many patients, although the onset of these symptoms may be delayed in distal obstructions because of the capacity of the small bowel to backfill before the stomach distends. Early bouts of emesis may reflect the nonbilious character of gastric contents, while emesis in more advanced states is typically more bilious. The green color indicates oxidation

of bile that has been stagnant. In more chronic obstructions, bacteria break down intraluminal contents, and the vomitus may take on a "feculent" or stool-like character. Abdominal distension is common in distal obstructions in which the small bowel distends diffusely, while patients with proximal SBO may have little to no distension. Inability to pass stool (constipation) or flatus (obstipation) may also ensue, with the latter signifying a higher grade obstruction. These symptoms may present later in the process, as stool and flatus distal to the point of obstruction may still pass.

Examination
Patients with SBO typically present with pain, nausea and vomiting, and fluid and electrolyte disturbances. Patients may appear acutely distressed in the early coliclike phase, or may appear lethargic in the presence of dehydration and acid-base or electrolyte disturbances. Tachycardia, dry mucous membranes, oliguria, decreased skin turgor, and relative hypotension may be seen in more advanced cases. Abdominal distension is present in advanced cases of distal SBO. Surgical scars and areas of potential herniation should be carefully examined. In patients with obesity, areas of focal contour change, erythema, or tenderness near a surgical scar may be the only clue to bowel incarceration within an otherwise occult hernia. On auscultation, high-pitched sounds may be noted early in the process as compensatory increases in motility attempt to overcome the obstruction. With progression of ineffective peristalsis, proximal distension of the small bowel continues and bowel sounds decrease. The abdomen will be tympanic if the bowel is distended with gas, or dull to percussion if the bowel is fluid filled or ascites has developed. In the absence of bowel ischemia, diffuse mild tenderness is common and may improve substantially after decompression via a nasogastric tube (NGT). Patients with generalized or focal peritonitis, rebound tenderness, and fear of movement may have bowel ischemia, necrosis, or perforation and should undergo urgent surgical exploration.

TABLE 13-1. Symptoms and Signs of Bowel Obstruction

Symptom or Sign	Proximal Small Bowel (Open Loop)	Distal Small Bowel (Open Loop)	Small Bowel (Closed Loop)	Colon and Rectum
Pain	Intermittent, intense, colicky, often relieved by vomiting	Intermittent to constant	Progressive, intermittent to constant, rapidly worsens	Continuous
Vomiting	Large volumes, bilious and frequent	Low volume and frequency; progressively feculent with time	May be prominent (reflex)	Intermittent, not prominent, feculent when present
Tenderness	Epigastric or periumbilical; quite mild unless strangulation is present	Diffuse and progressive	Diffuse, progressive	Diffuse
Distension	Absent	Moderate to marked	Often absent	Marked
Obstipation	May not be present	Present	May not be present	Present

Reprinted with permission from Saund M, Soybel DL. Ileus and bowel obstruction. In: Mulholland MW, Lillemoe KD, Doherty GM, et al, eds. *Greenfield's Surgery: Scientific Principles & Practice*. 4th ed. Lippincott Williams & Wilkins; 2006:770. Adapted from Schuffler MD, Sinanan MN. Intestinal obstruction and pseudo-obstruction. In: Sleisenger MH, Fordtran JS, eds. *Gastrointestinal Disease*. 5th ed. WB Saunders; 1993:898.

Laboratory Data

Laboratory abnormalities are not specific to SBO but may help exclude other disease processes and guide resuscitation. Leukocytosis, thrombocytosis, high serum ferritin, and elevated C-reactive protein are acute phase reactants and suggest systemic inflammation. Patients who have been experiencing emesis or copious diarrhea should undergo prompt laboratory testing for electrolyte and acid-base disturbances. Hypokalemic ("contraction") alkalosis occurs in patients with advanced dehydration. Urinalysis is important in evaluating for urinary tract infection, calculus, or ketosis. Lactic acidosis, particularly in the setting of adequate volume administration, indicates an anaerobic metabolic process and, in the context of SBO, is worrisome for bowel ischemia. Bowel infarction may occur without acidosis; therefore, other clinical parameters taken together should guide consideration of when to operate.

Radiographic Studies

An abdominal series, including supine and upright abdominal and upright chest radiographs ("plain films"), are expeditious initial studies. These studies may demonstrate renal or biliary calculi, pneumoperitoneum ("free air"), pneumatosis intestinalis, pneumobilia, ascites, portal venous gas, or pneumonia. Typical findings of SBO on plain films include gaseous bowel distension (highlighting the contour of the intestinal valvulae conniventes) proximal to the point of obstruction, with air-fluid levels evident on upright films (Figure 13-2). A "fixed loop" of the small bowel refers to the finding of a distended loop of the small bowel that appears unchanged on serial images. This finding is more likely to result in surgical correction than one in which the bowel changes shape and position on serial images. It is important to recognize that fluid-filled loops of obstructed bowel may blend in with other soft tissues on x-ray (XR) and that an obstructive pattern may not be clearly evident despite the presence of an SBO.

CT imaging produces a cross-sectional representation of the abdominal contents in three dimensions, which is useful in identifying points of transition between dilated (proximal to obstruction) and decompressed (distal to obstruction) small bowel and differentiation among stomach, duodenum, jejunoileum, and colon (Figure 13-3). CT also assesses other conditions such as nephrolithiasis, diverticulitis, hernias, perforated appendicitis, pancreatitis, or mesenteric vascular disease. Swirling of the small bowel mesentery (the "whirlpool sign") is highly suggestive of volvulus, closed-loop obstruction, or internal hernia.

Contrast studies of the small intestine are useful in a patient with persistent partial obstructive symptoms, or when it is difficult to distinguish SBO from other conditions of bowel dysmotility, such as paralytic ileus. Small bowel follow-through (SBFT) serves as a diagnostic and potentially therapeutic study. In it, water-soluble contrast is administered (either swallowed or administered via nasoenteric tube), and a series of plain radiographs demonstrate passage of contrast through the alimentary tract over time. The osmotic properties of the contrast medium may result in the passage of luminal contents beyond the point of obstruction, and this can help resolve the SBO, particularly if the obstruction is due to adhesions. If investigating suspected colonic obstruction with a contrast enema or

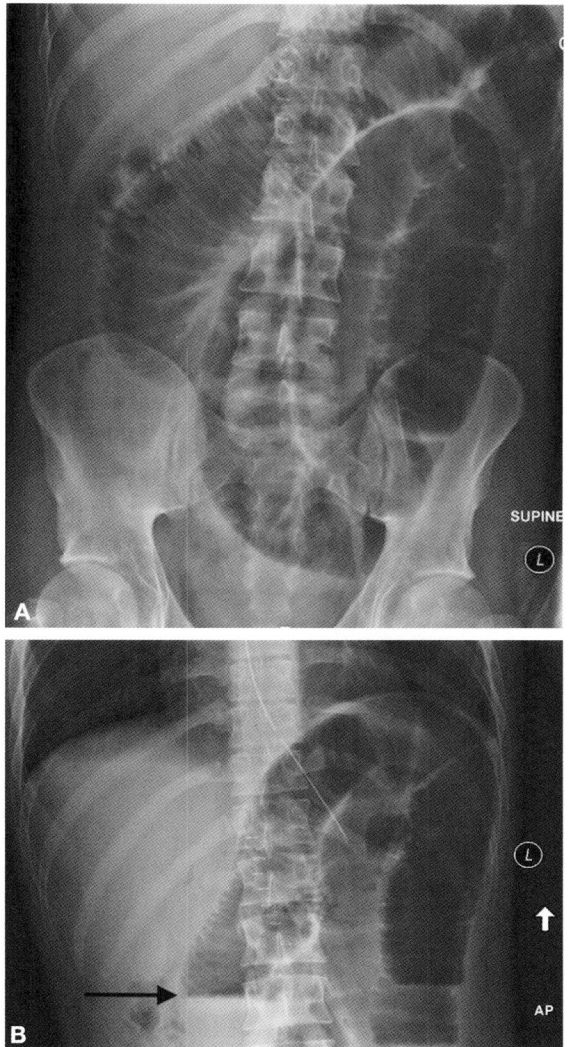

Figure 13-2. Mechanical small intestinal obstruction. A. Supine abdominal radiograph. There are many centrally located loops of air-filled small intestine and a paucity of gas in other parts of the abdomen. Valvulae conniventes are shown. B. Upright abdominal radiograph, showing an air-fluid level (black arrow). White arrow signifies cranial orientation.

mesenteric occlusive disease with angiography, these studies should be performed prior to SBFT, as the presence of contrast within the small bowel may interfere with a radiologic assessment of other structures containing contrast.

Differential Diagnosis

Paralytic (adynamic) ileus is the most common differential diagnosis in the setting of possible SBO. In the ileus, bowel motility is secondarily diminished due to a separate condition. The bowel may become distended because of stasis, and symptoms may mimic those of a mechanical SBO. Opioid medications, bed rest, trauma, hypothyroidism, electrolyte deficiencies (especially potassium, calcium, magnesium, and phosphate), anesthesia, psychotropic medications, and systemic or intraperitoneal inflammatory illnesses or sepsis are all common causes of ileus. XR and

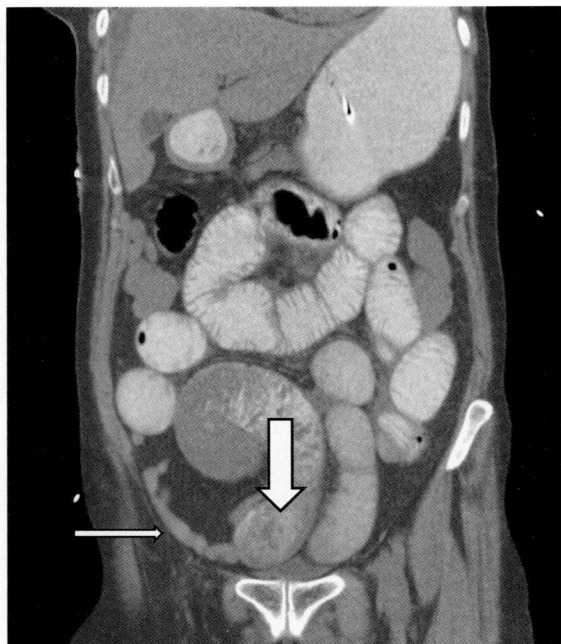

Figure 13-3. Computed tomography scan demonstrating mechanical small bowel obstruction. The thick, vertical arrow points to dilated bowel proximal to the point of obstruction. The thin, horizontal arrow points to the decompressed distal small bowel, with a clear transition point between these two segments.

CT imaging will demonstrate diffuse bowel dilation without evidence of a transition point between dilated and decompressed bowel (Figure 13-4). Contrast enema, SBFT, and CT of the abdomen and pelvis with intravenous (IV) contrast may all be used to differentiate between paralytic ileus and SBO. In those with chronic bowel dysmotility, a review of prior imaging studies will demonstrate similar diffuse bowel dilation.

Postoperative ileus (POI) is common following major abdominal surgery. The cause of POI is multifactorial but is related to the systemic stress of general anesthesia and surgery, direct mechanical irritation of the bowel wall, fluid and electrolyte fluctuations, fluid shifts, and pain management (especially with opioids). After major GI surgery, bowel peristalsis may be slow to return. To minimize POI, many institutions have introduced Enhanced Recovery After Surgery (ERAS) protocols. ERAS typically implements care pathways that avoid routine placement of perioperative NGTs, encourage early ambulation, prevent fluid overload, and advance regular diets following major GI surgery. ERAS protocols, as well as selective opioid antagonists such as alvimopan and methylnaltrexone, are associated with decreased duration of POI.

Treatment

The treatment of SBO begins with fluid resuscitation and electrolyte repletion. Typically, this includes IV volume replacement with isosmotic solutions, such as normal saline or lactated Ringer solution. It is important to establish euvolemia before aggressively replacing electrolytes such as potassium, as rapid rises in the serum level may cause

adverse events (eg, cardiac arrhythmias) if renal perfusion is impaired. End points of resuscitation include normalization of vital signs (heart rate, blood pressure [BP]) and physical examination findings (good skin turgor, visualization of superficial veins, moist mucous membranes, and production of tears and fontanel characteristics in infants). For all patients with SBO, it is critical to measure strict fluid intake and output. Frequent assessment of urine output is a reliable way to assess adequacy of volume resuscitation. If urine output is difficult to quantify, a Foley catheter should be placed. In adults, an hourly urine output of at least 0.5 mL/kg is usually indicative of adequate volume resuscitation.

During initial management, patients typically require a period of bowel rest, in which they receive nothing by mouth and are followed closely for response to fluid resuscitation. The advantages of NGT decompression include prevention of emesis, strict monitoring of ongoing fluid and electrolyte losses, and, potentially, decompression of the small bowel. The latter effect may assist in quicker resolution of the SBO, as the small bowel may relax into a configuration that allows more effective passage of obstructed contents. Theoretical disadvantages of NGT decompression include an increased risk of aspiration due to suppression of the gag reflex and stenting open the gastroesophageal junction in cases of inadequate gastric decompression. If the obstruction is partial, low grade, and there is a history of prior abdominal surgery (with no palpable hernia), the obstruction is likely due to adhesions and will resolve approximately 80% of the time with bowel rest, NGT decompression, and SBFT.

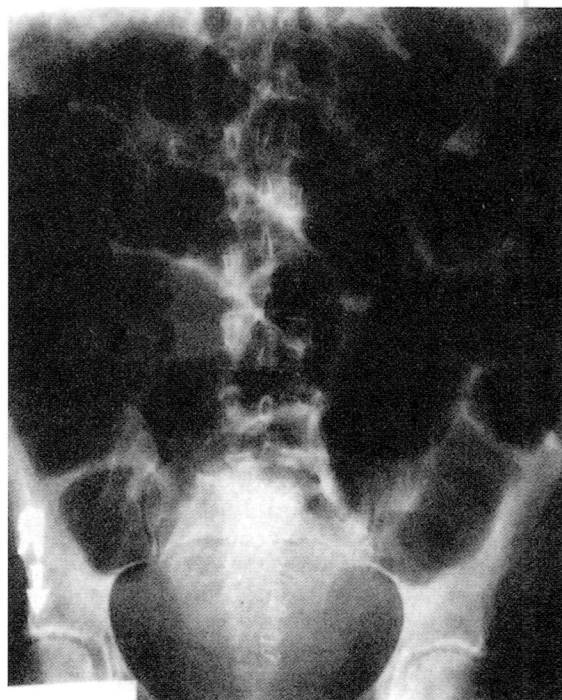

Figure 13-4. Abdominal radiograph showing paralytic ileus of the small bowel. Note the presence of gas diffusely throughout dilated small bowel and sigmoid colon.

In the absence of skin changes or peritoneal signs, patients with an obstructing hernia should undergo attempted reduction followed by observation for resolution of the SBO. If the symptoms of SBO fail to resolve following hernia reduction, this may indicate that the bowel may have ongoing ischemia, the hernia was not the cause of the SBO, or that the reduction was ineffective. Rarely, a *reduction en masse* occurs, in which the hernia sac still constricts its contents after reduction. This is due to reduction of the sac together with the hernia contents through the fascial defect. Repair of the hernia should follow the resolution of SBO to prevent recurrence. Hernias that cannot be reduced, those in association with skin erythema and exquisite tenderness, and those with peritoneal signs should be emergently repaired following immediate resuscitation.

Patients with SBO who are more likely to require operative exploration and correction include the following: (1) patients who have no hernias and no prior surgical history are more likely to have neoplastic lesions or internal hernias; (2) patients with complete or high-grade SBO have greater risk of bowel ischemia and failure of nonoperative management than those with partial or low-grade SBO; or (3) patients with persistent symptoms and signs of SBO despite efforts at resuscitation and more prolonged bowel rest.

Patients who experience early postoperative SBO following a major abdominal operation may require up to 6 weeks of observation and supportive measures as bulky adhesions and bowel edema gradually resolve. In some patients with early postoperative SBO, some surgeons will reoperate more expeditiously if there is a concern that waiting 5 weeks will be of less benefit and more problematic for the patient or family. That said, reoperations between 2 and 4 weeks after an abdominal operation are especially difficult. At this phase of the inflammatory process, normal tissue planes are less identifiable, and operating during this time frame is associated with a higher risk of enterotomies and injury to other abdominal organs. Patients with "hostile abdomens" are those with peritoneal carcinomatosis, recurrent obstructions in the setting of multiple prior operations, or radiation enteritis. These patients are also at substantially higher risk of surgical complications, and it may be safer to avoid an operation unless absolutely necessary under emergent or life-threatening conditions.

If an operation is required for SBO, perioperative antibiotics are given to cover gram-negative organisms and anaerobes. The operation may be performed laparoscopically, depending upon the level of risk, space for visualization despite dilated bowels, and the surgeon's level of experience. Otherwise, an open laparotomy is undertaken. Adhesions are divided, hernias reduced and repaired, and the bowel carefully inspected to ensure integrity of its blood supply. Surgeons are reassured about bowel viability if there is pink color, presence of bleeding at cut surfaces, and peristalsis. If there is uncertainty about whether the bowel is viable, intraoperative assessments may be performed via IV administration of fluorescein dye and visualization of fluorescence of the bowel wall with a Wood (ultraviolet) lamp, or via Doppler ultrasound evaluation of mesenteric and bowel wall blood flow.

When there is nonviable or necrotic bowel, it is resected. The goal of small bowel resection should be removal of all nonviable tissue and preservation of the greatest amount of healthy bowel as possible. Patients with Crohn disease are expected to have future episodes of small bowel fistulae or strictures that may require future operations and resections. In addition, those who have undergone extensive small bowel resections are at high risk of developing intestinal failure, for which they may require total parenteral nutrition (TPN) and intensive intestinal rehabilitation. In these cases, it is crucial to avoid removing any bowel unless it is necessary to preserve life.

If the surgeon has significant concern and cannot reach a conclusion about whether bowel is viable using any of the assessments listed earlier, they may leave the questionable bowel in situ, place a temporary abdominal closure device, and plan for a second-look operation in 24 to 48 hours. This strategy allows for a period of further resuscitation and demarcation of nonviable tissue. In the absence of infection or poor tissue viability, it is possible to anastomose the cut ends of the bowel. Diversion of succus through a temporary ostomy may be the safest approach in complicated circumstances.

Complications
Wound infection, anastomotic leak, abscess, peritonitis, and fistula formation may all complicate operations for SBO, especially when bowel infarction and/or resection have occurred. Overall, mortality is less than 1% for laparotomy in the setting of uncomplicated SBO but may exceed 25% when strangulation or perforation has occurred. Recurrent obstruction may also occur. Implantable agents to prevent the formation of adhesions are the subject of development and study. While compounds such as sodium hyaluronate and carboxymethylcellulose are effective in reducing adhesions after laparotomy, data from prospective studies are insufficient to conclude whether these agents prevent SBO.

Crohn Disease of the Small Intestine
Significance and Incidence
Crohn disease, first described in 1932, has a worldwide prevalence of 10 to 70 cases per 100,000 population, with the North American prevalence reported as high as 200 cases per 100,000. Its underlying cause remains elusive. It occurs primarily in industrialized nations and appears to be related to both genetic and environmental factors. First-degree relatives of affected patients have a 30-fold higher risk of developing the disease than the general population, and disease concordance is significantly higher in monozygotic than in dizygotic twins, suggesting a genetic predisposition. Thus far, more than 200 genes have been associated with Crohn disease. One of the first genes identified was *IBD1*, encoding the protein NOD2, which takes part in immune signaling in reaction to bacterial peptides; this gene is mutated in 40% of young patients with Crohn disease. Many of the other genes involved are also related to immune function. Environmental factors that have been implicated include NSAID use and smoking. It is generally accepted that, in the context of predisposing genetic and environmental factors, sustained mucosal immune responses to luminal microflora are responsible for the disease.

The timing of the onset of disease has a bimodal distribution, with an early peak in the late teens and early 20s, and a later one in the sixth and seventh decades. The distribution of the disease can be anywhere in the alimentary tract from the mouth to the anus, although small intestinal and colonic involvement is most common. The ileocecal area is involved in 40% to 50% of patients, localized to the small intestine only in 30% to 40%, and isolated to the colon in 20%. The disease may go into prolonged remission but tends to have a recurring course with intermittent flares, and it is not curable. As such, it is a significant public health problem.

Pathophysiology

Crohn disease is a chronic, transmural inflammatory condition of the alimentary tract and may include extraintestinal manifestations that affect the skin, eyes, mouth, joints, and biliary system (see also section "Clinical Presentation"). Patients with IBD, including those with Crohn disease, appear to have an increased number of bacteria adherent to and within the bowel's epithelial cells and likely have abnormal immune responses. The inflammatory process is mediated by a range of cytokines, arachidonic acid metabolites (including prostaglandins), and reactive oxygen metabolites. Sustained inflammation leads to tissue destruction and manifestations of clinical disease.

Crohn disease is distinguished from ulcerative colitis (UC) by several clinical features, although 10% to 15% of cases remain "indeterminate" after careful investigation. Namely, Crohn disease may involve segments of the GI tract other than the colon, with areas of sparing ("skip lesions") between the affected areas. Transmural involvement and the associated tendency to develop fistulae, as well as the presence of noncaseating granulomata on histology, are also characteristic of Crohn disease. UC, on the contrary, is confined to the mucosal layer, always involves the rectum, and may spread proximally to affect the rest of the colon, but without skip lesions. It does not affect the small intestine (except as the so-called "backwash ileitis"). Despite these differences, patients with Crohn disease may not have signs or symptoms that specifically distinguish it from UC, even after they are treated for UC for years. Some may even undergo major, irreversible operations for UC before they show definitive signs of Crohn disease.

On inspection in the operating room, the bowel involved with Crohn disease may appear thickened (Figure 13-5) and erythematous. The mesentery is often thickened and shortened, with enlarged mesenteric lymph nodes and fat "creeping" onto the bowel serosa. There may be adhesions of inflamed loops of bowel to the abdominal wall, bladder, adjacent bowel, or solid organs. Fistulae and abscesses may also be found in the abdomen, pelvis, or retroperitoneum. Because of its transmural nature and tendency to have periods of remission and exacerbation, Crohn disease may also lead to the development of fibrotic strictures and SBO. When visualized through an endoscope or if removed and sectioned, the bowel mucosa may have areas of aphthoid ulceration, fissures, and crypt abscesses. Noncaseating granulomata are seen on the histologic section in 60% of cases, although they may be missed with mucosal sampling alone.

Clinical Presentation and Diagnosis

The common presenting triad of Crohn disease includes abdominal pain, diarrhea, and weight loss. The symptoms

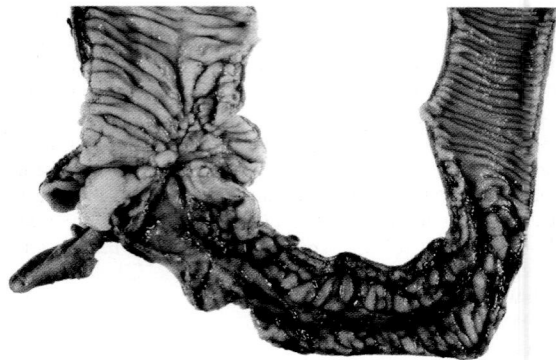

Figure 13-5. Right colon and terminal ileal specimen from a patient with Crohn disease demonstrating narrowing of the diseased segment.

are typically gradual in onset and progressive over time, although a waxing and waning of symptom severity is common. The pain can be related to partial obstruction caused by edema and, in more established cases, fibrotic strictures. In such settings, patients may have associated nausea and vomiting. Right lower quadrant pain may reflect ileocecal involvement, although other areas may also be affected. Bleeding is a rare symptom of Crohn disease, while in UC, bloody diarrhea is relatively frequent. Constitutional symptoms including malaise, fatigue, fever, weight loss, and anorexia are more common with disease progression.

Perianal disease, including atypical and multiple anal fistulae, is concerning for Crohn disease. Fissures and abscesses may also occur. Perianal manifestations are most common in patients with colonic involvement but may also occur in patients who appear to have isolated small bowel disease. Occasionally, a surgical incision on a simple perianal abscess or fistula may lead to poor wound healing or an incomplete response to treatment, which may be a sign of Crohn disease.

Extraintestinal manifestations of Crohn disease are more common when colonic disease is present and may include ocular (conjunctivitis, iritis, uveitis, iridocyclitis, episcleritis), skin (pyoderma gangrenosum, erythema nodosum), joint (ankylosing spondylitis, hypertrophic osteoarthropathy, arthritis), and biliary (sclerosing cholangitis, pericholangitis, granulomatous hepatitis) manifestations, as well as vasculitis and aphthous stomatitis. Often, these manifestations will respond to the treatment of IBD.

Nutritional losses, such as hypoalbuminemia and deficiencies of fat-soluble vitamins (A, D, E, and K) and vitamin B_{12}, are common in Crohn disease. These losses are due to diminished oral intake and impaired absorption, particularly with disease of the terminal ileum. Loss of bile salt reabsorption in the terminal ileum also may lead to reduced cholesterol emulsification and gallstone formation. Delays in growth and development are also common in younger patients with Crohn disease. Supplemental nutrition to correct these deficiencies is a critical part of early treatment in the patient with more advanced disease.

Although some patients present with acute urgent issues such as SBO or abscess, most patients present with more indolent symptoms. A careful history and physical examination are crucial to the diagnosis, as there are no laboratory studies specific for Crohn disease. In the ambulatory setting, endoscopic and contrast evaluations of the GI tract will often help establish the diagnosis. Esophagogastroduodenoscopy (EGD), colonoscopy with visualization of the terminal ileum, or barium enema with inspection of the terminal ileum, and small bowel contrast studies (Figure 13-6) are the most useful diagnostic evaluations. Findings may include ulceration, edema, stricture, or fistula formation. A contrast CT may be helpful in identifying abscesses, SBO, and other associated disease processes. An enteroclysis study of the small intestine may be helpful when standard SBFT is inconclusive. This test involves intubation of the small intestine and instillation of air and contrast to outline mucosal detail precisely. Endoscopic biopsies may be helpful, but because they sample primarily mucosa, they often fail histologically to prove the diagnosis of Crohn disease. EGD and/or upper GI contrast examination are important in evaluating patients with suspected foregut involvement. Capsule endoscopy may be used in the absence of stricture when standard

endoscopic and radiologic assessments are inconclusive. Cystography, cystoscopy, and vaginal examination are also useful in evaluating a patient with suspected urinary or vaginal fistula.

Differential Diagnosis

Acute flares of Crohn disease, UC, acute appendicitis, acute regional ileitis caused by *Yersinia* infection, pelvic inflammatory disease, and tuberculosis of the bowel are all diagnoses that may manifest similarly.

Treatment
Medical Therapy

Medical management of Crohn disease can include a variety of measures that control the inflammatory process. Symptom palliation can include analgesics, antimotility agents, and local measures for fistulae. IV fluids, enteral nutrition, or parenteral nutrition with complete bowel rest may be administered depending on the extent of fluid losses and malabsorption in severe disease. Several

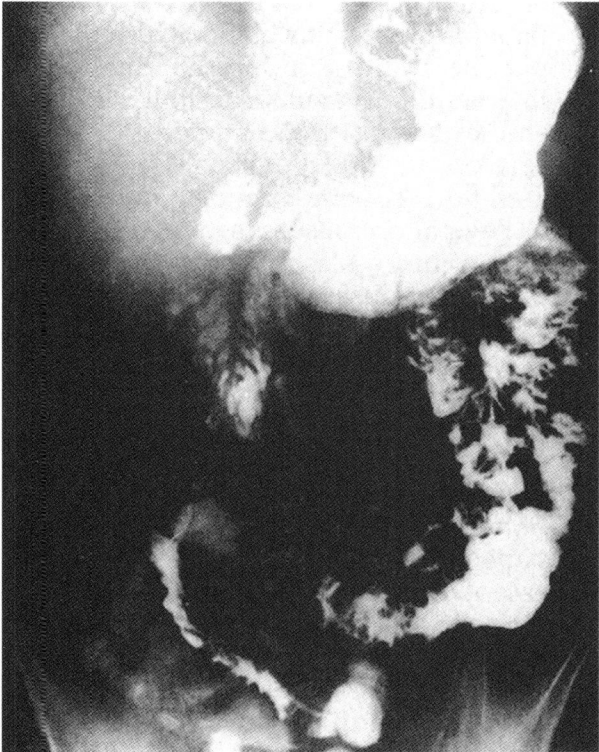
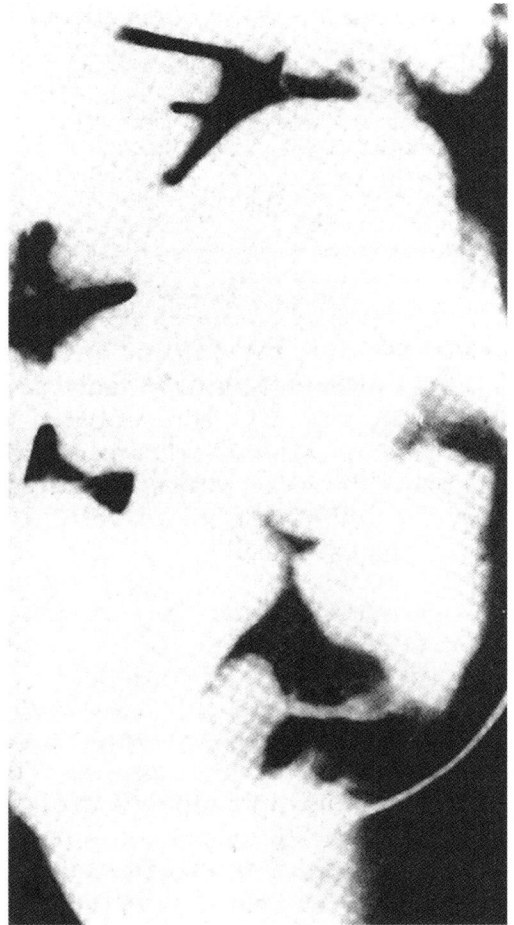

A **B**

Figure 13-6. A. Small bowel study showing narrowing in a segment of distal small bowel and in the antrum of the stomach. The mucosal pattern of the bowel is altered by pseudopolyps, and the valvulae conniventes are absent. Contrast fills some segments of the small bowel, suggesting skipped areas of Crohn disease involvement, while distally the bowel is narrowed. B. Small bowel study showing the "string sign of Kantor" in the terminal ileum adjacent to the cecum, with proximal dilation of the ileum.

pharmacologic agents may be used to mitigate inflammation. Historically, patients received therapy that escalated from anti-inflammatories and corticosteroids to immunomodulators and biologic agents (ie, "bottom-up" therapy) to achieve and maintain remission. More commonly now, patients receive more aggressive medical modalities upfront to minimize relapse or failure of acute flare control (ie, "top-down" therapy). The following paragraphs review the classes of medications commonly used in top-down approaches to treatment.

Biologic agents, or "biologics," are bioengineered medications made from living organisms and their products. The first approved biologic agent for Crohn disease was infliximab, a chimeric monoclonal antibody directed against tumor necrosis factor-α. Infliximab has demonstrated efficacy as treatment for steroid-resistant moderate-to-severe active disease, for enterocutaneous and perineal fistulae, and as maintenance therapy. Its major side effect is immune-mediated infusion reaction, likely due to the component of the antibody derived from mice. Because of the risk of these reactions, infusions must be performed in a relatively high-cost monitored setting. Adalimumab is a fully human-derived monoclonal antibody directed against tumor necrosis factor-α, which has lower risk of immune-mediated reaction compared with infliximab. Furthermore, adalimumab may be administered subcutaneously at home. Certolizumab is also a subcutaneously administered agent with a longer half-life, therefore requiring less frequent doses. Patients may have different responses to each biologic agent; therefore, it is reasonable to trial a different biologic if response to one agent begins to diminish.

Immunosuppressive and immune-modulating agents include azathioprine, 6-mercaptopurine, methotrexate, cyclosporine, tacrolimus, and mycophenolate. Azathioprine and 6-mercaptopurine take approximately 3 to 6 months to achieve full effect. They are valuable in preventing relapse of disease once remission has been achieved. Side effects of these agents include GI upset, hepatocellular injury, pancreatitis, and bone marrow toxicity. Methotrexate may also aid in sustaining remission. Cyclosporine is used frequently to treat Crohn fistulae that are refractory to steroids and metronidazole, though nephrotoxicity and susceptibility to *Pneumocystis carinii* pneumonitis are known side effects.

Corticosteroids are effective in Crohn disease. Suppositories and enemas are useful for disease limited to the distal colon, but they do not treat small bowel disease effectively. Prednisone in doses up to 60 mg/day can be used orally for severe disease. Clinical response occurs in a majority of patients within 7 to 10 days of initiation. IV steroids such as hydrocortisone or methylprednisolone are used when patients are unable to tolerate enteral administration. Budesonide is subject to first-pass metabolism in the liver and minimizes systemic toxicity, yet its efficacy may be slightly lower than other corticosteroids. The risk of side effects of corticosteroids is proportional to the dose and duration of therapy and includes hypertension, cataracts, osteoporosis, weight gain, striae, and adrenal suppression.

Pharmacologic agents used in the management of Crohn disease include anti-inflammatories and immunomodulators. Sulfasalazine was one of the first agents used, particularly for colonic disease, and was discovered when patients taking this drug for arthritis noted an improvement in their colitis symptoms. In the distal ileum and colon, intestinal bacteria remove the sulfonamide moiety of sulfasalazine, releasing the pharmacoactive 5-aminosalicylate metabolite. This metabolite may inhibit nuclear factor-κB, which is a potent inflammatory cytokine. It may also limit the production of prostaglandins and leukotrienes and assist as a scavenger of reactive oxygen species. The formulations of 5-aminosalicylic acid (mesalamine) commonly used today are deployed in the proximal small bowel and activated by a slow-release pH-dependent mechanism.

For those with chronic and subacute Crohn disease, enteral nutrition supplementation is preferred over parenteral nutrition, as it preserves mucosal and hepatic cellular structural integrity and function, costs less, and is associated with lower risk of complications. Elemental diets were thought to minimize the work of digestion, but are not palatable, require administration by tube, and have not demonstrated superiority over standard enteral formulas. Patients with persistent SBO, severe disease, and fistulae (especially those in the proximal small bowel) will often require parenteral nutrition. Supplementation with vitamins is frequently necessary. Refeeding syndrome may affect those with severe malnutrition when either of enteral feeds or parenteral nutrition is initiated. Serum electrolytes, especially phosphate, must be followed closely as the sudden need to process and store intracellular energy substrates increases demand upon electrolyte flux.

Antidiarrheal agents, including loperamide, diphenoxylate, codeine, and cholestyramine, may treat symptoms. Adverse effects of these agents include adynamic ileus, bacterial overgrowth, and toxic megacolon. Cholestyramine is effective in treating diarrhea from poorly reabsorbed bile salts when the distal ileum is diseased or absent following resection. Diarrhea may also be treated by lactose avoidance and/or the use of lactase supplementation.

Surgical Therapy

Operative interventions in patients with Crohn disease are reserved for complicated disease and disease refractory to medical management (Table 13-2). The likelihood of recurrence of Crohn disease after surgery is as high as 40% within 5 years and 75% within 15 years of operation. As such, the surgical strategy is one of conservative management rather than radical extirpation. Bowel resections are performed only when absolutely necessary, and resection margins are limited to tissue that appears grossly normal. Overly aggressive resection in the hope of achieving microscopically normal margins may predispose the patient long term to short bowel syndrome (SBS), given the propensity for recurrent disease. Enteric fistulae, high-grade SBO, and perforation are indications for an operation. Many types of fistulae may be managed medically, but

TABLE 13-2. Indications for Surgery, Crohn Disease

Perforation
Fibrotic stricture
Acute complete bowel obstruction
Chronic partial bowel obstruction
Fistula (eg, enterocutaneous, enterovesical, enterovaginal)

enterovesical fistulas usually require surgical correction to prevent recurring urosepsis and development of renal dysfunction. In the setting of fibrotic, chronic strictures, stricuroplasty may relieve symptoms of SBO and minimize bowel resection.

Patients with Crohn disease often have bacterial colonization of the small intestine, and septic, anastomotic, and surgical site infectious complications are relatively common. When a bowel resection is performed, primary anastomosis is usually possible, although temporary stomas may be performed in the setting of advanced peritonitis, sepsis, or immunosuppressed state from medical therapy. Historically, appendectomy was performed at the time of laparotomy to prevent future diagnostic confusion between Crohn flare and appendicitis; however, if appendectomy is performed in the setting of active disease involving the cecum or base of the appendix, the risk of fistula development is relatively high.

Patients with fistulae who fail to respond to medical management are usually managed with surgical resection of the involved loop of bowel and excision of the fistula tract. Patients with large abscesses are treated with percutaneous drainage and antibiotic therapy. If perianal fistulas fail to respond to medical management, surgical options include drainage of abscesses and placement of noncutting setons to promote continuous drainage. In refractory cases, fecal diversion via enterostomy creation or even proctectomy may be performed. As a general rule, surgical intervention is limited to the least aggressive intervention possible. Nearly all patients will require perioperative nutritional support. At the time of any operative intervention, the surgeon must inspect the entire bowel for skip lesions and document the length of bowel resected and the length of small bowel remaining for future reference. Patients with 100 cm of healthy small bowel (or 50 cm with an intact ICV are expected to recover without prolonged parenteral nutrition.

Complications

The most common complications of Crohn disease include malnutrition, obstruction, fistulae, and electrolyte disturbances. Surgical treatment can be complicated by wound infection, intestinal failure (SBS), impaired wound healing, and fistulae. Anal incontinence can complicate advanced perianal disease or aggressive surgical approaches that compromise sphincter integrity.

Acute Mesenteric Ischemia

Acute mesenteric ischemia (AMI) is a surgical emergency resulting from vascular compromise of the midgut. The SMA is a direct anterior branch of the aorta that supplies the small bowel and proximal colon, and the superior mesenteric vein (SMV) drains the same territory into the portal vein. There are extensive arterial collaterals to the branches of the SMA primarily originating from the celiac axis, and to a lesser extent from the inferior mesenteric artery. These collaterals protect the midgut from an acute drop in SMA blood flow. In AMI, blood flow is impaired and the poorly perfused bowel becomes ischemic and then necrotic. Unfortunately, it is difficult to diagnose AMI, and delayed recognition often results in extensive loss of bowel and even death.

Pathophysiology

There are four general categories of AMI. First, emboli to the SMA usually originate from the heart and are frequently associated with atrial fibrillation. In this scenario, mural thrombus forms within the atrium, becomes dislodged, and travels to the proximal SMA, where it will occlude arterial blood flow (usually distal to the middle colic artery as the artery narrows). Second, primary SMA thrombosis is caused by chronic narrowing of the SMA. It is frequently associated with other vascular diseases, such as atherosclerosis, coronary artery disease, peripheral vascular disease, and chronic renal insufficiency. Patients classically report a history of pain with eating ("intestinal angina"), food fear, and weight loss. If the vessel thromboses completely, AMI may occur. In contrast to SMA embolism, SMA thrombosis usually begins at the origin of the SMA and is more likely to lead to complete infarction of the midgut (the entire bowel from the ligament of Treitz to the proximal transverse colon). The third category is mesenteric venous thrombosis, which often reflects a hypercoagulable state, such as antithrombin III deficiency or factor V Leiden. Thrombosis of the SMV obstructs venous outflow, resulting in venous hypertension, bowel wall edema, and, ultimately, decreased arterial perfusion. The final category is nonocclusive mesenteric ischemia (NOMI), which occurs due to a systemic state of poor blood flow. This scenario occurs in patients with shock, heart failure, or those undergoing hemodialysis. Patients in severe shock may shunt blood flow away from the GI tract to preserve cerebral blood flow. In all categories, acute ischemia lasting longer than 12 hours is likely to progress to bowel necrosis.

Clinical Presentation

The pain associated with AMI is rapid and severe, though early in the process there may not be any impressive findings on physical examination. This presentation of "pain out of proportion to examination" may delay diagnosis, resulting in bowel necrosis. It is important to recognize this pattern of pain and associated risk factors for AMI. By the time a patient develops peritoneal signs, bowel infarction has probably already occurred, and the risk of mortality is relatively high.

In contrast to arterial occlusion, SMV thrombosis tends to have a more insidious onset. Patients may have pain for several days to weeks prior to diagnosis. The pain may be diffuse and nonspecific. Bowel ischemia symptoms in patients with NOMI may be difficult to assess in the context of other complex systemic pathophysiology. The predominant clinical feature of NOMI is hemodynamic compromise.

Diagnosis

Rapid diagnosis and treatment are crucial in AMI. Unfortunately, laboratory studies are nonspecific for AMI, and normal lab values do not exclude the diagnosis. Although some patients may develop an elevated white blood cell (WBC) count, increased lactic acid, and metabolic acidosis, these findings may be late indicators of bowel ischemia or infarction. The gold standard diagnostic test is a mesenteric arteriogram, a fluoroscopic evaluation of contrast filling the mesenteric arterial and venous systems. Sites of arterial or venous occlusion will be readily apparent, and narrowing or sluggish filling of the vessels suggests NOMI. Mesenteric arteriograms are commonly performed as part of high-resolution CT scans, as they provide excellent visualization of the vessels and intra-abdominal organs, and can diagnose nonvascular causes of abdominal pain. Furthermore, the CT scan can identify other ominous signs of bowel infarction, such as bowel wall thickening, pneumatosis intestinalis (gas within the bowel wall), or portal venous gas.

Treatment

The initial treatment of AMI is immediate fluid resuscitation and correction of metabolic abnormalities. Antibiotics are frequently administered due to the risk of contamination from necrotic bowel. Primary goals of treatment include restoration of blood flow to the gut, resection of necrotic bowel, and minimization of reperfusion injury following restoration of blood flow. For patients with an SMA embolism, emergent embolectomy and assessment of bowel viability are performed via laparotomy. The SMA is controlled proximally and distally, and an arteriotomy is performed. A balloon catheter is placed into the artery distal to the embolus, and the balloon is inflated as the catheter is removed, which evacuates the embolus from the vessel. In primary SMA thrombosis, the SMA is often narrowed by severe chronic atherosclerotic disease. The bowel is revascularized by either placement of an endovascular stent or creation of a conduit that bypasses the occluded segment of the SMA. SMV thrombosis is treated with pharmacologic anticoagulation. The treatment for NOMI is directed at the underlying pathology causing the low-perfusion state. Vasospasm contributes to bowel ischemia in NOMI, and so vasoconstrictors such as α-adrenergic agonists should be avoided. Invasive monitoring of cardiac output may also be performed. In all cases of AMI, suspicion of bowel necrosis should prompt an emergent exploratory laparotomy or laparoscopy, and necrotic bowel should be resected.

In some cases, it is unclear whether the bowel will be viable after blood flow is restored surgically. The bowel that remains ischemic appearing or is of questionable viability may be left in situ, and the surgeon may perform a second-look operation within 48 hours. During this time, the patient receives resuscitation and supportive care in the intensive care unit (ICU). Upon returning to the operating room, the time interval allows the bowel to demarcate margins of viability, and the surgeon can decide whether to resect additional bowel, perform a primary anastomosis, or create an enterostomy.

Complications

Patients with AMI are often quite ill, and complications include respiratory distress syndrome, acute kidney injury, multisystem organ failure, septic shock, and impaired wound healing (including fascial or anastomotic dehiscence). A prolonged ICU stay may be necessary. Complications are often compounded by the patient's comorbid conditions. In cases of massive small bowel necrosis, surgeons must decide whether to aggressively resect and risk intestinal failure or to minimize further invasive maneuvers. In these cases, it is critical to engage with the patient's family in candid multidisciplinary discussions of anticipated prognosis and goals of care. Rapid recognition and initiation of treatment predict the most favorable outcomes for AMI; however, mortality remains high.

Small Bowel Tumors

A variety of tumors arise from the small bowel. Tumors of the small bowel are much less common than those of the colon and rectum. Small bowel tumors may present with obstructive symptoms, bleeding, or symptoms of metastatic disease. They may also act as lead points for intussusception. These tumors may be identified by contrast studies, endoscopy, enteroclysis, or CT enterography.

Endoscopy is limited by the length and navigability of the bowel with a flexible fiber optic scope. Capsule endoscopy may assist in the visualization of luminal small bowel tumors. With this technique, the patient swallows a capsule-sized, camera-equipped device that transmits images for later interpretation as it passes through the bowel. While the capsule does not perform biopsies or therapeutic interventions, the minimally invasive nature of this diagnostic modality is favorable. Specialized double-balloon enteroscopy is a technique in which a balloon-fitted endoscope repetitively progresses through the bowel and is capable of visualizing up to two-thirds of the length of the small bowel.

Benign Tumors

Benign small intestinal tumors are much more common than malignant lesions. Most are asymptomatic. The peak incidence of these lesions is in the sixth decade, with no observable differences among sexes. The most common of these lesions are GISTs, derived from the mesenchyme, arising from interstitial cells of Cajal (Figure 13-7). Lesions in this category are diagnosed by expression of c-kit proto-oncogene protein (CD117), in resected specimens.

Nonepithelial, benign tumors of the small bowel include lipomas, hemangiomas, hamartomas, lymphangiomas, and neurogenic tumors, such as schwannomas and neurofibromas. Lipomas are more common in men and occur most commonly in the duodenum and ileum. Hemangiomas can cause occult bleeding and constitute 5% of benign small bowel lesions. These lesions are often multiple, as in Osler-Weber-Rendu syndrome. Capsule enteroscopy may be useful in diagnosing hemangiomas, as they do not show up on standard contrast studies. For actively bleeding lesions, angiography may also be useful. Hamartomas are benign proliferations of mature cell types, and they are usually

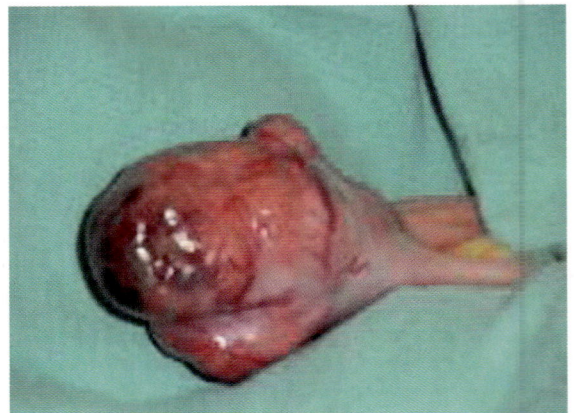

Figure 13-7. Operative photograph of a gastrointestinal stromal tumor arising from the antimesenteric aspect of the small bowel wall.

isolated and asymptomatic. They can be a cause of bleeding or intussusception, particularly in the pediatric population. Multiple hamartomas are associated with Peutz-Jeghers syndrome, an autosomal dominant condition that is also characterized by mucocutaneous hyperpigmentation.

Epithelial benign lesions of the small intestine include tubular, villous, and Brunner gland adenomas. Brunner gland adenomas occur primarily in the duodenum and are usually asymptomatic, as are most tubular adenomas. Villous adenomas should be excised, as they have a 30% risk of malignancy that increases with size.

Benign small bowel tumors are typically discovered incidentally and have an indolent course. As the tumor enlarges, it can cause obstruction or intussusception. Adenomas and submucosal lesions can have associated mucosal ulceration as they outgrow the capacity of their blood supply, which can lead to intraluminal hemorrhage. Less commonly, the tumor grows extraluminally and causes a palpable abdominal mass, intra-abdominal bleeding, or perforation.

Malignant Tumors

A variety of malignant tumors can affect the small intestine, although these constitute only 2% of all GI tract malignancies. Overall, malignant tumors are slightly more common in males than in females, and the mean age at presentation is in the sixth decade. The most common malignant disease that involves the small bowel is metastatic melanoma. The following sections outline the most common malignancies that arise primarily from the small bowel.

Adenocarcinomas

Adenocarcinomas account for approximately half of all primary small intestinal malignancies. They most commonly occur in the duodenum, and incidence decreases moving distally. Nearly half of small intestinal adenocarcinomas are diagnosed at the time of operation. Obstruction, often associated with weight loss, is the most common presentation. In adults, SBO in the absence of hernia or prior abdominal surgery should heighten one's concern for neoplasm. Occult bleeding and anemia may also be present. In younger patients, occult bleeding is a common manifestation of small bowel neoplasia. Massive bleeding is rare. Lesions in the periampullary region may present with painless jaundice due to biliary obstruction, and rarely with pancreatitis. Duodenal carcinoma of the periampullary region, typically arising from a preexisting benign adenoma, is the most common malignancy affecting individuals with familial adenomatous polyposis (FAP) after proctocolectomy. For this reason, routine surveillance endoscopy of the duodenum is required in these patients.

Operation for small bowel adenocarcinoma should include wide resection of the involved bowel and the mesenteric lymphatic drainage basin. Adjuvant therapies have little demonstrated efficacy, and the 5-year survival is approximately 10% to 30%. This poor prognosis likely reflects the advanced state of disease that manifests clinical symptoms at the time of diagnosis. For those with known risk factors, such as FAP, endoscopic screening may result in earlier diagnosis.

Carcinoid Tumors

Carcinoid tumors arise from Kulchitsky cells in the crypts of Lieberkühn. The risk of malignancy correlates with lesion size; metastasis occurs in only 2% of primary tumors less than 1 cm in size, but in 90% of those with primary tumors larger than 2 cm. Between 40% and 50% of all GI carcinoids originate in the appendix, and the small intestine is the second most common GI site. Small intestinal carcinoids are most common in the ileum and are multicentric in up to 30% of patients.

Obstruction is the most common presenting finding in patients with small intestinal carcinoid. This is usually due to an intense inflammatory (desmoplastic) reaction that characteristically occurs in the adjacent bowel mesentery rather than obstruction by the tumor, itself. Bleeding and intussusception are less common. Many patients experience nonspecific symptoms, including anorexia, fatigue, and weight loss. The diagnosis is often made at laparotomy, and surgical treatment consists of a wide excision of the bowel and mesentery. For lesions in the terminal ileum, right hemicolectomy may be necessary. Resectable liver metastases should also be removed if they are identified at the time of operation.

The carcinoid syndrome is characterized by episodic cutaneous flushing (especially of the head and trunk), bronchospasm, intestinal cramping and diarrhea, vasomotor instability, pellagra-like skin lesions, and right-sided valvular heart disease (Figure 13-8). These attacks may be spontaneous or triggered by exertion, excitement, alcohol, anesthesia, or tumor manipulation. Disease manifestations are related to the production of serotonin (5-hydroxytryptamine) by the tumor. This substance is degraded on delivery to the liver via the portal vein into 5-hydroxyindole acetic acid (5-HIAA), as well as other vasoactive peptides including 5-hydroxytryptophan, kallikrein, histamine, and adrenocorticotropic hormone (ACTH). It is not entirely clear which combination of these substances is responsible for the syndrome. The liver is highly effective in clearing serotonin and its metabolites from the bloodstream when received via the portal vein. For the syndrome to occur, these substances must be present in the systemic (and not the portal) circulation. Accordingly, a small bowel carcinoid tumor in association with carcinoid syndrome is assumed to have metastasized to the liver, or beyond. Otherwise, the primary tumor is located outside the portal circulation, such as the lungs, gonads, or rectum. The syndrome is confirmed by an elevated urine 5-HIAA level. Serum measurement of serotonin or chromogranin A may also be confirmatory. Treatment is via resection, when possible.

Lymphoma

The small bowel is the most common site of extranodal lymphoma, although only 5% of all lymphomas are found there. Lymphoma accounts for 10% to 15% of all small bowel malignancies. Peak incidence is in the fifth and sixth decades of life. The ileum is the most common site of involvement, given the concentration of lymphoid tissue in Peyer patches in that region. Although more commonly described in the stomach in association with chronic gastritis associated with *Helicobacter pylori* infection, mucosa-associated lymphoid tissue lymphomas may occur in the small intestine and are found in a subset of patients with small intestinal lymphoma. Although most patients present with nonspecific symptoms such as vague abdominal pain, weight loss, fatigue, and malaise, up to one in four may present as abdominal

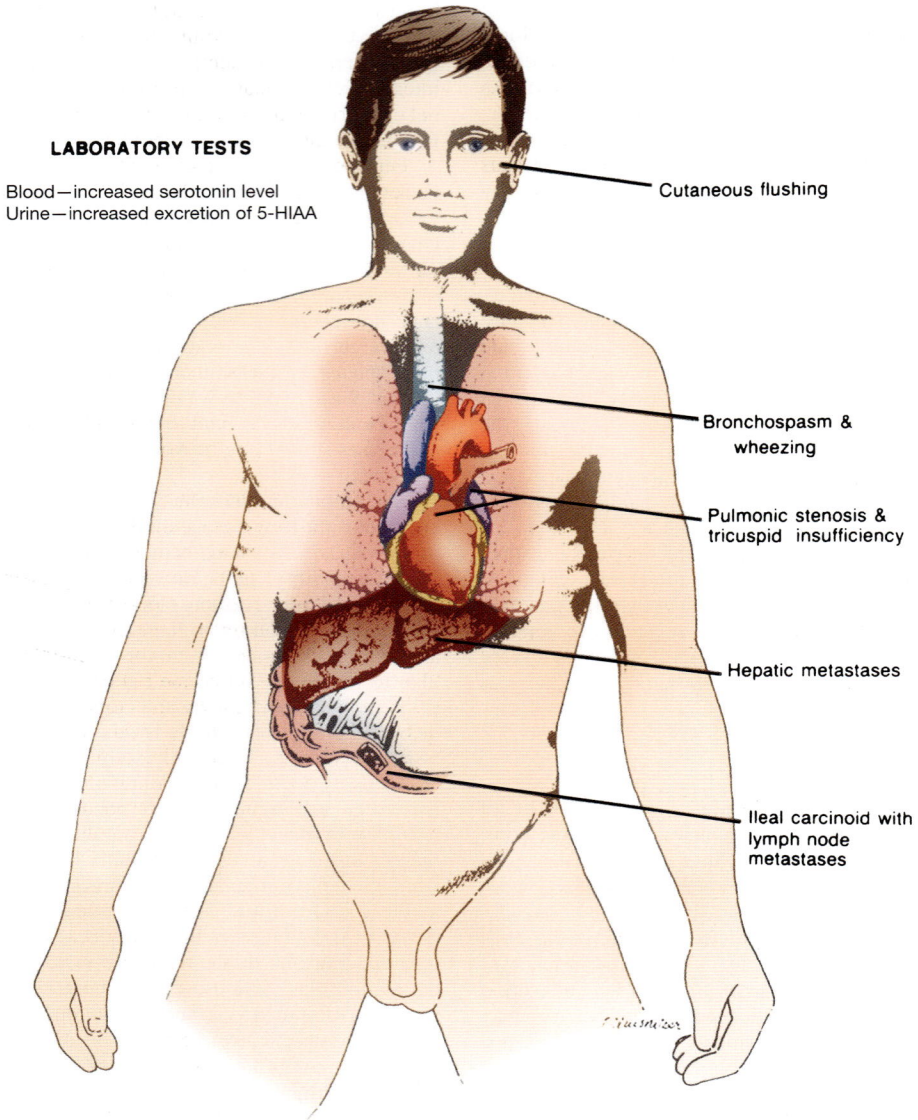

LABORATORY TESTS

Blood—increased serotonin level
Urine—increased excretion of 5-HIAA

Cutaneous flushing

Bronchospasm & wheezing

Pulmonic stenosis & tricuspid insufficiency

Hepatic metastases

Ileal carcinoid with lymph node metastases

Figure 13-8. **Clinical manifestations of malignant carcinoid syndrome.** 5-HIAA, 5-hydroxyindole acetic acid.

emergencies (eg, perforation, hemorrhage, obstruction, or intussusception). Nodularity and thickening of the bowel wall may be present on contrast studies or CT scan, often with associated mesenteric adenopathy. When diagnosed on imaging, patients generally undergo chemotherapy and sometimes radiation therapy. Rapid tumor lysis during treatment can cause intestinal perforation. Median survival exceeds 10 years. When patients present with a surgical emergency, resection is usually performed at the time of exploration, and subsequent adjuvant chemotherapy and/or radio therapy are administered, depending on the type of lymphoma and stage of disease. The 5-year survival in this condition is approximately 20% to 40%.

Gastrointestinal Stromal Tumors

GISTs can have a spectrum of clinical behaviors from benign to malignant. They have a peak incidence in the sixth decade, may occur anywhere in the GI tract, and can present with obstruction, bleeding, or perforation. Like their benign counterparts, malignant GISTs express c-kit protein. Malignant mesenchymal lesions that do not express c-kit are classified as leiomyosarcomas. Small bowel GISTs appear to have a worse prognosis than similar lesions of the esophagus and stomach. Surgical treatment includes wide excision of bowel and mesentery, and malignant behavior is determined by the number of mitoses per high-power field, evidence of tissue invasion, nuclear pleomorphism, and tumor necrosis. Approximately 50% of patients will have recurrent disease within 2 years. Some patients with metastatic GISTs have impressive responses to imatinib (Gleevec), a tyrosine kinase inhibitor that is also used to treat patients with chronic myelogenous leukemia. This agent may also be used as neoadjuvant treatment in patients presenting with advanced disease. If patients become refractory to or intolerant of imatinib, they may be transitioned to one of several tyrosine kinase inhibitors, such as sunitinib.

Congenital Abnormalities

Meckel Diverticulum

Significance and Incidence

Meckel diverticulum is the most common congenital anomaly of the small intestine and represents a remnant of the omphalomesenteric (vitelline) duct. They are present in approximately 2% of the population, usually 2 in long, twice as common in males, may have up to two types of mucosa, and are typically located within 2 ft of the ileocecal junction. These characteristics are collectively known as the "rule of twos." Symptoms caused by Meckel diverticula are rare and become less common with age. Accordingly, symptoms may develop in 5% of infants with Meckel diverticulum, 1.5% of individuals at age 40, and extremely rarely in older patients. Less than 4% of those with Meckel diverticulum will develop symptoms over their lifetimes.

Anatomy

Meckel diverticula result when there is incomplete obliteration of the vitelline duct, which arises from the midgut and provides communication between the yolk sac and the fetal midgut. It typically closes before the 10th week of gestation when the placenta becomes the primary source of fetal nutrition. The diverticulum arises from the antimesenteric border of the ileum, usually within 60 cm (2 ft) of the ileocecal junction (Figure 13-9). Its blood supply is from the omphalomesenteric (vitelline) vessels, which arise from the ileal branches of the SMA.

Pathophysiology

The cells lining the vitelline duct have pluripotent capabilities. As a result, it is not uncommon to find ectopic/heterotopic mucosa within the diverticulum. The most common type of mucosa is gastric (50%). Less frequently, pancreatic, duodenal, and colonic mucosa may be found.

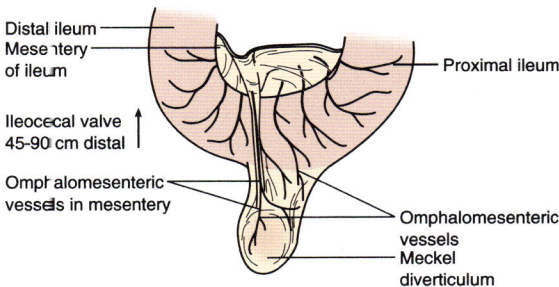

Distal ileum
Mesentery of ileum
Proximal ileum
Ileocecal valve 45-90 cm distal
Omphalomesenteric vessels in mesentery
Omphalomesenteric vessels
Meckel diverticulum

Figure 13-9. Anatomy of Meckel diverticulum.

Gastric mucosa in particular, because of its capacity to secrete acid in direct proximity to small bowel mucosa, may cause ulceration and hemorrhage. Benign tumors including lipomas, leiomyomas, neurofibromas, and angiomas have been described in diverticula as well. Such tumors may act as a lead point for intussusception and bowel obstruction.

Persistence of a patent omphalomesenteric duct can present as an enteric fistula, with drainage of succus entericus from the umbilicus. If the umbilical end of the duct remains patent with an obliterated mesenteric end, the result is an umbilical sinus, which may drain serous fluid or mucous. A persistent sinus or cyst may also develop bacterial overgrowth that can lead to infection. A Meckel diverticulum may itself become occluded and become inflamed, presenting in a manner that mimics acute appendicitis. If the duct obliterates but leaves a fibrous cord remnant, this cord can produce a "clothesline" phenomenon and may cause the normal bowel to volvulize around it.

Clinical Presentation and Evaluation

The most common presenting illnesses related to Meckel diverticula include SBO, hemorrhage, inflammation, and, rarely, umbilical fistula. Hemorrhage presents with painless bright red or maroon blood per rectum and is most common in infants under 2 years of age. Diagnosis can be made in some cases with technetium-99m pertechnetate "Meckel" scan, in which the radionuclide is taken up by gastric mucosa and shows its ectopic location within the diverticulum. The sensitivity of this scan may be enhanced by administration of cimetidine or pentagastrin.

SBO can occur because of volvulus of the small bowel around the diverticulum or remnant cord. Intussusception may also occur, with the diverticulum acting as a lead point. The inflammation of Meckel diverticulitis closely mimics the symptoms and signs of acute appendicitis, and so the surgeon should consider a Meckel diverticulum if a normal appendix is discovered when performing an appendectomy. Less common complications include iron deficiency anemia, malabsorption, foreign body impaction, perforation, and incarceration of a Meckel diverticulum within a hernia ("Littre" hernia).

Differential Diagnosis

Acute appendicitis, adhesive SBO, and regional enteritis are more common than Meckel diverticulum and have similar presenting symptoms and signs. Lower GI bleeding, except in a very young patient, is much more commonly caused by other pathologies, including diverticular disease of the colon and angiodysplastic lesions. In adult patients, endoscopic and contrast studies to exclude these more common conditions should be prioritized. In children with similar presenting symptoms, Meckel diverticulum should be more strongly considered. Patients who require operations for acute obstructive and inflammatory presentations will typically have the diagnosis established intraoperatively. Adults with atypical, subacute presentations and negative workup for other common diagnoses may require Meckel scans, small bowel contrast studies, or laparoscopy to establish the diagnosis.

Treatment

When a symptomatic Meckel diverticulum is discovered, resection is curative. A diverticulum with a narrow base that has no palpable ectopic mucosa may be divided at its base, preserving the adjacent small bowel. Ideally, the base of the diverticulum is closed without narrowing the small bowel lumen. When the diverticulum is broad based, segmental bowel resection may be required to remove all ectopic tissue. Laparoscopic resection is a safe option. There is controversy regarding the most appropriate management when an asymptomatic diverticulum is found incidentally at the time of surgery for other purposes. In younger patients, the low risk of morbidity may justify resection. However, this potential benefit is small and diminishes over time. With age, the likelihood of developing symptoms decreases. Resection is reasonable in adult patients when the diverticulum has a narrow base, when a large fibrous band is present, or when heterotopic tissue is evident or palpable. Resection may also be appropriate in patients who would be difficult to reexplore surgically (eg, recurrent adhesive SBO or pending radiation therapy).

Malrotation

Malrotation of the bowel may occur between the 4th and 10th weeks of gestation as bowel proliferation, rotation, and fixation occur. In normal development, an initial 90° counterclockwise rotation of the midgut places the duodenum in the retroperitoneum posterior to the superior mesenteric vessels. Next, a 180° counterclockwise rotation of the midgut places the cecum in the right lower quadrant, and the transverse colon anterior to the superior mesenteric vessels. When these two rotations are not completed correctly, a variety of anatomic abnormalities can occur. These anomalous configurations may be asymptomatic or present with symptoms at any age. Ladd bands are congenital adhesions that drape across the duodenum and affix the malpositioned cecum to the retroperitoneum in the right upper quadrant. Although Ladd bands may cause duodenal obstruction, the most common clinical manifestation of malrotation is midgut volvulus in an infant. Malrotation without midgut volvulus is usually diagnosed incidentally. Volvulus involves twisting of the small bowel around its mesentery. This occurs because the mesenteric root is narrow between the malrotated cecum and duodenum. Volvulus impairs blood flow through the mesenteric blood vessels, and this rapidly leads to ischemia and necrosis. Early symptoms include bilious emesis, which will progress to distension, tenderness, peritonitis, and septic shock. An infant with bilious emesis in the absence of peritonitis should undergo an emergent upper GI contrast study to exclude intestinal malrotation. Any suspicion of midgut volvulus requires emergent laparotomy and Ladd procedure, which includes detorsion of volvulized bowel, division of the Ladd bands, broadening of the mesentery, and replacement of the small bowel on the right and colon on the left side of the abdomen in a "nonrotated" state. This orientation decreases the risk of future volvulus, as the mesenteric root is no longer narrowed. Appendectomy may be performed during a Ladd procedure to avoid future misdiagnosis of appendicitis, as the appendix would otherwise be located in the left abdomen.

Short Bowel Syndrome

Intestinal failure occurs when a patient's bowel is incapable of maintaining fluid and nutritional needs. SBS is a cause of intestinal failure and, in an adult, is defined as less than 200 cm of continuous small intestine as measured from the duodenojejunal junction. SBS most commonly results from small bowel resection or tissue loss. Common predisposing conditions include Crohn disease, recurrent SBO, mesenteric ischemia, or hernia with strangulation. SBS in pediatric patients is defined as a small bowel length less than 25% of the expected size. The most common causes of SBS in infants are necrotizing enterocolitis, midgut volvulus, and gastroschisis. In SBS, the bowel adapts by dilating and increasing villous height. In some cases, increased feeding volume may be all that is required to maintain nutrition. The ileum is highly adaptive, but loss of the terminal ileum may result in an ability to absorb vitamin B$_{12}$ and bile salts.

An intact colon and ICV increase the absorptive capacity of the small bowel. The risk of requiring TPN is substantially increased when the bowel length is less than 100 cm or less than 50 cm with an intact ICV. TPN has many risks, including, but not limited to, central line-associated infections, hypoglycemia or hyperglycemia, cholestasis and hepatic failure, and gallstones. Intestinal rehabilitation is a long-term treatment strategy that includes dietary changes and supplements that support gut adaptation in hopes of decreasing the need for TPN over time.

In patients with intestinal failure that is refractory to rehabilitation, bowel lengthening procedures may provide some benefit. Lengthening may be accomplished surgically by the Bianchi procedure, where the dilated bowel is longitudinally divided into two tubularized segments, preserving each side of the mesenteric vessels, and anastomosing the segments end to end. Alternatively, the serial transverse enteroplasty (STEP) technique involves a series of stapled transverse hemisections of the dilated bowel. This creates a zigzag pattern of the intestinal lumen that theoretically increases the surface area-to-volume ratio. Neither the STEP nor the Bianchi procedure results in an increase of intestinal tissue, and both have mixed results in achieving TPN independence. Distraction enterogenesis is an experimental concept devised to regenerate intestinal tissue and absorptive capacity by applying a stretch force with an implantable device. This concept has shown promise in animal models. Small bowel or multivisceral transplant is the ultimate surgical option for patients with refractory or complicated intestinal failure, though it involves lifelong immunosuppression and is frequently complicated by chronic pain, diarrhea, malabsorption, enterostomal complications, and failure to thrive or malnutrition.

DISEASES OF THE APPENDIX

Acute Appendicitis

Significance and Incidence

In the United States, diseases of the appendix account for approximately 10,000 deaths annually. Appendectomy is the most common urgent operation performed by general surgeons. Approximately 8.7% of the global population will experience appendicitis, and there is an increasing trend of incidence between 1990 and 2019. Though appendicitis can occur at any age, most patients present between ages 5 to 35 years and within the first 48 hours of the onset of symptoms. Young children and older patients are more likely to present with atypical signs and symptoms, thereby delaying diagnosis. The risk of perforated appendicitis in these groups is nearly double that of the rest of the population.

Anatomy

The appendix is in the right lower quadrant at the confluence of the teniae coli at the apex of the cecum. It may be found in a variety of positions relative to the cecum. This position may dictate where periappendiceal inflammation causes tenderness on examination. The appendiceal artery is a branch of the ileocolic artery and travels within the mesoappendix. The appendix is rich in lymphatic follicles, which are most numerous in people between 10 and 20 years of age. Some hypothesize this may signify an immunologic role of the appendix, while others suggest the organ may serve to repopulate depleted or altered colonic flora.

Pathophysiology

Appendiceal luminal obstruction causes acute appendicitis. Lymphoid hyperplasia is seen in 60% of patients with appendicitis. An accumulation of fecal material, or fecalith, is noted histologically in 35% of patients. Viral illnesses that elicit lymphoid hyperplasia frequently precede appendicitis in young patients. With an obstructed lumen, mucus secretion by the appendiceal epithelium leads to distension. Venous outflow is compromised as the appendix is pressurized with mucus and bacterial overgrowth, and this leads to ischemia and bacterial infection. Bacterial toxins can produce further mucosal damage. Without treatment, transmural ischemia leads to gangrene, and perforation occurs in up to 20% of cases. Omentum or other adjacent visceral structures may adhere to the site of perforation to contain it, and this results in phlegmon/abscess formation and localized peritonitis. Diffuse peritonitis will develop if the perforation is not contained, and this commonly occurs in young children who lack a robust omentum. In advanced disease, gas-producing organisms may infiltrate the mesenteric venous system, and portal venous gas or liver abscesses may develop. The overwhelming infection may progress to septic shock, multisystem organ failure, and death.

Clinical Presentation and Evaluation

The initial discomfort of acute appendicitis is caused by luminal distension and is perceived as poorly localized, periumbilical visceral pain, which may be accompanied by anorexia, nausea, and vomiting. This presentation is attributed to the autonomic innervation of the appendix. As the disease progresses, inflammation in the adjacent parietal peritoneum results in more localized sharp pain and tenderness (usually in the right lower quadrant), which is conveyed by somatic nerves. Low-grade fever and leukocytosis are common but nonspecific, and either indicator may increase in severity as the disease progresses.

Classic examination findings include tenderness at McBurney point, located one-third of the distance from the anterior superior iliac spine to the umbilicus. If the inflamed appendix is positioned within the pelvis, tenderness may be elicited in the suprapubic area due to bladder irritation, or on rectal and/or pelvic examination. Signs of localized peritoneal irritation ("focal peritonitis") include rebound tenderness, guarding, and pain in the

right lower quadrant on deep palpation of the left lower quadrant (Rovsing sign). A positive Psoas sign describes pain on active flexion of the right hip against resistance, and this suggests a retrocecal position of the appendix with inflammation secondarily affecting the iliopsoas muscle. A positive Obturator sign describes pain with passive internal rotation of the right hip, and this suggests a pelvic position of the appendix, with inflammation affecting the adjacent obturator internus muscle.

When the appendix perforates, some report a temporary improvement in visceral pain as the appendix decompresses, but peritonitis will follow. Peritonitis becomes more likely as symptoms persist beyond 24 hours, and left untreated, sepsis develops with fever and leukocytosis. Small children with perforated appendicitis may present acutely with SBO, as secondary inflammation of the adjacent bowel may cause a kink or twist that obstructs its lumen.

The diagnosis of appendicitis may be difficult to make in a pregnant patient because the appendix is often displaced cephalad, and leukocytosis of pregnancy may mask the condition. A perforated appendix and peritonitis are associated with a 35% risk of fetal loss, and so early diagnosis is crucial. Appendectomy is acceptably safe when performed for acute appendicitis in any trimester, though surgeons must take care to avoid the gravid uterus during the operation. Perioperative and postoperative care should also include attention to the appropriate stage of pregnancy and may benefit from consultation with an obstetrician.

Differential Diagnosis and Diagnostic Evaluation

The differential diagnosis in a patient with a chief complaint of right lower quadrant abdominal pain includes a variety of GI, urologic, musculoskeletal, and gynecologic conditions. A careful and thorough history and physical examination must be performed. Common disease processes mimicking acute appendicitis include pelvic inflammatory disease, pyelonephritis, acute gastroenteritis, IBD, endometriosis, ovulatory pain (Mittelschmerz), ectopic pregnancy, tubo-ovarian abscess, and ruptured or hemorrhagic ovarian cyst. Right lower lobe pneumonia, Meckel diverticulitis, cecal or sigmoid diverticulitis, acute ileitis, cholecystitis, and perforated peptic ulcer disease may also have similar associated clinical symptoms and signs. Laboratory studies should include a complete blood count with differential and urinalysis.

For patients with equivocal clinical findings or atypical presentations, appendicitis is commonly diagnosed with cross-sectional imaging. Ultrasound is quite sensitive, especially among pediatric patients with low total body fat. The classic findings of appendicitis on ultrasound include a thickened, noncompressible, tubular structure with corresponding focal tenderness in the right lower quadrant. Secondary findings may include a luminal fecalith or free fluid around the tubular structure or in the pelvis. As with all ultrasound examinations, the reliability of the examination depends upon the levels of experience of the technician and the interpreting physician as well as the position of the appendix and amount of intraluminal gas obscuring the images. CT with IV contrast is both sensitive and specific in diagnosing appendicitis and may also clarify alternative differential diagnoses. Findings of appendicitis on CT scan classically include distension of the appendix with fluid, fecalith, inflammatory changes in the surrounding tissues (eg, fat stranding), abscess, and free fluid (Figure 13-10). MRI is an alternative modality with no risk of ionizing radiation, yet provides high diagnostic sensitivity and specificity, similar to those of CT. This profile makes MR an attractive choice for equivocal cases among children and pregnant patients; however, the need to lie still in a narrow space and the high cost or low availability may be prohibitive for some patients and hospitals.

The risk in failing to identify these differential diagnoses is a "negative appendectomy," in which an operation and general anesthesia are performed, but the diagnosis is incorrect. On the other hand, a missed diagnosis of appendicitis may lead to progression of perforation, sepsis, and threat to life. Weighing these competing risks, surgeons often have a difficult decision to make, and these risks must be addressed preoperatively during the informed consent discussion. Negative appendectomies comprise approximately 1% to 5% of all appendectomies performed in the United States.

Treatment

Acute appendicitis without perforation may be treated operatively or nonoperatively. Most operative approaches to appendectomy are laparoscopic, though an open approach is always reserved for cases that cannot proceed safely otherwise. Nonoperative management is appropriate for select patients, and this strategy has become more popular over time.

Several trials and systematic reviews support nonoperative treatment with intent to cure in patients with localized, mild disease. Treatment consists of resuscitation and antibiotics alone. Common antibiotics administered for this purpose are IV piperacillin with tazobactam (Zosyn) or ceftriaxone and metronidazole if remaining within the facility. Amoxicillin with clavulanate (Augmentin) or ciprofloxacin and metronidazole may be taken orally at home. They are carefully selected in these trials. Patients with fecalith on imaging, severe sepsis, obvious perforation, abscess, or higher risk comorbid conditions are generally not candidates for this strategy, though they will still initially receive IV fluid resuscitation and systemic antibiotics. Approximately 10% to 30% of well-selected patients will fail primary nonoperative treatment and undergo appendectomy, while about 20% more will have recurrent symptoms and receive an appendectomy within the next few years. In many cases, surgeons employ shared decision-making when reviewing these data and the patient's values in determining an operative or a nonoperative treatment pathway.

There are other states of disease that may be initially approached without an operation. Fluid resuscitation and antibiotics are the first lines of therapy for patients presenting with abscess, phlegmon, or severe sepsis/septic shock. Patients with a large abscess will then undergo urgent percutaneous image-guided drainage procedure. Those in septic shock receive supportive measures in a critical care setting and may require advanced or invasive measures to stabilize fluid shifts and hemodynamics. Adults with perforated appendicitis are often treated nonoperatively for the entire initial inpatient phase of care and are discharged following resolution of systemic signs of infection, such as fever, anorexia, tenderness on palpation, leukocytosis, and ileus. This process may take days to weeks to resolve.

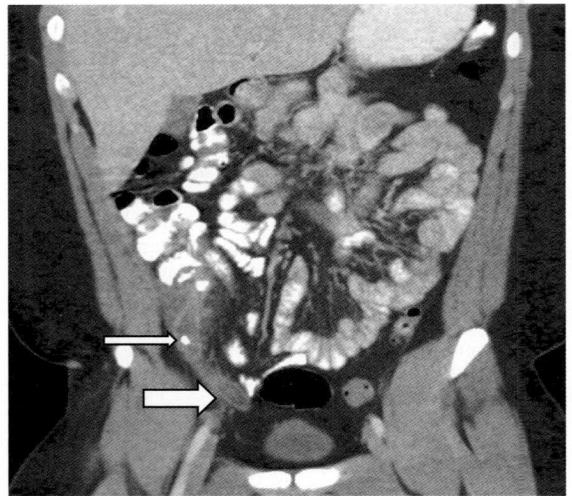

Figure 13-10. Computed tomography scan with intravenous and enteral contrast showing an enlarged appendix with thickening of the wall (large arrow) and a fecalith in the right lower quadrant (small arrow).

In a number of these cases, "interval appendectomy" is performed at least 6 to 8 weeks later, allowing the acute inflammatory process to subside. An operation is then performed on an elective basis when the perioperative risk is optimal. For patients over 40 years old, colonoscopy should be performed when safe, because in rare cases, perforated appendicitis may be the presenting sign of an intraluminal cecal neoplasm.

Appendectomy remains the gold standard approach for the treatment of appendicitis worldwide. Preoperative treatment includes IV fluid resuscitation and antibiotic coverage of gram-negative and anaerobic organisms. Common therapies include a second-generation cephalosporin, broad-spectrum penicillin, or a combination of fluoroquinolone or third-generation cephalosporin and metronidazole. If the appendix is not perforated, antibiotics are discontinued postoperatively. For cases of perforated appendicitis, antibiotics are typically continued until resolution of fever, leukocytosis, and ileus. Pediatric patients with perforated appendicitis, even those with abscesses, are more likely to undergo appendectomy urgently following initial resuscitation, as children and their families would otherwise have to make great sacrifices in school and at work while awaiting the effects of weeks-long inpatient medical therapy.

Historically, laparoscopic and open approaches to appendectomy were compared, and the laparoscopic approach was associated with lower postoperative pain scores, lower rates of wound infection, and increased operative time. Either approach is reasonable, depending upon the experience and discretion of the operating surgeon. The appendix is liberated from adherent tissues to expose it completely; the mesoappendix is divided, controlling the appendiceal artery; and the appendix is divided at its base. If present, free fluid is evacuated, purulent fluid is aspirated, and the incisions are closed.

Laparoscopy is useful for cases in which the diagnosis is uncertain because it allows inspection of the peritoneal cavity before committing to the rest of the operation. If the appendix appears normal, the surgeon must evaluate the remaining viscera and peritoneal cavity for another potential etiology. The surgeon evaluates the uterus, fallopian tubes, ovaries, entire length of the small bowel from the ligament of Treitz to the ileocecal junction, the entire colon, gallbladder, duodenum, and liver. In these cases, although the appendix may be free of disease, it is still removed, as future presentations of diagnostic uncertainty will otherwise lead to costly studies and delays in care ruling out appendicitis.

Complications

The most common postoperative complications of acute appendicitis are surgical site infections. Superficial infections involve only tissues above the fascial level, while deeper infections may take the form of intra-abdominal or pelvic abscesses. The risk of developing these infectious complications is extremely low in nonperforated acute appendicitis but is up to 20% to 30% in cases of perforated appendicitis. In the setting of severe inflammation, the appendiceal base may be difficult to identify, in which case appendiceal remnants may become a source of recurrent ("stump") appendicitis. Rarely, a cecal fistula may develop at the site of the transected appendiceal base, which indicates persistence of inflammation and raises suspicion for Crohn disease.

Incidental Appendectomy

An appendectomy performed during another surgical procedure is known as *incidental appendectomy*. This practice has fallen out of favor, as the benefit achieved did not meet historical expectations. Pediatric patients with complex congenital disease, intestinal malrotation, or comorbid conditions that are anticipated to develop diagnostic uncertainty later in life may still receive incidental appendectomies during other operations at the discretion of the surgeon, and with appropriate consent.

Appendiceal Tumors

Tumors commonly found in the appendix include carcinoids, adenocarcinomas, and mucoceles. Carcinoid tumors of the appendix account for approximately one-half of GI carcinoids. The majority of appendiceal carcinoids are benign, although they can be a source of luminal obstruction and appendicitis in rare cases. Lesions less than 2 cm in size and located in the distal appendix are usually treated adequately by simple appendectomy. As the size of the carcinoid increases, the possibility of malignancy and lymphatic spread also increases. For lesions greater than 2 cm in diameter, a formal right hemicolectomy with its lymphatic drainage basin is recommended to provide the most accurate diagnosis from the removed specimen.

Mucoceles may result from chronic luminal obstruction or may be associated with carcinoma in less than 1% of patients with appendiceal disease. When patients with this condition develop symptoms, they are very similar to those of acute appendicitis. Unexpected findings at the time of appendectomy in an adult patient should lead a surgeon to weigh the risks and benefits of a right hemicolectomy intraoperatively. The 5-year disease-free survival rate for appendiceal adenocarcinoma is 50% to 60%. Mucoceles and carcinomas, especially those that perforate, may develop pseudomyxoma peritonei (PMP), accumulations of gelatinous fluid within the peritoneal cavity. This condition is challenging to treat, with many receiving cytoreductive surgery (CRS) and hyperthermic intraperitoneal chemotherapy (HIPEC) to achieve cure. Those with more advanced disease receive therapies directed only to symptom palliation. The 5-year disease-free survival rate for PMP was approximately 35%; however, this has increased to more than 50% with CRS and HIPEC therapy.

SUGGESTED READINGS

Azagury D, Liu RC, Morgan A, Spain DA. Small bowel obstruction: a practical step-by-step evidence-based approach to evaluation, decision making, and management. *J Trauma Acute Care Surg*. 2015;79(4):661-668.

Cushing K, Higgins PDR. Management of Crohn disease: a review. *JAMA* 2021;325(1):69-80.

Harrnoss JC, Zelienka I, Probst P, et al. Antibiotics versus surgical therapy for treatment of uncomplicated appendicitis: systematic review and meta-analysis of controlled trials (PROSPERO 2015: CRD42015016882). *Ann Surg*. 2017;265(5):889-900.

Moris D, Paulson EK, Pappas TN. Diagnosis and management of acute appendicitis in adults: a review. *JAMA* 2021;326(22):2299-2311.

Strong S, Steele SR, Boutrous M, et al. Clinical practice guideline for the surgical management of Crohn's disease. *Dis Colon Rectum*. 2015;58(11):1021-1036.

Zielinski MD, Haddad NN, Choudry AJ, et al. Multi-institutional, prospective, observational study comparing the Gastrograffin challenge versus standard treatment in adhesive small bowel obstruction. *J Trauma Acute Care Surg*. 2017;83(1):47-54.

SAMPLE QUESTIONS

QUESTIONS

Choose the best answer for each question.

1. A 31-year-old woman presents to the emergency department with loss of appetite 2 nights ago followed by 1 day of progressively severe vomiting and right lower quadrant pain. She awoke yesterday morning with nausea, which led to vomiting and right lower quadrant pain developed over last night. The pain is exacerbated by movement and unrelieved by vomiting, which has reduced since yesterday. She is sexually active and had normal menses 2 weeks previously. She has had similar pains in the past but never this persistent or severe. Otherwise, she has been healthy, except for an open myomectomy for menorrhagia in her 20s.

She is lying quietly on the stretcher and appears ill and listless. Her temperature is 100.4 °F (38.0 °C), pulse is 91 beats/min, respiratory rate is 24, and BP is 125/60 mm Hg. Her abdomen has reduced bowel sounds, is mildly protuberant, and tender with fullness and focal right lower quadrant peritonitis. Pelvic and rectal examinations are tender on the right side but otherwise unremarkable. Her WBC is 13.7 with a normal basic chemistry panel, urinary β-human chorionic gonadotropin (β-HCG) is negative, and urinalysis is unremarkable.

The next best step is to

A. admit her for observation and IV broad-spectrum antibiotics.
B. obtain abdominal and pelvic ultrasounds.
C. obtain an abdominal and pelvic CT scan.
D. perform a diagnostic laparoscopy.
E. perform an open appendectomy through a McBurney incision.

2. At surgery on the patient in Question 1, a perforated necrotic appendix is found with a free fecalith in the right lower quadrant. The base of the appendix is healthy, and an appendectomy is performed with evacuation of pus and feculent fluid from the abdomen. Incidentally, a wide-based, soft, 6-cm long diverticulum is found approximately 50 cm from the ICV.

The most correct statement is that such a diverticulum

A. is usually located at the ileojejunal junction.
B. may contain heterotopic pancreatic tissue rather than gastric mucosa.
C. should be removed to prevent future symptoms.
D. should not be removed because the field is infected by the appendix.
E. is expected to be symptomatic in childhood.

3. The patient in Question 2 does well after surgery and, on postoperative day 2 (POD 2), has a WBC of 6.4 and has been afebrile for 24 hours. She is discharged home with pain medication and a scheduled follow-up appointment. On POD 7, she calls you to report that she is again febrile at 100.4 °F (38.0 °C). She feels well apart from some pelvic pain with urination.

You tell her that

A. because of the postoperative inflammation, she probably now has Meckel diverticulitis and should come to the emergency department.
B. mild fevers are not unusual after surgery, and you will see her next week.
C. she may have a pelvic abscess, and you will arrange immediate blood tests and a CT scan.
D. she probably has a urinary tract infection, and you will prescribe her an appropriate antibiotic.
E. you will prescribe her a broad-spectrum antibiotic for a possible infection and see her as scheduled next week.

4. A 49-year-old man presents with 3 days of vomiting large amounts of green liquid. He had a laparoscopic mesh repair of an epigastric hernia 1 year ago, and since then, he has been completely healthy, active, and without any pain. On examination, he appears tired and ill. He is afebrile and normotensive but mildly tachycardic with a slightly distended, quiet, and nontender abdomen. His laparoscopic scars are barely noticeable, and except for dry mucus membranes, his examination is otherwise unremarkable. His WBC is 12.3k, and his hemoglobin is 15.1.

The metabolic disturbance LEAST likely to be found is

A. acidosis.
B. hypocalcemia.
C. hypochloremia.
D. hypokalemia.
E. uremia.

5. For the patient in Question 4, which radiographic examination should you first order?

A. Abdominal ultrasound
B. CT scan of the abdomen and pelvis with rectal contrast
C. MRI of the abdomen
D. Supine XR and upright abdominal x-ray (AXR)
E. Upright chest XR

ANSWERS AND EXPLANATIONS

1. **Answer: C**

At this point, the differential diagnosis still includes right tubo-ovarian pathology, acute appendicitis or ruptured appendicitis with phlegmon or abscess, and less common infectious etiologies. Because several of these are managed with admission for antibiotics and possibly drainage rather than surgery, a diagnosis must be established before operative intervention. Although ultrasounds image the pelvic organs well and avoid ionizing radiation, they are less likely to clearly differentiate appendicitis from an appendiceal abscess. This is especially true in heavier, adult patients. For more information on this topic, see section "Acute Appendicitis."

2. **Answer: B**

In this clinical scenario, a Meckel diverticulum does not need to be removed because a symptomatic wide-based diverticulum has a miniscule chance of becoming symptomatic, not because of the infection from the appendix. While gastric mucosa is much more common, it may contain pancreatic or other tissue. Finally, although it is more frequently symptomatic in childhood than adulthood, Meckel diverticula are most commonly asymptomatic. For more information on this topic, see section "Meckel Diverticulum."

3. **Answer: C**

There is no such thing as a "normal" postoperative fever, and complications should be evaluated. An episode of Meckel diverticulitis is unlikely to be caused by perforated appendicitis. Although a urinary tract infection is possible, the characterization of pelvic pain rather than dysuria should point to a pelvic abscess. A CT scan with oral and IV contrast will diagnose a postoperative intra-abdominal abscess and exclude other less likely etiologies. For more information on this topic, see section "Complications" under the heading "Acute Appendicitis."

4. **Answer: A**

Persistent vomiting typically leads to a hypokalemic, hypochloremic, metabolic alkalosis because the kidney "wastes" hydrogen ions in the collecting ducts to preserve potassium and sodium ions. The dehydration will also typically lead to a prerenal azotemia. For more information on this topic, see section "Pathophysiology" under the heading "Small Bowel Obstruction".

5. **Answer: D**

Classic supine and upright AXRs are quick, inexpensive, and may be all that is required to diagnose adhesive SBO. It is important to specify "supine and upright" AXR because a supine XR will not reveal air-fluid levels.

A CT scan will show fluid as well as air-filled bowel loops, and it allows assessment of the bowel wall. However, it exposes the patient to more ionizing radiation, and rectal contrast is not indicated unless there is a suspicion for colorectal pathology.

MRI scans may give additional information about solid organs, but typically give less information about the bowel than a CT scan. There is no radiation exposure, and so it may be more useful and safe in pregnant and pediatric patients.

An upright chest XR may reveal distended loops of bowel and, in this clinical scenario, is used to identify free air under the diaphragm (signifying bowel perforation) or pulmonary pathology.

Abdominal ultrasounds do not image bowel well and are particularly unrevealing when large amounts of gas are present.

For more information on this topic, see section "Radiographic Studies" under the heading "Small Bowel Obstruction."

14 Colon, Rectum, and Anus

Patrick R. McGrew and Jacquelyn Seymour Turner

The colon, rectum, and anus are the terminal portions of the alimentary tract. Each has distinct anatomy and function and should be viewed as three separate entities. These organs are not biologically essential; one can live a virtually normal life without one's colon, rectum, and anus. Paradoxically, although the colon is much less vital for nutrition, fluid maintenance, and overall homeostasis than the small bowel, disease is far more common in the colon and rectum. The anus, anal canal, and anal sphincters play a critical role in continence, a function that is important for comfortable social interaction. Conditions of the colon and rectum such as diverticulosis coli, colon polyps, and adenocarcinoma of the colon and rectum and conditions of the anus such as hemorrhoids and anal fissures are frequent causes of office and emergency department visits. For these reasons, understanding colon, rectal, and anal anatomy, physiology, and pathology is important for all physicians.

ANATOMY

Beginning at the ileocecal junction, the colon is approximately 150 cm in length. The cecum and proximal transverse colon develop from the midgut. The distal third of the transverse, descending, and sigmoid colon and the rectum are hindgut structures. The anatomy of the colon differs from the small bowel in five key ways: its caliber, its degree of fixation, the appendices epiploicae, the teniae coli, and the haustra. The diameter of the colon is variable. The cecum has an average diameter of 7.5 cm, and the sigmoid colon has an average diameter of 2.5 cm. A considerable amount of the colon is retroperitoneal and fixed along the posterior abdominal sidewalls. In addition, the colon has appendices epiploicae, small fat tags on the serosal surface. There are no appendices epiploicae on the cecum, appendix, or rectum. The entire colon has three distinct longitudinal bands known as *teniae coli*. These bands are the condensation of the longitudinal muscle fibers in the outer layer of the bowel wall. The teniae coli converge at the appendix and at the rectum, making these structures void of teniae. Furthermore, the teniae coli are shorter than the colon itself. Therefore, the wall of the colon folds inward-forming small segmented pouches known as *haustra*. The bowel wall of the colon has the same layers as those of the small intestine: mucosa, submucosa muscularis, and serosa (Figure 14-1). The major histologic difference is that the colon has no villi (ie, mucosal crypts of Lieberkühn form a more uniform surface with less absorptive area).

Colon

The cecum is a blind-ending pouch and the most proximal part of the colon, which lies in the right iliac fossa. There is no formal location for the transition between the cecum and the ascending colon. The ascending colon extends from the ileocecal junction to the hepatic flexure, a fixed portion of the colon near the inferior surface of the right lobe of the liver. The ascending colon lies on the posterior abdominal wall and is covered by the parietal peritoneum anteriorly, making it normally a fixed retroperitoneal structure. The transverse colon begins just distal to the hepatic flexure and is suspended between the hepatic and splenic flexures; at the splenic flexure, it is also fixed retroperitoneally at the inferior surface of the spleen. The transverse colon is the most mobile portion of the colon. Attached to the antimesenteric transverse colon is the greater omentum. The descending colon is distal to the splenic flexure, and like the ascending colon, it lies on the posterior abdominal wall and is covered by the parietal peritoneum anteriorly, making it a fixed retroperitoneal structure. Conversely, the sigmoid colon becomes an intraperitoneal structure distal to the descending colon and forms a redundant loop of colon in the left lower quadrant. The sigmoid colon ends at the rectosigmoid junction, surgically known as a point where the teniae coli converge to form the rectum.

The blood supply to the colon is more complex than the blood supply to the small intestine. Like the small intestine, the ascending colon and proximal two-thirds of the transverse colon are supplied by the branches of the superior mesenteric arteries, whereas the distal third of the transverse colon, descending colon, and sigmoid colon are supplied by the branches of the inferior mesenteric artery. The importance of understanding this complex arterial blood supply is that in certain areas of the colon (eg, the splenic flexure where there is a junction of two separate

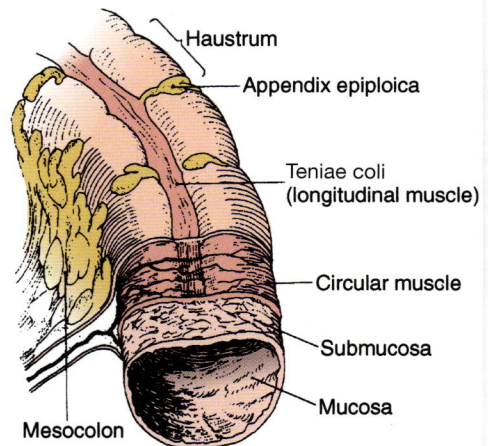

Figure 14-1. Oblique cross section showing the layers of the colon wall. (Reprinted with permission from Hardy JD. *Hardy's Textbook of Surgery.* 2nd ed. Lippincott Williams & Wilkins; 1983.)

blood vessel systems), the blood supply may be relatively poor, so the colon in this watershed area is at high risk for ischemic complications.

Another unique aspect of the arterial blood supply to the colon is the arc of Riolan and marginal artery of Drummond. The marginal artery runs parallel to and about 2 to 3 cm from the bowel wall; it commences at branches of the right colic artery and ends with the sigmoidal contributories, thus connecting the colic branches of the superior mesenteric artery and the inferior mesenteric artery (Figure 14-2). The arc of Riolan runs in a shorter loop inside the marginal artery. The venous drainage of the colon is less complex because most branches accompany the arteries and eventually drain into the portal system. The inferior mesenteric vein drains into the splenic vein, which joins the superior mesenteric vein to form the portal vein. Lymphatic drainage of the colon runs parallel to the arterial blood supply. In general, there are several levels of lymph nodes between the pericolic lymph nodes and the periaortic plexus.

Innervation of the colon is primarily through the autonomic nervous system. Sympathetic nerves pass from the spinal cord through the sympathetic chains and ganglia to postganglia that end in Meissner and Auerbach plexuses in the bowel wall. Sympathetic stimulation causes inhibition of colonic muscular activity. Parasympathetic innervation comes from the vagus nerve to the colon proximal to the mid-transverse colon. The distal transverse colon and beyond are innervated by branches from the S2 to S4 nerve roots. Parasympathetic activity results in the stimulation of colon muscular activity. However, the most important control of colon activity appears to be mediated by regional reflex activity that occurs in the submucosal plexuses. Thus, patients with spinal cord transection continue to have relatively normal bowel function.

Rectum

The rectum begins at the rectosigmoid junction and ends at the anorectal ring, a muscular structure that is made up of the puborectalis sling. The rectum is about 12 to 18 cm in length. It includes three submuscular folds called the "rectal valves" (of Houston) (Figure 14-3). The upper two-thirds of the rectum is covered by the peritoneum anteriorly and attached to the retroperitoneum posteriorly. The lower third of the rectum is completely extraperitoneal. Posteriorly, the rectum is separated from the sacrum at the level of S4 by an endopelvic fascia known as Waldeyer fascia. This fascia extends anteriorly to become Denonvilliers

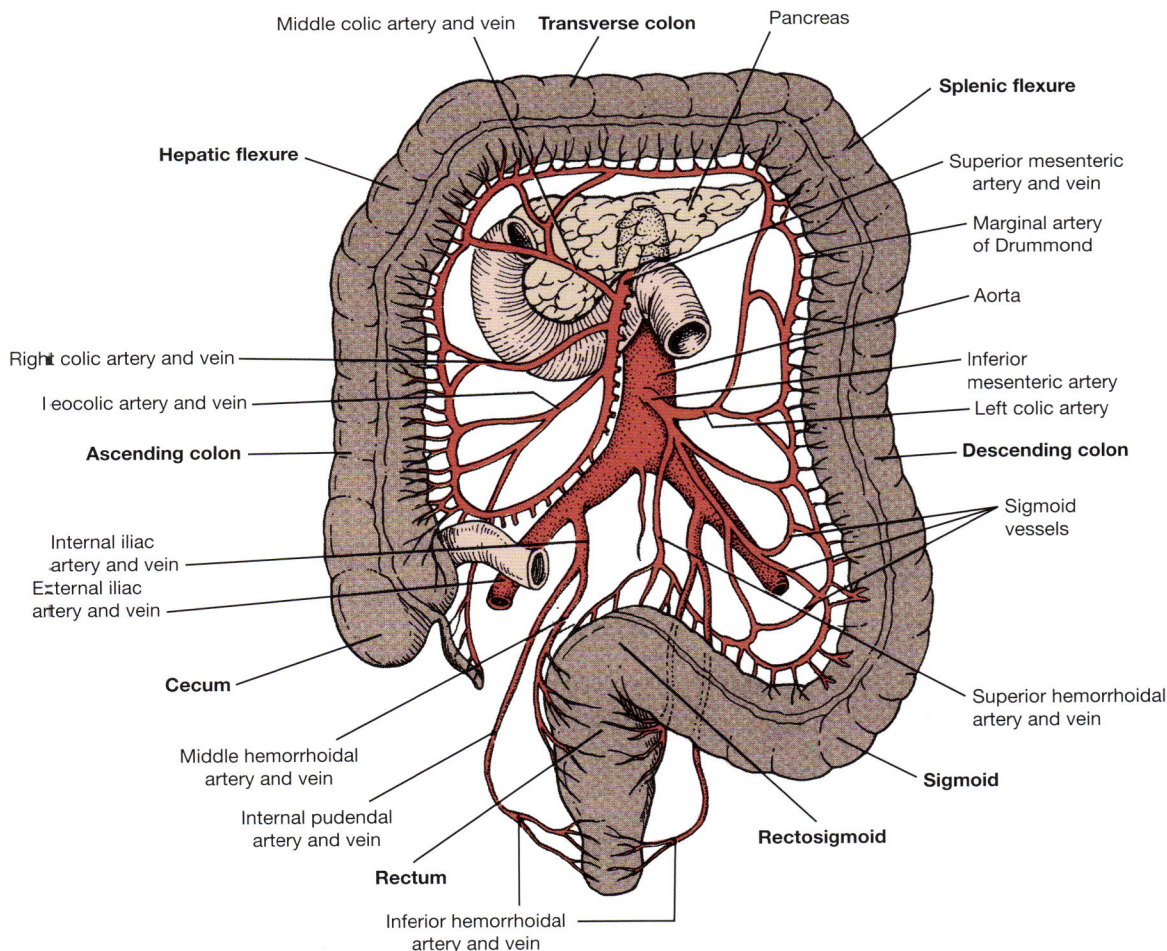

Figure 14-2. Normal anatomy and blood supply of the colon, rectum, and anus.

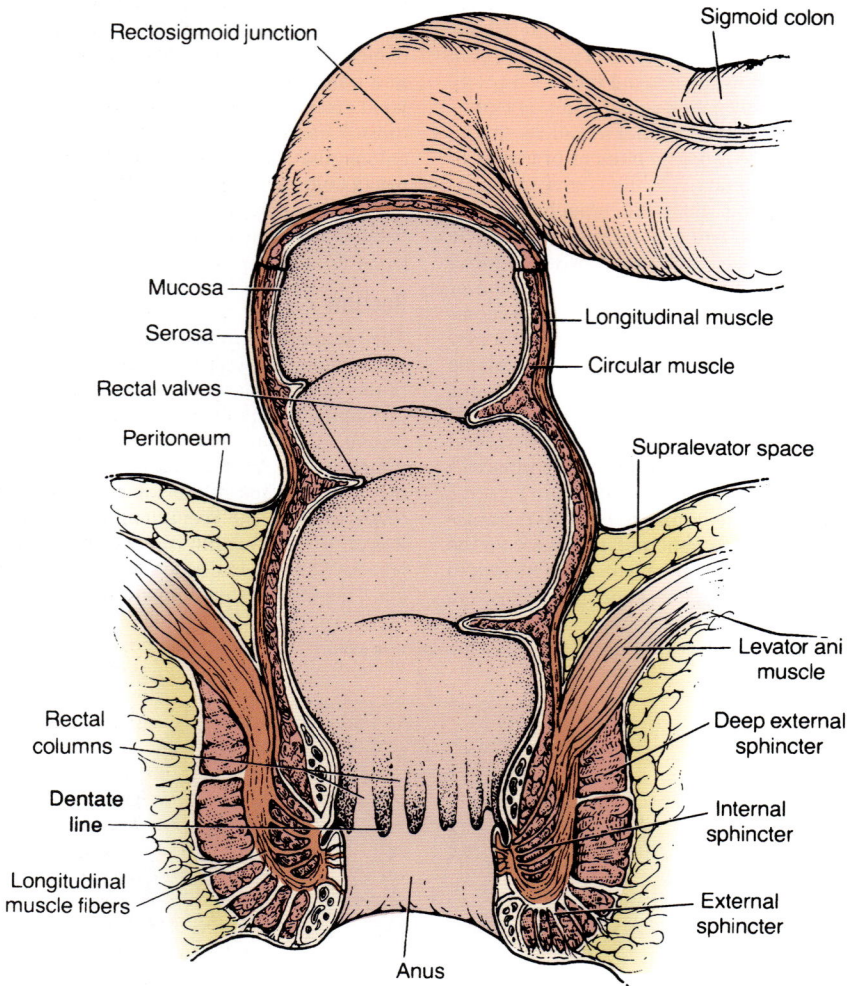

Figure 14-3. Normal anatomy of the rectum and anal canal.

fascia, which separates the rectum from the prostate and seminal vesicles in men and the vagina in women. This fascia encompasses perirectal adipose tissue called the "mesorectum." Mesorectum is a misnomer, as the rectum does not have true mesentery; however, the expression is still commonly used in surgical terminology. This fascia is important to identify as a plane of dissection for rectal cancer and clearing tumor margins. The rectum is supplied by the superior hemorrhoidal (also known as *rectal*) artery, which comes off the inferior mesenteric artery. The middle hemorrhoidal artery arises from the internal iliac artery to supply the distal rectum. The venous and lymphatic systems follow the arterial system, as they do in the colonic blood supply. The superior hemorrhoidal vein and lymphatics drain into the inferior mesenteric vein and lymph nodes, respectively, which ultimately drain into the portal system. The middle hemorrhoidal vein and lymphatics drain into the internal iliac veins and lymph nodes, respectively, which ultimately drain into the systemic system. This difference in venous drainage is critical to remember when considering rectal tumors and possible metastatic disease.

Sympathetic innervation of the upper rectum arises from L1, L2, and L3. After synapsing at the preaortic plexus, postganglionic fibers follow the inferior mesenteric artery and superior rectal artery. Sympathetic innervation of the lower third of the rectum is innervated by the presacral nerves, which form the hypogastric plexus and ultimately two hypogastric nerves. Parasympathetic innervation arises from S2, S3, and S4, which form the nervi erigentes.

Anus

The anus is the terminal portion of the alimentary tract. The anal sphincter complex is composed of an internal anal sphincter, which is an inner circular smooth muscle, and an external sphincter, which is an outer elliptical band of striated muscle. The internal sphincter is a continuation of the inner circular smooth muscle of the rectum and is involuntarily controlled. The external sphincter is a continuation of the levator ani muscle and has some voluntary control. The anal canal is 2.5 to 5 cm in length. This canal extends from the anorectal ring to the anal verge. The anal verge is the distal junction of the anal canal with skin that harbors hair follicles and glands. The anal verge is an important landmark used to localize pathology.

Within the anal canal lies the dentate line (see Figure 14-3). Immediately proximal to the dentate line are longitudinal folds called the "columns of Morgagni." Anal crypts terminate at the base of these columns, where secretions are discharged. A variable number of glands (6 on average) empty into each crypt. Above the dentate, the anal mucosa is insensate. The anus above the dentate line is innervated by both the sympathetic and parasympathetic systems. The anus below the dentate line is innervated by the somatic nervous system, which makes that portion of the anal canal sensate.

Venous and lymphatic drainage also vary according to the dentate line. Above the dentate line lies the internal hemorrhoidal plexus, which drains into the middle and inferior hemorrhoidal veins. In addition, the lymphatics above the dentate line drain into the inferior mesenteric and internal iliac nodes. The external hemorrhoidal plexus and lymphatic drainage below the dentate line drain into the inferior hemorrhoidal vein and lymph nodes and ultimately to the superficial inguinal lymph nodes, respectively. The arterial supply to the anal canal and anal sphincters is supplied by the inferior hemorrhoidal artery, which originates from the internal pudendal artery, a branch of the internal iliac artery (see Figure 14-2).

PHYSIOLOGY

The colon and rectum play a role in maintaining body homeostasis via three main functions: (1) they absorb water and electrolytes from liquid stool; (2) through fermentation they help digest some starches and protein that are resistant to digestion and absorption by the small bowel; and (3) they serve as storage for feces. In addition, the rectum and anus are key components for defecation.

The small bowel delivers 1 to 2 L of chyme to the cecum every day. Up to 90% of the water contained in chyme is absorbed, leaving less than 200 mL of fluid evacuated daily in solid stool. Digested material spends a significant amount of time in the cecum and ascending colon, where there is a mixing of the chyme and intestinal flora. The cecum and the ascending and transverse colon regulate sodium and water absorption. Ninety percent of sodium in the ileal effluent is actively absorbed in exchange for secretion of potassium. Chloride absorption occurs by both passive (75%) processes, created by a favorable electrochemical gradient from sodium absorption, and active (25%) processes through an active chloride-bicarbonate antiport where bicarbonate is secreted in exchange.

The colon harbors a greater number and variety of bacteria than any other organ in the body. It is host to more than 400 types of bacteria, most of which are anaerobes; *Bacteroides fragilis* is the most common anaerobic gram-negative rod. The colonic flora is also abundant in gram-positive organisms, such as enterococci and *Clostridium* species. Colonic bacteria perform a number of important functions for the host, including degradation of bile pigments and production of vitamin K. Colonic bacteria ferment undigested starches and proteins, producing short-chain fatty acids that are absorbed by the colon. Short-chain fatty acids are needed by the colonic epithelium for

metabolism, maintenance of low luminal pH, and an increase in regional blood flow, and they aid in the transport of sodium, bicarbonate, and water. Bacterial fermentation produces approximately 800 to 900 mL/d of colonic gas, which is mostly passed by flatus. The composition of gas is mostly nitrogen (70%) from swallowed air.

The digestive function of the colon represents only a small portion of the total digestion and absorption of nutrients that take place in the body. Therefore, surgical resection of the entire colon and rectum does not impact a person's capacity to maintain normal nutrition.

Colonic motility is unique among organs of the alimentary tract because of the multiple types of contraction patterns, including segmental and mass contractions. Slow waves are intermittent, low-frequency, segmental bidirectional contractions that aid in the mixing of fecal matter. Mass contractions produce strong, propulsive contractile movements that occur over a long length of the colon. They begin in the transverse colon and are useful for moving stool stored in the descending colon toward the rectum and anus. Mass contractions seem to occur after awakening and following the intake of food and are associated with the urge to defecate.

Defecation involves a complex interplay among the distal colon, rectum, and pelvic floor muscles, coordinating the relaxation and contraction of several muscle groups. Normal frequency of defecation can range from every 8 hours to every 72 hours, with an average of once a day. Frequency can be affected by the type and volume of food and fluid intake, physical activity, medications, and levels of stress. Severe or new-onset constipation (ability to pass flatus, but not stool) and obstipation (inability to pass stool or flatus) are examples of changes that must be evaluated.

The physiology of fecal continence is the result of complex interactions between sensory and involuntary and voluntary motor functions of the rectum, pelvic floor muscles, and anal sphincters. When stool distends the proximal rectum, the external anal sphincter contracts and the internal anal sphincter relaxes, allowing sampling of the rectal contents. If elimination is to proceed, there is voluntary inhibition of the external anal sphincter contractions. This very sensitive mechanism allows the passage of gas and stool to occur at an appropriate time. The inability to perform these functions and control the passage of gas and stool leads to incontinence.

EVALUATION

There are multiple modalities to evaluate the colon, rectum, and anus. The most important initial evaluation is still a complete history and a thorough abdominal and rectal examination. The abdominal examination should include all four key components: inspection, auscultation, percussion, and palpation. It is important to perform a digital rectal examination in patients with both anorectal and abdominal complaints. There is a tendency to defer the digital rectal examination because of patient embarrassment or physician inconvenience. However, deferring the rectal examination can result in missing a critical diagnosis and should not be forgone.

Endoscopy

Further investigation of the anal canal and rectum can be accomplished in the office using rigid and flexible endoscopes. An anoscope is a small rigid handheld scope that

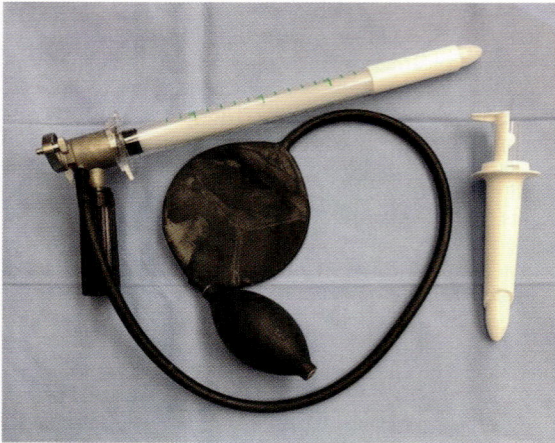

Figure 14-4. Disposable rigid proctoscope on the left and disposable anoscope on the right used to evaluate the rectum and anus, respectively. (Image courtesy of Jacquelyn Turner, MD.)

is available in several varieties to evaluate diseases in the anal canal and distal rectum. The rigid proctoscope is longer than the anoscope and is the best tool for evaluating rectal diseases and causes of rectal bleeding, such as rectal polyps, cancer, and proctitis (Figure 14-4). If possible, the patient should be advised to take a small-volume enema to aid in visualization of the rectal mucosa prior to the office visit. Rigid proctoscopy can be used intraoperatively to assess a colorectal anastomosis.

Some offices are equipped to perform flexible sigmoidoscopy. Otherwise, this examination is performed in an endoscopy suite or operating room. Patients should take an oral bowel preparation or an enema, if possible, prior to examination to aid in visualization. Flexible sigmoidoscopy allows for visualization of the last 30 to 65 cm of the colon and rectum. Sites of hemorrhage and obstruction in the rectum and sigmoid colon can be identified, and excessive colonic gas can be evacuated. If polyps or neoplasms are found, the patient should get a full colonoscopy.

Because colonoscopy allows for visualization of the entire colon and rectum, and the last few centimeters of the terminal ileum, it is the most accurate diagnostic tool for pathology in the distal alimentary tract. In addition to being a diagnostic tool, colonoscopy can also be used for endoscopic intervention with the ability to remove polyps, decompress the colon, dilate strictures, control bleeding, biopsy tumors or inflammatory conditions, and remove foreign bodies. An oral bowel preparation is needed prior to the examination. Once pathology is found, colonoscopy is the primary diagnostic modality for follow-up surveillance at variable intervals.

Diagnostic Radiologic Examinations

Plain films of the abdomen are a valuable initial radiologic test to obtain for the evaluation of anyone with abdominal pain. Specifically, an abdominal series includes an upright abdomen film to assess for air-fluid levels and an upright chest or left lateral decubitus abdominal film to assess for free intraperitoneal air. This series of films is not only useful for evaluating pneumoperitoneum but also useful for evaluating the bowel gas patterns and detecting large bowel obstruction. The haustral markings (Figure 14-5), associated with the large bowel, can be identified in radiographic studies, which help distinguish it from small bowel anatomy that has smaller, concentric folds known as *plicae circulares*.

A single-contrast barium enema assesses the lumen of the colon and rectum. This study can aid in diagnosing colonic strictures, diverticulosis, volvulus, and sites of colonic obstruction (Figure 14-6). Barium enemas can also be used to evaluate the patency of rectal stumps after colostomy procedures. Moreover, contrast enemas using Gastrografin can also be helpful in evaluating a colorectal anastomosis, especially if a leak is suspected.

Computed tomography (CT) scans of the abdomen and pelvis are useful in diagnosing and managing a wide variety of abdominal diseases. For example, the diagnosis of diverticulitis is best confirmed with an abdominal CT scan. Other uses include evaluation for metastatic cancer in patients diagnosed with colon and rectal cancer,

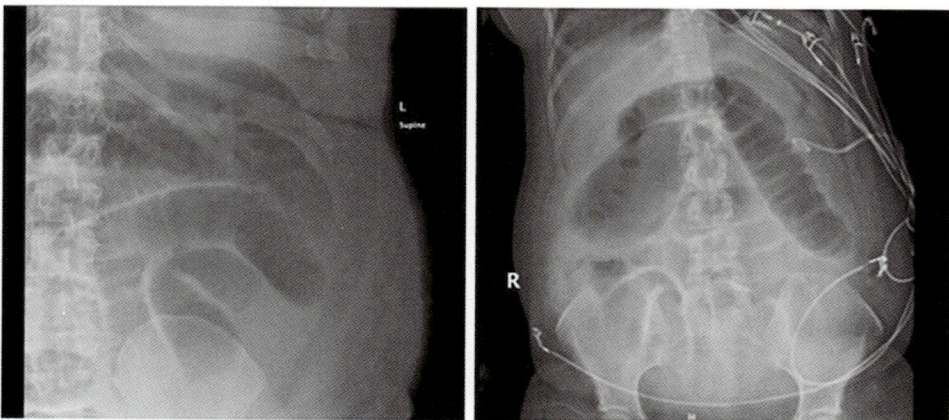

Figure 14-5. Left: radiograph demonstrating small bowel dilatation as evident by the plica circularis noted within the lumen of the distended bowel. Right: radiograph showing a gas-filled colon as evident by the haustral markings within the bowel lumen. (Image courtesy of Jacquelyn Turner, MD.)

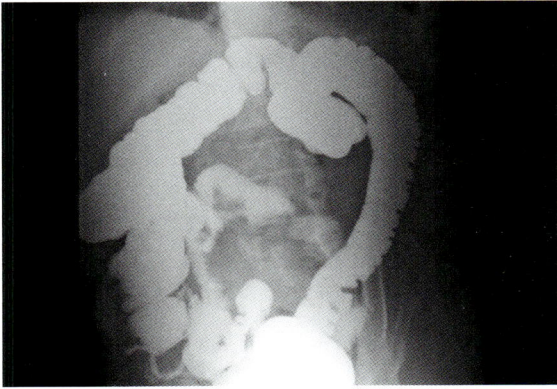

Figure 14-6. Single-contrast barium enema. (Image courtesy Jacquelyn Turner, MD.)

assessing the severity of colitis, determining the site of bowel obstruction, and distinguishing between a complete and partial bowel obstruction. CT scans of the abdomen and pelvis are often performed with intravenous (IV) and oral contrast. Rectal contrast is occasionally given to help opacify the lumen of the rectum and distal colon. Positron emission tomography (PET) is best used to determine recurrent and metastatic cancer.

More detailed evaluation of the rectum and anus can be accomplished with magnetic resonance imaging (MRI) or ano-rectal ultrasound. These examinations are useful for the assessment of complex perirectal/anal abscesses and fistulae and determination of the integrity of anal sphincters. When staging for cancer, MRI and rectal ultrasound are used to determine the depth of tumor invasion and to assess for enlarged perirectal and perianal lymph nodes. MRI is also useful for assessing the resectability of rectal tumors.

Lower gastrointestinal (GI) bleeding can be assessed with technetium-labeled red blood cell scanning and angiography (Figure 14-7). Technetium-labeled red blood cell nuclear scanning is indicated when bleeding is less rapid and the patient is stable. This nuclear medicine test can detect bleeding when the bleeding rate is less than 0.1 mL/min, but a positive scan does not localize the bleeding. A positive scan is most often followed by mesenteric angiography in an attempt to localize the bleeding site. Angiography is useful in detecting the source of moderate or rapid colonic bleeding (rate >0.5 mL/min). It is not helpful in patients with slow, chronic blood loss. Angiography is not only diagnostic but also therapeutic through endovascular interventions to occlude the offending vessel.

TERMINOLOGY

Understanding the treatment of colonic diseases requires familiarity with terms that are unique to this organ. Colostomy, for example, is a surgical procedure in which the colon is divided and the proximal end is brought through a surgically created defect in the abdominal wall (Figure 14-8). The distal end of the bowel is either closed and placed in the peritoneal cavity as a blind limb (Hartmann procedure) or brought out inferiorly to the colostomy through the abdominal wall as a mucous fistula. A loop colostomy is created by bringing

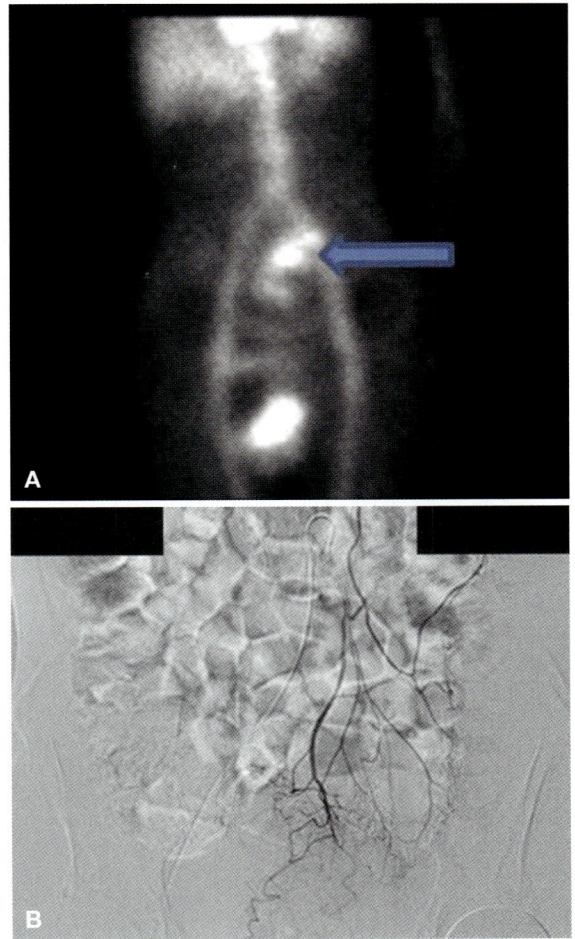

Figure 14-7. A. Technetium scan with activity in left lower quadrant (arrow). B. Normal inferior mesenteric arteriogram in the same patient. (Both images courtesy Jacquelyn Turner, MD.)

a loop of colon through a defect in the abdominal wall. The antimesenteric wall of the bowel is divided, leaving the posterior, mesenteric wall intact. This creates two limbs of the bowel, which are externalized to form the loop colostomy. The proximal limb allows for stool and gas to exit into the colostomy bag. The distal limb allows for decompression of gas in the bowel distal into the colostomy. An ileostomy is a similar procedure in which the ileum is brought through the abdominal wall.

Stomas, whether an ileostomy or a colostomy, can be temporary or permanent. Furthermore, stomas either divert content from distal intestinal diseases or become the terminal end of the GI tract after surgery. Diverting stomas are usually performed when stool needs to be redirected from the distal bowel for one of the following reasons: (1) a distal anastomosis needs to heal before bowel continuity is restored; (2) the ends of the bowel are not suitable for an immediate anastomosis after resection (eg, severely inflamed bowel, questionable vascular supply); (3) the conditions are not right for proceeding (eg, severe fecal peritonitis, patient too unstable or too sick to tolerate the

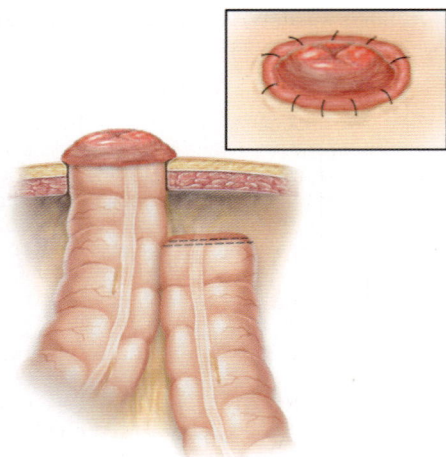

Figure 14-8. Lateral and anterior appearance of an end colostomy. (Reprinted with permission from Mulholland MW. *Operative Techniques in Surgery.* 1st ed. Wolters Kluwer Health; 2015.)

procedure); and (4) there is not enough bowel left for re-anastomosis (abdominoperineal resection [APR]).

Other terms that often confuse medical students include proctocolectomy, APR, and low anterior resection (LAR). *Procto* is the Greek word for the Latin word *rectum*. Proctocolectomy is operative removal of the entire colon and rectum (eg, for ulcerative colitis or polyposis syndromes). APR, a term used in the surgical treatment of very low rectal pathology, is the operative removal of the lower sigmoid colon and the entire rectum and anus, leaving a permanent proximal sigmoid colostomy. LAR, which is used to surgically treat pathology in the middle and upper sections of the rectum, is the removal of the distal sigmoid colon and a portion of the rectum, with primary anastomosis of the proximal sigmoid to the distal rectum.

BENIGN COLONIC DISORDERS

Diverticulosis

Diverticulosis of the colon is the most common anatomic abnormality of the colon. For years, it was considered to be a disease that affected the Westernized world; however, recent data have suggested an increase in its prevalence throughout the world. The prevalence of colonic diverticulosis increases with age. In the United States, one-third of the adults under the age of 50 have diverticulosis, and over two-thirds of the population over the age of 80 have colonic diverticula on colonoscopy. The majority (80%) of patients remain asymptomatic during their lifetime.

Factors associated with the development of diverticulosis include age and diet, but whether it is related to general relaxation of the colonic tissue or to lifelong dietary habits is not clear. Dietary influences have been implicated on the basis of comparative geographic epidemiology; these studies implicate the lower fiber diet found in Western Europe and the United States.

Most of the colonic diverticula are located in the sigmoid colon, but they can also be present on the right

side or throughout the entire colon. There are two types of diverticula found in the colon. Congenital or "true" diverticula have herniation of all three of the colonic wall layers and are usually present on the right side of the colon. Although these are infrequent among Western populations, they are common in Asia. Acquired or "false" diverticula are characterized by herniation of the colonic mucosa and submucosa through defects in the muscular layer at the weakest point in the colonic wall, which are the sites of penetration of blood vessels into the colon wall. It has been postulated that lower stool bulk results in slow transit times and the need for higher luminal pressures for propulsion, with the resultant increased force causing herniation of the mucosa and submucosa at the site of the vascular penetration of the bowel wall (Figure 14-9).

The term *diverticular disease* implies that the diverticula result in an illness, and it is defined as clinically significant and symptomatic diverticulosis. The symptoms can be due to diverticulitis, in which there is evidence of inflammation, or when there is no evidence of overt inflammation, but patients complain of various abdominal symptoms. This condition has now been defined as symptomatic uncomplicated diverticular disease (SUDD) (Figure 14-10). Symptoms of SUDD are thought to be due to visceral hypersensitivity in the absence of identifiable colonic inflammation. It is characterized by recurrent abdominal pain, often localized to the left lower quadrant, and functional changes in bowel habits, including bleeding, constipation, diarrhea, or alternating constipation and diarrhea. The physical examination is most often unremarkable, or it shows mild tenderness in the left lower quadrant. By definition, fever and leukocytosis are absent. Additional radiologic findings may include segmental spasm and luminal narrowing. Endoscopic evaluation of the colon generally does not show any mucosal abnormalities other than diverticulosis. The treatment of SUDD is adherence to a high-fiber diet or fiber supplementation.

Diverticulitis

Diverticulitis is an infection of one or more diverticula with extension into adjacent tissue. The condition is initiated by obstruction of the neck of the diverticulum by

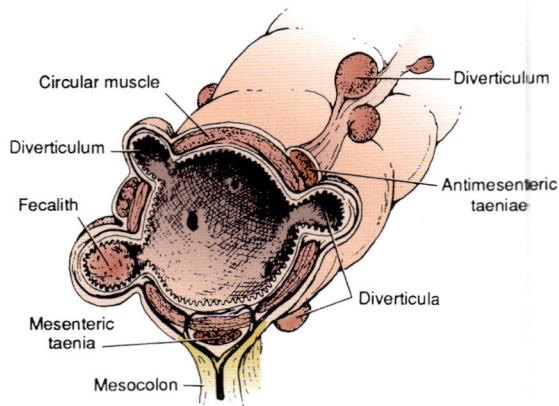

Figure 14-9. Mucosal herniation characteristic of diverticulosis. Most herniations occur at a site where the blood vessel penetrates the bowel wall.

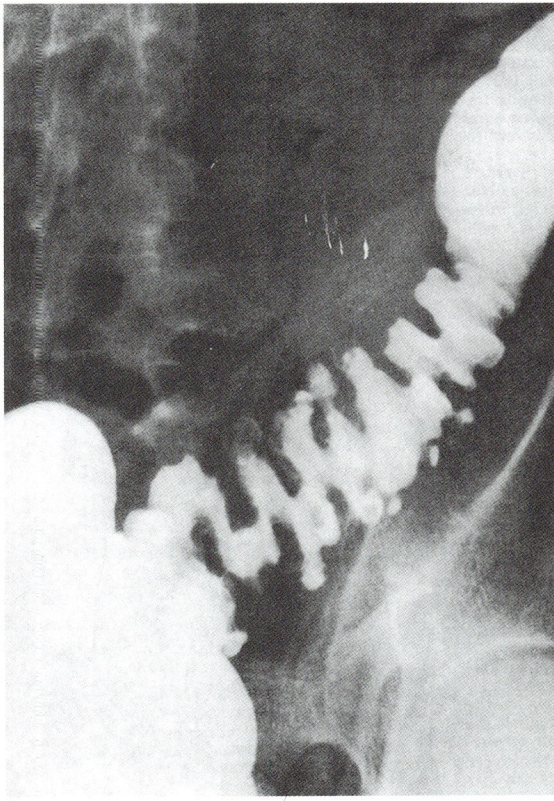

A

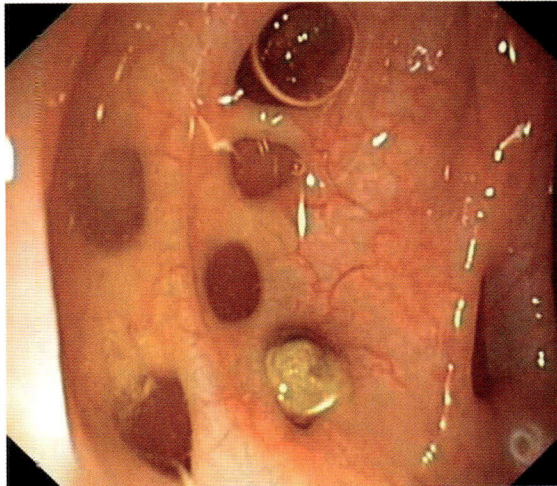

B

Figure 14-10. A. Sigmoid diverticulosis shown on barium enema. B. Diverticular openings seen during routine colonoscopy.

a fecalith. The obstruction leads to microperforation that results in inflammation in the colon wall or macroperforation that involves the pericolic tissues. Acute diverticulitis presents as a spectrum of severity ranging from uncomplicated diverticulitis to complicated diverticulitis. Uncomplicated diverticulitis is characterized by left lower quadrant abdominal pain (subacute onset), fever, alteration in bowel habits (constipation or diarrhea), and, occasionally, a palpable mass.

Clinical Presentation of Diverticulitis

The clinical presentation of complicated diverticulitis is due to the consequences of diverticular perforation, including abscess formation, fistula development, free perforation, and partial or total large bowel obstruction. Patients with an abscess will usually have left lower quadrant pain, fever, tenderness, and leukocytosis (Figure 14-11).

Colovesical fistula is the most common type of fistula caused by diverticulitis. It is more common in men than in women who have not had a hysterectomy, because the uterus acts as an anatomic barrier between the colon and the urinary bladder and vagina. However, women who have undergone a hysterectomy can develop a colovesical or colovaginal fistula. Fistula formation may be associated with diarrhea, stool per vagina (colovaginal fistula), pneumaturia and recurrent urinary tract infections (colovesical fistula), or skin rupture and associated stool drainage (colocutaneous fistula). The diagnostic workup includes a CT scan and colonoscopy to rule out other mucosal abnormities. The finding of air in the urinary bladder in the absence of recent bladder instrumentation supports the diagnosis of colovesical fistula. Cystoscopy is sometimes indicated to evaluate for primary bladder pathology. In the majority of cases, a definite fistulous communication is not identified and the diagnosis is based on clinical suspicion.

Patients with free perforation present with diffuse peritonitis and large amounts of free air or fluid on imaging studies. They may exhibit signs of septic shock and hemodynamic instability. Colonic obstruction from a diverticular stricture is usually an insidious process that may cause few symptoms until the degree of obstruction has become quite advanced. The patient will have symptoms of a large bowel obstruction, including abdominal distension and high-pitched bowel sounds.

Treatment of Diverticulitis

Treatment of the complications of diverticular disease is directed at the specific complication (Table 14-1). The treatment of acute diverticulitis is initially medical in 85% of cases. Although a proportion of patients can be managed as outpatients, patients with severe pain require hospital admission with IV hydration, giving the patient nothing

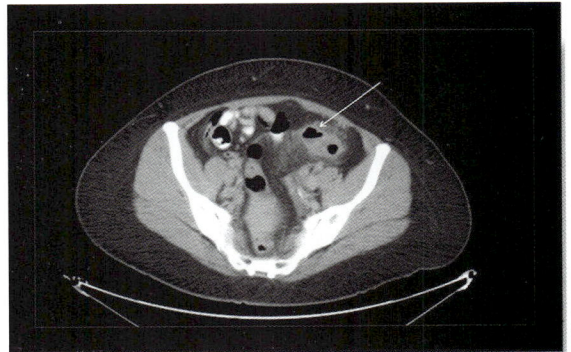

Figure 14-11. Computed tomography scan demonstrating abscess caused by diverticular perforation.

TABLE 14-1. Indications for Surgery in Diverticular Disease
Free perforation
Obstruction
Intractability
Bleeding
Fistula

by mouth (NPO), and administering IV antibiotics (usually broad coverage of gram-negative coliforms as well as coverage for anaerobes, particularly *B. fragilis*) for 5 to 7 days. Most patients respond to nonoperative treatment and do not require further therapy. However, a subset of this group has repeated bouts of acute diverticulitis, requiring subsequent hospitalization. In all cases of treated diverticulitis, follow-up colonoscopy is necessary to evaluate for other mucosal abnormalities such as malignancy or colitis.

For several decades, it was believed that any patient who has had two severe bouts of diverticulitis requiring hospitalization should undergo elective sigmoid colectomy (the site of the problem in 95% of cases). However, studies of the natural history of diverticulitis in large groups of patients have shown that although some patients have subsequent episodes of diverticulitis, it is the initial episode that is the most severe. Considering the costs and complications associated with resection of the sigmoid colon, this has prompted a shift in how many patients with diverticulitis are surgically treated. At present, most surgeons manage patients with uncomplicated diverticulitis on a case-by-case basis. A person who has one episode of diverticulitis every 3 years is most likely to be managed nonsurgically, while a patient who has episodes of uncomplicated diverticulitis requiring hospitalization several times a year is advised to consider elective sigmoid colon resection.

Small abscesses adjacent to the colon or within the colonic mesentery may respond to bowel rest and IV antibiotics. Larger abscesses (>5 cm) are treated with percutaneous drainage, along with bowel rest and IV antibiotics. These patients are also encouraged to consider sigmoid resection after abscess resolution, because up to 40% of patients will suffer recurrent abscess formation without surgery.

The primary treatment for fistulae from diverticular disease is surgery. For colovesical fistula, primary closure of the bladder and resection of the sigmoid colon with primary anastomosis is definitive. Similarly, colovaginal fistula is treated with fistula division and sigmoid colon resection and reanastomosis; the opening in the vagina is most often allowed to close by secondary intention. Most colovesical and colovaginal fistula surgery is done electively, because patients are rarely ill from these fistulas.

Patients who present with free perforation or large bowel obstruction are typically operated on emergently. The most common procedure is called a Hartmann procedure. The diseased sigmoid colon is resected, and an end colostomy is created. The rectum is left in place for possible colostomy closure and reestablishment of intestinal continuity at a later date (Figure 14-12).

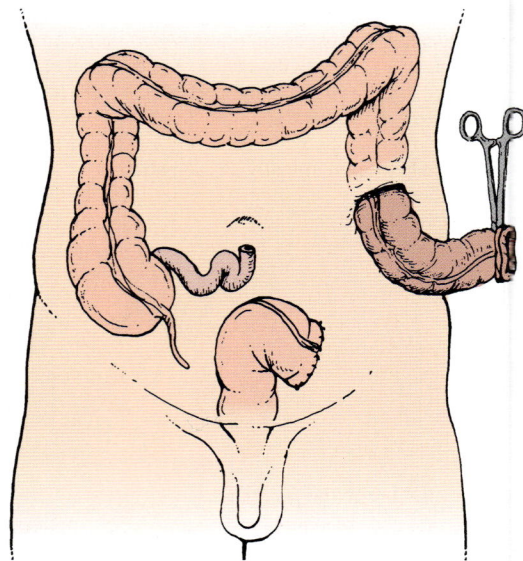

Figure 14-12. Operative therapy for diverticular disease usually involves resection of the sigmoid portion of the colon. If the operation is done for acute perforation or obstruction, the segment may be resected, a diverting end colostomy brought to the abdominal wall, and the distal rectal stump oversewn (Hartmann procedure). A second stage of the operation involves colostomy takedown and anastomosis to the rectal stump.

Diverticular Bleeding

Lower GI bleeding is defined as bleeding that comes from a source distal to the ligament of Treitz. Approximately 70% of lower GI bleeds are caused by diverticulosis, with bleeding as the primary presenting symptom in 5% to 10% of all patients with diverticular disease. Massive bleeding is defined as being sufficient to warrant transfusion of more than four units of blood in 24 hours to maintain normal hemodynamics. In one-fourth of diverticular bleeds, the bleeding is massive and can be fatal if not diagnosed and appropriately treated.

Clinical Presentation and Evaluation of Diverticular Bleeding

Patients with diverticular bleeding present with painless, profuse, bright, or dark red rectal bleeding. The volume of blood will determine whether the patient exhibits signs and symptoms of hemodynamic instability and shock, including hypotension and tachycardia. Several other colonic pathologies can present with similar symptoms, including angiodysplasia, malignancy, ischemic colitis (IC), and inflammatory bowel disease (IBD).

After resuscitation with volume expanders and blood transfusions, the diagnostic approach to the patient with lower GI bleeding includes insertion of a nasogastric tube with saline lavage and aspiration. A saline lavage will evaluate for an upper GI source. If bile is noted in the aspirate, then the source of bleeding is less likely to be from upper GI pathology. A rectal examination and anoscopy or proctoscopy are needed to rule out severe hemorrhoidal bleeding and other anorectal pathology.

There are several diagnostic algorithms to evaluate a lower GI bleed, the most common of which includes colonoscopy, because it is both diagnostic and can be therapeutic. Before a colonoscopy can be performed, a mechanical bowel prep should be used to clear the colon of stool and old blood. Colonoscopies for GI bleeding should only be performed in hemodynamically stable patients.

If the patient is hemodynamically unstable, the bleeding continues, or the bleeding cannot be controlled by colonoscopy, angiography is the next diagnostic procedure. Mesenteric angiography is useful in detecting the source of moderate or rapid colonic bleeding, defined as a bleeding rate of 0.5 mL/min or more. Identification of the bleeding site allows for segmental resection of the colon, if needed. In hemodynamically stable patients, a technetium-labeled red blood cell nuclear scan can also be used as the first diagnostic test because it may be more sensitive than colonoscopy and angiography.

Treatment of Diverticular Bleeding

Most diverticular bleeding will stop with supportive measures, including fluid resuscitation and reversal of anticoagulation, without invasive interventions. Invasive diagnostics and therapeutic interventions are indicated with ongoing bleeding and requirements for blood transfusion or hemodynamic instability despite adequate resuscitation.

When active bleeding is visualized from a diverticulum during colonoscopy, it can be controlled with clips, cauterization with the application of energy, or coagulation with injection of epinephrine. If the bleeding site cannot be identified or controlled, mesenteric angiography can be used therapeutically. Vasopressin can be instilled through the angiography catheter at the bleeding site, successfully stopping bleeding in over 80% of cases. However, because more than 50% will rebleed, vasopressin instillation is used as a temporizing measure, allowing patients to be resuscitated and then taken for a segmental colon resection when stable, usually within 8 to 12 hours. Similarly, transcatheter embolization with tiny coils can be done to stop bleeding acutely but is associated with a risk of ischemia and infarction of the involved bowel segment. For this reason, coil embolization is most often used to temporize, as described earlier, with surgical resection of the involved bowel segment after the patient is resuscitated and stabilized. If the bleeding does not cease spontaneously, surgical resection of the involved segment of the colon is indicated. If the bleeding has been determined to come from a lower GI source, but the segment of the colon has not been localized with diagnostic studies, a total abdominal colectomy is the surgical procedure of choice.

INFLAMMATORY BOWEL DISEASE: ULCERATIVE COLITIS AND CROHN DISEASE OF THE COLON

Chronic ulcerative colitis (CUC) and Crohn disease (CD) are the two most common forms of IBD. CUC and CD have many overlapping as well as distinguishing characteristics in their pathophysiology and management. Both diseases occur as a result of a combination of genetic and environmental factors that cause an immune-mediated dysregulation within the mucosa, resulting in acute and chronic inflammation.

CUC involves the mucosa and submucosa and affects only the colon and rectum. CD is a transmural disease that can involve any part of the alimentary canal, from the mouth to the anus. Approximately half the cases of CD involve the small and large bowel, usually at the ileocolic junction. Another 25% involve only the small bowel or large bowel. In about 10% of cases, there is only perianal disease, but most of these patients will also have proximal involvement of the small and large bowel. Stomach and duodenal involvement is uncommon, occurring in about 2% of cases. The age of presentation for CUC and CD is bimodal, with almost two-thirds of cases presenting in the second and third decades and one-third of cases occurring around the fifth decade of life.

Differences that may be used to distinguish CD from ulcerative colitis include rectal sparing, skip lesions (in which diseased segments alternate with normal segments), aphthous sores, and linear ulcers. In addition to the material contained here, refer to Chapter 13 for further discussion on CD.

The exact etiology of ulcerative colitis is unknown. Infections and immunologic, genetic, and environmental factors are implicated, but none are proven. The female-to-male ratio for CUC is 5:4. The disease is slightly more common in Western countries, and its annual incidence is 10 per 100,000 population. A family history of ulcerative colitis is present in 20% of patients. There is an increased incidence of the disease among certain Jewish ethnicities, but it is less common among African American and Native American patients.

Pathologic findings include involvement of the rectum (>90%) with variable proximal extension because the disease may involve the rectum (ulcerative proctitis), the left side of the colon (proctosigmoiditis or left-sided colitis), or the entire colon (pancolitis). The mucosa is initially involved, with lymphocytic and leukocyte infiltration that progresses to involve the submucosa with microabscess formation. The crypts of Lieberkühn are commonly affected (crypt abscesses), but muscle layers are rarely involved. These abscesses coalesce and erode the mucosa, leading to the formation of pseudopolyps, which are readily identified on endoscopic examination.

Clinical Presentation and Evaluation of Ulcerative Colitis

The initial clinical presentation of ulcerative colitis is variable, dependent on the extent of involvement of the colon and disease severity. The disease may have a sudden onset, with a fulminant, life-threatening course, or it may be mild and insidious. Most patients usually present with bloody, mucopurulent diarrhea, accompanied by cramping, abdominal pain, tenesmus, and urgency. To varying degrees, patients have weight loss, dehydration, pain, and fever. The presentation of fulminant colitis or toxic megacolon is often associated with massive colonic dilation secondary to the destruction of the myenteric plexus. Patients may have severe constitutional symptoms related to sepsis, malnutrition, anemia, acid-base disturbances, and electrolyte abnormalities. Fever can be indicative of multiple microabscesses or endotoxemia secondary to bacteremia from translocation across the inflamed colonic mucosa.

Extraintestinal CUC manifestations include ankylosing spondylitis, peripheral arthritis, uveitis, pyoderma gangrenosum, sclerosing cholangitis, pericholangitis, and pericarditis, each occurring in a small percentage of patients. Physical examination findings will depend on the acuity and severity of the disease process at the time of examination. If the patient is seen in a quiescent phase, there may be few or no findings; if the patient is seen in an acute phase, there may be findings of an acute abdomen with distension, tympany, tenderness, and guarding.

The mainstay of the diagnosis of CUC is endoscopy with biopsy. Typical endoscopic findings include friable, reddish mucosa with no normal intervening areas, mucosal exudates, and pseudopolyposis (Figure 14-13).

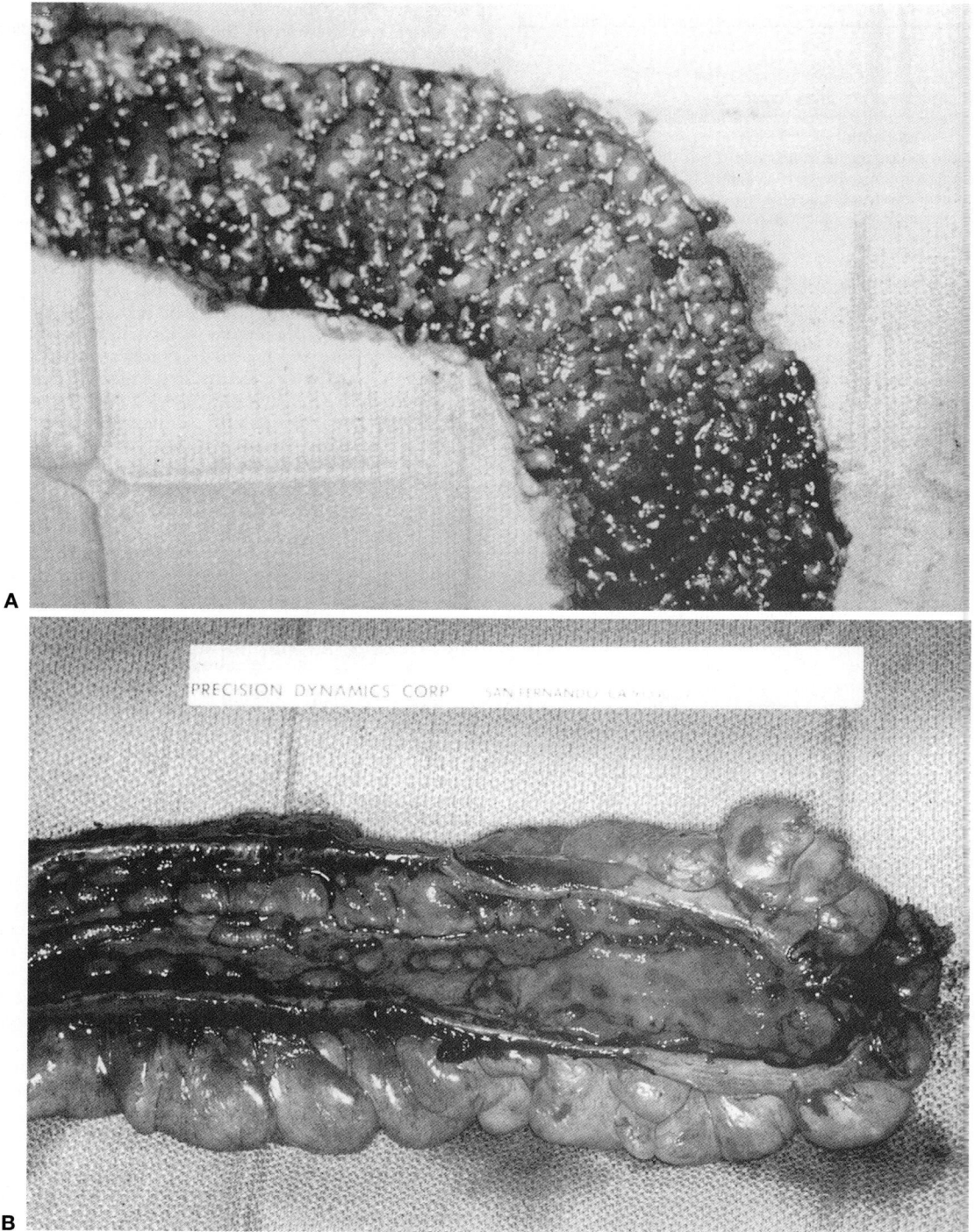

Figure 14-13. A. Severe ulcerative colitis showing pseudopolyps, deep ulceration, and friability. B. Severe Crohn colitis showing linear ulcers and "cobblestoning."

No specific laboratory tests are diagnostic of ulcerative colitis; however, leukocytosis and anemia may be present. Fecal calprotectin is a stool study used to detect intestinal inflammation and is often abnormal (95% sensitivity and 91% specificity) in IBD. Serologic markers, such as perinuclear antineutrophil cytoplasmic antibodies, a group of immunoglobulin G (IgG) antibodies commonly elevated in autoimmune disease, may corroborate the diagnosis.

The differential diagnosis includes other inflammatory or infectious disorders, including CD, infectious colitis, and pseudomembranous colitis. The disease that is most commonly confused with ulcerative colitis is CD of the colon. In approximately 10% of cases, there is an overlap of features; this type of colitis is called "indeterminate colitis." Its clinical behavior appears to be more like ulcerative colitis than CD. Table 14-2 shows the distinguishing characteristics of both disease processes.

Treatment of Ulcerative Colitis

The current medical therapies for CUC can be divided into the following categories:

1. Corticosteroids, including systemic (methylprednisolone, prednisone), oral (budesonide), and topical (hydrocortisone enemas) preparations
2. 5-Aminosalicylates, including mesalamine (oral, enemas) and sulfasalazine (which is a mesalamine prodrug)
3. Immunomodulators, including thiopurines (6-mercaptopurine, azathioprine), methotrexate, and cyclosporine
4. Antibiotics, including ciprofloxacin and metronidazole
5. Biologics, including antitumor necrosis factor agents such as infliximab, adalimumab, and certolizumab pegol

The goal of treatment is to induce remission and then maintain remission of the active disease while minimizing side effects from therapy. There are two main management strategies that are commonly used: (1) accelerated step-up approach in which advanced therapies such as biologics are introduced rapidly or (2) aggressive top-down treatment approaches in which advanced therapies are started and then tapered. Management of patients with CUC requires a multidisciplinary approach involving gastroenterologists, surgeons, nutritionists, pharmacists, nursing staff, and other members of the treatment team.

Surgical management is indicated for fulminant colitis, toxic megacolon, medically refractory disease, or the development of dysplasia or cancer. Patients with fulminant colitis and/or toxic megacolon are at risk of perforation, massive bleeding, and life-threatening sepsis. Therefore, these patients require aggressive inpatient medical care, including broad-spectrum antibiotics, IV steroids, IV administration of fluids, and nutritional support with hyperalimentation. The goal of this aggressive treatment is to convert these patients to a more stable condition so that they can tolerate an operative intervention that is associated with significant morbidity and even mortality.

Patients who have fulminant colitis who does not respond to medical therapy early in the course or those who have toxic megacolon (systemic symptoms of fever, tachycardia, and leukocytosis along with a dilated colon) should undergo a total abdominal colectomy with end ileostomy. Given the inflammation of the rectum and the added time to complete a potentially difficult pelvic dissection in this

setting, the rectum should not be removed during this operation but rather at a later, staged operation. In stable patients, despite optimal medical therapy, 10% to 20% of patients will not respond to medical therapy over time or will develop significant side effects.

TABLE 14-2. Comparison of Ulcerative Colitis and Crohn Colitis

	Ulcerative Colitis	Crohn Colitis
Symptoms and signs		
Diarrhea	Severe, bloody	Less severe, bleeding infrequent
Perianal fistulas	Rare	Common
Strictures or obstruction	Uncommon	Common
Perforation	Free, uncommon	Localized, common
Pattern of development		
Rectum	Virtually always involved	Often normal
Terminal ileum	Normal	Diseased in majority of patients
Distribution	Continuous	Segmented, skip lesions
Megacolon	Frequent	Less common
Appearance		
Gross	Friable, bleeding granular exudates, pseudopolyps, isolated ulcers	Linear ulcers, transverse fissures, cobblestoning, thickening, strictures
Microscopic	Inflamed submucosa and mucosa, crypt abscesses; fibrosis uncommon	Transmural inflammation, granulomas, fibrosis
Radiologic	Lead pipe, foreshortening, continuous, concentric	String sign in small bowel; segmental, asymmetric internal fistulae
Course		
Natural history	Exacerbations, remissions, dramatic flare-ups	Exacerbations, remissions, chronic, indolent
Medical treatment	Initial response high (>80%)	Response less predictable
Surgical treatment	Curative	Palliative
Recurrence	No	Common

The risk of developing cancer with CUC is dependent on the extent and duration of the disease. In patients with pancolitis, the risk increases 1% to 2% per year after the initial 10 years of disease. These patients who do not respond to medical therapy, have dysplasia not amenable to endoscopic excision, or have colon cancer should undergo total proctocolectomy.

In the past, the definitive operative procedure for ulcerative colitis was total proctocolectomy with permanent ileostomy. Proctocolectomy with ileoanal pouch anastomosis (Figure 14-14) is now considered the standard operative procedure. This involves removing the colon and rectum and constructing an ileal pouch from the small bowel that is connected to the anus, thereby sparing the patient a permanent ileostomy. This procedure can be performed as a one-stage procedure in which the colon and rectum are removed and a pouch is constructed without an ileostomy, as a two-stage procedure in which a pouch is constructed along with a diverting ileostomy that is later reversed (the

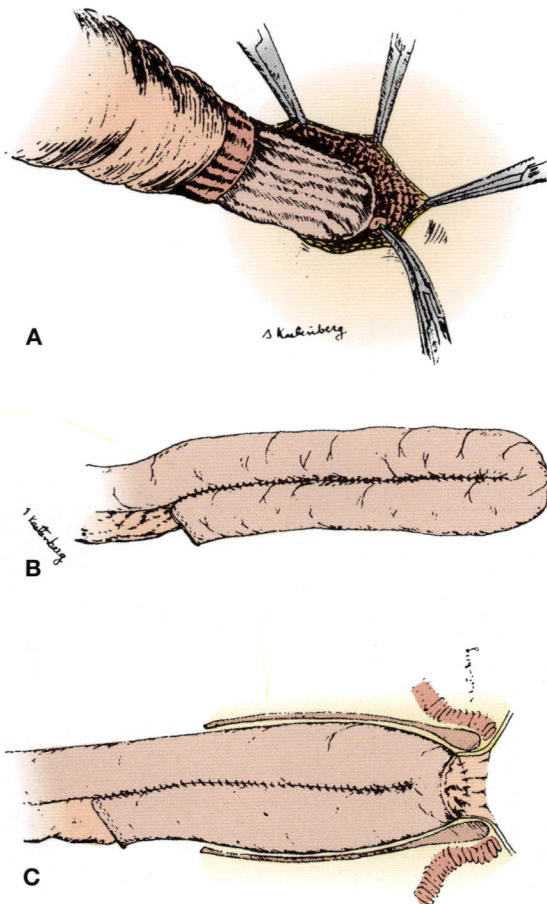

A

B

C

Figure 14-14. Ileoanal pouch anastomosis is the operation of choice for definitive treatment of ulcerative colitis and familial polyposis syndrome. A. The entire colon and rectum are removed. B. A small reservoir is constructed from the terminal ileum using a J-shaped configuration. C. This J-shaped pouch is then pulled through the muscular cuff and anastomosed to the dentate line to create a neorectum.

second stage), or as a three-stage procedure in which the colon is removed and an end ileostomy is constructed (first stage), followed by construction of the pouch with a diverting ileostomy (second stage), and then followed by ileostomy reversal (third stage).

COLITIS

Ischemic Colitis

IC results from a decrease in blood flow sufficient to cause injury to colonocytes and may be followed by a reperfusion injury and subsequent inflammation. It is the most common type of bowel ischemia and can be either occlusive or nonocclusive in etiology. Occlusive colonic ischemia results from interruption of the blood flow to the colon by thromboembolic phenomenon, trauma, surgical manipulation, or chronic or acute vessel occlusion, such as after aortic surgery. This is compared to nonocclusive disease, which is caused by a low-flow state. Nonocclusive IC can be precipitated by numerous factors, typically those that affect arterial vascular tone, volume status, and cardiac output. These include shock of any type, renal failure requiring dialysis, myocardial infarction, hypovolemia or hemorrhage, intense exercise, illicit drugs such as methamphetamines and cocaine, and prescription medications that affect volume status or blood pressure and cardiac output. The diagnosis of IC is made based on clinical, radiographic, and colonoscopy findings. Early in the course of disease, patients may present with crampy abdominal pain and hematochezia (bright red blood per rectum). Abdominal examination findings range from tenderness over the affected segments of the colon to peritonitis, which may herald full-thickness necrosis and perforation. Laboratory values are frequently nonspecific. Colonoscopy is the best technique to diagnose IC and can differentiate between gangrenous and nongangrenous IC, but there is a risk of perforation while doing the examination. CT scans of the abdomen are readily available and often performed prior to surgical consultation. CT findings can vary and are also nonspecific. A CT may demonstrate segmental involvement of the colon, with colon wall edema and pericolonic stranding. A discrete thrombus or occlusion is often not identified. Colonic pneumatosis or portal venous gas is ominous and can signify full-thickness necrosis, and free air indicates full-thickness perforation.

Treatment of IC without perforation or full-thickness infarction may respond to bowel rest and antibiotics. Gangrenous IC requires an operative procedure to resect necrotic segments of colon, and an ostomy is usually created. The bowel may be left in discontinuity, and a second-look operation planned if there is suspicion for worsening disease or the underlying precipitating factors have not been adequately controlled.

Pseudomembranous Colitis

Clostridioides difficile infection (CDI) is an infectious colitis resulting from colonization of the colon by *C. difficile* bacteria after alteration of the normal colonic microbiome. Exposure to antibiotics is the most important predisposing factor to infection. Toxins A and B lead to disruption in the colonic epithelium and necrosis. Diagnosis is made in the presence of diarrhea ($\geq$3 unformed stools in 24 hours) or ileus or megacolon demonstrated radiographically, detection of *C. diff* toxin or toxigenic *C. diff* in stool, or findings of pseudomembranous colitis on colonoscopy or by pathology.

Treatment of *C. diff* colitis has evolved along with the bacteria. In a 2021 update, the Infectious Diseases Society of America (IDSA) now suggests treatment of initial CDI be with fidaxomicin as the first-line agent. For patients with recurrent CDI in the past 6 months, concomitant treatment is with bezlotoxumab, a human monoclonal antibody against B toxin. Patients at an increased risk for recurrence during their first infection due to immune compromise, age greater than 65, or severe disease are also candidates for bezlotoxumab co-treatment. Oral vancomycin, IV metronidazole, and vancomycin enemas are recommended in fulminant CDI, which is defined as CDI with shock, hypotension, ileus, or megacolon.

Some patients with CDI who develop colonic necrosis or perforation, toxic megacolon, or who fail to improve or worsen despite maximum medical therapy will require surgery. Surgical consultation should be considered early in the disease process. The operation of choice is total abdominal colectomy or subtotal colectomy and end ileostomy. Early surgery performed prior to the development of shock or signs of end-organ failure is associated with improved mortality.

LARGE BOWEL OBSTRUCTION

Colonic obstruction is a serious condition that requires early identification and appropriate diagnosis. It is important to distinguish true mechanical obstruction from pseudo-obstruction and ileus, because treatment vastly differs. Large bowel obstruction in adults is most often caused by colon or rectal cancer, diverticular disease, and volvulus of the colon. Obstruction from colonic volvulus results from twisting of a redundant segment of the colon on its mesentery. Obstruction from adhesive bands, commonly seen in the small bowel, is extremely uncommon in the colon.

An important element of large bowel obstruction is the status of the ileocecal valve. If it is incompetent, signs and symptoms are indistinguishable from small bowel obstruction. If the ileocecal valve is competent, as in approximately 75% of patients, a "closed-loop" obstruction occurs between the ileocecal valve and the obstructing point distally in the colon or rectum. Massive colonic distension often results.

Evaluation of Large Bowel Obstruction

Similar signs and symptoms for all etiologies may include constipation, obstipation, and abdominal distension with nausea and vomiting. Symptoms that may be diagnostically significant include abrupt onset of symptoms (suggestive of an acute obstructive event), changes in stool caliber (raising suspicion for carcinoma), and history of the left lower quadrant pain over multiple episodes (suggestive of diverticulitis or a diverticular stricture). It is critical to distinguish between complete large bowel obstruction and partial large bowel obstruction; patients with complete obstruction have obstipation.

Physical examination should place special emphasis on the abdominal and rectal examination: abdominal inspection, auscultation, percussion, and palpation; evaluation of bowel sounds, tenderness, rigidity, guarding, any mass or fullness; or any signs of hernia. On rectal examination, an assessment should be made of the contents of the anal vault (presence of gas or feces or collapsed), stool consistency, and the presence of a mass or other lesion. A thorough history and physical examination will determine the most appropriate diagnostic studies to order.

Free air under the diaphragm on a chest radiography indicates perforation. Flat and upright abdominal films can distinguish constipation or impaction from bowel obstruction. Plain films may also help localize the site of obstruction (large vs small bowel). Sigmoid volvulus may have a coffee-bean appearance or a "bent-inner tube" sign on the abdominal films (Figure 14-15). Air seen within the bowel wall (pneumatosis) on radiographs is an ominous sign and suggests colonic ischemia.

The use of a water-soluble contrast enema can confirm the diagnosis of colonic obstruction and identify the exact location. Contrast enema with water-soluble contrast (eg, Gastrografin) revealing a column of contrast ending in a "bird's beak" is suggestive of colonic volvulus. Barium should never be given in the presence of suspected colonic obstruction or perforation.

CT scanning is often the imaging modality of choice if a colonic obstruction is clinically suspected; it can confirm the diagnosis and identify the cause of large bowel obstruction (Figure 14-16). Contrast-enhanced CT (oral and IV) can help delineate between partial and complete obstruction, ileus, and small bowel obstruction, as well as exclude large bowel obstruction. Because of the risk of aspiration and pneumonitis, oral water-soluble contrast should be used judiciously if a complete obstruction is suspected.

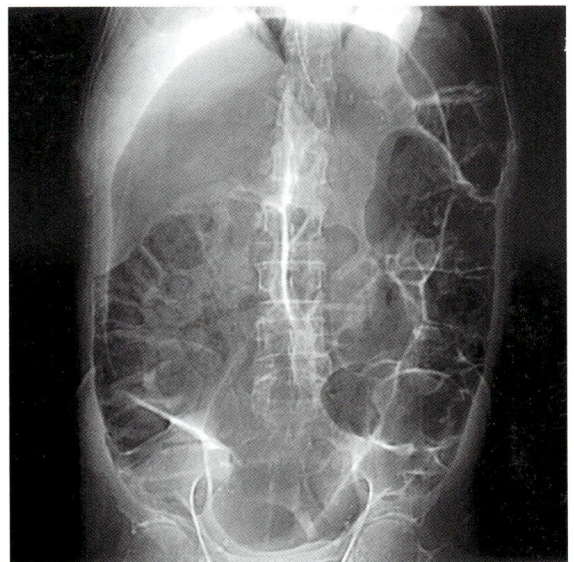

Figure 14-15. Volvulus of the sigmoid colon.

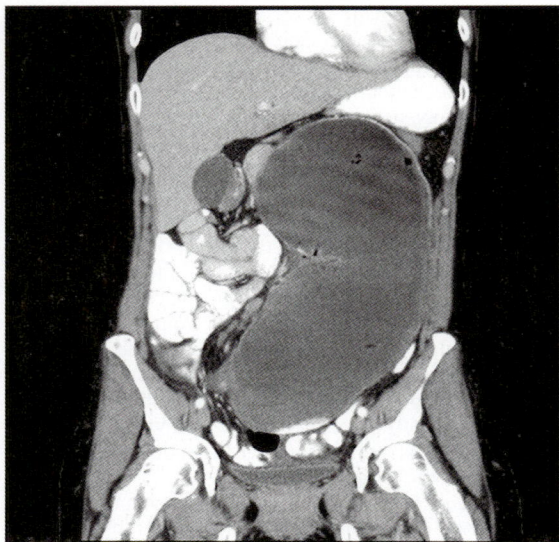

Figure 14-16. Computed tomography scan of a cecal volvulus.

Treatment of Large Bowel Obstruction

Initial therapy includes volume resuscitation and electrolyte repletion with timely surgical consultation. Surgical intervention is almost always indicated for patients with complete obstruction, while those with partial obstruction may be treated by nasogastric decompression, NPO, and IV fluids with resolution of the acute obstruction. This may allow patients with partial large bowel obstruction to be prepared for surgery and potentially avoid a colostomy.

Emergency laparotomy is mandatory for acute large bowel obstruction with cecal distension beyond 12 cm, severe tenderness, evidence of peritonitis, or generalized sepsis. Perforation caused by volvulus, obstructing cancers, or diverticular strictures often requires bowel resection and a diverting stoma. Patients with a large bowel obstruction due to cancer and without peritonitis may undergo endoscopic colonic stent placement that allows decompression without the need for urgent surgery and colostomy.

COLONIC VOLVULUS

Common presenting symptoms of both sigmoid and cecal volvulus include abdominal cramping, pain, nausea, vomiting, and obstipation. On physical examination, there is typically abdominal distension, tenderness, and often an empty rectum on digital examination. The duration of symptoms ranges from a few hours to several days, with an acute presentation more common with cecal volvulus and indolent presentations more common with sigmoid volvulus. Sigmoid volvulus classically presents in older patients, often with a history of constipation or dementia.

Imaging should occur early in the course of suspected volvulus because it may rapidly lead to a diagnosis. Plain abdominal radiographs are useful in the initial evaluation of suspected colon volvulus. Sigmoid volvulus may appear as a dilated colon loop arising from the pelvis and extending to the diaphragm in the shape of a coffee bean

or bent-inner tube. Typically, cecal volvulus produces large and small bowel obstruction. Radiographs reveal a markedly distended loop of bowel extending from the right lower quadrant to the left upper quadrant. The small bowel is distended, whereas the distal colon is decompressed

Contrast-enhanced CT imaging is currently the preferred confirmatory diagnostic study for both cecal and sigmoid volvulus because it is noninvasive, easily obtainable, accurate for both cecal and sigmoid volvulus, and may identify incidental pathology that may be missed with plain radiographs or fluoroscopic studies. In addition, abdominal CT may facilitate the diagnosis of colonic ischemia.

In the absence of colonic ischemia or perforation, the initial treatment of sigmoid volvulus is endoscopic detorsion, which is effective in 60% to 95% of patients. After successful detorsion of the sigmoid colon, a decompression tube should be left in place for a period of 1 to 3 days to maintain the reduction, allow for continued colonic decompression, and facilitate mechanical bowel preparation. Due to the high risk of recurrent volvulus, operative intervention should be strongly considered in appropriate patients during the initial admission. Of the elective operative interventions for sigmoid volvulus, sigmoid colectomy with anastomosis is the most effective at preventing recurrent episodes of volvulus. Urgent sigmoid resection is generally indicated when endoscopic detorsion of the sigmoid colon is not possible and in cases of nonviable or perforated colon.

Attempts at endoscopic detorsion of cecal volvulus are generally not recommended. Cecal resection is the most effective means of preventing recurrence.

ACUTE COLONIC PSEUDO-OBSTRUCTION

Acute colonic pseudo-obstruction (ACPO, also known as *Ogilvie syndrome*) is a functional condition that most often affects older, hospitalized, or institutionalized patients with severe comorbid conditions or infections, or those recovering from surgery or trauma. Abdominal pain, nausea and vomiting, abdominal distension, and dilation of the ascending and transverse colons on abdominal radiographs are typical findings but are nonspecific for ACPO. Abdominal CT or water-soluble contrast enema can reliably distinguish ACPO from a mechanical large bowel obstruction. Although most patients with ACPO have a nonemergent presentation, ischemia or perforation of the colon is reported in 3% to 15% of cases. Fever, significant leukocytosis, and cecal diameter greater than 12 cm are factors that may be indicative of colon ischemia or perforation in ACPO.

First-line treatment for ACPO without evidence of colon ischemia or perforation and cecal diameter less than 12 cm is noninvasive and includes correction of electrolyte abnormalities, fluid resuscitation, minimization of narcotics and anticholinergic medications, identification and treatment of any infection, bowel rest, and ambulation. The insertion of nasogastric and rectal tubes to facilitate intestinal decompression is also frequently used. Oral osmotic and stimulant laxatives should be avoided because they may worsen dilation of the colon via gas production and propulsion of gas into an already dilated colon. Supportive first-line treatment leads to a resolution of 70% to 90% of ACPO.

Pharmacologic treatment with neostigmine is an appropriate next step for ACPO that does not resolve with supportive therapy. Neostigmine is an antiacetylcholinesterase drug that transiently and reversibly increases acetylcholine levels in the muscarinic receptors of the parasympathetic nervous system. In patients with ACPO, trials of IV administration of neostigmine have shown that this drug leads to a resolution of colon dilation in approximately 90% of cases. Neostigmine therapy should be administered in a setting that allows for continuous monitoring of heart rate, oxygen saturation, and frequent blood pressure measurements and has glycopyrrolate or atropine readily available for rapid use in cases of bronchospasm or bradycardia. Neostigmine should not be used in colon ischemia or perforation or in the setting of pregnancy, uncontrolled cardiac arrhythmias, or severe active bronchospasm.

Endoscopic decompression of the colon should be considered in patients with ACPO in whom neostigmine therapy is contraindicated or ineffective. Endoscopic decompression of the colon has been shown to result in initial colon decompression in 61% to 95% of cases and sustained decompression in the 70% to 90% range. To prevent the recurrence of colon dilation, more than one endoscopic decompression procedure and/or endoscopic placement of a decompression tube is often required. Colonoscopy in ACPO has a reported perforation rate of 1% to 3% if it is performed without mechanical bowel preparation, with CO_2 or minimal air insufflation, and with minimal narcotics.

Surgery is reserved for cases of ACPO complicated by colon ischemia, perforation, or dilation refractory to non-operative management. Persistent colon dilation refractory to nonoperative measures can be estimated to occur in approximately 10% of patients. Intraoperative decisions in ACPO should be guided by the condition of the colon and the condition of the patient. With viable, dilated colon, cecostomy or tube cecostomy is successful in 95% to 100% of patients. Ileostomy and colostomy are also acceptable surgical alternatives. For ischemic or perforated colon, the choice of resection with end ostomy or resection with anastomosis with or without proximal diversion is determined on a case-by-case basis.

POLYPS AND CANCER OF THE COLON AND RECTUM

Colorectal Polyps

Polyp is a morphologic term that is used to describe small mucosal excrescences that grow into the lumen of the colon and rectum. A variety of polyp types have been described, all with different biologic behaviors (Table 14-3).

Inflammatory polyps (pseudopolyps) are common in IBD and have no malignant potential. Hamartomas (juvenile polyps and polyps associated with Peutz-Jeghers syndrome) similarly have very low malignant potential and often spontaneously regress or autoamputate. They may be safely observed. However, polyps that fall into the general category of "adenoma" are premalignant, and appropriate vigilance is indicated. Histologically, adenomas are described as (1) tubular, (2) tubulovillous, (3) villous, or (4) sessile serrated adenoma. Villous adenomas have the highest risk of becoming malignant. Evidence for the malignant potential of adenomas includes (1) the high incidence of cancer associated with the polyps in familial adenomatous polyposis (FAP) syndrome, (2) simultaneous occurrence of cancers and polyps in the same specimen, (3) carcinogens that experimentally produce both adenomas and cancers in the same model, and (4) lower cancer risks associated with those who have polyps removed.

Clinical Presentation and Evaluation of Polyps

Polyps are usually asymptomatic but occasionally bleed enough to cause the patient to seek medical evaluation. They are most commonly detected during routine colonoscopic surveillance (Figure 14-17). Occasionally, a family history of polyps causes the patient to seek endoscopic screening.

Treatment of Polyps

The treatment of colonic polyps involves colonoscopic polypectomy. This allows for pathologic analysis and correct diagnosis of polyp type. Occasionally, a large or flat polyp cannot be safely removed colonoscopically. In this case, a segmental resection of the colon is performed. For disease conditions that are characterized by extensive polyposis (eg, hereditary nonpolyposis colorectal cancer [HNPCC] syndrome), the operation most commonly performed is a total colectomy.

TABLE 14-3. Comparison of Colorectal Polyps				
Type	**Frequency**	**Location**	**Malignant Potential**	**Treatment**
Tubular adenoma	25% of adults over 50 y will have an adenoma.	Rectosigmoid in 20%	Low	Endoscopic excision
Villous adenoma		Rectosigmoid in 80%	High	Endoscopic excision
Hamartoma	Uncommon	Small bowel	Low; uncommon	Excise for bleeding or obstruction
Inflammatory	Uncommon, except in IBD	Colon and rectum	None	Observation
Hyperplastic	Fairly common	Stomach, colon, and rectum	None	Observation

IBD, inflammatory bowel disease.

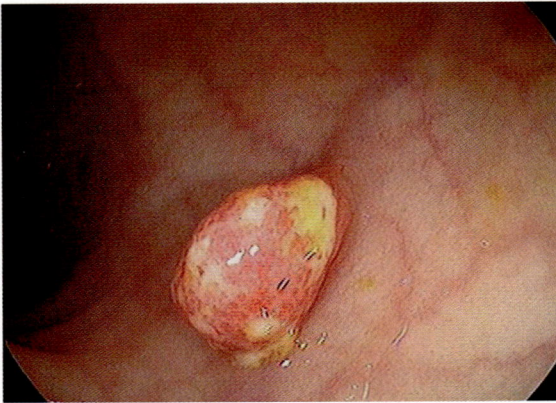

Figure 14-17. A polyp detected during colonoscopy.

Cancer of the Colon and Rectum

Cancer of the colon and rectum is a major cause of death in the United States. According to the American Cancer Society, it is the third most common cancer among men and women, and over 52,000 people die of this disease annually. Approximately 106,000 new colon cancer and 46,000 rectal cancer cases are identified every year. The great majority of colorectal cancers occur sporadically, without a known genetic mutation. Although a large number of factors are associated with the development of this disease, theories about its etiology center on the impact of intraluminal chemical carcinogenesis. There are various theories as to whether these carcinogens are ingested or are the result of biochemical processes that occur within the bowel lumen. Geographic epidemiologic studies show that certain populations have a very low incidence of cancer of the colon and rectum, apparently as a result of identifiable dietary factors (eg, high fiber, low fat), although, social customs and a lack of environmental carcinogens cannot be excluded. Certain health agencies promote a low-fat, high-fiber diet as protective against cancer of the colon and rectum. Chemoprevention by ingestion of agents such as carotenoids and other antioxidants has been suggested, but the efficacy of these is unproven. There is some evidence that prostaglandin inhibitors such as aspirin and sulindac significantly lower the risk of adenomatous polyp formation and colon cancer when taken on a regular basis.

Approximately 6% of all colorectal cancers are caused by a familial cancer syndrome with a known genetic mutation that may be inherited. FAP syndrome accounts for 1% of colorectal cancer and is caused by a mutation of the *APC* gene. Patients present with adenomas in adolescence and progress to carpeting of the colon with adenomas. Surgery can be performed to remove the colon and rectum and eliminate the risk of cancer. HNPCC, or Lynch syndrome, accounts for 5% of colon cancers. It is caused by mutations of the mismatch repair genes *MLH1*, *MSH2*, *MSH6*, and *PMS2*. Patients tend to develop right-sided colon cancers in their 30s or 40s and are at high risk for additional cancers, such as endometrial and urethral.

Most colorectal cancers occur on the left side of the colon, in the sigmoid, and rectum (Figure 14-18), although some studies suggest a slow shifting to right-side lesions.

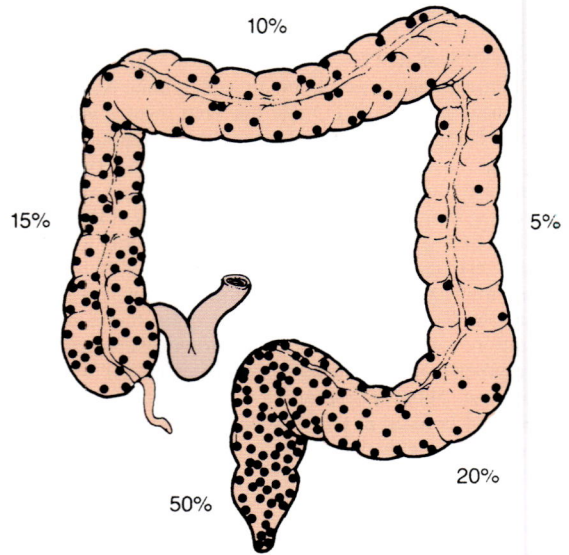

Figure 14-18. Frequency distribution of adenocarcinoma of the colon and rectum.

Synchronous (simultaneously occurring) tumors develop in 5% of patients, whereas 3% to 5% of patients have metachronous tumors (a second tumor developing after resection of the first). The peak incidence of colon cancers occurs at approximately 70 years of age. The incidence begins to increase in the fourth decade of life, and 90% of colorectal cancers develop after the age of 50.

Screening for Colon and Rectal Cancer

Of all GI cancers, more progress has been made in improving cure rates in colorectal cancer than in any other. Currently, according to the National Cancer Institute's Surveillance, Epidemiology, and End Results Program database, all stages included, the 5-year survival rate is 65%. There is little question that this improvement is partly due to effective screening that detects cancers at an early stage or prevents cancer by removing adenomatous polyps. For the purpose of colorectal cancer screening, patients are classified as average or high risk. High-risk patients have a family history of colorectal cancer in a first-degree relative, family history of precancerous polyps, a personal history of precancerous polyps, a personal history of colorectal cancer, a personal history of IBD, a personal history of abdominal or pelvic radiation, or a known familial cancer syndrome (FAP or HNPCC). Patients with none of these risk factors are determined to be at average risk.

Beginning at age 45, average-risk individuals should follow one of these screening options:

Tests that find both polyps and cancer

Flexible sigmoidoscopy every 5 years[a]

Colonoscopy every 10 years

CT colorography (virtual colonoscopy) every 5 years[a] (Figure 14-19)

Capsule colonoscopy every 5 years[a]

Tests that may find cancer
Fecal occult blood test (FOBT) every year[a]
Fecal immunochemical test (FIT) every year[a]
Stool DNA (sDNA) test every 3 years[a]

[a]Colonoscopy should be done if test results are positive.
(Recommendations based on the American Cancer Society, 2020.)

High-risk patients need to undergo colonoscopy. Patients with a first-degree relative with colon cancer will typically begin colonoscopy 10 years before the age of diagnosis of cancer for their family member or the age of 45, whichever comes first. Patients with a history of polyps will have colonoscopy at an interval shorter than 10 years and depending on the number, size, and histologic type of polyps. Patients with IBD for 10 years or more should begin annual colonoscopic surveillance.

Clinical Presentation and Evaluation of Colon and Rectal Cancer

The clinical signs and symptoms of colorectal cancer are determined largely by the anatomic location. Cancers of the right colon are usually exophytic lesions associated with occult blood loss, resulting in iron deficiency anemia (Table 14-4). Because of the liquid nature of stool in the right colon, the tumor may remain asymptomatic until quite advanced. Cancers that arise primarily in the left and sigmoid colon (Figure 14-20) are more likely to cause macroscopic rectal bleeding (see Table 14-4) and altered bowel habits with signs of partial obstruction (increased difficulty defecating, abdominal bloating, decrease in stool caliber, and increased frequency of small-volume bowel movements). Cancers of the rectum may cause a symptom complex of rectal bleeding, obstruction, and, occasionally, alternating diarrhea and constipation. Tenesmus (the continued or recurrent sensation of the need to have a bowel movement) occurs with advanced disease. Any patient older than 30 with a change in bowel

TABLE 14-4. Usual Symptoms of Colon and Rectal Cancers

Symptom	Site of Cancer		
	Right Colon	Left Colon	Rectum
Weight loss	+	+/0	+/0
Mass on abdominal exam	+	0	0
Rectal bleeding	0	+	+
Obstruction	0	+	+

habits, iron deficiency anemia, or rectal bleeding should undergo a complete examination of the colon and rectum by colonoscopy.

Patients who are diagnosed with adenocarcinoma of the colon or rectum undergo a staging workup. Staging is the phase at which the approach to colon and rectal cancer begins to diverge. Staging for both includes CT scans of the chest, abdomen, and pelvis to rule out distant metastatic disease. Common sites for metastasis are the liver and lung. Staging for rectal cancer includes an additional study, typically a pelvic MRI or endorectal ultrasound, to assess the depth of tumor invasion in the bowel wall and the involvement of lymph nodes. Preoperative assessment of the depth of tumor invasion and involvement of lymph nodes for colon cancer is difficult and, therefore, is determined postoperatively in the pathologic specimen. Management for both colon and rectal cancers should also include a carcinoembryonic antigen (CEA) level, a test that is used to help detect colorectal cancer recurrence. A baseline CEA should be obtained before

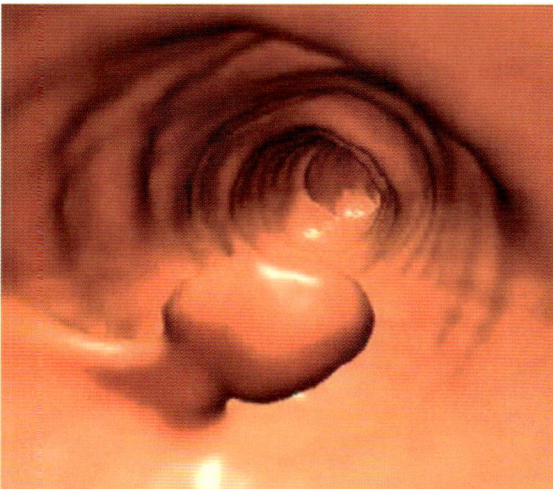

Figure 14-19. A polyp found on computed tomography colonography.

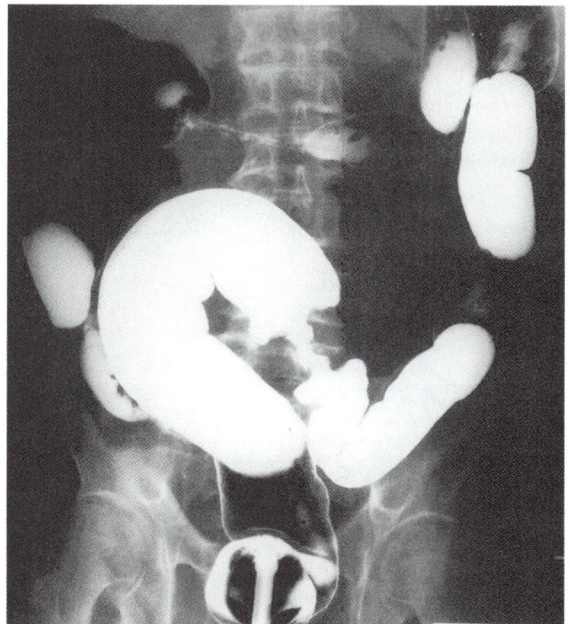

Figure 14-20. Barium enema demonstrating carcinoma of the sigmoid colon with a classic "apple core" lesion.

therapy starts. Results of the antigen study are elevated in many GI malignancies; therefore, it is not useful in diagnosis or staging.

Treatment of Colon and Rectal Cancer

The initial step in the treatment of colon cancer is surgery for nonmetastatic disease. The segment of the colon containing the cancerous lesion and a length of normal colon on either side is excised along with its mesentery. Inclusion of the mesentery allows for removal of the lymph nodes draining the segment of the colon containing the tumor (Figure 14-21). Removal of the lymph nodes is important because 30% of colon cancers will have spread to the regional mesenteric lymph nodes at the time of diagnosis. After the removal of the segment of the colon and mesentery, the bowel ends are anastomosed, typically without the need for a stoma.

Rectal cancers that are found on staging pelvic MRI or ultrasound to invade through the rectal wall (T3 or T4) or have lymph node involvement are initially treated with chemotherapy and radiation. The intent of this neoadjuvant (before surgery) treatment is to reduce the size of the tumor and lower the chance of local recurrence. There may also be a survival benefit to this approach. After a long course (up to 6 weeks) of neoadjuvant chemotherapy and radiation, the patient is allowed to recover for from 6 to 12 weeks. During this time, the cancer will often continue to regress and respond to the treatment it has received. Surgery is then performed.

Surgery for rectal cancer is an LAR with primary anastomosis. The rectum is removed with a gross margin distal to the tumor of 2 cm. Total mesorectal excision is an important part of this technique in which all perirectal fat-containing lymph nodes are removed with the cancer. The low-lying nature of the anastomosis and the effects of radiation make these anastomoses a high risk for leakage. Anastomotic leakage carries devastating consequences of sepsis, multisystem organ failure, and the possibility of permanent stoma. Therefore, most LAR anastomoses are protected with a temporary proximal diverting ileostomy. When rectal cancer invades the sphincters of the anal canal, an APR with permanent end sigmoid colostomy is indicated.

Recent developments in minimally invasive surgery involving the use of the laparoscope suggest that laparoscopic resection of colon cancers can be done safely and effectively, with an acceptable number of lymph nodes. The procedure is usually done with a small abdominal incision to facilitate removal of the bowel containing the tumor and to assist in the anastomosis. Further experience is needed to determine whether laparoscopy can be done safely and with the same oncologic results for rectal tumors.

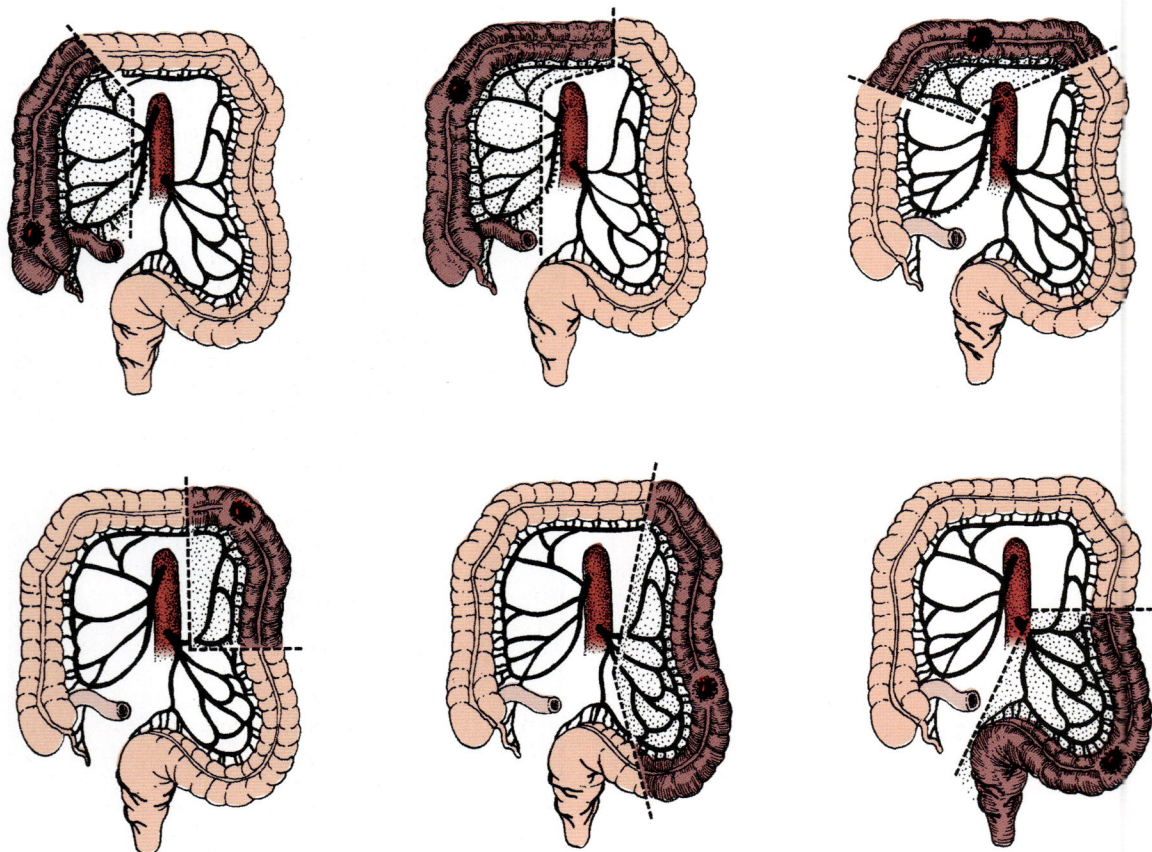

Figure 14-21. Indicated operative resection for colon cancer in different sites. The boundaries of the resection are dictated by lymphatic drainage patterns that parallel the blood supply.

Occasionally, patients may present with acute large bowel obstruction because of a colon or rectal cancer. In some of these cases, metallic stents can be placed endoscopically or with fluoroscopic guidance. When successfully placed, the stents prevent the need for emergency surgery and colostomy by opening the obstructed colon. This can serve as a bridge to elective resection or palliation if the patient has advanced metastatic disease. Alternatively, a diverting colostomy will allow the patient to get chemotherapy without being obstructed.

The specimen removed in the operating room for a colon or rectal cancer is sent to the pathologist for staging (Table 14-5). Stages 1 and 2 colon cancer are considered adequately treated with surgery alone. Adjuvant chemotherapy is typically recommended for patients with stage 3 colon cancer and stages 2 and 3 rectal cancer. The use of adjuvant therapies in the treatment of colon and rectal cancer has generated considerable research in the past several decades. Studies have demonstrated that 5-fluorouracil (5-FU) used in combination with levamisole or leucovorin lowers the mortality rate in patients with stage 3 tumors. Oxaliplatin appears to be twice as effective as 5-FU alone in reducing cancer recurrence in high-risk patients as well as in treating patients with metastatic colorectal cancer. Currently, 4 to 6 months of adjuvant (after surgery) 5-FU, leucovorin, and oxaliplatin (FOLFOX) is the standard of care. A number of new biologic agents (bevacizumab, irinotecan, and cetuximab) show promise in achieving even better results, especially with hepatic metastases.

TABLE 14-5. TNM Staging System

Primary tumor (T)	
TX	Primary tumor cannot be assessed.
T0	No evidence of primary tumor
Tis	Carcinoma in situ; intraepithelial tumor or invasion of the lamina propria
T1	Tumor invading the submucosa
T2	Tumor invading the muscularis propria
T3	Tumor invading through the muscularis propria into the subserosa, or into nonperitonealized pericolic or perirectal tissues
T4	Tumor directly invading other organs or structures or perforating the visceral peritoneum
Regional lymph nodes (N)	
NX	Regional lymph nodes cannot be assessed.
N0	No regional lymph node metastasis
N1	Metastasis in 1-3 pericolic or perirectal lymph nodes
N2	Metastasis in ≥4 pericolic or perirectal lymph nodes
Distant metastasis (M)	
MX	Presence of distant metastasis cannot be assessed.
M0	No distant metastasis
M1	Distant metastasis

Prognosis for Colon and Rectal Cancer

Once patients have recovered from surgery and adjuvant chemotherapy, they enter into follow-up surveillance. Most recurrences occur in the first 18 to 24 months, and surveillance is, therefore, front-loaded. Most guidelines recommend history, physical examination, and CEA every 3 months for the first 2 years and every 6 months for the next 3 years. Colonoscopy is routinely performed at 1 and 4 years postoperatively and then every 5 years thereafter. CT scans of the chest, abdomen, and pelvis are done 2 times in 5 years or annually in those patients at high risk for recurrence.

The use of CEA is well established, with recurrence suggested not only by the absolute level of this antigen but also by a progressive rise. A progressive rise mandates a complete evaluation of the patient, including CT of the chest, abdomen, and pelvis. PET scans should also be considered in patients with rising CEA levels. The prognosis of colon and rectal cancer depends on the stage detailed in Table 14-5. The most important prognostic variable is lymph node involvement. For patients who have recurrences, the combination of chemotherapy, embolization of liver metastases, and, occasionally, resection of isolated recurrences can lead to a median survival of 2 years.

ANUS AND RECTUM

Presentation and Evaluation of Anorectal Pathology

The anus and rectum are sites of many conditions that cause pain, protrusion, bleeding, discharge, or a combination of these. Most people who complain about hemorrhoids are unaware of pathology other than hemorrhoids (fissure, abscess, pruritus, fistula, condyloma, cancer, etc) that may affect the anal area. It is up to the physician to distinguish among various pathologies that present similarly. A complete history suggests the diagnosis in more than 80% of cases and guides the subsequent examination.

Examination of the perianal and rectal area is an integral part of every physical examination. The examination should be described in advance, and a chaperone should be offered. The importance of gentleness and empathy cannot be overemphasized. The patient may be placed in the lateral decubitus, knee-chest, or prone-jackknife position. The buttocks are spread, and any pain with spreading and any visible lesions are noted. The patient should be asked to Valsalva to simulate a bowel movement and to induce any prolapse. Gentle parting of the buttocks allows inspection that may show fissures, skin tags, hemorrhoids, fistulae, tumors, and dermatologic or infectious conditions. Gentle digital examination may reveal tumors, polyps, mucosal abnormalities, and sphincter weakness. Digital examination may be deferred in the presence of acute pain.

Anoscopic examination is mandatory because many visible lesions are not palpable. It may be deferred, however, in the presence of acute pain. The anoscope is a rigid instrument used to examine the anal canal. It allows better detection of more distal lesions than the rigid or flexible proctosigmoidoscope. Sigmoidoscopy and colonoscopy, however, are the instruments of choice for a proper evaluation of the rectum because they allow for proper assessment of middle and upper as well as distal rectal lesions. Preparation with an enema prior to examination is useful with anoscopy and sigmoidoscopy.

Rectal Prolapse (Procidentia)

Rectal prolapse is the intussusception of a full-thickness portion of the rectum through the anal opening. This condition occurs most commonly in thin, asthenic women who have weak rectal attachments and may involve from 4 to 20 cm of rectum protruding through the anal opening. The entity must be distinguished from mucosal prolapse, which is eversion through the anal opening of 2 to 3 cm of rectal mucosa that is not full thickness. They can be distinguished by the concentric, circumferential mucosal folds seen in true prolapse compared with the radial pattern of folds seen in mucosal or hemorrhoid prolapse (Figure 14-22).

Clinical Presentation and Evaluation of Rectal Prolapse

Symptoms of prolapse include rectal pain or pressure, mild bleeding, incontinence, mucous discharge, and a wet anus. On rare occasions, the prolapse cannot be reduced, and ischemia results. The prolapse commonly occurs after each bowel movement and must be manually reduced.

Treatment of Rectal Prolapse

Management of rectal prolapse involves an intra-abdominal procedure, including sigmoid resection of redundant bowel with rectopexy (suturing the bowel wall to the presacral fascia to immobilize it). Recurrence rates are less than 5% if the procedure is correctly performed. For high-risk patients, a procedure can be done in which the entire resection is done through the perineum, but recurrence rates are much higher. The treatment of mucosal or hemorrhoid prolapse is excisional hemorrhoidectomy.

Hemorrhoids

Hemorrhoids are normal vascular cushions that line the anal canal. Hemorrhoids are classified as either internal or external. Internal hemorrhoids are usually found in three constant positions: left lateral, right anterior, and right posterior. It is preferable to refer to the actual anatomic position of any anorectal process. With the "o'clock" system, 12 o'clock varies depending on the patient's position during an examination and the practitioner's conventions.

Internal hemorrhoids originate above the dentate line; external hemorrhoids are located below the level of the dentate line.

Hemorrhoid disease, which most often causes hemorrhoid protrusion or bleeding, is usually precipitated by constipation and straining at stool. Pregnancy, increased pelvic pressure (ascites, tumors), portal hypertension, and diarrhea may cause hemorrhoid symptoms.

Because the rectal mucosa above the dentate line is insensate, bleeding from internal hemorrhoids is usually painless. Conversely, external hemorrhoids are covered by richly innervated anoderm and usually cause pain when thrombosis occurs.

Clinical Presentation and Evaluation of Hemorrhoids

A careful history that delineates exactly what symptoms a patient is attributing to their hemorrhoids is essential. The relation of symptoms to bowel movements, the consistency of stool that is normally passed, the presence of pain, and prolapse of tissue should all be elucidated. The length of time a patient spends on the toilet and whether they strain can represent modifiable behavior that can substantially improve symptoms. The presence of blood, either with wiping, along the side of a hard stool, or mixed with the stool can help distinguish between hemorrhoid bleeding, bleeding from a fissure, or bleeding from a cancer.

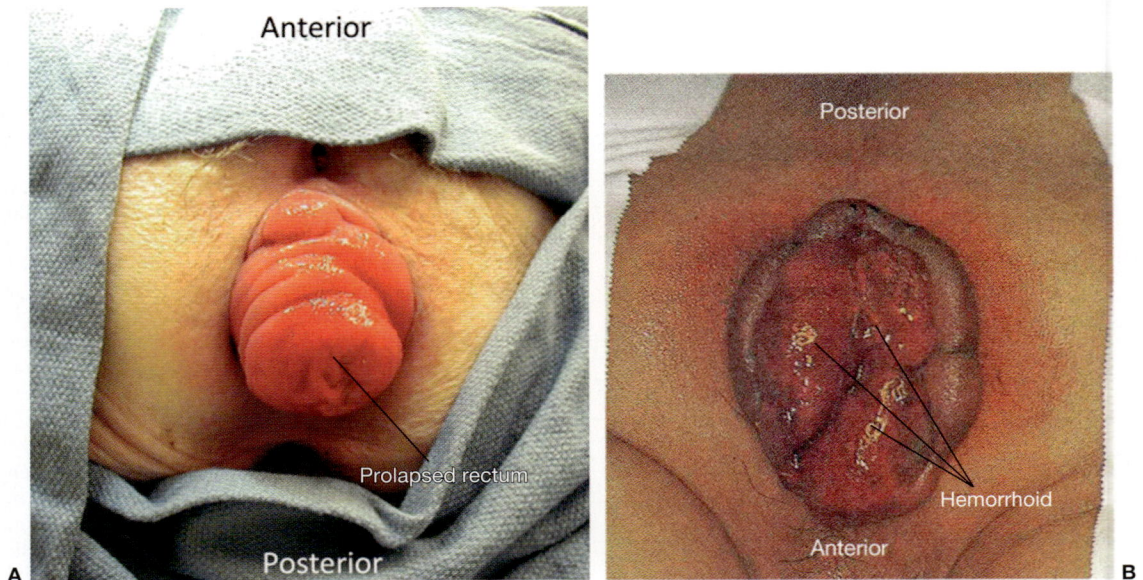

Figure 14-22. A. True rectal prolapse is characterized by concentric, circumferential mucosal folds. B. Mucosal prolapse is characterized by radial folds separating the mucosa. (Reprinted with permission from Albo D, Mulholland MW. *Operative Techniques in Colon and Rectal Surgery*. 1st ed. Wolters Kluwer Health; 2015.)

A patient with symptomatic internal hemorrhoids will typically complain of painless bright red bleeding, often seen with wiping or as drops of blood in the toilet. Rarely is the volume of blood enough to cause anemia. Patients may also have prolapse; first-degree internal hemorrhoids do not prolapse; the anoscope must be used to visualize them. Second-degree internal hemorrhoids prolapse with defecation and return spontaneously to their anatomic position. Third-degree internal hemorrhoids prolapse with defecation and require manual reduction. Fourth-degree hemorrhoids are not reducible (Figure 14-23). It can be helpful to examine a patient who is sitting on the toilet and straining; this allows for a more reliable assessment of the degree of internal prolapse or external engorgement that is occurring.

External hemorrhoids may become engorged and uncomfortable after bowel movements, but they do not bleed. Occasionally, blood may clot within the external hemorrhoids, and this thrombosis causes acute pain and a palpable, tender, tense, often purple-blue mass adjacent to the anal verge.

Treatment of Hemorrhoids

Treatment is based on the presence of symptoms and the degree of disease (Table 14-6). Asymptomatic hemorrhoids are best left alone; cosmetic treatment is not indicated. Bulk-forming agents (eg, psyllium derivatives), adequate water intake, avoidance of constipation, and limiting time seated on the toilet or straining are recommended. First-degree internal hemorrhoids are treated with topical agents or, if bleeding, with injection sclerotherapy or infrared coagulation. Tight rubber bands may be placed around the base of large first- or second- and some third-degree internal hemorrhoids. Banding is done in the ambulatory setting with an anoscope and induces ischemia and sloughing of the excess hemorrhoid tissue. Surgical hemorrhoidal artery ligation can be used for second-, third-, and some fourth-degree hemorrhoids. A mucopexy (lifting and fixing the hemorrhoid to the anal canal by suture) can be added to the hemorrhoid ligation procedure for symptomatic prolapsed hemorrhoidal cushions. Formal surgical hemorrhoidectomy is used for third-degree hemorrhoids (especially those mixed third-degree

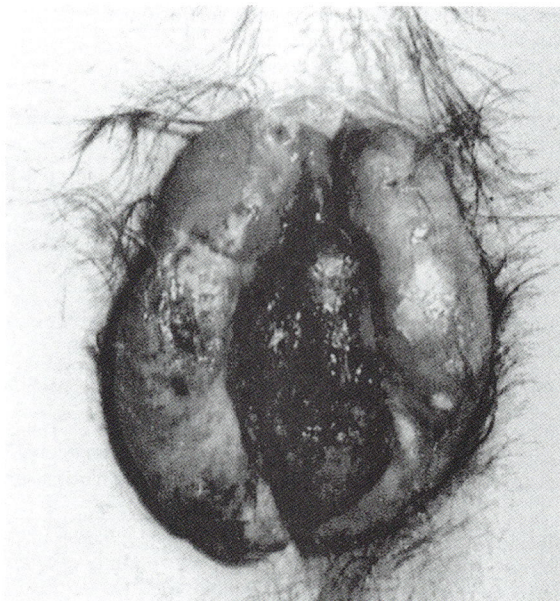

Figure 14-23. **Fourth-degree hemorrhoids associated with thrombosis.**

hemorrhoids with a large external component), for fourth-degree hemorrhoids, and in some emergency situations (eg, an acute hemorrhoid attack with gangrene, severe ulceration).

External hemorrhoids usually cause a few problems. Contrary to popular belief, hemorrhoids do not itch or burn; it is the perianal skin that is the site of pruritus ani. However, large external hemorrhoids may interfere with perianal hygiene and thus be indirectly associated with pruritus. In these cases, excision may be indicated. It is usually done under local anesthesia with sedation.

Thrombosed external hemorrhoids are self-limited and typically resolve over 7 to 10 days; creams, suppositories, and topical adjuncts provide no benefit. If the patient is seen in the first 24 to 48 hours after thrombosis, treatment

TABLE 14-6. Internal Hemorrhoids: Classification and Treatment		
Degree	**Definition**	**Treatment**
First	Bulge in the anal canal lumen; does not protrude outside the lumen Painless bleeding	*Asymptomatic*: conservative management—take bulking agents or stool softeners; increase water intake; avoid constipation, straining, and prolonged sitting on the toilet.
		Symptomatic: same treatment as asymptomatic; topical agents, rubber-band ligation
Second	Protrudes with defecation Reduces spontaneously	Conservative management (see earlier), topical agents, rubber-band ligation, and/or surgical hemorrhoid artery ligation with or without mucopexy
Third	Protrudes with defecation Must be reduced manually	Conservative management (see earlier), topical agents, surgical hemorrhoid artery ligation with or without mucopexy, or surgical hemorrhoidectomy *Selected cases*: rubber-band ligation
Fourth	Unable to be reduced	Surgical hemorrhoidectomy Select cases: surgical hemorrhoidal artery ligation with or without mucopexy

consists of excision of the thrombosed hemorrhoid under local anesthesia. If the patient is seen later in the course of the disease, spontaneous resolution is usually underway and conservative treatment is indicated. Sitz baths, nonsteroidal anti-inflammatory drugs (NSAIDs), acetaminophen, and application of ice are recommended. Donut cushions are to be avoided because they simply increase the pressure at the anus and result in increased swelling and pain. Rarely, the skin overlying the thrombus will ulcerate. This is an indication for excision.

Anorectal Abscesses

Anorectal abscesses are infections that commonly occupy the perianal and ischiorectal spaces and infrequently in the intersphincteric, supralevator, and deep postanal regions. Anorectal abscesses occur at any age, with a peak incidence among 20- to 40-year-olds. In general, the abscess is treated with incision and drainage, either at the bedside or in the operating room. Fistula-in-ano is a subcutaneous tunnel or tract that communicates between the perineal skin and the anal canal. In patients with an anorectal abscess, some will present with a concomitant fistula-in-ano. Approximately one-third will be diagnosed with a fistula in the months to years after abscess drainage.

Anorectal abscesses (Figure 14-24) are believed to start with obstruction of the glands located at the base of the columns of Morgagni, or anal crypts, at the dentate line. The term *cryptoglandular origin* distinguishes these from abscesses or fistulae related to CD, obstetric complications, or iatrogenic trauma.

Presentation and Evaluation of Anorectal Abscess

The diagnosis of anorectal abscess is based on history and physical examination. Anorectal pain and a palpable perianal mass or swelling are common with abscesses. The onset is usually insidious, with slow but progressive and relentless worsening pain over days or even weeks. Deeper abscesses may also present with pain that is referred to the perineum, to the low back, or down the legs or buttocks. Constitutional symptoms such as fever and chills

are uncommon. However, their presence may signify a more extensive infectious process and should be a cause for concern and more urgent intervention. Physical inspection and examination of the anus and perineum may reveal a mass with warmth, erythema, fluctuance, and exquisite tenderness to palpation. However, the perianal area may be normal in patients with deeper abscesses. Digital rectal examination is occasionally useful to clarify the diagnosis. Sedation or anesthesia may be needed when an examination is intolerable because of pain or tenderness. The differential diagnosis of anorectal abscess includes thrombosed hemorrhoids, pilonidal disease, hidradenitis, fissure, anal condyloma, malignancy, CD, sexually transmitted infections (STIs), and human immunodeficiency virus (HIV) proctalgia.

Laboratory studies are rarely required unless a secondary diagnosis or more complex infectious process is suspected. Superficial abscesses and simple fistulas, in general, do not require diagnostic imaging. Alternatively, imaging with MRI or anorectal ultrasound may prove useful in the assessment of occult anorectal abscess, unusual conditions (especially STIs), and perianal CD.

Treatment of Anorectal Abscess

The primary treatment of perianal and ischiorectal abscess is surgical drainage through the perianal skin. In general, the skin incision should be kept as close to the anal verge without damaging the anal sphincter muscles as possible. This minimizes the length of a potential fistula, while still providing adequate drainage. Studies have demonstrated that aggressive packing of the wound created by drainage is not only unwarranted but also delays resolution and may damage the anal sphincter muscles.

A variation of incision and drainage uses a small catheter (eg, Pezzer or Malecot) placed into the abscess cavity with the use of local anesthetic and a small stab incision. The drain is removed when the abscess cavity has closed, typically after 5 days. Intersphincteric, supralevator, deep postanal space, and horseshoe abscesses require individualized complex drainage procedures.

Antibiotics should be reserved for patients with anorectal abscess complicated by significant cellulitis, systemic signs of infection, or underlying immunosuppression.

Fistulae-in-Ano

Fistulae-in-ano are among the most varied and complex anorectal conditions encountered by the colorectal surgeon. An anorectal fistula is an abnormal communication between the anus at the level of the dentate line and the perirectal skin, through the bed of a previous abscess. Fistulae are named in relation to the involvement of the sphincter mechanism. Intersphincteric fistulae are the result of perianal abscesses, transsphincteric fistulae are the result of ischiorectal abscesses, and suprasphincteric fistulae are the result of supralevator abscesses. Extrasphincteric fistulae bypass the anal canal and the sphincter mechanism and open high up in the rectum. A history and physical examination are usually sufficient to diagnose simple fistulae. An examination of anus under anesthesia may be needed to confirm a suspected diagnosis. Endoanal ultrasound and pelvic MRI are the best studies to work up complex (fistulae associated with CD or with multiple extensions and/or openings) or recurrent fistulae.

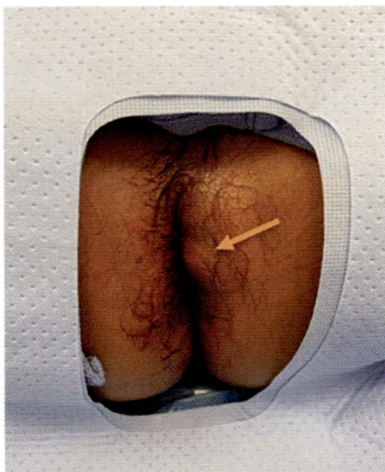

Figure 14-24. Perianal abscess. (Image courtesy of Jacquelyn Turner, MD.)

The course, depth, degree of muscular involvement, and the exact location of the fistula all play a part in the decision of the best surgical option. A simple fistula-in-ano (relatively straight and superficial with a readily identified internal opening) in a patient with normal anal sphincter function may be treated with primary fistulotomy or unroofing of the fistula tract, allowing the fistula to heal slowly by secondary intention. Fistulotomy is an effective treatment and results in healing in over 90% of patients. Fistulotomy failures have been associated with complex types of fistula, failure to identify the internal opening, CD, and other more complex anal diseases.

Simple and complex anal fistulae may be treated with the ligation of the intersphincteric fistula tract (LIFT) procedure. The LIFT procedure involves suture closure and division of the fistula tract in the intersphincteric groove. Meta-analyses report that the standard or "classic" LIFT has resulted in fistula healing in 61% to 94% of patients, with little morbidity.

Endoanal advancement flaps are recommended for the treatment of complex fistulae-in-ano. The flap is a sphincter-sparing technique that consists of curettage of the fistula tract, suture closure of the internal opening, and mobilization of a segment of healthy anorectal mucosa, submucosa, and muscle to cover the closed internal opening. Factors associated with failed repair include prior radiation, underlying CD, active proctitis, rectovaginal fistula, malignancy, obesity, and the number of previously attempted repairs.

When the fistula-in-ano presents with significant perianal infection, a draining Seton may be placed to control sepsis. This is typically followed by a secondary, definitive procedure. Healing rates have ranged from 62% to 100%, depending on the type of secondary procedure. Alternatively, the Seton may also be left in place and tightened at intervals to allow gradual division of the sphincter, a so-called *cutting* Seton. Although early data suggested high rates of incontinence with cutting Seton, other studies have suggested that the rates are similar to other treatments for fistula-in-ano.

Anal Fissures

Anal fissures (Figure 14-25) are the most common cause of anorectal pain that cause patients to seek medical attention. Anal fissures are longitudinal tears within the anal canal, typically from the dentate line toward the anal verge. Although external hemorrhoids may cause mild discomfort and associated symptoms such as itching and burning, they rarely cause the severe pain associated with fissures. The pain is described as sharp and knife-like. Patients often report the sense of "passing cut glass" with bowel movements. The pain is precipitated by a bowel movement and is usually accompanied by some bright red blood seen as a streak along the side of a stool, on toilet tissue when wiping, or as drops in the toilet bowl. Fissures are thought to be secondary to local trauma, either from constipation, instrumentation, or from excessive diarrhea.

The location of the fissure in the anal canal assists in the diagnosis. Greater than 80% will be located in the posterior midline, with the remainder in the anterior midline either as a free-standing fissure or in conjunction with a posterior midline fissure. The posterior and anterior

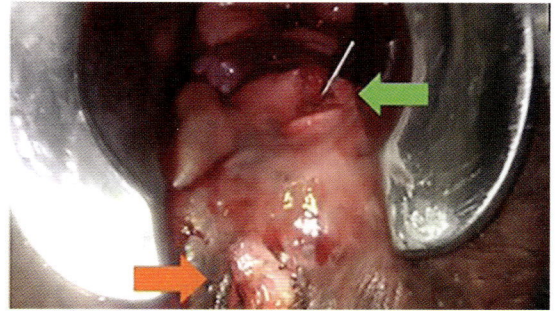

Figure 14-25. Anal fistula. Green arrow depicting the internal opening with probe. Orange arrow depicting the external opening. (Image courtesy of Jaquelyn Turner, MD.)

midlines are the watershed areas of blood supply in the anal canal, and thus, a component of ischemia is thought to participate in fissure pathogenesis. Multiple fissures or an eccentric, off-midline location suggest an alternate underlying diagnosis such as CD, STI (syphilis, lymphogranuloma venereum, and herpes), anal cancer, tuberculosis, HIV, or a hematologic malignancy.

The diagnosis of fissure can often be made solely by the patient's history and a brief anal inspection. Anorectal inspection for an acute fissure will reveal a longitudinal tear in the mucosa, occasionally with some mild inflammation. This can often be seen solely by gently spreading the buttocks while inspecting the posterior midline. Digital and anoscopic examination in the clinical setting is necessary if the diagnosis is unclear and the patient can tolerate it.

Endoscopic evaluation of the proximal colon should be instituted in patients with ongoing fissure symptoms, including pain or bleeding, and with patients who have concomitant abdominal symptoms or bowel irregularity. Colonoscopy is recommended in all patients aged 30 years and above, especially if there is family history of colorectal cancer or associated hematochezia. In the younger population, flexible sigmoidoscopy is likely sufficient unless the diagnosis of CD is suspected, when a full colonoscopy with intubation and possibly biopsy of the terminal ileum is ideal.

Once the initial diagnosis is made, immediate further workup is deferred secondary to the patient's discomfort. About 50% to 75% of patients who have an acute anal fissure will resolve their symptoms with simple conservative measures such as sitz baths and stool bulking agents and adequate fluid intake to ensure soft stools. Topical anesthetics or steroids may provide additional symptomatic relief. These interventions are well tolerated, with minimal to no side effects. Antibiotics are not warranted unless a concomitant infection is found. Topical calcium channel blockers (typically diltiazem or nifedipine) and topical nitrates (nitroglycerin) have been associated with healing rates of anal fissures of 65% to 95%. Side effects, particularly headaches, are less frequent with calcium channel blockers compared with nitrates.

The patient is reevaluated at approximately 1 month, unless symptoms worsen. If there is no resolution of symptoms, or if the patient is worsening, examination under anesthesia with biopsy is recommended. After approximately

8 weeks, the fissure may become chronic. On examination, chronicity is evidenced by a deeper fissure, with the underlying internal sphincter muscle fibers exposed. In addition, the development of a sentinel external skin tag and even a hypertrophied anal papilla will clarify the diagnosis of chronic anal fissure.

If conservative measures and topical treatments fail to resolve a patient's symptoms, more invasive options should be offered. Botulinum toxin (Botox) can be injected in the internal sphincter muscle. Botox has similar results as topical therapies, with slightly improved healing rates following failed topical treatments. This procedure is often performed in the operating room due to patient discomfort. Furthermore, a definitive surgical intervention should be offered if the other treatment options fail. The definitive surgical treatment for chronic anal fissure without fecal incontinence is the lateral internal sphincterotomy (LIS). Successful healing occurs after LIS, with 95% to 98% of patients reporting moderate to complete resolution of symptoms. Anorectal seepage and incontinence are reported in 5% to 10% of cases after LIS. For patients who are felt to be at a higher risk of incontinence, an anorectal advancement flap can be a safer option.

Anal Dysplasia and Anal Cancer

Human papillomaviruses (HPVs) are a group of more than 200 related viruses. HPV is the most common STI in the United States. HPV is so common that nearly all men and women get it at some point in their lives, and it can be spread when a person with infection has no signs or symptoms, by vaginal, anal, or oral sex.

Symptoms can develop many years after being infected, making it hard to know when it was acquired. Presenting complaints of perianal or anal condyloma accuminata (anal warts) may include a lump, pruritus, bleeding, drainage, pain, and difficulty with hygiene. Physical examination is generally definitive for the diagnosis and shows the characteristic fleshy, cauliflower-like growths of variable size. Anoscopy is a necessary part of the evaluation. In the anal canal, the lesions tend to be small papules. Examination should focus on the genitalia, including vaginal speculum examination and perineal examination. The goal of the treatment of HPV is destruction or removal of all obvious diseases while minimizing morbidity, although this process does not definitively eradicate infection. Excision, cryotherapy, topical treatment with chemicals such as podophyllin or imiquimod, or fulguration of small lesions can be performed. Larger lesions are treated by surgical excision. Lesions in patients with HIV and recurrent, flat, or suspicious lesions must be sent for histologic evaluation to assess for the presence of dysplasia also known as anal intraepithelial neoplasia (AIN). HPV "cure" rates for surgical excision range from 60% to 90%.

The role that HPV plays in the development of squamous cell carcinoma (SCC) of the anus is slightly less well defined than it is in cervical cancer. Parallels can be drawn between the anal canal and the cervix, both embryologically and via epidemiology studies, but a cause and effect are still incompletely proven. At-risk patients include those with large or suspicious lesions, recent history of AIN 3 lesions, recurrent lesions, lesions resistant to treatment, anoreceptive intercourse, prior history of anal cancer or anal dysplasia, and all patients with HIV. Both high-resolution anoscopy with biopsy and anal Pap smears are used as screening and surveillance tools. Lugol solution and acetic acid are often used to help identify lesions during high-resolution anoscopy. Excisional biopsy may be used in patients with a questionable diagnosis.

SCC of the anus has a well-defined treatment algorithm. Once biopsies and staging are completed, the primary treatment for most SCCs of the anal canal should be combined modality chemotherapy with mitomycin-c and fluorouracil and external beam radiation therapy (the Nigro protocol). This treatment approach cures 80% of patients. APR is reserved for patients whose tumors do not completely resolve with chemoradiation or recur. Selected cases of tumors less than 2 cm for which clear margins can be achieved and that do not invade the sphincter mechanism may be treated by local excision alone.

SUGGESTED READINGS

Ahmed M. Ischemic bowel disease in 2021. *World J Gastroenterol.* 2021;27(29):4746-4762.

Alavi, K, Poylin V, Davids J, et al. The American Society of Colon and Rectal Surgeons clinical practice guidelines for the management of colonic volvulus and acute colonic pseudo-obstruction. *Dis Colon Rectum.* 2021;64:1046-1057.

American Cancer Society. *American Cancer Society Guideline for Colorectal Cancer Screening.* American Cancer Society; 2020.

American Cancer Society. *Key Statistics for Colorectal Cancer.* American Cancer Society; 2023.

Foxx-Orenstein AE, Umar SB, Crowell MD. Common anorectal disorders. *Gastroenterol Hepatol.* 2014;10(5):294-301.

Hall J, Hardiman K, Lee S, et al. The American Society of Colon and Rectal Surgeons clinical practice guidelines for the treatment of left-sided colonic diverticulitis. *Dis Colon Rectum.* 2020;63:728-747.

Holubar SD, Lightner AL, Poylin V, et al. The American Society of Colon and Rectal Surgeons clinical practice guidelines for the surgical treatment of ulcerative colitis. *Dis Colon Rectum.* 2021;64:783-804.

Johnson S, Lavergne V, Skinner AM, et al. Clinical practice guideline by the Infectious Diseases Society of America (IDSA) and Society for Healthcare Epidemiology of America (SHEA): 2021 focused update guidelines on management of *Clostridioides difficile* infection in adults. *Clin Infect Dis.* 2021;73(5):e1029-e1044.

Vogel JD, Felder SI, Bhama AR, et al. The American Society of Colon and Rectal Surgeons clinical practice guidelines for the management of colon cancer. *Dis Colon Rectum.* 2022;65:148-177.

You YN, Hardiman KM, Bafford A, et al. The American Society of Colon and Rectal Surgeons clinical practice guidelines for the management of rectal cancer. *Dis Colon Rectum.* 2020;63:1191-1222.

SAMPLE QUESTIONS

QUESTIONS

Choose the best answer for each question.

1. A 52-year-old woman has never undergone any colorectal cancer screening. Her mother had colon cancer at the age of 53. What screening test would be most appropriate for the patient?

   A. FOBT
   B. Fecal DNA testing
   C. CT colonography
   D. Flexible sigmoidoscopy
   E. Colonoscopy

2. A patient with rectal cancer undergoes LAR with primary anastomosis and temporary proximal diverting stoma. The purpose of a temporary proximal diverting stoma is

   A. to reduce local recurrence of the cancer.
   B. to avoid further surgery.
   C. to reduce the complications of anastomotic leak.
   D. to avoid the need for chemotherapy after surgery.
   E. to reduce the use of radiation.

3. A patient undergoes right colectomy for cancer. The pathologic staging reveals T3N1 (invasion of the muscularis propria with 2 of 26 lymph nodes positive for cancer). What is the most appropriate next step in treatment?

   A. Colonoscopy
   B. Chemotherapy
   C. Radiation
   D. CT scan of the chest, abdomen, pelvis
   E. PET scan

4. A 39-year-old man complains of 6 months of intermittent blood in the stool, fatigue, and vague right-sided abdominal pain. The most appropriate next test would be

   A. CEA.
   B. flexible sigmoidoscopy.
   C. FOBT.
   D. CT colonoscopy.
   E. colonoscopy.

5. A 38-year-old woman undergoes normal spontaneous vaginal delivery. One day later, she notes the acute onset of an excruciatingly painful bump next to the anal opening. Examination of the perineum reveals a tense, blue, tender, 2-cm mass adjacent to the anus. The best treatment would be

   A. NSAIDs.
   B. topical hydrocortisone.
   C. sitz baths.
   D. excision.
   E. biopsy.

ANSWERS AND EXPLANATIONS

1. **Answer: E**

   Patients with a history of colon cancer in a first-degree relative are at high risk for colon cancer. High-risk patients must be screened with colonoscopy. The other screening options would be appropriate for an average-risk patient (negative family history of cancer, negative personal history of polyps or IBD, or known inherited familial cancer syndrome). For more information on this topic, see section "Screening for Colon and Rectal Cancer."

2. **Answer: C**

   The most feared complication after bowel resection is anastomotic leak. Anastomotic leak usually requires reoperation and creation of a stoma that may be permanent and usually results in sepsis and multisystem organ failure. Anastomoses created after LAR are usually low in the pelvis and attached to radiated tissue; these factors make them at high risk for leak. Temporary proximal diverting stoma reduces the risks of complications from an anastomotic leak but does require further surgery to close. Temporary stoma has no impact on the need for radiation or chemotherapy, or on the risk of local recurrence. For more information on this topic, see section "Treatment of Colon and Rectal Cancer."

3. **Answer: B**

   This patient has positive lymph nodes, which makes the cancer stage 3. Patients with stage 3 cancer benefit from adjuvant chemotherapy. Adjuvant chemotherapy, typically with FOLFOX, increases 5-year survival by 10% to 15% to approximately 75%. Colonoscopy and CT scans of the chest, abdomen, and pelvis are important parts of cancer surveillance but are not done until 1 year after surgery. Radiation is part of the treatment for rectal cancer, not colon cancer. A PET scan is not part of the treatment or surveillance for colon cancer. For more information on this topic, see section "Treatment of Colon and Rectal Cancer."

4. **Answer: E**

   This patient has symptoms concerning for a right-sided colon cancer. Colonoscopy would locate a tumor and allow for biopsy. A flexible sigmoidoscopy would not assess right-sided colon pathology. A CEA may be needed as part of a preoperative workup but is not the next test to perform. With visualized blood in the stool, there is no use in getting an FOBT, and a negative result could be falsely reassuring. CT colonoscopy might demonstrate a lesion in the colon but would not allow for a biopsy and would, therefore, be an extra, unnecessary test. For more information on this topic, see section "Clinical Presentation and Evaluation of Colon and Rectal Cancer."

5. **Answer: D**

Thrombosed external hemorrhoids can develop after vaginal delivery. This has been diagnosed in the first 48 hours, and the best treatment would be excision. NSAIDs and sitz baths can be used for symptom relief when the diagnosis is made after 48 hours or after excision. Topical hydrocortisone has not been shown to provide any benefit for hemorrhoidal disease. Biopsy is indicated for lesions that are suspicious of malignancy. Malignant lesions typically develop gradually, not acutely. For more information on this topic, see section "Treatment of Hemorrhoids."

Biliary Tract

O. Joe Hines and Saad Shebrain

Diseases of the gallbladder (GB) and bile ducts are common in the adult population of North America. These conditions can be life threatening and may require a detailed understanding to effectively triage patients. Approximately 15% of adults have gallstones, and more than 800,000 cholecystectomies are performed annually in the United States, accounting for more than $5 billion in health care costs. Accurate clinical assessment, including pertinent history and accurate physical examination, yields valuable information about the diagnosis of common diseases of the biliary tract. Laboratory tests are helpful in distinguishing among various causes of jaundice, and imaging studies play a pivotal role in confirming the diagnosis of biliary tract disease. To minimize the risk of iatrogenic injury during biliary procedures, the surgeon must possess the skills to recognize common variations in the anatomy of the biliary tract and to perform careful dissection of the vital structures during surgery. This dictum has been reemphasized in recent years with the meteoric rise in the popularity of minimally invasive cholecystectomy (MIC) using laparoscopic or robotic approaches, which have replaced open cholecystectomy as the preferred operation for most patients with gallstone disease.

ANATOMY

The origin of the biliary tree is an outgrowth from the foregut. Three endodermal buds from this diverticulum become the liver, ventral pancreas, and GB. Ultimately, the GB is located in the right upper quadrant (RUQ) of the abdomen under the anatomic division of the right and left lobes of the liver. Normally, it is a thin-walled, contractile, and pear-shaped organ measuring 5 to 10 cm and consists of the fundus, body, and neck, which narrows joining the cystic duct. Histologically, the GB wall consists of three layers: mucosa, muscularis, and serosa. The GB does not have submucosa. It contains approximately 50 mL of bile when distended and is mostly covered by the peritoneum, whereas the remainder is attached to the liver.

The right and left hepatic ducts join to form the common hepatic duct (CHD), which is connected to the cystic duct to form the common bile duct (CBD). The cystic duct is lined by the spiral valves of Heister, which provide some resistance to bile flow from the GB. In the hepatoduodenal ligament, the CBD lies to the right side of the patient, the proper hepatic artery to the left side, and the portal vein posterior to both of these. Anatomic variations of the hepatic artery are common and include the replaced right hepatic artery (from the superior mesenteric artery) and aberrant left hepatic artery (from the left gastric artery). The right hepatic artery gives off the cystic artery before traversing into the right hepatic lobe. The cystic artery

lies in the triangle of Calot, which is the anatomic area that is bound by the inferior margin of the liver superiorly, the CHD medially, and the cystic duct laterally. The CBD passes through the head of the pancreas, usually joins the pancreatic duct within 1 cm of the wall of the duodenum to form a common channel, and then empties into the second portion of the duodenum through the ampulla of Vater. Bile flow into the duodenum is regulated in part by the sphincter of Oddi, which encircles this common channel. The most common anatomic configuration of this region is shown in Figure 15-1, which demonstrates the usual relations of the important ductal and arterial structures.

GALLSTONE DISEASE

Epidemiology of Gallstones

The incidence of gallstones increases with age, and women are affected approximately 3 times more often than men. The prevalence of gallstone disease among White women who are younger than 50 years is 5% to 15%; in older women, it is approximately 25%. Among White men who are younger than 50 years, the prevalence is 4% to 10%; in older men, it is 10% to 15%. Gallstone disease also tends to cluster in families. Native Americans have an extremely high prevalence of gallstones; more than 50% of men and 80% of women have mixed stones by 60 years of age. Obesity (excessive cholesterol biosynthesis), multiparity (altered steroid metabolism, lithogenic bile, GB hypomotility), high-dose estrogen oral contraceptives, some cholesterol-lowering agents (alteration of cholesterol and bile acid biosynthesis), rapid weight loss (increased bile saturation index and GB stasis), and prolonged total parenteral nutrition (TPN) (hyperconcentration of bile and GB stasis) all predispose to the formation of stones. Patients who have had rapid weight loss following bariatric surgery may form gallstones. Diseases that diminish the bile acid pool, such as Crohn disease involving the terminal ileum or resection of the terminal ileum, increase the incidence of gallstones. Patients with hemolytic disorders and alcoholic cirrhosis tend to form pigment stones.

Patients may be able to prevent gallstone formation by avoiding obesity, following a high-fiber diet to diminish the enterohepatic circulation of dehydroxylated bile acids, eating meals at regular intervals to diminish GB storage time, and eating foods with low levels of saturated fatty acids to diminish the nucleation of lithogenic bile.

Pathogenesis of Gallstones (Cholelithiasis)

The most common type of gallstones in the Western population is mixed and contains a high proportion of cholesterol (see Figure 15-4) along with bile acids and lecithin.

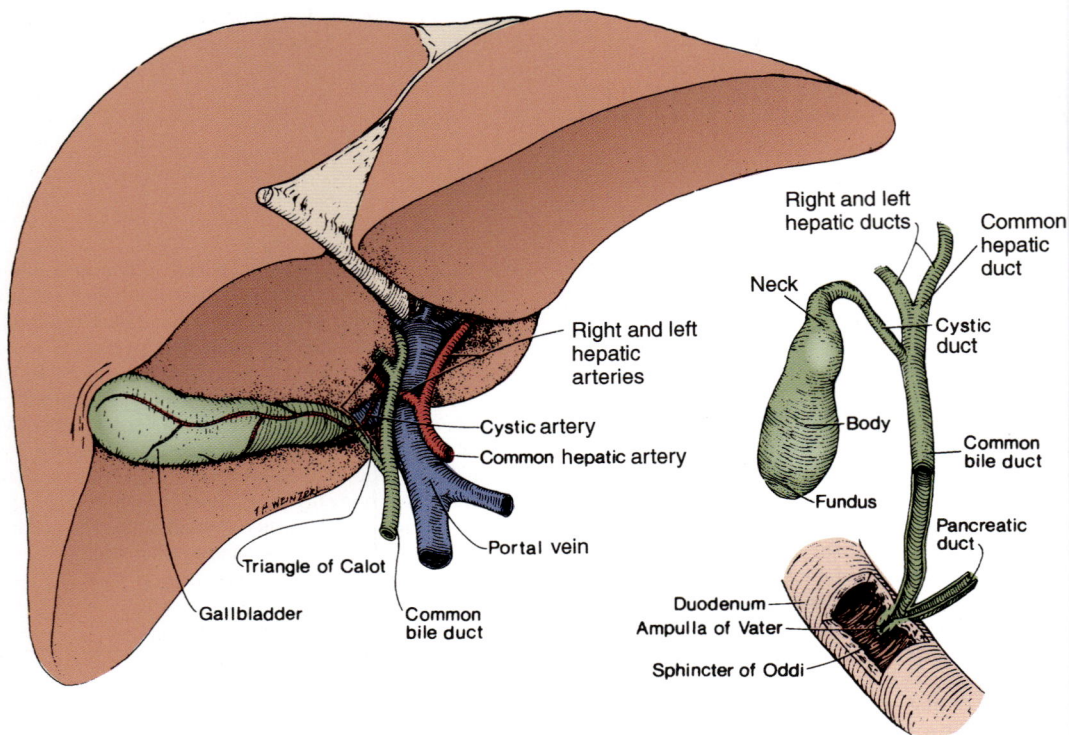

Figure 15-1. Anatomy of the gallbladder, porta hepatis, and extrahepatic bile ducts.

These stones account for approximately 75% to 80% of all types of gallstones. The relative concentrations of cholesterol, bile acids, and lecithin (phospholipids) must remain within a limited range to maintain the cholesterol in solution. A change in their relative concentrations favors the formation and precipitation of cholesterol crystals. Precipitation of cholesterol as crystals tends to occur if the bile is lithogenic (promoting the formation of calculi) and supersaturated with cholesterol. These crystals, in the presence of enucleating factors, may agglomerate to form gallstones and entrap other components of bile, including bilirubin, mucus, and calcium, in the process. Most mixed stones do not contain enough calcium to make them radiopaque. Occasionally, a single large stone forms and is composed almost entirely of cholesterol (cholesterol solitaire).

Incomplete emptying of the GB affords ideal conditions for agglomeration; for this reason, most stones form in the GB rather than in the other parts of the biliary tree. The source of most stones found in the biliary ducts (choledocholithiasis) is the GB. However, bile stasis and infection involving the bile ducts may predispose individuals to the formation of primary bile duct calculi within the ducts, although this is uncommon.

Pigment stones are of two types: black and brown. Black pigment stones account for approximately 20% of all biliary stones and are generally found in the GB. They typically form in sterile GB bile and are commonly associated with hemolytic diseases and cirrhosis. In chronic hemolysis, there is hypersecretion of bilirubin conjugates in the bile and greater secretion of monoglucuronides compared with diglucuronides, which favors the precipitation

of pigment stones. In contrast, brown stones are associated with infected bile. They are found primarily in the bile ducts and are soft. Pigment stones often contain enough calcium to render them radiopaque.

GB sludge is an amorphous material that contains mucoprotein, cholesterol crystals, and calcium bilirubinate. It is often associated with prolonged TPN, starvation, or rapid weight loss. GB sludge may be a precursor of gallstones.

Diagnostic Evaluation

History and Physical Examination

The identification of biliary tract disease requires a focused history and careful physical examination. Narrowing the differential diagnosis and determining the cause of the biliary tract disease can be accomplished by gathering valuable clues that point to either an acute or a chronic condition. If the patient is jaundiced, the history can suggest either obstructive, hemolytic, or hepatocellular disease and may also indicate an underlying malignancy. Specific physical findings may also yield useful information that can help with the evaluation.

The hallmark of gallstone disease is pain referred to as biliary colic. The pain is usually steady, fairly severe, and located in the RUQ or, less commonly, in the epigastrium of the abdomen, sometimes radiate to the back at the same level. The pain is visceral, often described as dull or aching, and may last from 1 to 4 hours. The pain is thought to be secondary to increased pressure in the GB that results from contraction against a stone that is impacted in the cystic duct. Typical biliary colic is caused by obstruction and is not associated with acute inflammation or infection. The pain tends to occur postprandially, possibly after a large or fatty meal, but it may have no relation to meals and awaken the patient at night. The patient may seek urgent evaluation in an emergency room to address the pain. Nausea and vomiting may accompany biliary colic. The pain is seldom relieved by anything but time and potent analgesics. The patient is most commonly well before the onset of pain and then again within minutes to a few hours after the pain subsides.

Acute cholecystitis is the acute inflammation and infection of the GB. These patients experience tenderness that is steady or increasing in nature and is localized to the RUQ of the abdomen or in the epigastrium. The pain lasts longer than 3 to 4 hours and may continue for several days. It is mediated by somatic sensory nerves because the parietal peritoneum is usually irritated. It may be accompanied by nausea, vomiting, and systemic manifestations of an inflammatory process including fever, tachycardia, and, in more severe cases, hemodynamic instability.

In patients with jaundice, the presence of light-colored stools and dark, tea-colored urine suggests extrahepatic biliary obstruction. Patients with malignancies (eg, carcinoma of the pancreas) generally have dull, vague, or insignificant upper abdominal pain. A history of significant weight loss is often present in patients with malignant conditions. Pruritus is believed to be caused by high tissue concentrations of reabsorbed conjugated bile acids and is often present in patients with obstructive jaundice.

On physical examination, a patient with biliary colic usually appears uncomfortable and restless, whereas a patient who has pain associated with inflammation and acute cholecystitis tends to be still because the pain is aggravated by movement. The pulse rate may be high secondary to pain, inflammation, or infection. Fever often accompanies acute cholecystitis but not biliary colic, and high fever may be present with gangrene of the GB or if the patient has cholangitis. Low blood pressure signifies severe dehydration or septic shock. The abdomen of patients with biliary colic is soft, but some tenderness may be found in the RUQ. Once the pain subsides, the abdomen is nontender between episodes of colic. In acute cholecystitis, examination of the abdomen may show a positive Murphy sign. A Murphy sign is the cessation of inspiration because of pain on deep palpation of the RUQ when the visceral peritoneum overlying the GB is inflamed. Once the inflammation spreads to the adjacent parietal peritoneum, abdominal examination shows localized guarding and may demonstrate rebound tenderness. A tender mass representing the inflamed GB may also be palpable in the RUQ of the abdomen in acute cholecystitis. The presence of a nontender, palpable GB with jaundice suggests underlying malignant disease, such as carcinoma of the pancreas, and is known as the *Courvoisier sign* (see Chapter 16). In the presence of a malignant obstruction of the CBD, the GB is passively distended as a result of back pressure and is palpable in the RUQ. If a stone is the cause of the distal ductal obstruction, the site of origin of the stone is generally a diseased thick-walled GB, which is incapable of passive distension.

Laboratory Tests

A number of laboratory tests aid in the diagnosis and management of biliary tract disease. Liver function tests are helpful in detecting hyperbilirubinemia and providing information about the underlying disease process. The serum level of unconjugated (indirect) bilirubin increases in hemolytic disorders, whereas the conjugated (direct) fraction is elevated with extrahepatic biliary obstruction or cholestasis. Alkaline phosphatase (ALP) is synthesized by the biliary tract epithelium. Serum ALP levels increase as a result of overproduction in conditions that cause extrahepatic biliary obstruction or, less commonly, from cholestasis resulting from a drug reaction or primary biliary cirrhosis. The serum level of this enzyme is moderately elevated in hepatitis, and it may also be elevated as a result of bone disease. The ALP of hepatobiliary origin may be differentiated from that originating from bone by confirming its heat stability. The concomitant elevation of γ-glutamyl transferase (GGT) also indicates that the source of the elevated ALP is the biliary tract. Aspartate aminotransferase (AST) and alanine aminotransferase (ALT) are released from hepatocytes, and serum levels of both enzymes are increased significantly in various types of hepatitis. AST and ALT are also often elevated with biliary obstruction, particularly when it is acute. As a rule, however, the increase in ALP and GGT is greater than the increase in the levels of AST and ALT in biliary obstruction. The converse suggests hepatitis. If the biliary ductal system is partially obstructed (eg, by a primary or metastatic neoplasm), ALP is released into the serum from the obstructed ducts, but the serum bilirubin may be normal. The international normalized ratio is often elevated (prothrombin time is often prolonged) in patients with obstructive jaundice as a result of the malabsorption of vitamin K. In obstructive jaundice, the water-soluble conjugated (direct) bilirubin is excreted in the urine. On the other hand, urobilinogen is produced in the intestine as a result of bacterial metabolism of bilirubin. Then it is reabsorbed from the intestine and secreted in the urine. Bile duct obstruction leads to the reduction of urobilinogen in the urine because the excretion of bilirubin into the intestine is blocked.

Hemoglobin or hematocrit may be elevated if the patient is dehydrated. Leukocytosis with a shift to the left suggests acute inflammation and infection. Serum amylase and lipase may be slightly elevated in both acute cholecystitis and acute cholangitis, but marked elevations suggest acute pancreatitis (AP).

Imaging Studies

Imaging studies are very helpful in establishing the definitive diagnosis in patients who have clinical features that suggest biliary disease. They are also useful in a variety of therapeutic interventions.

The initial study of choice for patients with biliary disease is ultrasonography. The study is noninvasive, quick, and relatively inexpensive and does not entail the use of radiation. Ultrasonography has replaced the oral cholecystogram for routine workup of patients with biliary colic. For stones in the GB, both the sensitivity and the specificity of this study are approximately 95%. Ultrasonography can successfully detect stones as small as 3 mm in diameter, and sometimes smaller stones and debris like GB sludge may be seen (Figure 15-2). Ultrasonography is highly sensitive for detecting dilatation of the bile ducts and may provide information on whether the site of biliary obstruction is intrahepatic or extrahepatic. The bile duct is generally considered dilated if it is larger than 7 mm. However, the ultrasound is less helpful for visualizing stones in the bile ducts because of the overlying structures like the

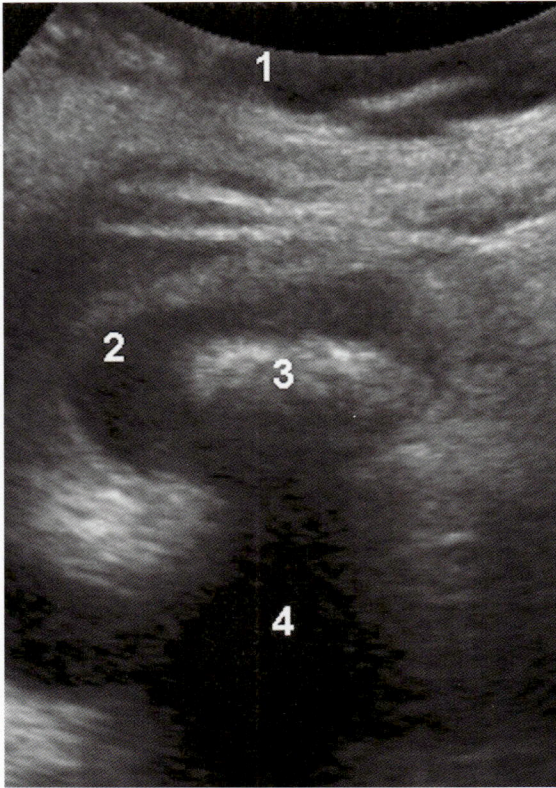

Figure 15-2. Ultrasound of the gallbladder showing gallstones. (1) Anterior abdominal wall. (2) Gallbladder. (3) Stones. (4) Acoustic shadow.

duodenum, which can contain air. If the GB is distended and the ducts are dilated, the site of obstruction is likely to be distal to the junction of the cystic duct and the CHD. The finding of a thickened GB wall or pericholecystic fluid supports the diagnosis of acute cholecystitis. Although ultrasonography provides additional information about the liver and pancreas, it remains an operator-dependent tests.

Rarely, gallstones are visible utilizing plain radiographs. Approximately 10% to 15% of gallstones contain sufficient calcium to render them radiopaque. Other findings on a plain x-ray include air in the biliary tree that is present as a result of communication between the biliary and gastrointestinal (GI) tracts secondary to a pathologic fistula or a connection created by a previous procedure. Also, air in the lumen or wall of the GB may be seen in acute emphysematous cholecystitis.

Computed tomography (CT) is not the preferred test for the diagnosis of cholelithiasis because of the lower sensitivity in detecting gallstones, the higher cost compared with ultrasonography, and the risks of radiation. A CT scan may be useful to assess patients with severe acute biliary disease, to rule out other causes of biliary obstruction or to identify an alternate diagnosis. Recently, the advent of CT cholangiography has been shown to reliably display anatomic detail of the biliary tree. For some patients, CT scan can be used to guide percutaneous needle aspiration for Gram stain, cytology, or core needle biopsy for histology to establish a definitive diagnosis.

Magnetic resonance cholangiography (MRC) refers to selected MR imaging of the biliary and pancreatic ducts, which is helpful in demonstrating common duct stones and other biliary tract abnormalities. It is commonly utilized as a first test now before percutaneous transhepatic cholangiogram (PTC) or an endoscopic retrograde cholangiopancreatogram (ERCP). An MRC may be all that is needed, but it usually provides preliminary data before a more invasive imaging test. The obvious advantages of this diagnostic procedure are that it is noninvasive and it does not involve the use of radiation.

Radionuclide biliary scanning (hepatobiliary iminodiacetic acid [HIDA] scan) involves the intravenous injection of a technetium-99m-labeled derivative of iminodiacetic acid. The radionuclide is excreted by the liver into the bile in high concentrations. Then it enters the GB (if the cystic duct is patent) and duodenum. The normal GB begins to fill within 30 minutes. Visualization of the CBD and duodenum without filling of the GB after 4 hours indicates cystic duct obstruction, which supports the diagnosis of acute cholecystitis. The sensitivity and specificity of the HIDA scan for diagnosing acute cholecystitis are 95% to 97% and 90% to 97%, respectively. False-positive results may occur in patients who are receiving TPN or those who have hepatitis. The scan is also of value in identifying a suspected bile leak after surgery, but it is rarely used for this now. The HIDA scan is not useful for showing stones in either the GB or the CBD. The sensitivity of a HIDA scan is reduced in patients with high bilirubin (>4.4 mg/dL).

In patients with obstructive jaundice with evidence of extrahepatic obstruction on ultrasonography, detailed radiographic visualization of the biliary ductal anatomy may be helpful in confirming the diagnosis and planning therapy. Direct injection of contrast agents into the ducts is necessary in these cases. This may be achieved by performing a PTC or ERCP. PTC involves inserting a thin needle through the skin and body wall, into the liver parenchyma, and injecting a contrast medium directly into the intrahepatic bile ducts. Dilated bile ducts facilitate this procedure, yielding a success rate of more than 95%. If the ducts are of normal caliber, the test is successful only 70% to 80% of the time. PTC is particularly valuable for visualizing the proximal ductal system. It can also be used to obtain a cytologic diagnosis, extract stones, and aid in the placement of a biliary drainage catheter into the obstructed bile ducts. ERCP requires a skilled endoscopist, who cannulates the sphincter of Oddi and injects contrast medium to obtain a picture of the biliary and pancreatic ductal anatomy. In addition, ERCP can be used to perform a sphincterotomy, which involves cutting the sphincter of Oddi with an electrosurgical current through a wire attached to the ERCP catheter. This facilitates the extraction of biliary calculi and placement of a stent through an area of bile duct obstruction. If coagulopathy is present, it must be corrected before either PTC or ERCP.

Figure 15-3 shows an algorithm for the evaluation of a patient with jaundice.

Clinical Presentation and Treatment of Gallstone Disease

Asymptomatic Gallstones

The majority of patients with gallstones remain asymptomatic. Of these individuals, approximately 1% to 2% per year

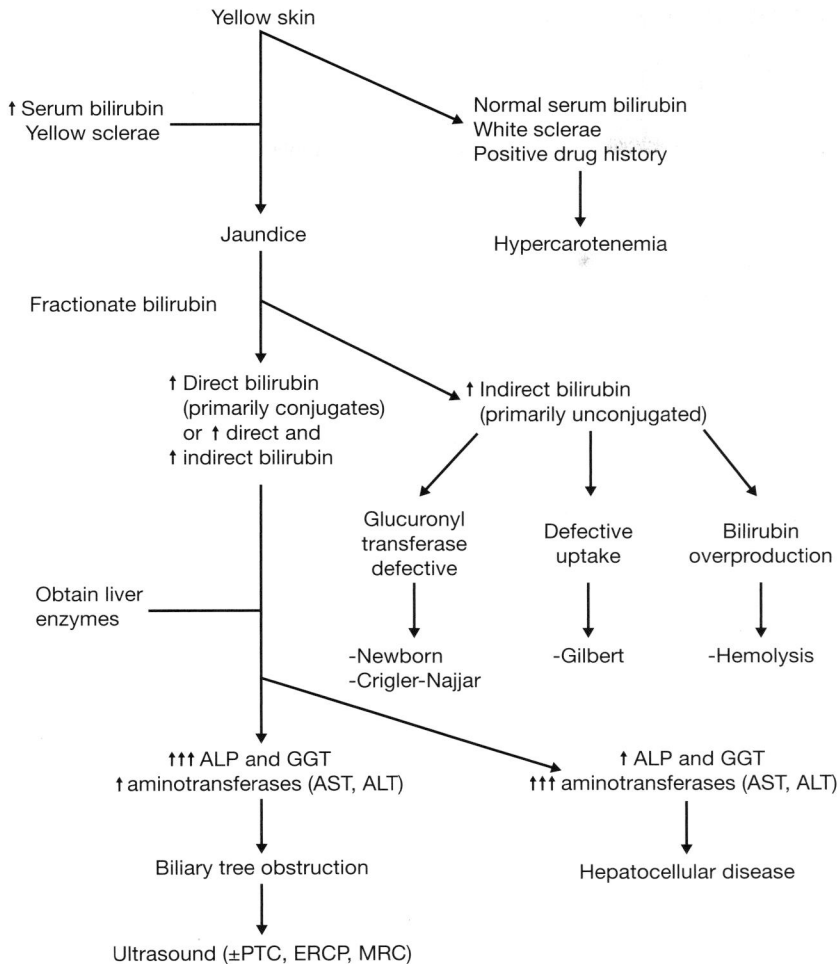

Figure 15-3. Algorithm for the evaluation of a patient with jaundice. ALP, alkaline phosphatase; ALT, alanine aminotransferase; AST, aspartate aminotransferase; ERCP, endoscopic retrograde cholangiopancreatogram; GGT, γ-glutamyl transferase; MRC, magnetic resonance cholangiography; PTC, percutaneous transhepatic cholangiogram.

will develop symptoms or complications of gallstone disease. Thus, two-thirds of individuals remain free of symptoms or complications after 20 years. Although complications secondary to gallstones may occur at any time, most patients experience symptoms for some time before a complication develops. Thus, in adults, prophylactic cholecystectomy is not indicated for asymptomatic gallstones. However, after patients have symptoms of biliary colic, they are at an increased risk for complications and should consider elective cholecystectomy. The risk of GB carcinoma in patients with gallstones is too low to justify cholecystectomy for asymptomatic gallstones. Porcelain GB and large gallstones may be associated with a higher risk of GB carcinoma, but recent studies suggest this is lower than previously thought.

Acute Cholecystitis

Acute cholecystitis can occur in the presence of gallstones (calculous cholecystitis) or without gallstones (acalculous cholecystitis). In the cases with gallstones, sustained obstruction of the cystic duct leads to bile stasis in the GB with subsequent inflammation and infection. The inflammation extends beyond the visceral peritoneum overlying the GB to involve the parietal peritoneum. Left untreated, complications of empyema (Figure 15-4) (pus in the GB), gangrene, or perforation of the GB may result from progression of the disease process. Clinically, acute cholecystitis is characterized by RUQ abdominal pain, which is constant, and may radiate to the back, shoulder, or scapula. The pain is associated with nausea, fever, and leukocytosis secondary to inflammation of the GB. Most patients with acute cholecystitis have a history of biliary colic, dyspepsia, or fatty food intolerance. On physical examination, the patient has tenderness in the RUQ and a positive Murphy sign. Once inflammation progresses to involve the parietal peritoneum, the patient has rebound tenderness and guarding. A tender mass is palpable in the RUQ in approximately 20% of cases. Rarely, generalized peritonitis with rebound tenderness may be present if the disease has progressed to free perforation.

The differential diagnosis is long but should include acute hepatitis, AP, perforated peptic ulcer, and acute

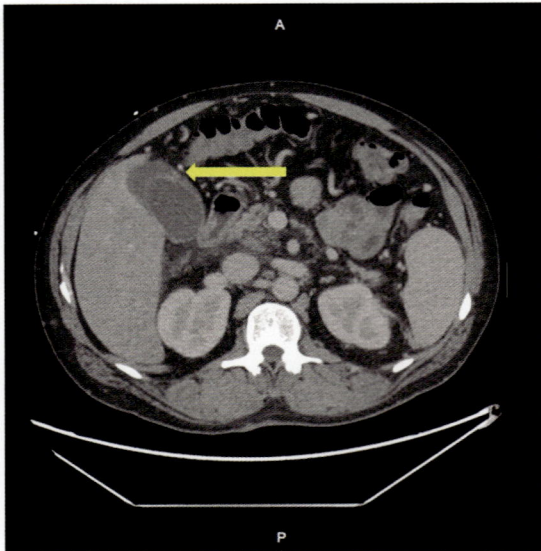

Figure 15-4. Computed tomography scan of a patient with acute cholecystitis. The gallbladder has a thick wall, small perforation with pericholecystic fluid (yellow arrow).

appendicitis along with extraabdominal conditions like myocardial infarction or pneumonia. A careful history, physical examination, and diagnostic evaluation will lead to an accurate diagnosis in most patients. Laboratory studies demonstrate a leukocytosis and a left shift. Mild increases in AST, ALT, and ALP are common. Patients may have a mild hyperbilirubinemia (mostly direct), but a significant elevation in the serum bilirubin suggests a CBD stone. On occasion, the patient will demonstrate a slight elevation of the serum amylase.

Ultrasonography is very helpful in making a definitive diagnosis. In addition to detecting gallstones with a high degree of accuracy, the study often shows specific characteristic findings of acute cholecystitis, such as a distended GB, thickened GB wall (>3-4 mm), pericholecystic fluid collection, and ultrasonographic Murphy sign. This sign is elicited by demonstrating the presence of the tenderest spot directly over the sonographically localized GB with the ultrasound probe. This sign is present in 98% of patients with acute cholecystitis. Ultrasonography can also provide additional information about the liver, intrahepatic bile ducts, CBD, and pancreas.

If there is any suspicion of an intestinal perforation, that is, peptic ulcer perforation, plain radiographs of the chest and abdomen should be obtained. Upright views are necessary to exclude pneumoperitoneum from another underlying cause of the acute abdomen. Plain x-rays may also show gallstones if they are radiopaque. However, finding stones alone does not establish the diagnosis of acute cholecystitis. Sometimes the patient will undergo evaluation for abdominal complaints by CT scan in equivocal cases. The CT can show GB wall thickening and pericholecystic stranding (Figure 15-4), but this imaging test can sometimes miss subtle inflammation of the GB and may miss small stones.

While the HIDA scan is considered the gold standard for diagnosing acute cholecystitis when the ultrasound results are inconclusive, it is rarely utilized to establish the diagnosis. Occasionally, a HIDA scan is used in the case of acalculous cholecystitis or when the diagnosis is uncertain. Nonvisualization of the GB after 4 hours of the study indicates cystic duct obstruction and is interpreted as positive for acute cholecystitis. However, certain patients (eg, individuals receiving TPN, those who have fasted for a long time or who are on narcotics such as morphine, which may cause spasms of the sphincter of Oddi) may demonstrate nonvisualization of the GB on HIDA scan, yielding a false-positive result.

The management of acute cholecystitis depends on the severity at presentation and entails the administration of antibiotics combined with either surgery or drainage of the GB, followed by interval cholecystectomy. However, generally, the initial management of acute cholecystitis includes nil per os status (nothing by mouth), administering intravenous fluids and starting antibiotic therapy. The bacteria commonly associated with acute cholecystitis are *Escherichia coli*, *Klebsiella pneumoniae*, and *Streptococcus faecalis*. In most cases antibiotics targeting gram-negative aerobes and enterococci are sufficient. Parenteral analgesics may be administered judiciously after the diagnosis is confirmed and further plans for therapy are made. A nasogastric tube is rarely required but is recommended when vomiting occurs.

Most patients are best served by early cholecystectomy within a few days of presentation. Once the patient has benefited from some hydration and antibiotic treatment, surgery is indicated. This approach prevents the potential complications of gangrene, perforation, and sepsis, and makes the surgical procedure easier than if it were performed later in the course of the disease, when the inflammatory reaction is more severe. However, the procedure should be delayed if major medical problems must be addressed and performed earlier if perforation or abscess is suspected. MIC and selective open cholecystectomy are indicated for acute cholecystitis. The most common reason for conversion is bleeding and severe inflammation, when poor definition of the anatomy leads to technical difficulty. A subtotal cholecystectomy can be performed when there is increased risk of bile duct injury (BDI). As with all urgent or emergent operations, surgery for acute cholecystitis is associated with slightly higher mortality and morbidity rates compared with those for elective cholecystectomy, often as a result of underlying cardiovascular, pulmonary, or metabolic disease.

Patients with acute cholecystitis who are too ill to undergo cholecystectomy may require cholecystostomy. This procedure involves the percutaneous placement of a tube under ultrasound guidance through the liver into the GB. This allows for the decompression of the GB by draining the contents of the GB. It is an effective approach for patients who are poor candidates for surgical management and should not be used as a bridge to cholecystectomy for patients who are otherwise good surgical candidates.

Acute gangrenous cholecystitis is associated with a morbidity rate of 15% to 25% and a mortality rate of 20% to 25%. Patients with this condition tend to be older and generally have more serious comorbid conditions than patients with simple acute cholecystitis. Often, these patients will present with a more serious systemic illness with higher leukocytosis. Treatment includes stabilization of the medical condition, administration of broad-spectrum antibiotics, and performance of emergency cholecystectomy. **Acute emphysematous cholecystitis** results from gas-forming bacteria and is associated with a higher risk of gangrene and perforation compared with nonemphysematous cholecystitis. It generally affects older individuals, and diabetes mellitus is present in 20% to 50% of these patients. The classic findings on plain radiographs include air within the wall or lumen of the GB, an air-fluid level within the lumen of the GB, or air in the pericholecystic tissues. Air in the bile ducts may also be seen. Patients with acute emphysematous cholecystitis should receive fluid resuscitation, broad-spectrum antibiotics with coverage for anaerobes, and undergo emergency cholecystectomy. If left untreated, this condition can result in death.

Acute acalculous cholecystitis may complicate the course of a patient who is being treated for other conditions in a medical or surgical intensive care unit. Many patients receive TPN and mechanical ventilatory support and are immunosuppressed. Establishing the diagnosis of acute acalculous cholecystitis can present significant difficulty. The clinical features resemble those of acute calculous cholecystitis; however, the patient often cannot give a coherent history, and the associated conditions result in complex physical findings that are less revealing and more difficult to interpret. Ultrasonography or CT scan can be helpful in establishing the diagnosis. Ultrasonography may show GB distension, a thickened GB wall, pericholecystic fluid, and a sonographic Murphy sign if the patient is responsive. A HIDA scan may help establish the diagnosis, but it often yields a false-positive result and is associated with a specificity of only 38% in such cases. After the diagnosis is established, the management is similar to that of patients with acute calculous cholecystitis.

Chronic Cholecystitis

Chronic cholecystitis is the most common form of symptomatic cholelithiasis. It results from repeated minor episodes of cystic duct obstruction with subsequent inflammation and fibrosis of the GB wall. Hydrops of the GB, which occurs when the cystic duct is chronically obstructed by a stone and the GB fills with mucinous or watery fluid, can also result in chronic cholecystitis. Clinically, biliary colic is the most common symptom associated with chronic calculous cholecystitis. The pain is colicky and located in the RUQ and epigastric area. The pain comes in mild to moderate or even severe attacks, usually within hours of eating, and lasts 30 minutes to several hours. Nausea and vomiting may accompany the pain. Because the condition is not associated with acute infection, fever and chills are absent. Other associated symptoms include intolerance to fatty foods, flatulence, belching, and indigestion. These symptoms are encompassed by the collective term "dyspepsia." However, the symptoms of dyspepsia are nonspecific and may be secondary to other diseases. Physical examination may demonstrate mild RUQ tenderness, especially during the attacks, but there may be no overt signs of peritoneal irritation. Between episodes of biliary colic, the abdomen shows no specific abnormality. Jaundice is not caused by cystic duct obstruction, and if present, other causes, such as CBD stone, should be excluded. The differential diagnosis includes peptic ulcer disease, gastroesophageal reflux, ureteral obstruction, irritable bowel syndrome, and angina pectoris, among others.

Laboratory tests including the total and differential leukocyte counts and liver function tests may be entirely normal. Typically, biliary colic is distinguished from acute cholecystitis by the presence of the characteristic clinical features described previously and by the absence of leukocytosis. Ultrasonography is the initial test of choice and can confirm the presence of gallstones in more than 95% of cases.

Initial management of biliary colic includes pain control and observation. Elective MIC is the standard of care in patients with symptomatic cholelithiasis. Previous history of multiple abdominal surgeries is not an absolute contraindication to MIC. However, open cholecystectomy remains an option. In selected patients, intraoperative cholangiogram (IOC) is performed to evaluate the biliary ducts for stones and to delineate anatomy. When stones are identified in the CBD, the duct should be explored at the time of surgery, or postoperatively via ERCP and sphincterotomy to extract the stones.

Nonoperative management of symptomatic gallstones is rarely used because of the safety, efficacy, and availability of MIC. Dissolution therapy is an option in 15% of patients with cholelithiasis who are poor operative candidates and in those who refuse surgery. Unfortunately, this approach is not effective. Options include dissolution with or without extracorporeal shock wave lithotripsy (ESWL). Ursodeoxycholic acid is the most commonly administered agent. It reduces the cholesterol saturation of bile by inhibiting cholesterol secretion. The resulting undersaturated bile dissolves the solid cholesterol in the gallstones. It is taken for at least 6 months and is more likely for a year. This therapy yields a dissolution rate of 90% for stones smaller than 5 mm and 60% for calculi smaller than 10 mm. However, there is a 50% recurrence of gallstones within 5 years of discontinuing the therapy. ESWL has been used in the past to manage gallstone disease in selected patients, but support for this procedure has waned because these patients are at an increased risk for postprocedural pancreatitis and may form new stones following the procedure.

Choledocholithiasis and Acute Cholangitis

CBD stones or choledocholithiasis can be either primary or secondary. Primary stones are very rare and develop de novo within the CBD (5%). Secondary stones (95%) are the most common and originate from the GB (usually cholesterol stones) and pass through the cystic duct to enter the CBD. Although the smaller stones that enter the CBD can progress further into the duodenum, choledocholithiasis may lead to biliary colic, obstruction, cholangitis, or pancreatitis.

Presentation of choledocholithiasis varies from asymptomatic (50% of cases) to biliary colic, obstructive jaundice, ascending cholangitis, and septic shock to pancreatitis. Patients may present with biliary colic as described earlier. The jaundice along with light-colored stools and dark, tea-colored urine associated with choledocholithiasis may fluctuate in intensity compared with the progressive jaundice caused by malignant disease. In the presence of concomitant infection, usually with *E. coli* or *K. pneumoniae*, acute cholangitis develops. It is characterized by jaundice, RUQ abdominal pain, and fever associated with chills (Charcot triad). A patient with severe acute suppurative cholangitis may develop septic shock. In this condition, the patient may be hypotensive and demonstrate mental confusion in addition to the Charcot triad. These five features together constitute Reynold pentad. Acute cholecystitis is differentiated from acute cholangitis by the lack of biliary obstruction and jaundice. Abdominal examination may be unremarkable in a patient with choledocholithiasis or may reveal tenderness in the RUQ if cholangitis is present. Rebound tenderness is not usually found, even in the presence of acute cholangitis. Other than choledocholithiasis, obstructive jaundice or cholangitis can be caused by periampullary malignancy and stricture, most commonly iatrogenic after cholecystectomy or secondary to chronic pancreatitis. Mirizzi syndrome, a condition in which a large stone in the GB compresses the CHD, can also lead to obstructive jaundice.

The diagnostic evaluation of jaundice associated with probable choledocholithiasis starts with laboratory studies described previously. In patients with cholangitis, the leukocyte count is usually elevated. Bile duct obstruction, partial or total, leads to elevation in total bilirubin, with a predominance of the direct fraction, marked elevation of serum ALP and GGT, and mild elevations of AST and ALT. Serum amylase and lipase may be elevated in cases of pancreatic duct obstruction. Ultrasonography is the best initial imaging study in patients with choledocholithiasis and cholangitis. It often shows dilated intrahepatic and extrahepatic ducts along with the presence of GB stones, suggesting that stones are the likely cause of the common duct obstruction. As stated previously, stones in the CBD are frequently missed on ultrasonography. Magnetic resonance cholangiopancreatography (MRCP), ERCP, or PTC are the best studies to define the specific site and determine the source of the bile duct obstruction. The advantage of ERCP is that not only can the diagnosis be established, but the stones can also be extracted. Figure 15-5 shows an MRCP with a stone in the distal CBD.

The management of **choledocholithiasis** depends on available experience and the clinical situation. A patient with choledocholithiasis without evidence of cholangitis should undergo MIC and IOC, possibly followed by laparoscopic or robotic CBD exploration if stones are seen. If the bile duct cannot be cleared of stones by laparoscopic exploration, open bile duct exploration or postoperative ERCP and sphincterotomy may be required. **Acute suppurative cholangitis** is a potential life-threatening condition and requires *urgent intervention*. Initial management includes resuscitation with intravenous fluids and antibiotics.

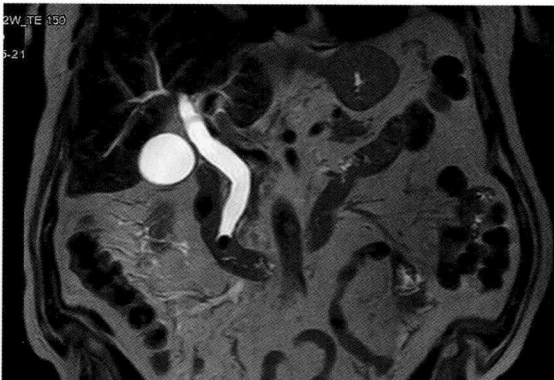

Figure 15-5. Magnetic resonance cholangiopancreatogram illustrating the common bile duct with a stone impacted distally.

The patient should be monitored closely in an intensive care unit. Blood cultures are obtained, and broad-spectrum antibiotics targeting gram-negative rods should be initiated. Any coagulation abnormalities should be corrected by giving parenteral vitamin K or administering fresh frozen plasma (FFP) before an invasive procedure. More than 70% of patients with cholangitis respond to this treatment algorithm, especially if the CBD stone passes to the duodenum. When the patient has recovered from the acute episode, a cholecystectomy should be performed. Patients who do not respond to the initial therapy should have an urgent biliary decompression through ERCP, percutaneous transhepatic tube placement, or surgery.

The success rate with ERCP and sphincterotomy in removing stones from the CBD is greater than 90%, with a complication rate of approximately 5% to 10% (eg, pancreatitis, duodenal perforation, and bleeding). Endoscopic intraluminal lithotripsy can be used to break up large stones. The fragments can then pass spontaneously or be removed with ERCP and sphincterotomy. If the stones cannot be removed by these methods, a CBD exploration is warranted.

Acute Biliary (Gallstone) Pancreatitis

AP is commonly caused by gallstones (40% of cases, more in women) and alcohol (40%, more in men). When caused by gallstones, it is called *gallstone* or *biliary pancreatitis*. This occurs because of transient or persistent obstruction of the pancreatitis duct, usually at the ampulla of Vater, by a large stone or the passage of small stones and biliary sludge. Patients with AP present with acute upper abdominal pain, often radiating to the back with tenderness usually in the upper abdomen. Severe cases may present with peritoneal signs, simulating other causes of an acute abdomen. Nausea, vomiting, and a low-grade fever are frequent, as are tachycardia and hypotension secondary to hypovolemia. Severity of AP can be predicted on the basis of clinical, laboratory, and radiologic risk factors. Some of these can be performed on admission to assist in a triage of patients (eg, Ranson criteria), whereas others can be obtained only after the first 48 to 72 hours or later. Regardless of the cause or the severity of the disease, the cornerstones of treating AP are aggressive fluid resuscitation, correction of electrolyte derangement, pain control, supportive care, and early nutrition. Once the acute episode of pancreatitis has resolved, the GB should be removed as expeditiously as possible to avoid recurrent pancreatitis from gallstones. If the pancreatitis is mild to moderate in severity, an MIC can be performed safely, often within the first 48 to 72 hours of admission. By this time, the abdominal pain has largely resolved and the serum amylase level is returning to normal. Without a same-admission cholecystectomy, as many as 60% of patients will experience recurrent gallstone pancreatitis within 6 months. A longer delay may be justified in patients who have had severe pancreatitis and in whom local inflammation or systemic illness contraindicates surgery. In these cases, ERCP with endoscopic sphincterotomy may reduce the incidence of recurrent pancreatitis to a range of 2% to 5% over 2 years. An IOC should be performed at the time of the cholecystectomy to confirm that the bile duct is free of stones.

Antibiotics are added for severe pancreatitis and for the management of septic complications. If acute cholecystitis is present, an interval cholecystostomy (6-8 weeks) may be required. Emergent endoscopic sphincterotomy with stone extraction may be lifesaving in some patients with severe biliary pancreatitis. It should be used when a patient with pancreatitis is known to have gallstones, when a high suspicion of choledocholithiasis is present, and when the clinical course does not improve within 24 to 36 hours with normal resuscitative efforts.

Severe AP can occur in up to 15% of patients with gallstone pancreatitis. This condition can result in necrosis of the pancreas along with organ failure or death. Management of this condition is multidisciplinary and may include care in the intensive care unit. In this case, a cholecystectomy is delayed sometimes often when the complications have been fully addressed and the patient has recovered.

Gallstone Ileus

Gallstone ileus (mechanical bowel obstruction caused by a gallstone) accounts for less than 1% of all cases of intestinal obstruction. It is an uncommon complication that results from a gallstone eroding through the wall of the GB into the adjacent bowel (usually duodenum), creating a cholecystoenteric fistula. The stone migrates until it lodges in the narrowest portion of the small bowel, just proximal to the ileocecal valve.

It occurs more commonly in women than in men (3.5:1 ratio). A history of biliary colic or gallstone disease is common. Patients present with the clinical picture (symptoms and signs) of small intestinal obstruction including nausea, vomiting, abdominal pain, and distension. Occasionally, the intermittent nature of the obstruction in the early stages (before impaction of the stone) often results in delay in the diagnosis.

Plain radiographs of the abdomen show findings of small intestinal obstruction and may show air in the biliary tree. Occasionally, a large stone has sufficient calcium to be seen in the intestine. Ultrasonography is useful in documenting gallstones. CT with oral contrast is the preferred diagnostic test, because it can demonstrate air in the biliary tree, a biliary-enteric fistula, the site of obstruction, and the obstructing stone. The CT scan in Figure 15-6 shows images of a patient with gallstone ileus and the intraoperative findings.

Gallstone ileus is managed initially as a small bowel obstruction, and this includes the placement of a nasogastric tube for gastric decompression and intravenous

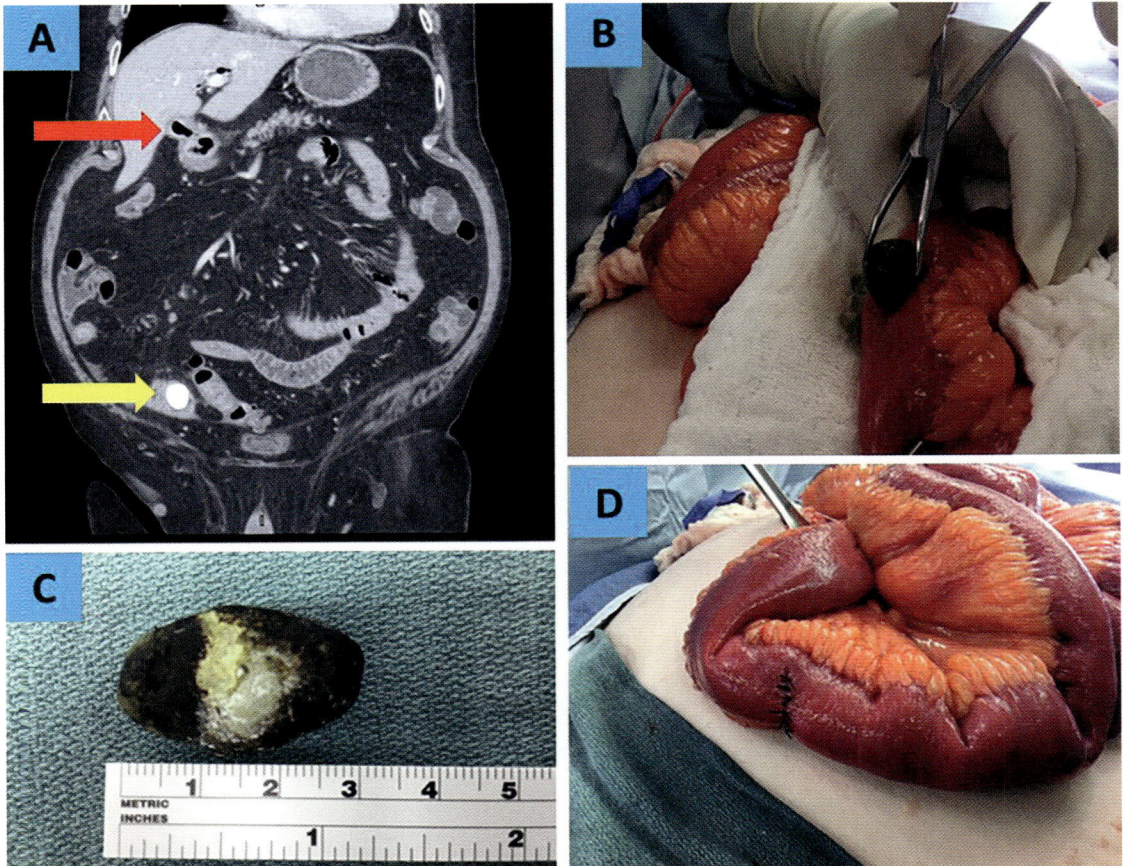

Figure 15-6. Gallstone ileus. A. This computed tomography scan shows air in the gallbladder and biliary tree (red arrow), and stone in the distal small bowel (yellow arrow), with proximal bowel distension, distal bowel collapse. B. Enterotomy (longitudinal) with stone extraction from distal small bowel. C. Extracted stone. D. Repaired enterotomy (transverse).

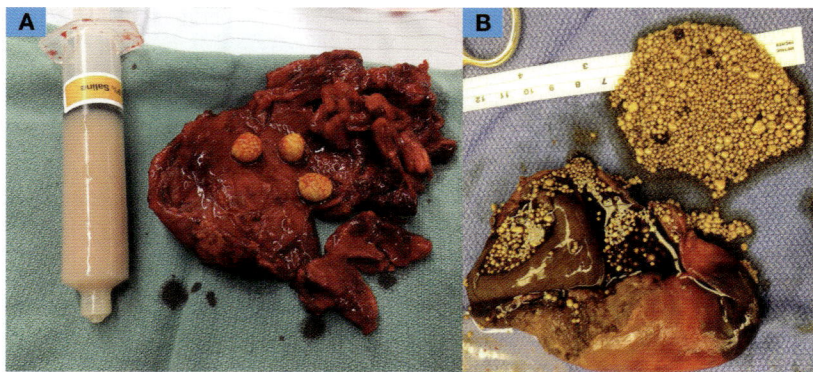

Figure 15-7. Intraoperative findings. A. Empyema of gallbladder. B. Gallstones (cholesterol stones).

hydration, and correction of electrolyte derangement. This should be followed by exploratory laparotomy (or laparoscopy) and removal of the obstructing gallstone by milking it back to an enterotomy made in the healthy intestine (Figure 15-7). The entire bowel should be searched diligently for other stones. Many of these patients are older and may not tolerate prolonged operations, but in a few select patients who are otherwise healthy, cholecystectomy and definitive correction of the internal fistula may be performed.

Table 15-1 summarizes the common clinical syndromes and complications that can result from cholelithiasis.

TABLE 15-1. Summary of the Common Clinical Syndromes That Result From Cholelithiasis and the Complications of Cholelithiasis

Syndrome	Etiology	Findings
Biliary colic	Transient cystic duct obstruction	Episodes of upper abdominal pain Nonspecific physical findings Ultrasound: cholelithiasis
Acute cholecystitis	Sustained cystic duct obstruction Acute inflammation of gallbladder	Constant, severe RUQ pain Elevated temperature Murphy sign Rebound tenderness Leukocytosis Mild elevation of liver function tests—ultrasound: cholelithiasis, with or without other signs of gallbladder inflammation HIDA scan: nonvisualization of gallbladder
Choledocholi-thiasis	Stone in the CBD	History of abdominal pain, jaundice, light stool, dark urine Laboratory findings: obstructive jaundice picture Ultrasound: cholelithiasis with dilated ducts CT, MRC, PTC, ERCP—ductal stones
Acute cholangitis	Infected bile; septicemia	History same as choledocholithiasis but acutely ill patient with abdominal pain, jaundice, fever, chills; may also have hypotension and change in mentation (in acute suppurative cholangitis) Stone impacted in the CBD Stricture of the CBD (previous biliary surgery) Tumor obstructing the CBD (especially after an invasive diagnostic procedure that might have seeded the bile with bacteria) Laboratory findings: same as choledocholithiasis, plus elevated white blood cell count Ultrasound: same as choledocholithiasis, but gallbladder may have been removed previously if the etiology is a stricture.
Biliary pancreatitis	Acute pancreatitis	Acutely ill, severe constant epigastric pain, with or without radiation through to the back Passage of small stones or sludge through the sphincter of Oddi Tenderness, guarding in upper abdomen markedly elevated serum amylase/lipase Ultrasound, CT scan, MRC cholelithiasis, with or without inflammatory mass in pancreas

TABLE 15-1. Summary of the Common Clinical Syndromes That Result From Cholelithiasis and the Complications of Cholelithiasis (*continued*)

Syndrome	Etiology	Findings
Gallstone ileus	Cholecystoenteric fistula Very large gallstone(s) Stone obstructing intestine (usually distal ileum)	Older debilitated patient Incomplete bowel obstruction Radiograph shows bowel obstruction (usually distal small bowel). May show air in biliary tree and may see large stone obstructing small intestine Ultrasound: ±stone in gallbladder and air in biliary tree CT: all of the above
Mirizzi syndrome	Obstruction of common hepatic duct caused by extrinsic compression from an impacted stone in the cystic duct or infundibulum of the gallbladder	Older populations Obstructive jaundice picture Ultrasound: dilated intrahepatic ducts, normal CBD Magnetic resonance cholangiopancreatography (MRCP) Endoscopic retrograde cholangiopancreatogram (ERCP) should be performed by a gastroenterologist. Percutaneous transhepatic cholangiogram (PTC)

CBD, common bile duct; CT, computed tomography; HIDA, hepatobiliary iminodiacetic acid, a radionuclide biliary scan; MRC, magnetic resonance cholangiography; RUQ, right upper quadrant.

GALLBLADDER CANCER

GB cancer is the most common cancer of the biliary tract and the fifth most common cancer of the GI tract. The incidence peaks at in the sixth and the seventh decade of life, with a 3:1 female-to-male ratio. There are a number of risk factors for GB cancer. Gallstones are the most common risk factor (especially with stones >3 cm). Up to 75% of patients with GB cancer have cholelithiasis. Patients with GB polyps 1.5 cm or larger in diameter have a 46% to 70% risk of cancer. An anomalous junction of the pancreaticobiliary duct has been noted in approximately 10% of patients with GB cancer. Another risk factor for GB cancer is a porcelain GB, which is characterized by calcification of the GB wall, but the contribution of this to the formation of cancer may be overestimated. Prophylactic cholecystectomy may be recommended for any finding of GB wall calcification on imaging studies. Other risk factors include primary sclerosing cholangitis (PSC), GB infection with *E. coli* and/or *Salmonella* species, and exposure to certain industrial solvents and toxins.

Thirty percent of these tumors are diagnosed incidentally during cholecystectomy, and cancer is found in 0.3% to 1% of all cholecystectomy specimens. Symptoms of early-stage disease are often directly caused by gallstones rather than the cancer. The most common presenting symptom is RUQ pain similar to previous episodes of biliary colic but more persistent. Patients with more advanced cancer have vague RUQ pain, weight loss, and malaise. Jaundice is present in approximately 50% of such patients because these cancers tend to spread early through direct extension into the liver and adjacent structures in the porta hepatis causing biliary obstruction and by metastasizing to the regional lymph nodes.

Physical examination may show a mass in the RUQ of the abdomen, which may not be recognized as a neoplasm if the patient has acute cholecystitis.

Laboratory tests generally are not helpful except to identify signs of advanced disease, such as anemia, hypoalbuminemia, leukocytosis, and elevated alkaline phosphate or bilirubin levels. Carcinoembryonic antigen (CEA) and carbohydrate antigen 19-9 (CA 19-9) may be elevated.

Ultrasound findings of GB cancer include thickening or irregularity of the GB, heterogeneous mass in the GB lumen, and asymmetrically thickened GB wall, a polypoid mass, or diffuse wall calcification indicative of porcelain GB. CT scan and MRCP accurately identify the extent of disease and are important imaging modalities to evaluate for metastatic disease. The correct diagnosis is made preoperatively in only 10% of cases. Early and mucosal adenocarcinoma confined to the GB wall is often identified after routine MIC. Because the overall 5-year survival rate is as high as 80%, cholecystectomy alone with negative resection margins (including the cystic duct margin) is adequate therapy. Patients with a preoperative suspicion of GB cancer should undergo open cholecystectomy. Larger tumors abutting or growing into the liver parenchyma are treated with a liver wedge resection of the GB fossa and a regional lymphadenectomy. Advanced tumors may require a formal liver resection. Porta hepatis lymphadenectomy lacks the standardization associated with other abdominal lymphadenectomies because of the proximity of vital structures and the organ's lack of a mobile mesentery. Moreover, despite radical approaches, the 5-year survival rate remains poor (<5% at 5 years) unless the cancer is detected incidentally as a small focus within a GB removed for symptomatic stone disease.

BILE DUCT MALIGNANCIES

Cancer of the bile ducts, called *cholangiocarcinoma*, accounts for approximately 3% of all GI malignancies. Anatomically, cholangiocarcinomas are classified as intrahepatic (arising proximal to the bifurcation of the left and right hepatic ducts) and extrahepatic. Extrahepatic cholangiocarcinoma is further divided into perihilar (including the confluence of the left and right hepatic ducts to the insertion of the cystic duct into the CBD) and distal segments (from the insertion of the cystic duct into the common duct to the ampulla of Vater). Extrahepatic cholangiocarcinoma is by far the most common, with 50% of cases having perihilar disease and 40% of cases having distal segment disease. Intrahepatic cholangiocarcinoma represents only about 10% of all bile duct malignancies.

Bile duct cancer occurs with equal frequency in both sexes, usually affecting individuals between 50 and 70 years of age. As with GB cancer, chronic inflammatory processes often precede the development of overt malignancy. The risk of bile duct malignancy is significantly higher in patients with PSC (which is strongly associated with ulcerative colitis). Other risk factors include choledochal cysts, infection with the parasitic liver flukes *Opisthorchis viverrini* or *Clonorchis sinensis*, toxic exposures, chronic liver disease, obesity, and genetic disorders (specifically, Lynch syndrome and biliary papillomatosis). Approximately one-third of patients with bile duct carcinoma have associated gallstones. Many patients with cholangiocarcinoma do not have a specific risk factor.

Histologically, the lesions are usually mucin-producing adenocarcinomas. In general, bile duct cancers are slow-growing, locally advanced tumors that rarely metastasize to distant sites. However, because of the anatomic relationships of the extrahepatic ducts to the liver, portal vein, and hepatic artery, curative resection of these lesions is the exception rather than the rule.

Common symptoms relate to local growth resulting in biliary obstruction. This leads to jaundice, pruritus, dark urine, and clay-colored stools. Other common presenting symptoms include weight loss, abdominal pain, and fever; cholangitis is rare. In contrast to the fluctuating jaundice that is often seen in patients with common duct calculi, the jaundice associated with bile duct cancers is progressive. On physical examination, hepatomegaly may be found. A palpable, nontender GB in a patient with jaundice (Courvoisier sign) indicates that the site of the obstructing tumor is distal to the junction of the cystic duct with the common duct, although this finding is not specific to bile duct malignancy. Distal cholangiocarcinomas presenting in this manner thus mimic the symptoms of pancreatic tumors.

Laboratory studies show a typical picture of cholestasis and biliary obstruction. Initial studies should include measurement of fractionated bilirubin, ALP, and serum aminotransferases. Abdominal ultrasound is typically the most helpful initial radiographic study. Although the cancer itself may not be visualized, ductal dilatation in the absence of stones suggests the diagnosis. Follow-up with CT or magnetic resonance imaging (MRI) is helpful in determining the extrahepatic extent of the tumors and providing information about the resectability and invasion of adjacent structures. PTC and ERCP are very helpful in demonstrating lesions, assessing intraductal tumor extent, and obtaining cytologic specimens. PTC is particularly useful for the evaluation of the proximal lesions and establishing antegrade access for stenting these lesions.

Prognosis for cholangiocarcinoma is poor, with a 5-year survival of only 5% to 10%. Surgery provides the only possibility for cure, but achieving tumor-free margins can be challenging, and local recurrence is common. The surgical approach depends on the location of the lesion. Intrahepatic cholangiocarcinomas are typically treated with liver resections, but negative margins are achieved in less than 30% of patients. If resection is not possible, the tumor may be traversed with a guide wire and a stent passed through it to relieve the biliary obstruction. Perihilar tumors, also called *Klatskin tumors*, are best treated by resection and Roux-en-Y hepaticojejunostomy, often with the addition of a hepatic resection. The 5-year survival rate after resection of middle-third lesions is approximately 10%. If resection is not possible, the bile duct may be stented with an endoscopic or transhepatic approach. The operation of choice for distal CBD tumors is the Whipple procedure (pancreaticoduodenectomy), which involves resecting the distal CBD, including the tumor, the pancreatic head, and the duodenum. Three anastomoses, connecting the pancreatic remnant, the hepatic duct, and the proximal GI tract in sequence to a mobilized length of jejunum, must be performed after the resection. The 5-year survival rate after a Whipple procedure for a lesion of the distal third of the CBD is approximately 12% to 25%. If distal lesions are unresectable, palliation can be achieved through a surgical bypass or biliary stent.

CONGENITAL CHOLEDOCHAL CYSTS

Very uncommonly, cystic enlargements of the bile ducts occur that are thought to be congenital. These are more frequent in females (4:1 female-to-male ratio) and among the Asian population. Morphologically, five types have been described: Type I: most common variety (80%-90%) involving dilatation of the entire CBD with normal intrahepatic duct, Type II: isolated diverticulum protruding from the CBD, Type III or choledochocele: Type IVa: multiple dilatations of the intrahepatic and extrahepatic biliary tree, Type IVb: multiple dilatations involving only the extrahepatic bile ducts, and Type V or Caroli disease: cystic dilatation of the intrahepatic biliary duct. Patients may present as asymptomatic after an imaging study performed for other reasons, or in the late teens or early 20s with pain and jaundice and rarely an upper abdominal mass. Choledochal cysts are best evaluated by CT scan initially and the specific anatomy is further delineated by MRC or ERCP. Except for those limited to the intrahepatic ducts, it is generally recommended that these cysts be resected to address symptoms, the associated risk of bile duct cancer (20- to 30-fold increased risk over the general population), and pancreatitis. Following resection, a Roux-en-Y hepaticojejunostomy is performed to reestablish bile flow. Continued follow-up of these patients is important because anastomotic structures can occur, and patients should be surveyed for malignancy.

BILE DUCT INJURY AND STRICTURE

Iatrogenic BDIs after cholecystectomy remain a substantial problem in GI surgery. More than 80% of BDIs occur during cholecystectomy and involve the division of the bile duct and its vasculature close to the liver. The bile duct is especially susceptible to this because of a limited blood supply with no redundancy. This underscores the importance of recognizing the anatomic variations of the biliary tree correctly and proceeding in a cautious, systematic fashion, even during routine cholecystectomy. Injuries can involve the common duct, the hepatic duct, or the left and right hepatic ducts. Although low, the incidence of BDIs associated with MIC (0.3%-0.6% which is translated into 3,200-4,800 BDIs annually) is about 4 times higher than that associated with open cholecystectomy. This incidence decreases with individual surgeon experience and is higher in operations performed for acute cholecystitis rather than those performed for biliary colic electively. The error leading to BDI is misperception of the biliary anatomy, where the CBD is mistakenly transected instead of cystic duct. Unfortunately, many iatrogenic injuries go unrecognized intraoperatively and declare themselves later as a subhepatic collection, iatrogenic occlusion, or delayed stricture formation.

When BDI or anomaly is suspected intraoperatively, cholangiography should be performed to delineate the anatomy and suspected injury. Injuries to accessory ducts smaller than 3 mm that drain a small amount of liver parenchyma may be ligated. Otherwise, the operation should be converted to an open procedure and an operative repair be performed. If the injury involves less than 50% of the circumference of the duct, and the duct has not sustained significant devascularization, primary repair may be performed. A T-tube stent is placed and brought out through another location in the common duct to decompress the duct and stent the repair open. In more significant injuries involving more than 50% of the circumference or with obvious devascularization, a Roux-en-Y hepaticojejunostomy should be performed in order to avoid stricturing of a primary repair.

In the early postoperative period, previously unrecognized BDIs may cause severe abdominal pain, jaundice, and drainage of bile from an operatively placed drain or through the wound, as well as signs of acute abdomen or sepsis. Ultrasonography or CT scan may be obtained to detect or exclude an intra-abdominal bile collection, which is called a *biloma*. Definition of the exact location of the ductal injury requires either ERCP or MRCP. A minor leak from an accessory hepatic duct is likely to heal spontaneously and merely requires the placement of a percutaneous drainage catheter in the subhepatic space under CT or ultrasound guidance. Leakage from a cystic duct is typically treated with ERCP placement of a stent. If major ductal injury is detected postoperatively, surgical reconstruction will need to be performed but should be delayed until the anatomy is defined, any sepsis has resolved, and the local inflammation induced from the bile leak has improved.

Late development of stricture leads to obstructive jaundice and recurrent cholangitis. Long-standing strictures may result in biliary cirrhosis and portal hypertension. Diagnosis of strictures is confirmed by MRC, ERCP, or PTC. Cholangitis should be managed with antibiotics and the stricture treated by bypassing the dilated proximal bile duct to a Roux-en-Y loop of the jejunum. In the hands of experienced surgeons, excellent outcome of the operative repair is achieved in 70% to 90% of patients. For high-risk surgical candidates, stenting is an option.

BRIEF DESCRIPTION OF SELECTED PROCEDURES

Minimally Invasive Cholecystectomy

Laparoscopic or robotic cholecystectomy has replaced open cholecystectomy as the preferred approach to the management of gallstone disease in most elective and many emergent situations. When performed electively in an otherwise healthy patient, most procedures can be done as day surgery. Even if the patient has serious comorbidities or if the surgery is done for acute cholecystitis, the postoperative hospital stay is usually only 24 to 48 hours. The main advantages of MIC are a short hospital stay and the greatly reduced postoperative incisional pain when compared with that of open cholecystectomy. In addition to decreased postoperative pain and shorter length of stay, the advantages of this approach are reduced wound, pulmonary complications, and rapid recovery from the procedure with early return to normal activity.

The main risks associated with the MIC are related to injury to the bile ducts, intestine, and major vessels, usually resulting from blind trocar insertion or the injudicious use of electrocautery. With greater experience of the operating surgeon, the risk of complications diminishes significantly. If anatomy is obscured because of the pathologic process or technical difficulties encountered with this approach, the procedure must be converted to an open approach. There is some controversy as to whether cholangiography should be performed routinely or selectively at the time of MIC. Most surgeons utilize a selective approach. If stones are found in the CBD on intraoperative cholangiography, they may be removed laparoscopically or robotically through the cystic duct or an incision in the CBD during the same operation depending on the surgeon's experience. Alternatively, ERCP with stone extraction and sphincterotomy may be performed postoperatively. Only if these options were not available would the MIC be converted to an open CBD exploration to extract the stones.

Open Cholecystectomy and Common Bile Duct Exploration

Open cholecystectomy is generally performed through a right subcostal incision. After the abdomen is opened, the GB is exposed and the GB is dissected out of the GB fossa. An IOC may be performed through the cystic duct at any time to define the anatomy and confirm or exclude suspected choledocholithiasis. Both the cystic duct and artery are individually identified and ligated.

A common duct exploration is sometimes performed during a cholecystectomy. Absolute indications for this include a palpable common duct stone and common duct stones visualized on preoperative or IOCs. Relative indications include jaundice, acute biliary pancreatitis, ductal dilatation, and small GB stones. An operative cholangiogram is performed to confirm or exclude stones in the bile duct when only relative indications for bile duct exploration are present.

The procedure for open CBD exploration involves mobilizing the duodenum with a Kocher maneuver, identifying the duct, and making a small longitudinal incision in the CBD. Then the lumen is irrigated with saline using flexible catheters to help flush out stones and debris from the duct. Inflatable balloon catheters are passed both proximally and distally in an attempt to extract stones. A small endoscope (choledochoscope) may be advanced through the opening and the duct thus carefully visualized both proximally and distally to determine whether residual stones are present. A variety of instruments, including stone forceps and collapsible wire baskets, are available to remove stones that remain impacted and resist removal by the previous maneuvers. All stones, mucus, and debris are removed from the bile duct, and the duct is irrigated with saline. A T tube is then placed in the lumen of the duct, and the opening in the duct is closed around the T tube. A completion cholangiogram is obtained to ensure that no stones remain in the duct and that contrast flows freely in the duodenum. A closed drainage catheter is often left in the subhepatic space. When there are multiple stones, or the physician believes that there are stones left in the bile duct, it is prudent to perform an anastomosis between the bile duct and the GI tract (choledochoduodenostomy or choledochojejunostomy), so that residual stones may pass easily from the duct into the intestine. Of note, the blood supply to CBD runs along the duct at the 3- and 9-o'clock positions. These vessels can be damaged and leave the bile duct at risk for ischemic injury if there is close dissection of the areolar tissue surrounding the bile duct.

The peritoneal drainage catheter is removed within 24 to 48 hours after the T tube has been clamped. Drainage of significant amounts of blood or bile requires further investigation. The typical T tube is left in place for 3 weeks, after which an injection of contrast material in the radiology department is obtained. If the dye flows freely into the duodenum and demonstrates no filling defects, the T tube may be removed. T tubes are typically pulled after an established track is present (3-6 weeks). If there is any concern about the interpretation of the cholangiogram, the T tube is left in place for a longer period of time and the x-ray study is repeated.

Occasionally, despite thorough common duct exploration, a filling defect is noticed on the postoperative T-tube cholangiogram, indicating a missed or retained stone. In approximately 20% of patients, these stones pass spontaneously, especially if they are small. Under such circumstances, the T tube is left in place for 4 to 6 weeks, and the cholangiogram is repeated. If stones remain, they may be extracted with the use of ERCP techniques. Alternatively, the T-tube tract can be used to advance a wire basket into the duct under fluoroscopy, so that the stones might be retrieved. In the rare circumstances where none of these methods is successful, operative reexploration of the duct is necessary.

Endoscopic Extraction of Common Bile Duct Stones

Most CBD stones are removed by ERCP and sphincterotomy. Sphincterotomy of the sphincter of Oddi is performed by a special cautery wire passed through the duodenoscope into the sphincter. The common duct is then cleared of stones and debris using special balloon catheters or wire baskets are also passed through the duodenoscope. When performed electively, this is usually an outpatient procedure. Any coagulopathy should be corrected before the procedure. If a stone cannot be extracted, jaundice can be relieved by inserting a stent with one end above the stone and the other in the duodenum. This stent is left in place, providing biliary decompression until ERCP extraction can be attempted again or surgical stone removal can be arranged. Potential complications of ERCP with sphincterotomy and stone manipulation are postprocedure pancreatitis, GI bleeding (1%-2%), and duodenal or common duct perforation (0.3%).

SUGGESTED READINGS

Buxbaum JL, Abbas Fehmi SM, et al. ASGE guideline on the role of endoscopy in the evaluation and management of choledocholithiasis. *Gastrointest Endosc.* 2019;89(6):1075-1105.e15. doi:10.1016/j.gie.2018.10.001

Gallaher JR, Charles A. Acute cholecystitis: a review. *JAMA.* 2022;327(10):965-975.

Hines OJ, Pandol SJ. Management of severe acute pancreatitis. *Br Med J.* 2019;367:l6227.

Mayumi T, Okamoto K, Takada T, et al. Tokyo Guidelines 2018: management bundles for acute cholangitis and cholecystitis. *J Hepatobiliary Pancreat Sci.* 2018;25(1):96-100. doi:10.1002/jhbp.519

Narula VK, Fung EC, Overby DW, Richardson W, Stefanidis D; SAGES Guidelines Committee. Clinical spotlight review for the management of choledocholithiasis. *Surg Endosc.* 2020;34(4):1482-1491. doi:10.1007/s00464-020-07462-2

Valle JW, Kelley RK, Nervi B, Oh D-Y, Zhu AX. Biliary tract cancer. *Lancet.* 2021;397(10272):428-444.

SAMPLE QUESTIONS

QUESTIONS

Choose the best answer for each question.

1. The blood supply to the GB is a branch of the
    A. gastroduodenal artery.
    B. proper hepatic artery.
    C. right hepatic artery.
    D. right gastric artery.
    E. superior mesenteric artery.

2. Bile consists of
    A. albumin, bile acids, and triglycerides.
    B. bile acids, triglycerides, and phospholipids.
    C. albumin, cholesterol, and bile acids.
    D. bile acids, lecithin, and cholesterol.
    E. lipopolysaccharide, bile acids, and albumin.

3. A 74-year-old male with multiple comorbidities was admitted to the medical intensive care unit for treatment of acute pneumonia and required mechanical ventilation for 2 days. On hospital day 5, the patient developed RUQ pain. Laboratory tests showed elevated AST, ALT, ALP, and mild hyperbilirubinemia. RUQ ultrasound showed distended GB with pericholecystic fluid, GB wall thickening, and no stones. After resuscitation, the next step in management is
    A. urgent open cholecystectomy.
    B. MIC.
    C. cholecystostomy tube.
    D. antibiotics only.
    E. interval laparoscopic cholecystectomy.

4. A 60-year-old male who is status post open repair of abdominal aortic aneurysm rupture has been in the intensive care unit for the past 2 weeks since on a ventilator with TPN. He is responsive and able to communicate. He complains of upper abdominal pain that he locates in the RUQ epigastric area. White blood cell count is now 12,500 and ALP, AST, and ALT are elevated. Total bilirubin is normal. The best test to use to diagnose this patient's condition is a(an)

A. CT scan of abdomen.
B. HIDA scan.
C. ultrasound of the RUQ.
D. MRCP.
E. abdominal series.

5. A 72-year-old man comes to the clinic because his wife noticed that his eyes are yellow. Recently, he has found that his urine is dark and his stool is light in color. He also has a diminished appetite but otherwise is feeling well without other complaints. His past medical history is unremarkable. He smoked cigarettes for 30 years but quit 15 years ago. On examination, he is afebrile and his vital signs are normal. He is deeply jaundiced and when examining the abdomen, a nontender smooth globular mass is found in the RUQ. The rest of his examination is normal. Which of the following is the most likely diagnosis in this patient?

A. Bile duct cancer
B. Choledocholithiasis
C. Choledochal cyst
D. Biliary stricture
E. Gallstones

ANSWERS AND EXPLANATIONS

1. **Answer: C**

The cystic artery is a branch of the right hepatic artery. The cystic artery branches into an anterior and posterior branch before joining the GB. Both of these branches will require ligation when performing a cholecystectomy. For more information on this topic, see section "Anatomy."

2. **Answer: D**

The three components of bile (bile acids, lecithin, and cholesterol) are normally balanced, but when one component of bile is present in a higher concentration, the formation of gallstones (cholesterol, bile, mixed) can occur. For more information on this topic, see section "Pathogenesis of Gallstones (Cholelithiasis)."

3. **Answer: C**

This patient has typical presentation of acalculous cholecystitis and requires treatment. Given his comorbidities, and the acuteness of situation, a cholecystostomy drain under ultrasound guidance is appropriate. For more information on this topic, see section "Acute Cholecystitis."

4. **Answer: C**

The presentation is consistent with possible cholecystitis. This clinical presentation is typical for acalculous cholecystitis in a sick patient who has been nil per os (NPO). A HIDA scan in this situation would have a high false-positive rate because the patient is NPO. A CT scan would not be as definitive as ultrasound but would be the test of choice if you were considering other possible etiologies. MRCP and an abdominal series would not be helpful. For more information on this topic, see section "Imaging Studies."

5. **Answer: A**

When a patient presents with jaundice and acholic stools, a bile duct obstruction is likely present. The other diagnoses listed may be associated with obstructed jaundice. Given the patient's age and the presentation along with a distended GB (Courvoisier sign), the most likely diagnosis is a pancreaticobiliary malignancy. For more information on this topic, see section "Bile Duct Malignancies."

INTRODUCTION

The pancreas is responsible for a variety of endocrine and exocrine functions. Diseases affecting the pancreas are common and include congenital, inflammatory, infectious, traumatic, and neoplastic processes, which may affect both the endocrine and exocrine functions. This chapter does not intend to reintroduce details of pancreatic embryology, anatomy, and physiology. Yet, an appreciation of this information is paramount to understanding pancreatic disease and surgical interventions that deal with pancreatic pathology. Important variations of the pancreatic anatomy are discussed in the following sections. Otherwise, we recommend referring to the first-year medical school textbooks to review essential information regarding pancreatic anatomy and physiology.

ANATOMY

The pancreas is a retroperitoneal gland that is divided into four distinct parts: head, neck, body, and tail (Figure 16-1). The head of the pancreas is located within the "C-loop" of the duodenum. The superior mesenteric vein (SMV) defines the junction of the head and neck of the gland. The neck of the gland is the part directly overlying the SMV, and the body extends to the left of the SMV. The uncinate process makes up a part of the posterior and inferior head. The tail is the most distal part of the gland and extends toward and/or abuts the splenic hilum. The anatomic dividing line between the body and the tail is ill defined, with lesions of the body or tail usually managed similarly.

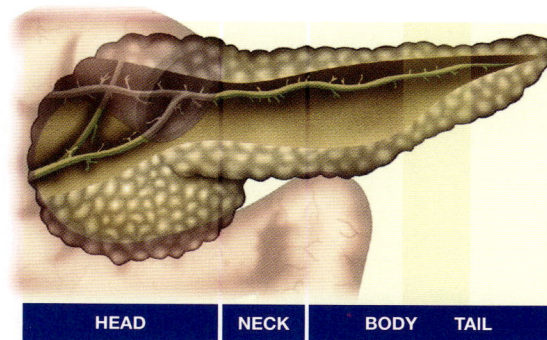

Figure 16-1. The pancreatic gland is divided into four parts: the head, neck, body, and tail. The superior mesenteric vein runs under the neck of the gland. The diagram is taken from the Internet Encyclopedia of Science. (Drawing by Matthew Campbell.)

Embryology and Ductal Anatomy

Understanding pancreatic embryology and development provides excellent insights into pancreatic ductal anatomy. At 30 days' gestation, the endoderm lining the duodenum forms the ventral and dorsal pancreatic buds. As the second part of the duodenum forms a C-shape, the ventral pancreatic bud, which will become the uncinate process, rotates clockwise to lie inferior to the dorsal bud, which forms the head, body, and tail (Figure 16-2). By 6 weeks' gestation, the dorsal and ventral pancreatic buds are contiguous with each other, and during the eighth week, the parenchyma and ducts of the dorsal and ventral pancreatic buds fuse. Most commonly, the duct of Wirsung (main pancreatic duct) is formed by the fusion of the distal part of the dorsal and ventral pancreatic ducts. The duct of Wirsung typically forms a common channel with the common bile duct. It enters the duodenum at the ampulla of Vater and the sphincter of Oddi (the major papilla) surrounds the duct. The distal part of the dorsal pancreatic duct may persist as the duct of Santorini (accessory pancreatic duct; Figure 16-3A) or be totally obliterated (Figure 16-3B).

There are a number of variations in the normal pancreatic ductal anatomy (Figure 16-3A, B). In approximately 10% of the population, the ventral and dorsal pancreatic ducts do not fuse completely (Figure 16-3C–E), which results in a persistent dominant dorsal duct. These variations, where most of the dorsal pancreas empties into the duodenum via the accessory duct of Santorini and a part of the pancreatic head and uncinate process empties via the major papilla, are often grouped together and are called "pancreas divisum." About 90% of patients with pancreas divisum are asymptomatic, yet some patients with this embryologic anomaly develop recurring attacks of acute pancreatitis. It is suspected that the minor duct orifice in patients with symptomatic pancreatic divisum is too small for the volume of pancreatic secretions coming from the body and tail of the pancreas. This relative obstruction at the minor papilla can lead to excessively high intrapancreatic dorsal ductal pressure during active secretion, resulting in ductal distension, pain, and in some cases, pancreatitis. Figure 16-4 shows endoscopic retrograde cholangiopancreatography (ERCP) images obtained from both major and minor pancreatic ducts. The major and minor pancreatic ducts are shown in Figure 16-5.

A second pancreatic developmental anomaly is called "annular pancreas." Less common than pancreas divisum, annular pancreas results from the incomplete rotation of the ventral pancreatic bud, thereby encircling the second part of the duodenum by a ring of pancreatic tissue. It is a rare cause of duodenal obstruction seen in infants and children. Treatment involves surgical bypass of the pancreatic tissue causing the obstruction (duodenojejunostomy) and specifically avoids division of the pancreatic parenchyma, which would result in a high rate of pancreatic fistula.

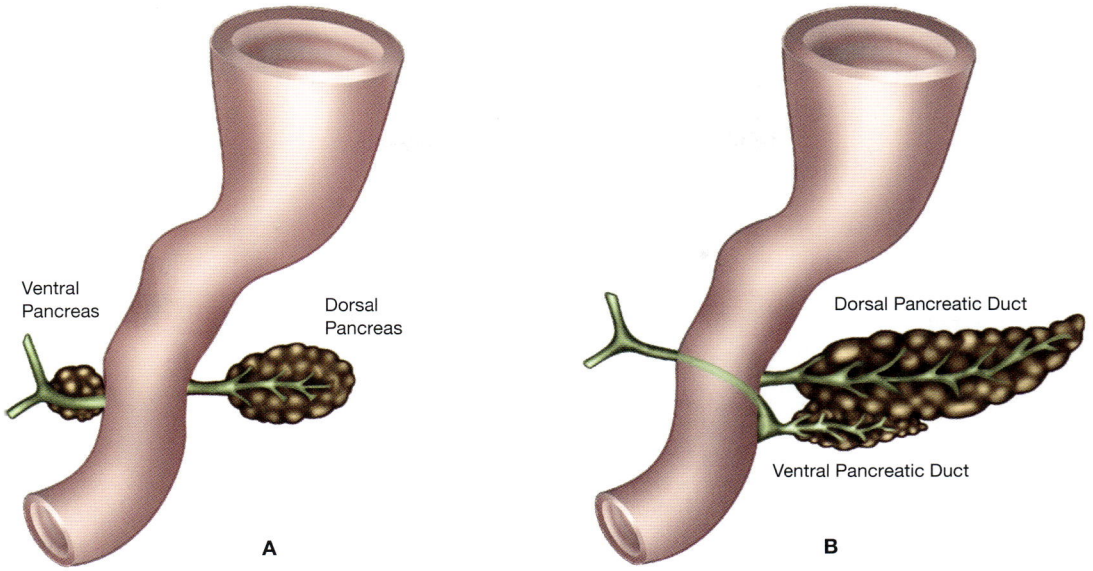

Figure 16-2. **Dorsal and ventral pancreatic buds.** A. Before migration. B. After migration. (Drawing by Matthew Campbell.)

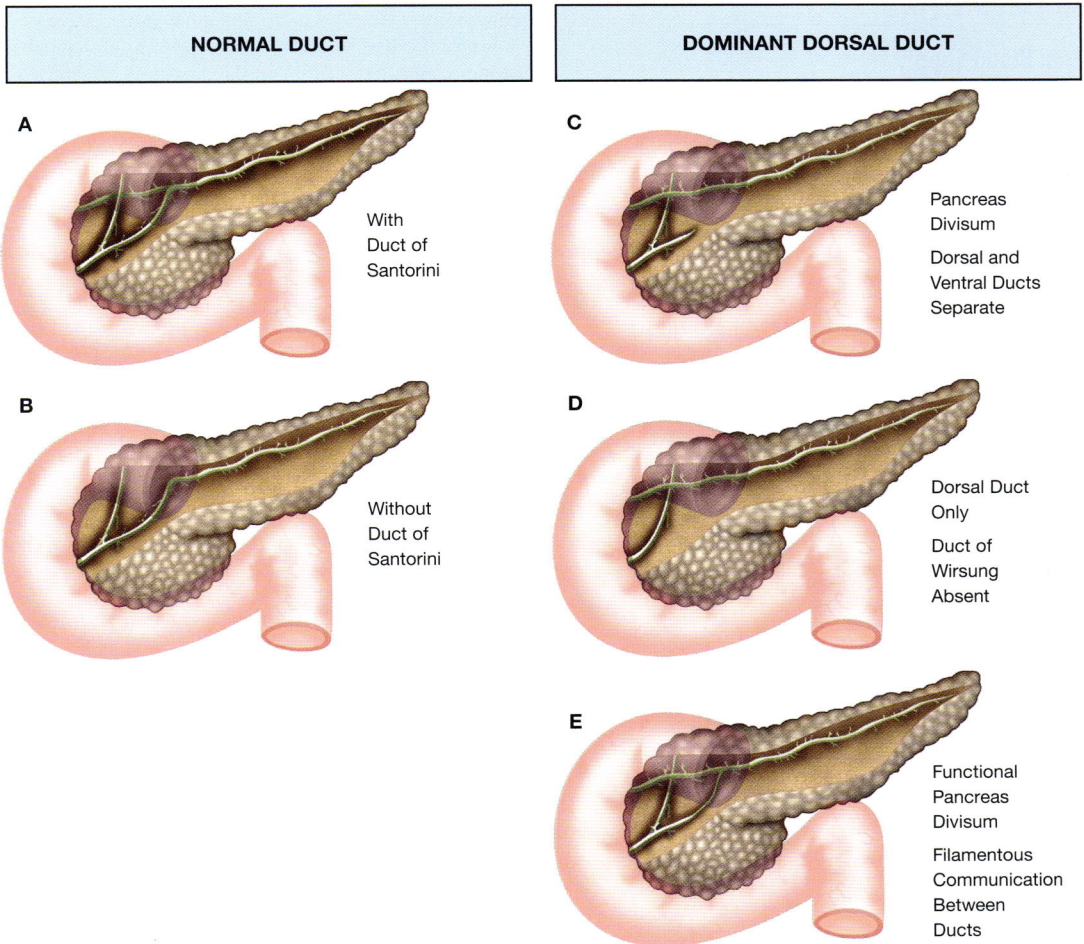

Figure 16-3. **Common pancreatic ductal anatomic variations.** (Drawing by Matthew Campbell.)

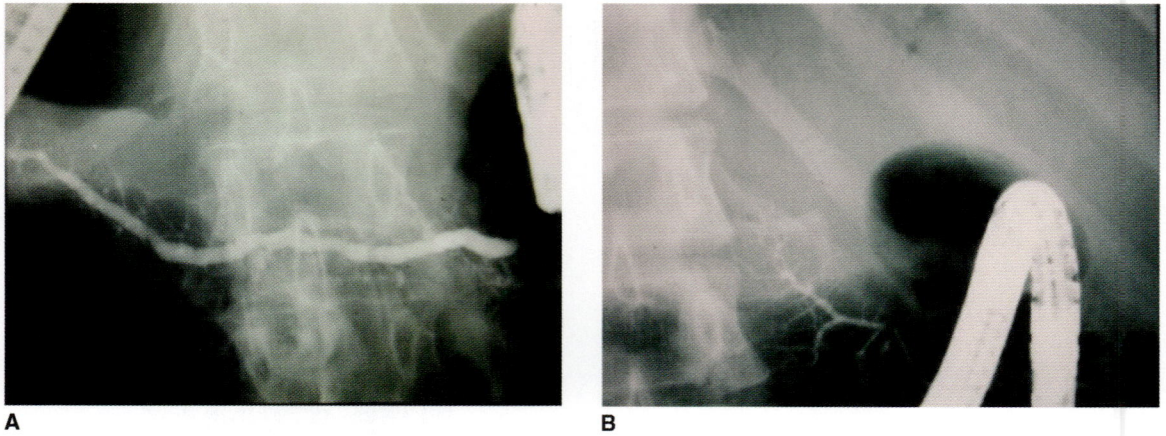

A   **B**

Figure 16-4. Endoscopic retrograde cholangiopancreatography study demonstrating pancreas divisum. Both the major and minor ducts have been imaged independently. A. Major pancreatic duct. B. Minor pancreatic duct. (Reprinted with permission from Gold SB, Carey LC. Pancreas divisum. In: Cameron JL, ed. *Current Surgical Therapy*. 8th ed. Elsevier Mosby; 2004:473.)

PANCREATIC VASCULAR ANATOMY AND INNERVATION

Arterial Blood Supply

Patient outcomes following any operation often rely upon correctly identifying normal and common vascular variations. Therefore, a thorough understanding of vascular anatomy is paramount, especially in pancreatic operations. The practicing pancreatic surgeon must know the basic anatomy and common variations.

Celiac Artery

The celiac artery supplies the embryologic foregut and classically trifurcates into the left gastric, splenic, and common hepatic arteries. There are multiple common anatomic variations of this classic anatomy of the celiac artery. Figure 16-6 details the arterial and venous anatomy surrounding the pancreas. The celiac artery contributes to the perfusion of the head of the pancreas, and for the duodenum, it is via the gastroduodenal artery (GDA) and its pancreaticoduodenal arcade, namely the superior anterior and posterior pancreaticoduodenal arteries. Perfusion to

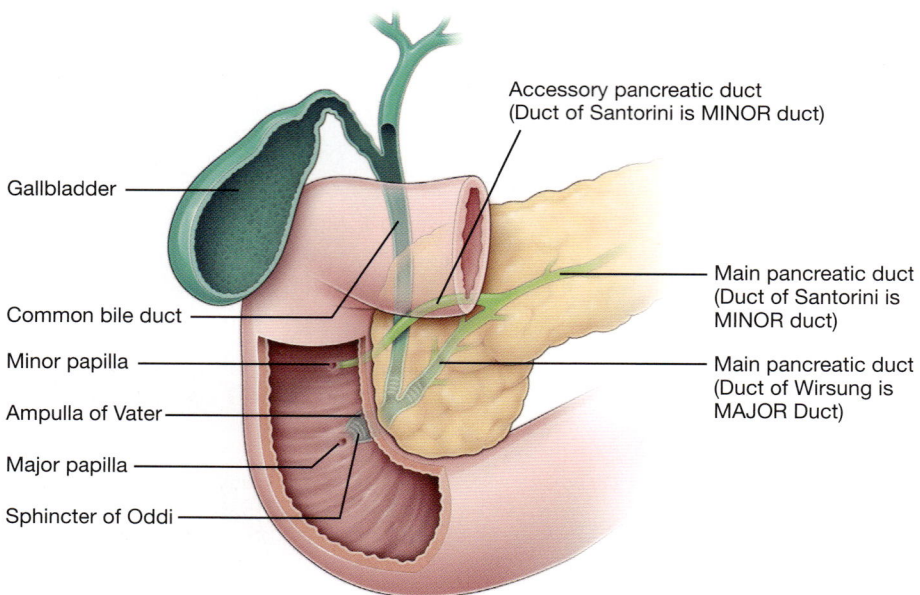

Figure 16-5. Major and minor pancreatic ducts.

| | ARTERIES | | VEINS |

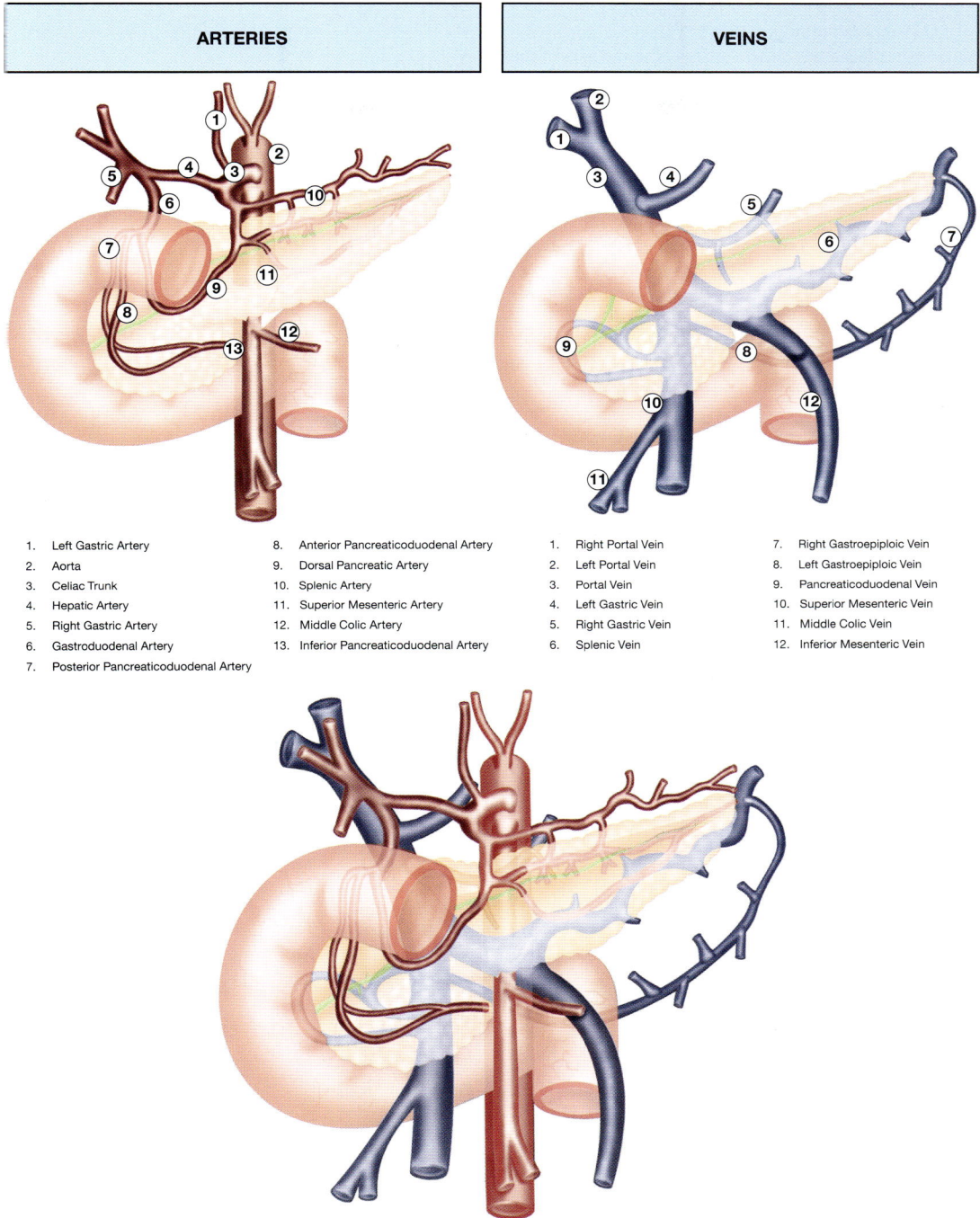

1.	Left Gastric Artery	8.	Anterior Pancreaticoduodenal Artery
2.	Aorta	9.	Dorsal Pancreatic Artery
3.	Celiac Trunk	10.	Splenic Artery
4.	Hepatic Artery	11.	Superior Mesenteric Artery
5.	Right Gastric Artery	12.	Middle Colic Artery
6.	Gastroduodenal Artery	13.	Inferior Pancreaticoduodenal Artery
7.	Posterior Pancreaticoduodenal Artery		

1.	Right Portal Vein	7.	Right Gastroepiploic Vein
2.	Left Portal Vein	8.	Left Gastroepiploic Vein
3.	Portal Vein	9.	Pancreaticoduodenal Vein
4.	Left Gastric Vein	10.	Superior Mesenteric Vein
5.	Right Gastric Vein	11.	Middle Colic Vein
6.	Splenic Vein	12.	Inferior Mesenteric Vein

Figure 16-6. Arterial vascular arcades supplying the duodenum and pancreas. (Drawing by Matthew Campbell.)

the body and tail of the pancreas originates from the pancreatic branches of the splenic artery and the dorsal pancreatic artery, often coming from the GDA. A relatively common and critically important variation in the anatomy of the hepatic artery is that the right hepatic artery does not originate from the celiac axis in approximately 20% of individuals. In this case, the blood supply to the right lobe of

the liver via the hepatic artery originates from the superior mesenteric artery (SMA) and is called a "replaced right hepatic artery." If both a right hepatic artery and a second vessel from the SMA supply the right liver, the latter vessel is termed a "recurrent" or "accessory" right hepatic artery. The replaced right or accessory vessels can easily be injured or ligated during a pancreaticoduodenectomy if their presence is not carefully assessed on preoperative contrasted computed tomography (CT) scans or during the operation. A replaced left hepatic artery, seen in 20% of the population, originates from the left gastric artery.

Superior Mesenteric Artery

The SMA supplies blood to the entire embryologic midgut. It arises anteriorly from the aorta and is directly posterior to the pancreas. The artery passes inferiorly, just medial and anterior to the uncinate process, giving off its first branch, that is, the inferior pancreaticoduodenal artery. This vessel splits into the anterior and posterior branches that anastomose with pancreaticoduodenal branches of the superior pancreaticoduodenal artery previously described. After passing the duodenum, the SMA enters the root of the mesentery, where it supplies the entire small bowel and the right and transverse colon.

Celiac Axis—Superior Mesenteric Arterial Collaterals

Many people have significant celiac artery stenosis. Yet, most of these individuals have no symptoms of chronic mesenteric ischemia because of the rich and extensive collateral vascular supply joining the celiac artery and SMA. The most common collateral pathways involving the celiac artery and SMA surrounding the duodenum and pancreas are shown in Figure 16-6 and involve the pancreaticoduodenal vessels. The celiac artery and SMA communicate via collateral circulation, and the inferior mesenteric artery communicates with the SMA via the arc of Riolan and the marginal artery of Drummond.

Venous Drainage

The venous drainage of the pancreas, duodenum, and spleen corresponds to the arterial supply (see Figure 16-6). The venous drainage of the body and tail of the pancreas is through draining branches that enter the splenic and inferior pancreatic veins. The inferior mesenteric vein may join the portal system anywhere along the splenic vein, including the splenic vein–SMV junction. Remember that all blood flow from the small and large bowel returns via the portal system, and injury to this venous structure may result in bowel infarction.

Innervation

The pancreas receives sympathetic (greater splanchnic) and parasympathetic (vagus) innervation, which are important in the gland's endocrine functions. Sensory signals are indicative of pancreatic pain travel by afferent autonomic sensory nerve fibers. Pancreatic pain may result from neoplastic infiltration, inflammatory processes, or ductal obstruction. Two major theories are thought to explain the pain experienced by patients with pancreatitis, including increased intraductal or intraparenchymal pressures and a neurogenic theory where immunologically activated cells or noxious substances irritate exposed nerve cells resulting in excruciating pain. Treatment of severe pain in patients with chronic pancreatitis may involve blocking the afferent nerves by celiac plexus neurolysis, which may be performed by alcohol or neurolytic injection. Neurolysis may be carried out percutaneously using CT, intraoperatively, or endoscopically using ultrasound (US).

PHYSIOLOGY

Exocrine

The pancreas plays a major role in digestion and secretes 500 to 800 mL/d of isotonic, alkaline fluid containing electrolytes and digestive enzymes. The sodium and potassium concentrations are equal to those in plasma. Chloride concentrations vary inversely with bicarbonate secretion, which is important in digestion. When acidic gastric contents (pH <3) enter the duodenum, there is a release of secretin from the mucosa of the duodenum that stimulates the pancreas to secrete large volumes of bicarbonate-rich fluid (pH >8).

Cholecystokinin (CCK) also weakly stimulates bicarbonate production. Intraluminal peptides, amino acids, and free fatty acids stimulate the release of duodenal CCK, which causes gallbladder contraction so that bile enters the duodenum to mix with pancreatic secretions and chyme to facilitate digestion and absorption.

There are numerous tests to assess the exocrine function of the pancreas. The pancreas also secretes three types of digestive enzymes, namely amylases, lipases, and proteases. These are secreted via neural and hormonal factors such as CCK, acetylcholine, vasoactive intestinal polypeptide (VIP), and secretin. Approximately 20 different digestive enzymes are secreted as inactive precursors (eg, trypsin and chymotrypsin are secreted as trypsinogen and chymotrypsinogen) and activated upon contact with the duodenal contents. Amylase is the only enzyme secreted in its active form, but it functions best at pH 7.0.

Endocrine

The islets of Langerhans are populated with many different cell lines that produce a variety of peptide hormones, including insulin, glucagon, somatostatin, pancreatic polypeptide (PP), VIP, galanin, serotonin, amylin, pancreastatin, and chromogranin A (CgA). The islets are abundant in the tail of the pancreas. The main endocrine role of the islet cells is to control glucose homeostasis with a feedback mechanism based on glucose levels. The α cells secrete glucagon in response to low glucose levels, which results in glycogenolysis and increased blood glucose levels.

PATHOPHYSIOLOGY

Acute Pancreatitis

Acute pancreatitis is due to acinar cell injury, which allows the activation of pancreatic enzymes outside of the pancreatic ducts and digestive tract. This results in the destruction of pancreatic and peripancreatic tissue. The gland may become swollen, edematous, hemorrhagic, or even necrotic. Histologic changes range from interstitial edema and inflammation to hemorrhage and necrosis. Even when imaging fails to show necrosis, glandular destruction does occur at a microscopic level. The disease ranges in severity from mild and self-limited to severe and life threatening. The Atlanta Classification defines acute pancreatitis as an acute inflammatory process of the pancreas with variable involvement of other regional tissues or remote organ systems. The diagnosis of acute pancreatitis is secured when at least two of the following three criteria are met: The patient's presenting signs and symptoms are consistent with the diagnosis (see signs and symptoms discussed later), the serum amylase or lipase is elevated, and the CT scan shows typical radiographic findings. The Atlanta Classification system introduces uniformity in the terminology used to describe acute pancreatitis, as outlined in Table 16-1.

Etiology

Alcohol ingestion and biliary calculi account for 85% of cases of acute pancreatitis. Other etiologies of pancreatitis include metabolic, mechanical, postoperative, traumatic, vascular, infectious, genetic, and autoimmune (Table 16-2) factors. In patients with pancreatitis related to alcohol consumption, the first episode of pancreatitis is usually preceded by 6 to 8 years of heavy alcohol ingestion. These patients often experience recurring acute attacks related to continued alcohol consumption. After multiple episodes of acute pancreatitis, the pancreatic ductal system becomes permanently damaged, leading to chronic pancreatitis. Alcohol may contribute by causing secretions with a high protein content that precipitate and block small pancreatic ductules. The mechanism by which hyperlipidemia, hypercalcemia, and medications such as corticosteroids, thiazide diuretics, furosemide, estrogens, and azathioprine cause the disease is unknown.

The mechanical causes of pancreatitis can be anything that may obstruct the pancreatic duct. This includes gallstones, tumors, trauma, and parasitic diseases. Gallstones are the most common mechanical cause of pancreatitis, and it is estimated that 60% of nonalcoholic patients with pancreatitis have gallstones. How choledocholithiasis causes pancreatitis is not fully understood but may be due to the reflux of bile into the pancreatic duct or markedly increased pancreatic ductal pressures. In experiments, bile did not cause pancreatitis when introduced into the pancreatic duct at physiologic pressures. It could be that mixing bile and pancreatic juice led to the formation of a highly toxic substance in the pancreas. Post-ERCP pancreatitis can develop in as many as 1% to 5% of patients, and it may be caused by an acute increase in intraductal pressure during injection of contrast.

Approximately 8% to 10% of cases of pancreatitis have no recognizable etiology (idiopathic pancreatitis); however, most of these cases are believed to be associated with biliary tract sludge (microlithiasis), congenital causes (pancreatic divisum), or autoimmune IgG4 pancreatitis.

Clinical Presentation and Evaluation

Patients with acute pancreatitis have noncrampy, constant, and severe epigastric abdominal pain that typically radiates to the back. The pain may be alleviated by sitting or standing. It is associated with nausea and vomiting. Physical examination shows fever, tachycardia, and upper abdominal tenderness with guarding. Patients may develop an adynamic ileus with abdominal distension. Generalized abdominal and rebound tenderness suggestive of an acute abdomen may also occur in severe pancreatitis. When there

TABLE 16-1. Definition of the Grades of Severity of Acute Pancreatitis

Term	Definition
Mild acute pancreatitis	No local complications No systemic complications
Moderately severe acute pancreatitis	Moderate local complications that resolve (acute fluid collections causing pain, fever, or an inability to eat) Transient organ failure of <48 h
Severe acute pancreatitis	Intense local complications (necrosis, infected necrosis, pseudocysts) Persistent MSOF
Local Peripancreatic Complications of Acute Pancreatitis	
Acute fluid collections	Ill-defined collection of sterile fluid located in or about the pancreas, appearing early in the course of acute pancreatitis; lack of a wall of granulation of fibrous tissue; spontaneous regression usually occurs; if it persists, it develops into a pancreatic abscess or pseudocyst.
Pancreatic necrosis	Diffuse or focal area(s) of nonviable pancreatic parenchyma typically associated with peripancreatic fat necrosis; nonenhanced pancreatic parenchyma
Acute pseudocyst	Collection of pancreatic juice enclosed by a wall of fibrous granulation tissue, which arises as a result of acute pancreatitis, pancreatic trauma, or chronic pancreatitis, occurring at least 4 wk after the onset of symptoms, is round or ovoid and most often sterile; when pus is present, the lesion is termed a pancreatic abscess.
Pancreatic abscess	Circumscribed, intra-abdominal collection of pus, usually in proximity to the pancreas, containing little or no pancreatic necrosis, which arises as a consequence of acute pancreatitis or pancreatic trauma; often 4 wk or more after onset; pancreatic abscess and infected pancreatic necrosis differ in clinical expression and the extent of associated necrosis.

MSOF, multisystem organ failure.

Sarr MG, Banks PA, Bollen TL, et al. The new revised classification of acute pancreatitis 2012. *Surg Clin N Am.* 2013;93:549-562. https://www.sciencedirect.com/sdfe/pdf/download/eid/1-s2.0-S0039610913000327/first-page-pdf.

TABLE 16-2. Etiologic Factors of Acute Pancreatitis	
Metabolic	Alcohol, hyperlipidemia, hypertriglyceridemia, hypercalcemia (hyperparathyroidism), uremia, pregnancy, and scorpion venom
Mechanical	Cholelithiasis, pancreas divisum, duct obstruction (ascaris, tumor, etc), ERCP, ductal bleeding, duodenal obstruction, duct obstruction from scar secondary to prior episodes of pancreatitis, and sphincter of Oddi dysfunction
Postoperative and traumatic	0.8%-17% gastric procedures, 0.7%-9.3% biliary procedures, direct pancreatic injury or trauma, injury to the pancreatic blood supply, obstruction of the pancreatic duct at the duodenum, and cardiopulmonary bypass (ischemia)
Vascular	Periarteritis nodosa, lupus erythematosus, and atheroembolism
Infectious	Mumps; coxsackie B virus; cytomegalovirus; *Cryptococcus*; *Enterovirus*; hepatitis A, B, or C; Epstein-Barr virus; herpes simplex virus; echovirus; and *Ascaris* infestation
Hereditary, genetic	Hereditary form of autosomal dominant, cystic fibrosis, pancreas divisum, familial pancreatitis, and tropical pancreatitis
Autoimmune	Autoimmune pancreatitis
Medications	Many medications may cause pancreatitis.
Idiopathic	Unknown

ERCP, endoscopic retrograde cholangiopancreatography.

is retroperitoneal bleeding from severe acute pancreatitis, blood may dissect into the posterior retroperitoneal soft tissue, causing a flank hematoma known as Grey Turner sign or up the falciform ligament resulting in a periumbilical ecchymosis called Cullen sign.

Laboratory evaluation usually reveals leukocytosis with elevated serum amylase and lipase. An elevation of the serum amylase level 1.5 times the normal limit with a lipase value of 5 times the normal limit has 95% sensitivity in confirming this diagnosis. Used individually, a serum amylase level 3 times the normal value has a specificity of 95% but a lower sensitivity of 61%. The serum amylase rises quickly within the first 12 hours after admission and usually returns to normal after 3 to 5 days. Severe cases of pancreatitis can initiate a systemic inflammatory response syndrome (SIRS) with the activation of inflammatory mediators (cytokines, lymphocytes, and the complement cascade). This SIRS response may look like severe sepsis and cause injury to other organs, such as acute kidney injury, acute respiratory distress syndrome (ARDS), and cardiovascular instability, in addition to hyperglycemia and hypocalcemia, elevated blood urea nitrogen (BUN) and creatinine levels, and hypoxemia as a result of injury to the liver, lungs, and kidneys.

The differential diagnosis of acute pancreatitis includes acute cholecystitis, perforated peptic ulcer, acute mesenteric ischemia, esophageal perforation, and myocardial infarction. It is important to note that not all patients with an acute abdomen and elevated amylase have pancreatitis, as outlined in Table 16-3.

Patients with suspected acute pancreatitis should be evaluated radiographically with (1) a chest x-ray to exclude free air (pneumoperitoneum); (2) plain and upright abdominal x-rays to look for possible calcifications (indicating chronic pancreatitis) or bowel obstruction; and (3) ultrasonography to look for gallstones, common duct dilatation, pancreatic enlargement, and peripancreatic fluid collections. Ultrasonography may be of limited value in

patients who are obese or patients with significant amounts of bowel gas overlying the pancreas.

In most cases, a CT scan is not required to diagnose acute pancreatitis (see the Atlanta definition). When the diagnosis remains unclear, the CT scan may resolve uncertainty and provide the diagnosis. Typical radiographic findings on CT scans range from peripancreatic fluid and pancreatic edema which are present in nearly all patients at the time of presentation, to pancreatic necrosis, which is most commonly seen days to weeks after the initial presentation in the setting of severe acute pancreatitis.

Pancreatic tissue that does not enhance with intravenous (IV) contrast is diagnostic of pancreatic necrosis. However, the radiographic diagnosis of pancreatic necrosis is not an indication for surgical intervention, and most patients with necrosis without infection recover without surgery. Other imaging modalities, including magnetic resonance cholangiopancreatography (MRCP), may be beneficial in selected cases by noninvasively visualizing the bile duct and pancreas.

Prognosis

A patient's outcome following an episode of acute pancreatitis is directly related to the severity of pancreatitis and the

TABLE 16-3. List of Disease Processes That May Result in Hyperamylasemia	
Perforated Ulcer	**Ovarian Tumor or Cyst**
Ischemic bowel	Lung cancer
Small bowel obstruction	Prostate cancer
Renal failure	Diabetic ketoacidosis
Salivary gland infection	Macroamylasemia
Ectopic pregnancy	

SIRS reaction. The Atlanta Classification discussed previously provides definitions for the different levels of severity of acute pancreatitis and its complications (see Table 16-1). Grading systems for the severity of pancreatitis at the time of presentation are used to predict the risk for subsequent complications. Ranson developed one of the first clinical grading systems for pancreatitis, which relies upon readily measured laboratory and clinical variables (Ranson criteria) when the patient presents to the hospital (Table 16-4). Five variables are measured on admission, and six additional variables are measured over the ensuing 48 hours. The presence of three or more criteria indicates severe pancreatitis and is associated with an increased incidence of local and systemic complications. Clinically, this is very useful because it identifies those patients who require more aggressive resuscitation, care, and monitoring at the time of admission to the hospital. It should be emphasized that neither serum amylase nor lipase is included in the Ranson criteria, indicating that neither reflects the severity of pancreatitis nor the likelihood of developing complications; they are only markers of acinar cell damage.

Finally, CT scans also yield prognostic information. Baltazar et al. developed a grading system based on CT findings, shown in Table 16-5. The severity of the attack is directly related to the development of pancreatic fluid collections. It is important to understand that acute pancreatitis is not a static disease, so a single CT scan at any one point in time might not reflect the severity of the disease at all timepoints. In other words, although the typical case proceeds with a rapid resolution of signs and symptoms

TABLE 16-5. CT Grading System for Acute Pancreatitis

Grade	CT Finding
A	Normal pancreas
B	Pancreatic enlargement
C	Pancreatic inflammation and/or peripancreatic fat
D	Single peripancreatic fluid collection
E	Two or more fluid collections and/or retroperitoneal air

CT, computed tomography.

and improvement in laboratory studies, there are certain patients whose pancreatitis worsens over time because of an exaggerated SIRS response. These patients fail to improve, or even deteriorate further, and serial CT scans can monitor the patient for surgically correctable complications.

Treatment
Medical
Medical therapy for acute pancreatitis can be divided into general supportive therapy and the specific treatment of pancreatic inflammation or its complications. Efforts to reduce pancreatic secretion are achieved by withholding food until pain and tenderness resolve and the serum amylase and white blood cell (WBC) count return to normal. A rising or persistently elevated amylase level indicates ongoing acinar injury due to continued leakage, which is usually secondary to persistent ductal obstruction.

Following more severe episodes of pancreatitis (ie, those with a Ranson score >2), it is important to maintain adequate tissue perfusion by monitoring hemodynamic parameters and maintaining adequate intravascular volume. Massive fluid sequestrations can occur in the retroperitoneum because of the peripancreatic inflammatory process, similar to patients with a third-degree burn. In severe cases, resuscitation with several liters of isotonic fluid may be required. Fluid management is aided by measuring urine output, checking central venous pressures, or performing an echocardiogram to assess inferior vena cava diameter and atrial filling. Electrolytes and blood glucose should also be monitored in severe pancreatitis.

Respiratory function must be monitored with pulse oximetry because sympathetic pleural effusions, atelectasis, ARDS due to SIRS, hemidiaphragm elevation, and fluid overload may impair oxygenation. Intubation and aggressive ventilatory support are sometimes required.

All pharmacologic attempts at reducing pancreatic secretion, including anticholinergics, somatostatin analogues, inhibitors of the inflammatory cascade, specific enzyme inhibitors (eg, aprotinin—a proteolytic enzyme inhibitor), and antacids, have not demonstrated a significant benefit. Nasogastric suction is only indicated in patients with significant nausea, vomiting, or abdominal distension, where its use might reduce the risk of aspiration. Numerous studies have shown that prophylactic antibiotics are not effective in mild or moderate pancreatitis. Prophylactic antibiotic use in severe disease (more than three of Ranson criteria) does not alter mortality but does prolong the time

TABLE 16-4. Ranson Criteria—Prognostic Factors for Major Complications or Death

	Nonbiliary	Biliary
On Admission		
Age	>55	>70
WBC count	>16	>18
Glucose	>200 mg/100 mL	>220 mg/100 mL
LDH	>350	>400
SGOT (AST)	>250	>250
During the Initial 48 h		
Hematocrit decrease	>10%	>10%
BUN increase	>5 mg/dL	>2 mg/dL
Calcium	<8 mg/dL	<8 mg/dL
Arterial P_{O_2}	<60 mm Hg	—
Base deficit	>4 mEq/L	>5 mEq/L
Fluid sequestration	>6 L	>4 L

AST, aspartate aminotransferase; BUN, blood urea nitrogen; LDH, lactate dehydrogenase; SGOT, serum glutamic oxaloacetic transaminase; WBC, white blood cells.

from presentation to infection at the expense of altering resistance patterns of the infecting pathogens. Therefore, prophylactic antibiotics are not indicated even in those patients with sterile necrosis. Antibiotics are essential once an infection is identified.

Nutritional support must also be provided to malnourished patients and patients with severe disease who may not eat for a prolonged period. Early enteral nutrition is preferred over parenteral nutrition, but there is no difference in outcome between nasogastric and nasojejunal feeding. Total parenteral nutrition may be required in patients without a functional gastrointestinal tract.

Surgical

Surgical indications for acute pancreatitis are divided into operations that prevent further episodes of pancreatitis and those required to deal with local peripancreatic complications.

First, patients with mild or moderate pancreatitis caused by cholelithiasis should undergo cholecystectomy during the initial phase but after the resolution of symptoms. Cholecystectomy for gallstone pancreatitis reduces the risk of developing another bout of pancreatitis from approximately 50% to around 5% but does not affect the episode of pancreatitis itself. If imaging or laboratory values suggest choledocholithiasis or the patient develops acute ascending cholangitis, an ERCP with sphincterotomy and stone extraction should be performed to clear the common bile duct.

ERCP with sphincterotomy and stone extraction is advisable only in patients with severe pancreatitis and a suspected gallstone impacted at the ampulla of Vater, often evident by cholangitis or a persistently rising amylase. These patients should then be allowed to recover before cholecystectomy and following the resolution of pancreatitis. Early cholecystectomy should not be performed in patients with severe gallstone pancreatitis because of the significant morbidity and mortality of this procedure in critically ill patients and the fact that this operation will not alter the course of pancreatitis itself.

Early operative intervention in patients with sterile pancreatic necrosis carries prohibitive risks. Therefore, every effort should be made not to operate on patients with sterile necrosis until at least 2 to 3 weeks after its occurrence. Indications for pancreatic necrosectomy for uninfected disease include persistent pain, enteric or biliary obstruction, or ongoing signs of SIRS. One should proceed with surgical intervention only when infected pancreatic necrosis or surgical complications in other organs are present (see the next section).

Complications

Complications of acute pancreatitis can be local (peripancreatic) and/or systemic (multisystem organ failure; Table 16-6) and are directly related to the intensity of each patient's SIRS response. Local peripancreatic complications should be suspected when there is persistent or worsening abdominal pain and subsequent increases in serum amylase, indicative of ongoing acute inflammation. Other local complications include common bile duct obstruction or gastric outlet obstruction due to compression by a fluid collection or inflammation within the head of the pancreas. Gastric outlet obstruction is treated by nasogastric decompression, fluid and electrolyte

TABLE 16-6. Systemic Complications Associated With Severe Pancreatitis	
Shock	Systolic blood pressure < 90 mm Hg
Pulmonary insufficiency	$PaO_2/FIO_2 < 300$
Renal failure	Creatinine $\geq$177 µmol/L or >2 mg/dL after rehydration
Gastrointestinal bleeding	500 mL in 24 h
Disseminated intravascular coagulation	Platelets $\leq$100,000/mm^3, fibrinogen <1.0 g/L, and fibrin split products >80 µg/L
Severe metabolic disturbances	Calcium $\leq$ 1.87 mmol/L or $\leq$7.5 mg/dL

repletion, and possible surgical intervention to drain a compressing fluid collection. Another common complication of severe pancreatitis is splenic vein and/or portal vein (PV) thrombosis, due to inflammation and edema in the pancreatic head, body, or tail. This may result in left-sided (sinistral) portal hypertension with the formation of large gastric varices that may hemorrhage. Splenectomy is the definitive treatment for bleeding gastric varices resulting from sinistral portal hypertension. Another consequence of PV thrombosis is acute mesenteric ischemia. Long-term complications may also affect the exocrine function and require pancreatic enzyme replacement.

The systemic complications of acute pancreatitis are thought to be a function of the cytokine storm and the consequential SIRS response. Multiple organ systems can be adversely affected in this situation, the most common being pulmonary insufficiency (ARDS), acute kidney injury, and cardiovascular instability. Each organ-specific complication is potentially life threatening, and management requires meticulous supportive care.

Infected Pancreatic Necrosis

Infected pancreatic necrosis is the number one cause of mortality, which may occur in over 40% of patients. Pancreatic necrosis develops only in about 20% of patients with acute pancreatitis, and only about 5% develop a secondary infection. The risk of infection is directly related to the extent of necrosis and usually occurs 2 to 3 weeks after the onset of severe necrotizing pancreatitis. Infected pancreatic necrosis should be suspected in those patients with fever with worsening organ dysfunction and a rising leukocytosis. A CT scan demonstrating edema surrounding the pancreas and retroperitoneal air or air within the lesser sac, as seen in Figure 16-7, is diagnostic.

Infection by some organisms, however, does not produce air in the retroperitoneum. If the suspicion of infection is high, CT-guided needle aspiration of the fluid collection may be diagnostic. The fluid obtained should be sent for Gram stain and culture, including yeast. Prior prophylactic use of antibiotics, which is discouraged, may have substantially affected the organism resistance spectrum. If an infection is identified, debridement, large-scale drainage, antibiotics, and supportive care are required.

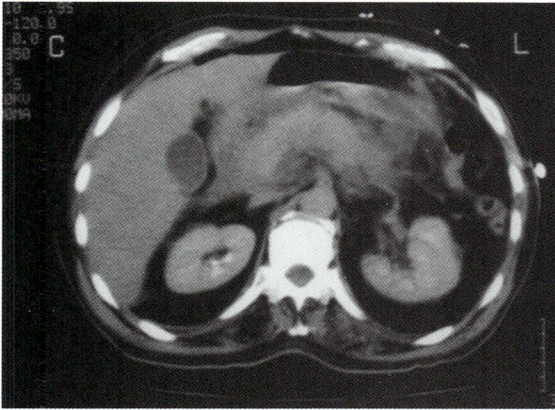

A

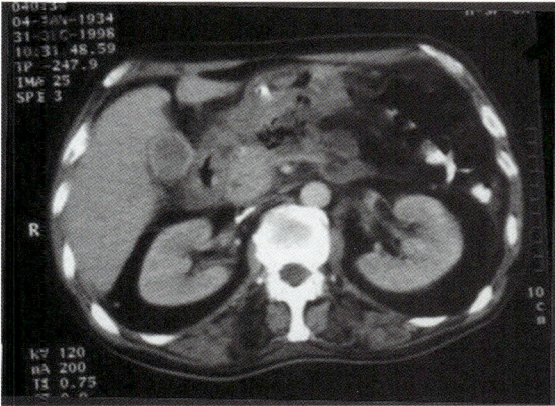

B

Figure 16-7. A. Computed tomography (CT) scan shows edema and inflammation surrounding most of the pancreas. B. CT scan after 30 days in the same patient. Air is present within the lesser sac signifying infected pancreatic necrosis.

The traditional invasive approach is associated with high rates of complications (34%-95%), death (11%-39%), and a risk of long-term pancreatic insufficiency. More recently, a minimally invasive step-up or endoscopic approach to pancreatic necrosectomy has been introduced. Compared with open necrosectomy, it reduces the rate of significant complications or death among patients with necrotizing pancreatitis and infected necrotic tissue.

Peripancreatic Fluid Collections and Pseudocysts

The most common complication of pancreatitis is the development of an acute fluid collection in the peripancreatic area or, in more severe cases, at distant locations in the retroperitoneum. This complication is caused by disruption of the pancreatic duct and the leakage of activated pancreatic enzymes into the mesentery and retroperitoneum, causing edema formation. These persistent fluid collections around the pancreas are walled off or contained by surrounding viscera and inflammatory tissue. Patients with peripancreatic fluid collections risk developing complications specific to the collection location. Therefore, a cystic mass should be followed closely for symptoms of biliary obstruction or gastric outlet obstruction. Most acute fluid collections

resolve spontaneously, but in those that persist, a collagen wall containing the fluid thickens or matures over time to form a well-defined pseudocyst, typically appearing some 3 to 4 weeks after the onset of acute pancreatitis. Defined as a collection of peripancreatic fluid contained in a cyst-like structure without an epithelial lining, pseudocysts may be either communicating or noncommunicating depending on whether or not the cyst is directly connected to the pancreatic duct. Pseudocysts may grow to a large size and can commonly cause symptoms related to the compression and obstruction of adjacent structures (mass effect), especially of the stomach, duodenum, or common bile duct. Therefore, internal or external drainage, depending on ductal anatomy evident on MRCP or ERCP, of these symptomatic pseudocysts is recommended.

Asymptomatic small pseudocysts may be followed, but those that persist for more than 1 year or are already larger than 5 cm tend to enlarge and eventually cause obstructive symptoms, so pseudocyst drainage of these asymptomatic pseudocysts is indicated.

CT scans are the best imaging studies for pseudocyst evaluation (Figure 16-8). CT scans allow delineation of the cyst wall thickness and its relationship to the surrounding structures. This is critically important when planning for surgery to address the pseudocyst. Mature pseudocysts, generally those more than 4 weeks "old," have thick walls suitable for suturing and may be treated in various ways. External drainage of a communicating pseudocyst is contraindicated because doing so would lead to a chronic pancreatic fistula or secondary infection. Communicating pseudocysts require internal drainage into the stomach, duodenum, or Roux limb because they communicate directly with the pancreatic duct. Internal drainage is accomplished by anastomosing the mature cyst wall directly to the stomach or other recipient drainage organ. During the procedure, a part of the cyst wall should be sent for frozen section pathologic evaluation to ensure that the cyst is not a neoplasm. Internal drainage is successful in over 90% of cases. Noncommunicating pseudocysts may be aspirated or drained percutaneously with little risk of re-formation or fistula formation. In centers with advanced endoscopic

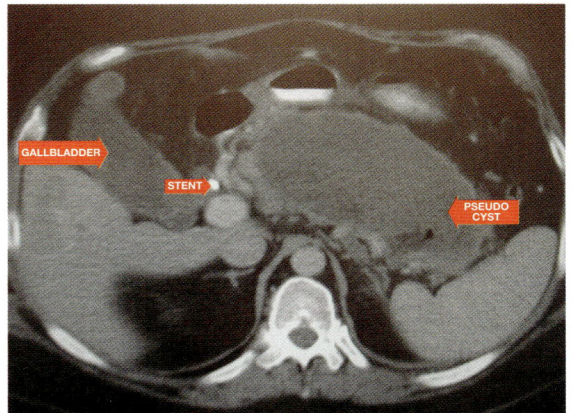

Figure 16-8. Computed tomography scan showing a large pancreatic pseudocyst. The wall of the pseudocyst is enhanced and thickened. An endostent is also present within the common bile duct because of a stricture formed in the bile duct due to the episode of pancreatitis.

facilities, other forms of treatment are available, such as pancreatic stenting and transgastric decompression.

Chronic Pancreatitis

Etiology

Alcohol consumption is related to approximately 70% of cases of chronic pancreatitis. Less common causes include anatomic variations (pancreatic divisum) and specific genetic causes such as cystic fibrosis. It differs from acute pancreatitis in that the glandular damage is no longer reversible and is usually progressive. Each recurring episode of pancreatitis contributes to forming a scarred, fibrotic gland with an abnormal ductal system that drains poorly and is easily clogged with debris.

Clinical Presentation and Evaluation

The most common symptom of chronic pancreatitis is chronic pain. The pain is usually dull and epigastric in location and radiates to the back. The pain is initially intermittent, but with the progression of the disease, it becomes constant and unrelenting. Any retroperitoneal neoplasm (sarcoma) can also present with similar features. Food often makes the pain worse. Self-medication of pain by increased alcohol ingestion and/or narcotic use with drug dependency is common. When 90% of the gland has been damaged or replaced with scar, endocrine and exocrine insufficiencies are manifested by malabsorption, diabetes, and deficiencies in fat-soluble vitamins, causing malnutrition. Oral pancreatic enzyme replacement generally aids in treating steatorrhea.

Unless a pancreatic pseudocyst is palpable, the abdominal examination of these patients tends to be unremarkable. Likewise, laboratory blood studies tend to be normal unless the chronic inflammation has led to biliary duct obstruction, in which case typical lab values of obstructive jaundice are evident.

Depending on the clinical situation, patients with chronic pancreatitis should undergo various imaging studies. If the etiology of the disease is not understood, CT, MRCP, and ERCP may play a role in determining other non–alcohol-related causes. CT usually shows atrophy, inflammation, tumors, fluid collections or pseudocysts, pancreatic ductal dilation, or calcifications (Figure 16-9). MRCP and ERCP may identify pancreas divisum (Figure 16-10), obstructing

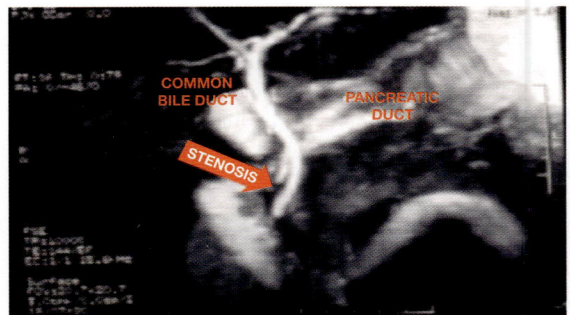

Figure 16-10. Magnetic resonance cholangiopancreatography shows stenosis of the minor duct and a dilated main pancreatic duct.

pancreatic duct stones, or pancreatic ductal strictures. ERCP is an invasive test with a small risk of exacerbating pancreatitis or biliary or pancreatic sepsis. ERCP is most sensitive for defining the pancreatic and bile ductal architecture, including the duct size and whether there are strictures, fistulas, or obstruction, which are essential to know before any operative intervention.

Treatment

Medical treatment is the mainstay for patients with chronic pancreatitis but rarely resolves the pain. It includes treatment of alcoholism and narcotic dependence, as well as a low-fat diabetic diet with pancreatic enzyme replacement to minimize steatorrhea and hyperglycemia. Surgery is indicated for those patients with chronic pain and other complications of the disease in which discreet and anatomically correctable abnormalities are identified. Preoperative imaging with CT, ERCP, or MRCP helps identify pancreatic ductal obstructions, strictures, calculi, masses, duct ectasia, pseudocysts, and the surrounding vascular anatomy. CT and MRCP are noninvasive tests but usually do not show sufficient detail to plan operative intervention. ERCP and/or MRCP are frequently required to outline ductal anatomy when planning any surgical intervention. Occasionally, isolated obstructing lesions within the pancreatic duct or at the level of the ampulla can be managed with endoscopic stenting.

Surgical options for treating chronic pancreatitis fall into two main categories: drainage or resectional procedures. The benefit of drainage procedures includes preserving any remaining functional pancreatic tissue, thereby delaying the onset of both exocrine and endocrine insufficiency. Drainage procedures work best on those with a dilated pancreatic duct (>4 mm). In contrast, resectional procedures are used in patients with nondilated ducts and disease that can be localized to a specific location within the gland. Patients with dilated ducts, including those with segmental ductal obstructions ("chain of lakes"), can undergo internal ductal decompression into a loop of jejunum, which is called a lateral pancreaticojejunostomy (Puestow procedure). This drainage procedure results in approximately 70% of patients achieving lasting pain relief. When the ductal system is not dilated, and no focal disease is identified, resectional procedures such as pancreaticoduodenectomy, distal pancreatectomy, and duodenum-preserving pancreatic head resections (Beger or Frey

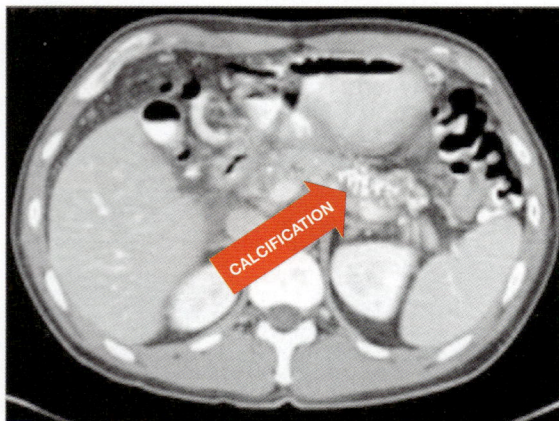

Figure 16-9. Computed tomography scan demonstrating multiple calcifications throughout the body and tail consistent with chronic pancreatitis.

procedures) are indicated. Total pancreatectomy has been utilized but is not recommended because of the severe exocrine and endocrine dysfunction that follows. Another option for pain relief in this group may be attempted via splanchnicectomy (neurolysis), which can be performed percutaneously, endoscopically, or surgically, but results have been disappointing, with poor long-term durability.

Pancreatic Neoplasms (Excluding Neuroendocrine Tumors)

General Considerations

Pancreatic neoplasms may be malignant, premalignant, or benign, as shown in Table 16-7. Over 90% of pancreatic cancers are adenocarcinomas originating from the ductal epithelium, with the remainder being islet cell tumors, lymphomas, and metastatic lesions. Benign neoplasms are significantly less common than malignant or premalignant tumors.

Pancreatic adenocarcinoma is the fourth most common cause of cancer death in the United States. The principal risk factors include increasing age and cigarette smoking, which doubles the risk of developing pancreatic cancer. The etiologic roles of diabetes, pancreatitis, and alcohol in pancreatic carcinoma remain controversial. Despite multimodality treatment, approximately 98% of patients diagnosed with pancreatic adenocarcinoma die from the disease. Two-thirds of the cases of pancreatic carcinoma occur in the head of the gland, but these adenocarcinomas may also be multicentric.

Genetic Mutations Associated With Pancreatic Cancer

Pancreatic cancer has been associated with three main genetic abnormalities: (1) oncogene activation, (2) tumor suppressor gene inactivation, and (3) overexpression of growth factors or their receptors (Table 16-8).

It is generally believed that pancreatic cancer evolves in a progressive, stepwise fashion, much like that

TABLE 16-7. Pancreatic Neoplasms Excluding Neuroendocrine Tumors of the Pancreas

Malignant

Adenocarcinoma
Mucinous cystadenocarcinoma
Mucinous noncystic carcinoma
Lymphoma
Metastatic disease

Premalignant

Mucinous adenoma
Mucinous cystic neoplasm
IPMN
Solid pseudopapillary neoplasm (Hamoudi tumor)

Benign Neoplasms

Serous cystadenoma (microcystic adenoma)
Pseudocyst
Simple cyst

IPMN, intraductal papillary mucinous neoplasm.

TABLE 16-8. Genetic Mutations Associated With Pancreatic Cancer

Type of Mutation	Name of Gene or Growth Factor
Oncogenes	K-*ras* (Kirsten rat sarcoma)
Tumor suppressor genes	p53
	p16
	SMAD4/DPC
	DCC
	APC
	DNA mismatch repair
	RB gene
Growth factors	EGF receptor
	HER2, HER3, and HER4 receptors

APC, adenomatous polyposis coli; DCC, deleted in colorectal carcinoma; DPC, deleted in pancreatic cancer; EGF, epidermal growth factor; HER, human epidermal growth factor; RB, retinoblastoma; SMAD4, small Mad domain 4.

observed in colon cancer. Precursor ductal lesions have been identified, and the stepwise progression toward invasive cancer and metastasis has been related to the accumulated presence of multiple genetic abnormalities. The most commonly expressed, earliest-appearing genetic mutation in malignant pancreatic neoplasms occurs in the K-*ras* (Kirsten rat sarcoma) oncogene that serves as a growth-promoting oncogene. Other mutations lead to the inactivation of tumor suppressor genes during the later stages of cancer progression and are found almost exclusively in invasive lesions.

The incidence of pancreatic cancer is increased in families with hereditary nonpolyposis colon cancer, familial breast cancer (associated with the *BRCA2* mutation), Peutz-Jeghers syndrome, and the familial atypical multiple mole–melanoma (FAMMM) syndrome. Patients with a paternal relative having pancreatic cancer are at a 75% risk for developing pancreatic cancer.

Clinical Presentation and Evaluation

The signs and symptoms of pancreatic carcinoma are related to the location of the tumor and its effects on surrounding structures. Periampullary carcinomas, such as those of the duodenum and ampulla of Vater, often present with painless jaundice earlier than those of the head of the pancreas and hence have a better prognosis. Constant back pain or epigastric pain radiating to the back without evidence of the patient having jaundice is the classic presentation of pancreatic cancer in the body or tail. Being remote from the common bile duct and producing no biliary obstruction, back pain is the usual first complaint of these patients because of tumor cells invading the retroperitoneal nerves of the celiac plexus. The absence of symptoms until the disease is advanced accounts for its poor prognosis. A palpable nontender gallbladder associated with painless jaundice is more commonly associated with malignancy (Courvoisier sign).

The evaluation of patients with jaundice includes serum chemistries. Along with elevated total and direct bilirubin levels, markedly elevated alkaline phosphatase and γ-glutamyl transferase (GGT) levels, significantly higher than a slight elevation in transaminase, are suggestive of obstructive jaundice.

Liver function studies suggesting obstructive jaundice demand further imaging studies, beginning with ultrasonography. US is useful in identifying the location of the ductal obstruction and possible etiologies, such as choledocholithiasis and cholangiocarcinoma, most commonly located at the confluence of the common hepatic ducts. In patients with a history and physical findings suggestive of a pancreatic neoplasm, CT scans are the best modality for examining the pancreas. CT provides information about the level of biliary tract obstruction, delineates masses and their relation to vital structures, and identifies liver metastases. A high-quality, contrast-enhanced CT scan is required to stage the lesion preoperatively and to determine tumor resectability, as defined by the absence of distant spread of disease, ascites, and lack of involvement of the SMV, PV, SMA, hepatic artery, vena cava, or aorta. Figure 16-11A shows a normal CT scan of the SMV and SMA, vena cava, and aorta. Figure 16-11B shows a CT scan demonstrating an unresectable pancreatic mass involving the SMV–PV junction, as seen by contrast, ending abruptly in the splenic vein at the pancreatic mass. MRCP, ERCP, and percutaneous transhepatic cholangiography can also delineate biliary and pancreatic ductal anatomy; each has its unique indication. A preoperative biopsy of a

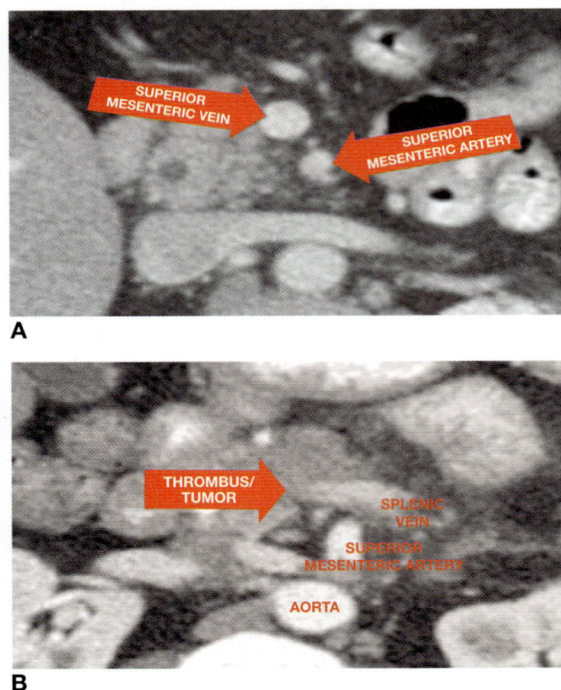

Figure 16-12. Algorithm for the evaluation of a pancreatic mass. CT, computed tomography. (Drawing by Matthew Campbell.)

resectable pancreatic mass is not always indicated because of a high false negative rate, difficulty establishing the diagnosis, or postprocedural bleeding, all of which can delay resection. The diagnostic algorithm for evaluating a pancreatic neoplasm is shown in Figure 16-12.

Treatment

Obstructive jaundice may result in vitamin K-related coagulopathy because of interruption of the enterohepatic circulation; associated malnutrition should also be corrected before any major operation. Baseline laboratory studies to evaluate hepatic function and nutritional status include albumin, transferrin, prealbumin, and prothrombin times. Patients with preoperative studies suggesting resectability should undergo surgical exploration with a curative intent to proceed. Preoperative drainage of the biliary system is not indicated when imaging studies suggest a resectable pancreatic tumor. These preoperative biliary drainage procedures increase the risk of infectious complications after pancreatic resection.

Pancreatic head or periampullary lesions are best approached with pancreaticoduodenectomy (Whipple procedure) whereas body and tail lesions are treated with a distal pancreatectomy, which usually includes a splenectomy. Pancreaticoduodenectomy involves resection of the distal common bile duct, duodenum, and head of the pancreas, as seen in Figure 16-13. In the classic Whipple operation, the gastric antrum, the head of the pancreas, and the entire duodenum are removed. Reconstruction includes a choledochojejunostomy, pancreaticojejunostomy, and gastrojejunostomy. Although mortality for the procedure is less than 5%, complications are common, but most can usually be managed without reoperation. The most feared complication is an anastomotic leak, with the highest rate at the pancreaticojejunostomy site, which can lead to abscess formation, possible sepsis, or a pancreatic fistula. An anastomotic leak or disruption is usually managed by drainage and optimization of nutrition. Other procedure-related complications include delayed gastric emptying, leak from the other anastomoses, and diabetes. Minimally invasive methods of pancreaticoduodenectomy involving laparoscopic or robotic approaches are being developed.

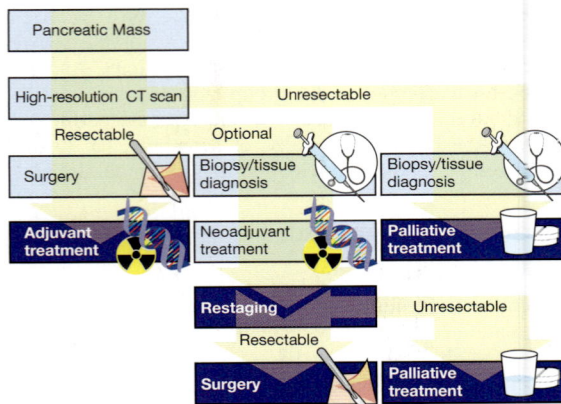

Figure 16-11. A. Computed tomography (CT) scan showing a patent portal and superior mesenteric vein (SMV). Neither the superior mesenteric artery nor SMV is encroached upon by the tumor. B. CT scan of an unresectable pancreatic mass secondary to portal-SMV replacement by tumor. An endostent is present in the common bile duct.

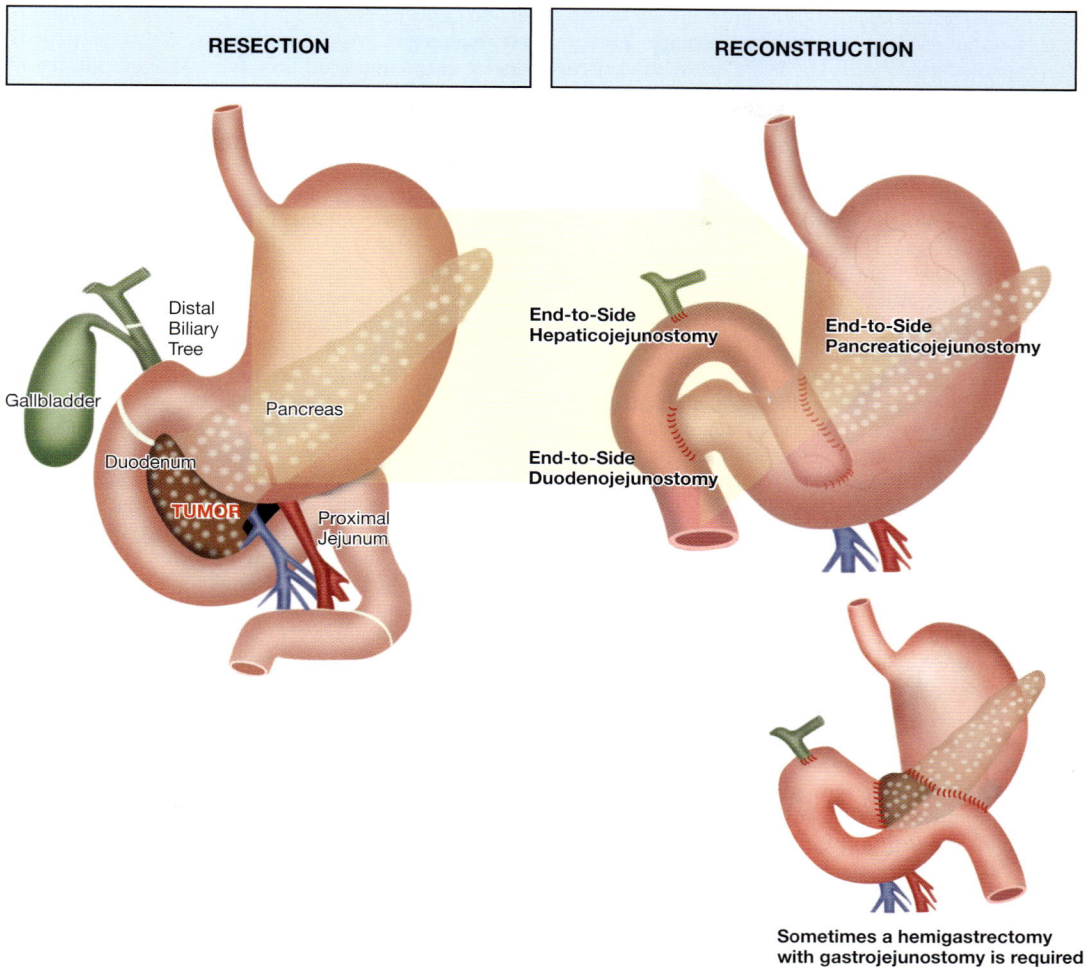

RESECTION

RECONSTRUCTION

Distal
Biliary
Tree

Gallbladder

Pancreas

Duodenum

TUMOR

Proximal
Jejunum

End-to-Side
Hepaticojejunostomy

End-to-Side
Duodenojejunostomy

End-to-Side
Pancreaticojejunostomy

**Sometimes a hemigastrectomy
with gastrojejunostomy is required**

Figure 16-13. Pancreaticoduodenectomy. The resection is shown on the left, and on the right reconstruction with a pancreaticojejunostomy, choledochojejunostomy, and a duodenojejunostomy above or gastrojejunostomy below is shown. The top reconstruction is used for pylorus-preserving pancreaticoduodenectomies, and the bottom approach is used when a hemigastrectomy is required. (Drawing by Matthew Campbell.)

Laparoscopy is sometimes performed before celiotomy to search for metastatic disease not visualized by preoperative imaging studies. A palliative biliary bypass is typically carried out if unresectable disease is found during exploration. Gastric outlet obstruction (early satiety, bloating, and emesis of undigested nonbilious gastric contents) develops in approximately 10% of patients with unresectable pancreatic cancer and requires a palliative gastrojejunostomy. Back pain can be improved with celiac axis neurolysis. For patients whose preoperative evaluations show unresectable disease, palliation of pruritus due to hyperbilirubinemia can usually be achieved by endoscopically stenting the biliary tract.

Prognosis

Most patients with pancreatic cancer present with unresectable disease and have a median survival of approximately 6 months, even with chemotherapy. Surgical resection extends life to approximately 19 months if negative margins are obtained and adjuvant chemoradiation is tolerated.

These patients, however, usually die from this disease, with approximately 20% surviving 5 years. Poor prognostic indicators include lymph node metastasis, tumor size larger than 3 cm, and perineural invasion.

Adjuvant and Neoadjuvant Treatment for Pancreatic Cancer

Pancreatic cancer has a low resectability rate, a high recurrence rate after surgical resection, and poor long-term survival rates, presumably because of the presence of micrometastatic disease after surgical resection. Because of these facts, efforts have been directed toward developing neoadjuvant and adjuvant therapies to improve survival. Neoadjuvant therapy is the treatment given to patients preoperatively to enhance the curative resection rates and survival. Presently, studies are underway to determine whether neoadjuvant therapy is efficacious in converting marginally resectable lesions (those tumors abutting the SMA or partially encasing the SMV) into resectable ones. Proponents hypothesize that neoadjuvant therapy reduces the chance of leaving behind microscopic or gross disease during resection. Neoadjuvant regimens also allow radiation delivery to well-oxygenated cancer cells and avoid delays in chemotherapy administration related to complications after resection. A tissue diagnosis is mandatory before neoadjuvant therapy is initiated, and endoscopic US (EUS) with biopsy provides this information. Pruritus can be alleviated due to hyperbilirubinemia by endoscopically stenting the biliary tract while the patient receives this neoadjuvant treatment. Until large randomized trials comparing neoadjuvant therapy to adjuvant therapy or resection alone are carried out, the utility of neoadjuvant therapy in pancreatic cancer will remain unknown.

Adjuvant strategies include systemic chemotherapy and chemoradiation, based on the belief that chemoradiation and chemotherapy are better than surgery alone. A recent Mayo Clinic study has shown a survival benefit with the addition of chemoradiation therapy (radiation to the area of the pancreatic resection combined with IV gemcitabine or 5-fluorouracil [5-FU] and leucovorin) after an R0 resection. In contrast, two recent randomized trials from Europe have supported the use of systemic chemotherapy alone in the adjuvant setting. Large clinical trials are needed to resolve these differences.

Pancreatic Endocrine Tumors

Pancreatic neuroendocrine tumors (pNETs) are known by various synonyms, including pancreatic islet cell tumors and neuroendocrine neoplasms. They are much less common than pancreatic adenocarcinoma and comprise approximately 7% of all pancreatic malignancies. There is no gender predilection, and pNETs may occur at any age, with the peak incidence occurring between the ages of 30 and 60 years.

Depending on whether they are associated with a clinical syndrome secondary to peptide secretion, pNETs are categorized as functional or nonfunctional (Table 16-9). Approximately 50% of pNETs are nonfunctional. Although nonfunctional pNETs may secrete peptides such as PP, CgA, neurotensin, or ghrelin, these increased hormone outputs are not associated with a clinically recognizable syndrome. Most pNETs occur sporadically, and symptoms are directly related to predominant hormone production by the pNET. Following a CT or positron emission tomography (PET) scan, identification of these lesions and treatment involve pancreatic resection for all pNETs. Metastatic disease is often identified with octreotide scans.

Insulinoma

Insulinomas comprise 20% to 30% of all pNETs and are the most common functional pNETs. Majority (85%-90%)

TABLE 16-9. Pancreatic Neuroendocrine Tumors

Benign (Majority)
Insulinoma

Malignant (Majority)
Gastrinoma
Glucagonoma
Somatostatinoma
VIPoma
PPoma
Nonfunctional islet cell

PP, pancreatic polypeptide; VIP, vasoactive intestinal polypeptide.

are benign whereas the majority (60%) of all other pNETs are malignant. Most insulinomas are solitary and less than 2 cm in diameter, and about 75% are located in the body and tail of the pancreas whereas majority of all other functional pNETs are located in the head of the pancreas. About 10% of patients with insulinoma have multiple endocrine neoplasia 1 (MEN 1) syndrome.

Insulin hypersecretion causes hypoglycemia manifested by sweating, hunger, weakness, anxiety, irritability, headaches, blurry vision, incoherence, confusion, personality changes, amnesia, psychosis, peripheral distal neuropathy, palpitations, diaphoresis, tremors, seizure, and coma. Patients eat frequent meals with a high sugar content and often gain weight attempting to prevent hypoglycemic symptoms. These patients are also frequently diagnosed with psychiatric conditions or epilepsy before receiving the correct diagnosis because of the vagueness of their symptoms and erratic behavior often observed.

Insulinoma is confirmed during a monitored 72-hour fast and thin-cut enhanced CT scan of the pancreas. The Whipple triad ([1] symptoms of hypoglycemia, [2] a low blood glucose level [40-50 mg/dL], and [3] relief of symptoms following the IV administration of glucose) is suggestive of insulinoma. There are, however, six diagnostic criteria of insulinoma: (1) documented blood glucose of 45 mg/dL or less, (2) concomitant serum insulin levels of 36 μU/L or more, (3) plasma/serum C-peptide levels of 200 pmol/L or more, (4) serum proinsulin levels of 5 pmol/L or more, (5) serum β-hydroxybutyrate levels of 2.7 mmol/L or less, and (6) the absence of sulfonylurea in the plasma and/or urine. When results are indeterminate, a secretin injection test may help make the diagnosis. Normally, secretin stimulates the release of insulin from β-cells, but insulinomas do not release insulin in response to secretin and also inhibit the normal response of β-cells to secretin. Thus, patients with insulinoma do not show increased insulin production in response to secretin. Certain insulinomas may be surgically enucleated when small and remote from the main pancreatic duct. When larger and adjacent to the pancreatic duct, formal pancreatectomy is indicated. Diazoxide or streptozotocin can be used for patients with unresectable or metastatic disease.

Gastrinoma

Zollinger and Ellison initially identified gastrinomas, which account for approximately 20% of the functional pNETs. Three-quarters occur sporadically, and one-fourth occur as part of MEN 1 syndrome. In patients with MEN 1 syndrome, gastrinomas are the most common functional islet cell tumor. Many gastrinomas are not found in the pancreas, with over 50% located within the duodenal wall. Between 60% and 90% are found within the gastrinoma triangle (Figure 16-14), defined by the junction of the common bile and cystic ducts, the neck and body of the pancreas, and the second and third parts of the duodenum.

Gastrinomas are multicentric in half of the cases and tend to metastasize to lymph nodes and the liver (50%). Gastric acid hypersecretion is responsible for most symptoms, including intractable abdominal pain, severe esophagitis, persistent diarrhea resulting from small bowel mucosal injury, inactivation of lipase, and precipitation of bile salts. Thus, when gastric acid secretion is controlled, symptoms resolve regardless of the gastrin level.

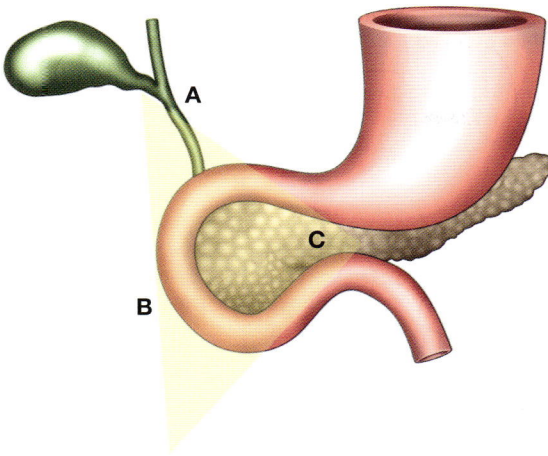

Figure 16-14. The gastrinoma triangle. Approximately 90% of gastrinomas are located within the region bounded by the confluence of the cystic duct and common bile duct (A), the junction of the second and third parts of the duodenum (B), and the junction of the neck and body of the pancreas (C). (Drawing by Matthew Campbell.)

The diagnosis should be considered in all patients with peptic ulcers and diarrhea, particularly when peptic ulcers are identified by esophagogastroduodenoscopy (EGD) in unusual locations and in patients who develop recurrent peptic ulcers that are resistant to treatment. A fasting serum gastrin level should be measured in patients requiring gastric surgery for peptic ulcer disease. Gastrin levels greater than 1,000 pg/mL in a patient with a gastric pH less than 2 is diagnostic. Two-thirds of patients with gastrinoma, however, have gastrin levels less than 1,000 pg/mL and require additional testing. In this group, an elevated fasting gastrin level greater than 200 pg/mL and a positive secretin stimulation test, defined as an increase in gastrin greater than 200 pg/mL after secretin injection, are diagnostic. (Note that secretin normally causes a decrease in the gastrin level.) All patients found to have a gastrinoma must have a serum calcium level drawn to rule out MEN 1 syndrome.

Gastrin levels may also be elevated for a variety of reasons besides a gastrinoma. Hypergastrinemic states include patients with pernicious anemia or atrophic gastritis, chronic renal failure, use of proton-pump inhibitors, *Helicobacter pylori* infection, postvagotomy syndromes, G-cell hyperplasia, retained antrum, short bowel syndrome, and gastric outlet obstruction. Before diagnosing gastrinoma, these conditions should be considered in the differential diagnosis for any patient with an elevated gastrin level.

Glucagonoma

Glucagonomas arise from pancreatic α cells. They are more commonly located in the body or tail of the gland. Patients usually present with large lesions and metastatic disease. Symptoms include mild glucose intolerance and, in over half of the cases, necrolytic migratory erythema, which is a characteristic skin rash. Patients develop frequent deep vein thromboses, thrombophlebitis, weight loss, anemia, cachexia, and psychiatric disorders. A serum glucagon level of 500 to 1,000 pg/mL is diagnostic.

Octreotide provides symptomatic relief for those with metastatic disease.

Vasoactive Intestinal Polypeptidoma

Vasoactive intestinal polypeptide (VIP) tumor (VIPomas) cause watery diarrhea, hypokalemia, and hypochlorhydria. This triad is called the watery diarrhea, hypokalemia, and achlorhydria (WDHA) syndrome, pancreatic cholera, endocrine cholera, or Verner-Morrison syndrome. The diarrhea is chronic, unresponsive to medical management, large in volume (6-8 L/day), and present despite fasting. Patients experience dehydration, weight loss, and metabolic acidosis. VIP also inhibits gastric acid output and stimulates bone resorption, glycogenolysis, and vasodilatation, which can cause hypochlorhydria, hypercalcemia, hyperglycemia, and flushing. A serum VIP level greater than 75 to 150 pg/mL is diagnostic. Octreotide helps control diarrhea in patients with metastatic disease.

Somatostatinoma

Somatostatinomas may arise in the pancreas, ampulla, duodenum, jejunum, cystic duct, or rectum. Somatostatin inhibits the production of various hormones, including growth hormone, gastrin, insulin, and glucagon. Somatostatin also inhibits intestinal absorption, gastrointestinal motility, and gallbladder contraction. Patients can present in various manners and may develop diabetes, gallstones, and diarrhea, resulting in hypochlorhydria with steatorrhea. Most patients' symptoms are nonspecific and include pain, weight loss, and a change in bowel habits. Somatostatinomas are usually located in the pancreatic head (60%) and are large solitary lesions at the time of diagnosis (>5 cm, range 0.5-10 cm), and up to 90% are malignant. Because of their size and malignant nature, enucleation is not indicated here; instead, resection should be performed. A fasting somatostatin level greater than 160 pg/mL and a pancreatic or duodenal mass are diagnostic.

Evaluation

All patients with pNETs should undergo a CT or magnetic resonance imaging (MRI) for localization, determination of resectability, and evaluation for metastatic disease. Functional tumors often present earlier than nonfunctional tumors because of their clinical symptoms of excess hormone production. Hence, they are typically smaller and can be more challenging to image. Radiographically, most pNETs look like solid hypervascular lesions. Imaging findings of calcification, necrosis, and invasion of retroperitoneal structures suggest malignancy. EUS may help identify small pancreatic lesions.

When an insulinoma is suspected, and CT, MRI, and EUS cannot localize the lesion, selective arterial calcium stimulation and hepatic venous sampling (ASVS [arterial selective venous sampling]) can be performed. Insulinoma cells increase the secretion of insulin in response to calcium. Calcium gluconate is injected separately into the GDA, mid and proximal splenic arteries, and SMA whereas insulin levels are obtained from the right hepatic vein. Depending on the location of the selective arterial calcium injection, the finding of an elevated hepatic vein insulin level would suggest that the insulinoma is located in the pancreatic tissue where the calcium was intraarterially infused. It does not show the insulinoma but allows for surgery to be targeted to a specific area of the pancreas needing resection. Intraoperative US can also be helpful in combination with ASVS in identifying the lesion.

Somatostatin scintigraphy (octreoscan) should also be carried out for all pNETs, except for insulinoma, because it is not readily detected with a sensitivity of less than 50%. Octreoscan is also very useful for evaluating metastatic pNETs. PET may also be complementary to octreoscan. Should localizing studies fail to identify the location of a gastrinoma, a selective arterial secretagogue injection test with the arterial injection of calcium or secretin can be used similarly to the ASVS test with measurement of gastrin levels in venous tributaries to localize the gastrinoma to a specific area in the patient.

Treatment

Curative treatment of pNETs requires complete surgical extirpation of the primary and all metastatic disease. Resection should not be undertaken if extraabdominal or bony metastases are identified. Overall survival is significantly better than with adenocarcinoma, and long-term survival with metastatic disease is possible for patients with these typically slow-growing tumors. Surgical debulking procedures for liver metastases are also appropriate if at least 90% of the tumor can be removed.

The symptoms of pNETs should be controlled preoperatively using somatostatin analogues and proton-pump inhibitors. Surgery for small gastrinomas can be aided by intraoperative duodenoscopy with transillumination, as many of these are located within the duodenal wall. Pancreatic head lesions are best treated by pancreaticoduodenectomy whereas body or tail lesions are treated with distal pancreatectomy. Metastases should be resected, if possible, to help control the systemic effects of excess hormone production.

Nonoperative palliative treatment includes symptom control and ablative modalities, including radiofrequency ablation, cryotherapy, hepatic artery embolization, and chemoembolization using cisplatin and doxorubicin, or combinations of these with systemic chemotherapeutic agents.

Chemotherapy with streptozocin, 5-FU, and doxorubicin can be used as salvage therapy for malignant insulinomas but has poor efficacy and significant toxicity. Somatostatin analogues can control symptoms in almost 100% of patients. These analogues are well tolerated and may briefly stabilize disease progression but not prolong survival.

Staging and Prognosis

The malignant potential and staging of pNETs are determined by several features such as the tumor's cytologic and histologic characteristics, mitotic index, nuclear pleomorphism, the Ki-67 index along capsular extension, focal vascular invasion, and tumor invasion into adjacent organs or overt metastatic disease. In 2004, the World Health Organization DEVELOPED a classification system for pNETs and placed them into three risk groups (Table 16-10) based on these histologic criteria. This staging system is useful for determining the prognosis.

Pancreatic Cystic Lesions

Although ductal adenocarcinoma is the most common neoplasm, an increasing number of pancreatic cystic lesions are being identified on CT scans of the abdomen. In addition to previously discussed pseudocysts, there are both benign and malignant pancreatic cyst tumors, as outlined in Table 16-11. Each of these may be asymptomatic and incidentally discovered on CT scans. These lesions can cause abdominal pain, nausea, vomiting, weight loss, jaundice, or gastric outlet obstruction when symptomatic. Differentiating these lesions from each other can be difficult, but it is important because the management of each varies. Often, the CT scan characteristics provide precise diagnostic help, but, on occasion, EGD-directed ultrasonography with fluid aspiration and wall biopsy are required to arrive at the exact final diagnosis (Table 16-11). Serous cystadenomas are benign and do not need formal resection.

Although very rare, when identified, serous cystadenocarcinomas should be resected. The mucinous cystic

---

TABLE 16-10. Classification of Neuroendocrine Tumors of the Pancreas

1. Well-differentiated neuroendocrine tumor
   - Benign: confined to pancreas, <2 cm in size, nonangioinvasive, ≤2 mitoses/HPF, and ≤2% Ki-67-positive cells
     - Functional insulinoma
     - Nonfunctional
   - Benign or low-grade malignant (uncertain malignant potential): confined to the pancreas, ≥2 cm in size, >2 mitoses/HPF, >2% Ki-67-positive cells, or angioinvasive
     - Functional: gastrinoma, insulinoma, VIPoma, glucagonoma, somatostatinoma, or ectopic hormonal syndrome
     - Nonfunctional
2. Well-differentiated neuroendocrine carcinoma
   - Low-grade malignant: invasion of adjacent organs and/or metastases
     - Functional: gastrinoma, insulinoma, glucagonoma, VIPomas, somatostatinoma, or ectopic hormonal syndrome
     - Nonfunctional
3. Poorly differentiated neuroendocrine carcinoma
   - High-grade malignant

HPF, high-power field; VIP, vasoactive intestinal polypeptide.

From DeLellis L, Heitz PU, Eng C, eds. Tumors of the endocrine pancreas. In: DeLellis L, Heitz PU, Eng C, eds. *Pathology and Genetics: Tumors of the Endocrine Organs.* WHO Classification of Tumors. IARC Press; 2004:175-208 (Table 71). Used with permission.

TABLE 16-11. Pancreatic Cystic Lesions: Differentiation Based on EGD US Cyst Fluid Aspiration and Biopsy

Pancreatic Cystic Lesion	Cyst Fluid Analysis	Pathology
Serous cystadenoma	Serous cystadenoma	No mitoses
Serous cystadenocarcinoma	Low amylase, CEA, and 19-9	+mitoses
Mucinous cystadenoma	High CEA, 19-9	No mitoses, +ovarian stroma
Mucinous cystadenocarcinoma	Higher CEA, 19-9	+mitoses, +ovarian stroma
IPMN	High CEA	Dysplasia, no ovarian stroma

CEA, carcinoembryonic antigen; EGD, esophagogastroduodenoscopy; IPMN, intraductal papillary mucinous neoplasm; US, ultrasound.

neoplasms are seen almost only in middle-aged women, are frequently symptomatic, and contain ovarian stroma on histology, unlike the other cystic lesions. About 40% are invasive malignancies at the time of diagnosis and are most commonly located in the body and tail of the pancreas. These lesions should be resected. Intraductal papillary mucinous neoplasms (IPMNs) are a type of mucinous neoplasm of the pancreas that does not contain ovarian stroma. More commonly seen in men, IPMNs involve either the main pancreatic or side branch ducts. Main-duct involvement, suggested by main-duct dilation greater than 5 mm, is much more commonly found to be malignant and invasive than small-duct IPMNs. Nearly all main-duct IPMNs should be resected. Branch-duct IPMNs should be observed with serial CT scans unless symptomatic, greater than 3 cm in size, or are found to have worrisome features on CT scans (nodules) or cytology.

SUGGESTED READINGS

Banks PA, Bollen TL, Dervenis C, et al. Classification of acute pancreatitis—2012: revision of the Atlanta Classification and definitions by international consensus. *Gut*. 2013;62(1):102-111.

Balthazar EJ. Acute pancreatitis: assessment of severity with clinical and CT evaluation. *Radiology*. 2002;223(3):603-613. doi: 10.1148/radiol.2233010680.

Karakas Y, Lacin S, Yalcin S. Recent advances in the management of pancreatic adenocarcinoma. *Expert Rev Anticancer Ther*. 2018;18(1):51-62.

Lewis A, Li D, Williams J, Singh G. Pancreatic neuroendocrine tumors: state-of-the-art diagnosis and management. *Oncology*. 2017;31(10):e1-e12.

Parekh D, Natarajan S. Surgical management of chronic pancreatitis. *Indian J Surg*. 2015;77(5):453-469.

Working Group IAP/APA Acute Pancreatitis Guidelines. IAP/APA evidence-based guidelines for the management of acute pancreatitis. *Pancreatology*. 2013;13:e1-e15.

SAMPLE QUESTIONS

QUESTIONS

Choose the best answer for each question.

1. A 20-year-old man comes to the emergency department with severe epigastric pain. He has a history of postprandial right upper quadrant discomfort and fatty food intolerance. He has otherwise been healthy. He does not smoke or drink alcohol. He takes no medications. His vital signs are temperature of 37 °C, blood pressure (BP) of 130/80 mm Hg, pulse of 110/min, and respirations of 18/min. He has severe epigastric tenderness with guarding. There is no scleral icterus. A US shows gallstones. The bile ducts are not dilated. Laboratory studies show the following:

   Lipase: 20,000 U/L
   Amylase: 800 U/L
   Total bilirubin: 0.9 mg/dL
   Alkaline phosphatase: 20 mg/dL

   Which of the following should be part of his treatment plan?

   A. Foley catheter and diuretics to maintain urine output greater than 40 mL/h
   B. Exploratory laparotomy to evaluate acute abdomen findings
   C. Immediate ERCP
   D. Supportive treatment and cholecystectomy before discharge
   E. MRCP

2. A 50-year-old woman has severe gallstone pancreatitis. She receives IV fluid and nothing by mouth to slow pancreatic secretions and reduce the amount of active pancreatic enzymes leaking into the disrupted glandular tissue. Which of the following enzymes is produced by the pancreas and secreted in its active form?

   A. Amylase
   B. Trypsin
   C. Chymotrypsin
   D. CCK
   E. Gastrin

3. A 42-year-old man comes to the emergency department with severe abdominal pain. He takes no medications. He drinks a quart of vodka daily and smokes one to two packs of cigarettes daily. His temperature is 38 °C, BP is 110/90, pulse is 20/min, and respirations are 24/min. He has severe epigastric tenderness. Which of the following variables is included in Ranson criteria *on admission* to predict the severity of this patient's illness?

   A. Calcium
   B. Arterial P_{O_2}
   C. WBC
   D. Base deficit
   E. Total bilirubin

4. A 70-year-old woman is brought to the clinic by her family because of jaundice. She has also had weight loss of 20 lb over the past few months and has recently noticed very dark urine and light-colored stools. She does not have any pain. She is thin. There is a nontender, globular mass in the right upper quadrant. A US shows dilated intrahepatic and extrahepatic bile ducts with a dilated pancreatic duct and a mass in the head of the pancreas. Which one of the following mutations is most likely associated with this patient's diagnosis?

   A. p53
   B. p16
   C. K-*ras*
   D. DNA mismatch repair
   E. Retinoblastoma gene

5. A 66-year-old man presented to the clinic with painless jaundice. Further evaluation with CT imaging and EUS showed a small resectable tumor in the head of the pancreas with no evidence of metastatic disease. EUS-guided biopsy confirmed the diagnosis of pancreatic adenocarcinoma. Pancreaticoduodenectomy is planned. Which of the following statements regarding the role of adjuvant or neoadjuvant therapy for this patient is true?

   A. Adjuvant and neoadjuvant strategies can include radiation and/or chemotherapy.
   B. There is no role for chemotherapy in the adjuvant or neoadjuvant setting.
   C. Neoadjuvant strategies are the standard of care for patients with pancreatic cancer.
   D. The use of neoadjuvant and adjuvant strategies is usually not indicated because of the low recurrence rates in patients with resected disease.
   E. Neoadjuvant therapy is given postoperatively.

ANSWERS AND EXPLANATIONS

1. Answer: D

X-rays are needed only to rule out a perforated peptic ulcer, which can present with hyperamylasemia. However, immediate laparotomy is not indicated at this time, with a diagnosis of uncomplicated gallstone pancreatitis. IV fluids are necessary to maintain perfusion, as indicated by adequate urine output. MRCP is unnecessary, and ERCP may be detrimental in cases without suspicion of impacted common bile duct stone, such as a dilated common bile duct or elevated hepatic enzymes. Cholecystectomy should be performed as soon as the pancreatitis resolves to prevent the next attack. For more information on this topic, please see section "Surgical" under "Acute Pancreatitis."

2. Answer: A

The pancreas secretes digestive enzymes, namely amylases, lipases, and proteases. Most enzymes, including trypsin and chymotrypsin, are secreted in their inactive form (trypsinogen and chymotrypsinogen). Amylase is secreted in its active form. CCK is secreted by the duodenum and leads to the secretion of several pancreatic enzymes, whereas gastrin is a hormone primarily produced in the antrum. For more information on this topic, please see section "Exocrine."

3. Answer: C

Ranson criteria is one of the grading systems for the severity of pancreatitis that relies on clinical and laboratory values on admission and during the initial 48 hours. It is predictive of later complications such as respiratory failure, infection, sepsis, multiorgan failure. On admission, the criteria include age, WBC count, serum glucose, serum lactate dehydrogenase, and serum glutamic oxaloacetic transaminase. Arterial Po_2, calcium, and base deficit are three of six criteria measured during the initial 48 hours. Total bilirubin, although often measured, is not part of the criteria. For more information on this topic, please see section "Prognosis" under "Acute Pancreatitis."

4. Answer: C

The most commonly expressed genetic mutation in pancreatic cancer occurs in the K-*ras* oncogene. It is present in at least 75% of pancreatic carcinomas. Mutations in the p53 tumor suppressor gene are the second most common mutation in pancreatic cancer and the most common genetic event in all human cancers. Mutations in other genes, including p16, the retinoblastoma gene, and DNA mismatch repair genes, also occur but are less common. For more information on this topic, please see section "Genetic Mutations Associated With Pancreatic Cancer."

5. Answer: A

Unfortunately, even after successful surgical resection, most patients with pancreatic cancer will develop a recurrence of their disease—both locally and systemically. Because of the high recurrence rates, efforts to develop adjuvant and neoadjuvant strategies have been pursued. Treatment can consist of either chemotherapy alone or radiation. Treatment can be given preoperatively (neoadjuvant) or postoperatively (adjuvant). For more information on this topic, please see section "Adjuvant and Neoadjuvant Treatment for Pancreatic Cancer."

17

Breast

Ted A. James and Mediget Teshome

Gaining familiarity with breast evaluation and an understanding of breast disease are critically important for primary care physicians and surgeons. This chapter focuses on the evaluation of the patient who is undergoing routine screening as well as the patient who has a breast concern. Breast surveillance and the appropriate treatment of breast problems have become prominent aspects of health care because breast cancer is common, often curable, and almost always treatable. Among women in the United States in 2023, there were an estimated 297,790 new cases of invasive breast cancer, 55,720 new cases of breast carcinoma in situ, and approximately 43,700 women had died from breast cancer (Breast Cancer Facts and Figures, American Cancer Society). The rate of breast cancer in women has shown a slow but steady rise over the past 25 years; presently, it is estimated that women in the United States have a one in eight (or about 12%) lifetime risk of developing breast cancer. For men, approximately 2,800 new cases of invasive breast cancer were diagnosed and approximately 530 men died from breast cancer in 2023. The survival rate of breast cancer has increased steadily over the past several decades and is thought to reflect earlier diagnosis and advances in systemic therapy.

ANATOMY

The breast is a heterogeneous structure consisting of skin, subcutaneous tissue, parenchyma, and stroma. Contained within this architecture are glandular, ductal, and connective tissues, as well as blood vessels, nerves, and a rich lymphatic system. The breast parenchyma is divided into 15 to 20 segments that converge at the nipple in a radial pattern. Collecting ducts drain each segment into terminal lactiferous sinuses in the subareolar space. Each segment or lobe is further subdivided into 20 to 40 lobules, which are further divided into 10 to 100 alveoli or tubulosaccular secretory units. The upper outer quadrant of the breast contains a greater amount of glandular tissue.

The breast may extend from the clavicle superiorly to the sixth rib inferiorly and from the midsternal line medially into the axilla laterally (Figure 17-1). Breast tissue often extends into the anterior axillary fold known as the tail of Spence. The breast is located within the superficial fascia of the anterior thoracic wall continuous with the superficial abdominal fascia (Camper fascia). It rests on the deep posterior fascia overlying the muscles of the pectoralis major, serratus anterior, external oblique, and the rectus sheath. Cooper ligaments are fibrous bands connecting the deep layer to the superficial layer and provide a suspensory function to the breast. Skin dimpling, produced by retraction of Cooper ligaments, may be associated with underlying malignancy.

The nipple contains numerous sensory nerves as well as sebaceous and apocrine sweat glands. The areola is a pigmented dermal region surrounding the nipple containing sebaceous glands (Montgomery glands).

The breast is a well-vascularized organ and derives its main blood supply from perforating branches of the internal mammary and lateral thoracic arteries. Additional supply is provided from pectoral branches of the thoracoacromial artery and branches of the intercostal, subscapular, and thoracodorsal arteries. The axillary, subclavian, and intercostal veins receive venous drainage from the breast. Lymphatics of the breast are confluent with the subepithelial lymphatics over the surface of the body and ultimately communicate with the subdermal lymphatic vessels and subareolar lymphatic plexus of Sappey (Figure 17-2). Lymph flows from the superficial lymphatics into the deep subcutaneous and perilobular lymphatics. The vast majority of lymphatic flow goes to the axilla, with only a minor amount directed to the internal mammary chain.

The concept of lymphatic flow from the breast to axilla forms the basis for sentinel lymph node staging. Following injection into the breast of a radioactive tracer and/or blue dye, lymphatic drainage of the breast is thought to follow an orderly pattern so that drainage is first to the sentinel lymph node(s) and subsequently to the nonsentinel lymph nodes. Consequently, in early-stage clinically node-negative breast cancer, if the sentinel lymph node(s) is negative for malignant cells, involvement of any other nodes is rare and axillary dissection can be avoided.

The axilla is a pyramidal-shaped region located between the upper extremity and thorax. It contains a rich complex of neurovascular and lymphatic structures within a layer of dense connective tissue known as the "axillary sheath." Contained within the axilla are two motor branches of the brachial plexus: the long thoracic and thoracodorsal nerves. The long thoracic, thoracodorsal, and intercostobrachial nerves are intimately associated anatomically with the breast and the axillary space. The long thoracic nerve courses vertically along the superficial surface of the serratus anterior muscle in the axilla. It provides motor innervation to the serratus anterior muscle, which abducts and laterally rotates the scapula and holds it against the chest wall. Injury to this nerve, which can occur during mastectomy or axillary dissection, results in a winged scapula. The loss of the serratus anterior muscle holding the scapula against the posterior chest wall results in a limiting of the overhead elevation of the arm above the shoulder. The thoracodorsal nerve, which is located posteriorly in the axillary space, innervates the latissimus dorsi muscle, which adducts, extends, and medially rotates the arm. This nerve is also potentially at risk during axillary surgery. The medial pectoral nerve, named for its origin from the medial cord of the brachial plexus, most commonly pierces the

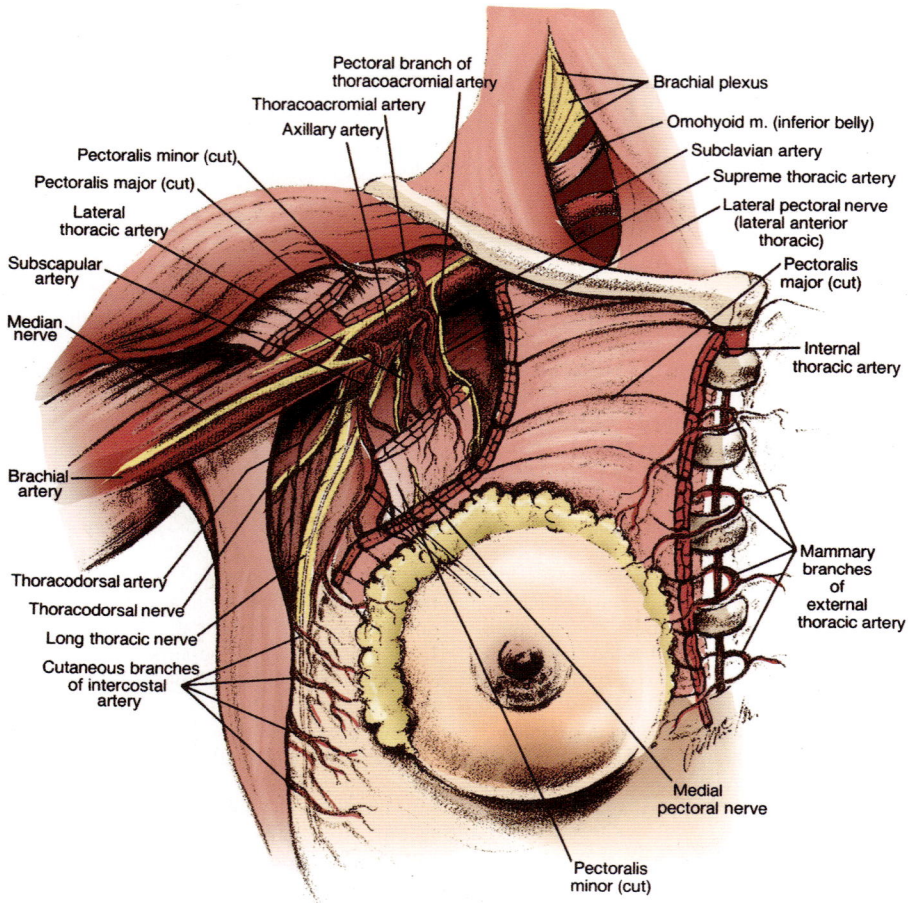

Figure 17-1. Normal breast anatomy showing vascular and neural origins.

pectoralis minor en route to the pectoralis major while innervating both. The nerve may pass *lateral* to the pectoralis minor muscle, and for this reason, it is vulnerable to injury during axillary dissection. The intercostobrachial nerves, which are the lateral cutaneous branches of the first and second intercostal nerves, course across the axillary space to provide cutaneous innervation to the inner aspect of the upper arm and the axilla. Attempts should be made to identify and preserve the intercostobrachial nerves during an axillary dissection; however, it is acceptable to sacrifice these sensory nerves if they are in the direct path of the specimen. Patients will have a resultant loss of sensation or paresthesia at the medial portion of the upper arm, which often resolves over time.

PHYSIOLOGY

The female breast is a modified apocrine gland that undergoes considerable structural and physiologic changes during a woman's lifetime. The mammary glands have evolved as a milk-producing organ for breastfeeding children. The paired glands develop along the milk lines. A wide range of congenital abnormalities in breast

development exists. Polythelia (accessory nipple) can occur anywhere along the milk line from the axilla to the inguinal region. A more rare condition—polymastia (accessory breast tissue)—occurs in the axilla. Congenital absence of the breast is called "amastia" whereas a lack of breast tissue development with perseverance of the nipple is termed "amazia."

The development of the breast from childhood to adulthood has been categorized into the five Tanner phases. Increased hormonal production by the ovary at puberty causes ductal budding and the initial formation of acini, which are proliferations of the terminal ducts lined with secretory cells for milk production. Periductal connective tissue increases in volume elasticity, vascularity, and in the amount of adipose deposition. The synergistic physiologic effect of both estrogen and progesterone results in the full maturation of the ductal and lobular components of the breast. With each menstrual cycle, preovulatory estrogen production stimulates the proliferation of the breast ductal system. After ovulation, decreased estrogen and progesterone levels cause a decrease in ductal proliferation. In pregnancy, when estrogen and progesterone levels remain relatively high, there is continued hypertrophy and budding of the ductal system, with associated acinar

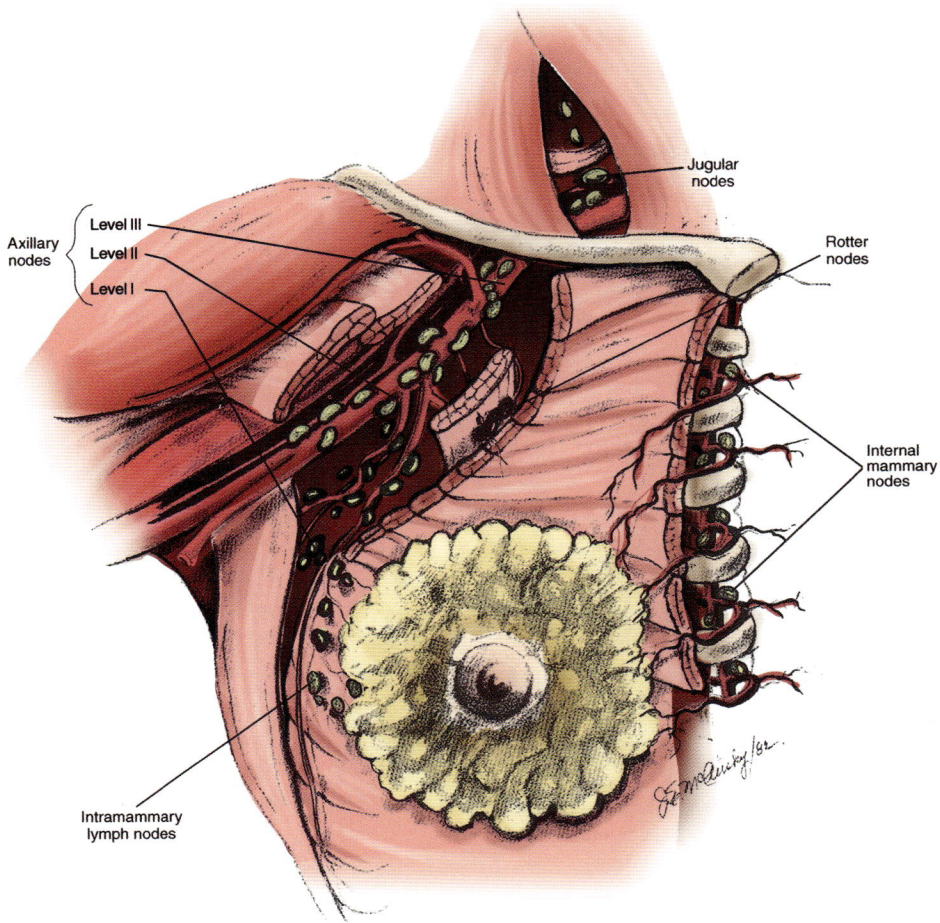

Figure 17-2. Lymphatic drainage of the breast.

development. The sudden decrease in hormone levels in the postpartum period, associated with prolactin secretion from the pituitary gland, precipitates the onset of lactation. Postmenopausally, in the absence of the hormonal stimulus for cyclic proliferation of the breast ductal system, breast parenchyma is progressively lost and replaced by adipose tissue. The male breast is anatomically composed of the same heterogeneous tissue as the female breast, but it does not undergo cyclic hormonally related changes.

Physiologic gynecomastia occurs in over one-half of adolescent males. For these young patients, the enlarged breasts may be asymmetric and tender secondary to a physiologic excess of plasma estradiol relative to plasma testosterone. This adolescent gynecomastia usually resolves by age 20. In young girls, adolescent or juvenile hypertrophy is a postpubertal persistence of epithelial and stromal growth that can result in very large breasts. Often, this occurs in the absence of any systemic hormonal imbalances. Physiologic gynecomastia is also prevalent in a significant percentage of aging men. This is manifested by either bilateral or unilateral breast enlargement often associated with breast tenderness. This gynecomastia is secondary to a relative hyperestrinism with falling plasma testosterone levels and increasing conversion of androgens

to estrogens in peripheral tissues. In the absence of a palpable mass or of significant symptoms, this condition does not require clinical evaluation. A thorough history and careful physical examination will often be all that is required for most asymptomatic patients without features suggestive of possible malignancy. Less frequently, gynecomastia may be associated with certain drugs or result from pathologic conditions such as hepatic, renal, or endocrine disorders. The treatment of gynecomastia is tailored to the underlying etiology and symptoms.

CLINICAL PRESENTATION AND EVALUATION: ASSESSMENT OF BREAST CANCER RISK

A complete medical history, risk assessment, and focused physical examination should be obtained from any woman with breast complaints. Table 17-1 summarizes the essential elements of the history. Risk assessment is useful primarily in women without active breast-related concerns because diagnostic and therapeutic approaches in women who do have active breast-related concerns are determined

TABLE 17-1. Key Elements in the History of a Patient With a Breast Concern
History of current problem (duration, timing, intensity)
Previous breast problems including biopsies
Results of recent mammography
Family history of breast cancer, ovarian cancer
Age at onset of menses and natural or surgical menopause
Age at first full-term pregnancy, number of pregnancies
Use of birth control pills, HRT
Current medications
Past medical and surgical history

HRT, hormone replacement therapy.

TABLE 17-2. Breast Cancer Risk Factors	
Relative Risk	**Factor**
>4.0	Female
	Age (65+ vs <65 y, although risk increases across all ages until age 80)
	Certain inherited genetic mutations for breast cancer (BRCA1 and/or BRCA2)
	Two or more first-degree relatives with breast cancer diagnosed at an early age
	Personal history of breast cancer
	High breast tissue density
	Biopsy-confirmed atypical hyperplasia
2.1-4.0	One first-degree relative with breast cancer
	High-dose radiation to chest
	High bone density (postmenopausal)
1.1-2.0	
Factors that affect circulating hormones	Late age at first full-term pregnancy (>30 y)
	Early menarche (<12 y)
	Late menopause (>55 y)
	No full-term pregnancies
	Never breastfed a child
	Recent oral contraceptive use
	Recent and long-term use of HRT
Other factors	Obesity (postmenopausal)
	Personal history of endometrium, ovary, or colon cancer
	Alcohol consumption
	Height (tall)
	High socioeconomic status
	Jewish heritage

HRT, hormone replacement therapy.
Adapted with permission from BS, Moorman PG. Breast cancer: hormones and other risk factors. *Maturitas*. 2001;38(1):103-113; discussion 113-106.

by the nature of the problem rather than by the level of risk. In other words, concerns should not be disregarded because the risk is low. Many women who develop breast cancer *do not* have significant risk factors.

Abnormalities occurring in young women, those under the age of 30, are likely to be related to benign pathologies such as fibrocystic changes, cysts, and fibroadenomas, although malignancy remains a possibility. Abnormalities in postmenopausal women, such as pain, nipple discharge, and new masses, are much more likely to be related to malignancies. A solid mass in a postmenopausal woman should be considered suspicious for cancer until proven otherwise.

Breast cancer risk factors are statistical associations and do not define causality. A greater number of risk factors (Table 17-2) suggest greater risk, but the nature of these interactions is not fully delineated and requires further study.

Hormone replacement therapy (HRT) has been studied in relation to its risk of breast cancer, particularly in the Women's Health Initiative (WHI) whose results were released in the early 2000s. The risk associated with HRT depends on the type of HRT and the duration of its use. HRT has long been known to be associated with an increased risk of breast cancer. Recent data have demonstrated that combination HRT increases breast cancer risk by approximately 75%. The risk increases the longer a woman uses combined HRT and decreases over time after discontinuation. There have been conflicting data on the risk of estrogen-only HRT with some studies showing a small increased risk, especially with long-term use, and others showing no risk. Studies have also shown that HRT may reduce bone loss and benefit treatment of menopausal symptoms; however, it may increase the risk of heart disease.

Major risk factors for breast cancer include female sex, increasing age, family history, increased breast density, postmenopausal obesity, large amounts of radiation exposure early in life (eg, radiation treatment to the chest area for childhood cancer), and proliferative pathology with atypia on biopsy (ie, atypical ductal or lobular hyperplasia). As women age, they are more likely to be diagnosed with breast cancer, but they become less likely to die from it (Table 17-3). Breast cancer in families featuring an early age of onset (premenopausal) and in multiple close

relatives, bilateral disease, male breast cancer, and breast cancer in combination with ovarian cancer are all more suggestive of a hereditary predisposition (eg, *BRCA*).

It is estimated that approximately 5% to 10% of breast cancers are related to specific genetic mutations inherited from family members. Certain genes linked to an increased susceptibility to breast cancer have been identified, including, most notably, *BRCA1* and *BRCA2* gene mutations. *BRCA1* has been mapped to the long arm of chromosome 17

TABLE 17-3. Age-Specific Probability of Breast Cancer

If Current Age Is:	The Probability of Developing Breast Cancer in the Next 10 y Is (%):	Or 1 in:
20	0.05	1,837
30	0.43	234
40	1.43	70
50	2.51	40
60	3.51	28
70	3.88	26
Lifetime risk	12.28	8

From American Cancer Society. *Surveillance Research. Cancer Facts & Figures 2007*. American Cancer Society; 2007.

and *BRCA2* to the long arm of chromosome 13. The lifetime risk of penetrance (disease expression) in *BRCA* mutation carriers is 36% to 85% for breast cancer and 16% to 60% for ovarian cancer. In order to best provide options for high-risk screening and prevention, patients suspected to have a hereditary mutation predisposing them to breast cancer should be offered further assessment with a genetic counselor and genetic testing (Table 17-4). Both maternal and paternal sides of the family history should be collected. Other familial cancer syndromes, such as Li-Fraumeni and Cowden, have also been associated with an increased risk of breast cancer.

TABLE 17-4. Guidelines: Referral for Genetic Counseling

The National Comprehensive Cancer Network (NCCN), the American College of Medical Genetics and Genomics, and the National Society of Genetic Counselors provide detailed criteria for identifying candidates for genetic counseling and possible testing for hereditary breast and ovarian cancer (HBOC). The NCCN guidelines are updated at least annually on the basis of evidence-based reviews of published studies. Key criteria for hereditary cancer risk evaluation and possible testing are as follows:

Patients with:
- Female breast cancer diagnosed ≤45 y
- Triple-negative breast cancer diagnosed ≤60 y
- Two or more primary breast cancers
- Invasive ovarian or fallopian tube cancer, or primary peritoneal cancer
- Male breast cancer
- Any HBOC-associated cancers, regardless of age at diagnosis, and of Ashkenazi (central or eastern European) Jewish ancestry
- Patients with breast cancer and first-degree, second-degree, or third-degree relatives with breast cancer diagnosed ≤50 y in one or more relatives
- Invasive ovarian, fallopian tube, or primary peritoneal cancer in one or more relatives
- Breast, prostate, and/or pancreatic cancer, diagnosed at any age in two or more relatives

Management of high-risk patients, with or without confirmation of a genetic mutation, often requires the coordination of a multidisciplinary team. High-risk screening with a clinical breast examination every 6 months, annual mammography, and annual magnetic resonance imaging (MRI) can begin at age 25 or be individualized on the basis of the earliest age of breast cancer onset in the family. Although controversial for normal-risk patients, high-risk patients may also benefit from regular breast self-exam (BSE). Randomized controlled trials have demonstrated the benefit of chemoprevention with agents tamoxifen and raloxifene. The use of these drugs in high-risk individuals reduces the incidence of breast cancer by approximately 50%. The potential risks and side effects of these drugs need to be taken into consideration and discussed with the patient before initiating chemoprevention. Patients should also have a careful discussion about risk-reducing (ie, prophylactic) bilateral mastectomy as well as risk-reducing bilateral salpingo-oophorectomy. Prophylactic mastectomy is associated with approximately 90% risk reduction of breast cancer. The addition of prophylactic oophorectomy in premenopausal women yields approximately 95% risk reduction of breast cancer whereas prophylactic oophorectomy alone is associated with approximately 50% risk reduction of breast cancer and 90% risk reduction of ovarian cancer. Patients electing to undergo prophylactic bilateral mastectomy should be offered the opportunity to explore breast reconstruction options versus aesthetic flat closure. Patient education is an essential component of risk management, and it is important that all risks including psychosocial, benefits, and alternate approaches are thoroughly discussed with the patient.

Physical Examination of the Breasts

A systematic approach to the physical examination of the breasts includes both inspection and palpation. Important elements in the breast examination should be performed thoroughly while maintaining patient comfort. The examination begins with the patient in the seated position. Both breasts should be exposed to allow for full inspection and assessment for any breast asymmetry, skin changes (eg, retraction or erythema), or nipple-areolar abnormalities (eg, scaling of the nipple or nipple inversion). The breasts are inspected first with the arms at the patient's side and then pressed firmly at the waist in order to contract the pectoralis muscle. This maneuver may accentuate skin retraction associated with a mass. Other maneuvers such as elevating the arms above the head and leaning forward are not routinely necessary; however, they can be utilized as needed (ie, large pendulous breasts). With the patient still in the seated position, both axillae are examined, with the patient's arm resting over the forearm of the examiner to relax the shoulder musculature, allowing for full assessment of axillary contents. Lymph nodes are best detected as the examiner gently presses superiorly in the axilla and then moves the fingertips inferiorly against the chest wall, trapping lymph nodes between the finger and the chest wall. A careful lymph node examination also involves palpation in the supraclavicular fossae. Palpation of the breasts in the sitting position alone is discouraged because it often yields inaccurate findings for the examiner (as well as for the patient during self-examination). The breasts should also be palpated with the patient supine and the arm resting comfortably above the head. This position evenly distributes the breast tissue out over the chest wall, allowing more accurate detection of abnormalities.

There are several different methods of palpating the breast; however, the vertical strip technique is a reliable, evidence-based method shown to have the lowest incidence of missed abnormalities. Palpation of the breast should encompass all breast tissue and cover the perimeter bordered by the clavicle, sternum, axilla, and inframammary crease. The examination should be performed with a vertical strip pattern covering the entire breast using overlapping dime-sized circular motions of increasing pressure (light, medium, deep). The pads (not the tips) of the index, middle, and ring fingers are used for palpation. Irregularities are palpated between the skin and the chest wall, not between the two hands of the examiner. The size of any palpable abnormality should be described with the use of a measuring instrument. The examiner should note additional features including mobility, texture, and whether or not there is associated tenderness. The precise location of any abnormality should be described. When annotating location, using the clock-face position and distance from the nipple is helpful (ie, right breast mass in the 12 o'clock position, 4 cm from the nipple). It is not necessary to squeeze the nipples during a breast examination because typically only spontaneous nipple discharge (especially bloody or serous) requires further evaluation. Unilateral nonspontaneous discharge is frequently benign, particularly in younger women. With a history of spontaneous nipple discharge, the source of the discharge should be localized with systematic palpation from the outer breast to the nipple circumferentially around the areola. If discharge is identified, the color should be noted, as well as whether it is bloody, whether more than one duct orifice is involved, and whether it is bilateral. Unilateral bloody single-duct spontaneous discharge is more likely to result from an underlying malignancy, especially if it is associated with a mass in the breast. However, the most common cause of unilateral spontaneous bloody nipple discharge is a benign papilloma.

Diagnostic Evaluation

The foundation of breast cancer screening is the annual mammogram. Large prospective studies evaluating the impact of screening mammogram on breast cancer mortality demonstrate a 40% to 45% reduction in breast cancer deaths in a screened population compared with the years before screening. Monthly BSE in addition to mammography does not yield additional improvement in breast cancer survival, yet the fact remains that among patients not engaged in screening, such as those under age 40, the majority of breast cancers are diagnosed after a patient reports a self-detected mass or change in the appearance of the breast. Therefore, women should be encouraged to seek medical attention if a new breast mass or other abnormality is found. (The current recommendations for breast cancer screening from the American Cancer Society are shown in Table 17-5.)

Mammography

Screening mammography is an x-ray image with two views of each breast: craniocaudal (CC) and median lateral oblique (MLO), with identifiable markers placed on the nipple and any visible or palpable lesions. Film labels are by convention located on the lateral aspect of a CC view and the superior aspect of an MLO view, allowing the reader to determine the quadrant wherein an abnormality is located (Figure 17-3). The x-ray modality can demonstrate

TABLE 17-5. American Cancer Society Guidelines for Breast Cancer Screening

American Cancer Society screening recommendations for women at average breast cancer risk

These guidelines are for women at **average risk** for breast cancer. For screening purposes, a woman is considered to be at average risk if she doesn't have a personal history of breast cancer, a strong family history of breast cancer, or a genetic mutation known to increase the risk of breast cancer (such as in a *BRCA* gene), and has not had chest radiation therapy before the age of 30. (See below for guidelines for women at high risk.)

- **Women between 40 and 44** have the option to start screening with a mammogram every year.
- **Women 45-54** should get mammograms every year.
- **Women 55 and older** can switch to a mammogram every other year, or they can choose to continue yearly mammograms. Screening should continue as long as women are in good health and are expected to live at least 10 more years.
- **All women** should understand what to expect when getting a mammogram for breast cancer screening—what the test can and cannot do.

Clinical breast exams are not recommended for breast cancer screening among average-risk women at any age.

American Cancer Society Recommendations for the Early Detection of Breast Cancer. ©American Cancer Society 2023. Used with permission.

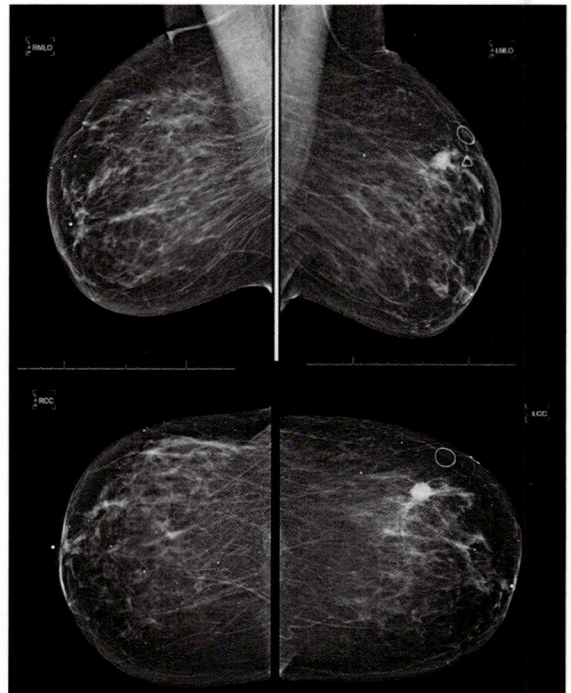

Figure 17-3. Median lateral oblique and craniocaudal views of right and left breasts showing a left spiculated lesion.

TABLE 17-6.	Breast Imaging Reporting and Data System Classification for Mammogram Findings
Category 0	Needs additional imaging evaluation
Category 1	Negative
Category 2	Benign finding
Category 3	Probably benign finding—short interval follow-up suggested
Category 4	Suspicious abnormality—biopsy should be considered.
Category 5	Highly suggestive of malignancy— appropriate action should be taken.
Category 6	Known malignancy

differences in the density of breast tissue, architectural distortion of the tissue planes, asymmetry such as unilateral nipple retraction, and calcifications ranging from those associated with benign involutional changes to suspicious microcalcifications that can be described as pleomorphic, clustered, linear, or branching. The findings are scored for the level of suspicion according to the Breast Imaging Reporting and Data System classification (Table 17-6), which corresponds to the need for additional studies or interval follow-up. The assigned score is inherently subjective to the radiologist and includes a comparison with mammograms from previous years.

Additional diagnostic views involve tissue compression and magnification, which can resolve summation artifacts, eliminate a perceived density, or enhance the spiculated contours of an actual mass lesion or a cluster of microcalcifications.

Although mammography is an effective tool for screening, it is not a definitive diagnostic study. The false-negative rate of mammography is 10% to 20%. Any physical finding or mammographic abnormality must be further evaluated on clinical grounds as well as with additional diagnostic studies, usually combined with a biopsy.

Technologic advances in mammography include computer-assisted detection software, which highlights potentially suspicious patterns on a digital image, and digital mammography, which is a technique that eliminates photographic film and creates digital images that can be processed to enhance contrast in dense soft tissue. Both techniques increase sensitivity and the breast cancer detection rate. Digital mammography, or digital breast tomosynthesis (DBT), offers greater sensitivity in dense breast tissue, results in fewer callbacks for false positives, and is more accurate in premenopausal or perimenopausal women.

Ultrasound

Ultrasonography of the breast is a diagnostic adjunct to mammography. It is particularly valuable in characterizing a mammographic density or palpable mass as cystic or solid, and in guiding core-needle biopsy. Benign sonographic features of masses include well-demarcated borders, posterior enhancement, and absence of internal echoes (characteristic of cysts). Features suspicious for malignancy include poorly demarcated borders, posterior shadowing, heterogeneous internal echoes, and a "taller than wide" orientation that invades across tissue planes.

Magnetic Resonance Imaging

MRI uses the physical characteristics of fat, water, and intravenous gadolinium contrast in magnetic fields to produce breast images with improved resolution of soft tissues. Dense breast tissue, scars, and implants, which may make mammography less sensitive, do not interfere with MRI diagnosis. In addition to such "problem-solving" applications, MRI has been shown to be a more sensitive screening test than mammography and is appropriate in women who carry a deleterious *BRCA1* or *BRCA2* mutation or who by family history and other risk factors, carry at least a 20% lifetime risk of breast cancer. The development of biopsy equipment compatible with magnetic fields allows MRI-directed breast biopsy when a suspicious lesion is detected by MRI.

Tissue Sampling Techniques

The definitive diagnosis of breast lesions depends on microscopic examination of tissue by either cytology (individual cells obtained by fine needle aspiration) or histology (samples of tissue obtained by core-needle or surgical biopsy). Cytology specimens can be air dried and stained in minutes, providing rapid diagnosis of a suspected malignancy; however, this method is not as accurate as core-needle biopsy. Histologic specimens obtained from a core-needle biopsy (preferred) or surgical excision provide tissue that can be processed for special staining techniques to demonstrate invasive versus in situ carcinoma, the type of cancer, and the expression of estrogen, progesterone, and human epidermal growth factor 2 receptor (HER2/*neu*).

The majority of lesions are detected radiologically and must be biopsied under radiologic guidance. Mass lesions are efficiently biopsied by ultrasound guidance, but microcalcifications and subtle abnormalities require stereotactic localization in the mammography suite (Figure 17-4).

Any needle biopsy must be regarded as only a sampling and verification that a lesion is benign requires the so-called triple test: concordance between clinical examination, radiographic appearance, and pathology. If the needle biopsy results are discordant, an excisional biopsy is usually necessary. Open excisional biopsy without a prior needle biopsy can lead to less-than-optimal management of a malignancy because of possible positive margins, cosmetically unfavorable incision placement, and the need to go back to the operating room for lymph node staging in the case of invasive disease.

Evaluation of the Patient With a Breast Mass

The evaluation of a patient presenting with a breast mass depends on the patient's age and physical findings. If physical and radiographic examinations show typical areas of fibroglandular tissue without a discrete mass, the patient should be reevaluated in 6 to 12 weeks. If there is a question as to whether the physical findings reveal a specific area of thickening or discrete mass, a workup should be initiated along the lines of the presented algorithm (Figure 17-5). Most patients felt that having a discrete, solid, and persistent mass requires tissue diagnosis.

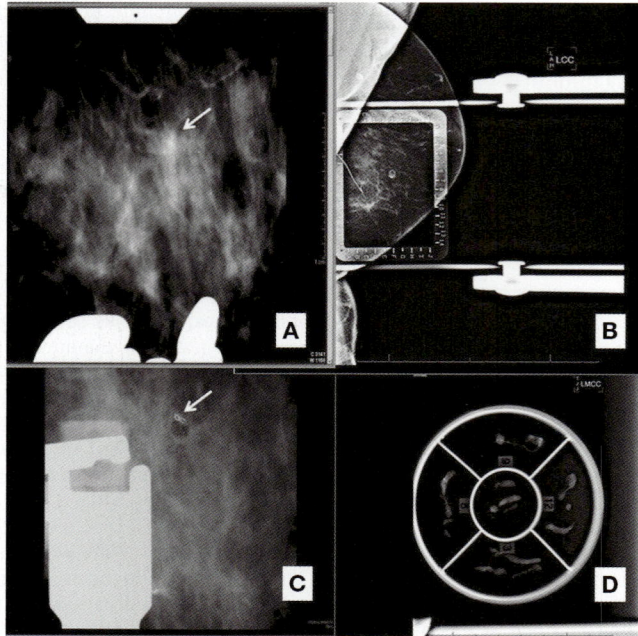

Figure 17-4. Stereotactic biopsy of mammographically detected lesion. A. Suspicious microcalcifications (arrow). B. With the patient positioned on a stereotactic biopsy table, the lesion is localized for a core-needle biopsy. C. A clip (arrow) is deployed at the site of biopsy for future reference. D. The specimen cores are radiographed to demonstrate targeted microcalcifications.

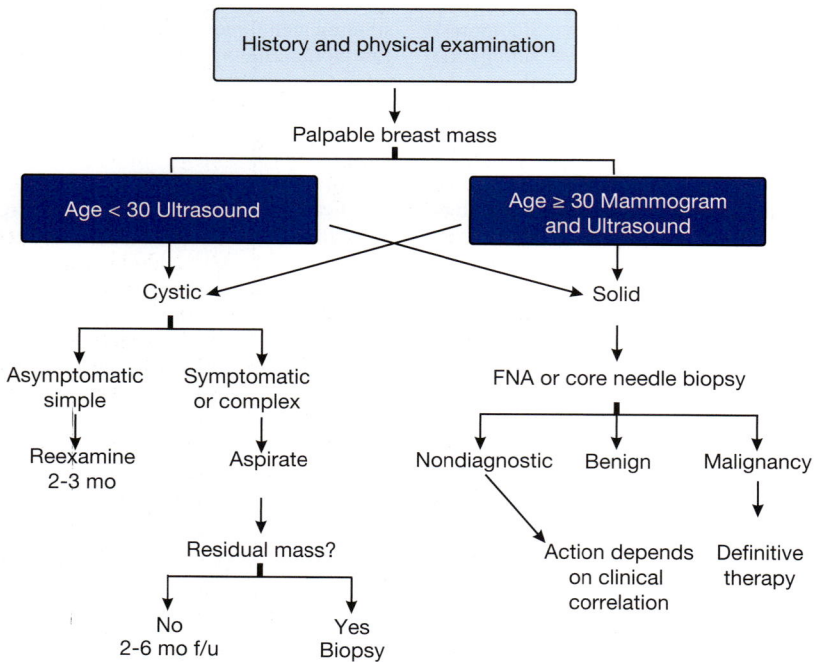

Figure 17-5. Algorithm for evaluation of a palpable mass. f/u, follow-up; FNA, fine needle aspiration.

BENIGN CONDITIONS OF THE BREAST

Breast Pain

Mild, cyclic bilateral breast tenderness and swelling are common a few days before menstruation and rarely prompt medical consultation. Although it is distinctly unusual for the presence of breast cancer to be signaled by pain, persistent or unilateral pain and tenderness can be a cause of alarm. A thorough clinical evaluation and appropriate diagnostic workup should be performed. Musculoskeletal causes and angina should be considered, and breast imaging such as mammogram and ultrasound should be used to rule out a malignancy. In the absence of any physical or radiologic abnormality, reassurance and a follow-up examination in a few months often provide adequate relief.

Hormonal stimulation of glandular breast tissue is thought to be the underlying cause of mastalgia. Discontinuing HRT in postmenopausal women with breast pain is recommended. Other therapeutic measures include using a compressive elastic style of bra (sport or minimizer bra), nonsteroidal anti-inflammatory analgesics, and evening primrose oil capsules, and reducing caffeine consumption. Danazol, an androgen analogue, and tamoxifen have been shown to be effective in relieving breast pain and tenderness but should be used only after failure of the previous measures because of adverse effects, including deepening of the voice and hirsutism (danazol), and night sweat, hot flashes, and thromboembolic and endometrial risks (tamoxifen).

Fibroadenoma

Fibroadenoma is a very common benign tumor of the breast. It usually occurs in young women (late teens to early 30s), although it may develop at any age. Typically, fibroadenomas are 1 to 3 cm in size and palpated as a freely movable, discrete, firm, and rounded mass in the breast. Histologically, fibroadenomas are composed of fibrous stromal tissue and tissue clefts lined with normal epithelium. Fine needle aspiration or core biopsy (preferred) can establish the diagnosis. Fibroadenomas resemble normal mammary lobules in that they exhibit lactation during pregnancy and involution during menopause. This similarity supports the concept of aberrancies in normal development and involution, which advocates for observation rather than excision.

For young women with a typical clinical presentation and histologic diagnosis of fibroadenoma, excision is not required if the fibroadenoma is small (<3 cm). In this group, approximately 50% of fibroadenomas involute within 5 years. Stable fibroadenomas may be followed. Hormonal stimulation during pregnancy may cause rapid growth of a fibroadenoma and require its excision. Giant fibroadenoma is an uncommon benign tumor in adolescent girls. Core-needle biopsy should be performed before excision to distinguish the relatively rare phyllodes tumor, a usually benign (90%) tumor of the stromal elements requiring wide margins of resection to prevent local recurrence.

Breast Cyst

A cyst is the most common cause of breast mass in women in their fourth and fifth decades of life. Cysts may be solitary or multiple, and present as firm, mobile, slightly tender

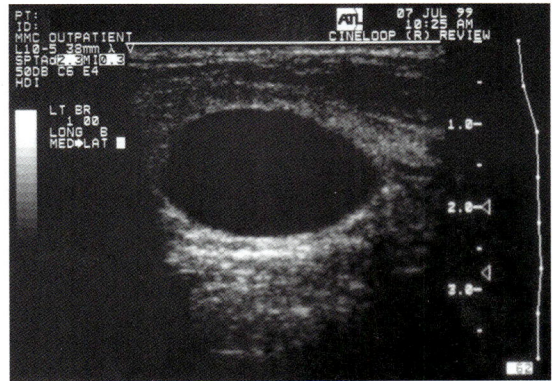

Figure 17-6. Sonogram of a simple breast cyst.

masses, often with less well-defined borders compared with fibroadenomas. Unlike fibroadenomas, the size and degree of tenderness of a cyst typically fluctuate with the menstrual cycle. Screening mammography will frequently detect nonpalpable cysts. Ultrasonography is very useful in demonstrating a simple cyst as a well-demarcated, hypoechoic mass with a posterior enhancement of transmission (Figure 17-6).

Such an appearance is diagnostic and does not require biopsy. Aspiration may be performed on large, symptomatic cysts. The resulting fluid may be straw colored or greenish, and cytologic analysis is unnecessary. If blood is present in the aspiration or residual mass remains, it is suspicious and warrants further assessment. The ultrasound appearance of complex cysts shows internal echoes or an associated solid component. Mammography and core-needle biopsy are warranted before excision, so that if a malignancy is diagnosed, an appropriate resection may be planned.

Nipple Discharge

The most common cause of nipple discharge is duct ectasia, a nonneoplastic condition characterized by multiple dilated ducts in the subareolar space. The nipple discharge may be clear, milky, or green-brown. The discharge can be applied to occult blood test paper and further evaluation performed when blood is present. Persistent, spontaneous discharge from a single-duct and bloody discharge are considered pathologic. The incidence of malignancy is 10% to 15% in unilateral, bloody nipple discharge. An intraductal papilloma is the usual cause in the remaining instances. An intraductal papilloma is a local proliferation of ductal epithelial cells that typically presents in women in their fourth or fifth decade of life.

Systematic palpation around the nipple-areolar complex can frequently identify the discharging duct. A ductogram is a technically difficult study that rarely alters the surgical management and thus can be avoided. Mammography is important to evaluate for malignancy, and breast ultrasound with or without biopsy may prove diagnostic. MRI offers excellent sensitivity for pathologic nipple discharge compared to conventional imaging. In the absence of clinical or radiologic evidence of malignancy, duct excision through a circumareolar incision allows definitive histologic diagnosis and eliminates the discharge with a cosmetically acceptable result.

The Erythematous Breast

When a woman presents with a breast that is warm, edematous, and erythematous, the differential diagnosis primarily consists of an infectious process, such as mastitis or breast abscess, versus malignancy presenting as inflammatory breast cancer. A careful history must be taken to assess risk factors and onset and the time course of symptoms. Mastitis is most commonly associated with lactation. In nonlactating women, especially those who smoke or have nipple piercings, recurrent retroareolar abscesses may occur with chronic inflammation and fistula formation between the skin and the duct. In a postmenopausal woman, the likelihood of breast cancer is higher. The patient may report having a breast lump that was asymptomatic and only comes to attention because of the redness, but inflammatory breast cancer can occur with diffuse breast swelling and no discrete mass.

Physical findings include erythema spreading in a lymphangitic pattern from areola toward the axilla, skin thickening with accentuation of the pores (*peau d'orange*), lymphadenopathy, overall breast enlargement and heaviness, and a mass that may be fluctuant. Breast malignancy typically does not present with pain whereas abscesses are exquisitely tender. However, it is important to note that inflammatory breast cancer can be associated with pain, tenderness, or burning. The nipple can be distorted in either cancer or recurrent retroareolar abscess. Diagnostic imaging includes mammography and ultrasound. In cases where no mass is demonstrated by these modalities, breast MRI is useful. Punch biopsy of the skin may show dilated lymphatic channels carrying malignant cells, but it is not necessary to demonstrate these in order to make a clinical diagnosis of inflammatory breast cancer. Fine needle aspiration of a mass can establish the presence of malignancy in minutes, but core-needle biopsies should also be obtained for immunohistochemical studies to plan primary systemic therapy.

Ultrasound demonstrates drainable fluid collections when an abscess is present. Repeated aspiration of a breast abscess combined with antibiotics may allow resolution of the abscess without open drainage. Chronic retroareolar inflammation and mammary duct fistula require antibiotics with coverage of anaerobic organisms followed by excision of the subareolar ducts including the fistula tract. Mastitis in lactating women is usually caused by staphylococci or streptococci. Appropriate antibiotics such as dicloxacillin or clindamycin should bring prompt relief. Breastfeeding may continue on the unaffected breast whereas the use of a breast pump is helpful in reducing congestion of the infected breast.

BREAST CANCER

Women in the United States have a one in eight approximate lifetime risk of breast cancer. It is the most frequently diagnosed female cancer and the second leading cause of cancer death in women. Although incidence rates have been increasing, the rate of increase has slowed in the past decade. Approximately 25% of new cancers are in situ. The rise in the detection of ductal carcinoma in situ is a result of the increased use of screening mammography, which detects breast cancers before they are palpable.

The earliest sign of a breast cancer is usually an abnormality on a mammogram. As breast cancers grow, they can produce a palpable mass that is often hard and irregular. Other signs may include thickening, swelling, skin irritation, or dimpling. Nipple changes caused by breast cancer can include scaliness and dryness, ulceration, retraction, or discharge.

In most cases of breast cancer, the cause is unknown, but many risk factors such as hormonal, environmental, and lifestyle factors have been identified. About 5% to 10% of cancers are related to genetic factors. Approximately 1% of breast cancers occur in men.

Histologic Types of Breast Cancer

Ductal cancer in situ (DCIS), also known as intraductal carcinoma, is a preinvasive form of ductal cancer. If not treated adequately, invasive cancer may develop in 30% to 50% of patients over 10 years (Figure 17-7). The typical appearance of DCIS on mammography is microcalcifications; there is rarely a mass on physical examination or mammography. The histologic types of DCIS include solid, cribriform, micropapillary, and comedo. DCIS can be classified as low, intermediate, or high grade, with low grade being the most favorable. Patients with comedo-type necrosis and/or high-grade lesions have an increased risk of recurrence and of the lesion developing into invasive cancer.

Infiltrating ductal carcinoma constitutes approximately 80% of invasive breast cancers. It produces the characteristic firm, irregular mass on physical examination. These masses are characteristically better defined both mammographically and histologically compared with infiltrating lobular cancers.

Infiltrating lobular carcinoma makes up approximately 10% of breast cancers and is often difficult to detect mammographically and on physical examination because of its indistinct borders. It is characterized by a higher incidence of multicentricity and bilateral presentation.

Tubular carcinoma, a very well-differentiated form of ductal carcinoma, constitutes approximately 1% to 2% of breast

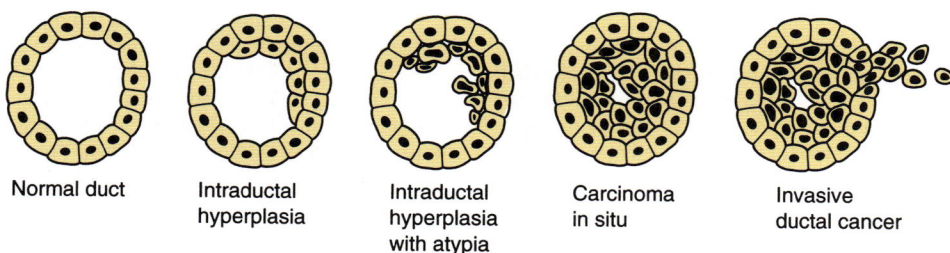

Figure 17-7. The evolution from normal duct to invasive cancer. (Adapted with permission from Love SM. *Dr. Susan Love's Breast Book.* Addison-Wesley Longman; 1990:192. Copyright © 1990, 1991 by Susan M. Love, MD. Reprinted by permission of Addison-Wesley Longman, Inc).

Normal duct   Intraductal hyperplasia   Intraductal hyperplasia with atypia   Carcinoma in situ   Invasive ductal cancer cancers. It is so named because it forms small tubules, randomly arranged, each lined by a single uniform row of cells. This subtype tends to occur in women who are slightly younger than the average patient with breast cancer. The prognosis is more favorable than other infiltrating ductal carcinomas.

Medullary carcinoma, another variant of infiltrating ductal cancer, is characterized by extensive tumor invasion by small lymphocytes and is slightly less well differentiated than tubular carcinoma. It constitutes approximately 5% of breast carcinomas. At diagnosis, it tends to be rapidly growing and large, and it is often associated with DCIS. It less commonly metastasizes to regional lymph nodes and has a better prognosis than the typical infiltrating ductal carcinoma. Medullary carcinomas or medullary features are more likely to be associated with *BRCA* mutation.

Colloid or *mucinous carcinoma* is also a variant of infiltrating ductal cancer and accounts for approximately 2% to 3% of breast carcinomas. It is characterized histologically by clumps and strands of epithelial cells in pools of mucoid material. It grows slowly and occurs more often in older women. The pure type has a relatively favorable prognosis.

True papillary carcinoma accounts for approximately 1% of breast carcinomas. These tumors can be difficult to distinguish histologically from intraductal papilloma, a benign lesion. They tend to be quite small, and even when they metastasize to regional nodes, they have a better prognosis than ductal carcinomas because of their slower rate of growth.

Inflammatory carcinoma accounts for 2% to 6% of all breast cancers and presents with skin edema (peau d'orange) and erythema. The skin edema is secondary to involvement of the dermal lymphatics with malignant cells that are generally ductal in origin. Inflammatory carcinoma of the breast has a poor prognosis, with a 5-year survival rate of approximately 40% to 50%.

Paget disease of the nipple is a cutaneous nipple abnormality, which may be moist and exudative, dry and scaly, erosive, or just a thickened area. The patient may note itching, burning, or sticking pain in the nipple. As time passes, the lesion spreads out from the duct orifice. Histologically, the dermis is infiltrated by Paget cells, which are of ductal origin, large and pale, with large nuclei, prominent nucleoli, and abundant cytoplasm. Paget disease of the nipple is seen in approximately 3% of breast cancers and is usually, but not always, associated with an underlying malignancy, which is palpable in half of cases. It may originate in DCIS or in an invasive cancer.

Paget disease of the nipple is often misdiagnosed as a simple dermatologic eruption and treated with ointments and creams for prolonged periods, during which time the cancer progresses. If a lesion is clinically suspicious for Paget disease, a nipple biopsy should be done.

Malignancies that rarely occur in the breast include sarcomas, lymphomas, and leukemia.

Staging

The treatment for breast cancer depends on the likelihood of local recurrence and distant spread. The most common areas of distant metastasis of breast cancer are bone, lungs, liver, and brain. The risk for distant spread is related to tumor grade, size, and lymph node involvement, as well as to molecular features (eg, HER2 positive, triple negative) and tumor genomic biomarker assays. These elements define the patient's stage of disease according to tumor, node, and metastasis (TNM). (TNM staging for breast cancer can be found at https://urldefense.com/v3/—https://www.facs.org/media/u4djjc4v/breast-8th-ed .pdf—;!!F9wkZZsI-LA!FRzJZkFsNBsppeN7 rxsU-7pD8_ytr_wEg2CJbiymmQRnNDb7qu-dJ-6uGO GwJ7gMrnNq9eeguqriiv1grtPd_XXVtg2DtK07wGo$)

Besides TNM status, other factors are taken into account when planning therapy for breast cancer. These include the estrogen receptor (ER), progesterone receptor (PR), and HER2/*neu* status, the histopathologic grade of the tumor, and the mitotic index. HER2/*neu*, an oncogene produced by some tumors, predicts a more aggressive form of breast cancer, as well as the likelihood of a response to herceptin, a monoclonal antibody, and other medications targeting the HER2 protein receptor.

When the patient's risk for metastatic disease is low (tumor size <5 cm, no palpable lymphadenopathy, and no symptoms), extensive staging evaluation is not required. Patients with more advanced disease or concerning systemic symptoms should have comprehensive staging (eg, computed tomography [CT], bone scan, positron emission tomography [PET]) before surgical treatment.

Prognosis

The most important prognostic factors for breast cancer are related to the stage of disease (Table 17-7). Important factors determining disease-free and overall survival include axillary node status, tumor grade, tumor size, hormone-receptor (ER and/or PR) status, HER2 receptor status, and tumor genomic assays. The risk of developing a second primary breast cancer is approximately 1% per year for the first 15 years. The risk of recurrence, while never reaching 0%, reduces over time.

Follow-Up

Patients treated for breast cancer are generally advised to undergo a bilateral mammogram about 6 months postradiation therapy following lumpectomy, with subsequent annual screenings thereafter. After a unilateral mastectomy, contralateral breast mammogram is typically performed annually. Physical examination should be done every 3 to 6 months for 3 years and then annually. Other studies to detect metastasis (eg, CT scan, PET) should primarily be based on clinical indications, such as symptoms or physical findings, as routine staging imaging may not be effective and risks false-positive findings.

TABLE 17-7. Five-Year Relative Survival Rates for Breast Cancer

SEER Stage	Five-Year Relative Survival Rate (%)
Localized[a]	99
Regional	86
Distant	31
All SEER stages combined	91

- These numbers are based on women diagnosed with breast cancer between 2013 and 2019.
- [a]Localized stage only includes invasive cancer. It does not include ductal carcinoma in situ (DCIS).

From *Survival Rates for Breast Cancer*. American Cancer Society; 2024. https://urldefense.com/v3/__https://www.cancer.org/cancer/types/ breast-cancer/understanding-a-breast-cancer-diagnosis/breast-cancer- survival-rates.html__;!!F9wkZZsI-LA!FRzJZkFsNBsppeN7rxsU-7pD8_ytr_ wEg2CJbiymmQRnNDb7qu-dJ-6uGOGwJ7gMrnNq9eeguqriiv1grtPd_ XXVtg2DylagoT0$

Treatment of Breast Cancer

Cancer is a disorder of individual cells, and treatment, whether local or systemic, is directed at eliminating these abnormal cells. Early-stage breast cancer, stages 0, I, and II, is regarded as potentially curable, meaning that once the cancer is treated, it may never recur. Later-stage breast cancer, stage III, has a lower survival rate. Stage IV breast cancer is treatable but rarely curable.

Breast cancer treatment is a multidisciplinary effort that draws on the expertise of many specialties, including radiologists, breast surgical oncologists, plastic and reconstructive surgeons, medical oncologists, radiation oncologists, pathologists, gynecologists, oncology nurses, social workers, physical therapists, and mental health professionals. It typically encompasses both local and systemic therapies, aiming to achieve a cure, minimize recurrence, and enhance both survival rates and quality of life. Local-regional treatments include surgery and radiation. Systemic treatments consist of intravenous and oral medicines.

Local Treatments

Surgery

The best surgical option should consider the severity of the disease, the potential side effects of the treatment, and the patient's preferences and priorities. The primary goal of surgical treatment in breast cancer is to completely remove the malignancy and provide pathologic and regional staging when appropriate. However, in some circumstances, the objective might be palliation to alleviate symptoms and improve quality of life. Additionally, surgery can be employed for prophylactic risk reduction in individuals with a high predisposition to breast cancer.

Surgical options for breast cancer broadly consist of breast-conserving surgery (ie, partial mastectomy, lumpectomy) and mastectomy. When breast-conserving surgery is paired with adjuvant radiation, its efficacy in preventing local recurrence is essentially equivalent to mastectomy with no significant difference in overall survival between the two surgical approaches.

Partial mastectomy, lumpectomy, wide excision, and segmental resection are all forms of breast-conserving surgery. Each involves removing the malignancy along with a surrounding margin of microscopically normal tissue while preserving the majority of the breast. Breast-conserving surgery may be used in the treatment of DCIS and invasive carcinoma. It is usually feasible in tumors under 4 cm, depending on the size of the breast. The histologic type of breast cancer (ductal vs lobular cancer) and tumor subtype are not major factors in the choice of surgical treatment.

A total, or simple, mastectomy removes the entire breast with the pectoralis major fascia. A modified radical mastectomy consists of a total mastectomy with an axillary lymph node dissection (ALND). This differs from the radical mastectomy, which also involves the removal of the pectoralis muscle. The radical mastectomy is largely historical and is no longer routinely performed. In certain cases, a skin-sparing or nipple-sparing mastectomy may also be a surgical option, offering improved cosmetic results for breast reconstruction.

Dermal lymphatic involvement, as seen in inflammatory breast cancer, widespread disease or multiple tumors, challenges in achieving clear margins, constraints or aversion to radiation therapy, and anticipated cosmetic concerns, such as a significant tumor-to-breast size ratio, are all factors that may indicate a mastectomy. All patients undergoing mastectomy should be informed about breast reconstruction options, which include prosthetic implants or using their own tissue (autologous flap reconstruction). Reconstruction can be performed simultaneously with the mastectomy or in a delayed fashion. Options include saline or silicone implants, or autologous tissue from areas like the abdomen, latissimus, or gluteal regions. The Women's Health and Cancer Rights Act mandates insurance coverage for mastectomy to also cover certain breast reconstruction procedures. Alternatively, some women may opt for an aesthetic flat closure, resulting in a smooth chest contour without reconstruction.

Assessment of the axilla is essential in staging and treating breast cancer. Since its initial pilot study in 1993, sentinel node biopsy has emerged as the standard of care for axillary staging in early-stage breast cancer, supplanting the routine use of ALND. In a clinically negative axilla, injecting a radioactive colloid or blue dye into the breast allows surgeons to identify the initial lymph node(s) draining the breast. Typically, only two to three nodes, known as sentinel nodes, absorb the tracer. These can be extracted with a smaller incision, reduced dissection, and a lower risk of affecting axillary nerves and the arm's lymphatic drainage compared to an ALND. Staging of the regional nodes is then based on the histopathologic analysis of the sentinel node(s). Noninvasive disease (DCIS), typically, does not require axillary staging. However, if a patient is undergoing a mastectomy for DCIS, it is advisable to address the axillary nodes. This is because if any invasive disease is discovered after the surgery, performing a sentinel lymph node biopsy becomes challenging without the breast present for injection.

Axillary dissection is typically indicated for positive sentinel nodes or a clinically involved axilla, which refers to patients presenting with physical examination or imaging findings confirmed to be metastasis to the axillary lymph nodes. The procedure involves removal of lymph nodes from Level I (located in the axillary fat pad lateral to the pectoralis minor muscle), Level II (situated beneath the pectoralis minor muscle), and occasionally Level III (positioned superomedial to the pectoralis minor muscle). Level III nodes are only removed if suspected of cancer involvement, which is a rare occurrence in most breast cancers and is typically based on palpability during surgery or suspicious imaging findings.

Recent clinical trials indicate that in certain specific scenarios, patients with early-stage clinically node-negative breast cancer and limited pathologic involvement in only one to two sentinel nodes may undergo axillary radiation instead of axillary dissection. Additionally, neoadjuvant chemotherapy has shown potential in converting some clinically node-positive patients to node-negative status, allowing for sentinel node biopsy as an alternative to axillary dissection. Additionally, emerging data highlight the potential of immediate lymphatic reconstruction as a strategy to prevent lymphedema following ALND.

Radiation Treatment

In early-stage breast cancer, adjuvant radiation therapy reduces the local recurrence rate following breast-conserving surgery from approximately 30% to less than 10%. Adjuvant radiation is not usually given after mastectomy for early-stage breast cancer, as the local recurrence rate following mastectomy alone is already less than 5%. However, for more advanced breast cancer, adjuvant radiation may be given even after mastectomy if the risk of local recurrence is thought to be high. Postmastectomy radiation is considered for inflammatory breast cancer, locally advanced disease, node-positive breast cancer, and positive margins despite mastectomy.

Pregnancy and previous radiation to the same field are absolute contraindications to radiation therapy. Relative contraindications include previous radiation to the same general area, underlying pulmonary disease or cardiomyopathy, significant collagen vascular disease (eg, scleroderma, systemic lupus erythematosus), and inability to be positioned for radiation treatment. Omitting radiation may be considered if the patient is at least 65 years old, has a single cancer of size less than 2 cm completely excised with wide margins, and has negative lymph nodes, especially if the tumor is lower grade and hormone-receptor positive. Studies have also successfully investigated the omission of radiation in low-risk DCIS (eg, low grade, ER-positive, wide margins).

Whole-breast external beam radiation treatments each take only a few minutes and are given 5 days a week for a period of at least 4 to 6 weeks, usually including a "boost" to the tumor bed. Tangential fields (giving the treatments from multiple angles across the chest) spare underlying organs such as the heart and lungs.

Partial breast irradiation, in which only the local area of the lumpectomy is radiated, provides a shorter treatment duration, potentially fewer acute adverse events, and greater convenience. Studies are ongoing, and whole-breast radiation is still the standard of care.

Systemic Treatments

The development of an increasingly effective array of adjuvant systemic treatments is thought to be largely responsible for the recent gradual improvement in breast cancer survival. This remains an area of rapid innovation and frequent change.

Hormonal Therapy

Hormonal therapy is generally used after surgery, chemotherapy, and radiation have been completed. However, in some situations, it may be used in neoadjuvant therapy or as a sole therapy. Selective ER modulators, particularly tamoxifen, act as ER antagonists in breast tissue and as estrogen agonists in bone and uterus. They are used to treat ER-positive (ER+) tumors, reducing the incidence of recurrence as well as contralateral breast cancer. Tamoxifen is also used for prophylaxis in high-risk women, reducing the risk of breast cancer by approximately 50%. Aromatase inhibitors (AIs), such as letrozole, anastrozole, and exemestane, are used as an alternative to tamoxifen in postmenopausal women. As a class of drugs, they have been shown to decrease circulating estrogen levels by approximately 90% in postmenopausal women, and they may be superior to tamoxifen in prolonging disease-free survival. Multiple regimens are currently in use and in trial. The use of tamoxifen or AI therapy is typically of 5 to 10 years duration.

Chemotherapy

The primary goal of chemotherapy for breast cancer is to provide systemic treatment, targeting cancer cells throughout the body, thereby reducing the risk of distant organ recurrence and improving overall survival. It can be used preoperatively as neoadjuvant therapy or postoperatively as adjuvant therapy.

Numerous chemotherapy regimens have been introduced, with more under investigation. When administered as the initial treatment, neoadjuvant chemotherapy can reduce or downstage breast tumors and axillary nodes, aiding subsequent surgery and potentially enabling more conservative operative interventions. Conversely, adjuvant chemotherapy is provided after the initial cancer surgery. Indications to consider chemotherapy include node-positive disease, triple-negative breast cancer (TNBC), HER2-positive breast cancer, locally advanced disease, and high-grade tumors. Multigene assays can now predict recurrence and treatment response, helping determine which patients with early-stage ER+ breast cancer with node-negative or limited nodal involvement (one to three positive nodes) will likely benefit from chemotherapy in addition to hormonal therapy and which patients can safely omit chemotherapy.

Chemotherapy involves cytotoxic agents that destroy cancer cells, and different drugs within this category operate through varied mechanisms to disrupt the growth and division of these cells. It is rarely ever given as a single agent in the treatment of breast cancer. A commonly used chemotherapy regimen for breast cancer includes an anthracycline, a taxane (such as paclitaxel and docetaxel), and an alkylating agent like cyclophosphamide. Advances in systemic therapy are reshaping the landscape of breast cancer treatment. While biologic, targeted therapies like trastuzumab, a monoclonal antibody, have been pivotal in targeting the HER2 receptor and improving survival in HER2-positive tumors, newer strategies are emerging. The success of immune checkpoint inhibitors, especially in TNBC, highlights the potential of harnessing the immune system against cancer. These therapies, including PD-1/PD-L1 (programmed cell death protein 1/programmed death-ligand 1) inhibitors, work by enhancing the body's natural defense mechanisms against breast cancer. As the field advances, a combination of immunotherapies with conventional treatments is being explored, and novel immunotherapeutic strategies, such as cancer vaccines and CAR-T (chimeric antigen receptor T) cells, are under investigation.

Treatment of Male Breast Cancer

Male breast cancer accounts for approximately 1% of all breast cancer cases. Mastectomy is the usual surgical treatment of operable breast cancer in men because the breast is typically small in volume, and the tumors are located in the subareolar position. Most of these cancers are hormone-receptor positive. Evidence-based treatment regimens are difficult to develop because of the rarity of the disease. In general, treatment is similar to that for women with breast cancer, including the use of radiation, antiestrogen therapy, chemotherapy, and targeted therapy like trastuzumab, based on the tumor subtype. Additionally, genetic testing is indicated for all men with breast cancer and in women with a family history of male breast cancer.

Treatment of Recurrence and Metastasis

Local tumor recurrence in the breast after breast-conserving surgery and radiation is typically treated with mastectomy. If radiation was never given, a small recurrence may be treated with partial mastectomy and radiation.

Local recurrence after mastectomy is treated with surgical excision, if possible, and radiation to the area, if not contraindicated.

In addition to surgery and possibly radiation, systemic therapy may be involved in the treatment of local recurrence, as recurrence can suggest an aggressive form of the disease or the presence of microscopic disease that was not eliminated by the initial treatment. Systemic therapy, which can include chemotherapy, hormonal therapy, targeted therapy, or a combination thereof, aims to address any cancer cells that might have spread beyond the original site. The specific treatment approach is always individualized based on the patient's specific circumstances and the characteristics of the recurrence. The goal is to control the disease and prevent further spread while also managing symptoms and maintaining quality of life.

Metastatic disease is treated primarily with systemic therapy, which can consist of antiestrogen therapy, chemotherapy, and biologic treatments. Although there are some conflicting data, the prevailing evidence suggests that there is no survival advantage associated with surgery in the setting of stage IV breast cancer. As such, surgical interventions are primarily reserved for palliative purposes when deemed necessary. For patients presenting with brain metastases, frequently characterized by multiple lesions, radiation to the brain can be a key component in treatment alongside systemic therapy. In specific scenarios, such as isolated breast metastasis from another malignancy, surgical resection may also have a role. Bony metastases are treated with radiation and surgical fixation if there is associated pain or a high risk of fracture. Prior studies reported that radioactive strontium (^{89}Sr) could be used for widespread and painful bony metastases. Bisphosphonates support bone strength, lessen the risk of fracture, and may reduce bone pain.

Complications of Treatment
Surgery
Most patients undergo treatment of breast disease without complications. It is important, however, to be aware of the potential problems that may arise as a consequence of surgical and nonsurgical therapy in the management of breast disease.

Adverse effects of breast surgery may include bleeding, infection, development of seroma, inflammation, pain and tenderness, swelling, and cosmetic deformity. Some cosmetic problems can be corrected at least in part by plastic surgery. In addition, mastectomy can be complicated by flap necrosis.

Complications from axillary surgery may include seroma, infection, cording, hematoma, and nerve or musculoskeletal issues. Postoperative shoulder movement may initially be limited; however, mobility is usually fully restored with home exercises or physical therapy. Lymphedema is a risk in 25% to 30% of patients undergoing ALND. New axillary lymphatic reconstructive procedures have been introduced with the potential to reduce the risk of lymphedema when an axillary dissection is performed. Long-term results are pending. The proximity of the intercostobrachial nerves to the nodes frequently leads to sensation loss in the inner upper arm. Motor nerve complications are less common, particularly outside the context of reoperative or completion ALND. Sentinel node biopsy, due to its less-invasive dissection, generally has a lower incidence of these complications.

Reconstruction with implants has a somewhat higher risk of infection and in the long term may develop contracture of the capsule. All methods may result in chronic pain; however, the incidence of this is rare. With silicone breast implants, rupture and leakage can cause problems and require further surgery. All implants may eventually fail with time. Musculocutaneous flaps from the abdomen, latissimus, or gluteal region may cause weakness or deformity in the donor area. The deep inferior epigastric perforator (DIEP) flap procedure, which uses natural tissue from the abdomen as a free flap for breast reconstruction, can mitigate these complications. However, the procedure is technically demanding and requires specialized expertise. The DIEP flap offers advantages over the transverse rectus abdominis myocutaneous (TRAM) flap surgery, as it preserves the abdominal muscle and generally presents fewer risks. These flaps are also at risk for ischemic necrosis.

Radiation Treatment
Radiation treatment for breast cancer can lead to a range of side effects. In the early stages posttreatment, patients often experience symptoms akin to severe sunburn, such as breast erythema, skin damage, and edema. Altered sensation of the breast and fatigue may also occur. Over time, these acute symptoms can evolve into chronic changes like hyperpigmentation, poor wound healing, fat necrosis, and potential fibrosis. Radiation can also accentuate differences in the size and shape of the breasts, often leading to some contraction in the radiated breast. Rare complications include pneumonitis, cardiac disease, and bone necrosis. The risk of secondary cancers, notably angiosarcoma, is very low. Partial breast irradiation targets a smaller area and is administered over a shorter duration compared to whole-breast radiation. Though this may result in fewer acute side effects, the overall effects are largely similar.

Systemic Treatments
The adverse effects listed here are only the most common or dramatic.

Common side effects of tamoxifen are fatigue, night sweats, hot flashes, fluid retention, vaginitis, and thrombocytopenia (rare). Serious side effects are much less common and include deep vein thrombosis, pulmonary embolism, stroke, hepatotoxicity, and endometrial cancer. AIs cause fewer blood clots than tamoxifen and do not cause endometrial cancer. Adverse reactions from AIs include hot flashes, muscle and joint pains, osteoporosis, and potential fractures.

Chemotherapies in general are cytotoxic and act on cell division and growth. Normal, necessary cells are also affected, and those in the bone marrow and the lining of the gut are particularly vulnerable. Common adverse effects of chemotherapy include nausea, vomiting, bone marrow suppression, stomatitis, and alopecia. Adverse effects of taxanes specifically include, but are not limited to, hypersensitivity reactions, myelosuppression, and neuropathy. Anthracyclines can cause dose-dependent cardiotoxicity. Adverse effects of trastuzumab are usually mild but may include significant cardiac, especially when combined with adriamycin.

The common adverse effects of nausea and vomiting can be treated effectively with modern antiemetic therapy. Recombinant erythropoietin and granulocyte colony-stimulating factors have made it possible to keep hematocrit and neutrophil counts at acceptable levels.

Summary of Treatment

The treatment of patients with breast cancer is a multidisciplinary approach tailored to the tumor type, stage, and individual patient. Core modalities include surgery, radiation, and systemic therapy. Advances in targeted and immune therapies are revolutionizing breast cancer outcomes. Surgical options range from breast-conserving surgery to mastectomy, often accompanied by axillary evaluation. Radiation and systemic treatments are chosen based on tumor characteristics and potential benefits. Emerging techniques and therapies continue to evolve, aiming to improve oncologic outcomes and reduce side effects. Routine follow-up and surveillance are crucial for early detection of recurrences and managing long-term complications. The treatment of breast cancer is nuanced and benefits from a comprehensive, multidisciplinary team approach. A breast cancer diagnosis can be emotionally, psychologically, and physically challenging for the patient. It involves many complex choices with sometimes unpredictable outcomes. Patient education and engagement in shared decision-making is critical. Well-coordinated, patient-centered care not only enhances the patient experience but also leads to improved clinical outcomes.

SUGGESTED READINGS

American Cancer Society. *Breast Cancer Facts & Figures 2024-2025 Report.* American Cancer Society; 2024. https://urldefense.com/v3/__https://www.cancer.org/content/dam/cancer-org/research/cancer-facts-and-statistics/breast-cancer-facts-and-figures/2024/breast-cancer-facts-and-figures-2024.pdf__;!!F9wkZZsI-LA!FRzJZkFsNBsppeN7rxsU-7pD8_ytr_wEg2CJbiymmQRnNDb7qu-dJ-6uGOGwJ7gMrnNq9eeguqriiv1grtPd_XXVtg2DapQogvE$

Barton MB, Harris R, Fletcher SW. The rational clinical examination. Does this patient have breast cancer? The screening clinical breast examination: should it be done? How? *JAMA.* 1999;282(13):1270-1280. doi:10.1001/jama.282.13.1270

Fisher CS, Margenthaler JA, Hunt KK, Schwartz T. The landmark series: axillary management in breast cancer. *Ann Surg Oncol.* 2020;27(3):724-729. doi:10.1245/s10434-019-08154-5.

Fraker JL, Clune CG, Sahni SK, Yaganti A, Vegunta S. Prevalence, impact, and diagnostic challenges of benign breast disease: a narrative review. *Int J Women's Health.* 2023;15:765-778. doi:10.2147/IJWH.S351095

Giaquinto AN, Sung H, Newman LA, et al. Breast cancer statistics 2024. *CA Cancer J Clin.* 2024;74(6):477-495. doi:10.3322/caac.21863. https://urldefense.com/v3/__https:/acsjournals.onlinelibrary.wiley.com/doi/full/10.3322/caac.21863__;!!F9wkZZsI-LA!FRzJZkFsNBsppeN7rxsU-7pD8_ytr_wEg2CJbiymmQRnNDb7qu-dJ-6uGOGwJ7gMrnNq9eeguqriiv1grtPd_XXVtg2DoD9IZmc$

Giuliano AE, Edge SB, Hortobagyi GN. Eighth Edition of the AJCC Cancer Staging Manual: Breast Cancer. *Ann Surg Oncol.* 2018;25(7):1783-1785. doi: 10.1245/s10434-018-6486-6

Gradishar WJ, Moran MS, Abraham J, et al. NCCN Guidelines® Insights: Breast Cancer, Version 4.2023. *J Natl Compr Canc Netw.* 2023;21(6):594-608. doi:10.6004/jnccn.2023.0031

Waks AG, Winer EP. Breast cancer treatment: a review. *JAMA.* 2019;321(3):288-300. doi:10.1001/jama.2018.19323

SAMPLE QUESTIONS

QUESTIONS

Choose the best answer for each question.

1. A 35-year-old woman comes to the clinic because of right breast pain for the past 3 months. The pain is cyclical in nature. Her mother and two maternal aunts were all diagnosed with breast cancer in their 30s. There are no abnormal findings on examination, and a recent diagnostic mammogram and ultrasound are normal. Which of the following would be the most appropriate option for management?

   A. Prophylactic right breast mastectomy
   B. Chemoprevention with an oral contraceptive
   C. High-risk screening and genetic counseling
   D. Reassurance and routine observation
   E. Prophylactic hysterectomy

2. A 35-year-old woman comes to the clinic because of a 2-month history of thickening in the upper outer quadrant of her left breast. The patient's mother had breast cancer at age 48. Physical examination shows a slight retraction of the skin in the upper outer quadrant when the patient is upright. The breast tissue in that quadrant is rather firm, with the impression of a poorly demarcated thickening. A mammogram also shows dense tissue with no distinct mass or suspicious microcalcifications. What is the next step in the evaluation?

   A. Reexamination in 3 months
   B. Ultrasound of the palpable area
   C. Excisional biopsy
   D. Stereotactic biopsy
   E. Giving a 2-week course of the antibiotic clindamycin

3. A 51-year-old woman comes to the clinic because of a mass in the left breast for 2 weeks. She has no previous history of breast problems. Her last menstrual period was 1 week ago, menarche was at age 12, and she had her first child at age 30. She has no history of any major medical illness. Her paternal aunt had breast cancer at age 75. On physical examination, she has a 1-cm mass in the upper outer quadrant of the left breast. The mass is firm and freely movable with indistinct borders. There is minimal tenderness and skin dimpling over the mass. There is no nipple discharge and no axillary lymphadenopathy. The mammogram and breast ultrasound are normal. A biopsy shows cancer. Which of the

following is the most likely histologic type of cancer causing these findings?

A. Inflammatory
B. Infiltrating ductal
C. Infiltrating lobular
D. Lobular carcinoma in situ
E. Paget disease

4. A 45-year-old woman is seen in the clinic because of skin nodules on the upper portion of the breast and over the clavicle. One year ago, she underwent lumpectomy and sentinel node biopsy for stage IIA invasive ductal carcinoma, ER+, PR−, and HER2/neu−. She then received a full course of whole-breast radiation with a boost to the tumor bed. After four cycles of cytotoxic chemotherapy, she was started on tamoxifen by her oncologist and continues to tolerate this endocrine therapy well. Physical examination shows several clusters of firm nodules in the skin over the clavicle and along the upper portion of the left breast. Biopsy of one of these nodules shows metastatic breast cancer. What is the best treatment now?

A. An AI
B. Cytotoxic chemotherapy
C. Immediate mastectomy
D. Radiation treatment to the affected area
E. Trastuzumab

5. A 52-year-old woman comes to the clinic because of a bloody nipple discharge. She has noticed spontaneous bloody nipple discharge from her left breast every 2 to 3 days for the last month. She has no pain and takes no medications. Menarche was at age 12. She has four children and was 22 years old when her first child was born. There is no family history of breast cancer. There are no palpable breast masses, but a small amount of bloody discharge can be expressed from the upper inner quadrant of the left nipple. A mammogram done earlier today was read as normal. Which of the following is the most definitive step in diagnosis?

A. Breast MRI
B. Ductography
C. Duct excision
D. Cytology of the discharge
E. Additional mammographic views with focus on the retroareolar region

ANSWERS AND EXPLANATIONS

1. **Answer: C**

High-risk screening and genetic counseling are the best options for this patient, not reassurance and observation, as she has multiple first-degree and second-degree relatives with breast cancer. A unilateral prophylactic mastectomy would not be appropriate for achieving risk reduction, as both breasts are at risk. Evidence from clinical trials has demonstrated successful chemoprevention with an approximately 50% reduced risk of breast cancer; however, no trials demonstrating the role of oral contraceptives in breast cancer prevention exist. Hysterectomy alone has not been associated with a reduced risk of breast cancer. For more information on this answer, please see section "Clinical Presentation and Evaluation: Assessment of Breast Cancer Risk" and Table 17-4.

2. **Answer: B**

Ultrasound is an adjunct to mammography that is useful to characterize palpable masses. The radiographic finding is discordant with suspicious clinical presentation; therefore, further diagnostic workup is required. Excisional biopsy without prior attempted needle biopsy can lead to suboptimal management of a breast cancer. Stereotactic biopsy can be performed only on a lesion demonstrated by mammography. A breast abscess is exquisitely tender and demonstrable by ultrasonography. For more information on this answer, please see section "Evaluation of the Patient With a Breast Mass," and Figure 17-5.

3. **Answer: C**

Infiltrating lobular cancer often presents as described in this patient. It is frequently not apparent on mammogram because of weak desmoplastic response, low opacity, and lower likelihood of forming calcifications. Inflammatory breast cancer presents with red edematous skin. Infiltrating ductal carcinoma is hard with irregular borders and is usually seen on mammogram and ultrasound. Lobular carcinoma in situ does not usually present as a mass. Paget disease involves the nipple. For more information on this answer, please see section "Histologic Types of Breast Cancer."

4. **Answer: B**

Cytotoxic chemotherapy should be started as soon as possible. An AI is not indicated, because the patient failed hormonal treatment and her cancer advanced while she was taking tamoxifen. This is not a single-skin nodule but rather several clusters extending beyond the breast. Mastectomy may be considered, including excision of the entire area of the involved skin and possible skin graft, if she responds well to cytotoxic chemotherapy. The breast has already been radiated once and should not be radiated again. Trastuzumab is effective only in HER2 neu-positive breast cancers. For more information on this answer, please see sections "Systemic Treatments" and "Treatment of Recurrence and Metastasis."

5. **Answer: C**

MRI may have an emerging role in the evaluation of nipple discharge; however, it will not provide as definitive and reliable a diagnosis as a tissue specimen. Likewise, cytology and ductography may not avoid the need for duct excision to confirm the diagnosis. A significant percentage of patients with nipple discharge have no mammographic abnormalities. For more information on this answer, please see section "Nipple Discharge."

18

Surgical Endocrinology

Abbey L. Fingeret, Benjamin C. James, Adam S. Kabaker, Hadley E. Ritter, and Meredith J. Sorensen

THYROID GLAND

ANATOMY

The thyroid is a butterfly-shaped gland that sits in the lower part of the neck, at approximately the level of the second tracheal ring. It has left and right lobes connected by a narrow bridge of tissue called the "isthmus" (Figure 18-1). The sternohyoid and sternothyroid muscles lie in front of the gland. The trachea, larynx, and esophagus lie deep to it, and on either side are the carotid arteries.

The adult thyroid gland, weighing 10 to 20 g, is one of the most vascular organs in the body. The superior and inferior thyroid arteries, branches of the external carotid artery and the thyrocervical trunk, respectively, form the arterial supply. Venous drainage occurs through the superior, middle, and inferior thyroid veins. The recurrent laryngeal nerves that supply sensory and motor innervation to the larynx run in the tracheoesophageal grooves posterior to the thyroid lobes. The parathyroid glands, usually two on each side, typically lie on the posterior aspect of the thyroid gland although parathyroid anatomy can be variable.

The thyroid gland is derived mainly from the endoderm. It appears at approximately 24 days after conception as a thickening on the floor of the pharynx at the site of the foramen cecum in the adult tongue. This endodermal thickening grows caudally into the neck, as the thyroglossal duct, passing ventral to the embryonic hyoid bone and thyroic cartilage. The duct usually disappears by the 50th day of gestation but may persist anywhere along its migratory

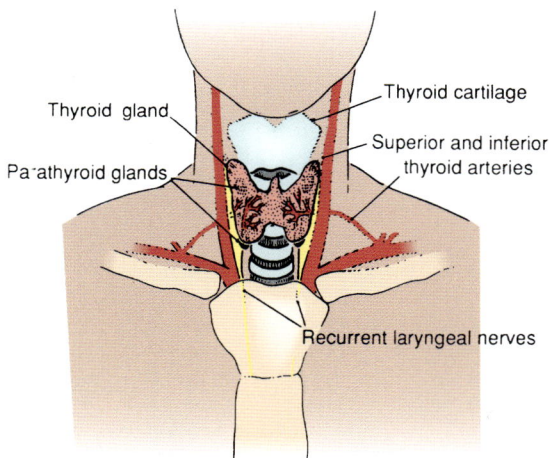

Figure 18-1. The thyroid gland.

pathway as the pyramidal lobe of the thyroid (present in up to 50% of adults) or as a thyroglossal duct cyst. The C cells of the thyroid gland originate from the ultimobranchial body, which is derived from the ectoderm.

PHYSIOLOGY

The thyroid gland has two distinct groups of hormone-producing cells. Follicular cells produce, store, and release thyroxine (T4) and triiodothyronine (T3), the two biologically active thyroid hormones and major regulators of the basal metabolic rate. Parafollicular cells, or C cells, secrete calcitonin, a hormone that has a minor role in maintaining calcium homeostasis.

Thyroid hormone synthesis is a multistep process that depends on iodine, which can only be obtained through diet or dietary supplements. Iodide is transported into follicular cells via a sodium iodide transporter. The iodide (I^-) is then oxidized to I^+ or iodine (I^0), catalyzed by the membrane-bound enzyme thyroid peroxidase. Thyroglobulin is a large-molecular-weight glycoprotein synthesized by the follicular cells and secreted into the extracellular storage spaces called the "follicles." Tyrosine residues of thyroglobulin are iodinated by the I^0 or I^+ species, forming mono- and di-iodotyrosine, which couple to form the iodothyronines T3 and T4. This iodinated thyroglobulin is the storage form of the thyroid hormones within the follicle (Figure 18-2). When thyroid-stimulating hormone (TSH), which originates in the anterior pituitary gland, stimulates the thyroid gland, iodinated thyroglobulin is transported back into the follicular cells by endocytosis. Here, it is hydrolyzed to T3 and T4, the active forms of the hormone, and released into the circulation. Eighty percent of the circulating hormone is T4, but T3, generated by the peripheral conversion of T4 to T3, is the most active form.

TSH, derived from the anterior pituitary gland, controls follicular cell function. It stimulates follicular cells to increase thyroglobulin synthesis, increases iodide transport efficiency, and stimulates the thyroid to release T3 and T4. Thyrotropin-releasing hormone (TRH), secreted by the hypothalamus into the hypothalamic-pituitary portal venous system, increases TSH release. If excessive concentrations of T3 and T4 are present, however, a negative feedback system shuts off the secretion of TSH and probably TRH (Figure 18-3).

The other hormone-producing cells in the thyroid are the parafollicular cells, or C cells, which make up only 0.1% of the total thyroid mass. When these cells are stimulated by high-serum calcium levels, they secrete the hormone calcitonin, which inhibits osteoclast activity, decreasing the calcium level. Calcitonin secretion, also affected by serum estrogen and vitamin D levels, does not

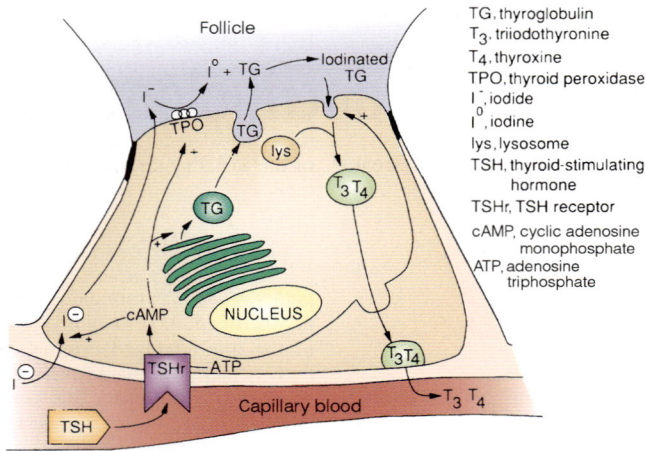

Figure 18-2. Iodinated thyroglobulin stored as thyroid hormones in the follicle.

normally play a major role in regulating serum calcium levels. Its function probably is to protect the skeleton from excessive scavenging during times of high calcium demand (eg, growth, pregnancy, lactation). The absence of calcitonin production (eg, after total thyroidectomy) appears to have no demonstrable negative physiologic effect.

PATHOPHYSIOLOGY

Thyroid Nodule

Thyroid nodules are extremely common. While clinically apparent thyroid nodules occur in approximately 6.5% of women and 1.5% of men, ultrasound studies have suggested that nodules are found in up to three-quarters of women and up to one-third of men. At autopsy, 37% to 57% of thyroid glands are noted to have one or more nodules. Thyroid nodules are often detected by the patients themselves, by health care providers during routine physical examinations (PEs), or increasingly by radiographic tests, such as neck ultrasound, computed tomography

(CT), or magnetic resonance imaging (MRI) performed for some other indication. Only about 5% of all thyroid nodules are cancerous; however, because of the high prevalence of thyroid nodules in the general population, a clear strategy is required to evaluate nodules.

Clinical Presentation and Evaluation

Evaluation should begin with a thorough history and physical (H&P) examination. History should include the duration of the nodule, any increase in size or changes over time, and the presence of symptoms. Symptoms can be caused by compression of adjacent structures, leading to globus sensation (lump in the throat or choking sensation), dysphagia (difficulty swallowing), or difficulty breathing. Symptoms can also be caused by excess thyroid hormone levels, such as heat intolerance, anxiety, or weight loss.

It is important to note that H&P examination has a low accuracy in predicting thyroid cancer. Features associated with a higher risk for cancer include rapid growth of the nodule, hoarseness, young age, a history of radiation exposure especially as a child, and a family history of thyroid cancer

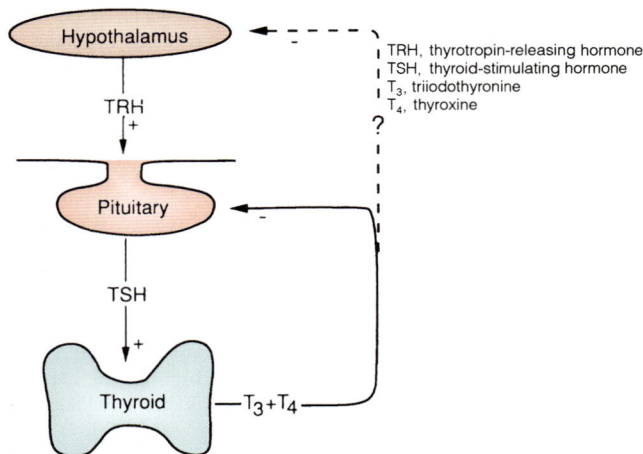

Figure 18-3. The hypothalamus-pituitary-thyroid axis.

or thyroid cancer syndromes (multiple endocrine neoplasia [MEN] type 2, familial adenomatous polyposis, etc).

The PE should include careful palpation of the entire thyroid gland and cervical lymph nodes to determine whether a nodule is solitary or dominant (in a multinodular goiter), the number and size of nodules, the consistency (soft, rubbery, or hard), and the involvement of adjacent structures, often indicated by fixation. Thyroid nodules should be mobile when the patient swallows. PE findings that may indicate malignancy include a hard, fixed mass and the presence of cervical lymphadenopathy. Indirect or direct laryngoscopy is indicated when there is voice hoarseness or when there is concern for local invasion of a malignancy, based on clinical presentation and/or imaging findings.

After H&P, serum TSH, T3, and T4, as well as thyroid ultrasound, are the initial diagnostic steps for any patient with a thyroid nodule, whether clinically palpable or incidentally noted. If the TSH is low, suggesting a hyperfunctioning gland or nodule, a radionuclide thyroid scan is the next step. If the TSH is high or normal (meaning the patient is either hypothyroid or euthyroid) and the nodule meets ultrasonic criteria for biopsy, fine needle aspiration (FNA) is the next step (Figure 18-4).

Other laboratory evaluations are of limited utility in thyroid nodule workup and should only be carried out in special circumstances. Medullary thyroid cancer (MTC) is the only thyroid cancer that reliably expresses a tumor marker (calcitonin) measurable in the serum. This should be checked preoperatively if MTH is suspected but should not be included for routine nodule workup. Serum thyroglobulin levels may be elevated in follicular or papillary carcinomas but may also be elevated in benign diseases, reducing its diagnostic significance for nodules. Patients with a history of radiation exposure or a family history of one of the MEN syndromes should have serum calcium levels measured. Patients who have a known rearranged during transfection (RET) mutation or a relative with MEN2 syndrome should also have plasma metanephrines evaluated to screen for functional pheochromocytoma (PHEO).

Ultrasound of the neck is the mainstay of imaging for thyroid nodules. It can determine the exact number and location of nodules, whether a nodule is cystic or solid, and detect enlarged or abnormal cervical lymph nodes. There are several ultrasound features associated with a higher risk of cancer, including solid composition, hypoechogenicity (compared with normal thyroid), irregular borders, microcalcifications, and nonspherical shape. These findings can help guide the selection of nodules for FNA. Nonfunctional thyroid nodules that do not meet the sonographic criteria for FNA are monitored with periodic ultrasonography. The frequency of evaluation, ranging from 6 to 24 months, depends upon the size and sonographic features of the nodule.

Except in patients who are hyperthyroid, radionuclide thyroid scanning is of limited utility in the management of thyroid nodules because no scan pattern is diagnostic of thyroid cancer nor can scan findings exclude thyroid

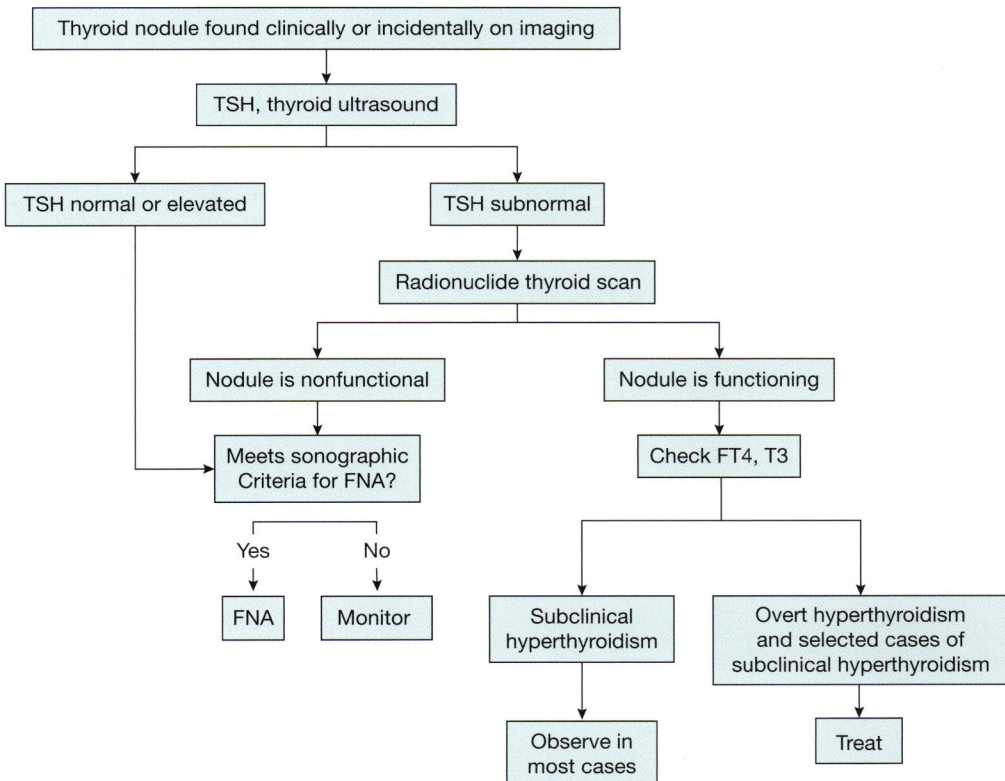

Figure 18-4. Initial evaluation of a patient with a thyroid nodule. FNA, fine needle aspiration; FT4, free thyroxine; T3, triiodothyronine; TSH, thyroid-stimulating hormone. (Reproduced with permission from Ross DS. Diagnostic approach to and treatment of thyroid nodules in adults. In: Connor RF, ed. UpToDate. Wolters Kluwer. Accessed January 10, 2025. Copyright © 2025 UpToDate, Inc. and/or its affiliates. All rights reserved.)

cancer. However, radionuclide scanning may be valuable in patients with nodular disease who are hyperthyroid to help distinguish toxic adenoma versus toxic multinodular goiter versus a nonfunctional nodule in the setting of Graves disease.

For nodules meeting the criteria, FNA provides specific information about the cytology of a nodule, which is the basis for subsequent management decisions. It is usually an easy and safe outpatient procedure. A 25-gauge needle is commonly used to aspirate the nodular material, with or without local anesthetic, under palpation or ultrasound guidance.

FNA cytology results are reported in six major categories (Bethesda Classification) (Table 18-1):

1. **Nondiagnostic (Bethesda 1):** The sample does not have an adequate number of follicular cells necessary to make a cytologic diagnosis. It is important not to interpret these biopsies as negative. The risk of malignancy is 5% to 10% (the incidence of malignancy in any thyroid nodule).

2. **Benign nodules (Bethesda 2):** normal-appearing cells with abundant colloid, usually obtained from colloid, adenomatous, or hyperplastic nodules, or autoimmune thyroiditis. There is a 0% to 3% risk of malignancy.

3. **Atypia of undetermined significance (AUS) or follicular lesion of undetermined significance (FLUS) (Bethesda 3):** Cells from these samples have enough atypical features that they cannot be called benign, but they are not highly suspicious for malignancy. The risk of malignancy is 6% to 18%.

4. **Follicular neoplasm (Bethesda 4):** These samples typically show microfollicles, cellular crowding, and scant colloid—patterns that can be seen in both benign and malignant lesions. The risk of malignancy is 10% to 40%.

TABLE 18-1. Bethesda System Diagnostic Categories for Reporting Thyroid Cytopathology

Bethesda Class	Diagnostic Category	Cancer Risk (%)
I	Nondiagnostic (unsatisfactory)	5-10
II	Benign	0-3
III	AUS or FLUS	10-30
IV	Follicular neoplasm (or suspicious for follicular neoplasm)	25-40
V	Suspicious for malignancy	50-75
VI	Malignant	97-99

AUS, atypia of undetermined significance; FLUS, follicular lesion of undetermined significance.

Data from Cibas ES, Ali SZ. The 2017 Bethesda system for reporting thyroid cytopathology. *Thyroid*. 2017;27:1341-1346; Haugen BR, Alexander EK, Bible KC, et al. 2015 American Thyroid Association Management guidelines for adult patients with thyroid nodules and differentiated thyroid cancer: the American Thyroid Association guidelines task force on thyroid nodules and differentiated thyroid cancer. *Thyroid*. 2016;26(1):1-133.

5. **Suspicious for malignancy (Bethesda 5):** Lesions have some features suggestive of, but not definitive for, thyroid cancer. The risk of malignancy is 50% to 75%.

6. **Malignant nodule (Bethesda 6):** This includes papillary thyroid cancer, medullary thyroid carcinoma (MTC), thyroid lymphoma, anaplastic cancer, and cancer metastatic to the thyroid gland. Follicular thyroid cancers cannot be diagnosed using FNA because the diagnosis is based on the presence of capsular or vascular invasion, which cannot be determined by cytology.

Bethesda 3 and 4 are often described as "indeterminate." Before the introduction of molecular testing, patients with indeterminate cytology required diagnostic surgery (usually thyroid lobectomy), but the majority of these lesions (60%-94%) were benign. The advent of molecular testing (mutational analysis, measurement of mRNA genomic expression, or both) has reduced the need for diagnostic surgery because they have very high negative predictive values.

Management of indeterminate nodules depends on institutional practices and availability of molecular testing. In some centers, an extra FNA sample is collected at the time of the initial biopsy that can be sent for molecular testing in the event of a Bethesda 3 or 4 cytology result. In other clinical settings, a repeat FNA is offered 6 to 12 weeks later. If the repeat aspiration is indeterminate again, molecular testing can be sent at that time or the patient may be referred for diagnostic surgery. Molecular testing is expensive, and the optimal use of these tests should be guided by clinical and local practice factors.

Treatment

The optimal therapy for patients with thyroid nodules depends on whether the patient is symptomatic or not, the specific type of lesion, and most importantly, the FNA result and the possibility of malignancy (Figure 18-5).

1. **Nondiagnostic (Bethesda 1):** Patients should have a repeat FNA in about 4 to 6 weeks, ideally under ultrasound guidance. If two repeat FNAs are nondiagnostic, the options are diagnostic surgery (usually thyroid lobectomy) or observation, depending upon the size of the nodule, the ultrasound features, and patient characteristics.

2. **Benign nodules (Bethesda 2):** This is the most common FNA result. Patients with benign nodules are usually followed up without surgery. Thyroid suppressive therapy is not recommended. Periodic ultrasound is performed to monitor for growth in size or other changes in the nodule. The monitoring interval is 12 to 24 months initially and is increased or decreased thereafter on the basis of clinical progress. FNA is repeated if there is a substantial increase in size or the appearance of suspicious ultrasound features, or if new clinical symptoms arise. Even in the setting of a benign FNA, patients with compressive symptoms attributable to the thyroid nodule(s) can be offered surgery in the form of thyroid lobectomy or total thyroidectomy for symptom relief.

3. **Indeterminate nodules (Bethesda 3 and 4):** If available, the aspirate should be tested further using various molecular markers, which may or may not require repeat FNA (see under Bethesda 2). If molecular testing

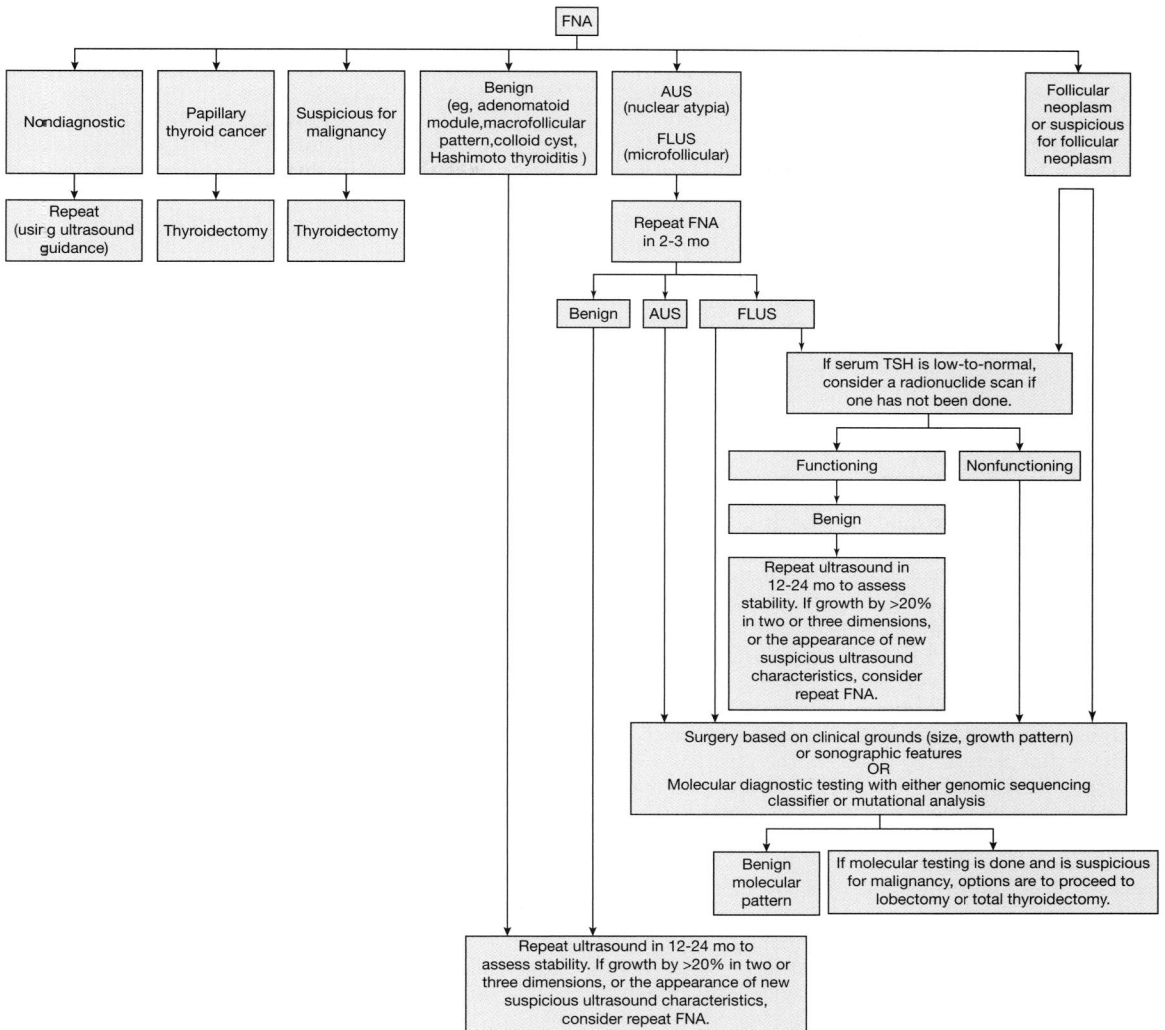

Figure 18-5. Management of thyroid nodules based upon results of fine needle aspiration. AUS, atypical cells of undetermined significance; FLUS, follicular lesion of undetermined significance; FNA, fine needle aspiration; TSH, thyroid-stimulating hormone. (Reproduced with permission from Ross DS. Thyroid biopsy. In: Post TW, ed. UpToDate. Accessed July 3, 2018. Copyright @2018 UpToDate, Inc. For more information, visit www.uptodate.com.)

is not available or if the molecular testing result is suspicious, diagnostic surgery (usually thyroid lobectomy) is performed. Patients undergoing diagnostic lobectomy may require completion thyroidectomy if an intermediate- or high-risk thyroid cancer is found.

4. **Suspicious for malignancy (Bethesda 5):** Nodules in this category have a high risk of malignancy and are typically referred for surgical evaluation. Molecular testing is not indicated in this group.

5. **Malignant nodules (Bethesda 6):** These patients should all be referred for surgical evaluation. For well-differentiated thyroid cancers (papillary and follicular), thyroid lobectomy is recommended for tumors smaller than 1 cm, and total thyroidectomy is recommended for tumors larger than 4 cm or with evidence of extrathyroidal extension or metastatic disease. For tumors of size between 1 and 4 cm, with no extrathyroidal

extension, and no evidence of lymph node involvement, the initial surgical procedure can be either a thyroid lobectomy or a total thyroidectomy. Patients with MTC should undergo total thyroidectomy with central neck dissection.

Thyroid surgery is usually safe, with low complication rates, especially when performed by experienced endocrine surgeons. It is typically performed under general anesthesia and as either an outpatient procedure or a one-night stay. A complete lobectomy is the minimum acceptable extent of thyroid surgery. Partial lobectomies or "nodulectomies" are not performed because of the risk of inadequate resection, disease recurrence, scar tissue formation, and the need for reoperations. Patients who undergo total thyroidectomy will be permanently dependent on thyroid hormone replacement that should be initiated after surgery.

After lobectomy, only about one-third of patients will require thyroid hormone supplementation. These patients are not routinely started on any thyroid medication postoperatively, and their need for thyroid hormone replacement is determined by TSH levels measured approximately 6 weeks after surgery.

One of the challenges of thyroid surgery is parathyroid preservation. The four parathyroid glands are closely associated with the thyroid gland, and it is important to identify them and preserve their blood supply during thyroidectomy. Hypocalcemia resulting from damage to the parathyroid glands can lead to symptoms ranging from paresthesias in the lips, hands, and feet to muscle twitching and tetany whereas permanent hypoparathyroidism is rare after total thyroidectomy (2%-13%), and transient hypoparathyroidism affects up to 49% of patients after thyroidectomy. Some surgeons recommend empiric calcium supplementation to all patients who have undergone thyroidectomy to prevent symptoms of hypocalcemia whereas others prefer selective calcium supplementation based on measurement of postoperative parathyroid hormone (PTH) levels. If injury to a parathyroid gland's blood supply is recognized during the procedure, the parathyroid can be autotransplanted into a nearby muscle, usually the ipsilateral strap or sternocleidomastoid muscle.

Preservation of the recurrent laryngeal nerve and the external branch of the superior laryngeal nerve is also essential. Injury to the recurrent laryngeal nerve causes paralysis of the ipsilateral vocal cord, which becomes immobile in the paramedian position. The other cord may not be opposable, leaving the patient with a weak, breathy voice. Bilateral injury causes total loss of speech and airway control, and requires tracheostomy. Injury to the external branch of the superior nerve results in a loss of voice quality with deficits in high pitch and projection. Transient neurapraxia of the nerves caused by stretch or traction injuries is more common than permanent injury and usually resolves without sequelae within 6 months.

Meticulous hemostasis must be maintained during thyroid surgery to prevent hematoma formation. Bleeding in the central neck can cause tracheal compression, even when the hematoma is small. The surgical wound should be opened, at the bedside if necessary, to evacuate the hematoma and avert an airway emergency.

Hyperthyroidism

Hyperthyroidism or thyrotoxicosis is caused by excessive secretion of thyroid hormone. The signs and symptoms are those of a hypermetabolic state (Table 18-2). Serum TSH levels in thyrotoxicosis can determine whether the hyperthyroidism is pituitary dependent or independent. A low level of TSH in the presence of high thyroid hormone levels establishes thyroid-dependent hyperthyroidism—the most common situation. Elevated TSH levels are seen in pituitary causes. The most common cause of thyroid-dependent hyperthyroidism is Graves disease or diffuse toxic goiter. Less commonly, hyperthyroidism is caused by one (toxic adenoma) or more (toxic multinodular goiter) hyperfunctioning nodules. History, PE, radionuclide scan, and thyroid ultrasound findings can differentiate these three etiologies of hyperthyroidism. A diffusely enlarged, soft gland with a homogeneously increased radionuclide uptake, with or without nodules, is seen in Graves disease. A

TABLE 18-2. Symptoms and Signs of Hyperthyroidism

Central Nervous System	Cardiovascular and Respiratory Systems	Other Systems
Nervousness	Tachycardia	Lid lag
Restlessness	Palpitations	Proptosis or exophthalmos
Emotional lability	Arrhythmias	Ophthalmopathy
Fast speech	Dyspnea	Increased sweating
Fine tremor		Fatigue
		Weakness
		Hair loss
		Leg swelling
		Pretibial myxedema

solitary nodule with increased uptake against a background of suppressed uptake in the remaining thyroid characterizes toxic adenoma. The features of toxic multinodular goiter are a diffusely multinodular gland, heterogeneous radionuclide uptake, and multiple nodules of varying sizes on ultrasonography.

The lifetime risk of hyperthyroidism is approximately 5% for women and 1% for men. Graves disease occurs predominantly in young women (8:1 ratio). Toxic nodular goiter is more common in older women.

Graves Disease
Clinical Presentation and Evaluation

Graves disease (named for Robert J. Graves, an Irish physician, 1797-1853) is a syndrome of diffuse goiter with hyperthyroidism, sometimes accompanied by eye disease or an infiltrative dermopathy. The ophthalmologic effects of Graves disease cover a continuum from a stare with lid lag to proptosis, and may progress to deformity of the periorbital tissues with optic nerve involvement and complete loss of vision.

Patients with Graves disease have circulating thyrotropin receptor autoantibodies (TRAb), or thyroid-stimulating immunoglobulin (TSI), which activate the TSH receptors on the follicular cells, stimulating the thyroid to generate and secrete excessive T3 and T4. The sensitivity to the negative feedback system that controls normal thyroid function is lost. The presence of TRAb/TSI in serum is diagnostic of Graves disease. The exophthalmos and the pretibial myxedema associated with Graves disease result from the expression of TSH receptors by retroorbital and adipose tissues.

Treatment

There are three possible treatments for Graves disease: (1) antithyroid drugs, (2) radioiodine ablation, and (3) surgery (total thyroidectomy). The choice of therapy is determined by the severity of hyperthyroidism and shared decision-making between the clinician and patient.

Antithyroid drugs (thionamides) can be used for initial symptom control before definitive therapy, as a 1- to 2-year strategy to try to achieve remission, or as long-term treatment. β-Blockers are used for initial symptom control in patients who are severely hyperadrenergic. Remission rates after 1 to 2 years of antithyroid drug therapy are less than 40% but can exceed 80% after 5 to 10 years. Thionamides (methimazole and propylthiouracil [PTU]) interfere with the synthesis of thyroid hormones by inhibiting iodide organification and iodotyrosine coupling. PTU also reduces the rate of peripheral conversion of T4 to T3. Both thionamides can cause significant side effects, including skin reactions (rash, urticaria), agranulocytosis, and hepatotoxicity. Methimazole is teratogenic, so PTU must be used during the first trimester of pregnancy instead of methimazole. Otherwise, methimazole is most commonly used due to its longer duration of action and less severe toxicity. If medical management is unsuccessful, or if a more durable long-term solution is desired, there are two options for definitive treatment: radioiodine ablation or surgery.

Radioiodine ablation is a safe and effective treatment. It is administered as a capsule or an oral solution of sodium I-131, which gets rapidly absorbed by the gastrointestinal (GI) tract and concentrated in the thyroid. The tissue damage caused by the radioiodine results in ablation of the thyroid in 6 to 18 weeks. However, for as many as 20% of patients, a second or even a third dose may be necessary. Over a period of 5 to 10 years, 50% to 70% of patients develop hypothyroidism. Radioiodine ablation is contraindicated in pregnant or lactating women, those who desire immediate childbearing, or in patients with significant orbitopathy, which can be worsened by radioiodine.

Total thyroidectomy provides immediate control of the disease. Surgery is indicated in patients who are allergic to thionamides or have contraindications to, or are unwilling to get, radioiodine ablation. Patients with severe hyperthyroidism, significant orbitopathy, and very large goiters or nodular thyroid disease are also suitable candidates for surgery.

None of the antithyroid therapies significantly affects the exophthalmos or pretibial myxedema that is associated with Graves disease. These manifestations may respond to local or systemic cortisol treatment, and external beam radiation therapy is occasionally used for severe ophthalmopathy. However, stabilization and regression of these signs and symptoms are reported most consistently after total thyroidectomy. This effect is thought to occur by lessening the generalized autoimmune response by removing all thyroid tissue.

Toxic Adenoma

Toxic adenoma is a solitary tumor of the thyroid gland that produces excessive amounts of thyroid hormone and causes overt hyperthyroidism. Malignancy in a toxic nodule is rare. The presentation of hyperthyroidism is similar to that seen in Graves disease. However, patients do not have associated ophthalmopathy or pretibial myxedema because toxic adenoma is not an autoimmune phenomenon like Graves disease.

Clinical Presentation and Evaluation

Serum thyroid hormone levels show high T3 and T4 and suppressed TSH, consistent with an autonomous thyroid source of excessive thyroid hormone production. Unlike the diffuse goiter in Graves disease, the thyroid gland is normal or small, with a nodule that is "hot" or functional on a thyroid scan.

Treatment

The initial treatment is similar to that for Graves disease, but definitive treatment requires surgery because resolution after treatment with thionamides is rare. After symptom control, usually with propranolol or one of the thionamides, the lobe with the "hot" nodule is excised by thyroid lobectomy. Surgery is also the optimal therapy for a toxic multinodular goiter (Plummer disease). Total thyroidectomy is indicated, especially if the goiter is large and associated with symptoms such as compression. Radioactive iodine ablation is not considered appropriate therapy for toxic adenoma or Plummer disease. Although the overactive thyroid elements can be ablated, recurrence is more common than with Graves disease because of the intrinsic autonomy of the thyroid tissue. In addition, solitary toxic adenoma that is surgically treated preserves the normal lobe, reducing the likelihood that the patient will need thyroid hormone replacement.

Thyroid Carcinoma

Thyroid cancer represents 2.3% of all new cancer cases in the United States and about 0.4% of all cancer-related deaths. From the 1990s to 2000s, the incidence of thyroid cancer more than doubled, possibly due to increased incidental detection. However, the incidence of tumors of all sizes increased, suggesting another cause for the increasing incidence besides simply an overdiagnosis phenomenon. The death rate did not increase commensurately. Since 2010, age-adjusted rates for new thyroid cancer cases have remained stable. In 2022, the annual incidence and death rates were 13.8 and 0.5 people per 100,000 people, respectively. Approximately 1.2% of people will be diagnosed with thyroid cancer in their lifetime. It is 3 times as common in women as in men and affects all age groups. In general, the prognosis is excellent, with a 5-year survival rate of 98% for all stages combined.

Thyroid cancers can arise from any of the cells that make up the gland. Follicular cells give rise to papillary and follicular thyroid carcinomas, termed together as *well-differentiated thyroid cancers*. Parafollicular cells give rise to medullary carcinoma, and lymphoid cells can give rise to lymphoma. When analyzed by electron microscopy and immunohistochemistry, anaplastic tumors appear to arise from follicular cells, although they have dedifferentiated to the point that they are no longer recognizable by light microscopy.

Treatment

Surgery is the therapy of choice for well-differentiated thyroid cancer (papillary and follicular) and MTC. The extent of the disease including tumor size, suspicion for extrathyroidal extension, lymph node involvement, patient's age, and comorbid conditions determines the extent of surgery: typically lobectomy or total thyroidectomy. Cervical lymph node status should be evaluated in all patients by preoperative ultrasound. Other preoperative imaging is usually not indicated except in selected patients with locally advanced disease. Suspected lymph node metastases from thyroid cancer should be confirmed by FNA preoperatively so that the patients may undergo a therapeutic neck dissection of the relevant compartments (central and/or lateral) at the time of thyroidectomy.

Several stratification systems are available to assess the risk of residual and recurrent disease. The American Thyroid Association's system is commonly used. This system is primarily based on certain pathologic features, including extrathyroidal extension, regional metastases, worrisome histologies, or vascular invasion. Following surgery, patients with high and intermediate risks for recurrence receive radioactive iodine treatment. The goal of adjuvant radioiodine is to destroy any residual subclinical tumor deposits after surgical resection of all grossly apparent diseases.

After completion of treatment, patients are monitored for residual or recurrent disease using neck ultrasound, TSH, and serum thyroglobulin. Since most differentiated thyroid cancer cells are TSH responsive, postoperative thyroid replacement is dosed to maintain TSH in the low-to-normal range, or even the subnormal range in high-risk patients. The frequency of monitoring and need for additional imaging are based on the initial risk stratification and response to treatment.

Papillary Carcinoma
Papillary carcinoma is the most common thyroid malignancy in the United States, accounting for approximately 80% to 90% of cases.

Clinical Presentation and Evaluation
Papillary cancers usually present as nodules, detected on routine PE or incidentally noted on imaging. FNA is usually diagnostic. Characteristic cytologic features on FNA include cytoplasmic pseudoinclusions, nuclear grooves, and psammoma bodies (concentric layers of calcium found in stalk formations that give this cancer its name). Tumors with a mix of papillary and follicular features on FNA (follicular variant of papillary carcinoma) are classified with the papillary cancers because they have similar biologic behavior.

Treatment
Surgery is the primary mode of therapy, followed by radioactive iodine therapy when indicated. Metastatic disease to regional lymph nodes is common in patients with papillary thyroid cancer. Palpable nodal disease is present in approximately 5% to 10% of patients and in 20% to 30% of patients on preoperative neck ultrasound, so preoperative ultrasound of both the thyroid and the cervical lymph nodes is essential. Patients with known nodal disease at the time of presentation should undergo total thyroidectomy with therapeutic neck dissection of the involved compartment(s). Microscopic metastatic disease to central neck lymph nodes is very common, found in up to 80% of patients with papillary thyroid carcinoma (PTC), but it is rarely of clinical significance. Consequently, routine prophylactic central neck dissection in patients presenting without nodal disease is not recommended but may be carried out selectively in high-risk patients.

Papillary cancers usually grow slowly and most patients have an excellent prognosis even in the presence of metastatic involvement of lymph nodes at the time of presentation. Worse prognosis is associated with male sex, age older than 55 years, a primary tumor larger than 4 cm, less well-differentiated cells, and locally invasive or distant metastatic disease.

Follicular Carcinoma
Follicular thyroid carcinoma (FTC) is the second most common thyroid cancer, accounting for 5% to 10% of cases. It is more common in iodine-deficient areas of the world. Compared with papillary carcinoma, it is more common in older patients and may have a more aggressive clinical course.

Clinical Presentation and Evaluation
Patients typically present with a thyroid nodule. On FNA, follicular carcinomas have a monotonous, relatively uniform appearance of microfollicles. FNA cytology alone cannot distinguish between follicular adenoma and follicular carcinoma. The actual diagnosis requires histologic evaluation of a surgical specimen for capsular and/or vascular invasion. FNA specimens are often indeterminate: AUS (Bethesda 3) or follicular neoplasm (Bethesda 4). Molecular testing may allow avoidance of diagnostic surgery in this patient population. Unlike PTC, lymph node metastases are uncommon, found in only 8% to 13% of follicular cancers. Hematogenous metastatic spread, usually to bone and lungs, is seen in 10% to 15% of patients with FTC.

Treatment
Surgery is the primary treatment option, in some cases followed by radioactive iodine therapy and thyroid suppression, as described earlier. Metastatic lesions may concentrate iodine and be amenable to radioiodine therapy after the thyroid gland is removed. Follicular carcinomas also grow slowly, and the prognosis is good for younger patients with small, minimally invasive tumors. Factors associated with worse prognosis include age older than 55 years, extensive angioinvasion, local invasion, oncocytic variant (formerly classified as Hurthle cell carcinoma), and distant metastases.

Medullary Carcinoma
MTC is a neuroendocrine tumor (NET) of the C cells of the thyroid gland and constitutes less than 5% of all thyroid cancers. Calcitonin production is a characteristic feature. Most MTCs are sporadic in nature, but approximately 20% have a genetically transmitted, autosomal dominant inheritance pattern associated with MEN2 syndrome (discussed later in the chapter). Patients with MTC have a worse prognosis than patients with well-differentiated papillary or follicular carcinoma; only 50% of patients survive for 10 years.

Clinical Presentation and Evaluation
The usual presentation is in an older patient, typically in the fourth to sixth decades of life, with a solitary thyroid nodule. Clinically detectable cervical lymph node involvement is common at presentation. Patients may also present with signs of invasion (hoarseness or dysphagia) or with distant metastases. Patients with advanced disease may present with diarrhea or facial flushing because of hormonal secretion by the tumor.

The diagnosis is usually suspected on FNA. Further evaluation includes measurement of serum calcitonin, carcinoembryonic antigen (CEA), biochemical evaluation for coexisting tumors, especially PHEO, and genetic testing for RET mutations. Preoperative cervical ultrasound is essential for adequate local staging. Patients with local lymph node metastases or preoperative serum calcitonin levels greater than 500 pg/mL require additional cross-sectional imaging, specifically evaluating the neck, chest, liver and bones.

Treatment

The primary treatment for MTC is complete surgical resection (total thyroidectomy) and prophylactic central lymph node dissection. If lateral lymph node metastases are suspected preoperatively based on either examination or imaging, FNA should be carried out and modified radical lymph node dissection should also be performed. Because MTC is a tumor of the C cells, which do not concentrate iodine, adjuvant radioactive iodine is not effective. There is a limited role for external beam radiation therapy in locally advanced tumors. In patients with progressive or symptomatic metastatic disease, systemic treatment with kinase inhibitors can stabilize the disease and delay progression.

Anaplastic Carcinoma

Unlike the well-differentiated thyroid cancers, anaplastic carcinoma of the thyroid gland is an extremely aggressive neoplasm with rapid progression and nearly 100% disease-specific mortality. Almost all patients present with a rapidly growing neck mass. Prognosis is dismal, with a median survival of 3 to 7 months. Approximately 90% of patients have metastatic disease at the time of presentation. All anaplastic cancers are considered Stage IV cancers.

Anaplastic cancer arises from the follicular cells but is nearly totally dedifferentiated. Core needle biopsy may be necessary to establish the diagnosis and to obtain adequate tissue for molecular testing, which should be carried out expeditiously to guide treatment. All patients should have an ultrasound of the neck (if not already taken), a positron emission tomography (PET)/CT scan, brain imaging (either MRI or CT), and skeletal evaluation if bony metastases are suspected. CT neck/chest may be helpful to assess surgical resectability. For tumors confined to the thyroid without metastatic disease (Stage IVA), complete surgical resection should be performed. Survival can be prolonged for more than 2 years. Depending on molecular testing results, neoadjuvant targeted therapy can be attempted in patients with initially unresectable disease, followed by surgery if there is good response. For patients with metastatic anaplastic thyroid cancer, the disease is uniformly fatal. Chemoradiation and/or targeted therapies may delay progression. Regardless, palliative care and end-of-life planning are an integral part of anaplastic thyroid cancer care.

Lymphoma

Lymphoma can present as a rapidly enlarging thyroid mass and, on ultrasound, looks similar to chronic thyroiditis. To distinguish a lymphoma from florid Hashimoto thyroiditis, a core needle or open biopsy may be necessary. The treatment is not surgical; rather, it is treated with chemotherapy and radiation similarly to lymphoma presenting at other sites.

PARATHYROID GLANDS

ANATOMY AND MORPHOLOGY

Normal parathyroid glands are yellow-brown, ovoid, and fatty glands that are usually positioned on or near the posterior aspect of the thyroid gland. Each gland normally weighs 30 to 50 mg and measures about 5 mm in its greatest dimension. Most adults have four glands; however, 10% to 15% can have additional normal-sized glands or additional parathyroid "rests" from fragmentation of the glands during development. The embryologic development also determines the position of the parathyroid glands. The superior parathyroid glands develop from the fourth branchial pouches whereas the inferior parathyroid glands develop from the third branchial pouches and migrate caudally together with the thymus. Arterial supply is normally from inferior thyroid artery branches, and venous drainage is to the internal jugular, subclavian, and innominate veins. The superior glands generally lie posterior and lateral to the recurrent laryngeal nerve and superior to the inferior thyroid artery. The inferior glands are typically anterior and medial to the recurrent laryngeal nerve between the inferior thyroid pole and the superior aspect of the cervical thymus at the thyrothymic ligament. Any of the parathyroid glands can be ectopically positioned because of alterations in migration during embryologic development, although inferior glands are more often ectopic because of the longer path of migration. Ectopic locations are still along the path of migration often associated with other structures that develop with the third and fourth branchial pouches. These locations include the carotid sheath, intrathyroidal, retrotracheal, or retroesophageal, within the thymus and in the superior mediastinum (see Figure 18-2). As parathyroid glands pathologically enlarge, they become darker brown, firm, and less fatty.

PHYSIOLOGY AND PATHOPHYSIOLOGY

The parathyroid glands are the sole source of PTH, an 84-amino-acid peptide. Plasma PTH is rapidly cleaved into active N-terminal and inactive C-terminal fragments. The active fragment half-life is about 3 minutes compared with about 18 hours for the C-terminal fragment. The short half-life of the active fragment allows rapid and tight control of serum calcium levels. This characteristic is also used in parathyroid surgery to be able to confirm adequate excision by testing the change in intraoperative PTH (ioPTH) levels before and after the removal of abnormal glands. PTH is closely related to serum calcium levels through a sensitive and rapid inverse feedback loop. Hypocalcemia stimulates PTH secretion and hypercalcemia inhibits PTH secretion. Dysregulation of this feedback system with autonomously secreted PTH is the basis of primary and tertiary hyperparathyroidism. Other major regulators of calcium homeostasis are renal calcium excretion, bone turnover, intestinal calcium absorption, and vitamin D. Secondary factors include magnesium and calcitonin. Serum magnesium usually fluctuates with serum calcium

Site	Vitamin D

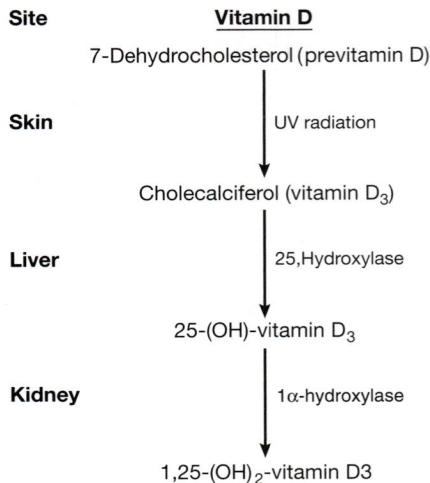

Figure 18-6. Vitamin D synthesis.

in an inverse relationship with PTH, but severe hypomagnesemia paradoxically inhibits PTH secretion. Therefore, hypomagnesemia must be corrected when it coexists with hypocalcemia. Calcitonin is produced in the parafollicular cells of the thyroid. High-dose calcitonin inhibits osteoclastic bone reabsorption, but the physiologic role of calcitonin in calcium homeostasis is unclear and does not significantly affect serum calcium levels.

The summary effect of PTH is to increase serum calcium levels to a normal level.

This is achieved by three distinct mechanisms:

1. Directly affecting the kidneys to increase calcium resorption and increase phosphate clearance
2. Directly mobilizing calcium from bone and stimulating osteoclast activation and bone reabsorption
3. Indirectly increasing GI calcium absorption by stimulating 1α-hydroxylase activity of vitamin D production to produce 1,25-dihydroxy-cholecalciferol ($1,25(OH)_2$-D3), which directly enhances GI absorption of calcium (Figure 18-6).

Vitamin D is fat soluble and is formed in three steps. Previtamin D is converted to cholecalciferol when skin is exposed to sunlight. Cholecalciferol undergoes 25-hydroxylation in the liver. Renal hydroxylation, catalyzed by 1α-hydroxylase, yields the most active form: $1,25(OH)_2$-D3. Low vitamin D levels increase PTH secretion and thereby increase 1α-hydroxylase activity. Once normal calcium levels are achieved, calcium negatively feeds back to decrease PTH secretion. $1,25(OH)_2$-D3 has slight inhibitory function on PTH, but PTH secretion is not influenced by serum phosphate levels.

Primary Hyperparathyroidism

In primary hyperparathyroidism (PHP), the inverse relationship between PTH and serum calcium is disturbed by one or more parathyroid glands autonomously secreting PTH, and the negative feedback loop is lost. Although calcium may be elevated or remain within upper normal limits, PTH is elevated relative to the serum calcium level. Serum phosphate is often low and renal function is normal. PHP may be caused by parathyroid adenoma (85%),

parathyroid hyperplasia (15%), or parathyroid carcinoma (<1%). PTH secretion is increased and the homeostatic set point for calcium is reset at a higher value in all three conditions. By exerting its normal effects as listed earlier, excess PTH secretion leads to increased GI calcium absorption, increased urinary calcium excretion, and net bone loss. Adenoma refers to one or two enlarged glands and is a benign process. Because of the softness and mobility of parathyroid glands, the abnormal gland is rarely palpable preoperatively. Typical adenomas measure about 1 to 2 cm in size and weigh 500 to 1,000 mg. Hyperplasia, or multiglandular disease, is diagnosed when all glands are grossly abnormal. Hyperplasia is also a benign process affecting all glands, but gland enlargement is usually asymmetric. PHP from hyperplasia is most often sporadic but may be inherited, either alone or as part of a MEN syndrome.

Secondary and Tertiary Hyperparathyroidism

Secondary hyperparathyroidism most often occurs in patients with renal failure (renal hyperparathyroidism). Impaired glomerular filtration causes phosphate retention and decreased serum calcium levels. Reduced functional renal mass is available to hydroxylate 25-OH-vitamin D. The resultant lower 1,25-dihydroxy-vitamin D levels lead to lower GI absorption of calcium and further hypocalcemia. PTH secretion by all glands is stimulated to restore calcium and phosphorus homeostasis. Continued nephron loss produces chronic overstimulation of PTH secretion, elevated PTH levels, parathyroid hyperplasia, and hyperphosphatemia (Figure 18-7). The multiple abnormalities in calcium, phosphate, and vitamin D metabolism have extremely deleterious effects on bone mineralization and may also lead to soft-tissue calcium deposition and damage, such as tendon rupture or skin necrosis.

Secondary hyperparathyroidism can also occur because of low vitamin D levels or low calcium absorption related to nutritional deficiencies (eg, malabsorptive disorders, bariatric surgery, obesity) or a lack of sun exposure. An important role for vitamin D is emerging in cardiovascular health, malignancy, and autoimmune disorders, yielding

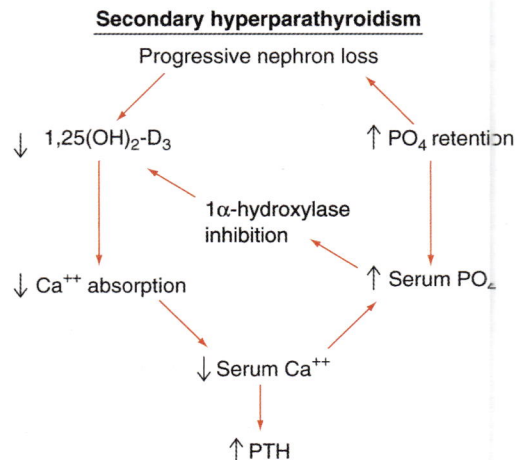

Figure 18-7. In secondary hyperparathyroidism, progressive nephron loss leads to phosphate retention, decreased calcium absorption, inhibition of 1α-hydroxylase, and decreased activation of vitamin D. These factors lead to decreased serum calcium and increased secretion of PTH. PTH, parathyroid hormone.

upward revisions of existing normal ranges and dietary recommendations. Since vitamin D is fat soluble, levels should be checked before high-dose replacement. Once the secondary cause of the hyperparathyroidism is corrected, the PTH levels should return to normal.

In tertiary hyperparathyroidism, the hyperplastic glands in a patient with secondary hyperparathyroidism become an autonomous producer of PTH after the chronic stimulation of the glands from the secondary etiology has resolved. Despite the corrected secondary cause of hyperparathyroidism, the parathyroid glands continue to overproduce PTH. In patients with renal disease, most are identified with tertiary hyperparathyroidism when their PTH levels remain high despite successful renal transplantation. The remaining patients are those who remain on dialysis and spontaneously progress from secondary to tertiary hyperparathyroidism, usually marked by the onset of hypercalcemia. Tertiary hyperparathyroidism behaves in most ways like PHP from hyperplasia.

Parathyroid Cancer

Parathyroid cancer is quite rare and may be suspected preoperatively with critically high calcium and significantly elevated PTH levels. There may be a suggestion of invasion on imaging or intraoperatively by adjacent tissue invasion. The difference between an adenoma and a carcinoma is determined pathologically by the presence of gross or microscopic invasion.

Clinical Presentation and Evaluation

Historically, patients with PHP have classically presented with the complaints suggested in the mnemonic, "stones, bones, groans, moans, and psychiatric overtones." Most patients developed urolithiasis ("stones") or bone diseases including bone resorption with cyst (osteitis cystica) and brown tumor formation ("bones"). Less commonly seen symptoms were abdominal pain from peptic ulcers, constipation or pancreatitis ("moans"), diffuse joint and muscle pains, fatigue and lethargy ("groans"), and neuropsychiatric abnormalities including depression or worsening psychosis ("psychiatric overtones").

Currently, most patients with PHP are found when unrelated laboratory testing reveals incidental hypercalcemia. The most common cause of outpatient hypercalcemia is PHP and the most frequent source of inpatient hypercalcemia is malignancy, either via paraneoplastic syndrome and primary bone malignancy or bony metastases. Additional causes include medications (eg, hydrochlorothiazide, lithium, and calcium supplements), inherited hypercalcemia syndromes, and sarcoidosis (Table 18-3).

History taking should target not only the classic complaints of PHP but also the now more common, poorly defined constitutional or neuropsychiatric symptoms such as a reduced sense of well-being, fatigue, insomnia, malaise, lack of mental clarity, or behavioral changes. Negative drug and family histories, plus negative system reviews focused on the most common occult malignancies, support a working diagnosis of sporadic PHP. Further workup begins by assessing the relationship between calcium and PTH as well as assessing vitamin D and renal function. These should be drawn simultaneously. Standard PTH assays measure the whole PTH peptide by double antibody techniques and are known as "intact" or "biointact" assays (Figure 18-8). Table 18-3 lists diseases associated with

TABLE 18-3.	Differential Diagnosis of Hypercalcemia	
Diagnosis	**PTH**	**PTHrP**
Primary hyperparathyroidism	High	Low
Tertiary hyperparathyroidism	High	Low
Familial hypercalcemic hypocalciuria	High, normal, or low	Low
Lithium therapy	High or normal	Low
Paraneoplastic syndrome (humoral hypercalcemia of malignancy)	Low	High
Osteolytic metastases	Low	Low
Multiple myeloma	Low	Low
Drug-induced hypercalcemia[a]	Low	Low
Granulomatous disease	Low	Low
Hypervitaminosis D	Low	Low
Milk-alkali syndrome	Low	Low
Nonparathyroid endocrine disease	Low	Low
Immobilization	Low	Low
Idiopathic	Low	Low

[a]Except lithium induced; see text.
PTH, parathyroid hormone; PTHrP, parathyroid hormone-related peptide.

hypercalcemia arranged into those associated with or without elevated PTH. Elevated intact PTH plus hypercalcemia occurs only with primary and tertiary hyperparathyroidism, familial hypercalcemic hypocalciuria (FHH), vitamin D deficiency, or lithium-induced hypercalcemia. Urinary calcium and serum vitamin D levels may help differentiate among the causes of increased PTH. FHH is a very rare autosomal dominant asymptomatic disease with lifetime elevated calcium levels and additional affected family members. Distinguishing PHP from FHH is necessary before surgical intervention because patients with FHH will not benefit from surgery. Urinary calcium excretion should be obtained to differentiate this patient population. A genetic analysis for FHH mutations in the calcium-sensing receptor should be carried out to confirm the diagnosis.

Malignancy can also cause hypercalcemia but will not cause an elevated PTH, except for a parathyroid cancer. Obtaining a serum parathyroid hormone-related peptide (PTHrP) level might be useful when occult malignancy is a concern and the PTH level is suppressed, indicating a paraneoplastic syndrome. The most common malignant causes of hypercalcemia are bronchial squamous cell carcinoma, bone destruction by primary cancers (eg, multiple myeloma), or lytic bony metastases causing hypercalcemia without PTHrP elevation (Table 18-3). Vitamin D analogues are secreted by some tumors (eg, lymphoma) and can produce hypercalcemia without PTH or PTHrP elevations.

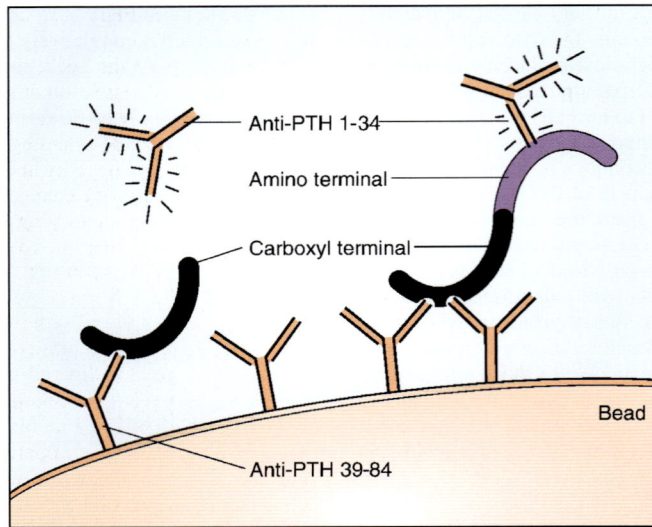

Figure 18-8. Intact parathyroid hormone (PTH) assay. An antibody recognizing PTH 39-84 binds carboxyl fragments in the midpoint and C-terminus of the molecule. A second antibody recognizes the amino-terminal region of PTH (1-34).

Increased activation of 25-OH-vitamin D by macrophages in granulomatous lesions (eg, sarcoidosis) can lead to hypercalcemia without increased PTH or PTHrP. A normal chest radiograph makes sarcoidosis unlikely. Lithium appears to interfere with the calcium-PTH feedback loop; a history of bipolar disorder or a therapeutic lithium level should point to this possibility.

Secondary hyperparathyroidism is present to some degree in most patients with end-stage renal disease. Intact PTH levels are often elevated, but serum calcium is usually normal. An elevated serum calcium level raises concern for tertiary disease. Serum phosphorus and creatinine are increased whereas vitamin D levels are often low. PTH fragments, especially C-terminal ones, have prolonged half-lives and are increased in chronic renal failure. Typical manifestations of the disease are bone pain, soft-tissue calcifications with calcinosis or uremic calcific arteriolopathy, and pruritus.

Treatment
Medical
Acute, severe hypercalcemia is managed by large-volume saline infusion to restore intravascular volume and to initiate a saline diuresis, which in turn triggers calciuresis. Loop diuretics (eg, furosemide) are used adjunctively. Drugs may be added to decrease bone turnover (eg, bisphosphonates, calcitonin). Acute dialysis is rarely required. Treatment directed at any underlying malignancy or other precipitating condition is added where appropriate (eg, glucocorticoids for sarcoidosis).

Currently, there is no definitive medical treatment for primary or tertiary hyperparathyroidism. Bisphosphonates (eg, alendronate) and selective estrogen receptor modulators (eg, raloxifene) can help slow down and sometimes prevent bone loss. Because these drugs are relatively ineffective in primary and tertiary hyperparathyroidism, they are generally reserved for patients who have prohibitive operative risk. For patients with end-stage renal disease,

improved techniques of dialysis, vitamin D supplements, and effective oral phosphate binders have markedly enhanced the medical control of secondary hyperparathyroidism and reduced the incidence of significant bony disease. Cinacalcet, a calcimimetic that lowers calcium by activating the calcium-sensing receptor, is available for use in secondary disease but is ineffective for primary or tertiary disease.

Surgical
For patients with objective symptoms or signs of PHP (eg, urolithiasis, osteoporosis, or fragility fractures), the operation is clearly indicated. In the absence of major, life-limiting comorbidities, patients with metabolic derangements caused by PHP are also best served by surgery. Operative indications for patients with no or minimal symptoms are somewhat less clear. Outcome data are confounded by the overlap between the constitutional symptoms of PHP and the aches and pains of aging. It is important to note that the extent of calcium elevation does not reliably correlate with the severity of symptoms. Patients with age-related vague symptoms may show improvement with correcting a mildly elevated calcium levels from PHP. Current less-invasive parathyroid operations offer a low-risk, lower-cost procedure with rapid convalescence. When compared with the inconvenience and cost of observation with serial metabolic evaluations and the inherent risks of prolonged hyperparathyroidism, surgery is increasingly being recommended for minimally symptomatic patients. Patient selection criteria for parathyroidectomy as developed by the National Institutes of Health include asymptomatic patients younger than 50 years, signs of renal impairment, urolithiasis, and bone loss, and a calcium level greater than the one above the upper limit of normal (Table 18-4).

For patients with end-stage renal disease, renal transplantation remains the most effective long-term treatment for both renal disease and secondary hyperparathyroidism. Subtotal parathyroidectomy is indicated for ongoing bone

TABLE 18-4. National Institutes of Health Criteria for Parathyroidectomy

Age <50 or any age with any of the following:

Nephrolithiasis
Osteitis fibrosa cystica
Serum calcium >1.0 mg/dL above reference range (typically >11.2)
Hypercalciuria (>400 mg/d)
Bone mineral density T score reduced by >2.5 SD measured at ≥1 sites
Creatinine clearance reduced by 30% compared with age-matched normal range
History of an episode of life-threatening hypercalcemia
Neuromuscular symptoms: documented proximal weakness, atrophy, hyperreflexia, and gait disturbance

SD, standard deviation.

loss, soft-tissue calcifications, or severe pruritus, particularly for patients who are not transplant candidates. Parathyroidectomy is occasionally indicated for patients on lithium who develop hypercalcemia and who cannot be managed with alternate medications.

Although most surgeons use preoperative localization studies to help guide the type of operation, the decision to operate should be made on the biochemical diagnosis of the disease and the patient's indications for an operation. The goal of any parathyroid operation is to remove any abnormal glands while leaving the appropriate amount of functional parathyroid tissue.

Classic four-gland exploration for sporadic PHP includes visualization of all cervical glands, characterization of the disease by the surgeon on the basis of operative observations of the presence of adenoma or multiglandular hyperplasia, and resection of sufficient parathyroid tissue to restore long-term eucalcemia without creating hypoparathyroidism. This is appropriate for all patients. Exploration is typically performed under general anesthesia although some patients are candidates for cervical block and heavy sedation. Single-gland resection is performed for parathyroid adenoma, while hyperplasia is most often treated by subtotal resection (removing three and a half gland). Familial syndromes (see section "Multiple Endocrine Neoplasia Syndromes") introduce other considerations, and alternatives such as total parathyroidectomy with autotransplantation and cryopreservation of excised tissue are often performed. Autotransplantation is commonly performed into the forearm (brachioradialis) so that if there is a recurrence, the graft in the arm can more easily be removed. Cervical thymectomy is also appropriate in hyperplasia to remove any parathyroid "rests" that can be associated with the thymus. This can be performed through a small incision and is most often confirmed to be an adequate excision with ioPTH assay monitoring.

Directed operative strategies, also known as minimally invasive, focal, or targeted, are applicable but only to localized sporadic PHP. If an abnormal parathyroid gland can be identified preoperatively to guide the surgeon to the appropriate side of the neck, that gland can be removed, with no additional dissection of the other glands. Preoperative localization may be performed using ultrasonography, sestamibi radionuclide scanning, or four-dimensional CT. Each technique has benefits and limitations, so a combination of tests is used by some surgeons. One unique benefit of ultrasound is identifying intrathyroidal parathyroid glands as well as ruling out coexisting thyroid pathology that may need attention during the same operation.

For the minimally invasive focused ioPTH-directed strategy, peripheral blood is drawn for ioPTH assay, which is an intact PTH assay modified to shorten the turnaround time to 20 minutes. A limited incision is made sufficient to expose and excise the preoperatively localized abnormal parathyroid gland. Serial blood samples for ioPTH are drawn after excision for comparison with a baseline drawn after anesthetic induction. An ioPTH level at 10 minutes post excision that has fallen into the normal range and has declined by more than 50% from baseline indicates sufficient parathyroid resection to restore long-term eucalcemia. Ideally, the level should also fall within the normal reference range to increase confidence that a second adenoma is not present. Time criteria may be modified when PTH degradation kinetics are impaired (eg, renal disease). Failure of the ioPTH level to drop appropriately necessitates continued neck exploration to evaluate the remaining glands.

With either a four-gland exploration or a directed parathyroidectomy by either method, most patients can be discharged in 24 hours or less. Minimal analgesics are required, and convalescence is typically brief. Patients are sometimes discharged on calcium supplements to be weaned as outpatients, depending upon how suppressed the remaining parathyroid glands are and how depleted the patient is of calcium. Most patients are total-body depleted of calcium despite elevated serum levels. Short-term calcium supplements are often used to prevent symptoms of low calcium, including peripheral and facial paresthesias and muscle spasms.

Some abnormal parathyroid glands are located low in the mediastinum and are not accessible via a cervical incision. These can usually be removed thoracoscopically or via an open approach.

If a parathyroid cancer is suspected, an en bloc resection is performed. This operation includes resection of the primary tumor and the ipsilateral thyroid lobe plus adherent soft tissue and regional lymph nodes. For parathyroid cancer diagnosed postoperatively on the basis of final histopathology only, reoperation may not be indicated. Serum calcium and PTH levels are followed in patients with parathyroid cancer to detect recurrences. There is no effective adjuvant radiotherapy or chemotherapy. Recurrences are treated by medical control of hypercalcemia plus cinacalcet and by resection of tumor whenever feasible.

Because secondary hyperparathyroidism is always multiglandular, at least subtotal parathyroidectomy (of three and a half glands) should be performed. Total parathyroidectomy with autotransplantation is preferred by some surgeons. Published results are similar for both procedures. More recently, some surgeons have employed total parathyroidectomy without autotransplantation, because patients often have residual rests of cervical parathyroid tissue that suffice for calcium homeostasis. Cervical thymectomy is typically performed with operations for secondary disease because the inferior glands and many parathyroid rests are near to or within the thymus.

Operations for tertiary hyperparathyroidism are guided by the intraoperative findings, which is most often multiglandular disease leading to either total parathyroidectomy with autotransplant or subtotal parathyroidectomy. As in PHP with hyperplasia, autotransplantation in secondary and tertiary hyperparathyroidism is usually performed in the forearm.

Complications

Parathyroid surgery is usually very safe with the benefit of eucalcemia outweighing the risks. The most serious complication of cervical parathyroidectomy, recurrent laryngeal nerve injury, is extremely rare. Factors that increase the risk are previous cervical operations or radiation, concomitant thyroid surgery, and parathyroid cancer. Some surgeons employ nerve monitoring techniques to help manage this risk. Persistent hypercalcemia because of failure to identify or adequately resect the adenoma or the hyperplastic glands can occur in 1% to 5% of patients. Transient, early postoperative hypoparathyroidism sometimes occurs because of chronic preoperative suppression of the remaining normal parathyroid tissue by the hyperfunctioning gland(s). Patients with established bone disease appear to be at an increased risk for early hypoparathyroidism. Permanent hypoparathyroidism is rare with an occurrence of less than 1%. Phosphorus as well as calcium should be measured postoperatively because a successful operation typically corrects hypophosphatemia. In the "hungry bone" syndrome, phosphorus is taken up by the bone with calcium, and serum phosphorus remains low. Such patients require supplemental calcium postoperatively until the syndrome resolves.

In the event of persistent or recurrent hypercalcemia, repeat laboratory testing is performed first to confirm the diagnosis of hyperparathyroidism. Radionuclide and anatomic imaging studies are then repeated. When conventional imaging is negative, some institutions utilize transfemoral selective venous sampling for PTH in the neck and mediastinum, which may localize the side of the disease. Most persistent abnormal tissue is found in the neck. Cervical reoperation carries greater risks of recurrent nerve injury and permanent hypoparathyroidism.

In those patients who have had an autotransplantation into their forearm, labs should be drawn simultaneously from both arms, with the graft side being drawn above the level of the implant. This can help differentiate between recurrence from a gland in the neck and overgrowth of the transplanted graft.

ADRENAL GLANDS

ANATOMY

The adrenal glands are small (3-5 g each), yellow, and triangular glands located behind the peritoneum of the posterior abdominal wall, closely associated with the upper poles of the kidneys (Figure 18-9). The right adrenal gland lies posterior to the liver and posterior and lateral to the inferior vena cava. The left adrenal is lateral to the aorta and just behind the superior border of the pancreatic tail.

The arterial blood supply to the adrenal glands is from three main arteries: the superior adrenal artery branches from the inferior phrenic artery, the middle adrenal artery arises from the aorta, and the inferior adrenal artery is a branch from the renal artery. The adrenal veins are remarkably consistent in their location and drainage but different by side. The right adrenal vein drains directly into the inferior vena cava whereas the left adrenal vein drains into the left renal vein.

The adrenal gland is divided into two primary areas on the basis of embryologic development of the tissue types:

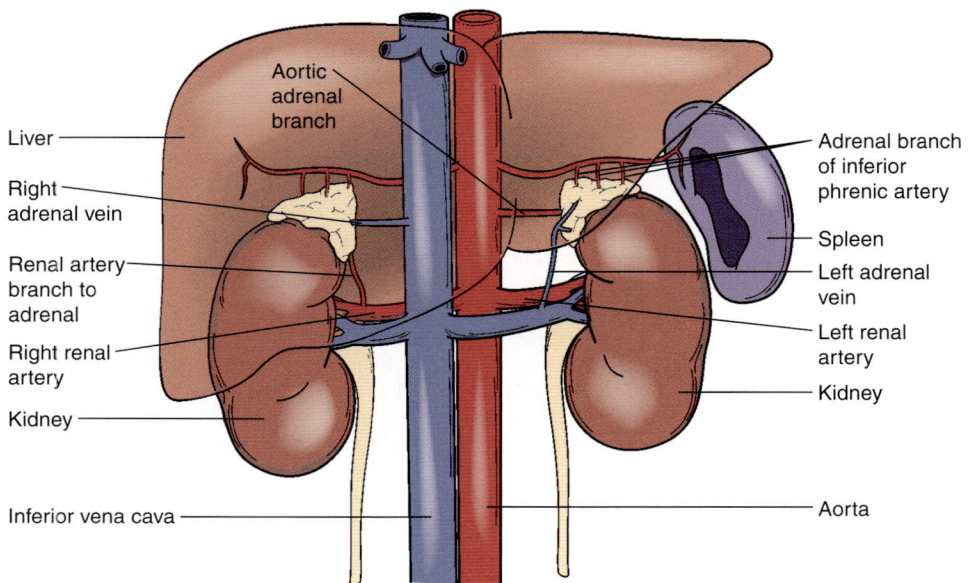

Figure 18-9. Anatomy of the adrenal glands showing their relations to the adjacent structure and their blood supply.

the cortex, which is derived from the mesoderm, and the medulla, which arises from neural crest cells. The medulla is the only endocrine organ gland whose activity is controlled entirely by nervous impulses. The innervation of the adrenal medulla is unusual in that there are no post-ganglionic cells.

PHYSIOLOGY

The adrenal cortex has three layers: the outer zona glomerulosa, the middle zona fasciculata, and the inner zona reticularis. Each zone produces its own distinct hormones derived from cholesterol, which is converted to pregnenolone. The latter serves as the precursor for the glucocorticoids, mineralocorticoids, and androgenic steroids produced by the cortical cells (Table 18-5).

The zona glomerulosa produces and secretes mineralocorticoids, of which the most predominant is aldosterone. Secretion of aldosterone is primarily regulated by the renin-angiotensin system in a negative feedback fashion and is also influenced by plasma potassium concentration. In response to a decrease in renal blood flow, the juxtaglomerular cells within the kidneys produce renin, which cleaves angiotensinogen into angiotensin I, which is then converted by the angiotensin-converting enzyme in the lungs to angiotensin II. Angiotensin II directly stimulates aldosterone release from the zona glomerulosa, which increases the exchange of sodium for potassium and hydrogen ions in the distal nephron. Aldosterone stimulates renal sodium reabsorption while promoting potassium wasting to modulate the body's electrolyte composition, fluid volume, and blood pressure.

The cells within the zona fasciculata secrete the glucocorticoid cortisol, stimulated by circulating adrenocorticotropic hormone (ACTH) from the anterior pituitary and suppressed by cortisol feedback inhibition. Cortisol is involved in the intermediate metabolism of carbohydrates, proteins, and lipids. It increases blood glucose levels by decreasing insulin uptake and stimulating hepatic

TABLE 18-5. Correlation of Adrenal Zones With Disease Syndromes and Abnormal Adrenal Function

Adrenal Zone	Hormone Produced	Normal Function	Hypersecretory Syndrome	Symptoms	Pearls
Zona glomerulosa	Aldosterone	Electrolyte metabolism	Conn syndrome	Hypokalemia	Insuppressible hyperaldosteronism and suppressed plasma renin
				Hypertension	
				Muscle weakness	
Zona fasciculata	Cortisone	Protein and carbohydrate metabolism	Cushing syndrome or disease	Buffalo hump	Exclude exogenous intake of glucocorticoids.
	Hydrocortisone			Violaceous striae	
				Moon facies	
				Truncal obesity	
				Hypertension	
Zona reticularis	Progesterone	Sexual differentiation	Adrenogenital syndrome	Virilism/feminization	Presents in early childhood
	Androgen			Hyponatremia	
	Estrogen			Hypertension	
Medulla	Epinephrine	Sympathetic response	Pheochromocytoma	Episodic hypertension	10% are:
				Malignant	
				Bilateral	
				Familial	
				Extra-adrenal	
	Norepinephrine			Headache	
				Sweating	
				Palpitations	

gluconeogenesis. Cortisol also slows amino acid uptake and peripheral protein synthesis while increasing peripheral lipolysis. Prolonged effects of high levels of cortisol include the induction of a catabolic state, proximal muscle wasting, truncal obesity, insulin-resistant diabetes, impaired wound healing, and immunosuppression.

The cells of the zona reticularis respond to ACTH by converting pregnenolone to 17-hydroxypregnenolone, which is then converted to dehydroepiandrosterone (DHEA), the major sex steroid produced by the adrenal glands. DHEA is converted by local tissues into testosterone. Adrenal production of sex hormones is responsible, in part, for the development of male secondary sexual features. Abnormal production can cause virilization in women.

Finally, the adrenal medulla secretes catecholamines. The secretions of the adrenal cortex flow through the medulla and bathe the cells in high levels of cortisol before draining into the venous system, which induces expression of the enzyme phenylethanolamine-N-methyltransferase (PNMT) that converts norepinephrine (NE) to epinephrine (EPI). The secretion of EPI and NE is regulated primarily by descending sympathetic signals from the brain in response to various forms of stress. Because the adrenal medulla is directly innervated by the autonomic nervous system, adrenomedullary responses are very rapid.

DISEASE STATES

Cushing Syndrome

Cushing syndrome (CS) refers to the signs and symptoms of hypercortisolism and can be caused by a variety of disease processes. CS is classified as either ACTH dependent or ACTH independent. ACTH-independent hypercortisolism most commonly results from exogenous corticosteroid administration but can also be caused by adrenocortical tumors including adenomas in 10% to 25% of patients, adrenal cortical carcinomas (ACCs) in 8% of patients, and bilateral adrenal hyperplasia in 1% of patients. ACTH-dependent CS can be caused by excessive ACTH production secondary to the hypothalamus releasing excessive amounts of corticotrophin-releasing hormone, pituitary adenomas (Cushing disease [CD]) which produce excessive amounts of ACTH, or extrapituitary ACTH-producing tumors, such as bronchial carcinoids and small-cell lung cancer in 5% to 10% of cases.

Clinical Presentation

CS usually presents in the third and the fourth decades, and it has a 4:1 female-to-male preponderance. Some of the classic clinical features include truncal obesity (90%), hypertension (80%), diabetes (80%), weakness (80%), purple striae (70%), hirsutism (70%), moon facies (60%), and lipodystrophy of the dorsocervical fat pad, which is described as a "buffalo hump." A number of other symptoms can be seen, including depression, mental changes, osteoporosis, kidney stones, polyuria, fungal skin infections, poor wound healing, menstrual disturbances, and acne. However, patients may also present with subclinical disease. In patients with CS, the diurnal variation in glucocorticoid secretion (high levels in the morning, declining during the day, with lowest levels in the evening) and the ability of the adrenal gland to increase cortisol secretion in response to ACTH stimulation are either lost or blunted. When CS is caused by ectopic ACTH and pituitary tumors, melanotropins are also secreted, leading to increased skin pigmentation.

Diagnosis

In patients with suspected CS, a complete H&P examination looking for the abovementioned symptoms is critical. It is particularly important to rule out sources of exogenous glucocorticoid exposure and to be aware of medications that might interfere with some screening tests. There are three main screening tests: urinary-free cortisol (at least two measurements), late-night salivary cortisol (two measurements), and low-dose 1-mg overnight dexamethasone suppression test (DST). One of these tests should be performed, and if there is any abnormal result, with serial testing, one or two of the other tests should also be performed.

If CS is confirmed by one of the abovementioned tests, a workup is performed to determine the subtype of CS affecting the patient. Plasma ACTH measurement segregates patients into ACTH-dependent or ACTH-independent subtypes. In patients with a suppressed ACTH level <5 pg/mL), the CS etiology is caused by a primary adrenal tumor. CT scan or MRI of the abdomen should be performed to localize the mass.

If the ACTH level is normal or increased, then the patient should have a pituitary MRI to evaluate for a pituitary tumor.

Treatment

Solitary, unilateral, and benign adenomas are the cause of primary adrenal hypercortisolism in 80% to 90% of patients. The treatment of choice is laparoscopic unilateral adrenalectomy. All of these patients should receive perioperative doses of steroids. Biochemical evaluation of adrenal function should be performed postoperatively to determine if exogenous supplementation is necessary until the remaining adrenal tissue regains function.

Patients with bilateral cortisol-secreting adenomas are often treated in a staged fashion with the larger gland being removed first. However, patients with more severe disease may ultimately require bilateral adrenalectomy resulting in permanent adrenal insufficiency requiring lifelong steroid replacement.

Primary Aldosteronism

Primary aldosteronism (PA), termed *Conn syndrome*, is defined as inappropriate hypersecretion of aldosterone in the absence of activation of the renin-angiotensin system. The syndrome is twice as common in women as in men and most commonly occurs between the fourth and the sixth decades of life. Patients with PA produce excess aldosterone that is not responsive to the renin-angiotensin axis and that is not suppressed by salt loading. PA has been reported in more than 10% of patients with hypertension and 20% of patients with resistant hypertension. Although the classic presentation of PA is hypertension and hypokalemia, only 30% of patients have hypokalemia on presentation. The importance of diagnosing PA is that it may be surgically curable, and these patients have higher cardiovascular morbidity and mortality than matched patients with hypertension due to other etiologies.

Clinical Presentation

The vast majority of patients present without clinical symptoms but will often have a history of poorly controlled hypertension. Excess aldosterone increases total-body sodium, decreases potassium levels, and increases extracellular volume, resulting in metabolic alkalosis and hypertension. The classic biochemical findings include persistently elevated plasma and urinary aldosterone levels and reduced plasma renin activity unresponsive to stimulation.

Diagnosis

The diagnosis is suspected in patients with moderate or severe hypertension or drug-resistant hypertension, hypertension and hypokalemia, hypertension and an adrenal lesion, or hypertension in a patient with a family history of PA, early-onset hypertension, or the sequelae of hypertension. Fifty-five to sixty percent of these patients have bilateral hyperplasia whereas 35% to 45% have an adrenal adenoma.

An aldosterone-to-renin ratio (ARR) is the best initial screening test. Before testing, hypokalemia should be corrected and sodium intake should not be restricted; certain medications like spironolactone, potassium-wasting diuretics, and chewing tobacco should be stopped 4 weeks before testing. The diagnosis is confirmed in patients with significantly elevated aldosterone concentrations over 30 ng/dL along with low renin levels. In patients with laboratory findings suspicious of PA but not diagnostic, further testing should be performed to confirm inappropriate aldosterone secretion. The confirmatory testing involves loading the patient with either oral or intravenous (IV) saline and testing the aldosterone response. If the patient demonstrates persistently elevated aldosterone levels despite sodium loading, then the diagnosis is confirmed. Once PA has been confirmed, all patients should undergo a CT scan of the abdomen. Adrenal vein sampling for aldosterone levels in the bilateral adrenal veins is used to confirm that a lesion found on cross-sectional imaging is the source of hypersecretion.

Treatment

Patients with unilateral aldosteronomas should have their hypertension and hypokalemia normalized before surgical intervention, often with a mineralocorticoid receptor antagonist (like spironolactone). Laparoscopic unilateral adrenalectomy is the treatment of choice in these patients. When adenomas are removed, the blood pressure becomes normal in 70% of patients; the remainder will require modest antihypertensive therapy. Patients with hyperaldosteronism that cannot be localized to one adrenal gland are managed with medical therapy. In most of these patients, bilateral adrenal hyperplasia (diffuse disease) is the cause of the hyperaldosteronism, and bilateral adrenalectomy is not recommended.

Pheochromocytoma

PHEOs are tumors arising from catecholamine-producing chromaffin cells in the adrenal medulla. Most are hormonally active, producing NE and EPI. A few produce EPI only, which can be seen in heritable causes such as MEN2. Vasoconstriction occurs from α-adrenergic stimulation, and increased cardiac output occurs from β-adrenergic

stimulation, all resulting in hypertension. The incidence of PHEOs among patients with hypertension is 0.1% to 2%. Extra-adrenal lesions are classified as "paragangliomas." These extra-adrenal sites may be anywhere along the sympathetic chain from the base of the skull to the pelvis but are most often para-aortic.

Ninety-eight percent of PHEOs are located in the abdominal cavity. In order to convert NE to EPI, PNMT must be induced. Extra-adrenal tumors do not have this activated enzyme and thus usually secrete only NE. Plasma normetanephrine levels are elevated in 97% of patients with adrenal PHEO and 100% of patients with extra-adrenal PHEOs.

Clinical Presentation

Although patients with PHEOs may have extremely variable presentations, most have episodic hypertension associated with palpitations, headache, and sweating. These symptoms are a direct result of sustained or paroxysmal secretion of NE and/or EPI. Patients may also experience a sense of impending doom, significant anxiety, weight loss, and constipation. Physical signs of an attack may include pallor, flushing, and sweating. Most attacks are short-lived, lasting 15 minutes or shorter, and can be precipitated by trauma including invasive medical procedures, physical activity, exertion, changes in position, alcohol intake, micturition, smoking, or labor. Hypertension can be episodic, sustained or widely fluctuating, and superimposed on sustained hypertension. Fifty percent of these patients have sustained hypertension; however, some patients exhibit only mild clinical symptoms, making the diagnosis difficult. PHEO most commonly presents as a sporadic tumor but may also be found as a part of MEN 2A and 2B syndromes. PHEOs are also associated with many familial disorders, including von Recklinghausen disease, von Hippel-Lindau, Sturge-Weber syndrome, and succinate dehydrogenase deficiencies.

Diagnosis

Evaluating patients for PHEO or functional paraganglioma includes measuring plasma-free metanephrine and normetanephrine levels with confirmatory 24-hour urine catecholamines and metanephrines, and chest and abdominal CT or MRI. All patients diagnosed with a PHEO should undergo genetic counseling. If CT imaging is negative or there is a suspicion of multiple tumors or malignancy, then total-body nuclear imaging is indicated using either DOTATATE Gallium-68 PET scan or metaiodobenzylguanidine (MIBG) scan. MIBG is a compound resembling NE that is taken up by adrenergic tissue.

Treatment

Once the diagnosis of PHEO is confirmed, patients should be started on α-blockers (phenoxybenzamine or doxazosin). Doses of phenoxybenzamine should be increased until adequate α-blockade is achieved as demonstrated by orthostatic hypotension. During this period, the patient must be kept adequately hydrated to maintain adequate intravascular volume. After the patient is α blocked, β-blockade is used 2 to 3 days before surgery or if the patient is tachycardic. It is critical to initiate β-blocker therapy only after achieving adequate α-blockade to avoid unopposed α-adrenergic receptor stimulation. Patients with PHEO have severe peripheral vasoconstriction, increased systemic vascular resistance, and increased cardiac afterload. In order to maintain perfusion, patients compensate by increasing the heart rate and stroke volume.

If the PHEO is resectable, laparoscopic adrenalectomy is the procedure of choice. Patients must have long-term follow-up after resection as PHEO recurs in 10% to 15% of patients.

Adrenal Cortical Carcinomas

ACCs are rare tumors with a worldwide incidence of 2 per million people annually and 70% of patients presenting with metastatic disease. Although they can occur at any age, ACCs demonstrate a peak and are most commonly diagnosed in the fourth and fifth decades. They are usually unilateral, and symptoms are most often related to hormone hypersecretion found in 40% to 60% of patients. The prognosis is generally poor, with a 50% survival at 5 years. Poor prognosis is related to advanced stage and incomplete surgical resection, and there is debate about the prognostic significance of tumor grade, hormonal hypersecretion, age, gender, and tumor size.

Most ACCs are large, often more than 6 cm in size, encapsulated, friable, and having extensive central necrosis and hemorrhage. It is often difficult to differentiate large benign adrenal neoplasms from malignant lesions purely on the basis of cellular characteristics; therefore, preoperative biopsy is rarely indicated. Venous or capsular invasion and distant metastases are the most reliable signs of malignancy. However, tumor necrosis, intratumoral hemorrhage, marked nuclear and cellular pleomorphism, and the presence of many mitotic figures under a high-power field all strongly support the diagnosis of ACC.

Clinical Presentation

Over 50% of patients with ACCs present with CS; 15% present with virilizing, feminizing, and purely aldosterone-secreting carcinomas; and 10% of tumors are found to be hormonally active only by biochemical studies. However, in the majority of cases, ACCs present as an incidental finding on imaging. An abdominal mass is a common finding. Women with virilizing tumors have hirsutism, temporal balding, increased muscle mass, and amenorrhea. Boys present with precocious puberty. Men with virilizing tumors typically present with gynecomastia, testicular atrophy, impotence, or decreased libido.

Diagnosis

CT scan is the imaging modality of choice for adrenal lesions. Features on abdominal CT that suggest that an adrenal mass is a carcinoma include large size, irregular borders, heterogeneity, evidence of central necrosis, stippled calcifications, regional adenopathy, invasion of adjacent structures, and the presence of metastases. ACCs have a predilection for extension through the adrenal vein.

Treatment

The treatment of choice is surgical excision with total gross tumor removal. Resection is possible in 80% of cases. If patients present with early disease, adrenalectomy and excision of involved regional lymph nodes may be all that is necessary. If there is a presence of local invasion or visceral metastases, ipsilateral nephrectomy and resection of contiguous structures or hepatic metastases are indicated. When ACC is suspected preoperatively, an open adrenalectomy is the recommended surgical approach because recurrence rates and long-term survival related to oncologic resection are improved when compared with a laparoscopic approach.

The overall prognosis of ACC is poor. Unadjusted 5-year observed survival is 30% and ranges from 24% to 44%, with worse survival in older patients. Patients with negative resection margins have a median survival of 51 months compared with 7 months in patients who had positive resection margins. Survival has been relatively unchanged for the past 30 years.

Treatment of Complications After Adrenalectomy

The morbidity and complications associated with adrenalectomy are typically a consequence of the underlying adrenal pathology. For example, among patients who are undergoing adrenalectomy for CS, the increased susceptibility to infection, deep vein thrombosis, poor wound healing, and mild glucose intolerance are primarily the consequences of hypercortisolism.

Intraoperative complications include hypertension and hemorrhage secondary to inadvertent injury to the adrenal vein, especially during right adrenalectomy. The surgeon should secure control of the venous drainage of the adrenal gland and divide the adrenal vein before manipulating any tumors. The risk of significant changes in blood pressure during adrenalectomy for PHEO is minimized with adequate preoperative preparation that includes volume replacement and adrenergic blockade. Intraoperative hypertension, usually associated with manipulation of the PHEO, is managed with nitroprusside.

Perhaps the most important postoperative complication of adrenalectomy is the onset of occult adrenal insufficiency or Addisonian crisis as a result of inadequate glucocorticoid (cortisol) replacement. Patients who undergo unilateral adrenalectomy for an adrenal cause of CS are treated with hydrocortisone perioperatively because the contralateral adrenal gland is assumed to be suppressed until proven otherwise. Patients who undergo unilateral adrenalectomy for PA, PHEO, or a nonfunctional adrenal tumor (eg, adrenal cyst, myelolipoma) do not need cortisol replacement.

Postural hypotension or dizziness, nausea, vomiting, abdominal pain, weakness, fatigability, hyperkalemia, hyponatremia, and fever are common symptoms and signs of adrenal insufficiency. When adrenal insufficiency is suspected in a patient who is unstable, it is appropriate to draw blood to measure cortisol and then immediately give the patient parenteral steroids (100 mg hydrocortisone IV).

It is important to establish that the patient has adequate adrenal reserve (ie, demonstrate the ability of the remaining adrenal gland to respond appropriately to ACTH). This can be achieved with an ACTH stimulation test, which involves administering 250 mg of synthetic ACTH by IV bolus or intramuscular injection after a baseline plasma cortisol level is drawn. Plasma cortisol is then measured at 30 and 60 minutes. The test should be performed before 9:00 AM, and only if there are no known contraindications.

Incidentally Discovered Adrenal Mass

With the increasing use of CT, MRI, and ultrasound, adrenal masses are most commonly discovered incidentally. These so-called adrenal "incidentalomas" are typically asymptomatic and therefore present a unique challenge for the managing physician. The prevalence of an adrenal incidentaloma has been estimated at 0.6% to 5% when upper abdominal CT scans are evaluated. Incidental adrenal lesions are noted in 8.7% of patients on autopsy.

For all incidentalomas larger than 1 cm in size, it is essential to assess for functionality with clinical and laboratory evaluation regardless of the presence or absence of symptoms because some patients may present with subclinical disease.

Approximately 80% of incidentally discovered adrenal masses are nonfunctioning adenomas, 5% are subclinical cortisol-secreting CS, 5% are PHEO, 1% are aldosteronoma, less than 5% are adrenocortical carcinomas, and 2.5% are metastases to the adrenal gland.

Diagnosis

To assess for CS, the 1-mg overnight DST is a good initial screening test to evaluate for excess cortisol (subclinical CS). PHEO should be assessed with serum metanephrines and follow-up 24-hour urine catecholamines when results are positive or equivocal. Hyperaldosteronism should be assessed with serum ARR in patients with a history of hypertension (see sections "Cushing syndrome," "Pheochromocytoma," and "Primary Aldosteronism").

It is also important to determine if the lesion has radiographic findings concerning for malignancy. If the lesion is smaller than 4 cm with heterogeneous, regular borders, the patient should be tested for a hormonally active tumor. If there is no evidence of an aberrant hormonal milieu, the patient should be followed. If there is evidence of a hormonally active tumor, the patient should undergo adrenalectomy. If the CT scan shows a lesion that is 4 cm or larger and has features that are indeterminate or consistent with malignancy, a hormonal workup should be completed and the tumor surgically removed as is appropriate on the basis of the suspected etiology.

Finally, if the lesion does not meet any of the above-mentioned criteria and occurs in a patient with a history of cancer, a metastatic lesion should be considered. It is very rare that the diagnostic workup necessitates an adrenal biopsy; however, if a biopsy is indicated, the practitioner must be sure that the lesion is not a PHEO before performing a biopsy.

Treatment

If there is no evidence of an adrenal tumor requiring surgical excision, patients should undergo follow-up radiographic imaging in 6 to 12 months and then annually for 1 to 2 years with evaluation for hormonal disturbances at the time of diagnosis and then each year for 3 years.

All PHEOs should be resected after appropriate preoperative treatment (see section "Pheochromocytoma"). In patients with PA whose venous sample shows a unilateral source of aldosterone, laparoscopic adrenalectomy is indicated. Patients with hyperaldosteronism that is bilateral, or in patients who are not surgical candidates, can be managed with mineralocorticoid receptor blockers. Any tumor with concerning findings on CT, and most lesions larger than 4 cm, should be resected because of the risk for adrenal cancer. In patients with isolated adrenal metastasis, resection may be warranted depending on the underlying primary malignancy.

MULTIPLE ENDOCRINE NEOPLASIA SYNDROMES

The hereditary syndromes of the endocrine and neuroendocrine glands are collectively referred to as MEN syndromes and encompass MEN1, MEN2—including 2A and 2B—and MEN4. These syndromes are a group of heritable tumors that may be benign or malignant. MEN1, also known as *Wermer Syndrome*, is associated with PHP, duodenopancreatic NETs, and pituitary tumors, and is caused by a germline mutation in the *MEN1* gene. The MEN2 syndromes include MTC, PHEO, and parathyroid adenomas or hyperplasia. MEN2 is caused by germline mutations in the *RET* gene. MEN2 is further divided into type 2A, type 2B, or familial medullary thyroid carcinoma (FMTC).

MULTIPLE ENDOCRINE NEOPLASIA SYNDROME TYPE 1

MEN1 occurs due to a mutation in the *MEN1* gene inherited in an autosomal dominant fashion, with an estimated prevalence of 1 in 30,000 people. The *MEN1* gene is located on chromosome 11q13 and encodes the protein menin. Over 1,300 pathogenic variants have been identified in the *MEN1* gene to date. The manifestations of MEN1 have variable penetrance and include the following: PHP, duodenopancreatic NETs, and pituitary tumors. Clinical features are used to diagnose MEN1 with two of the three manifestations. Familial MEN1 is defined as at least one of the features with one first-degree relative who has one or more of these tumors, or two first-degree relatives with a known germline mutation. Patients typically present with initial symptoms between 20 and 30 years of age. The age-related penetrance of MEN1 is 45% to 73% by age 30, 82% by age 50, and 96% by age 70.

Primary Hyperparathyroidism

The most common manifestation and frequently the first presenting sign of MEN1 is PHP with parathyroid hyperplasia. PHP occurs in 80% to 100% of patients with MEN1 by the age of 50. Unlike sporadic PHP, which typically presents as a solitary parathyroid adenoma in the fifth or sixth decade of life, patients with MEN1 have multigland parathyroid hyperplasia and are present in the third decade of life. In sporadic PHP, women have higher rates of disease but MEN1-associated PHP is equally distributed between men and women. In individuals with an apparently sporadic PHP, occurrence of MEN1 is less than 5%, but the prevalence is higher in individuals diagnosed with these tumors before age 30. Parathyroid carcinoma is rare in MEN1. Patients, especially those with a known family history, may present with incidental hypercalcemia and elevated PTH levels. Symptoms may include neurocognitive dysfunction with fatigue, lethargy, depression, sleep disturbance; renal dysfunction with nephrolithiasis; GI dysfunction with constipation, nausea, bloating, abdominal pain; and skeletal effects of increased bone resorption with decreased bone mineral density or fragility fracture. Surgery for PHP in patients with MEN1 should include exploration of all parathyroid glands, subtotal (3-3.5 gland removal) parathyroidectomy or total parathyroidectomy with a reimplantation of parathyroid in the sternocleidomastoid or brachialis muscle. Although total parathyroidectomy with reimplantation has lower recurrence rates, it has the added risk of permanent hypoparathyroidism rendering the necessity for multiple daily doses of calcium and calcitriol to maintain eucalcemia. Additionally, cervical thymectomy should be performed during the index operation to mitigate the risk of recurrent PHP and thymic carcinoid in the future. Recurrence rates for PHP in MEN1 are high and patients may require remedial parathyroidectomy.

Duodenopancreatic Neuroendocrine Tumors

Duodenopancreatic NETs are the second most common endocrine manifestation in MEN1, occurring in up to 80% of patients by age 40 years. These tumors may be nonfunctional or hypersecreting with gastrinoma, insulinoma, vasoactive intestinal peptide tumor (VIPoma), glucagonoma, or somatostatinoma (Table 18-6). Gastrinomas are the most common functional NETs in MEN1 and account for the majority of morbidity and mortality. Typically, these tumors are small and multifocal and are located throughout the duodenum in the so-called "gastrinoma triangle." These gastrinomas cause Zollinger-Ellison syndrome (ZES) of peptic ulcer disease and up to half are malignant. Although ZES may be sporadic, approximately one-third of patients with ZES carry

an *MEN1 m*utation. Nonfunctional NETs are increasing in prevalence with the accuracy of high-resolution CT and MRI as well as endoscopic ultrasonography for surveillance in individuals known to have MEN1, with a frequency as high as 55% by age 40. These nonfunctional tumors may be malignant and metastases are correlated with tumor size, with tumors larger than 2 cm having higher rates of metastases and disease-specific mortality. Glucagonomas, VIPomas, and somatostatinomas are rare but have higher rates of malignancy than other NETs. Insulinomas are typically benign but have higher rates of metastases for patients with MEN1 than sporadic tumors. Although they can be located throughout the pancreas, insulinomas are common in the tail. Selective arterial calcium stimulation can help determine the location of insulinoma in patients with multiple NETs.

The timing and extent of surgery for NET depend on the symptoms of hormonal secretion as well as size, extent, and location of disease. Preoperative evaluation with cross-sectional imaging CT or MRI as well as Gallium Ga 68-DOTATATE NET PET may be used to localize tumors. NET PET is more sensitive and specific than octreotide nuclear imaging. Intraoperative ultrasound may also be used to identify small tumors. NETs may be amenable to enucleation or may require distal or subtotal pancreatectomy or pancreaticoduodenectomy (Whipple procedure), and in some cases, total pancreatectomy. Surgery is typically recommended for hormonally active tumors or those with a size larger than 2 cm. The goals of surgery are to alleviate symptoms of hormonal secretion and lower the risk of distant metastases and disease-specific mortality. Laparoscopy, when appropriate for the tumor size and location, may be safely employed. Medical management includes long-acting somatostatin analogues that can suppress hormonal activity.

Pituitary Tumors

Approximately 15% to 50% of patients with MEN1 develop a pituitary tumor. Two-thirds are microadenomas (<1.0 cm in diameter), and the majority of these tumors are prolactin secreting with an estimated penetrance of 20%. Prolactinomas may cause symptoms of galactorrhea, amenorrhea/dysmenorrhea, or hypogonadism. Other pituitary tumors can include somatotropinomas and corticotropinomas, or they may be nonfunctioning.

Medical therapy to suppress hypersecretion is the first line of therapy for MEN1-associated pituitary tumors. Surgery is often necessary for patients who are resistant to this treatment or who develop macroadenomas or symptoms of compression. Radiation therapy may be used for patients with incomplete surgical resection.

Other Multiple Endocrine Neoplasia Syndrome Type 1-Associated Tumors

Manifestations of MEN1 may also include carcinoid tumors primarily of the foregut, bronchi, thymus, or stomach, and these can be found in 5% to 10% of patients with MEN1. Skin and soft-tissue lesions are also common findings, including lipomas in 30% and facial angiofibromas or collagenomas in 75% to 80%. Adrenal lesions may be found in up to 50% of patients with MEN1 including benign cortical adenomas, nodular hyperplasia, or adrenocortical carcinoma. Thyroid adenomas, thyroid carcinoma, and PHEO are found less frequently but have also been associated with MEN1.

TABLE 18-6.	Multiple Endocrine Neoplasia Type 1 Duodenopancreatic Neuroendocrine Tumors: Penetrance and Clinical Features	
Tumor Type	**Estimated Penetrance (%)**	**Symptoms**
Gastrinoma	≤70	Peptic ulcer disease Diarrhea Abdominal pain Weight loss
Nonfunctioning	20-55	Symptoms from local compression or obstruction
Insulinoma	10	Whipple triad: fasting symptomatic hypoglycemia, relieved by glucose
Vasoactive intestinal peptide	1	Watery diarrhea Hypokalemia Achlorhydria
Glucagonoma	1	Diabetes mellitus Diarrhea Depression Necrolytic migratory erythema Thromboembolic disease
Somatostatinoma	<1	Diabetes mellitus Diarrhea Cholestasis Hypochlorhydria Weight loss

Making the Diagnosis of Multiple Endocrine Neoplasia Syndrome Type 1

The diagnosis of MEN1 may be challenging in the absence of a significant family history because of the unrelated presenting symptoms of MEN1-associated tumors which can lead to a delay in diagnosis upward of 10 years in many patients. Subsequent generations of *MEN1* carriers in known familial cohorts are diagnosed at an earlier age, but still many nonindex family members already have MEN1 manifestations at the time of diagnosis. Genetic counseling is recommended for the following: gastrinoma at any age, multifocal NET at any age, PHP before age 30, recurrent PHP, the presence of one major tumor manifestation of MEN1 and one other MEN1-associated tumors, two or more MEN1-associated tumors, and a family history of PHP, pituitary adenoma, NET, or carcinoid tumor. For individuals meeting diagnostic criteria, the rate of detecting an MEN1 gene mutation is 75% to 90%.

MULTIPLE ENDOCRINE NEOPLASIA SYNDROME TYPE 2

The MEN2 syndrome pathology includes MTC, PHEO, and PHP with parathyroid adenoma or hyperplasia. MEN2 is inherited in an autosomal dominant fashion with a defect in the *RET* proto-oncogene on chromosome 10q11.2, which encodes a tyrosine kinase receptor. The prevalence of MEN2 is estimated as 1 in 35,000 with the majority of cases subtype 2A. The MEN2 syndrome has subclassifications based on the additional clinical characteristics in the patient or the family cohort. MEN2A, or Sipple syndrome, includes MTC, PHEO, and/or PHP with additional features of cutaneous lichen amyloidosis or Hirschsprung disease. Features of MEN2B are mucosal neuromas of the lips and tongue, thickening of corneal nerve fibers, distinctive facial appearance with enlarged lips, Marfanoid body habitus, and MTC. An additional subtype of MEN2 is FMTC, which includes a *RET* mutation and MTC but no family or personal history of PHEO or PHP.

Medullary Thyroid Carcinoma

MTC represents up to 3% of thyroid carcinomas, of which about 75% are sporadic. Patients with MEN2-associated MTC present at an earlier age than those with sporadic carcinomas, which typically occur in the fifth or sixth decade of life. MEN2 should be suspected when MTC occurs at an early age or is multifocal or bilateral. Up to 95% of patients with MEN2A will develop MTC.

Survival is correlated with the stage at diagnosis, and reduced survival in MTC can be accounted for in part by a high proportion of late-stage diagnosis. Survival rates for MTC with disease confined to the thyroid gland approach 96% at 10 years and are the rationale for risk-reducing thyroidectomy in MEN2. Patients with MEN2 undergoing thyroidectomy for MTC should be screened for PHEO with plasma metanephrine and normetanephrine assays.

MTC is typically the first presentation of MEN2. In MEN2 familial cohorts, the biochemical manifestations of MTC with elevated calcitonin and/or nodular disease of the thyroid gland generally appear between the ages of 5 and 25 years. In patients who do not undergo screening and risk-reducing thyroidectomy, MTC typically presents as a palpable neck mass by age 20 and more than half of these patients will have cervical lymph node metastases at the time of diagnosis. Patients with locally advanced bulky cervical disease or hepatic metastases may present with diarrhea, which is a poor prognostic indicator.

Risk-reducing thyroidectomy is the preferred treatment strategy for patients with MEN2. The timing of surgery depends on the risk classification based on specific *RET* codon mutation as well as surveillance thyroid ultrasound and calcitonin assay. Children with moderate risk mutations should have a PE, ultrasound of the neck, and measurement of the serum calcitonin beginning around age 5. Children with negative calcitonin may be followed at semiannual or annual intervals. The timing of surgery should be determined by a multidisciplinary group of pediatricians, endocrinologists, and surgeons in conjunction with the child's parents on the basis of the findings of screening evaluations. Total thyroidectomy with or without central neck lymph node dissection is indicated in these patients.

Genetic counseling for *RET* mutation testing is recommended for all patients with MTC, regardless of family history suggestive of MEN2.

Primary Hyperparathyroidism

PHP in MEN2 has less severe manifestations than in MEN1, often with only mild hypercalcemia. The pathology is more likely from solitary adenoma than multigland hyperplasia in MEN1, but patients still have higher rates of multigland disease (50%) than the sporadic population (85%). PHP is rarely the initial manifestation of MEN2. Most patients with MEN2-related PHP are incidentally diagnosed at the time of thyroidectomy for MTC. Otherwise, surgical indications for MEN2-associated PHP are similar to those for sporadic disease. Because of the high rates of multigland hyperplasia, a four-gland exploration is recommended. Recurrence rates for PHP after parathyroidectomy are lower for MEN2 than for MEN1 but still higher than the sporadic population.

For known patients with MEN2, screening for PHP should be considered by age 11 for high-risk mutations and age 16 for moderate risk with periodic serum calcium and PTH assays.

Multiple Endocrine Neoplasia Syndrome Type 2B

The MEN2B subtype, mucosal neuroma or Wagenmann-Froboese syndrome, accounts for about 5% of patients with MEN2 and is characterized by oral mucosal neuromas, a Marfanoid body habitus, and early-onset aggressive MTC with complete penetrance. PHEOs occur in about 50% of MEN2B cases; about half are multiple and often bilateral. Symptomatic PHP is very uncommon in this cohort. Nearly half of patients with MEN2B will also have diffuse ganglioneuromatosis of the GI tract.

Genetic testing can classify individuals at the highest risk of MTC on the basis of the *RET* variant detected. Those with MEN2B and *RET* codon M918T are associated with the youngest age of MTC and highest disease mortality, which can inform the timing of thyroidectomy. Total thyroidectomy should be considered by 1 year of age in the highest risk patients with M918T mutations. Children with other high-risk mutations may undergo prophylactic thyroidectomy at age 5 or earlier, on the basis of serum calcitonin levels. A central neck dissection is typically performed only if there is radiographic evidence of metastatic lymph node involvement or if the serum calcitonin level is greater than 40 pg/mL to lower the risk of permanent hypoparathyroidism.

Multiple Endocrine Neoplasia Syndrome Type 4

MEN4 is a novel, rare syndrome with clinical features that overlap with the other MEN syndromes. MEN4 is caused by a mutation in the tumor suppressor gene *CDKN1B* on chromosome 12p13.1 with autosomal dominant transmission. The most common manifestation of MEN4 is PHP followed by pituitary adenoma. The age at diagnosis for PHP is typically later onset compared with patients with MEN1.

SUGGESTED READINGS

Bilezikian JP, Brandi ML, Eastell R, et al. Guidelines for the management of asymptomatic primary hyperparathyroidism: summary statement from the Fourth International Workshop. *J Clin Endocrinol Metab*. 2014;99:3561-3569.

Eidman KE, Wetmore JB. The role of parathyroidectomy in the management of secondary hyperparathyroidism. *Curr Opin Nephrol Hypertens*. 2017;26(6):516-522.

Haugen BR, Alexander EK, Bible KC, et al. 2015 American Thyroid Association management guidelines for adult patients with thyroid nodules and differentiated thyroid cancer. The American Thyroid Association Guidelines Task Force on Thyroid Nodules and Differentiated Thyroid Cancer. *Thyroid*. 2016;26:1-133.

Wilhelm SM, Wang TS, Ruan DT, et al. The American Association of endocrine surgeons guidelines for definitive management of primary hyperparathyroidism. *JAMA Surg*. 2016;151:959-968.

SAMPLE QUESTIONS

QUESTIONS

Choose the best answer for each question.

1. A 20-year-old woman is seen in the clinic because of a thyroid nodule. She is asymptomatic, and her past medical history is unremarkable. She takes no medications. There is a 2-cm firm, solitary nodule in the lateral aspect of the left lobe of the thyroid. TSH is normal. Ultrasonography shows a solid, hypoechoic 2-cm mass. FNA cytology shows a suspicious for follicular neoplasm (Bethesda 4) cytology. What is the next best step in management?

   A. Irradiation (radioactive iodine)
   B. Thyroid suppression with T4
   C. Incisional biopsy and enucleation if benign
   D. Total thyroidectomy
   E. Left thyroid lobectomy

2. A 50-year-old woman is seen in the clinic because of weight loss, restlessness, and palpitations. She also has noted leg swelling and excessive hair loss. Her past medical history is unremarkable. She takes no medications. She is afebrile. On examination, she is tachycardic and has a fine tremor. She has mild exophthalmos. Her thyroid is smooth and uniformly enlarged. TSH levels are low, and T3 and T4 levels are elevated. Serum TRAb is positive. What is the next best step in management?

   A. Radioactive iodine
   B. Early operation
   C. Propranolol
   D. Antithyroid medication
   E. T4 suppression

3. Which of the following statements is true?

   A. Papillary carcinoma is the most common and the most aggressive form of thyroid cancer.
   B. FNA biopsy can be diagnostic for follicular carcinoma.
   C. Anaplastic carcinoma is the least common and the most aggressive form of thyroid cancer.
   D. FTC may be associated with flushing and diarrhea.
   E. MTC arises from follicular cells.

4. A 55-year-old man with a history of end-stage renal disease is successfully managed medically for secondary hyperparathyroidism. He subsequently undergoes a renal transplant and is taken off cinacalcet. He shows a moderate decrease in PTH; however, it is still elevated at 250 pg/mL (normal 10-65), and his calcium increases to 11.2 mg/dL (normal 8.5-10.5). Creatinine level is higher than his new baseline at 1.7 mg/dL (normal 0.6-1.2). His sestamibi scan does not show clear uptake, but his ultrasound shows two vague hypoechoic soft-tissue masses near the thyroid that are typical for enlarged parathyroids. What is the best treatment plan for this patient?

   A. Resume cinacalcet
   B. Observation
   C. Four-gland parathyroid exploration with subtotal parathyroidectomy/thymectomy
   D. Focal parathyroidectomy with ioPTH monitoring
   E. Resume dialysis to protect his renal transplant

5. A 40-year-old healthy woman is found to have a serum calcium level of 11 mg/dL during a preventive medicine visit. She is otherwise healthy and takes no medications. There is no family history of endocrine disease. Serum phosphorus is 2.4 mg/dL, and the PTH level is 90 pg/mL. Sestamibi scan shows persistent uptake in the region of the inferior lobe of the thyroid on the right. Cervical ultrasonography demonstrates a 15-mm ovoid hypoechoic solid soft-tissue mass immediately adjacent and lateral to the inferior pole of the right thyroid lobe. Which of the following is the most appropriate treatment recommendation for this patient?

   A. Observation and repeat laboratory studies in 6 months
   B. Begin daily oral furosemide.
   C. Begin saline and bisphosphonates IV.
   D. Begin daily cinacalcet.
   E. Targeted parathyroidectomy with ioPTH monitoring

6. A 35-year-old woman is seen in the clinic because of weight gain and abnormal hair growth. She has gained 15 kg in 6 months, most notably in her torso. She denies increased appetite and has not changed her daily activity patterns. She has been emotionally labile, and her previously regular menses have become irregular (periods are shorter or missed altogether). On examination, she has truncal obesity and hirsutism. The most likely primary cause of her symptoms is due to hyperfunction of which one of the following?

   A. Pituitary basophils
   B. Pulmonary enterochromaffin (Kulchitsky) cells
   C. Adrenal medullary cells
   D. Adrenal cortical cells
   E. Ovarian epithelial cells

7. A 54-year-old woman presents to the hospital for removal of her 3-cm right adrenal mass associated with hypercortisolism. The procedure was uneventful, and the patient was transferred to the floor postoperatively. The next day the patient becomes unstable with hypotension, low urine output, lethargy, and nausea. The patient's morning labs are significant for hyponatremia and hyperkalemia. The next step in the management of this patient would be:

   A. Transfuse packed red blood cells (PRBCs).
   B. Return to the operating room.
   C. Administer IV corticosteroids.
   D. Laboratory testing for cortisol and ACTH.
   E. Administer IV fludrocortisone.

8. A 33-year-old man presents to the emergency department after a fall from an 8-ft ladder with no loss of consciousness. He reported vague abdominal pain, and a contrast-enhanced CT scan was obtained which showed no intra-abdominal organ damage but revealed an incidental 2-cm left adrenal mass. The patient is otherwise healthy with no past medical or surgical history. Laboratory testing reveals normal serum metanephrine levels. What is the next step in the management of this patient?

   A. Surgical removal of the left adrenal gland
   B. No further testing warranted
   C. 1-mg overnight DST
   D. Serum aldosterone and renin levels
   E. Core biopsy of the left adrenal mass

9. A 58-year-old woman with a history of hypertension and diabetes presents to the clinic with a newly diagnosed left adrenal mass. The patient initially complained of left flank and back pain, which prompted a CT scan of the abdomen and revealed the large 8-cm left adrenal mass with concern for invasion into the left kidney. The patient reports recent weight loss and anorexia; however, she otherwise has been in her usual state of health. She has no previous surgical history and no family history of endocrine tumors. The patient completed a full hormonal workup including plasma metanephrines, renin, aldosterone, and a 1-mg overnight DST which were all normal. The next step in management would be:

   A. Biopsy of the left adrenal mass
   B. Left adrenalectomy and left nephrectomy
   C. External beam radiotherapy
   D. Neoadjuvant chemotherapy
   E. Minimally invasive laparoscopic removal of the left adrenal gland

10. A 32-year-old man presents to the emergency department with left flank pain. A CT scan demonstrates a nonobstructing ureteral stone. Which of the following would not be consistent with a diagnosis of MEN1?

   A. Serum calcium level of 11.3 mg/dL with a PTH of 220 pg/mL
   B. Marfanoid body habitus
   C. CT findings of multiple 1- to 2-cm masses in the head, body, and tail of the pancreas
   D. Review of systems positive for galactorrhea
   E. Family history of PHP

ANSWERS AND EXPLANATIONS

1. **Answer: E**

   This patient should undergo a thyroid lobectomy. Even though FNA showing follicular cells is only 5% likely to be a malignancy, most endocrine surgeons would recommend excision because of that concern. Radioactive iodine is inappropriate because it would destroy normal thyroid tissue and leave the nodule. Suppression with levothyroxine to lower TSH to below-normal limits is associated with accelerated osteoporosis and cardiac irregularities. Suppression to within normal range could be a temporizing maneuver. Incisional biopsy and enucleation are inappropriate because neither will allow examination of the interface between the nodule and normal thyroid and potentially not allow the diagnosis of a follicular variant of PTC. Total thyroidectomy is unnecessarily aggressive. For more information on this topic, please see section "Thyroid Nodule."

2. **Answer: D**

The patient has Graves disease. Initial treatment should be with antithyroid medication (thionamides) to suppress T4 production. Radioactive iodine as the first line of treatment is inappropriate because as many as 75% of patients have been reported to have sustained remission after 3 to 6 months of treatment with antithyroid drugs. Early operation is too aggressive when nonoperative methods of treatment are available. Propranolol may be used as an adjunct to antithyroid medications but used alone does not help suppress the thyrotropin receptor antibodies that are responsible for Graves disease. The highest rates of remission are associated with the elimination of these antibodies. T4 suppression will be ineffective because the patient already has high levels of T4. For more information on this topic, please see section "Treatment" under the heading "Graves Disease."

3. **Answer: C**

Papillary carcinoma is the most common thyroid cancer, accounting for approximately 85% of cases, with the least aggressive course. Follicular carcinoma is the second most common, accounting for approximately 10% of cases, with a slightly more aggressive course. FNA cytology alone cannot distinguish between follicular adenoma and carcinoma. The diagnosis requires histologic evaluation of a surgical specimen. MTC is a NET of the C cells of the thyroid gland. Patients with advanced disease may present with flushing or diarrhea secondary to hormone secretion by the tumor. Medullary carcinoma is the only thyroid cancer that reliably expresses a tumor marker, calcitonin. Thyroglobulin levels may be elevated in benign thyroid disease and are not reliably elevated in follicular or papillary carcinomas, and therefore not useful as a tumor marker. Anaplastic carcinoma is the least common but the most aggressive form of thyroid cancer with a dismal prognosis. For more information on this topic, please see section "Thyroid Carcinoma."

4. **Answer: C**

This patient has tertiary hyperparathyroidism after a renal transplant. The condition progressed from secondary hyperparathyroidism due to renal failure to tertiary hyperparathyroidism once the secondary cause was corrected with a renal transplant. He now has autonomously functioning parathyroid tissue causing hypercalcemia. Treatment should focus on curative intent. Cinacalcet is effective only in secondary hyperparathyroidism. Hypercalcemia is not severe enough to warrant resuming dialysis but does put stress on the transplanted kidney, so observation is not recommended. An operation is indicated, with four-gland exploration and subtotal parathyroidectomy, with thymectomy being the operation of choice. All parathyroid glands are abnormal, so even if only two are identified on preoperative imaging, the rest need to be identified and removed, except for a small part of one. For more information on this topic, please see section on "Clinical Presentation and Evaluation" under the heading "Secondary and Tertiary Hyperparathyroidism."

5. **Answer: E**

This patient has early sporadic PHP. Although she is asymptomatic, she meets the National Institutes of Health consensus criterion for parathyroid operation due to being under 50 years old. She localized preoperatively to an abnormal right inferior parathyroid gland, so she is a candidate for a targeted approach to parathyroidectomy using a focal exploration and ioPTH monitoring. Four-gland exploration would also be an appropriate answer if this had been an option and would be the appropriate next step if the ioPTH did not decrease as expected. For more information on this topic, please see section "Primary Hyperparathyroidism."

6. **Answer: A**

This patient has symptoms and signs of hypercortisolism (CS). The most common cause of CS in adults is an ACTH-secreting tumor of the pituitary basophils (CD). Women in the third and fourth decades of life are the typical patients. CD accounts for 70% of cases of CS. Bronchial carcinoid tumors (arising from Kulchitsky cells) are a source of ectopic ACTH production. Ectopic ACTH syndrome causes about 15% of CS in adults. The adrenal medulla does not produce glucocorticoids; tumors of the medulla are PHEOs and produce excess catecholamines. A tumor of ovarian epithelial cells could lead to menstrual irregularities through excess sex steroid production but would not produce hypercortisolism. For more information on this topic, please see section "Diagnosis" under the heading "Cushing Syndrome."

7. **Answer: C**

This patient has signs and symptoms of adrenal insufficiency after removal of her adrenal gland. The function of the remaining adrenal gland in patients with long-standing hypercortisolism is often initially suppressed, and patients can develop adrenal insufficiency after surgery unless they are given perioperative corticosteroids. The patient is unstable, so treatment is initiated with IV corticosteroids first, and then laboratory testing is performed to confirm the diagnosis, despite the potential delay in treatment associated with waiting for the lab results. There are other possibilities for the onset of this patient's shock, including hemorrhage, which will need to be assessed if the patient does not respond to the infusion of corticosteroids. For more information on this topic, see section "Treatment of Complications After Adrenalectomy."

8. **Answer: C**

The patient is asymptomatic from his incidental adrenal mass and has no history suggesting it is a metastatic lesion. All patients with incidental adrenal masses need to be screened for subclinical PHEO and hypercortisolism but only patients who present with hypertension need to be screened for hyperaldosteronism. The patients with unilateral disease and abnormal hormone levels are candidates for adrenalectomy; however, they must undergo functional testing before consideration of surgery. A biopsy of the adrenal gland is reserved for very select cases where metastatic disease is suspected. For more information on this topic, see section "Incidentally Discovered Adrenal Mass."

9. **Answer: B**

The patient is presenting with a likely ACC, and the treatment of choice is surgical excision. The best chance of survival is the removal of all of the tumor and any involved structures. There is no effective chemotherapy for these tumors, and radiotherapy is not useful either. A biopsy is not indicated, as it can increase the risk of recurrent disease after resection. These operations should be performed in an open fashion to ensure complete removal of the tumor and avoid tumor spillage. For more information on this topic, see section "Adrenal Cortical Carcinoma."

10. **Answer: B**

This patient presents with nephrolithiasis. The MEN1 syndrome includes PHP, pituitary adenoma, and duodenopancreatic NETs. With PHP, the serum calcium and PTH levels are elevated. In MEN1, NETs can be found in the duodenum and pancreas and are frequently multifocal. A prolactin-secreting pituitary tumor can cause galactorrhea. PHP is the most highly penetrant manifestation of MEN1 and would be expected in the family history. A Marfanoid body habitus is characteristic of MEN2B and would not be consistent with a diagnosis of MEN1. For more information on this topic, please see section "Multiple Endocrine Neoplasia Syndrome Type 1."

19 Liver and Spleen

Jesse Clanton and Adnan Alseidi

LIVER ANATOMY

Although anatomy remains pivotal to the treatment of almost any surgical disease, nowhere does this relationship become as crucial as when approaching surgical liver disease. The liver is the largest single gland in the body. In the average adult, it weighs approximately 1,200 to 1,600 g. It is located below the diaphragm, with its greatest mass to the right of the midline but extends to a variable degree into the left upper quadrant. In the cranial-caudal axis, the liver extends from about the fourth to fifth intercostal space on both sides to just below the costal margin on the right. It is covered by a tough, fibrous Glisson capsule, which extends into its parenchyma along penetrating vessels, such as the porta hepatis. The liver is invested in the peritoneum except for the bare area, located over its posterior surface near the vena cava, and the gallbladder bed. Folds or reflections of this peritoneum are named "ligaments." These ligaments, such as the falciform, coronary, and triangular ligaments, attach the liver to the diaphragm and the anterior abdominal wall. Another reflection of the peritoneum is the gastrohepatic ligament (lesser omentum), which extends from the liver to the lesser curvature of the stomach and the first part of the duodenum.

The liver enjoys dual blood supply from the hepatic arterial and portal venous systems. Most (between two-thirds and three-quarters) of the blood flow to the liver comes from the portal vein, while the remainder comes from the hepatic arterial system. As the arterial blood contains significantly higher amounts of oxygen, this results in roughly half of the oxygen delivered from each system. The hepatic arterial system is known to be quite variable; up to 40% of cases have some variation from the "traditional" branching of the arterial system (Figure 19-1). These variations can be either accessory vessels (an aberrant vessel in addition to the normal branching vessel) or replaced vessels (an aberrant vessel that is present in the absence of the normal branching vessel), or both. The portal vein represents the confluence of drainage from the bowel (superior mesenteric vein) and the spleen (splenic vein). The liver itself has right, middle, and left hepatic veins, which drain directly into the inferior vena cava.

In 2000, the International Hepato-Pancreato-Biliary Association adopted a coherent and universal terminology for liver anatomy on the basis of the work of James Cantlie and the anatomists Couinaud and Healey. This classification divides the liver into right and left hemilivers, further dividing the right hemiliver into anterior and posterior

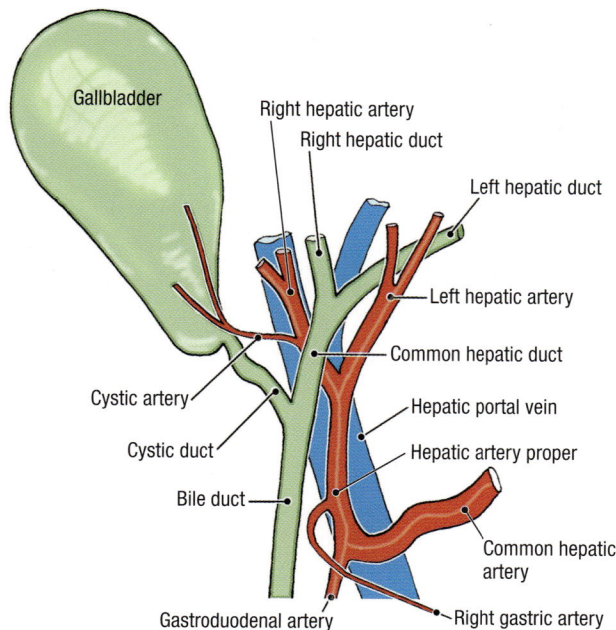

Figure 19-1. Arterial anatomy of the liver. Closeup of structures contained in the hepatoduodenal ligament. Tributaries of bile duct and branches of common hepatic artery. (Reprinted with permission from Sauerland EK, ed. *Grant's Dissector.* 14th ed. Lippincott Williams & Wilkins; 2008.)

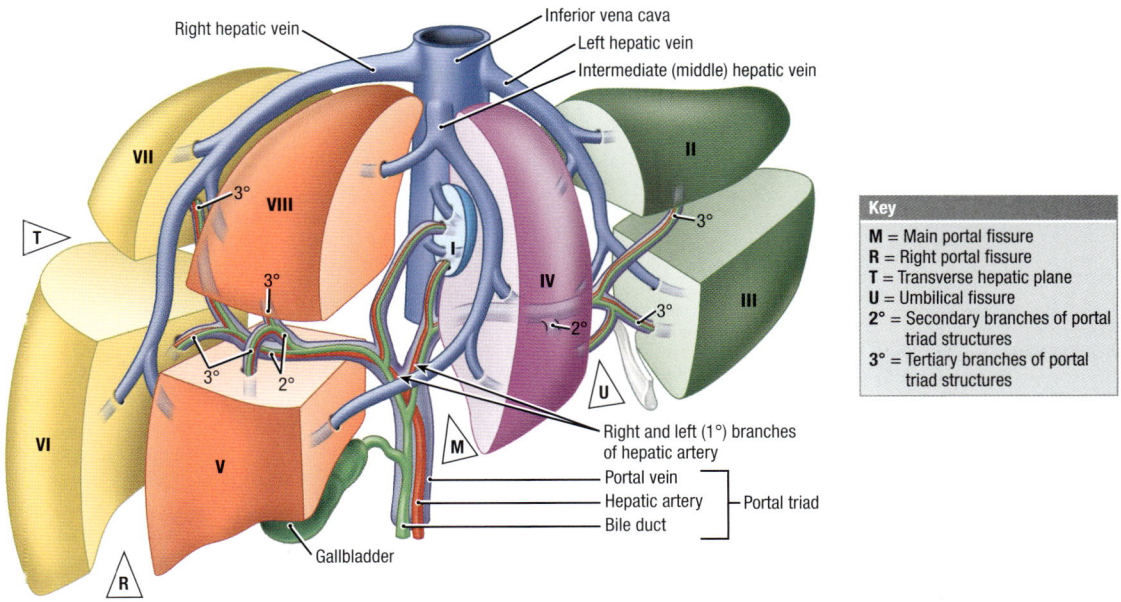

Figure 19-2. Couinaud segmental anatomy, anterior view. (Reprinted with permission from Agur AMR, Dalley AF. *Grant's Atlas of Anatomy*. 14th ed. Wolters Kluwer; 2017:344.)

sections and the left hemiliver into medial and lateral sections (Figures 19-2 and 19-3). The liver is thus divided into eight separate segments, each with its own circulation and biliary drainage. The terminology for hepatic resections was also standardized (Figure 19-3).

LIVER PHYSIOLOGY

The functional unit of the liver is the lobule. On the periphery of each lobule lie the hepatic arterial and portal venous branches. Centrally lies a draining hepatic vein. Blood from the terminal portal venules and hepatic arterioles converges in the hepatic sinusoids, with which each hepatocyte has intimate contact, and drains centrally into the hepatic venule (Figure 19-4).

Major hepatic functions include protein synthesis, energy metabolism, detoxification, bile production, and immune reticuloendothelial function. However, many other functions, some not very well understood, also exist. The hepatocyte, which is the principal cell of the liver, accounts for most metabolic activities. These cells continually divide and can potentially reproduce the entire cell mass of the liver every 50 days. The cells are aligned in a single layer along the hepatic sinusoids and transport essential substrates and hormones intracellularly. The hepatocytes then transport metabolic products back into the plasma or the bile canaliculus, which is positioned on the opposite side of this single layer of cells. In this way, the hepatocyte monitors and regulates plasma levels of proteins and ensures that metabolic requirements are met.

The liver also performs many important immunologic functions. Kupffer cells line the vascular endothelium and are in close proximity to hepatocytes. These macrophages represent 80% to 90% of the fixed macrophages of the body and are subject to frequent turnover.

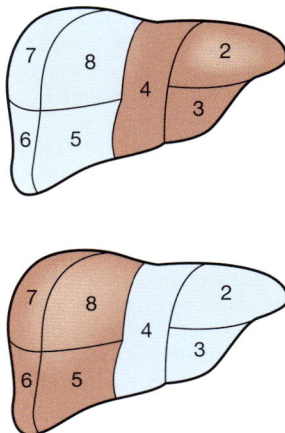

Figure 19-3. First-order division. Top, Left hepatectomy or left hemihepatectomy (seg 2-4). Bottom, Right hepatectomy or right hemihepatectomy (seg 5-8) (Courtesy of Dr. Steven Strasberg.)

LIVER INJURIES

Despite the substantial protection afforded by the ribs and abdominal musculature, the liver can be injured by penetrating trauma or blunt force injury. A focused assessment is made to detect liver injury, with sonography in trauma, ultrasound study, or computed tomography (CT) scan being the usual modalities utilized for the purpose whereas hemodynamic instability is the major reason for operative intervention (see Chapter 7).

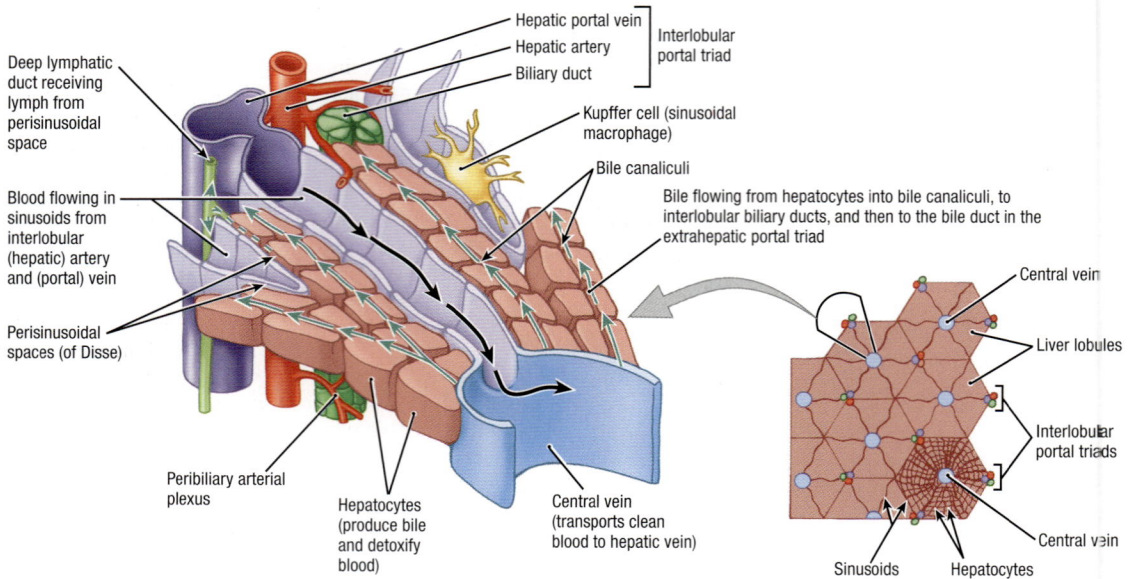

Figure 19-4. Flow of blood and bile in the liver. (Reprinted with permission from Agur AMR, Dalley AF. *Grant's Atlas of Anatomy*. 14th ed. Wolters Kluwer; 2017:345.)

HEPATIC TUMORS, CYSTS, AND ABSCESSES

With the increased availability and the use of abdominal imaging techniques, including CT scanning, asymptomatic and incidental liver abnormalities are discovered with greater frequency. Careful patient assessment is needed because incidental benign liver tumors and cysts are common and typically require no specific therapy. On the other hand, some benign liver tumors are resected, if feasible, even in the asymptomatic patient. An important principle is to avoid liver biopsy early in the workup of a newly discovered liver mass in an otherwise asymptomatic patient. Needle biopsy is usually not necessary to determine the most likely diagnosis. It is subject to sampling error and may introduce the additional risks of bleeding or tumor seeding in a patient who might undergo tumor resection regardless of the biopsy result. Needle biopsy may be appropriate when the nature of an unresectable tumor remains unknown despite imaging and laboratory tests.

Benign Tumors

Hemangioma

Cavernous hemangioma of the liver is the most common benign liver tumor and occurs in as many as 1% to 20% of the general population. These are probably congenital lesions and are embryologic hamartomas (benign tumors with two distinct cell types). Microscopic evaluation shows endothelial vascular spaces separated by fibrous septa. These lesions may enlarge over the lifetime of an individual. They are 5 times more common in women, and some findings suggest hormonal responsiveness, including enlargement during pregnancy. Cavernous hemangiomas that are larger than 10 cm are defined as giant hemangiomas. Hemangiomas are often incidental findings and require no

specific therapy. Liver function tests are usually normal. Ultrasonography may be diagnostic, showing characteristic focal hyperechoic abnormalities. Contrast-enhanced CT imaging usually shows a progressive peripheral-to-central prominent enhancement and a central hypodense region.

Most patients are asymptomatic at presentation and remain so in follow-up. Longitudinal studies assessing long-term (>10 years) follow-up in patients with giant cavernous hemangiomas confirm the absence of spontaneous hemorrhage and/or rupture in most. Patients with very large hemangiomas occasionally have pain, and surgical resection may be considered.

Focal Nodular Hyperplasia

Focal nodular hyperplasia (FNH) is a well-circumscribed benign lesion, usually found incidentally. Classic findings are a central scar with fibrous septae and nodular hyperplasia. Unlike hepatic adenoma, bile ducts are scattered throughout. Liver function tests are usually normal. These tumors do not have malignant potential and are rarely associated with rupture or hemorrhage.

The major issue in managing FNH lies in differentiating it from hepatic adenoma and hepatocellular carcinoma (HCC). Ultrasonography or CT scanning may demonstrate the classic central stellate scar in only one-third of cases. Magnetic resonance imaging (MRI) scans, especially when utilizing gadolinium-based contrast agents such as Eovist, allow for better evaluation reaching a sensitivity and specificity above 95%. Core-needle biopsy may distinguish this tumor from hepatic adenoma in some but not all cases.

As FNH is a benign, regenerative process, it should be treated conservatively when the diagnosis is established by imaging. Its growth is not altered by hormonal or oral contraceptive use. When symptoms such as abdominal pain are present, evaluation should be carried out to exclude other causes.

Hepatic Adenoma

A hepatic adenoma is a benign epithelial tumor that usually occurs in women between ages 30 and 50 years. Although many of these tumors are not clinically significant, there is a small but real risk of hemorrhage or malignant transformation. Most patients have a history of estrogen exposure, usually in the form of long-standing use of oral contraceptives or occasionally from estrogen replacement therapy. Anabolic steroid use, obesity, diabetes mellitus, glycogen storage diseases, and aplastic anemia are additional risk factors. Microscopically, it appears as sheets of hepatocytes without portal triads or bile ducts.

CT imaging typically shows a solid iso- or hypodense mass but can be variable depending on the fat content and any associated hemorrhage (Figure 19-5). ^{99m}Tc sulfur colloid scan has been utilized to make the diagnosis, as these tumors do not contain Kupffer cells and do not take up this tracer. This has been largely replaced now by MRI, with liver-directed contrast such as Eovist showing excellent sensitivity and specificity. Core-needle biopsy is generally not required after adequate imaging but may be useful in certain instances to establish the subtype and for risk stratification.

Discontinuation of oral contraceptives may result in the shrinkage or even complete regression of these tumors and is often attempted first in asymptomatic and incidentally found lesions. Women with a history of hepatic adenoma should use alternate methods of contraception and avoid further use of oral contraceptives. Others will need close follow-up or even excision. Spontaneous hemorrhage can often be initially managed with transarterial embolization. Surgical resection is generally considered in patients deemed high risk for complications, including all men and those women with tumors larger than 5 cm. The risk of malignant transformation is 5% to 10%, with the β–catenin-activated subtype being especially high risk. Surgical resection is determined by weighing the risks and benefits of the tumor versus the complexity of the resection. Radiofrequency (RFA) or microwave ablation (MWA) is also an option for select individuals at experienced centers.

Malignant Tumors

Hepatocellular Carcinoma

HCC, or hepatoma, accounts for more than 90% of all primary liver malignancies. This tumor usually occurs in patients with an underlying liver disease (70%-80%).

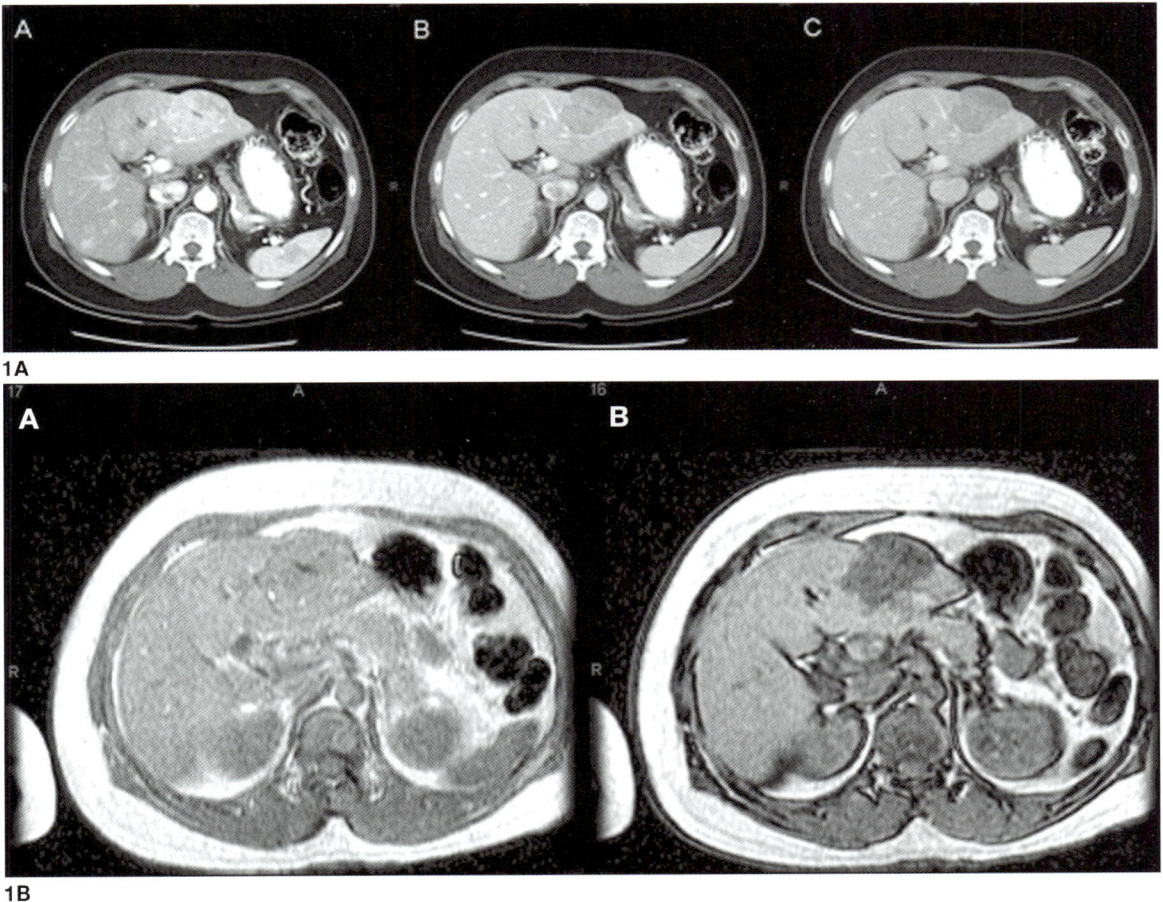

Figure 19-5. 1A. Three-phase CT scan of a hepatic adenoma. (A) Arterial phase; (B) portal phase; (C) venous phase. 1B. In-phase (A) and out-of-phase (B) MRI scan of the same hepatic adenoma. As a result of the high-fat content of the lesion, the signal cancels out on the out-of-phase image. The lesion, therefore, appears to be nonenhancing. (Reprinted with permission from Mulholland MW, Lillemoe KD, Doherty GM, et al, eds. *Greenfield's Surgery.* 4th ed. Lippincott Williams & Wilkins; 2006:962.)

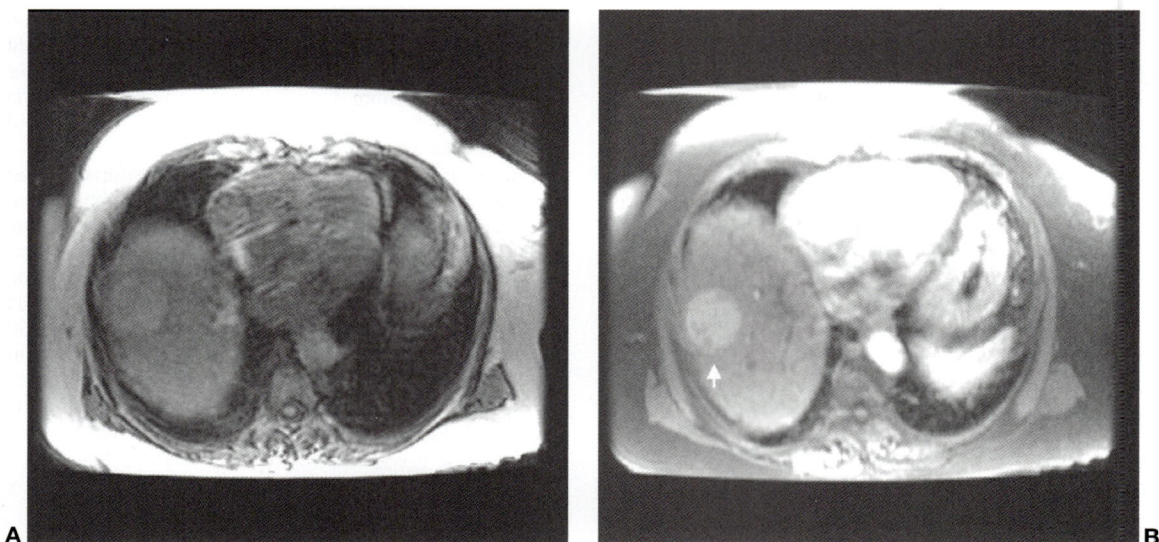

Figure 19-6. Hepatocellular carcinoma. A 4-cm lesion in hepatic segment 8 seen before (A) and after (B) the administration of gadolinium contrast on T1-weighted MR images. Arrow depicts the lesion. (Reprinted with permission from Schiff ER, Sorrell MF, Maddrey WC, et al, eds. *Schiff's Diseases of the Liver*. 10th ed. Lippincott Williams & Wilkins; 2007:chap 4.)

It occurs at high rates in areas where hepatitis B is endemic. Although cirrhosis from any cause appears to be associated with the development of HCC, noncirrhotic, chronic carriers of hepatitis B and hepatitis C show increased rates, too. Alcohol intake and obesity-related nonalcoholic steatohepatitis are other risk factors. As the risk of developing HCC is high in cirrhotics, they are recommended to undergo a biannual screening ultrasound to evaluate for new liver lesions.

HCC is suspected in any patient with known cirrhosis and sudden clinical decompensation, including worsening jaundice, encephalopathy, or increasing ascites. HCC should be included in the differential diagnosis for any solid liver tumor. α-Fetoprotein (AFP) is an α_1-globulin serum marker that is elevated in 60% to 80% of patients with HCC. This tumor marker may also be elevated to 200 to 400 mg/dL in patients with cirrhosis who do not have a hepatoma. Values of 500 to 1,000 mg/dL or higher are almost always associated with HCC.

Any mass larger than 1 cm in a patient with cirrhosis must be investigated for possible HCC. When HCC is suspected, ultrasound, CT, or MRI may show the tumor mass. A typical vascular pattern of contrast enhancement on early arterial phase images followed by washout with residual ring enhancement on delayed imaging is diagnostic (Figure 19-6). The use of contrast, specifically liver directed contrast such as gadoxetate disodium, in MRI has been very helpful in the identification and diagnosis of liver tumors; the Liver Imaging Reporting and Data System (LI-RADS). A biopsy should be considered only if the typical pattern is not seen or if a mixed-type variant, such as HCC–cholangiocarcinoma, is suspected.

The treatment for HCC depends on the number and size of the tumors and the extent of underlying liver disease (Table 19-1). There are multiple different treatment guidelines for the treatment of HCC, including those from the National Comprehensive Cancer Network, Barcelona Clinic Liver Cancer Group, and American Association

for the Study of Liver Disease, as well as several other European and Asian organizations, with no single set of guidelines being universally accepted. For patients with a single, small (<2 cm) tumor, ablation is now the first-line treatment. Examples of such technologies include RFA and MWA, which heat the tumors above 100 °C for cellular destruction. This can be performed surgically via an open approach or using minimally invasive techniques, or even percutaneously with imaging guidance by radiologists or surgeons depending on the tumor location and experience of the facility and involved physicians. For larger tumors in patients without cirrhosis, liver resection with clear margins is the standard. Unfortunately, surgical resection is often highly risky because of the underlying cirrhosis common in patients with HCC. Although it is possible to

TABLE 19-1. Treatments for Hepatocellular Carcinoma
Resection
Transplantation
Transarterial chemoembolization
Ablation
Cryoablation
Radiofrequency ablation
Laser photocoagulation
Microwave ablation
Ethanol injection
Chemotherapy
Observation/supportive care

remove as much as 70% of the normal hepatic parenchyma on resection, cirrhosis limits the liver's regenerative capacity. No specific studies conclusively determine the extent of hepatic parenchyma that can be safely resected in a patient with cirrhosis, and most surgeons attempt smaller resections in this setting.

Liver transplantation is appropriate for some patients with HCC because it removes the malignant tumor, eliminates possible sites of recurrence in the remaining diseased liver, and provides hepatic replacement in patients who usually have severely limited hepatic reserve in addition to their tumor. Limitations to the use of liver transplantation in the treatment of patients with HCC include the limited number of donor livers for transplantation and the high cost of this treatment modality. Strict criteria (Milan criteria: single tumor <5 cm or up to three tumors all ≤3 cm; no vascular invasion) have been developed to guide the use of transplantation for HCC. An AFP value above 1,000 ng/dL is also used by many centers as a cut-off value to exclude liver transplantation.

Noncurative strategies include liver-directed therapies that administer cytotoxic chemotherapy agents (transarterial chemoembolization or TACE) or radioactive microspheres (selective internal radiation therapy or SIRT) via the hepatic arterial system. Chemoembolization involves the infusion of chemotherapy (usually doxorubicin [Adriamycin]) combined with embolic particles, either gelatin foam or glass microspheres, administered directly to the tumor through the hepatic artery, whereas radioembolization involves the delivery of Y90 (yttrium 90) using glass beads. The latter is not a true embolization, as the beads are small enough that the arterial supply is not occluded. This approach takes advantage of the preferential arterial blood supply of HCC, whereas normal hepatocytes receive 70% of their blood and 50% of their oxygen delivery from the portal venous system. Directly administering these therapies allows for higher doses of chemotherapy or radiation with fewer side effects, as the liver breaks down metabolites before they enter the systemic circulation.

When patients with HCC and cirrhosis undergo successful tumor resection, the remaining liver is the most common site of future recurrence (≥50% of patients), probably because similar etiologic factors are present in the remaining liver (eg, hepatitis with the formation of second primary lesions) and also from satellite lesions that were not detected at initial resection. The other sites of tumor metastasis include the lungs and bone. Brain and intraperitoneal metastases are less common.

Cholangiocarcinoma

Cholangiocarcinoma arises from the mucosa of the biliary tree (see Chapter 15) and may present in the periphery of the liver, centrally within the liver, or in the extrahepatic bile ducts. The location determines the nature of the symptoms experienced by the patient. Peripheral tumors may be asymptomatic whereas central or hilar tumors (Klatskin tumor) may cause obstructive jaundice from biliary obstruction. There is often no visible tumor mass on CT scan whereas magnetic resonance cholangiopancreatography may show missing segments of the central biliary tree, and endoscopic retrograde cholangiopancreatography may only demonstrate a bile duct stricture. Jaundice with dilated intrahepatic ducts and a small gallbladder strongly

suggest a hilar or central cholangiocarcinoma. These cancers are treated by liver resection. Other rare primary tumors of the liver include angiosarcoma and epithelioid hemangioendothelioma.

Metastatic Tumors

The most common malignant tumors found in the liver are metastatic, most commonly from a gastrointestinal (GI) source. Among all patients with cancer, 30% to 40% have hepatic metastases at autopsy. When hepatic metastases are the only site of metastatic disease, treating the tumors in the liver often confers a survival benefit. This approach is clearly established for colorectal carcinoma, where successful resection of metastatic foci can result in 5-year survival rates of 55% to 65% in properly selected patients. Other cancers that may exhibit a liver-only metastatic pattern are neuroendocrine tumors and GI stromal tumors. On rare occasions, hepatic metastases from other sites (breast, melanoma) may be resected for cure in highly selected patients.

With colorectal cancer metastases, patients with fewer and smaller tumors, low carcinoembryonic antigen levels, a longer (>1 year) disease-free interval, no extrahepatic disease, and node-negative primaries have the best outcomes from liver resection. Surgeons are now more aggressive in treating colorectal metastases because hepatic resection for colorectal cancer now carries a very low mortality rate, and, with the advent of several new and effective chemotherapy drugs, long-term survival is reported with multiple tumors in both lobes and even extrahepatic disease.

Although resection of hepatic metastases may afford long-term survival, most patients (60%-70%) have a recurrence of colorectal carcinoma, and the residual liver is the most common site of recurrence. For this reason, patients who have undergone resection require careful selection and close follow-up. Ablative therapy techniques (MWA and RFA) have been used for metastatic tumors. The precise role of ablative therapy in the management of hepatic tumors remains to be fully defined and, although generally considered inferior to hepatic resection, remains an option for tumors not amenable to surgical excision.

Hepatic Cysts

Simple Cysts and Polycystic Liver Disease

Cysts of the liver are common and are identified more frequently with the increased use of CT to investigate many abdominal conditions. Liver cysts may be congenital or acquired; the latter may be neoplastic or infectious. Simple cysts occur in as many as 10% of patients. Most are small, asymptomatic, contain clear serous fluid, and do not communicate with the biliary tree. When multiple, they typically number three or four and are scattered throughout the liver.

Simple cysts (Figure 19-7) may occasionally become quite large and be associated with pain, early satiety because of the mass effect, or segmental biliary obstruction from pressure effects. Intracystic bleeding may occur with larger cysts, resulting in symptoms and difficulty differentiating this entity from neoplastic or infectious cysts. Needle aspiration may provide temporary relief of symptoms from simple cysts, but the cyst almost always recurs. For this reason, standard treatment for clearly symptomatic cysts includes surgical unroofing.

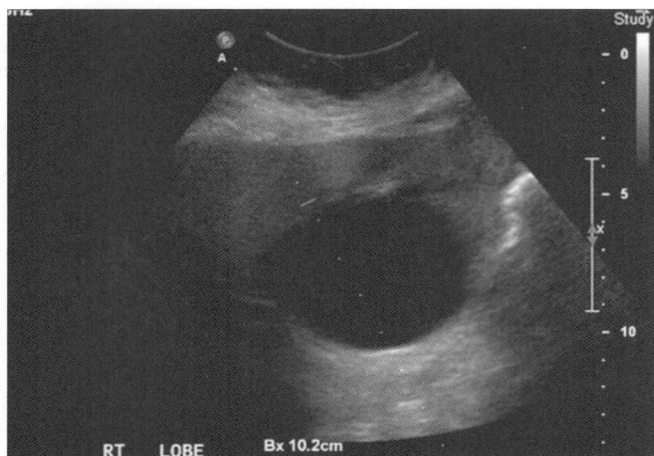

Figure 19-7. Simple liver cyst.

Polycystic liver disease (Figure 19-8) is an autosomal dominant disorder that causes multiple cysts that are microscopically similar to simple cysts. Unlike simple cysts, however, these cysts are numerous, and progressive enlargement is the norm. Additionally, patients with polycystic liver disease often have polycystic kidney disease that may progress to end-stage renal disease. The hepatic cysts in this condition may be treated with the resection of the dominant area of cystic involvement. Simple cyst unroofing alone is rarely effective because of extensive involvement. In severe cases, especially when hepatic synthetic function is abnormal, transplantation is an option.

Cystic Neoplasms

Neoplastic cysts of the liver (cystadenoma) are rare. Cystadenomas occur mainly in women over 40 years, tend to recur, and have the potential for malignant transformation. These cystic tumors are usually single and large (>10 cm), have multiple septations and thin walls, and contain mucinous fluid. Ultrasound and CT scans may show internal echoes consistent with septations or papillary growths within the cyst. Mural nodules may be seen.

Cyst walls, septations, and mural nodules may enhance with contrast on CT scan.

Because of the malignant potential of these lesions, the preferred treatment is surgical excision. Nonresectional procedures, including marsupialization (creation of a pouch), drainage into the peritoneal cavity, and drainage into the GI tract, are contraindicated because of a high rate of cyst recurrence and infection, as well as the inability to completely eliminate the risk of malignant potential.

Hepatic Abscesses

Pyogenic Abscess

Patients with bacterial liver abscesses usually have right upper quadrant pain, fever, and leukocytosis. The alkaline phosphatase level is elevated in most patients. Ultrasound imaging usually shows a hypoechoic mass, often associated with a hyperechoic wall. CT usually shows a fluid-density lesion, which may have a hypervascular wall. Although hepatic abscess may develop as a consequence of hematogenous seeding from any site, most result from a GI (ie, diverticulitis or appendicitis) or biliary tract source of infection.

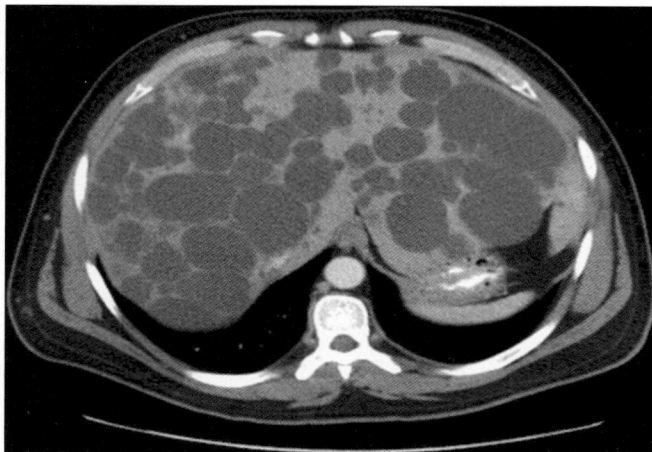

Figure 19-8. Polycystic disease.

Percutaneous aspiration and drain placement aid in diagnosing and resolving the infectious process; however, it is typically not needed in smaller lesions (<4-5 cm) or multifocal abscesses. In such cases, antibiotics are all that is needed. The results of blood and abscess cultures direct antimicrobial therapy. Biliary stenting may be required if biliary obstruction contributed to the abscess formation. The source of the bacteria should be identified and treated although no etiology is discovered in up to 20% of these cases.

Amebic Abscess

Although rare in the United States, amebic liver abscesses are relatively common in regions endemic for amebiasis, including Central and South America. For this reason, it should be considered in immigrants from, or travelers to, these regions. Liver abscess occurs in as many as 10% of patients with amebiasis; the liver is one of the most common sites of extraintestinal infection. Antiamebic antibodies can be found in almost all patients with infection and are a useful test in patients who are not from endemic areas (many patients from endemic areas without active amebiasis will test positive). Percutaneous aspiration shows a sterile fluid that has a characteristic "anchovy paste" appearance. These abscesses respond dramatically to metronidazole. Unlike pyogenic abscesses, they do not require percutaneous drainage.

Hydatid Cysts

Hydatid cystic disease occurs as a result of infection by a parasite, either *Echinococcus granulosus* or *Echinococcus multilocularis*. The normal life cycle of this parasite involves sheep and carnivores (wolves or dogs), but humans may become infected by contact with dog feces and become an accidental, intermediate host. Unilocular cysts may develop in any organ but occur within the hepatic parenchyma two-thirds of the time, and may grow as large as 10 to 20 cm. Within the larger cysts are multiple daughter cysts that contain innumerable protoscoleces. This disease may result in the compression of normal liver tissue, secondary pyogenic infection, or biliary fistula with an extension into the chest, bronchial tree, or peritoneal cavity.

The diagnosis should be suspected in any patient with a liver cyst (Figure 19-9) who has lived in an endemic region (Mediterranean countries, the Middle and Far East, East Africa, South America, and Australia). Calcifications may be seen on imaging and may be indicative of long-standing indolent infection. Eosinophilia may be seen in one-third to one-half of patients. The diagnosis of echinococcal infection is confirmed by serologic testing. Diagnostic needle aspiration or biopsy should be avoided because these approaches may result in the seeding of protoscoleces throughout the abdominal cavity as well as possibly anaphylaxis and shock. After the diagnosis is established, treatment is based on cyst characteristics, including location, size, and any complications caused by the cyst. Antiparasitic therapy with albendazole is initiated for small, unilocular cysts, and this therapy alone may be successful in controlling further growth and spread of the disease.

Surgery remains the most effective treatment for larger cysts with biliary communication. The goals of surgery are to remove the parasites and to treat the biliary complications of the disease (fistula). Conservative surgery may be performed to remove the cyst contents and inactivate protoscoleces through the use of scolicidal agents. The prevention of intraoperative spillage, which can lead to intraperitoneal recurrence of hydatid cyst disease, is the critical component of the procedure. PAIR (Puncture, Aspiration, Instillation with scolicidal agent, and Reaspiration) treatment has been shown to be successful in selected patients with unilocular cysts in the hands of experienced operators.

PORTAL HYPERTENSION AND ASSOCIATED COMPLICATIONS

Portal hypertension is defined as an abnormally high pressure (>10 mm Hg) in the portal vein or its tributaries estimated by the hepatic venous pressure gradient (HVPG). The portal circulation is shown in Figure 19-10. Portal hypertension may occur because of a variety of causes, which can be divided into prehepatic, hepatic, and posthepatic etiologies (Table 19-2), with cirrhosis responsible for approximately 90% of all portal hypertension in the United States. Portal vein thrombosis accounts for 50% of cases of portal hypertension in children, often the consequence of umbilical venous catheterization in infancy. The best-known example of outflow obstruction is the Budd–Chiari syndrome of hepatic venous occlusion, which can result from various thrombotic states or from vascular webs in the vena cava. Schistosomiasis is the most common worldwide cause of presinusoidal portal hypertension but is not found in the United States.

Compensation for elevated portal venous pressure occurs partly by the dilation of the portal venous tributaries and partly by the development of collateral channels to the systemic venous system. Collateral portosystemic channels form at sites where portal and systemic veins normally meet (Figure 19-11). These sites include the submucosal veins of the esophagus, the hemorrhoidal veins, the umbilical vein, and retroperitoneal veins. Surgery in patients with portal hypertension represents a formidable challenge and should be undertaken only for well-considered indications. Specific problems include bleeding from collateral vessels, hemodynamic abnormalities related to the drainage of large volumes of ascites, and postoperative hepatic decompensation related to general anesthesia. A number of scoring systems have been used to predict mortality from the complications of portal hypertension, with or without operative therapy; these include the Modified Child–Pugh Classification and Model for End-Stage Liver Disease (MELD) score (Table 19-3) and are discussed further in subsequent sections of this chapter.

Complications of portal hypertension include ascites, hepatic encephalopathy, GI variceal bleeding, hepatorenal syndrome (HRS), hydrothorax, spontaneous bacterial peritonitis (SBP), hepatopulmonary syndrome, and portopulmonary hypertension. The evaluation and management of variceal bleeding, ascites, and encephalopathy will be considered in detail.

Variceal Bleeding

Esophageal varices are submucosal veins in the short gastric and coronary to azygous collateral venous routes that become dilated and fragile in the presence of portal

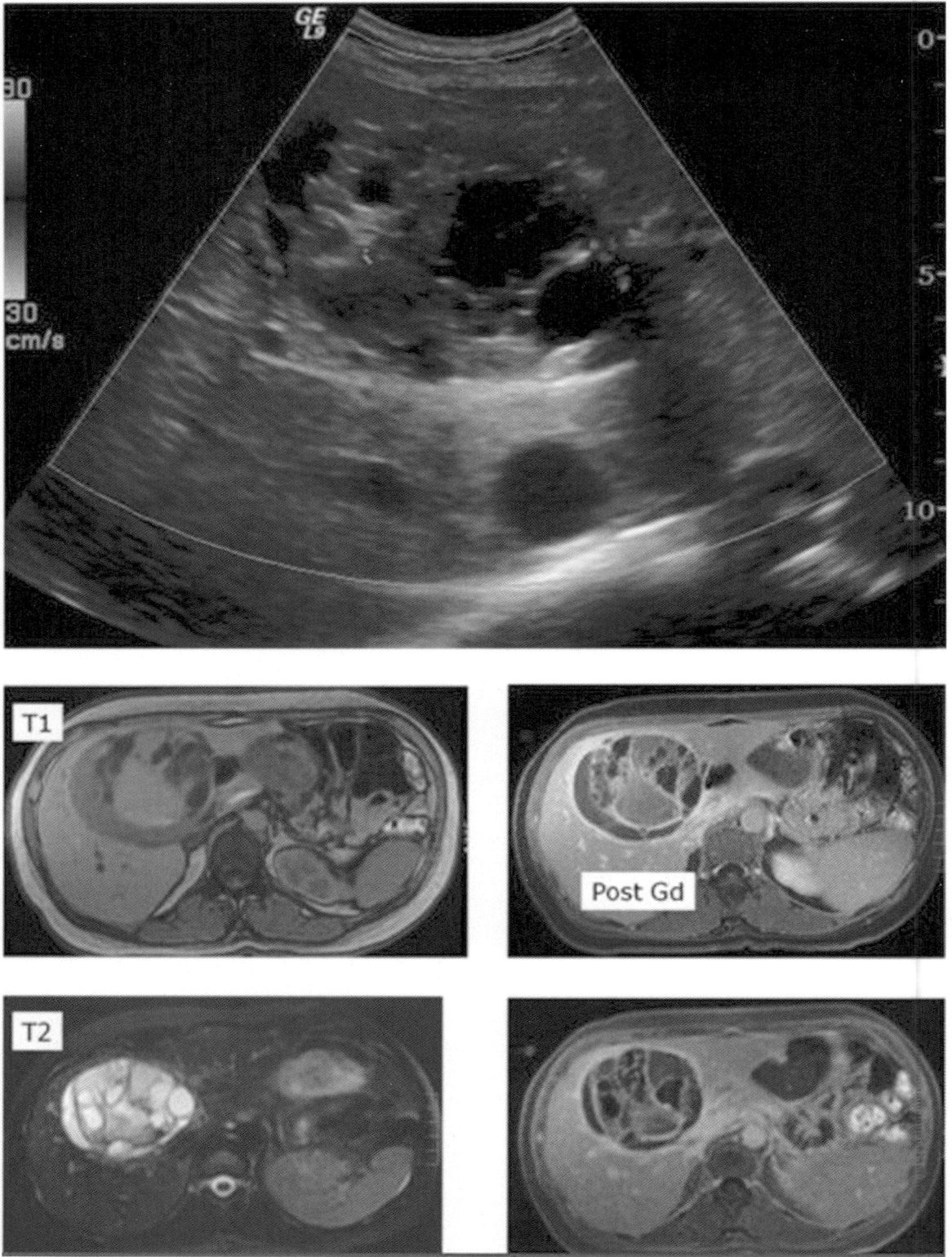

Figure 19-9. Hydatid liver disease. Hydatid cyst ultrasound (top row) and MRI (bottom two rows).

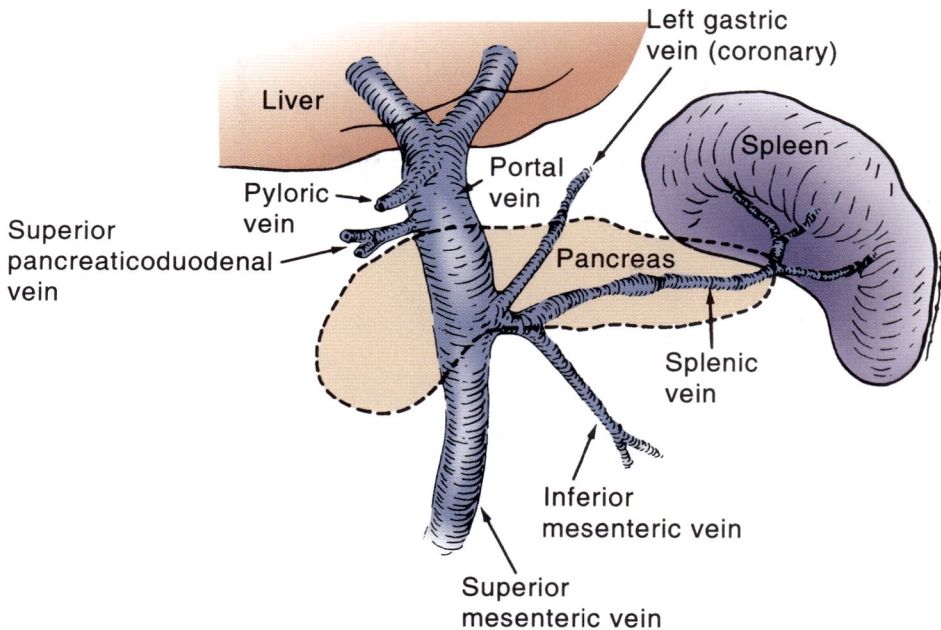

Figure 19-10.   Anatomy of portal circulation. (Reprinted with permission from Rikkers LF. Portal hypertension. In: Goldsmith HS, ed. *Practice of Surgery: General Surgery*. Vol 3. 1st ed. Harper & Row; 1981:chap 4.)

TABLE 19-2. Causes of Portal Hypertension

Prehepatic Etiologies

Portal vein thrombosis

Splenic vein thrombosis

Portal/splenic arteriovenous fistula

Splenomegaly

Hepatic Etiologies

Cirrhosis (viral, alcoholic, etc)

Viral hepatitis

Primary sclerosing cholangitis

Primary biliary cirrhosis

Nonalcoholic fatty liver disease

Schistosomiasis

Congenital hepatic fibrosis

Nodular regenerative hyperplasia

Hepatic toxicity (amiodarone, arsenic, methotrexate, copper, vitamin A, etc)

Infiltrative liver disease (sarcoidosis, amyloidosis, Gaucher disease, myeloproliferative disorders, etc)

Posthepatic Etiologies

Budd–Chiari syndrome

Inferior vena cava obstruction/web

Congestive heart failure

Constrictive pericarditis

Severe tricuspid regurgitation

hypertension. Bleeding from esophageal varices is the complication associated with the greatest mortality. The proportion of patients with cirrhosis with esophageal varices is unknown, but approximately 30% of patients with varices will experience bleeding. Therapy is directed at the cessation of acute bleeding and the prevention of recurrent bleeding.

When patients present with variceal bleeding, the ABCs (airway, breathing, and circulation) of acute resuscitation apply here as in any ill or injured patient. The airway is secured, oxygen is administered, and hemoglobin-oxygen saturation is monitored closely. The initial goal of treatment is volume resuscitation using large-bore intravenous (IV) lines to maintain tissue perfusion. Lost blood is replaced with its components to restore adequate circulatory volume while avoiding excessive crystalloid volume that may promote ascites formation and rebleeding because variceal pressure varies directly with central venous pressure. Short-term antibiotic prophylaxis is also utilized because of the risk of infection in these critically ill patients.

It is critical to establish the diagnosis of variceal bleeding and exclude other causes of GI hemorrhage so that therapy can be directed properly and specifically. Numerous studies show that as many as half of acute upper GI bleeding episodes in patients with cirrhosis originate from nonvariceal sources such as peptic ulcer disease and Mallory–Weiss mucosal tears at the gastroesophageal junction. For this reason, upper GI endoscopy is essential to determine the source of bleeding and is performed as early as possible. Endoscopic therapy should be performed within 12 hours of presentation and is effective in approximately 80% of patients with acute variceal hemorrhage. During endoscopy, the diagnosis is made by visualizing the bleeding varix or by documenting the presence of varices and the absence of other bleeding sources. Endoscopic

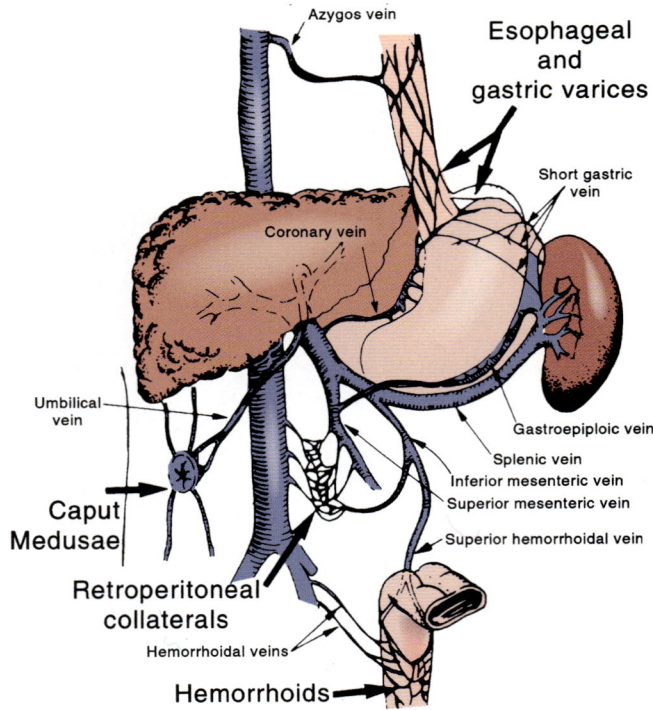

Figure 19-11. Sites of portal-systemic collateralization. (Reprinted with permission from Rikkers LF. Portal hypertension. In: Goldsmith HS, ed. *Practice of Surgery: General Surgery.* Vol 3. 1st ed. Harper & Row; 1981:chap 4.)

sclerotherapy and band ligation are the two principal procedures that are used.

As pharmacologic therapy for variceal hemorrhage is usually well tolerated with limited adverse effects, even if there is a nonvariceal cause of bleeding, treatment with vasoactive agents is initiated before the diagnosis of variceal bleeding is confirmed. IV somatostatin acts promptly to reduce variceal bleeding by splanchnic vasoconstriction and decrease portal venous flow. Somatostatin diminishes or halts variceal bleeding in more than 50% of patients and has few clinically significant side effects. IV vasopressin also acts by splanchnic vasoconstriction, but in prospective randomized trials they were not as effective as somatostatin in controlling variceal hemorrhage. Also, the vasoconstrictive effect of vasopressin is not limited to the splanchnic circulation and may cause serious ischemic complications, such as myocardial infarction and limb ischemia in patients with atherosclerotic disease. As the simultaneous infusion of nitroglycerin with vasopressin ameliorates these complications and may help stop variceal bleeding, the two drugs are usually used in combination.

When both pharmacologic and endoscopic treatments fail to control acute variceal hemorrhage, luminal tamponade can be used. The Sengstaken–Blakemore tube (Figure 19-12) is one specific device available for luminal tamponade, which has a distal port to evacuate the luminal contents of the stomach and balloons to provide tamponade to the submucosal veins at the gastric fundus as well as directly to the esophageal varices. When properly applied, luminal tamponade effectively controls variceal bleeding in approximately 90% of cases but a number of serious complications may occur, including aspiration,

airway obstruction, and esophageal injury (ulceration, necrosis, and rupture). Therefore, the placement and maintenance of these tubes require experience and a very strict protocol.

A transjugular intrahepatic portosystemic shunt (TIPS) is an interventional radiologic procedure used to treat various complications of portal hypertension by decreasing the portal pressure. It works by diverting blood from a portal vein branch to a hepatic vein, bypassing the liver and effectively creating a portacaval shunt within the liver. TIPS is accomplished successfully in approximately 95% of patients and, except in profoundly patients with coagulopathy, is highly effective in controlling acute variceal hemorrhage.

Options for the prevention of recurrent variceal bleeding include medical, endoscopic, radiologic, and surgical therapy. Medical therapy centers on the use of β-blockade to decrease portal venous flow and is commonly used as an adjunct to other treatments. Endoscopic therapy (Figure 19-13) is often used as the primary treatment regardless of the status of the hepatic reserve, and TIPS is used increasingly as definitive therapy, either primarily or after the failure of endoscopic therapy. Surgical shunts, despite excellent long-term patency with a low risk of recurrent bleeding, are now utilized far less frequently than in prior eras because of high morbidity and more readily available radiologic options. The choice among the more invasive options should consider the functional hepatic reserve, the reliability of the patient to return for additional studies and treatment, and the patient's ongoing access to prompt medical care.

Regardless of the choice of therapy for patients with bleeding varices, the most important predictor of

TABLE 19-3. Two Models Used for Predicting Survival in Patients With Liver Disease (Child–Pugh Score and Model of End-Stage Liver Disease)

Models for Predicting Survival in Patients With Decompensated Cirrhosis				
CPS				**MELD Score**
Points Given				MELD = 3.8 log^{e}TB + 11.2 log^{e}INR + 9.6 log^{e}Cr + 6.4
	1	**2**	**3**	**Variables**
Bilirubin (mg/dL)	<2	2-3	>3	TB = Serum total bilirubin (mg/dL)
Albumin (g/dL)	>3.5	2.8-3.5	<2.8	INR = International normalized ratio
Prothrombin time(s)	1-3	4-6	>6	Cr = Serum creatinine (mg/dL)
Ascites	None	Mild	Moderate	**Rules**
Encephalopathy	None	Grade I-II	Grade III-IV	Any lab value <1 is rounded to 1.
Classification				Serum creatinine >4 or hemodialysis is rounded to 4.
	A	**B**	**C**	Scores range from 6 (least ill) to 40 (most ill). All scores >40 are given a score of 40.
Total points	5-6	7-9	>9	For age ≤12, use the PELD score instead. A modification for patients with cancer exists.

CPS, Child–Pugh score; MELD, model for end-stage liver disease; PELD, pediatric end-liver disease.

Adapted from Pugh RN, Murray-Lyon IM, Dawson JL, et al. Transaction of the oesophagus for bleeding oesophageal varices. *Br J Surg*. 1973;60(8):646-649. Copyright © 1973 British Journal of Surgery Society Ltd. Reprinted by permission of John Wiley & Sons, Inc.

Adapted from Pugh RN, Murray-Lyon IM, Dawson JL, et al. Transaction of the oesophagus for bleeding oesophageal varices. *Br J Surg*. 1973;60(8):646-649. Copyright © 1973 British Journal of Surgery Society Ltd. Reprinted by permission of John Wiley & Sons, Inc.

Adapted with Kamath PS, Wiesner RH, Malinchoc M, et al. A model to predict survival in patients with endstage liver disease. *Hepatology*. 2001;33(2):464-470. Copyright © 2001 American Association for the Study of Liver Diseases. Reprinted by permission of John Wiley & Sons, Inc.

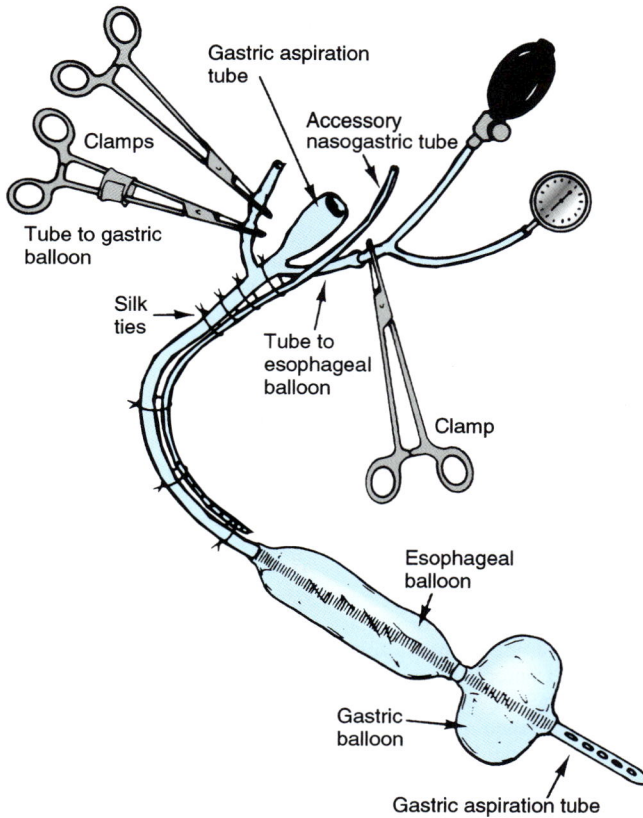

Figure 19-12. The Sengstaken–Blakemore tube.

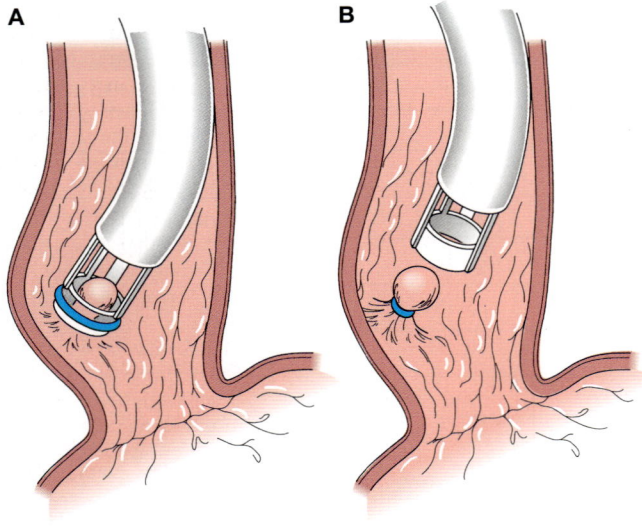

Figure 19-13. Endoscopic ligation of esophageal varices. The device used for ligation is based on the standard Barron-type ligator for the treatment of anal hemorrhoids. The esophageal varix is drawn up into the ligating device with suction (A) and the base of the varix is ligated with an O-ring (B). Up to six varices can be treated in a single session. (Reprinted with permission from Mulholland MW, Lillemoe KD, Doherty GM, et al, eds. *Greenfield's Surgery: Scientific Principles and Practice*. 6th ed. Lippincott Williams & Wilkins; 2017. Figure 59.6.)

long-term survival is the functional reserve of the liver. Because cirrhosis tends to progress relentlessly, only 50% of patients who have had variceal bleeding survive for 5 years without liver transplantation.

Ascites

Ascites is the accumulation of serous fluid in the peritoneal cavity. In portal hypertension, ascites forms due to increased hydrostatic pressure and decreased colloid oncotic pressure caused by deficient protein production. This situation favors transudation of fluid out of the vascular space, into the hepatic parenchyma, and ultimately into the peritoneal cavity. The renin-angiotensin-aldosterone system is involved, as are mediators, including nitric oxide, atrial natriuretic peptide, and prostaglandins. Ascitic volumes of 1,500 mL or more are detected with physical findings, including dependent dullness to percussion and the presence of a fluid wave whereas ultrasonography or CT can detect volumes as low as 100 mL.

Morbidity from ascites caused by portal hypertension may be substantial. Umbilical, groin, and other abdominal wall hernias can enlarge dramatically with the added pressure of ascites. The skin overlying hernias can become thinned and ulcerated; rupture of the skin may occur and has been associated with a high mortality rate. SBP occurs in approximately 10% of patients with cirrhosis with ascites. It is usually associated with an ascitic fluid white blood cell (WBC) count of more than 250 cells/mL and a predominance of neutrophils. Most infections are monomicrobial with enteric organisms. The mechanism of inoculation is unclear, with theories including gut bacterial translocation, seeding of ascites from other sources, and impaired reticuloendothelial clearance of portal bacteremia. Mortality rate is 50% within 1 year. SBP is treated with aggressive antibiotic therapy, and secondary peritonitis caused by perforation of an abdominal viscus or other etiology must be excluded.

Medical management effectively controls ascites in more than 90% of patients. Fluid intake is moderately restricted, and sodium intake is limited to less than 40 mEq/d. Diuresis begins with spironolactone, an aldosterone antagonist, to promote sodium excretion. If further diuresis is necessary, loop or thiazide diuretics are added. When the ascitic volume severely limits respiration or mobility and rapid decompression is needed, therapeutic paracentesis is performed. Large volumes of ascites (8-10 L) can safely be removed in one session. During paracentesis, albumin is administered IV (8 g/L removed) to replace protein and to avoid hypovolemia.

Rarely, more invasive treatment is required when medical measures and paracentesis fail. Portal-systemic shunts (TIPS or surgically created) provide control of ascites by reducing portal pressure. TIPS has now replaced surgical shunting but is not always successful in controlling ascites and may precipitate the development of encephalopathy. No survival advantages to the use of surgical shunts over medical measures have been shown.

Hepatic Encephalopathy

Hepatic encephalopathy is a neuropsychiatric disorder that occurs commonly in patients with severe hepatic insufficiency. Clinical features include confusion, obtundation, tremor, asterixis, and fetor hepaticus—a sweet, slightly feculent smell of the breath noted in advanced liver disease. Four stages of encephalopathy are recognized: stage I, mild confusion or lack of awareness; stage II, lethargy; stage III, somnolent but arousable; stage IV, coma. Even with normal consciousness, patients with advanced liver disease show impaired psychomotor testing.

The pathogenesis of encephalopathy is not understood. A number of theories have been advanced, including increased circulating levels of nitrogenous toxins, particularly ammonia; the presence of false neurotransmitters such as aromatic amino acids; and the concerted effect of two or more metabolic abnormalities such as alkalosis, hypoxia, infection, and electrolyte imbalances. Ammonia is believed to have a key role. Ammonia in the gut normally enters the portal circulation and is converted to urea by the liver; with hepatocellular dysfunction and portosystemic collaterals (or shunts), ammonia enters the systemic circulation, crosses the blood-brain barrier, and induces neuronal edema.

Certain factors are known to precipitate encephalopathy. including infection, GI bleeding, constipation, dehydration, sedatives and opioids, metabolic disorders, and portosystemic shunts. In some cases, the ingestion of even modest amounts of dietary protein will induce encephalopathy.

The diagnosis of hepatic encephalopathy is made clinically. The serum ammonia level is often elevated in patients with encephalopathy, but this test lacks sufficient specificity to be diagnostic. Certain electroencephalographic patterns are seen in encephalopathy but are also not diagnostic. Other causes of mental status alterations must be excluded, including acute intoxication, organic brain syndrome and infection, head injury, or central nervous system tumor.

Encephalopathy is usually reversible with medical measures. Much of the treatment is empiric and not consistently supported by controlled trials. Any precipitating causes of encephalopathy, such as infection, should be sought and corrected. A number of pharmacologic agents are used to treat encephalopathy. Lactulose, a nonabsorbable disaccharide, is administered by mouth, nasogastric tube, or enema. Lactulose acts as a cathartic and alters colonic pH, trapping ammonia in the lumen. Intraluminal antibiotics, including neomycin, metronidazole, and rifaximin, decrease ammonia production by reducing the urease-producing bacterial flora. Zinc supplementation, benzodiazepine receptor antagonists, and probiotics have shown benefit for the treatment of encephalopathy in some trials.

END-STAGE LIVER DISEASE AND LIVER TRANSPLANTATION

End-stage liver disease occurs after repeated damage to the liver resulting in a progression from inflammation to fibrosis and cirrhosis. Liver transplantation is now considered standard treatment for many causes of acute and chronic liver failure. However, the physician must be aware of not only the risks and costs of the surgical procedure itself but also the fact that there is limited organ availability and the procedure commits the transplant recipient to lifelong immunosuppressive therapy, with its own inherent risks. Thus, physicians must exercise careful judgment to determine which patients can be treated with medical measures or less complicated surgical procedures and which ones are likely to require transplantation because of disease progression.

Laboratory parameters may be altered depending on the etiology of liver disease. When cirrhosis has a hepatocellular cause, the prothrombin time is prolonged beyond 18 to 20 seconds (international normalized ratio [INR] ≥ 2.0). A serum albumin level of less than 2.5 to 3.0 g/L is associated with diminished hepatic synthetic reserve. Patients whose cirrhosis has a cholestatic etiology may have near-normal prothrombin times and serum albumin values of 3 g/L or greater. However, elevation of the serum bilirubin above 10 mg/dL suggests advanced liver disease in this group. Laboratory parameters are only guides to hepatic functional reserve and must be considered in the context of the individual patient's clinical condition.

Patients who are under consideration for liver transplantation usually have irreversible hepatic failure for which there is no suitable alternative therapy. Liver transplantation in adults is generally performed for chronic, progressive advanced liver disease, clinically significant portal hypertension, liver cancer, and acute fulminant hepatic failure, the latter being present for about 5% or less of all liver transplants. For most patients, medical measures are initially used to treat specific complications associated with cirrhosis and liver failure, with transplantation considered only if these measures are ineffective. Table 19-4 lists contraindications to liver transplantation. Living-donor liver transplantation offers an additional supply of suitable liver tissue to patients in need. This practice remains underutilized in the United States, accounting for 6% of all liver transplants, compared to 90% of liver transplantations in Asian countries. Despite the infrequent use, living-donor liver transplantation is considered safe when performed in experienced centers. Further strategies to expand the pool of available livers include expanding donor criteria to include those infected with hepatitis C virus (HCV) or human immunodeficiency virus (HIV) and donation after circulatory death, but the need for liver transplants still exceeds the supply both in the United States and worldwide.

Chronic and Progressive Advanced Liver Disease

Chronic liver disease usually results from either hepatocellular injury (eg, viral hepatitis, alcohol-induced injury) or cholestatic liver disease (eg, primary biliary cirrhosis, sclerosing cholangitis) (discussed later). Because of the risks and expenses associated with transplantation, patients are usually considered for this procedure when their 1- to 2-year survival rate is estimated at 50% or less. Although it is sometimes difficult to predict expected survival in patients with advanced liver disease, certain markers assist in this prediction. For example, in patients with chronic

TABLE 19-4. Absolute Contraindications to Liver Transplantation
Uncontrolled sepsis
Extrahepatic malignancy
Active alcohol or substance use
Advanced cardiac or pulmonary disease

liver disease, clinical factors that indicate advanced liver disease include nutritional impairment and muscle wasting, hepatic encephalopathy, difficult-to-control ascites, variceal hemorrhage, and renal insufficiency.

In an effort to predict the mortality risk (without transplant or other intervention) for patients with chronic endstage liver disease, MELD was developed (see Table 19-3). This scoring system utilizes only three objective parameters: serum bilirubin, INR, and creatinine. Using these variables, a MELD score is determined, ranging from 7 to 40, and this has been found to correlate with 3-month mortality without transplantation. Currently, patients are generally not considered for liver transplantation on the basis of chronic liver disease until their MELD score reaches 15.

Chronic Hepatitis C

Chronic hepatitis C infection is one of the most common indications for liver transplantation today. Hepatitis C was previously categorized under the heading non-A, non-B hepatitis, but molecular techniques allowed the identification of this single-stranded RNA virus in 1989. Although it was a common cause of transfusion-associated hepatitis in the past, this risk is now less than 0.05% per unit of blood product transfused with the current testing of banked blood. Many patients with chronic hepatitis C have such identifiable risk factors as previous drug use, previous transfusions, and multiple sexual partners, but up to 50% have no definable risk factors. Its course is usually slowly progressive, and most patients have chronic infections for 10 to 20 years before complications of liver disease occur or a liver transplant is needed. Only approximately 20% of patients clear the HCV in response to acute infection. Fortunately, hepatitis C has become a curable disease because of recent advancements in treatment. However, the new treatments remain costly, and patients with advanced disease and at a high risk of complications are prioritized for treatment.

After liver transplantation for chronic hepatitis C, reinfection of the transplanted liver is nearly universal, but fortunately, the course of hepatocellular injury is indolent in most patients. New strategies, including antiviral therapies, are under investigation, but no effective measures to prevent allograft infection have been established. Although the short-term results of liver transplantation for hepatitis C are satisfactory in most cases, cirrhosis in the allograft can develop, leading to graft failure.

Chronic Hepatitis B

Chronic hepatitis B infection, unlike hepatitis C infection, shows a marked propensity to cause significant hepatocellular injury in the transplanted allograft if untreated, with a high incidence of early graft loss and death of the transplant recipient. Although at one time hepatitis B infection was a contraindication to liver transplantation, the use of hepatitis B immunoglobulin to suppress viral expression along with antiviral therapy (eg, adefovir) has been very effective in preventing the recurrence of hepatitis B virus (HBV) in the posttransplant period in the majority of patients. Fortunately, the universal use of HBV vaccination in the United States has markedly reduced this as an indication for transplantation. Chronic hepatitis B infection is still endemic in many regions of the world and can be seen in immigrants to the United States.

Alcoholic Liver Disease

Transplantation for alcoholic liver disease is one of the most controversial indications for liver transplantation. With intensive pretransplant screening, including the completion of an alcohol rehabilitation program and a period of supervised abstinence (usually ≥6 months), the risk of recidivism is less than 10% to 15%. Of those who consume alcohol after transplantation, continued alcohol use to the point of causing liver disease in the allograft is extremely rare. For reasons that are not well understood, as many as one-third of patients with a history of alcohol misuse also have serologic markers for hepatitis C infection without other known risk factors.

Fulminant Hepatic Failure

Fulminant hepatic failure occurs when massive hepatocyte necrosis or severe impairment of liver function occurs without evidence of chronic liver disease. Common causes of fulminant hepatic failure include viral infection and hepatotoxic drugs (eg, anesthetic drugs, acetaminophen, isoniazid) or even mushroom poisoning in certain areas of the United States (Pacific Northwest) and Europe. Liver dysfunction occurs within 8 to 12 weeks of the onset of symptoms. In these patients, hepatic encephalopathy develops, progressing to coma, brain stem herniation, and death without liver replacement. The INR is usually significantly prolonged, and reversible renal insufficiency (HRS) may develop. Because these patients do not have chronic liver disease, muscle wasting and portal hypertension are usually not present. For this reason, liver transplantation is technically easier to perform than in the setting of chronic liver disease. Most patients die within 1 to 2 weeks of presentation without liver transplantation because of the rapidly advancing nature of liver dysfunction in this setting.

The rapid progression of fulminant hepatic failure necessitates an aggressive and accelerated workup in addition to aggressive supportive measures. Some patients with milder forms recover without liver transplantation, but the period of observation cannot extend for too long or it may not be possible to obtain a suitable donor liver in time to perform a successful transplant. Thus, the decision to proceed with liver transplantation requires careful judgment by the treating physicians who must weigh the risks of death without a transplant against the potential commitment to lifelong immunosuppression in a patient who might otherwise recover without this procedure. Clinical trials with extracorporeal liver support systems are underway. These systems may prevent cerebral injury while the injured liver recovers or until a suitable donor liver is located. In the future, these systems may successfully assist patients during this critical period.

ANATOMY AND PHYSIOLOGY OF THE SPLEEN

The normal adult spleen weighs between 75 and 150 g and is the largest mass of lymphoid tissue in the body. As such, it plays a key role in maintaining the integrity of an individual's immune status. The spleen resides in the left upper quadrant of the abdomen, bounded by the left hemidiaphragm superiorly and the lower thoracic cage anterolaterally and posteriorly (Figure 19-14). The spleen is intimately associated with a series of suspensory ligaments to nearby organs including the stomach (gastrosplenic ligament), left kidney (splenorenal), colon (splenocolic), and diaphragm (splenophrenic).

The spleen is an extremely vascular organ that receives approximately 5% of the cardiac output. The splenic artery, a branch of the celiac artery, provides the primary inflow and courses along the superior border of the pancreas. There are usually four to six short gastric arterial branches from the distal splenic artery as well as the left gastroomental or gastroepiploic artery. If the splenic artery becomes occluded, the short gastric arteries can provide collateral blood flow to the spleen (Figure 19-15A). Venous drainage of the spleen occurs through the splenic and short gastric veins. The splenic vein parallels the splenic artery and joins the superior mesenteric vein to form the portal vein (Figure 19-15B).

A variety of developmental disorders affect the spleen. The most common developmental anomaly is the presence of accessory spleens in addition to a normal spleen. Accessory spleens are found in 10% to 30% of the population and are believed to result from a failure of separate splenic masses in the dorsal mesogastrium to fuse. The most common sites for accessory spleens, in the order of decreasing frequency, are the splenic hilum, splenocolic ligament, gastrocolic ligament, splenorenal ligament, and omentum (Figure 19-16). Although these do not typically cause symptoms in most patients, failure to identify and remove accessory spleens may lead to a relapse of various hematologic disorders after splenectomy.

The spleen has several distinct functions, including hematopoiesis, blood filtering, and immune modulation. The function of the spleen is intimately related to its microstructure. Central to its microstructure is its microcirculation (Figure 19-17). A trabecular meshwork of fibrous tissue joins the fibroelastic capsule to the hilum of the spleen and surrounds the entering blood vessels. Blood enters the splenic parenchyma through central arteries that branch off the trabecular arteries. These central arteries course through the white pulp, where they are surrounded by periarterial lymphatic sheaths that consist primarily of T lymphocytes and macrophages that can process soluble antigens. Some blood flows into surrounding lymphatic follicles where B lymphocytes can proliferate in germinal centers. Mature antibody-producing cells (plasma cells) are found here. Blood that leaves the white pulp flows into a marginal zone, where it is directed either back to the white pulp or through terminal arterioles into the splenic cords of Billroth in the red pulp (open circulation). In the reticular network of the cords, which have no endothelial cells, blood percolates slowly and comes into contact with numerous macrophages before they enter the endothelial-lined sinuses that connect with the splenic vein branches. The red pulp is the site of removal of antibody-sensitized cells and particulate material. In some pathologic conditions, blood is shunted from the marginal zone directly into the sinuses (closed circulation) (depicted in the lower portion of Figure 19-17), bypassing much of the critical filtering function.

The spleen's role in extramedullary hematopoiesis is found in the fetus, but this activity usually ceases by birth in normal humans. In its role as a blood filter, the spleen culls abnormal and aged erythrocytes, granulocytes, and platelets from the nearly 350 L/d of blood that passes through it. As red blood cells (RBCs) near the end of their lives (normal RBC lifespan, 110-120 days), they are removed in the red pulp because they lose membrane integrity and the ability to deform appropriately when entering the splenic sinuses. In addition, as normal RBCs deform to enter the splenic sinuses, "pitting" occurs, which removes nuclear remnants (Howell–Jolly bodies) and inclusions such as denatured hemoglobin (Heinz bodies) and iron (Pappenheimer bodies).

The role of the spleen in the sequestration and destruction of granulocytes and platelets under normal circumstances is not well understood. Normally, one-third of the body's platelets are stored in the spleen. Abnormal splenic processing of platelets occurs in several diseases and

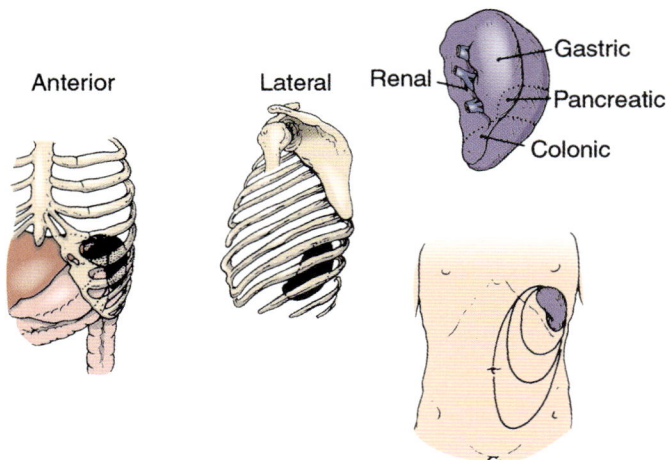

Figure 19-14. Normal external relations of the spleen. (Reprinted with permission from Mulholland MW, Lillemoe KD, Doherty GM, et al, eds. *Greenfield's Surgery*. 4th ed. Lippincott Williams & Wilkins; 2006:940.)

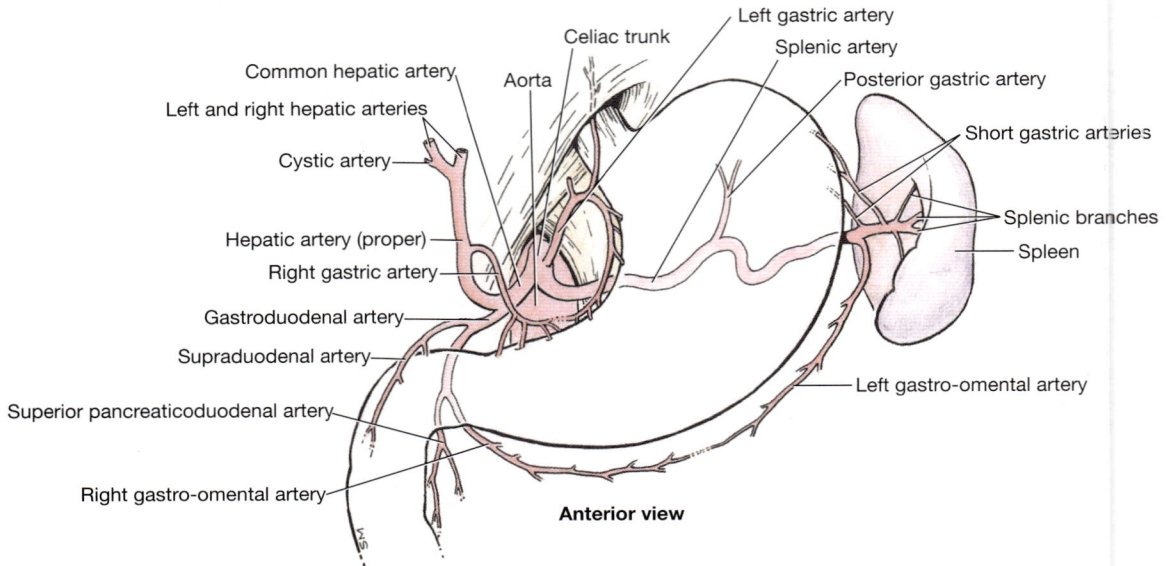

Anterior view

A

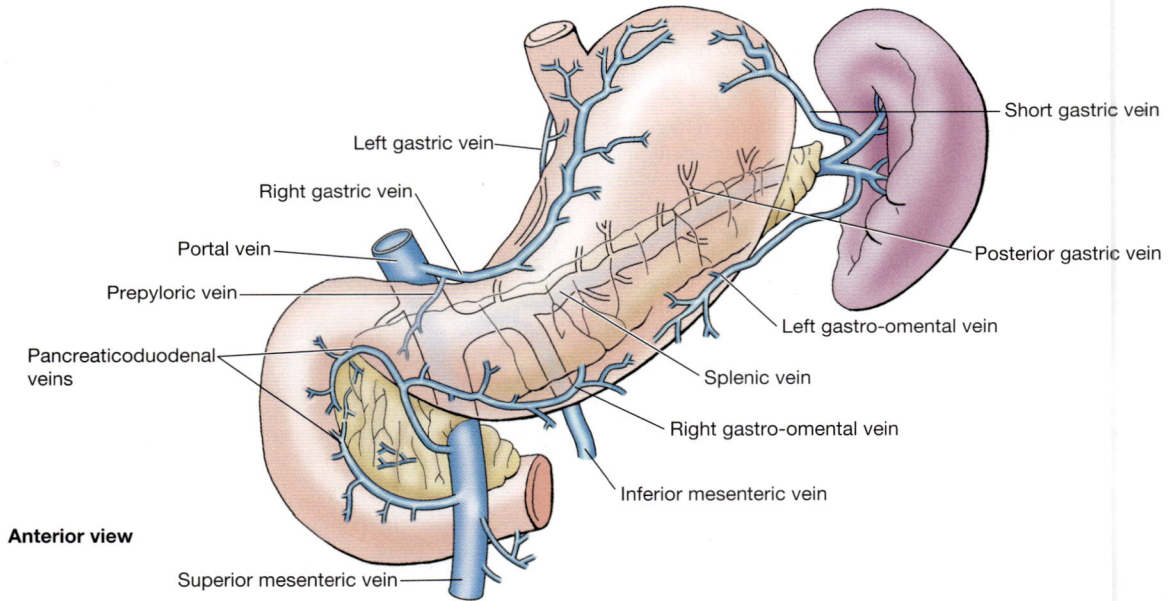

Anterior view

B

Figure 19-15. A. Arterial supply to the spleen. B. Venous supply to the spleen. (Reprinted with permission from Moore KL, Dailey AF, eds. *Clinically Oriented Anatomy*. 9th ed. Lippincott Williams & Wilkins; 2023.)

causes marked thrombocytopenia. Splenectomy is usually followed by transient thrombocytosis.

The spleen is a part of the reticuloendothelial system and plays an important role in the immune system. It provides both nonspecific and specific immune responses. The spleen is the body's largest source of immunoglobulin M (IgM), and splenectomy causes a marked decrease in IgM and opsonin production. Because of its mass and its position in the circulation, the spleen probably plays a major role in modulating the systemic cytokine response to infection. However, little is understood about this role.

APPROACHING DISORDERS OF THE SPLEEN—GENERAL DIAGNOSTIC CONSIDERATIONS

History and Physical Examination

When evaluating a patient with a possible surgical disorder involving the spleen, it is important to obtain accurate and pertinent personal and family history. The physician should ask if the patient has a history of easy or abnormal bleeding or bruising, including spontaneous nose bleeds,

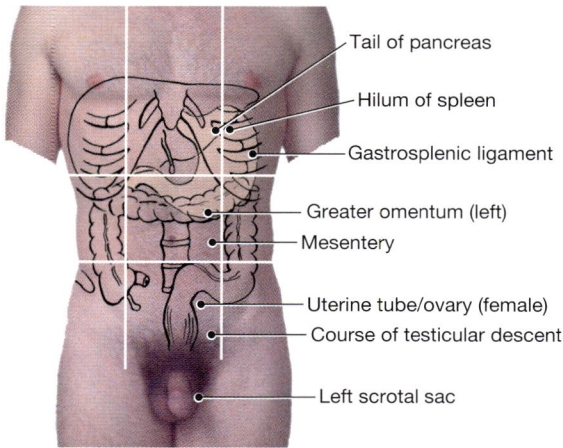

Figure 19-16. **Potential sites of accessory spleens.** The dots indicate where potential accessory spleens may be located. (Reprinted with permission from Moore KL, Dailey AF, eds. *Clinically Oriented Anatomy.* 5th ed. Lippincott Williams & Wilkins; 2005.)

bleeding from the gums, or excessively heavy menstrual cycles. Careful evaluation of medications includes any medication that may interfere with platelet function. A personal or family history of any blood disorders, as well as lymphoma or leukemia, is also important to making the diagnosis. If the patient already has a specific diagnosis, it is important to note what treatments, if any, have already been attempted and if the patient had a successful response.

Physical examination begins with the observation of the abdomen while the patient lies supine, paying careful attention to the patient during inspiration. An abnormally enlarged spleen may be identified below the costal margin or may even cause asymmetry of the abdominal wall. It is usually difficult to palpate a normal spleen. Palpation of the spleen is performed bimanually with the patient lying flat (Figure 19-18) or if this is unsuccessful then with Middleton method, whereby the examiner's fingers are "hooked" under the costal margin (Figure 19-19).

A spleen that is enlarged secondary to a hematologic condition is usually not tender. Therefore, discomfort on palpation alerts the clinician to the possibility of splenic infection, splenic infarction, or splenic rupture.

Radiographic Imaging

A variety of radiographic techniques are available to aid in the diagnosis and treatment of disorders of the spleen.

Plain Abdominal Roentgenogram

Plain films of the abdomen rarely show the normal spleen. However, splenomegaly is suggested when there is displacement of the colon inferiorly or the stomach medially, or when the left diaphragm is elevated. At times an enlarged splenic shadow is seen (Figure 19-20). Fractures of the lower left ribs suggest concomitant splenic rupture.

Ultrasound

Ultrasound is a useful tool for the evaluation of splenic size. Sonography may show splenomegaly, splenic cysts, or splenic abscesses (Figure 19-21). Abdominal ultrasound is one of the best ways to rapidly evaluate patients with trauma patients for the presence of blood within the abdomen (see discussion in the abdominal trauma section of Chapter 7). However, gas within the intestines may interfere with the visualization of the spleen and other abdominal structures. Sonography and Doppler imaging can be used to obtain information about the patency of splenic vessels.

Computed Tomography

CT scanning performed with IV and oral contrast agents is the most useful imaging technique to determine splenic size and detect splenic injury (Figure 19-22). CT scans also provide useful information about other potential disease processes or injuries in adjacent organs. Splenic cysts and abscesses are clearly shown by CT scans, and percutaneous drainage can be performed under CT guidance. CT scans can be used to follow splenic injuries and to obtain information about the patency of splenic vessels, but sonography is preferred, as it does not require radiation of the patient. Thin-slice rapid CT angiography has replaced splenic artery catheterization for evaluation of the

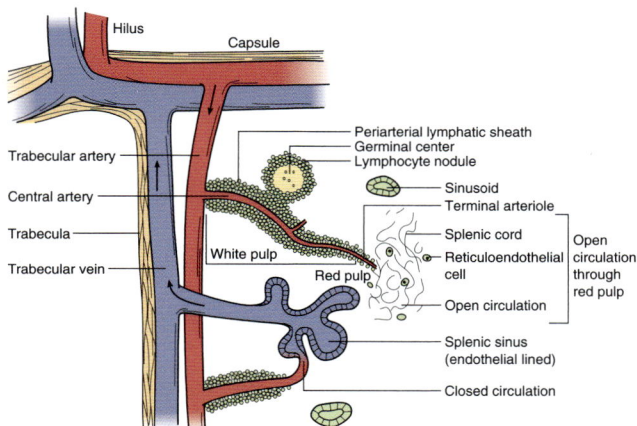

Figure 19-17. **Microanatomy of the spleen, with its functional components, showing both open and closed circulations.** (Reprinted with permission from Moore KL, Dailey AF, eds. *Clinically Oriented Anatomy.* 5th ed. Lippincott Williams & Wilkins; 2005.)

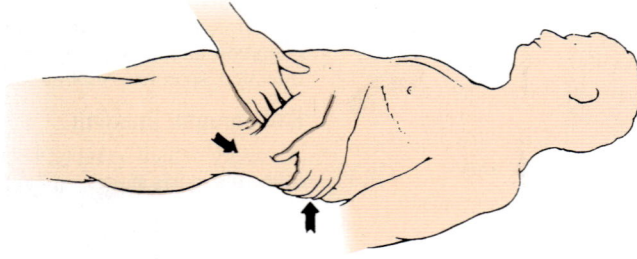

Figure 19-18. Bimanual palpation of the spleen.

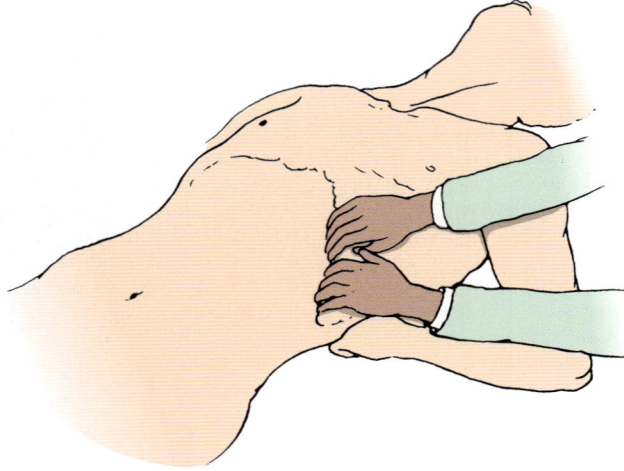

Figure 19-19. Palpation of the spleen by the Middleton method.

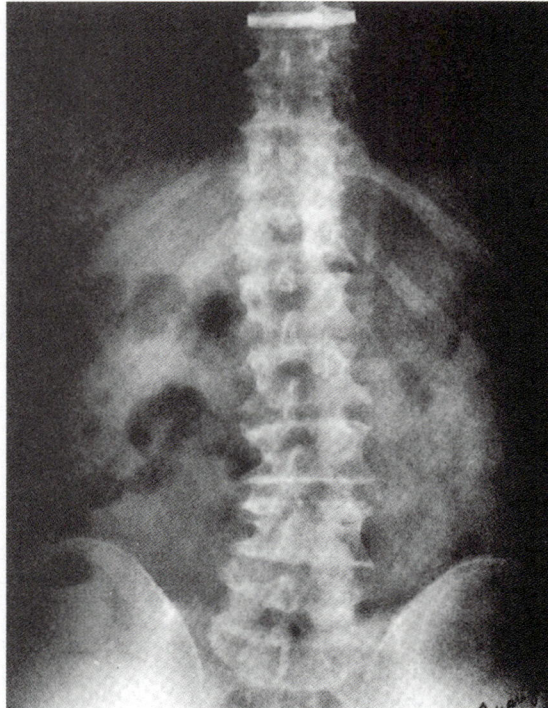

Figure 19-20. Plain film of the abdomen showing an enlarged spleen (radiopaque shadow in the left upper quadrant).

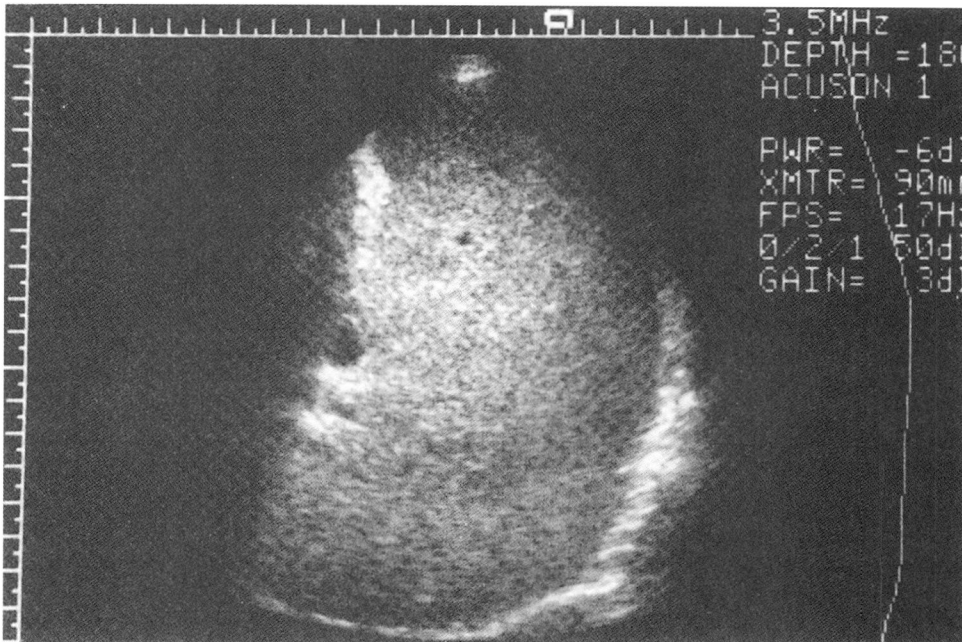

Figure 19-21. Ultrasound of the left upper quadrant showing an enlarged spleen. In this case, splenomegaly is secondary to myelofibrosis.

spleen in stable patients in cases of trauma, especially after sonography demonstrates intra-abdominal fluid. CT angiography has become the mainstay for noninvasive vascular assessment of the spleen and is also useful to help guide angiographic procedures.

Magnetic Resonance Imaging

Although not as prevalent as CT, the rate of MRI imaging of the spleen continues to steadily increase. MRI may more readily detect certain pathologies compared to CT such as microabscesses or small splenic infarcts, and may be able to provide more detailed information about certain disorders, such as the presence of septations within a splenic

cyst. Additionally, MRI may be more sensitive for detecting infiltrative processes involving the spleen, but guidelines regarding its use have not been established.

Radionuclide Scans

Colloid suspensions of technetium are taken up by the reticuloendothelial system, and subsequent imaging gives information about splenic size and function, commonly referred to as a liver/spleen scan. Although utilized less frequently since the widespread adoption of CT and MRI imaging, radionuclide scans can still be helpful in searching for missed accessory spleens in patients in whom splenectomy failed to control the underlying hematologic

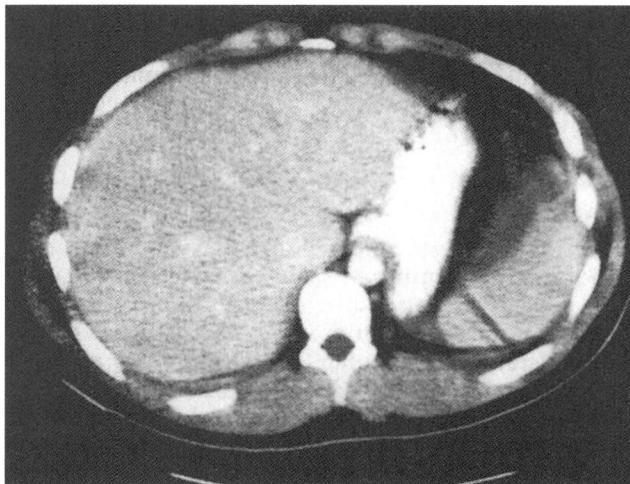

Figure 19-22. Computed tomography scan of the abdomen showing a subcapsular hematoma of the spleen.

disorder or in those with a later return of the hematologic disorder after a period of improvement. Radionuclide scans can also help differentiate an accessory spleen from a tumor in the tail of the pancreas. Splenosis results in uptake in aberrant positions.

SURGICAL DISORDERS OF THE SPLEEN

The spleen is subject to a variety of disorders that may require surgical intervention (see Table 19-5). Trauma is the most common reason for splenectomy and typically approached in an open fashion. Minimally invasive approaches to splenectomy, such as laparoscopic and robotic resection, have reduced the morbidity of this treatment for other conditions.

TABLE 19-5. Indications for Splenectomy
Splenic rupture (repair of the spleen is preferred in certain patients)
Trauma
Iatrogenic injury
Hematologic disorders
Hemolytic anemias
Hereditary spherocytosis
Hereditary elliptocytosis
Thalassemia minor and major (rarely)
Autoimmune hemolytic anemia not responsive to steroid therapy
Idiopathic thrombocytopenic purpura
Immunologic thrombocytopenia associated with chronic lymphocytic leukemia or systemic lupus erythematosus
Thrombotic thrombocytopenic purpura (rarely)
Hypersplenism associated with other diseases
Inflammation
Infiltrative diseases
Congestion
Leukemia and lymphoma (rarely)
Other diseases
Splenic abscess (often associated with drug use or AIDS)
Primary and metastatic tumors
Splenic cysts
Splenic artery aneurysm
Bleeding gastric varices secondary to splenic vein thrombosis

AIDS, acquired immunodeficiency syndrome.

If platelet counts are less than 20,000, platelets should be available for transfusion during the procedure. Transfusion of platelets should not be performed before the splenic artery is clamped because transfused platelets are rapidly destroyed in the spleen. Recurrence of disease may be related to persistent splenic tissue after splenectomy, either as overlooked accessory spleens or as splenosis in patients who have residual splenic tissue from a splenic capsule rupture. Alternatives to total splenectomy (eg, partial splenectomy, embolization to control bleeding, and image-guided percutaneous drainage procedures) are also used successfully depending on the pathology (see later).

Splenic Trauma

The spleen is the most commonly injured organ following blunt abdominal trauma and the second most commonly injured organ after penetrating abdominal trauma. Traditionally, injuries to the spleen were treated with prompt splenectomy. However, a recognition of overwhelming postsplenectomy infection (OPSI), coupled with a better understanding of the immunologic function of the spleen, has led to attempts at splenic preservation in patients who are hemodynamically stable when feasible. In patients who are unstable with ruptured spleens, expeditious splenectomy remains the standard of care (see Chapter 7).

Splenic Abscess

Splenic abscess is a rare but serious condition. Primary splenic abscess is quite unusual, and infection typically spreads hematogenously from another location. IV drug use remains a significant risk factor, but splenic abscesses can also be commonly seen in endocarditis, urinary tract infections, osteomyelitis, acquired immune deficiency syndrome, and after previous trauma. Direct spread can also occur secondary to an infection of the nearby kidney, colon, or pancreas. If left untreated, the mortality rate for splenic abscess can exceed 20% in a healthy patient but increases to 80% in the immunocompromised.

Symptoms of splenic abscess may be vague and nonspecific, including fevers, chills, left upper quadrant abdominal pain, nausea, and fatigue. Other patients may present with more acute symptoms, such as peritonitis or pleuritic chest pain. Diagnosis can be readily made with ultrasound or CT imaging. Treatment is based on the number and characteristics of the abscess. Single unilocular abscesses, even if large, are effectively treated with percutaneous drainage. Multiple and/or loculated abscesses are more difficult to treat percutaneously and may often require splenectomy.

Splenic Cysts

The incidence of splenic cysts has increased with more widespread use of CT imaging and includes both parasitic and nonparasitic cysts. Parasitic cysts are caused by *E. granulosus* infection, leading to hydatid disease. Cystic echinococcosis is present worldwide but especially endemic in parts of South America, East Africa, and Central Asia. Infection in the United States is uncommon, but all patients should be asked about possible travel to endemic areas. Ultrasound or CT imaging can identify cysts with identifiable imaging characteristics such as calcifications or daughter cysts, and serologic testing will confirm the diagnosis. Treatment of echinococcal cysts can include surgery, percutaneous treatment with a chemical agent such as ethanol (also known as PAIR), antiinfective drugs, or simply observation. Treatment depends on imaging characteristics and follows a stage-specific approach. When surgery is performed, care is taken not to rupture the cyst as it may cause an anaphylactic response or could lead to intraperitoneal dissemination of disease.

Nonparasitic cysts are divided into true cysts and pseudocysts. True splenic cysts, those lined with epithelium, account for only 10% of all splenic cysts and are considered congenital. The majority of nonparasitic splenic cysts are pseudocysts. Splenic pseudocysts are acquired and lack a true epithelial lining. More than 80% of splenic pseudocysts are due to a history of trauma, with other causes including infection, infarction, or local inflammation. Both true cysts and pseudocysts of the spleen are benign without any malignant potential.

The majority of nonparasitic splenic cysts remain asymptomatic and are discovered incidentally. Larger cysts may cause pain, not only left upper quadrant pain but also back pain, left shoulder pain, or pleuritic chest pain. Large cysts may also cause symptoms such as early satiety, nausea, shortness of breath, or abdominal fullness due to compression of nearby structures. Nonparasitic splenic cysts may present more acutely due to rupture, hemorrhage, or infection, although this is rare. Due to their benign nature, intervention for nonparasitic splenic cysts is typically pursued only when patients are symptomatic. Percutaneous aspiration of the cyst is often possible, but recurrence rates are very high (≥80%) and aspiration subjects the patient to complications such as bleeding or infection. Definitive management is surgical intervention, which can include total splenectomy, but more often partial splenectomy or cyst "unroofing" is utilized to preserve splenic function.

Disorders of Splenic Function

Disorders of the splenic function are classified as either functional or anatomic. Functional disorders are considered in terms of too little function (hyposplenism and asplenia) or excessive function (hypersplenism). Congenital asplenia or hyposplenism is extremely rare. Splenectomy is the most common reason for the asplenic state, although other conditions (eg, sickle cell anemia) may lead to a functional asplenic state. The size of the spleen is not related to its hematologic function. Splenomegaly (anatomic enlargement of the spleen) is caused by a variety of conditions (Table 19-6) and should not be confused with hypersplenism (excessive function of the spleen).

In three categories of disorders of splenic function, splenectomy may be helpful: hemolytic anemias, immune thrombocytopenia (ITP), and cytopenia associated with splenomegaly from other diseases (secondary hypersplenism).

Hemolytic Anemia

Hemolytic anemia may be hereditary or acquired. Hereditary hemolytic anemias are classified into three broad classes: membrane structural abnormalities, metabolic abnormalities, and hemoglobinopathies (Table 19-7).

Splenectomy can be most effective in hereditary spherocytosis, an autosomal dominant trait characterized by abnormally shaped, rigid red cells as a result of a deficiency

in membrane proteins (spectrin, ankyrin, or band 3). Splenectomy is usually indicated because it allows red cells to survive and hematocrit to reach near-normal values postoperatively. An intraoperative search for accessory spleens is integral to the procedure because the remaining accessory spleens can hypertrophy and reproduce the symptoms. Patients may present with symptomatic cholelithiasis, hemolytic episodes, or aplastic crisis. Because the risk of OPSI is much greater in young children, operation should be delayed until after 4 to 5 years of age.

Other hereditary and acquired hemolytic anemias respond less well to splenectomy. Patients with sickle cell anemia become functionally asplenic because of repeated splenic infarcts and fibrosis and therefore do not typically require splenectomy except in the rare case of splenomegaly in hemolytic crisis. Patients with thalassemia may benefit from splenectomy with a decreased need for transfusions, but patients who have thalassemia and undergo splenectomy are at the highest risk for OPSI. For this reason, alternatives to total splenectomy (eg, splenic embolization, partial splenectomy) are preferred. Acquired autoimmune hemolytic anemias can be classified based on the results of the Coombs test, a laboratory procedure used to detect the presence of antibodies against RBCs in the body. Coombs-negative hemolytic anemia is usually secondary to drugs, toxins, or infectious agents and is best treated by removing the responsible agent. Patients with Coombs-positive hemolytic anemia should receive corticosteroid therapy and treatment for any underlying disorders. Splenectomy is indicated when steroids are ineffective or the patient has side effects during treatment.

Thrombocytopenia

Thrombocytopenia disorders are usually characterized by the coexistence of a low platelet count, a normal or increased number of megakaryocytes in the bone marrow,

TABLE 19-6. Classification of Splenomegaly (Based on Degree of Enlargement)

Slight	Moderate	Great
Chronic passive congestion	Rickets	Chronic myelocytic leukemia
Acute malaria	Hepatitis	Myelofibrosis
Typhoid fever	Hepatic cirrhosis	Gaucher disease
Subacute bacterial endocarditis	Lymphoma (leukemia)	Niemann–Pick disease
Acute and subacute infection	Infectious mononucleosis	Thalassemia major
Systemic lupus erythematosus	Pernicious anemia	Chronic malaria
Thalassemia minor	Abscesses, infarcts	Leishmaniasis
	Amyloidosis	Splenic vein thrombosis
		Reticuloendotheliosis (hairy-cell leukemia)

TABLE 19-7. Hereditary Hemolytic Anemias

Type	Inheritance	Defect	Usefulness of Splenectomy
Abnormal Membrane Structure			
Spherocytosis	Autosomal dominant	Deficiency in spectrin (membrane component essential for deformability)	Usually
		Rigid erythrocytes cannot pass through splenic vasculature and are sequestered, leading to progressive splenomegaly.	Usually
Elliptocytosis	Autosomal dominant	Decreased levels of spectrin; relatively mild in most cases	Rarely
Pyropoikilocytosis	Autosomal recessive	Rare variant of spherocytosis	Usually
Xerocytosis	Autosomal dominant	Water loss leading to increased concentration of hemoglobin	Rarely
Hydrocytosis	Autosomal dominant	Abnormality in erythrocyte Na+/K+ transport	Often
Metabolic Abnormalities			
Pyruvate kinase deficiency	Autosomal recessive	Decreased ATP generation leads to membrane destruction.	Rarely
G6PD deficiency	Sex-linked recessive	Pentose phosphate shunt is blocked and membrane is injured by oxidation injury from certain drugs (eg, sulfamethoxazole, ASA, phenacetin, nitrofurantoin).	Never
Hemoglobinopathies			
Sickle cell	Autosomal recessive (homozygous more severe)	Valine substitute for glutamic acid at position 6 of β-chain of HbA; rigid, sickle-shaped cells at low O_2	Rarely
Thalassemias	Many varieties	Deficits in the synthesis of one or more subunits of Hb	Rarely

ASA, aminosalicylic acid; ATP, adenosine triphosphate; G6PD, glucose-6-phosphate dehydrogenase; Hb, hemoglobin.

and the absence of other hematologic disorders or splenomegaly. The medication history is important, particularly the history of the use of drugs that interfere with platelet function (eg, aspirin) or other therapeutic agents that are known to cause thrombocytopenia. Patients with thrombocytopenia often have multiple petechiae (pinpoint lesions that result from a breakage of small capillaries or increased permeability of the arterioles, capillaries, or venules). A confluence of petechiae results in purpura.

In these disorders, splenectomy is most often performed in idiopathic, immune-mediated thrombocytopenias (those in which a cause cannot be found). ITP, formerly known as idiopathic thrombocytopenic purpura, is an acquired disease typified by the immune destruction of platelets. Despite its name, the majority of patients do not have purpura at presentation. Primary ITP is associated with

antiplatelet antibodies or T-cell-mediated platelet destruction, and many patients also have impaired platelet production. Secondary ITP is associated with other autoimmune disorders or viral illnesses, such as HIV. The diagnosis of ITP is made by history and physical examination along with inspection of the peripheral blood smear. A course of corticosteroids remains the first-line treatment for ITP. The therapy for ITP continues to evolve, with decreasing incidence of splenectomy as a second-line therapy with the recently demonstrated efficacy of thrombopoietin receptor agonists. In patients who undergo splenectomy, long-term response rates are favorable, with 60% to 85% requiring no further therapy.

Thrombotic thrombocytopenic purpura (TTP) is a congenital or acquired disease of the arteries or capillaries characterized by thrombotic episodes and low platelet counts. The classic pentad of clinical features consists of fever, purpura, hemolytic anemia, neurologic manifestations with changes in mental status and renal disease. The complete pentad is not universally seen at presentation and the presumptive diagnosis is sufficiently made by the presence of microangiopathic anemia and thrombocytopenia. Mortality from untreated TTP is approximately 90%. Congenital TTP is treated with prophylactic plasma infusion. Plasmapheresis, a therapy aimed at removing plasma-derived factors that cause platelet aggregation, is usually successful, either alone or in combination with antiplatelet therapy, whole-blood exchange transfusions, and steroids. Splenectomy may be used if these measures fail.

Hypersplenism Associated With Other Diseases

Hypersplenism is characterized by cytopenia (anemia, leukopenia, and thrombocytopenia, alone or in combination), normal or hyperplastic cellular precursors in the bone marrow, and correction of cytopenia observed after splenectomy. Cytopenia results from an increased sequestration of the cells in the spleen, increased destruction of cells by the spleen, or the production of antibodies in the spleen, leading to increased sequestration and destruction of cells. Splenomegaly may or may not be present and is not part of the diagnosis. A number of clinical syndromes are characterized by the destruction of various formed elements of the blood. Both infiltrative and congestive forms of splenomegaly are associated with hypersplenism (Table 19-8).

Splenectomy is indicated for hypersplenism if the platelet count is less than 50,000, with evidence of bleeding; if the neutrophil count is less than 2,000, with or without frequent intercurrent infections; or if the patient has anemia requiring blood transfusion. With secondary hypersplenism, the underlying disease should be treated before considering splenectomy, as in most cases splenectomy does not completely alleviate the cytopenia. For instance, hypersplenism associated with congestive splenomegaly as a result of liver failure and the vascular consequences of portal hypertension requires treatment of the hypertension rather than splenectomy. In benign cases of infiltrative splenomegaly (eg, Gaucher disease, an autosomal recessive disorder that causes an abnormal accumulation of glucocerebrosides in the reticuloendothelial cells), partial splenectomy and splenic embolization are used instead of splenectomy to treat hypersplenism and abdominal discomfort caused by massive splenomegaly.

When splenectomy is undertaken for hypersplenism, a dramatic increase in the number of platelets may occur postoperatively and may be associated with thrombosis and thromboembolism, particularly in patients with myelofibrosis. Close postoperative monitoring of platelets is essential with the initiation of antiplatelet therapy if needed. Hydroxyurea is the treatment of choice when there is significant postsplenectomy thrombocytosis.

Malignancies

Despite being one of the most vascular organs in the body, the spleen is a rare site of primary or metastatic disease, with lymphoma being the most common tumor involving the spleen. The most common primary splenic tumors, either benign or malignant, are vascular neoplasms, such as hemangiomas, hamartomas, lymphangiomas, or angiosarcomas. Splenectomy can be considered and is effective for both the diagnosis and treatment of these tumors. Splenectomy has historically been explored as treatment for hematologic malignancies. In recent past, splenectomy was believed to be an important therapeutic intervention early in the treatment of hairy-cell leukemia, an indolent, progressive form of chronic leukemia. Splenectomy is now reserved primarily for palliating cytopenias and symptoms of splenomegaly. Although historically used frequently, splenectomy as part of a staging laparotomy is now rarely performed for Hodgkin disease because of improvements in imaging technologies and changes to better systemic forms of therapy. Splenectomy for non-Hodgkin lymphoma is rarely indicated, except in patients with primary splenic lymphoma or symptomatic massive splenomegaly or hypersplenism.

CONSEQUENCES AND COMPLICATIONS OF SPLENECTOMY

Hematologic Changes

In a normal patient, after the spleen is removed the WBC count increases by an average of 50% over baseline. In some cases, the number of neutrophils increases to 15,000 to 20,000 per mm^3 in the initial postoperative period. The WBC count usually returns to normal within 5 to 7 days. Elevation beyond this period suggests infection. In some patients, the elevation of the WBC count is permanent. In such cases, there is a normal differential count.

The peripheral smear of a patient who has undergone splenectomy routinely shows Howell–Jolly bodies (nuclear remnants), nucleated red cells, Heinz bodies (hemoglobin precipitates), Pappenheimer bodies, and pitted

TABLE 19-8.   Diseases Associated With Hypersplenism
Congestive diseases of the spleen
Portal hypertension
Splenic vein thrombosis
Infiltrative diseases of the spleen
Benign conditions (Gaucher disease, Niemann–Pick disease, amyloidosis, extramedullary hematopoiesis)
Neoplastic conditions (leukemias, lymphoma, Hodgkin disease, primary tumors, metastatic tumors, myeloid metaplasia)
Miscellaneous diseases
Felty syndrome (rheumatoid arthritis, splenomegaly, neutropenia)
Porphyria erythropoietica
Sarcoidosis

red cells on phase microscopy. Some RBCs may show abnormal morphology. The absence of these findings after splenectomy for hematologic disease suggests that an accessory spleen was missed. A radionuclide spleen scan may be useful for identifying retained splenic elements. The platelet count increases by 30% between 2 and 10 days after splenectomy and usually returns to normal within 2 weeks. Thrombocytosis (platelet count >400,000/mm^3) occurs in as many as 50% of patients. Theoretically, this increase predisposes the patient to thrombotic complications (eg, deep vein thrombosis in the lower extremities, thrombosis of the mesenteric veins, and possible pulmonary embolism). However, little evidence supports a correlation between absolute platelet count and thrombosis. Most thromboses and pulmonary emboli occur in patients who have myeloproliferative disorders. Postoperative therapy with platelet inhibitors (eg, aspirin, dipyridamole) has been used in patients who have myeloproliferative disease and platelet counts larger than 400,000/mm^3 and in all other patients after splenectomy if the platelet count is larger than 750,000/mm^3. Treatment continues until the platelet count returns to normal. Anticoagulation with heparin or warfarin therapy is not beneficial and should be avoided. For more extreme elevations of the platelet count, treatment with hydroxyurea is indicated.

Immune Consequences

The risk of OPSI varies with the age of the patient at the time of splenectomy and the reason for splenectomy. In otherwise normal children, the potential risk of OPSI is approximately 2% to 4%. In adults, it is approximately 1% to 2%. Patients who undergo splenectomy for hematologic disorders are at the highest risk. The overall incidence of OPSI in postsplenectomy patients is 40 times that of the general population. OPSI usually does not occur in the immediate postoperative period. Residual functioning splenic tissue may lessen the risk as evidenced by the lower incidence of postsplenectomy sepsis in patients with trauma in whom retained accessory spleens and the development of splenosis are likely to account for some residual immune protection.

Overwhelming infections are usually caused by encapsulated organisms. *Streptococcus pneumoniae* (pneumococcus) is the most common agent (75%), followed in decreasing frequency by *Haemophilus influenzae*, *Neisseria meningitidis*, β-hemolytic streptococcus, *Staphylococcus aureus*, *Escherichia coli*, and *Pseudomonas*. Viral infections, most commonly herpes zoster, may be severe in patients who have undergone splenectomy. Some parasitic infections (babesiosis, malaria) also overwhelm the host who has undergone splenectomy. Overwhelming infections with encapsulated bacteria (eg, pneumococcus) are insidious in onset, often mimicking a cold or flu. However, within a few hours, patients may become septic, and death may ensue rapidly (24-48 hours) despite vigorous antibiotic therapy. Adrenal infarction causing adrenal insufficiency is often associated with these infections (Waterhouse–Friderichsen syndrome).

Vaccinations against *H. influenzae* type B, *N. meningitidis*, and *S. pneumoniae* should be administered to all patients who have undergone splenectomy. Patients with splenic trauma who are managed nonoperatively may also benefit from vaccination. Neither the surgeon nor the patient should consider this vaccine as full protection against overwhelming postsplenectomy sepsis. Children who are younger than 2 years do not become effectively immunized and pneumococcal types that are not contained in the vaccine (or other bacteria) may cause overwhelming sepsis. The exact timing for immunization is unknown but 2 weeks before surgery is probably sufficient. However, if the patient undergoing splenectomy is being treated with steroids, this may lessen the immune response. In such patients, delayed immunization after steroids have been discontinued may be preferred. Additionally, it is wise to wait until the patient is nutritionally intact and recovers from other injuries before administering vaccinations.

Other Complications After Splenectomy

Morbidity and mortality rates after splenectomy are relatively low. Persistent hemorrhage after splenectomy occurs in less than 1% of patients, most commonly in those who undergo splenectomy for thrombocytopenia. Pulmonary complications include atelectasis and left pleural effusion. Injury to the pancreas occurs in 1% to 5% of patients who undergo splenectomy. It may be clinically unrecognized and cause mild hyperamylasemia or may cause clinical pancreatitis, pancreatic fistula, or pancreatic pseudocysts. Gastric injury may lead to the development of a subphrenic abscess or gastrocutaneous fistula. Subphrenic abscesses are usually apparent within 5 to 10 days after surgery. Signs include fever, left upper quadrant pain, left pleural effusion, prolonged atelectasis, pneumonia, and prolonged leukocytosis. Ultrasonography and CT scanning are useful for identifying abscesses. Once identified, they should be drained promptly either percutaneously with image guidance or operatively.

SUGGESTED READINGS

Garcia-Tsao G, Abraldes JG, Berzigotti A, et al. Portal hypertensive bleeding in cirrhosis: risk stratification, diagnosis, and management: 2016 practice guidance by the American Association for the Study of Liver Diseases. *Hepatology*. 2017;65(1):310-335.

Jackson WE, Malamon JS, Kaplan B, et al. Survival benefit of living-donor liver transplant. *JAMA Surg*. 2022;157(10):926-932. doi:10.1001/jamasurg.2022.3327

Reig M, Forner A, Rimola J, Ferrer-Fàbrega J, et al. BCLC strategy for prognosis prediction and treatment recommendation: the 2022 update. *J Hepatol*. 2022;76(3):681-693. doi:10.1016/j.jhep.2021.11.018.

Rodeghiero F. A critical appraisal of the evidence for the role of splenectomy in adults and children with ITP. *Br J Haematol*. 2018;181(2):183-195.

Tapper EB, Lok AS. Use of liver imaging and biopsy in clinical practice. *N Engl J Med*. 2017;377(8):756-768.

SAMPLE QUESTIONS

QUESTIONS

Choose the best answer for each question.

1. A 42-year-old woman presents to the emergency department after a motor vehicle accident. She sustains only minor injuries and is discharged in stable condition but is referred to your clinic for follow-up of a 3-cm mass in segment 6 of the liver found on CT scan in the emergency department. This mass was found to demonstrate progressive peripheral-to-central enhancement with a central hypodense region. She does not drink alcohol and does not have any history of hepatitis or cirrhosis. Her liver function tests are normal. She does not take oral contraceptive pills. She has no complaints at this time, including no pain, nausea, jaundice, or weight loss. What is your recommendation to this patient?

   A. Percutaneous biopsy for pathologic evaluation and diagnosis
   B. Surgical resection of this lesion
   C. Repeat imaging (CT or MRI) in 6 to 12 months
   D. Referral to oncologist for initiation of systemic chemotherapy
   E. MWA of this lesion

2. A 60-year-old woman with chronic hepatitis C is brought to an acute care clinic by her family because of increasing confusion. Physical examination identifies jaundice, spider angiomata, and splenomegaly. Neurologic examination shows the patient to be lethargic; asterixis is present. Which of the following pharmacologic agents is most appropriate for the treatment of this condition?

   A. Spironolactone
   B. Lactulose
   C. Somatostatin
   D. Ammonia
   E. Midodrine

3. A 46-year-old man presents to the emergency department with hematemesis. There have been no prior episodes. He admits to drinking a pint of hard liquor daily for more than 10 years. Upper GI endoscopy is performed and shows bleeding esophageal varices. Which of the following is the best management for this patient's bleeding?

   A. Emergency surgical portosystemic shunt
   B. Luminal tamponade
   C. Endoscopic rubber band ligation
   D. TIPS
   E. Peritoneovenous shunt

4. A 55-year-old man with known cirrhosis presents to the emergency department with severe abdominal pain. He appears ill. His blood pressure is 90/50 mm Hg, pulse is 110 beats/min, respirations are 24/min, and temperature is 38.8 °C. The abdomen is distended and tender; a fluid wave is present. Blood test results are Hgb of 13 g/dL, WBC count of 16,500/μL, normal electrolytes, urea nitrogen of

10 mg/dL, and creatinine of 1.1 mg/dL. A CT scan shows a small shrunken liver, an enlarged spleen, and a large volume of ascites. The ascites is sampled by paracentesis, and the results of this analysis show a WBC count of 750 cells/mL with 90% neutrophils; cultures are positive for a single gram-negative aerobic organism. Which of the following is the most likely diagnosis?

   A. Perforated viscus
   B. Carcinomatosis
   C. Mallory–Weiss tear
   D. SBP
   E. HRS

5. For the patient in question 4, which of the following is the most appropriate immediate therapy?

   A. Exploratory laparotomy
   B. Intraluminal antibiotics
   C. Protein restriction
   D. IV antibiotics
   E. Albumin

ANSWERS AND EXPLANATIONS

1. **Answer: C**

   The imaging characteristics of this lesion (progressive peripheral-to-central enhancement) and a lack of risk factors in this patient make a diagnosis of hemangioma most likely. These lesions are typically asymptomatic and remain benign. Biopsies should generally be avoided early in the workup of an asymptomatic patient and are often not necessary to determine the diagnosis. Surgical resection would not be necessary for this small asymptomatic hemangioma whereas surgical resection can be considered in patients with symptomatic hemangiomas or giant cavernous hemangiomas. It is reasonable at this stage to proceed with follow-up imaging to confirm the diagnosis and evaluate for any rapid change in growth. MWA or chemotherapy would not be indicated for treatment in this patient. For more information on this topic, please see section "Hemangioma."

2. **Answer: B**

   The answer is lactulose, a nonabsorbable disaccharide that acts to increase stool transit and convert ammonia to nonabsorbable ammonium (NH_4+). Increased levels of ammonia are associated with the development of hepatic encephalopathy, and therefore, additional ammonia administration would not be indicated. The goal of lactulose administration is for patients to have three to five soft stools per day. Spironolactone is a potassium-sparing diuretic used in patients with chronic liver disease and fluid retention (peripheral edema and ascites). Somatostatin is a GI peptide that regulates endocrine function, often used to decrease mesenteric blood flow in patients with portal hypertensive bleeding. Midodrine is a vasoactive antihypotensive oral peptide used in patients with symptomatic orthostatic hypotension. For more information on this topic, please see section "Hepatic Encephalopathy."

3. **Answer: C**

Endoscopic therapy with rubber band ligation has become the procedure of choice in patients with bleeding esophageal varices and should be performed as soon as the diagnosis is made and the patient initially stabilized. Emergency surgical portosystemic shunt procedures are associated with very high morbidity and mortality rates, especially liver failure. In addition, other measures are usually able to control bleeding so that invasive procedures can be performed on a semielective basis under optimized conditions. Luminal tamponade with a Sengstaken–Blakemore (or similar device) tube is usually employed as a last-ditch effort in patients who have failed medical management and endoscopic therapy. TIPS is associated with a high rate of liver failure when performed as an emergency procedure in unstable patients. For this reason, TIPS should be performed on an elective basis in patients with well-compensated liver disease. For more information on this topic, please see section "Variceal Bleeding."

4. **Answer: D**

This patient has SBP. This is thought to occur in the setting of ascites with immunosuppression (cirrhosis) and is a marker of advanced, end-stage liver disease. Bacterial translocation across the gut is thought to be the leading cause in most cases.

A perforated viscus is usually associated with free air on CT and plain films and will almost always show a polymicrobial infection on wound culture. In addition, the WBC count of the ascites in this setting would be much greater, typically higher than 10,000. Carcinomatosis can present with ascites, but this is usually gradual in onset and unassociated with severe pain. A Mallory–Weiss tear occurs following forceful vomiting and results in significant upper GI hemorrhage, with ascites not a typical finding. For more information on this topic, please see section "Ascites."

5. **Answer: D**

In cases of SBP, the culture of the ascitic fluid often shows a single organism but may not result in positive growth, and clinical treatment decisions are made on an empirical basis, with antibiotic selection usually targeted toward enteric organisms. Exploratory laparotomy is never required for SBP because the cause is bacterial contamination of the ascitic fluid, and this almost always resolves with appropriate antibiotic therapy. Intraluminal antibiotics (eg, neomycin) are sometimes used for the treatment of hepatic encephalopathy, but because they are not absorbed from the GI tract, they are ineffective for the treatment of systemic infection. Protein restriction is sometimes required for the treatment of hepatic encephalopathy but will have no effect on SBP. IV albumin has been shown to be beneficial for the treatment of associated renal insufficiency in patients with cirrhosis and SBP. However, this therapy would be considered an adjunct in their management and not primary treatment of the SBP per se. For more information on this topic, please see section "Ascites."

20 Transplantation

Amy R. Evenson and Vatche G. Agopian

Until the middle of the 20th century, the failure of any organ essential to life was uniformly fatal. However, technologies to sustain life despite transient organ failure were slowly developed. Two examples are early dialysis for acute renal failure and the refinement of respirators for respiratory insufficiency. The experimental techniques of organ and tissue transfer were attempted in humans, mostly in the form of kidney transplantation and skin grafting. Early attempts at kidney transplantation failed because the understanding of immunology did not evolve as rapidly as the surgical techniques for organ replacement. Now, because of an improved understanding of immunology and the evolution of modern-day organ and tissue preservation, end-stage failure of many organs essential to life no longer dooms the patient. In addition, tissues that are not vital to life (eg, cornea, bone, skin, dura) can be transplanted, improving the quality of many lives.

ORGAN AND TISSUE DONATION

Organ transplantation can be a lifesaving therapy for many patients with organ failure. Organs and tissues for transplantation come from deceased or living donors. Although grafts from living donors have the advantages of increased graft survival and immediate graft function, deceased donors are the major sources of graft tissues in the United States. The organ donation and transplantation community in the United States continues to undergo dramatic and sustainable change for better performance and quality. The United Network for Organ Sharing (UNOS), a private nonprofit group based in Richmond, Virginia, operates the Organ Procurement and Transplantation Network (OPTN) under contract with the federal government and is committed to increasing the number of donors. Over the past 30 years, the number of transplanted organs from deceased donors has steadily increased, whereas transplants from living donors have plateaued (Figure 20-1). The sharp increase in deceased donation starting in 2013 has been attributed, at least in part, to the increased number of deaths from opioid overdose.

The total number of organs transplanted has increased by 120% over the past 24 years (Table 20-1). This rise is most notable for an almost 6,000% increase in the number of donations after circulatory death (DCD) and a 500% increase in living liver donors. Both of these factors are reflective of the need to expand the donor pool to meet the demands of an increasing recipient waiting list. Vascularized composite allografts (VCAs) (ie, face, arm, penis) and uterus transplantation are relatively new areas of organ transplantation, reflecting the expansion of organ transplant principles to new types of recipients in need. Increasingly, some living donors are not related to

their intended recipients and may not even know them, a practice known as nondirected or altruistic donation. All potential living donors undergo a thorough medical and psychosocial evaluation to ensure they are suitable candidates for donation. Transplant centers are also required to have an independent donor advocate to ensure donor well-being throughout the evaluation and transplant process.

The recognition of a potential deceased donor is the initial step in organ donation. Solid organs can be transplanted if they remain perfused in situ until the time of retrieval. Therefore, any patient who has been pronounced dead using brain death criteria is a potential donor. The majority of organs recovered from deceased donors are from brain-dead donors. The diagnosis of brain death must be made before organ recovery is performed. The clinical neurologic examination remains the standard for the determination of brain death. The primary physician or a neurologic specialist usually makes this diagnosis. The President's Commission for the Study of Ethical Problems in Medicine and Biochemical and Behavioral Research defined brain death and endorsed criteria that are used as guidelines. These guidelines are separated into clinical criteria and confirmatory objective studies. Clinical criteria indicate that the individual is totally unresponsive to stimuli (Table 20-2). Clinical situations that mimic complete unresponsiveness (eg, barbiturate or opiate overdose, profound hypothermia) must be excluded or corrected. Confirmatory studies support the diagnosis of brain death, but this diagnosis may be made by clinical criteria only. Evaluation of the potential donor requires serial observations over a period of 6 to 24 hours. During this time, referral by the primary hospital staff to the organ procurement organization is initiated.

The most rapid increase in the rate of organ recovery from deceased persons has occurred in the category of DCD, that is, a death declared on the basis of cardiopulmonary criteria (irreversible cessation of circulatory and respiratory function) rather than neurologic criteria used to declare brain death (irreversible loss of all functions of the entire brain, including the brain stem). The process begins with the selection of a suitable candidate and the consent of the legal next of kin to the withdrawal of care and retrieval of organs. Subsequently, life-sustaining measures are withdrawn under controlled circumstances in the intensive care unit (ICU) or the operating room; organ donation after an unexpected fatal cardiac arrest is rare. When the potential donor meets the criteria for cardiac death, a physician independent from the transplant team declares the patient to be dead. The time from the onset of asystole to the declaration of death is generally 5 minutes to ensure no spontaneous resumption of cardiac activity occurs. Once the donor has been declared dead, a rapid recovery process

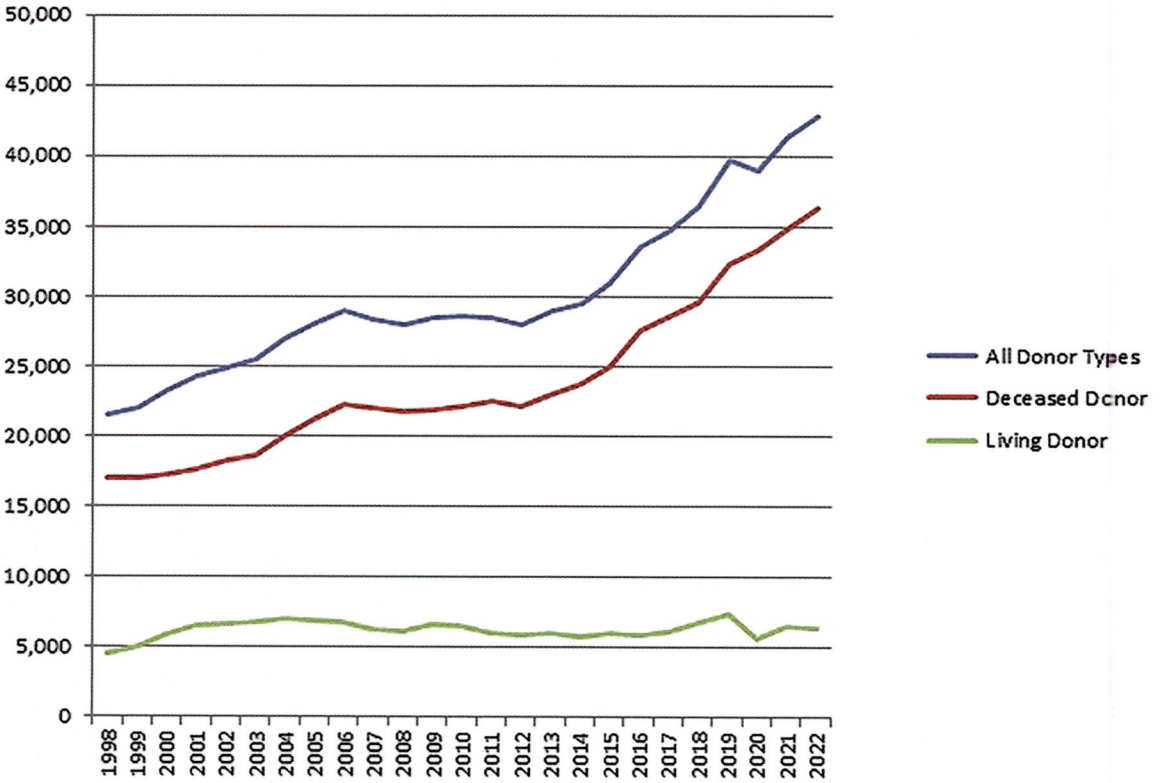

Figure 20-1. Total number of living and deceased donor organs transplanted, 1990 to 2022. (https://optn.transplant.hrsa.gov/data/view-data-reports/national-data/#. Accessed September 2, 2023.)

TABLE 20-1. US Transplants by Organ and Donor Type, 1998-2022

		1998	2022	Percentage Change (%)
All organs	Total	21,524	42,889	120
	Deceased	16,979	36,421	115
	Living	4,545	6,468	42
Kidney	Total	12,454	25,500	105
	Deceased	8,034	19,636	144
	Living	4,420	5,864	33
Pancreas	Total	245	108	−56
Kidney/pancreas	Total	972	810	−17
	Living	2	0	–
Liver	Total	4,519	9,528	111
	Deceased	4,427	8,925	101
	Living	92	603	555
Intestine	Total	70	82	30

TABLE 20-1. US Transplants by Organ and Donor Type, 1998-2022 (*continued*)

		1998	2022	Percentage Change (%)
Heart	Total	2,348	4,111	75
Heart/lung	Total	47	51	8
Lung	Total	869	2,692	210
Vascularized composite allograft	Total	0	81[a]	–
Uterus	Total	0	41[b]	–
All organs transplanted from donation after circulatory death (DCD) donors	Total	131	7,692	5,772

Data from Scientific Registry of Transplant Recipients. OPTN/SRTR Annual Data Reports. Accessed January 9, 2025. https://srtr.transplant.hrsa.gov/.
[a]Reflects entire US experience through August 2023 for abdominal wall, craniofacial, scalp, penile, and bilateral or unilateral upper limb allografts.
[b]Reflects total US experience through August 2023 with 17 deceased donor and 24 living donor allografts.

ensues to minimize the time the donor's organs are subject to warm ischemia. The organs most commonly recovered are the kidneys and liver; increasingly, the pancreas, lungs, and heart are recovered. To avoid obvious conflicts of interest, neither the surgeon who recovers the organs nor any other personnel involved in transplantation can participate in end-of-life care or the declaration of death.

The outcomes for organs transplanted after cardiac death are similar to those for organs transplanted after brain death. However, the length of time varies as to which organs can be subjected to cessation of circulation until the initiation of perfusion with cold preservation solutions and still be transplanted successfully. Livers transplanted after prolonged donor warm ischemic times are at increased risk for ischemic cholangiopathy as well as graft failure and death. If a potential donor does not reach circulatory death in a suitable time frame to permit organ recovery, end-of-life care

continues and donation is canceled. This may happen in up to 20% of cases. Recent advances in the development of both normothermic and hypothermic perfusion systems have helped broaden the use of organs recovered from DCD donors by mitigating some of these obligate ischemic changes.

Eligible donors are patients who have sustained irreversible central nervous system injury as a result of trauma, cerebrovascular accident, central nervous system tumors, or cerebral anoxia. Contraindications to donation include organ-specific chronic medical problems, many malignancies other than primary brain tumors, cardiac arrest that causes prolonged warm ischemia of organs, uncontrolled infection, and HIV infection, except under specific circumstances. Transplantation of livers (with acceptable biopsies) and kidneys from donors with hepatitis B into recipients with appropriate serologic profiles who are maintained on antiviral therapy poses minimal risk of posttransplantation morbidity and mortality from viral transmission or disease. Similarly, organs can be recovered and transplanted from donors who are infected with hepatitis C virus (HCV). With the advent of direct-acting antiviral agents, the use of hepatitis C–infected organs in non-hepatitis C–infected recipients has rapidly expanded. Clinical trials using organs from HIV-positive donors for recipients infected with HIV are increasing in the United States and have been used successfully in South Africa since 2008. The U.S. Public Health Service defines donors considered to be at increased risk of disease transmission on the basis of factors from their medical and social histories. Examples of such factors include men who have sex with men; nonmedical injection of drugs; people who have had sex in exchange for money or drugs; people who have had sex with a person known to have HIV, HBV, or HCV; people who have been incarcerated for more than 72 hours; patients for whom a medical or behavioral health history is unavailable or not obtainable; and patients involved in various other behaviors. Using data from national experience, the highest risk behavior (nonmedical injection of drugs) results in a disease transmission rate of 3 to 4 per 1,000 organs transplanted. Of note, per OPTN policy, both deceased and living donors are required to undergo antigen/

TABLE 20-2. Criteria to Determine Cessation of Brain Function

Clinical Findings

In the absence of intoxications or sedative medication use, hypothermia, or acute metabolic derangement:

Absence of spontaneous respirations

Absence of pupillary light reflex

Absence of corneal reflex

Sustained apnea when disconnecting respirator

Confirmatory Tests

Cerebral angiography

Electroencephalography

Transcranial Doppler ultrasonography

Cerebral scintigraphy (technetium [^{99m}Tc] exametazime)

antibody and/or nucleic acid testing for HIV, HBV, HCV, syphilis, cytomegalovirus (CMV), Epstein-Barr virus (EBV) prior to donation.

Potential recipients of both living and deceased donor organs need to be informed of the risks of disease transmission as part of their education and consent processes. The risk of significant complications from an unexpected disease transmission is generally considered to be lower than the risk of remaining on the transplant list until the next potential offer.

Acute or chronic diseases that affect certain organs may exclude them from consideration. Significant pre-existing renal disease excludes kidney donation, and diabetes mellitus precludes pancreatic donation. Cardiac trauma, coronary artery disease, pneumonia, and advanced age exclude cardiac and heart-lung donation. Donors who are older than 35 to 40 years may require coronary catheterization to rule out significant cardiac disease. Pulmonary trauma, pneumonia, and respiratory compromise may preclude lung donation. Bronchoscopy may be required to rule out infection. Minimal hypertension may not be a contraindication to kidney donation, although severe hypertension is a general contraindication to cardiac or renal donation. Laboratory studies, imaging studies, and biopsy are useful to determine the acceptability of donor organs (Table 20-3). Organs from donors

with a history of hepatitis B or hepatitis C may be used in selected cases either where the recipient has antibody protection or with a plan for treatment of a new infection after transplant.

All deceased donor kidneys are assigned a Kidney Donor Profile Index (KDPI) score that predicts the risk of failure on the basis of donor age, height, weight, race/ethnicity, history of hypertension or diabetes, cause of death, serum creatinine, HCV status, and whether the kidney is from a brain-dead donor or recovered after cardiac death. Kidneys with a KDPI score of over 85% have the worst predicted survival, require specific consent from potential recipients, and are used for patients who may not require a high-longevity kidney and would benefit from more rapid transplantation.

Consent for organ or tissue donation is obtained through a signed donor designation, driver's license designation, a consent statement, or a will. The US system of organ donation relies on obtaining written consent for donation from next of kin in the absence of a signed donor designation or driver's license. If a medical examiner is involved, their permission may also be required. Public education efforts emphasize the fact that the optimal situation for organ donation occurs when the family has previously discussed and agreed on organ donation.

Donor Management

After the donor is declared brain dead, treatment is directed toward optimizing the function of all transplantable organs. Ventilation is maintained with a mechanical respirator, and arterial blood gases are monitored. Because many patients who have closed head injuries are purposefully dehydrated to decrease cerebral edema, vigorous rehydration may be necessary. Donors who have massive diuresis because of diabetes insipidus may require vasopressin. If vigorous hydration with crystalloid or colloid is inadequate to maintain end-organ perfusion, a vasopressor is used. Vasoconstrictors are avoided because of their vasospastic effect on the renal and splanchnic beds. Monitoring of cardiac and pulmonary function is imperative when a heart, heart-lung, or lung donation is considered. Severe hypernatremia (serum sodium over ~160 mEq/L) is a risk factor for liver nonfunction after transplant, so appropriate management with vasopressin and fluids is required. Bone, skin, dura, fascia, and cornea donors do not need a functioning cardiovascular system, and the corresponding tissue can be procured 12 to 24 hours after the cessation of cardiac and respiratory function.

Organ Preservation

Effective preservation of whole organs after recovery enhances the success of deceased donor transplantation by providing time for distant transplant centers to retrieve the needed organs, perform precise tissue typing and cross-matching between donor and recipient, prepare the recipient, and work with national and international organ-sharing programs. The most critical steps in the preservation of solid organs are rapid organ cooling and sterile storage in a cold environment.

The kidney, heart, lung, liver, and pancreas are routinely flushed in situ with a cold solution to stop metabolism rapidly. Usually, hyperosmotic (325-420 mOsm/L) or hyperkalemic solutions are used. In some situations, a colloid is

TABLE 20-3. Laboratory Studies Used to Determine Acceptability of Organs for Transplantation

Laboratory Study	Evaluated Organ
Blood, urine, sputum culture	All
Hepatitis screen, EBV, CMV, RPR	All
HIV	All
Blood group	All
BUN, creatinine	Kidney
Glucose, hemoglobin A_{1c}	Pancreas
Liver function tests, INR, albumin	Liver
Cardiac catheterization, echocardiogram	Heart, heart-lung
Electrocardiogram	Heart, heart-lung
Chest radiograph	Heart, heart-lung, lung
Creatinine phosphokinase, MB, troponin	Heart, heart-lung
Bronchoscopy	Lung
Ultrasound, cross-sectional imaging	Liver, pancreas, kidney

BUN, blood urea nitrogen; CMV, cytomegalovirus; EBV, Epstein-Barr virus; HIV, human immunodeficiency virus; MB, creatine kinase muscle/brain; RPR, rapid plasma reagin.

added. The organs are subsequently removed, individually packaged in sterile containers, and placed in ice. Hypothermic (7-10 °C) continuous pulsatile machine perfusion with a colloid solution is used to extend renal preservation time. Pulsatile machine preservation is sometimes administered with an apparatus that includes a pulsatile pump, a membrane oxygenator, and tubing connected to the renal artery. In the past several years, both normothermic and hypothermic machine perfusion systems for liver, lung, and heart allografts have been utilized to expand the pool of potential organ donors by improving the function of marginal organs and avoiding ischemia-reperfusion injury. Additionally, the use of a period of normothermic regional perfusion (NRP) via an extracorporeal membrane oxygenation (ECMO) circuit is being investigated for DCD donors to improve organ function after transplant.

Organ and Tissue Allocation

UNOS, the national allocation system, coordinates the process of identifying and managing donors, notifying transplant centers of potential offers, coordinating the recovery of organs, and transportation of organs to recipient centers. All donors are registered with UNOS. As organs become available, the computer listing process matches the patients on the waiting list and the organs according to ABO compatibility. In addition, kidneys and kidney-pancreas combinations are distributed according to recipient factors, including age, prior transplantation, degree of sensitization to human leukocyte antigen (HLA), and waiting time. Hearts, livers, and lungs are shared primarily on the basis of ABO match and prioritized based on the recipient's medical condition. In addition, the Model for End-Stage Liver Disease (MELD) score is used for liver allocation with additional priority given to certain complications of liver disease, including early hepatocellular carcinoma (HCC), hepatopulmonary syndrome, acute liver failure, and other conditions. Allocation algorithms are updated periodically to optimize organ utilization while also balancing medical and ethical issues to share these scarce resources equitably. The transplant community and general public are encouraged to provide comments on pending changes to ensure transparency and the consideration of many perspectives during policy development.

IMMUNOLOGY

Transplantation involves a surgical procedure that transfers tissue from one site to another in the same individual or between different individuals. This tissue transfer can take a number of forms. An autograft is transplanted from one site of the body to another in the same individual (eg, skin graft removed from the leg and placed on a wound elsewhere). An isograft is transferred between genetically identical individuals (eg, renal transplant between monozygotic twins). An allograft is transplanted between genetically dissimilar individuals of the same species (eg, deceased donor renal transplant). A xenograft is a tissue that is transferred between different species (eg, porcine skin grafted onto a human burn victim). An orthotopic graft involves the placement of an organ in the normal anatomic position.

An orthotopic graft usually necessitates the removal of the native organ (eg, cardiac, lung, or liver transplantation). A heterotopic graft involves the placement of an organ at a site different from its normal anatomic position (eg, kidney, pancreas).

Components of the Immune System

The immune system is composed of cellular (T cells) and humoral (B cells/antibodies) components. T cells are derived from the thymus and play a central role in cellular immunity. They can be divided into CD4 and CD8 T cells and can recognize antigens presented by the major histocompatibility complex (also called HLA), through T-cell receptors (TCRs) expressed on their cell surface. B cells express a highly specialized form of antigen receptors, known as surface immunoglobulins, and are the precursors of plasma cells, which can secrete a soluble form of immunoglobulin, the antibody.

The highly polymorphic HLA loci are the primary targets of the alloimmune response. These genetic loci are located on the short arm of the sixth chromosome and are responsible for two classes of histocompatibility molecules. Class I antigens are single-chain glycoproteins and are cataloged as HLA, B, or C. These antigens are expressed on essentially all somatic cells and are recognized by CD8 T cells. Class II antigens are glycoproteins that have two polymeric chains, each with a common subunit. These antigens are present on B cells, dendritic cells, activated T cells, endothelial cells, and monocytes. Several series are found within this HLA locus, including the HLA-D locus and the HLA-DR, DQ, and DP loci. These class II HLA molecules are recognized by CD4 T cells.

The subloci are genetically transferred as haplotypes on a single segment of chromosome. Thus, a recipient shares one of two haplotypes with each parent. According to Mendelian genetics, a recipient has a 25% chance of sharing two haplotypes (called HLA identical), a 50% chance of sharing one haplotype, and a 25% chance of not sharing a haplotype with a sibling. Unrelated individuals randomly share similar antigens.

Antibodies may be present at birth (eg, ABO blood group antibodies), or they may be acquired. Successful transplantation generally requires transplantation of ABO blood group–compatible organs. Unless transplantation occurs as part of a donor-incompatible protocol with recipient pretreatment and desensitization, transplantation of incompatible organs that express ABO antigens (eg, kidney, heart) results in antibody-mediated killing of the endothelium, leading to thrombosis and organ necrosis, a process known as hyperacute rejection. Donor-specific anti-HLA antibodies (DSAs) can be present in a patient before transplantation because of sensitization events, including previous transplant, blood transfusion, or pregnancy. The presence of pretransplant DSAs can predispose grafts to a higher risk of acute and chronic antibody-mediated rejection.

Crossmatch

Sera from prospective transplant recipients are routinely screened for the presence of preformed anti-HLA antibodies to determine the extent of alloimmunization. Traditionally, the screening is performed against a panel of cells, representing most antigens encountered in the general population. A complement-dependent cytotoxicity assay (CDC) is utilized. Lymphocytes from a panel of donors are mixed with the sera of the recipient, and complement is added to determine whether the recipient has antibodies that bind to the donor cells and thus activate complement. The results are reported as a percentage of panel cells that are killed by reacting with the anti-HLA antibodies in a patient's serum; hence the term *panel-reactive antibody* (PRA). The same technique has been used for crossmatching recipients against potential donors to determine their suitability. Newer techniques, including single-antigen bead testing, are used to identify the specific alloantibodies present in recipient blood. The single-antigen bead testing allows the identification of all antibodies present in a recipient candidate and provides a measure of the intensity of the antibodies. This information can be used to determine whether a recipient candidate will have a positive crossmatch or increased risk of rejection with specific HLA antigens and monitor the response to attempts to decrease the levels of these antibodies (ie, desensitization).

The pretransplantation crossmatch test is the final immunologic screening step. Using the previously described HLA antibody screening assays, the potential donor's lymphocytes serve as the target cells for the patient's serum. There are two types of CDC crossmatch, depending on the type of donor lymphocytes used (T and B cells). A positive CDC crossmatch is generally a contraindication to transplantation. A more sensitive technique is the flow cytometry crossmatch, which can detect very low levels of circulating antibodies. Recipient patient sera are incubated with donor lymphocytes and stained with fluorescence-labeled anti-CD3 (T-cell marker) and anti-CD19 (B-cell marker). Positive flow cytometry crossmatches have been associated with a higher rate of early acute rejection. If certain organs are transplanted in the presence of a positive crossmatch, circulating anti-HLA antibodies attach to the endothelium of the donor organ. The effects of circulating preformed antibodies may be neutralized with the use of plasmapheresis and infusion of IV immunoglobulin G (IgG). ABO matching and crossmatching are the most common tests performed before renal, cardiac, lung, and pancreas transplantation. ABO matching alone is performed for liver transplantation in most circumstances. Bone, skin, dura, and other cryopreserved or lyophilized tissues usually do not require ABO typing and crossmatching because their immunogenic activity is very weak after preservation.

Immunologic Events After Transplantation

Transplantation tolerance is defined as immune unresponsiveness to graft alloantigens in the absence of ongoing therapy, but not to other (third-party) antigens. The functional characteristics of tolerance are lack of demonstrable immune reactivity to donor graft alloantigens, presence of immune reactivity to other alloantigens, and absence of generalized immunosuppression for graft maintenance. At this time, tolerance is not achieved by available immunosuppressive regimens.

Rejection is an immunologic attempt to destroy foreign tissue after transplantation. It is a complex and incompletely understood event. Four types of clinically identified rejection occur. The forms of allograft rejection are classified according to the time of occurrence and the immune mechanism involved (Table 20-4).

Hyperacute rejection occurs soon (minutes to hours) after graft implantation. The organ becomes flaccid, cyanotic, and, in the case of the kidney, anuric. Histologically, polymorphonuclear leukocytes are packed in the pericapillary area, and endothelial necrosis with vascular thrombosis occurs. Hyperacute rejection is associated with preformed antibodies in the recipient directed toward either the ABO blood group or

TABLE 20-4. Rejection: General Pathology

Rejection Type	Time	Pathology	Treatment
Hyperacute	Immediately to hours	Swollen, edematous organ Antibody-mediated vascular thrombosis and necrosis Polymorphonuclear infiltrates	Usually prevented by cross-matching and blood group matching
Accelerated	2-5 d	Swollen, edematous organ Arterial necrosis Lymphocyte infiltration	No effective treatment
Acute	7-10 d; may recur during subsequent years	Cellular: mononuclear cell infiltration into vascular and interstitial spaces Antibody-mediated: Cd4 deposition along vasculature	Increased immunosuppression or change to a different regimen Plasmapheresis, monoclonal antibodies
Chronic	Years	Obliterative vasculopathy Relentless deterioration Glomerular sclerosis, tubular atrophy, and interstitial fibrosis (kidney) Myocardial fibrosis and coronary obliteration (heart) Progressive bile duct loss (liver) Bronchiectasis, pleural thickening (lung)	No effective treatment

HLA antigens. It rarely occurs today because of the practice of crossmatching and blood group matching.

Accelerated acute rejection occurs during the first several days after transplantation. In the kidney, it is characterized by oliguria and may be accompanied by disseminated intravascular coagulation, thrombocytopenia, and hemolysis. The organ becomes swollen, tender, and congested. Histologically, extensive arteriolar necrosis and perivasculitis are present. Monocyte/macrophage infiltration of renal allografts has been shown to adversely affect graft survival. Intense CD4 deposition in the glomerular basement membrane and peritubular capillaries can be found by immunofluorescence staining. This type of rejection is believed to represent an immunologic memory response to prior sensitization.

Acute rejection can be T-cell mediated (acute cellular rejection or acute T-cell-mediated rejection) or mediated by antibodies (acute humoral rejection or acute antibody-mediated rejection). Biopsy is required when rejection is suspected based on worsening graft function. Findings of acute T-cell-mediated rejection include lymphocyte infiltration of the tubules of the kidney or portal triad of the liver. Antibody-mediated rejection is suggested by inflammation of the glomeruli of the kidney or peritubular capillaries. Special stains for C4d, a marker of complement deposition, also support a diagnosis of acute humoral rejection. Additionally, donor-specific antibodies in the recipient serum may be present. In the heart, the infiltrate is usually pericapillary and is associated with interstitial edema and myonecrosis. In the lung, perivascular and interstitial mononuclear cell infiltrates may be present. Rejection in the lung can lead to bronchiolitis obliterans.

Acute cellular rejection is treated with increased doses of immunosuppression. If it is reversed, the patient has an excellent chance of retaining the graft. In cases of antibody-mediated rejection, treatments are used to decrease the circulating antibodies (plasmapheresis) and eliminate memory B cells (often antibody therapies).

Chronic rejection is a slow, progressive process that occurs over a period of months to years. It is characterized by vascular intimal hyperplasia; lymphocytic infiltration; and atrophy and fibrosis of renal, cardiac, or hepatic tissue. Chronic rejection is mediated by both immune and nonimmune processes through poorly understood mechanisms. The healing process after repeated episodes of acute rejection, chronic graft injury by a delayed type of hypersensitivity response, chronic ischemia, antibody formation, calcineurin inhibitor toxicity, and enhanced transforming growth factor (TGF)-β production have been proposed as alternative stimuli for the development of chronic allograft dysfunction. In the kidney, this injury is now described as *interstitial fibrosis with tubular atrophy* (IFTA).

Immunosuppressive Drug Therapy

Currently, nearly all recipients of allografts require immunosuppressive therapy. The sole exception is a patient who receives a transplanted organ from an identical monozygotic twin (isograft). Establishment of tolerance to transplanted organs and tissues is a major focus of transplant and immunology research. Because of their lack of lymphatic drainage, the eyes are an immune-privileged site.

Thus, matching and systemic immunosuppression are rarely required for corneal transplants. However, when rejection occurs, topical steroids are used.

The role of immunosuppression is 3-fold: (1) to provide induction immunosuppression at the time of transplantation, (2) to provide maintenance suppression of the immune system to prevent rejection, and (3) to treat episodes of rejection if the recipient "breaks through" the maintenance program. Immunosuppressive agents are classified as biologic or pharmacologic (Table 20-5). Many medications used in immunosuppression for organ transplantation are not approved by the U.S. Food and Drug Administration (FDA) for these indications and represent "off-label use." Patients on long-term immunosuppression are at risk for skin cancers (both melanoma and nonmelanoma) and posttransplant lymphoproliferative disorder, a B-cell lymphoma commonly driven by EBV infection or reactivation.

Immunosuppressive agents are usually used in combination because no single agent or technique provides adequate therapy. For this reason, agents are often chosen to modulate the immune system at various times after transplantation and to complement each other by suppressing the immune system at different levels or by different mechanisms. Multimodal therapy reduces the toxicity and side effects of individual drugs by enabling lower doses of each while still maintaining an adequate level of immunosuppression (Table 20-6).

Pharmacologic Agents

Pharmacologic agents can be classified as corticosteroids, calcineurin inhibitors, inhibitors of nucleotide metabolism, inhibitors of the protein TOR (target of rapamycin), or lymphocyte-depleting agents or receptor blockers. The most commonly used immunosuppressive agents are corticosteroids (prednisone, methylprednisolone). These compounds are used to provide maintenance immunosuppression, and, in higher doses, to treat rejection. Glucocorticoids bind to a cytosolic receptor that translocates to the nucleus, where the complex binds to DNA regulatory sequences. Glucocorticoids decrease the transcription of key cytokines. Steroids are lympholytic—they kill T and B cells and inhibit the release of interleukin-1 (IL-1) from macrophages. Prednisone is the most common steroid

TABLE 20-5. Clinically Available Immunosuppressive Agents and Techniques in Organ Transplantation	
Pharmacologic	**Biologic**
Azathioprine	Polyclonal sera
Cyclosporine	Monoclonal sera (OKT3)
Tacrolimus	Daclizumab
Sirolimus	Basiliximab
Everolimus	Belatacept
Steroids	Alemtuzumab
Mycophenolic acid, mycophenolate mofetil	Rituximab

TABLE 20-6. Drugs Used for Immunosuppression

Name	Use	Mechanism of Action	Side Effects
Corticosteroids	Maintenance, rejection	Lympholysis, inhibition of IL-1 release	Cushing syndrome, dyspepsia, hypertension, osteonecrosis, posttransplant diabetes mellitus
Azathioprine	Maintenance	Inhibition of nucleic acid synthesis	Bone marrow depression, veno-occlusive hepatic disease, arthralgias, pancreatitis, red cell aplasia
Cyclosporine	Maintenance	Inhibition of secretion and formation of IL-2 (calcineurin inhibitor)	Nephrotoxicity, hypertension, hyperkalemia, hepatotoxicity, hirsutism, gingival hyperplasia, tremors
Tacrolimus	Maintenance, treatment of refractory rejection	Inhibition of production of IL-2 (calcineurin inhibitor)	Nephrotoxicity, glucose intolerance, neurotoxicity
Mycophenolic acid mycophenolate mofetil	Maintenance	Inhibition of inosine monophosphate dehydrogenase	Gastrointestinal intolerance, neutropenia
Sirolimus, everolimus	Maintenance	Inhibition of mTOR	Neutropenia, dyslipidemia, impaired wound healing; concern for hepatic artery thrombosis with sirolimus
OKT3 (monoclonal antibody, no longer available in the United States)	Treatment of rejection	Depletion of T cells Modulation of CD receptor from the surface of T cells	Fever, chills, pulmonary edema, lymphoproliferative disorder
Polyclonal antilymphocyte	Induction, treatment of rejection	Depletion of lymphocytes	Anaphylaxis, fever, leukopenia, thrombocytopenia, lymphoproliferative disorders, cytokine release syndrome
Daclizumab, basiliximab	Induction	Blockage of IL-2 receptor via CD25	Minimal
Belatacept	Induction, maintenance	Blockage of T-cell costimulation via CTLA-4	Minimal
Alemtuzumab	Induction	Depletion of lymphocytes via CD52	Hypotension, rigors, fever, shortness of breath
Rituximab	Treatment of rejection	Depletion of B cells via CD20	Cytokine release syndrome, hypotension, rigors, fevers

IL, interleukin; TOR, target of rapamycin.

preparation used in transplantation. Steroids are initially given at high doses intravenously during the transplant surgery and then tapered after transplantation. The complications of steroid use are variable and include dyspepsia, cataracts, osteonecrosis, Cushing syndrome, acne, capillary fragility, and glucose intolerance. Given the significant side effects of steroid therapy, there are many protocols that avoid steroids or withdraw them early in the posttransplant period.

Cyclosporine and tacrolimus are calcineurin inhibitors. They inhibit the expression of multiple genes involved in T-cell activation and proliferation, including IL-2 and other lymphokines. Cyclosporine binds to a cytoplasmic immunophilin called cyclophilin, thereby producing a complex that inhibits the calcium-sensitive phosphatase calcineurin.

It ultimately prevents the proliferation and maturation of cytotoxic T cells that cause graft rejection. Tacrolimus is a macrolide antibiotic. Its mechanism of action is similar to that of cyclosporine (inhibiting the production of IL-2 and other cytokines) except that it binds to the FK-binding protein. It is more potent than cyclosporine and is now the predominantly used calcineurin inhibitor in the United States. It is used for maintenance immunosuppression in combination with azathioprine or mycophenolate mofetil and sometimes steroids. Both agents cause dose-dependent nephrotoxicity, hypertension, tremors, and hyperkalemia. Cyclosporine may cause hyperlipidemia, hyperuricemia, hepatotoxicity, gingival hyperplasia, and hirsutism. Tacrolimus may cause glucose intolerance and alopecia. Trough levels of cyclosporine and tacrolimus are routinely monitored to ensure maximal therapeutic benefit and to minimize complications.

Since both calcineurin inhibitors are metabolized in the liver by the cytochrome P_{450} system, liver disease and drugs that interact with or are metabolized competitively by that system should be monitored closely for effects on drug levels and toxicity as well as for their own toxicities. Examples of such drugs are barbiturates, phenytoin, imidazole antifungals, macrolide antibiotics, and rifampin.

Azathioprine is an antimetabolite. It is metabolized to its active form, 6-mercaptopurine, by the liver. It acts principally to inhibit the synthesis of nucleic acid. Therefore, it is a relatively nonspecific agent, and it affects all replicating cells of the body. Its major side effect is bone marrow suppression manifested by leukopenia and thrombocytopenia. These effects are dose dependent. Other side effects include veno-occlusive hepatic disease, arthralgias, pancreatitis, and red cell aplasia. It is used for baseline immunosuppression but not to treat rejection directly. It is always used with other immunosuppressants. Recently, it has been largely replaced by mycophenolic acid or mycophenolate mofetil.

Mycophenolate mofetil and mycophenolic acid are noncompetitive, reversible inhibitors of inosine monophosphate dehydrogenase (the enzyme necessary to convert inosine monophosphate to guanosine monophosphate) and are specific T- and B-cell antimetabolites. Because only lymphocytes require the *de novo* synthesis of guanosine monophosphate, these agents profoundly inhibit T- and B-cell function. These drugs are used in combination with steroids and cyclosporine or tacrolimus for maintenance therapy. These compounds are particularly effective in transplant populations that are at high risk for rejection. Their major side effects are gastrointestinal intolerance and bone marrow suppression.

Sirolimus or rapamycin and everolimus are macrolide antifungals that interfere with the intracellular signaling pathways of the IL-2-dependent clonal expansion of activated T lymphocytes. Like the calcineurin inhibitors, they bind to a cytoplasm-binding protein (FKBP). The ligand engages a protein, mammalian target of rapamycin (mTOR), a key regulatory kinase, which, once inhibited, reduces cytokine-dependent cellular proliferation. Sirolimus is used as an adjunctive agent in combination with prednisone and calcineurin inhibitors. The major side effects seem to be impaired wound healing, myelosuppression, and hyperlipidemia. There is also evidence of pulmonary toxicity, proteinuria, and painful oral ulcers. Sirolimus has been associated with an increased risk of hepatic artery thrombosis and graft loss following liver transplantation. Everolimus does not have this association and may decrease the risk of HCC recurrence following liver transplantation for this indication.

Biologic Agents

Biologic agents are either polyclonal or monoclonal sera that are prepared by immunizing an animal (eg, horse, rabbit, mouse, and rat) with human lymphocytes or antibodies to specific cellular receptors. The polyclonal sera antithymocyte globulin and antilymphocyte globulin are beneficial when used as induction therapy during the first 1 or 2 weeks of therapy for solid organ transplant recipients or to treat acute cellular rejection. Induction agents are given in the early peritransplantation period to decrease the risk of acute rejection and possibly delayed graft

function. These agents are generally given to immunologically high-risk patients and those patients receiving early steroid withdrawal. These preparations are usually given intravenously and are never used for maintenance therapy. Monoclonal antibodies have been prepared against various cell surface receptors on the T cell and are directed against specific T-cell subsets, not against the entire T- or B-cell population. One of the earliest antibodies, OKT3, is directed against the CD3 receptor on the T cell and was used for prophylactic induction therapy as well as for the treatment of acute cellular rejection. It is no longer available in the United States. The humanized anti-TAC (anti-CD25) monoclonal antibody preparations, daclizumab and basiliximab, block the IL-2 receptor, thus preventing the upregulation of T cells. They are used in both induction and maintenance therapies. Alemtuzumab, a humanized anti-CD52 monoclonal antibody that depletes T and B lymphocytes, natural killer cells, and some monocytes and macrophages, has been used in renal transplantation, with good results. Belatacept is a fusion protein that blocks CD28-mediated costimulatory signals and is used in maintenance therapy. Rituximab causes lysis of B lymphocytes that express CD20. It is used to treat acute antibody-mediated rejection in combination with other medications and often with plasmapheresis. The success of a graft depends on the degree of genetic similarity between the donor and the recipient, on the ischemia-reperfusion injury induced by the cold storage, and on the effectiveness of the immunosuppressive means used to alter host response.

END-STAGE RENAL DISEASE AND KIDNEY TRANSPLANTATION

Dialysis

Treatment of end-stage renal failure often involves long-term hemodialysis or peritoneal dialysis to maintain life. Because of the availability of maintenance dialysis, kidney transplantation is usually a nonemergency procedure that allows preoperative preparation with tissue typing and matching, and survival after transplant rejection. The principle of dialysis is simple: on one side of the semipermeable membrane is the extracellular fluid of the patient and on the other side of the membrane is the material that is to be discarded. Products of normal metabolism that are not excreted by the failed kidney accumulate in the extracellular fluid, pass through the semipermeable membrane to the dialysate solution, and are discarded. Hemodialysis requires the connection of the patient's vascular space to a dialysis machine. In acute situations, large cannulae are inserted into the venous circulation through the femoral, jugular, or subclavian veins. For long-term hemodialysis, permanent access to the circulation is achieved by the creation of an autologous arteriovenous fistula, connecting an artery to a vein in an easily accessible and reusable area (eg, brachial artery and cephalic vein just above the anteromedial elbow joint). A conduit of an artificial graft may be placed in a subcutaneous tunnel, with one end sewn to an artery and the other to a vein to provide a large caliber shunt for hemodialysis. In peritoneal dialysis, access to the peritoneal membrane requires a transabdominal, indwelling catheter that is used for infusion and drainage of dialysate fluid using the peritoneum as the dialysis membrane.

In patients on dialysis who await a transplant for longer than 2 years, the risk of losing their new kidney is 3 times greater than those who wait less than 6 months. Patients on dialysis for a long time are often sicker at the time of the transplantation and thus may not do as well as those who are on dialysis for a short time. There is 22% mortality in the first year of dialysis and 60% mortality in 5 years. For patients on dialysis, the longer the wait is, the more complications they are likely to develop. For most patients, the only mechanism for a preemptive transplant (a transplant prior to starting dialysis) is to identify a living donor who is willing and able to donate a kidney. There are more than 100,000 people waiting for renal transplants. In 2022, there were 19,636 deceased donor renal transplants and 5,864 living donor renal transplants. Most patients who undergo deceased donor kidney transplantation wait 3 to 7 years for a transplant, depending on their location.

Renal transplantation is associated with significantly improved survival compared with hemodialysis in patients with end-stage renal disease. Although a significant selection bias exists, this improved survival is likely a result of a reduced incidence of cardiovascular complications after renal transplantation compared to those remaining on dialysis.

Indications for Transplant

Renal transplantation is regarded by most physicians as the preferred treatment for chronic renal failure. Transplantation is lifesaving and more cost-effective than other modalities of renal replacement therapy. According to the UNOS, the 1-year graft survival rate for a living donor renal transplant is 97.5% and for a deceased donor transplant is 93.2%. The recipient mortality in the first year is less than 5%. The donor shortage is the major obstacle to the routine application of renal transplantation. A patient who has end-stage renal failure from any cause may be a candidate for transplant, regardless of the type or duration of dialysis support required. The acceptable age range for kidney recipients is 1 to 70 years, although infants and patients who are older than 70 years of age can be successfully transplanted. The patient should be currently free of infections and free of cancer for 2 to 5 years, depending on the type, location, and stage of the tumor. Patients with localized or early-stage cancers may undergo transplantation after successful excision of the lesion or after a 2-year wait. Other chronic disease processes should be minor, self-limited, or under control (eg, a patient with known coronary artery disease should be optimally treated and show cardiovascular stability before undergoing renal transplantation).

Operative Considerations

The renal graft is usually transplanted heterotopically in the extraperitoneal iliac fossa of the pelvis (Figure 20-2). In most cases, the native kidneys are left intact. The right side is generally preferred as the external iliac vessels are more superficial on this side. In theory, the renal graft can be transplanted in any location that has a suitable recipient artery, vein, and urine conduit or reservoir. The renal artery and renal vein are anastomosed to the common or

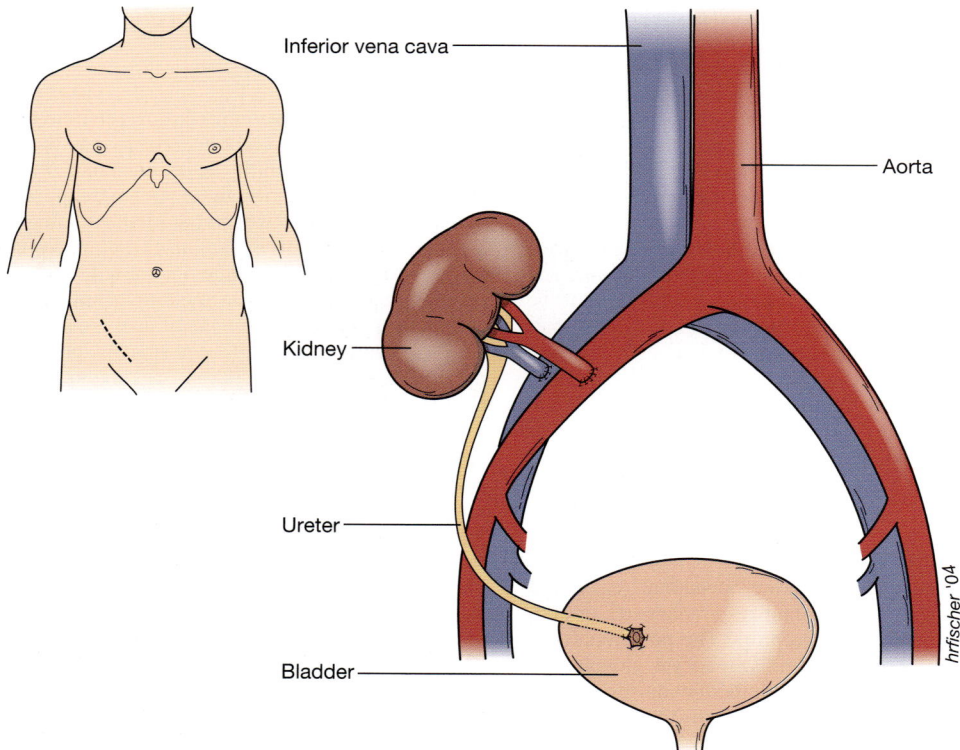

Figure 20-2. A heterotopic human renal allograft in the right extraperitoneal iliac fossa. The renal artery and vein anastomoses are end to side, respectively, to the common iliac artery and vein. A tunneled ureteroneocystostomy allows normal micturition.

external iliac artery and vein, respectively. The ureter is attached to the bladder or urinary conduit. Many surgeons use a temporary internal stent across the ureteroneocystostomy to decrease the risk of leak or obstruction of the ureter caused by edema. The bladder is decompressed with a urinary catheter to prevent excess tension on the ureteroneocystostomy and to allow accurate assessment of urine production. When recovering a kidney from a living donor, the left kidney is preferred because of the longer length of the renal vein as compared to the right kidney. In the case of an abnormality of the left kidney (ie, multiple arteries or veins), the right kidney of a living donor can be used, albeit with slightly more difficulty than a left kidney.

Complications

Wound infection is the most common complication after renal transplantation (Table 20-7). Contributory factors include obesity, diabetes, uremia with protein malnutrition, and immunosuppression. Typically, the characteristic findings of fever, local erythema, swelling, and drainage present 4 to 7 days after surgery. The prevalence of thrombosis of the transplant artery or vein is 1%. Clinically, acute anuria raises the concern for the presence of graft thrombosis. Doppler ultrasonography or radionuclide scanning shows greatly decreased or no flow to the graft. If the index of suspicion for thrombosis is high—for example, an uneventful live donor graft that does not diurese postoperatively—the patient should be taken back to the operating room for immediate exploration. Characteristically, significant bleeding requiring a return to the operating room presents in the early postoperative period with tachycardia, hypotension, and a falling hematocrit after volume resuscitation. Bleeding is more likely in renal transplant recipients than in normal patients because of decreased platelet adhesiveness secondary to uremia. The prevalence of urine leak is approximately 2%. A large urine leak at the ureter-to-bladder anastomosis caused by a technical flaw results in a rapid fall-off in urine output in the early postoperative period. Ureteral necrosis and leak may be due to procurement errors (eg, degloving) or ischemia from rejection-induced vasculitis and thrombosis

of periureteral blood supply. Obstruction occurs in about 2% of renal transplants. Decompression can be accomplished by percutaneous, endourologic, open operative approaches, or a combination of modalities. Delayed graft function, commonly defined as the need for dialysis in the first week following transplant, occurs in up to 30% of deceased donor renal transplants. Risk factors for delayed graft function include advanced donor age, donor acute kidney injury, prolonged cold storage time, and previous transplant in the recipient.

Nonrenal early complications include infections and cardiovascular events (eg, postoperative myocardial infarction, cerebrovascular accident, deep vein thrombosis). Kidney transplant recipients are usually treated prophylactically for ulcer disease with an H_2-receptor blocker. Infections are the most common complications (see Figure 20-3 for timing of infections in relation to transplantation). They may be common (eg, pneumococcal pneumonia) or unusual (eg, necrotizing fasciitis from a rare fungus). Organisms that cause clinical infection in the immunosuppressed host include CMV, common bacteria, fungi, and protozoa such as *Pneumocystis (carinii) jiroveci*. For this reason, all patients receive antifungals and prophylaxis for *Pneumocystis*, commonly with trimethoprim-sulfamethoxazole. CMV infection is one of the most common infections posttransplant. It is manifested by fever, malaise, weakness, gastrointestinal bleeding, and esophagitis. The disease results from the infection of a seronegative recipient by a positive donor or from the reactivation of the recipient's endogenous viral load by excessive immunosuppression, especially in the context of biologic agents. Prophylactic therapy with valganciclovir is commonly used.

Prognosis

The results of kidney transplantation have improved since 1975. Graft and patient survival are expected to exceed 90% at one year (Table 20-8). Rates of infection-related deaths have fallen drastically. These improvements are the result of a better selection of patients with end-stage renal failure and recognition of the limits of antirejection therapy. Overuse of immunosuppressive therapy does not result in better graft survival and is detrimental to patient survival. The loss of a renal allograft requires a return to dialysis, but second and subsequent renal allografts are often performed successfully.

PANCREAS AND ISLET CELL TRANSPLANTATION

Indications

Pancreatic transplantation is the only form of treatment for type 1 diabetes mellitus that establishes a long-term, insulin-independent, normoglycemic state. To achieve this end, whole-organ or, to a lesser extent, islet cell transplantation is offered to patients who have this disease. Increasingly, simultaneous kidney-pancreas transplantation is being offered to selected patients with type 2 diabetes already requiring kidney transplantation. Patients with renal failure may receive a simultaneous kidney-pancreas transplant (SPK) from a deceased donor. Patients with a living donor for a kidney transplant may receive a pancreas after kidney (PAK). Patients with preserved renal function who

TABLE 20-7. Complications of Renal Transplantation		
Type	**Early**	**Late**
Renal	Massive diuresis	Ureteric stenosis
	Delayed graft function	Vascular anastomotic stenosis
	Ureter anastomotic leak	Recurrent primary renal disease
	Hemorrhage	Rejection
	Lymphocele	Neoplasia
	Rupture	
	Thrombosis	
Nonrenal	Infection	Infection
	Cardiovascular event (MI, CVA)	Progressive atherosclerotic vascular disorders, hypertension
	Diabetes mellitus	
	Steroid-induced acne	Posttransplant lymphoproliferative disorder
	Peptic ulcer disease	

CVA, cerebrovascular accident; MI, myocardial infarction.

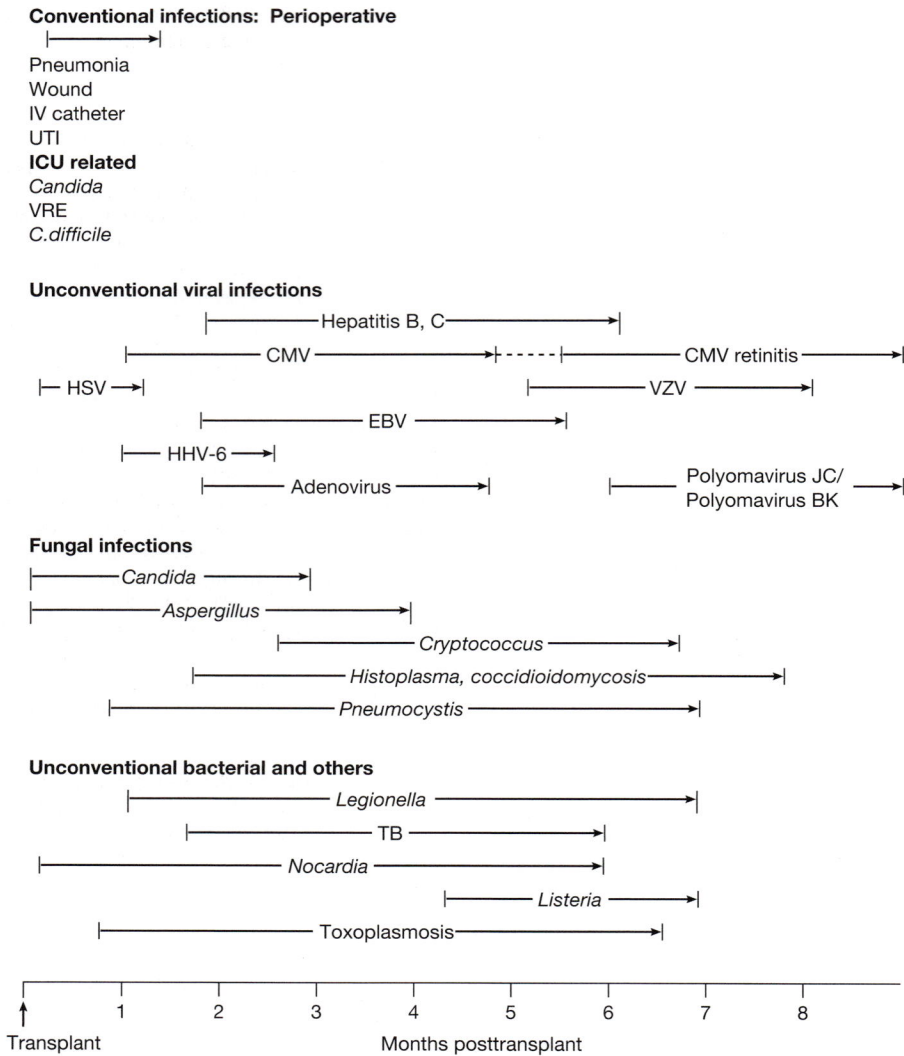

Figure 20-3. Timing of infections in relation to transplantation. CMV, cytomegalovirus; EBV, Epstein-Barr virus; HHV, human herpesvirus; HSV, herpes simplex viruses; ICU, intensive care unit; IV, intravenous; TB, tuberculosis; UTI, urinary tract infection; VRE, vancomycin-resistant enterococci; VZV, varicella zoster virus.

suffer complications of diabetes may receive a pancreas transplant alone (PTA). In 2022, there were 108 isolated pancreas transplants and 810 simultaneous kidney-pancreas transplants. Although successful whole-organ or islet cell–only transplantation affords the patient normoglycemia, the effect of pancreatic transplantation on the chronic complications of diabetes mellitus is less clear. However, peripheral neuropathy may improve, and diabetic retinopathy may stabilize. In patients who undergo simultaneous kidney-pancreas transplants, the kidney may be protected because glomerular and mesangial changes (signs of early diabetic damage) are absent from the kidney after simultaneous kidney-pancreas transplantation. Unfortunately, pancreatic transplantation does not seem to mitigate the main causes of morbidity and mortality in patients with diabetes (eg, vascular disease, infection). The last two decades of work in this field have shown that patients who have diabetes and functioning pancreatic grafts could enjoy perfect metabolic control and freedom from dietary restrictions.

Operative Considerations: Whole-Organ Pancreas Transplantation

Procedure

The donor pancreas and duodenal C-loop are transplanted together into the recipient (Figure 20-4). The operation is usually performed in an intraperitoneal location although a retroperitoneal approach in the pelvis may also be used. The arterial supply of the pancreas, including the splenic and superior mesenteric arteries, is reconstructed using a donor iliac artery Y-graft, which is anastomosed to the recipient iliac artery. The pancreatic venous drainage (donor portal vein) may be attached to the recipient's iliac vein (systemic drainage) or the recipient's superior mesenteric vein (portal drainage). The donor duodenal C-loop is used to drain the donor's pancreatic exocrine secretions. The donor duodenum may be drained to the recipient's jejunum (enteric drainage) or the recipient's bladder (bladder drainage). Enteric drainage is the more common practice despite the increased morbidity of a leak at this anastomosis. Although controversy exists

TABLE 20-8. 1- and 5-Year Graft and Patient Survival by Organ		
	Graft (%)	**Patient (%)**
Kidney: deceased donor, 1 y	93.2	96.3
5 y	74.4	83.6
Kidney: living donor, 1 y	97.5	98.8
5 y	85.6	92.2
Liver: deceased donor, 1 y	89.1	91.2
5 y	71.9	75.1
Liver: living donor, 1 y	88.0	92.3
5 y	77.3	83.9
Pancreas, 1 y	81.0	92.0
5 y	58.2	80.7
Intestine, 1 y	76.0	81.1
5 y	49.5	58.1
Heart, 1 y	90.5	90.8
5 y	76.8	78.0
Lung, 1 y	87.0	87.7
5 y	52.9	55.5

Data from https://optn.transplant.hrsa.gov/data/view-data-reports/national-data/, Accessed September 2, 2023.

regarding the optimal surgical technique, excellent survival rates and similar rates of complications are achieved with all techniques. There may be a physiologic advantage to portal drainage of the pancreas allograft, which replicates normal physiology and allows first-pass metabolism of insulin via the liver. Pancreas graft function and readmissions are similar, regardless of surgical technique.

Complications

The postoperative course of combined whole-organ pancreas or pancreas-kidney transplantation is more complicated than that of kidney transplantation alone. More episodes of rejection occur, and patients typically require more immunosuppression. Subsequently, the patients have more infectious complications and longer hospital stays. The frequency of early graft loss caused by thrombosis is reported as 5% to 10%. Urinary complications (eg, infection, leakage, minor bleeding) are greater in pancreas transplant patients if the anastomosis is performed to the bladder. In the long term, patients with bladder-drained pancreas grafts may suffer local complications from irritation of the bladder and perineum by pancreatic enzymes as well as large bicarbonate losses. Compared to SPK, pancreas-alone transplants have similar complications, including anastomotic leak, vascular thrombosis, and urinary complications, but rejection episodes are more difficult to monitor. Elevation of serum amylase or lipase should prompt investigation for local complications, pancreatitis, or rejection; hyperglycemia occurs only after a large proportion of islet cell mass has been lost and is a very late sign of rejection. When transplanted with a kidney, pancreas rejection may be suspected on the basis of concurrent kidney rejection and elevated serum creatinine. Discordant rejection (rejection of one organ but not the other) is possible but uncommon.

Prognosis

The success rates for whole-organ pancreas transplantation approach those for other solid organ transplantations. National data demonstrate patient survival rates of over 90%. Graft loss is more common than for kidney transplant with

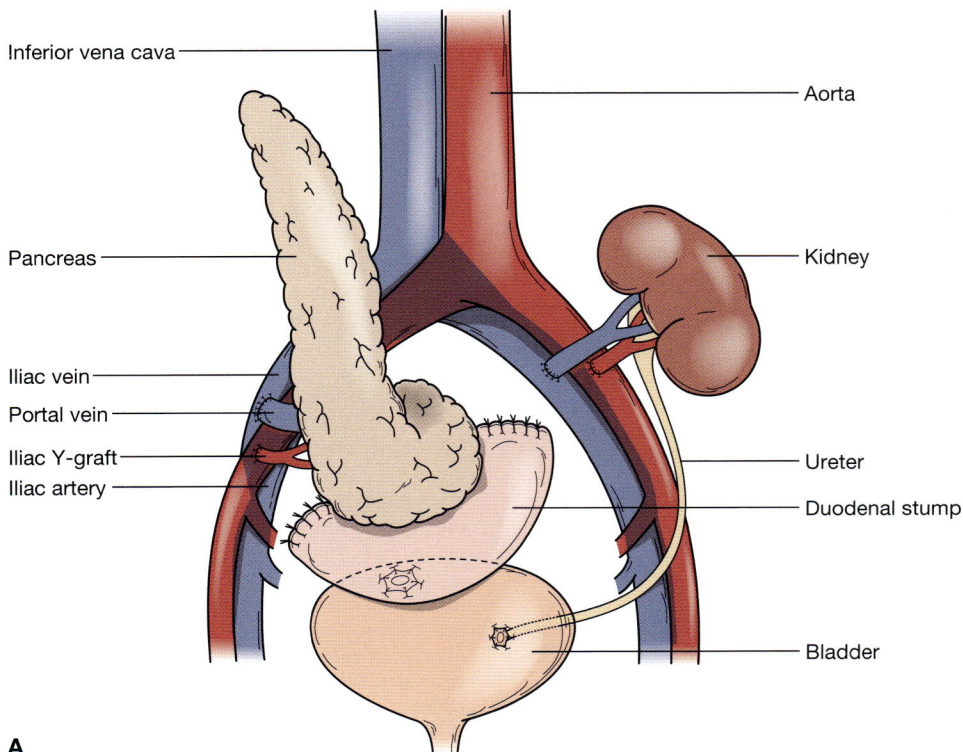

A

Figure 20-4. Pancreatic transplants using bladder (A) or enteric (B) drainage.

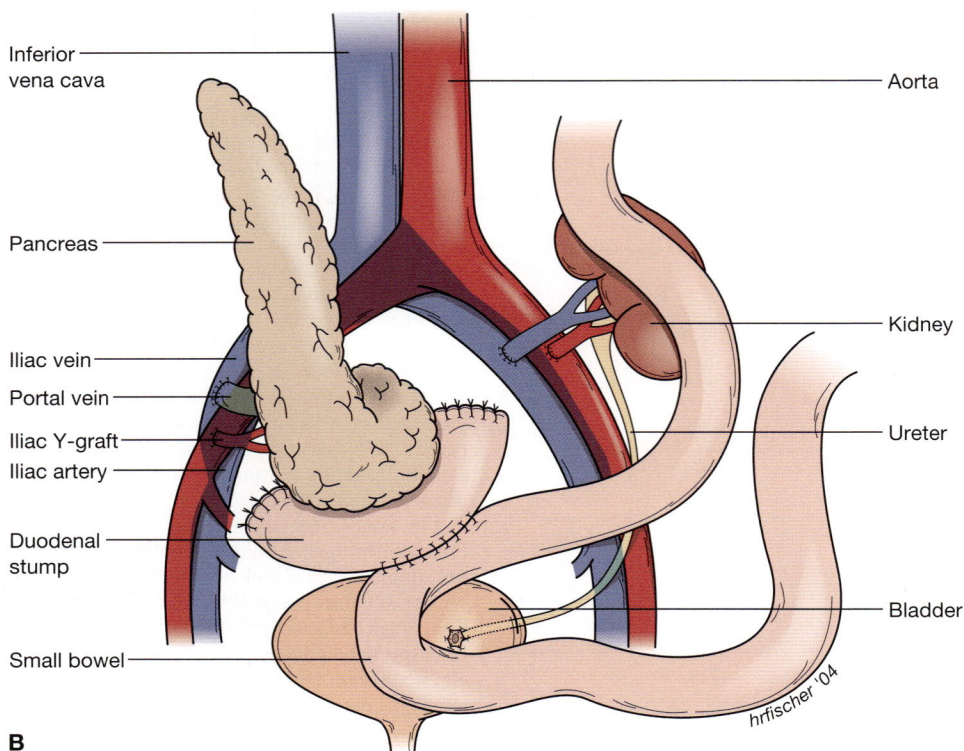

Inferior vena cava

Pancreas

Iliac vein

Portal vein

Iliac Y-graft

Iliac artery

Duodenal stump

Small bowel

Aorta

Kidney

Ureter

Bladder

hrfischer '04

B

Figure 20-4. (*continued*)

1-year graft survival around 80%. At 5 years, nearly 60% of pancreas allografts are still functioning.

Islet Cell Transplantation

Islet cell transplantation offers the potential for long-lasting strict glucose control. Recent strides have been made by increasing the number of viable islets from a donor pancreas with the use of new, gentler digesting agents. Techniques to culture or freeze the islets may eventually provide an islet banking and distribution system for elective transplantation. The proper delivery system for islets is still under investigation. Current options include injection into the portal vein, placement under the renal capsule, and encapsulation into immunoisolated chambers. The increased rejection rate, the need for large numbers of islets, and the small number of donors relative to the large potential recipient pool have held back the widespread implementation of islet cell transplantation. Initial trials have not resulted in complete or uniform insulin independence in recipients but work to optimize the processes continues.

LIVER TRANSPLANTATION

Indications

Liver transplantation is indicated in patients with acute or chronic liver failure. The most common indication for liver transplantation is for patients with decompensated liver disease who have failed medical therapy. Clinical signs of decompensated liver failure include ascites or spontaneous

bacterial peritonitis, hepatic encephalopathy, jaundice, coagulopathy, esophageal or gastric varices or bleeding, and peripheral edema. Early-stage HCC is another major indication for liver transplantation. Currently, liver transplantation for HCC is typically reserved for patients with early-stage HCC and a limited tumor burden, most commonly assessed by the Milan criteria (one tumor ≤ 5 cm, or up to three tumors with no tumor > 3 cm), and no evidence of radiographic large vessel invasion or extrahepatic disease. The prognostic value of high α-fetoprotein (AFP) levels is established, and current UNOS policy does not allow for MELD exception points to be granted to recipients with an AFP greater than 1,000, unless the use of locoregional therapy demonstrates a reduction of the AFP to less than 500. The best results are obtained if transplantation is carried out before the onset of terminal events associated with end-stage liver failure.

Acute liver failure may also be treated with urgent liver transplantation in selected cases. Acute liver failure is defined as the onset of encephalopathy within 8 weeks of the liver injury or inciting event. Patients with acute liver failure are at risk for cerebral edema and may require invasive intracranial pressure monitoring for treatment while awaiting urgent transplantation. Table 20-9 lists diseases that are treated by liver transplantation.

The most common indications for liver transplantation include alcoholic liver disease and acute alcoholic hepatitis, metabolic dysfunction–associated steatotic liver disease (MASLD), and metabolic dysfunction–associated steatohepatitis (MASH) (previously known as nonalcoholic steatohepatitis [NASH]), and chronic hepatitis C infection. Waiting times before transplantation may be

TABLE 20-9. Diseases Treated With Liver Transplantation

Chronic Liver Disease	Acute Liver Failure
Hepatitis C, hepatitis B	Toxic ingestion (acetaminophen, many others)
Alcoholic liver disease	Mushroom ingestion (*Amanita*, others)
Metabolic dysfunction–associated steatotic liver disease (MASLD) and metabolic dysfunction–associated steatohepatitis (MASH)	Acute Wilson disease
Cholestatic liver disease (primary biliary cirrhosis, primary sclerosing cholangitis)	Acute hepatitis B infection, other viral infections
Metabolic liver disease (Wilson disease, α1-antitrypsin disease, hemochromatosis)	
Vascular disease (Budd-Chiari syndrome)	
Hepatocellular carcinoma	
Autoimmune hepatitis	

1 year or longer, depending on the availability of organs and the condition of the recipient. Patients with cirrhosis are prioritized on the waiting list according to their MELD 3.0 score. The MELD 3.0 score is a numerical scale ranging from 6 to 40 (the higher the value, the more severely ill the patient) calculated using the patient's sex, bilirubin, international normalized ratio (INR), creatinine, sodium, and albumin.

Patients with acute liver failure receive priority on the liver waiting list (status 1). Status 1 patients have acute (sudden and severe onset) liver failure and a life expectancy of hours to a few days without a transplant. Less than 1% of liver transplant candidates fall into this category. All other liver transplant candidates aged 14 and older are prioritized by the MELD 3.0 system. Extra MELD 3.0 points are given to patients with conditions that increase their mortality but are not reflected in the laboratory-based score. Examples of MELD exception categories include patients with small HCCs, hepatopulmonary syndrome,

primary oxaluria, and portopulmonary hypertension. A patient's score may go up or down over time depending on the status of their liver disease. Candidates will have their MELD 3.0 score reassessed at set intervals while they are on the waiting list. This will help ensure that donated livers go to the patients in greatest need at that moment.

Operative Considerations

Liver transplantation is always performed in an orthotopic manner, with the removal of the native diseased liver and implantation of the liver allograft in the native position. Technical variations involve either removal of the recipient's entire retrohepatic inferior vena cava (IVC), necessitating a "bi-caval" anastomosis of the suprahepatic and infrahepatic IVC (Figure 20-5), or a "piggyback" technique, where there is retention of the recipient's retrohepatic IVC and the donor suprahepatic IVC is anastomosed to the native hepatic vein stumps. The donor portal vein

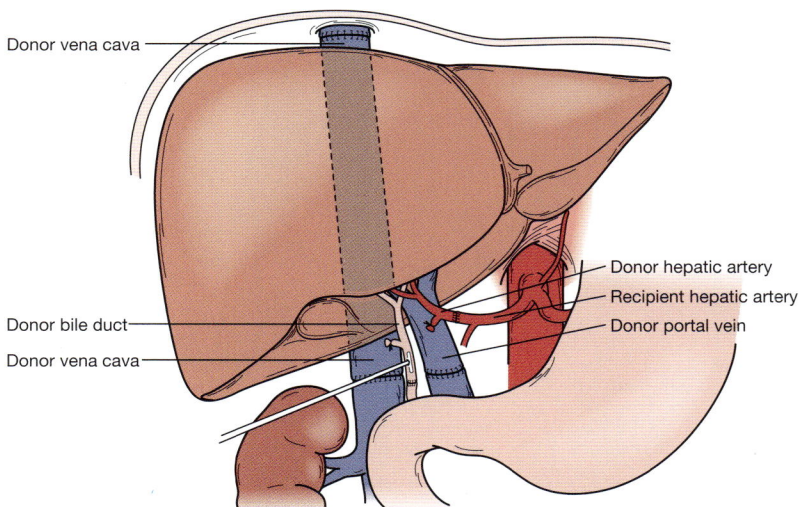

Figure 20-5. An orthotopic human hepatic allograft. End-to-end vascular anastomoses connect the donor and recipient hepatic artery, portal vein, and vena cava both suprahepatically and infrahepatically. The most commonly used common bile duct-to-duct anastomosis is shown.

is sewn to the recipient portal vein, and the donor hepatic artery is sewn to the recipient artery. Biliary drainage is commonly achieved either by duct-to-duct anastomosis or by Roux-en-Y choledochojejunostomy.

One requirement for hepatic transplantation is a size match between the donor and recipient livers. This match is particularly difficult to obtain in a timely manner in small children. This problem has led to the introduction of reduced-size livers, usually the left lobe or lateral segment. The resulting segment of the liver, its blood supply, and the bile duct are implanted into the recipient. The success rate with this procedure is equivalent to that of whole liver grafts, and it is even used for adult recipients. In fact, split livers are used to provide transplants to two recipients from a single deceased donor. In recent years, the demand for liver transplantation has exceeded the supply of cadaveric organs, leading to the introduction of living donor liver transplantation in adults as well as children. In adults, the right or left lobe of the liver is removed from a living donor and transplanted into the recipient (Figure 20-6). In children, the smaller left lobe or left lateral section is usually removed from the donor.

Complications

Complications of liver transplantation may be categorized as immunologic, technical, infectious, drug related, systemic, or related to poor graft function (Table 20-10). Acute rejection may occur, but it is usually less common than that seen in kidney transplantation. Chronic rejection may be an indication for retransplantation. Primary nonfunction is a condition in which the transplanted liver fails to function and is an indication for emergency retransplantation. Various degrees of graft dysfunction may occur and may usually be managed supportively. Untreated hepatic artery thrombosis occurring in the first week of transplantation is a devastating complication and is also an indication for urgent retransplantation. Unlike the native liver, the transplanted liver is almost totally dependent on blood supply from the hepatic artery in order to maintain the integrity of the biliary tree. Hepatic artery ischemia may therefore lead to biliary strictures. Cardiac, respiratory, and renal complications may occur after any major surgery, and liver transplantation is no exception. Late complications of liver transplantation include recurrent disease, chronic rejection, and toxicity from immunosuppressive drug therapy.

Prognosis

Patient and graft survival rates in liver transplantation approach 90% at 1 year and 70% to 85% at 5 years.

HEART AND HEART-LUNG TRANSPLANTATION

Heart Transplantation

Indications

The indication for heart transplantation is end-stage cardiac disease not amenable to other medical or surgical therapy (Table 20-11).

Age is not an absolute contraindication, although many centers are increasingly selective with candidates over 70 years of age. Oxygen consumption at maximal exercise, a peak $\dot{V}o_2$ of less than 12 to 14 mL/kg/min, has been used as an objective criterion for candidacy for transplantation. The patient must be free of infection and neoplasm and have full potential for rehabilitation. Specific indications for heart transplantation include idiopathic cardiomyopathy, viral cardiomyopathy, ischemic cardiac disease, postpartum

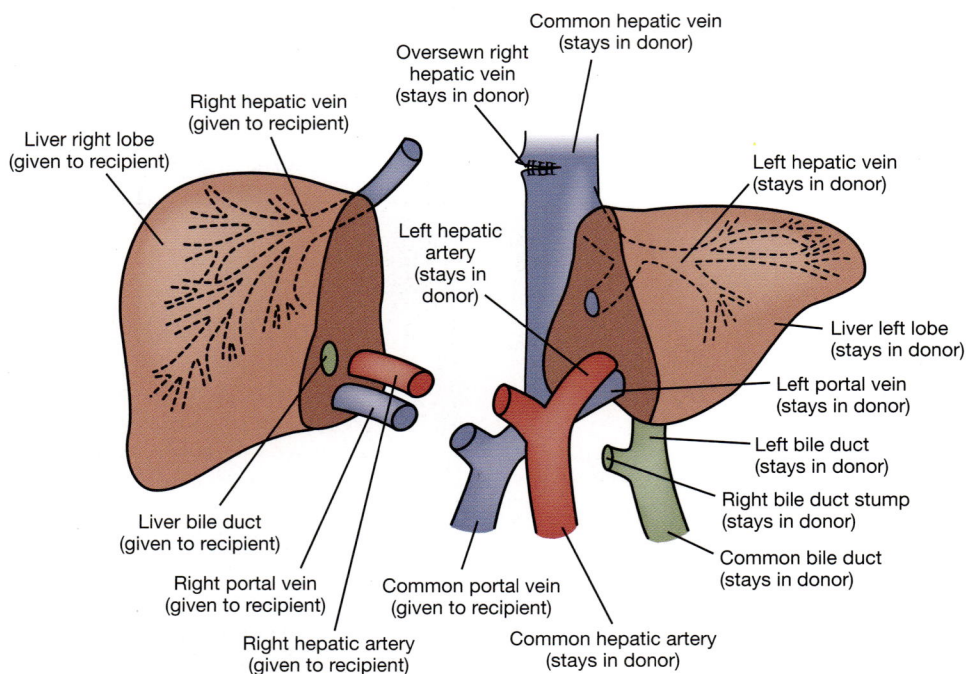

Figure 20-6. Living donor right hepatectomy. The right hepatic duct, hepatic artery, and right portal vein are divided after the division of the liver.

TABLE 20-10. Postoperative Complications of Liver Transplantation

	Complications
Immunologic	Acute rejection Chronic rejection
Technical	Bleeding Hepatic artery stenosis or thrombosis Portal vein stenosis or thrombosis Biliary leak or stricture
Graft function	Primary nonfunction Slow graft function or graft dysfunction
Infection	Bacterial Fungal Viral
Systemic	Cardiac event (ischemia, congestive heart failure) Respiratory failure Renal failure
Drug related	Nephrotoxicity Hypertension
Recurrent disease	HBV, HCV, autoimmune, PSC, PBC, alcohol

HBV, hepatitis B virus; HCV, hepatitis C virus; PBC, primary biliary cholangitis; PSC, primary sclerosing cholangitis.

cardiomyopathy, terminal cardiac valvular disease, and hypertensive cardiomyopathy. Many patients are maintained on ventricular assist devices as a bridge to transplantation. Severe pulmonary hypertension with a fixed pulmonary vascular resistance of greater than 3 Wood units at rest with optimal medical management is a contraindication to heart transplantation alone, and heart-lung transplantation should be considered. Cardiac transplantation is most often performed in adults because many congenital cardiac defects can be corrected surgically. However, neonatal and pediatric cardiac transplantation is also performed successfully.

Operative Considerations
The ideal cardiac preservation time is under 6 hours. Thus, donor and recipient surgeries are highly coordinated.

TABLE 20-11. Indications for Cardiac Transplantation

Adult
Cardiac ischemia/cardiac fatigue
Nonischemic cardiomyopathy
Valvular heart disease
Congenital heart disease (adult)
Pediatric
Cardiomyopathy
Congenital heart disease

Since the number of donors is far exceeded by the number of potential recipients, and cold time is an important consideration, hearts are distributed through the UNOS computer system to the sickest patients. These patients, who usually require mechanical or medical support in the ICU, are in a hospital that is close enough to the donor hospital to enable implantation within the prescribed cold ischemia limits.

The usual cardiac transplant is a size-matched, ABO-matched orthotopic allograft. The recipient's heart is removed, and the donor's heart is sewn into place by attaching the left and right atria of the donor's heart to the left and right atria of the recipient. The pulmonary artery and aortic anastomoses are completed (Figure 20-7). The heart is resuscitated and allowed to take over the support of the recipient. Heterotopic grafts (transplanted heart placed alongside the native heart) are rarely used.

Complications
The complications of cardiac transplantation are largely infection and rejection, with ensuing progressive cardiac failure. Early postoperative problems, in addition to infection, include respiratory, renal, and cerebrovascular complications. Late problems are limited to chronic allograft rejection and the long-term effects of immunosuppressive therapy, including calcineurin inhibitor–induced nephropathy. Accelerated coronary artery disease occurs in some patients and may be related to chronic rejection. Retransplantation and percutaneous transluminal angioplasty are performed for this problem. The most common cancers associated with cardiac transplants are skin cancers, posttransplant lymphoproliferative disorder, and lung cancer.

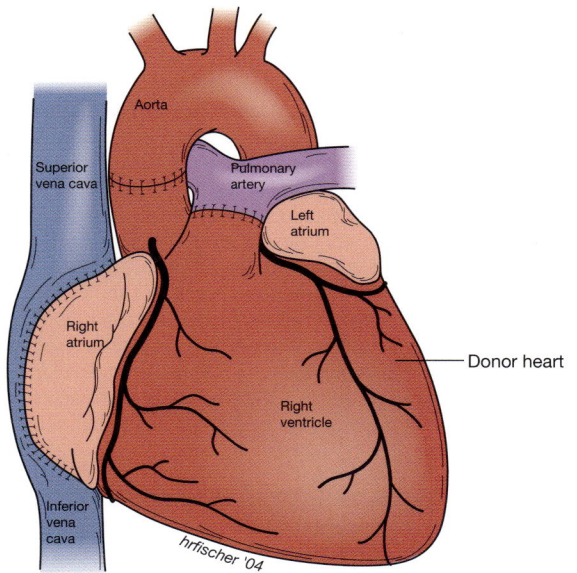

Figure 20-7. An orthotopic human cardiac allograft. The left and right atria of the graft are sutured to the most posterior atrial walls, which remain intact in the recipient. End-to-end anastomoses of the pulmonary artery and aorta are completed before the transplanted heart is resuscitated and cardiopulmonary bypass support is terminated.

Prognosis

Newer immunosuppressive agents and the serial use of endomyocardial biopsy to diagnose rejection have improved the outcome of cardiac transplantation. The current 1-year graft and patient survival rate is 90% or higher, and the 5-year rate is 70% to 80%. In the first year, mortality associated with cardiac transplants is often caused by graft failure, non-CMV infection, and multiorgan failure. Beyond 5 years, cardiac allograft vasculopathy, cancer, and non-CMV infection account for the majority of deaths.

Heart-Lung Transplantation

Heart-lung transplantation is performed when severe pulmonary hypertension accompanies cardiac disease. It is also performed for congenital heart diseases such as Eisenmenger syndrome. It may sometimes be used in a "domino procedure," where a donor's heart and lung are given to one recipient with cystic fibrosis, and the normal heart is given to someone else who requires a heart transplant. In addition to the complications of cardiac transplantation, complications of heart-lung transplantation include restrictive fibrosis of the lung. Acute and chronic rejection of the lung may be manifested by bronchiolitis. The 1-year survival rate for heart-lung transplant recipients is 80%.

LUNG TRANSPLANTATION

Indications

Single-lung and sequential double-lung transplantations are performed for patients with α_1-antitrypsin deficiency, interstitial pulmonary fibrosis, primary pulmonary hypertension, cystic fibrosis, and chronic obstructive pulmonary disease (Table 20-12). Single- or double-lung transplantation can provide total pulmonary function to patients with end-stage pulmonary disease without suppuration and concomitant cardiac failure.

A forced expiratory volume (FEV_1) of less than 25%, partial pressure of carbon dioxide ($Paco_2$) of greater than 55 torr, or an elevated pulmonary artery pressure in the presence of deteriorating clinical function are good indicators of the need for pulmonary transplantation. Severe coronary artery disease and lung cancer are contraindications to lung transplantation. Recipients must be free of infection and are usually younger than 65 years of age. The donor and the recipient must be of equivalent height and weight. Living donor lobar donation is possible, especially if the recipient is a child. Since the number of recipients is greater than the number of lungs available, a reasonably equitable system called the Lung Allocation Score (LAS) has been developed for potential recipients over 12 years. It takes into account patient disease, extent of diseased lung, functional status, and comorbidities to try to find a balance between urgency of need and likelihood of a favorable outcome.

Complications

Rejection is the most common complication. It is diagnosed by the appearance of infiltrates on chest x-ray and is confirmed with transbronchial or transthoracic needle biopsy and bronchioalveolar lavage, slowing infiltrating, mononuclear cells, endotheliitis, or alveolar necrosis. Breakdown of the bronchial anastomosis is a dreaded complication that occurs in 5% of transplants. For this reason, to enhance healing, the dose of steroids is kept as low as possible. The use of calcineurin inhibitors has enabled lower steroid use. In lung transplantation, acute and chronic rejection of the lung may be manifested by bronchiolitis. Obliterative bronchiolitis is the primary manifestation of chronic rejection and is the greatest cause of long-term mortality. It is diagnosed by biopsy. Early mortality is associated with unsuspected donor lung injury and reperfusion injury. Pulmonary infection with bacteria, fungi, or CMV is common in the postoperative period. Bronchioalveolar lavage is useful to direct antibiotic therapy.

Operative Considerations

The surgery is performed through a posterolateral thoracotomy for single-lung transplants and through a transverse thoracotomy for double-lung transplants. The donor pulmonary veins are sewn to a left atrial recipient cuff after the sleeve bronchial anastomosis is performed. Finally, the pulmonary arteries are anastomosed. Care must be taken to avoid fluid overload to minimize lung edema in the postoperative period.

Prognosis

Patient survival rates for lung transplantation are 87% at 1 year and 55% at 5 years. Bilateral lung transplant patients have better survival than single-lung recipients. Double-lung transplantation is preferred in situations where there has been chronic lung infection in cystic fibrosis or bronchiectasis. In single-lung transplantation, the residual infection may be transferred from the native to the transplanted lung. Also, in extensive emphysema where there is the possibility of air trapping in the native lung and mediastinal shift compressing the transplanted lung, a double-lung transplant is recommended.

INTESTINAL TRANSPLANTATION

Bowel transplantation was first attempted in humans during the 1960s. At that time, patients were dying of starvation after having a large portion of their bowel removed because of disease or trauma. Parenteral (intravenous) feeding was not yet available, and surgeons hoped that the transplanted bowel would function normally. These first intestinal transplant patients died, however, from technical complications, rejection, or infection. Successful intestinal transplants were not performed until the mid-1980s. Intestinal transplantation is often performed in centers with extensive experience managing intestinal failure and short-gut syndrome. Intestinal rehabilitation may include strategies to optimize nutritional support and offer other surgical interventions, including bowel lengthening and tapering procedures such as the serial transverse enteroplasty procedure (STEP). For patients who require transplantation, many patients have been able to stop total parenteral nutrition (TPN), resume a normal diet, and enjoy a healthy lifestyle after intestinal transplantation.

TABLE 20-12. Indications for Lung Transplantation
Chronic obstructive pulmonary disease
Pulmonary fibrosis
Cystic fibrosis
α_1-antitrypsin deficiency
Pulmonary artery hypertension

Indications

Short-gut syndrome, the primary indication for small intestinal transplantation, has an incidence of two to three per 1 million population. The syndrome is the result of many intestinal disorders, including intestinal strangulation or infarction from midgut volvulus, obstruction, or internal hernias; trauma; and vascular accidents of the mesenteric vessels. Other associated diseases include Crohn disease, low-grade tumors, and necrotizing enterocolitis. Candidates for transplantation must be dependent on parenteral nutrition. Some transplant centers perform multiorgan transplantation, including liver, pancreas, and small bowel, after upper abdominal exenteration.

The contraindications of intestinal transplantation are essentially the same as those in other types of transplants and include significant coexistent medical conditions that have no potential for improvement following transplantation and active uncontrolled infection or malignancy that is not eliminated by the transplant process.

The number of intestinal transplants performed peaked in the early 2000s at nearly 200 per year. Still, major issues remain, such as the extremely high mortality in patients on the waiting list and the organ shortage. Another issue is the difficult balance between appropriate immunosuppression in order to avoid rejection and overimmunosuppression with its devastating complications. This issue makes the development of biomarkers to detect early rejection imperative.

Operative Considerations

The donor bowel most often comes from a deceased donor, although segmental living donor intestinal transplants are performed very rarely. A segment of a small bowel at least 100 to 150 cm long is necessary to provide an adequate absorptive surface. The allograft may be heterotopic or orthotopic. The proximal end of the bowel is anastomosed to the recipient's proximal gastrointestinal (GI) tract, whereas the distal end is usually brought up to the abdominal wall as an ileostomy. The approach allows easy observation and biopsy to monitor rejection or ischemia. The venous anastomosis to the graft may be performed to the recipient vena cava or to the portal vein. The arterial anastomosis is performed to the abdominal aorta.

Complications

Complications include rejection, graft-versus-host disease, and sepsis from the translocation of bacteria through the bowel mucosal barriers.

Prognosis

The 1- and 5-year graft survival are 76% and 50%, respectively. The 1- and 5-year patient survival are 81% and 58%.

VASCULARIZED COMPOSITE ALLOGRAFT TRANSPLANTATION

Recognizing the success of solid organ transplantation and responding to the unique needs of patients who have suffered the loss of external body components, transplantation of VCAs has become more common in the past 5 years. VCAs include multiple types of tissues such as skin, bone, muscle, blood vessels, and nerves transplanted as a functional unit. Examples of transplanted VCAs include arm/hand, face, penis, and uterus allografts. These transplants often involve physicians with expertise in diverse fields, including plastic surgery, vascular surgery, solid organ transplantation, psychology/psychiatry, obstetrics and gynecology, and physical and occupational therapies. Given the small number of VCA transplants performed to date, meaningful statistical analysis of graft survival and functional status is not yet available. As an example, by late 2023, in the United States, there had been a total of 41 uterus transplants from both living and deceased donors with reports of successful pregnancies and deliveries. Transplanted uterus grafts are generally removed after the recipient has completed childbearing; thus, long-term graft survival statistics are not the most useful measure of the success of these transplants.

SUGGESTED READINGS

Al-Adra DP, Hammel L, Roberts J, et al. Pretransplant solid organ malignancy and organ transplant candidacy: a consensus expert opinion statement. *Am J Transplant.* 2021;21:460-474.

Kwong AJ, Ebel NH, Kim WR, et al. OPTN/SRTR 2021 Annual Data Report: liver. *Am J Transplant.* 2023;23;S178-S263.

Lentine KL, Smith JM, Miller JM, et al. OPRN/SRTR 2021 annual data report: kidney. *Am J Transplant.* 2023;23:S21-S120.

Roberts MB, Fishman JA. Immunosuppressive agents and infectious risk in transplantation: managing the "net state of immunosuppression." *Clin Infect Dis.* 2021;73:e1302-e1317.

The OPTN Web site offers a wealth of information about transplantation (http://optn.transplant.hrsa.gov).

SAMPLE QUESTIONS

QUESTIONS

Choose the best answer for each question.

1. Which of the following is a true statement about organ donation in the United States?

    A. Over the past 20 years, the number of transplanted organs has increased largely because of an increase in the number of living donors (both related and unrelated).

    B. Grafts from living donors and deceased donors have equivalent graft survival and immediate graft function.

    C. In the deceased donor pool, the most rapid increase in the rate of organ recovery has occurred in the category of donation after cardiac death.

    D. Because of the time-sensitive nature of organ recovery after cardiac death, the procurement team is intimately involved in the declaration of death.

    E. Pronouncement of brain death requires both clinical criteria and a confirmatory study to support the diagnosis of brain death.

2. A 37-year-old man is brought to the emergency department after he attempted suicide by hanging. Cardiopulmonary resuscitation was performed at the scene with return of spontaneous circulation, and he was intubated at the scene. He lacks pupillary light reflex and corneal reflex on exam, and computed tomography of the head is significant for findings of anoxic brain injury. What is the next best step to determine brain death?

   A. Check for sustained apnea when disconnecting the respirator.
   B. Perform transcranial Doppler ultrasonography.
   C. Perform electroencephalography.
   D. Check urine or serum drug screen for intoxication or sedative medication.
   E. Obtain a neurology consultation.

3. Which of the following statements is true concerning immunity for clinical transplantation?

   A. A patient with a history of prior transplant will have a low PRA.
   B. DSAs are formed within the first few hours after transplantation.
   C. HLA matching is important for heart, pancreas, and liver transplantation.
   D. A crossmatch assay determines if there are preformed antibodies in the recipient's serum, which will react with antigens on the cell surface of the potential donor's lymphocytes.
   E. Bone, skin, dura, and other cryopreserved or lyophilized tissues require ABO typing and crossmatching because their immunogenic activity is increased as a result of the preservation.

4. A 65-year-old man with end-stage renal disease underwent a deceased donor kidney transplantation. On postoperative day 2, he experiences tremors and has hyperkalemia despite good allograft function. His current immunosuppression regimen includes antithymocyte globulin, tacrolimus, mycophenolate mofetil, and prednisone. Which one of his drugs is the potential offending agent?

   A. Antithymocyte globulin
   B. Tacrolimus
   C. Mycophenolate mofetil
   D. Prednisone
   E. None of the above

5. A 45-year-old woman presents with end-stage liver disease due to chronic hepatitis C infection. You are trying to calculate her MELD 3.0 score. Which of the following is NOT a component of the MELD 3.0 calculation?

   A. Serum sodium
   B. Serum aspartate aminotransferase
   C. Serum bilirubin
   D. Serum creatinine
   E. INR

ANSWERS AND EXPLANATIONS

1. **Answer: C**

   The total number of organs transplanted has increased by 120% over the past 24 years, with the most rapid increase in the rate of organ recovery from deceased persons after circulatory death. To avoid obvious conflicts of interest, neither the surgeon who recovers the organs nor any personnel involved in transplantation can participate in end-of-life care or the declaration of death. Grafts from living donors have increased graft survival and immediate graft function compared to grafts from deceased donors. For more information on this topic, please see the section "Organ and Tissue Donation."

2. **Answer: D**

   Clinical criteria for determining cessation of brain function include absence of spontaneous respirations or sustained apnea when disconnecting the respirator, absence of pupillary light reflex, and absence of corneal reflex. However, clinical situations that mimic complete unresponsiveness such as barbiturate or opiate overdose, profound hypothermia, or severe metabolic derangements must be excluded or corrected prior to the clinical exam. For more information on this answer, please see section "Organ and Tissue Donation."

3. **Answer: D**

   A pretransplantation crossmatch test is the final immunologic screening step that utilizes a potential donor's lymphocytes as target cells for the patient's serum. ABO matching and crossmatching are the most common tests performed before renal, cardiac, lung, and pancreas transplantation, but ABO matching alone is performed for liver transplantation in most circumstances. For more information on this topic, please see section "Crossmatch."

4. **Answer: B**

   Tacrolimus is a calcineurin inhibitor. It inhibits the expression of multiple genes involved in T-cell activation and proliferation, including IL-2 and other lymphokines. It can cause dose-dependent nephrotoxicity, hypertension, tremors, hyperkalemia, glucose intolerance, and alopecia. For more information on this topic, please see section "Pharmacologic Agents."

5. **Answer: B**

   The MELD 3.0 score is a numerical scale ranging from 6 to 40 that is used to prioritize patients with cirrhosis on the waiting list for a liver transplantation. MELD 3.0 is calculated using the patient's sex, bilirubin, INR, creatinine, albumin, and sodium. For more information on this topic, please see section "Liver Transplantation."

21

Pediatric Surgery: Surgical Diseases of Children

Hayden W. Stagg, Jonathan Meisel, Andreana Butter, and Dan C. Little

PERIOPERATIVE MANAGEMENT OF THE PEDIATRIC SURGICAL PATIENT

Fluids and Electrolytes

Fluid and electrolyte management in pediatric patients must be extremely precise, given the narrow margin between dehydration and fluid overload. Compared with adults, infants and children have greater metabolic demands, and because they turn over body water and electrolytes so rapidly, pediatric patients may undergo rapid, major shifts in body fluid compartments. The immature neonatal kidney has limited concentrating and diluting capacities and therefore cannot be entirely relied upon to compensate for a deficiency or overabundance of fluids and electrolytes. Although a child's need may be estimated according to standard formulas, there is no substitute for frequent adjustments based on careful monitoring of the patient, including a review of nursing documentation of intake and output.

Neonates have a significantly greater proportion of total body water than adults because newborns have a larger pool of extracellular fluid (ECF) (Figure 21-1). This fluid compartment is increased further in extremely premature infants (<28 weeks' gestation). At birth, the ECF is even more expanded, and as much as 10% of birth weight is lost during the first week as this surplus water is excreted.

In calculating fluid and electrolyte requirements for children who cannot receive enteral feeds, the following quantities must be considered:

1. Maintenance requirements
2. Replacement of preexisting deficits
3. Replacement of ongoing abnormal losses

Maintenance Requirements

Maintenance fluids and electrolytes are the quantities that must be provided to compensate for normal renal excretion and insensible losses through the skin and lungs. Table 21-1 provides guidelines for calculating the amounts of water and electrolytes required. In addition, a minimal quantity of glucose is included to provide for some protein sparing and to avoid hypoglycemia, a common problem in the newborn population. These constituents can all be provided by 5% dextrose (D5%) in ½ normal saline + 20 mEq/L KCl in infants and D5% in normal saline + 20 mEq/L KCl in older children at the infusion rate calculated in Table 21-1. The patient's electrolytes should be monitored closely when there is an extended period of nil per os (NPO) and when there are significant gastrointestinal (GI) fluid losses as in the instance of a bowel

obstruction from an incarcerated hernia, volvulus, atresia, and so on.

Preexisting Deficits

Children with acute surgical illness may have significant fluid and electrolyte deficits from poor oral intake, vomiting, diarrhea, peritonitis, sepsis, burns, or hemorrhage. Intravascular volume must be rapidly restored to maintain adequate tissue perfusion for normal organ function. Most surgical diseases cause isotonic dehydration. Fluid deficits are best corrected empirically in stages, as outlined in Table 21-2.

Children who are significantly anemic or actively bleeding may require blood transfusions. There is no arbitrary value of hemoglobin below which a transfusion is indicated, and each child must be individually assessed to optimize oxygen delivery. Volumes used for pediatric "units" range from 10 to 20 mL/kg.

For the actively bleeding patient requiring blood product transfusion, a "balanced" transfusion with a ratio of 1:1:1 of packed red blood cells (PRBCs), fresh frozen plasma, and platelets should be used. This massive transfusion protocol (MTP) has been shown to reduce transfusion-associated coagulopathy and improve outcomes in severely injured patients. The more recent practice of using liquid plasma has decreased previous wait times associated with "thawing" fresh frozen plasma.

Abnormal Ongoing Losses

Abnormal losses include measurable and immeasurable third-space fluid losses. Measurable losses refer to abnormal external drainage. In the surgical patient, these losses usually arise from the GI tract or from various drainage tubes and are most accurately replaced on a volume-for-volume basis. Gastric drainage is approximated as D5% in ½ normal saline + 10 mEq/L KCl. Alimentary tract losses distal to the pylorus are replaced as lactated Ringer solution.

Immeasurable third-space losses are fluids and electrolytes that are pathologically sequestered within the body and are neither in equilibrium nor available to the intravascular space. In children with surgical diseases, such fluid can accumulate in the GI tract from obstruction and inflammation, in body cavities as ascites and pleural effusions, and diffusely as edema from the leaky capillary syndrome that accompanies shock. Operative manipulation can cause edema in tissues as a result of direct trauma. Because third-space losses cannot be measured directly, their intravenous (IV) replacement is approximated. Sequestered fluid is almost always isotonic and is replaced

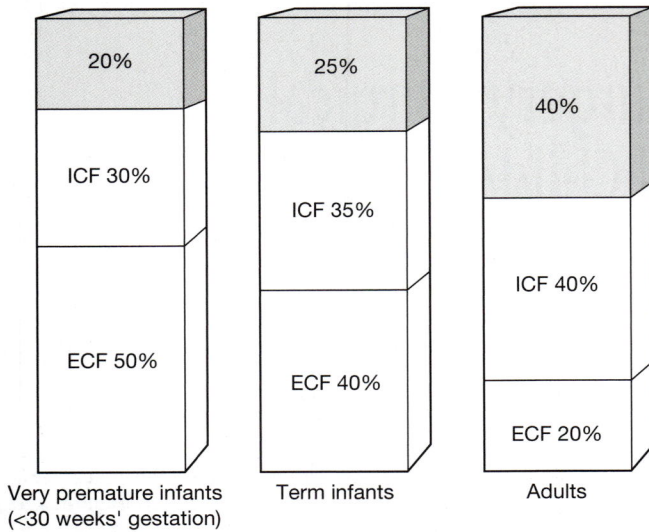

Figure 21-1. Body fluid compartments in very premature infants, term infants, and adults. Unshaded areas show the percentage of body weight as total body water. ECF, extracellular fluid; ICF, intracellular fluid. (From Lawrence PF. *Essentials of Surgical Specialties.* 3rd ed. Lippincott Williams & Wilkins; 2007.)

as a balanced salt solution. Clinicians can choose to run IV fluids at 1.5 to 2 times maintenance for the first 24 hours or to administer boluses of isotonic fluids in 10 to 20 mL/kg aliquots.

The adequacy of IV fluid therapy can be determined only by monitoring the patient's response. Useful parameters are the level of activity, color, skin turgor and temperature, heart rate, and blood pressure. Most helpful is the urine output, which should exceed 1 to 2 mL/kg/h in infants and 0.5 mL/kg/h in adolescents. Children who receive fluids solely as IV infusions should have periodic electrolyte measurements.

Nutrition

The well-nourished child who will be eating within a week does not need nutritional support other than basic fluids and electrolytes, as outlined earlier. On the contrary, if oral feedings are withheld longer, if the child is under significant stress, or if the child is premature, enteral or total parenteral nutrition (TPN) may be critical for survival. Compared with adults, growing children have increased

nutritional demands but often limited nutritional reserves. For example, 25 to 30 kcal/kg will generally meet adult nutritional demands, whereas an infant will typically require 100 kcal/kg. When compounded by the increased metabolic requirements imposed by surgical illness, the risks for malnutrition are considerable. Significant consequences of malnutrition include a lack of growth, impaired organ function, immunologic incompetence, and the inability to heal wounds.

Enteral Nutrition

The provision of nutrients through the intestinal tract is ideal. Compared with TPN, enteral feeding is more physiologic, less prone to complications, and far less costly. A lack of enteral feeds leads to atrophy of the intestinal microvilli and stagnation of the enterohepatic circulation. In critically ill patients, it can also lead to translocation of bacteria across the intestinal mucosa, resulting in sepsis. Even if full enteral feeds cannot be tolerated, the provision of small, "trophic" amounts of enteral nutrition may counterbalance some of these problems. The common enteral feeds used for infants are summarized in Table 21-3.

TABLE 21-1. Fluids and Electrolytes: Maintenance Requirements		
	Weight (kg)	**mL/24 h[a]**
Water	≤10	100 mL/kg
	11–20	1,000 + 50 mL/kg for each kg >10
	>20	1,500 + 20 mL/kg for each kg >20
Sodium	3 mEq/kg/d	
Potassium	2 mEq/kg/d	

[a]Exceptions: (1) Premature infants (<38 weeks' gestation) have increased evaporative losses because of their very thin skin and require up to twice the standard maintenance calculations; (2) fever and various disease states (eg, sepsis) elevate metabolic rate and increase fluid needs.

TABLE 21-2. Fluids and Electrolytes: Replacement of Deficits
Fluid Deficit
Resuscitation stage (for initial rapid correction of isotonic, hypotonic, and hypertonic dehydration): lactated Ringer solution[a] at 20 mL/kg every 10–20 min, with close monitoring, until clinical improvement occurs. Then:
Rapid infusion stage (for isotonic or mild hypotonic dehydration): D5% ½ normal saline at 2× the maintenance dose until the patient is clinically euvolemic.
Sodium Deficit
If significant (Na < 120), correct as: mEq Na required = (130 − serum Na) × 0.6 × weight (kg).
Potassium Deficit
May add up to 40 mEq of KCl to each liter of intravenous fluid.

[a]Normal saline may be used instead of lactated Ringer solution.

TABLE 21-3. Enteral Feeding in Infants	
Breast milk	The "gold standard"; may be collected and stored for later use in surgical patients
Enfamil, Similac	Commercially available cow's milk formulas
Isomil	Soy-based formula for infants with milk protein allergy or lactose intolerance
Pregestimil, Neocate	Elemental formulas with nutrients in their simplest form; indicated for short bowel syndrome

Infants should receive at least 150 mL/kg/d of these formulas to obtain 100 to 110 cal/kg/d.

If a baby cannot suck but has an otherwise functional intestinal tract, a small nasogastric or orogastric (OG) tube may be inserted for gavage feedings. Nasojejunal tubes may be used for individuals at high risk for aspiration (eg, those with delayed gastric emptying or gastroesophageal reflux [GER]). A child who requires prolonged tube feedings is best served by a gastrostomy tube because nasogastric tubes are irritating, are easily displaced, can promote aspiration, and contribute to oral aversion when used long term. A number of silastic low-profile tubes and buttons are available.

Parenteral Nutrition

Many children with major surgical disorders require TPN while the GI tract is temporarily nonfunctional. All nutrient requirements are supplied intravenously by the administration of carbohydrates, proteins, fats, electrolytes, trace elements, and vitamins. IV nutrition may be infused through either a peripheral or a central vein. Advantages of peripheral venous nutrition are ease of catheter placement and fewer catheter complications. Glucose can be administered peripherally up to a concentration of 12.5%. The rest of the required calories are supplied as emulsified fat. More hypertonic solutions (up to 25% glucose) may be delivered centrally through the superior or inferior vena cava. The glucose infusion rate will need to be calculated daily. The umbilical vein can often be utilized for the first 1 to 2 weeks following birth. Thin, silastic percutaneously inserted central catheters (PICCs) are placed centrally through a percutaneously accessed extremity vein, often with ultrasound guidance. Most children's hospitals now enjoy specialized vascular access teams who perform these procedures at the bedside. When peripheral veins are scarce, central access is achieved percutaneously through the subclavian vein, internal jugular vein, or rarely by a cut-down procedure in the neck or groin. A silicone catheter with a tunneled Dacron cuff (of the Hickman or Broviac type) is preferred because it is minimally thrombogenic and tends to resist infection.

The nutritional needs of each child who is receiving TPN are calculated daily, and the appropriate solution is prepared. TPN is infused at maintenance fluid rates by an infusion pump. Concentrations are gradually increased over several days until daily requirements are achieved. All children who receive TPN are monitored closely. Weight is recorded daily, and blood is analyzed periodically for glucose, electrolytes, lipids, bilirubin, and liver enzymes.

Registered dietitian nutritionists serve as a valuable resource for the surgical team when initiating and maintaining TPN.

Mechanical complications are most common with centrally placed catheters. Catheter sepsis is also a major hazard with central catheters, and it can be minimized by scrupulous surgical and nursing techniques. Bacterial contamination is often treated successfully with antibiotics administered through the catheter, whereas life-threatening infections or fungal sepsis usually necessitate immediate catheter removal. Liver damage may occur in any patient who is receiving long-term TPN, but preterm infants are most susceptible. The association of lipids and hepatocyte injury has been well-documented, and minimizing exposure to IV lipids and using fish oil–based lipids have shown promise in both preventing and reversing cholestasis and hepatotoxicity. Cholestasis is initially identified by rising serum bilirubin and alkaline phosphatase levels. It usually reverses when TPN is discontinued but may progress to cirrhosis and hepatic failure.

Respiratory Management

Respiratory failure is common in surgically ill children. Infants have high oxygen requirements, are obligate nasal breathers, and depend almost exclusively on their diaphragms rather than on chest wall muscles for air movement. As a result, they have a limited safety margin before respiratory insufficiency develops. Even moderate increases in intra-abdominal pressure can cause respiratory distress.

Endotracheal intubation provides the most secure airway. The size of the tube to be inserted may be estimated from the diameter of the child's external nares or little finger, or for children over 2 years of age, using the formulas: Age (years)/4 + 4 for uncuffed tubes or Age (years)/4 + 3 for cuffed tubes. Routine use of capnography and chest x-ray (CXR) is recommended. To avoid inserting the tube into a bronchus, bilateral equality of the breath sounds must be verified. Difficult intubation may be predicted on the basis of short thyromental distance, a Mallampati score of 3 or 4, micrognathia, and syndromic children (such as Pierre Robin sequence) with craniofacial asymmetry. In these instances, video laryngoscopy and consultation with pediatric anesthesia are essential.

The two types of mechanical ventilators available are the volume and pressure-modulated varieties. Volume ventilators deliver a preset tidal volume, regardless of pulmonary compliance, and are used in most patients beyond the newborn period. Pressure ventilators deliver breaths up to a preset pressure and are preferred for infants, in whom the very low lung volumes involved compared with the dead space would prevent accurate delivery of a preset volume to the lungs. The ventilator should be adjusted to its lowest possible settings consistent with adequate gas exchange. Concepts of permissive hypercapnia are increasingly popular as this strategy reduces barotrauma from the positive pressure ventilator. Oxygen levels must not be excessive, particularly in preterm neonates, who are at high risk for retinal damage and pulmonary toxicity that can lead to bronchopulmonary dysplasia.

Pneumothorax occurs in children who receive positive pressure ventilation and should be suspected whenever there is a sudden deterioration in the respiratory status. The diagnosis is confirmed by CXR or ultrasound by looking for the lung slide of the parietal and visceral pleura. Definitive treatment is the placement of an intercostal chest tube, but expeditious needle aspiration can provide immediate relief. When suspecting a tension pneumothorax, a provider should place a chest tube expeditiously and without the delay of a confirmatory x-ray.

High-frequency oscillatory ventilation is an innovation in which very low tidal volumes are directed down the trachea at extremely rapid rates (150-900 breaths/min). When very high ventilatory settings are needed, this technique may allow adequate gas exchange to occur at lower airway pressures than with conventional rates, producing less trauma to the lungs.

Extracorporeal membrane oxygenation (ECMO) is a form of prolonged cardiopulmonary bypass in which gas exchange occurs in an external circuit that contains the patient's flowing blood and is utilized only when all forms of positive pressure ventilation are inadequate. ECMO can provide complete respiratory support, independent of the lungs, and thereby allows the lungs to rest and recover while organ function is well maintained. ECMO should only be considered in cases that are felt to be reversible. ECMO is reserved for the most desperately ill infants and children because it requires cannulation of major vessels and systemic anticoagulation. Veno-venous ECMO is recommended for pure respiratory support, while veno-arterial ECMO is preferred for children with combined respiratory and cardiovascular failure. Given the ability to predict mortality, the oxygen index is often calculated as decisions for ECMO cannulation are weighed. Overall survival in newborn infants treated with ECMO is approximately 80%, depending on the cause of respiratory failure. The survival rate for older children and adults is approximately 50%.

Preoperative Evaluation and Preparation

All children who undergo surgery require a careful history and a thorough physical examination, but laboratory studies are not necessary in healthy children undergoing routine procedures. Labs, including complete blood count (CBC), blood type, crossmatching, and supporting imaging and echocardiogram, are ordered for complicated, lengthy procedures. Recent preliminary work is raising concern about worsening neurodevelopmental outcomes in children undergoing multiple general anesthetics. Thus, when possible, procedures should be grouped and overall operative time be minimized.

Children must be in the best possible condition at the time of operation. A child with an upper respiratory infection should have elective surgery postponed for 4 to 6 weeks to minimize the chance of intraoperative bronchospasm. A patient who is in shock should be resuscitated as completely as possible before even an urgent operation.

Many operations on infants can be performed on an outpatient basis, starting at 3 months of age for term babies and at approximately 52 weeks after conception for premature infants. Because the respiratory center is immature before that time and there is a risk of apnea after general anesthesia, elective operations should be delayed. After emergency procedures, close postoperative apnea monitoring in the hospital for 24 hours or longer is mandatory.

Preoperative NPO guidelines differ from those of adults and are outlined in Table 21-4.

TABLE 21-4. Preoperative NPO Guidelines for Children

Type of Feeding	Hours NPO
Clear liquids	2
Breast milk	4
Formula	6
Solids, all else	8

Guidelines will vary by institution.
NPO, nil per os.

Operative Care and Monitoring

The ability to perform major surgery successfully on preterm infants is a recent development and is largely the result of an increased understanding of neonatal physiology and advances in technology. Even extremely premature neonates can be safely brought through surgery, provided that the pediatric anesthesiologist is knowledgeable and attentive to their special needs and the surgeon handles the fragile tissues with the utmost gentleness and skill. Minimizing time in the operating room (OR) is essential in this population. Many procedures are best performed at the bedside in the neonatal intensive care unit (NICU).

Although general anesthesia is used for almost all children who undergo operations, supplementation with regional or local blocks (such as epidural, ilioinguinal/iliohypogastric, penile, and intercostal infusions) can lower intraoperative requirements of potent general agents and diminish postoperative pain and discomfort. Epidural catheters can be left in place for several days. Thoracic cryoablation for children undergoing thoracotomies or pectus repairs is showing increasing promise with superior pain control and decreased length of stay.

During the course of an operation, the clinical condition of a small child who is almost completely covered with drapes can change rapidly. The endotracheal tube can become blocked, slip out of the trachea, or migrate down a mainstem bronchus. Close monitoring is essential and should always include an electrocardiogram (ECG), precordial or esophageal stethoscope, blood pressure cuff, temperature probe, pulse oximeter, and end-tidal CO_2 monitor for measurement of the adequacy of ventilation. Additional options can include a urinary catheter and arterial access (usually with an umbilical artery catheter in neonates) for frequent blood sampling and arterial pressure measurement.

Infants can rapidly become hypothermic in the OR, leading to greatly increased metabolic demands, peripheral vasoconstriction, acidosis, and even death. Premature infants have a surface area that is up to 10 times that of adults per unit weight and have significant transepithelial water loss because of skin immaturity leading to evaporative heat loss. In addition, they have little subcutaneous tissue for insulation and rely on the metabolism of brown fat for heat generation, which may be rendered inactive by anesthetic agents or depleted by poor nutrition. In the OR, heat loss is exacerbated because body cavities are exposed and anesthesia abolishes muscular activity and causes vasodilatation. Children are kept warm by adequately heating the OR, using radiant heaters and warming mattresses, circulating warm air, covering the extremities and head, and warming all solutions and IV fluids used to prepare them for surgery.

Allowable blood loss is generally 15% to 20% of estimated blood volume, depending on patient stability. Greater losses generally require transfusions with PRBCs.

Postoperative Care and Pain Management

Close monitoring is most essential during the immediate postanesthesia recovery period. Although most children can be extubated at the conclusion of the operative procedure, those who are critically ill or prone to apnea should remain ventilated until stabilized. Following extubation, supplemental oxygen should be given and pulse oximetry monitored to prevent hypoxia.

The most common cause of hypotension or oliguria in the postoperative period is hypovolemia secondary to inadequate resuscitation or third-space losses. A fluid challenge of 10 to 20 mL/kg of isotonic fluid should be given, and the clinical response should be monitored.

Nutrition must be started postoperatively as soon as possible. In many situations, a regular diet may be offered as soon as the child is awake. Following GI surgery or if the child is critically ill, parenteral nutrition should be considered if the anticipated time for resumption of full enteral feeds is greater than a week. It is important to remember that many children have had poor nutritional intake for several days before presentation. Nasogastric tube decompression may avoid gastric distention, which can compromise respiration and lead to aspiration.

Postoperative pain is often inadequately managed because children may be unable to clearly express their complaints. Narcotics should be administered intravenously. Patient-controlled analgesia is a viable alternative for children aged 8 years or older. Because apnea is a concern in children younger than 6 months of age, narcotics should be given only in a carefully monitored setting. Recent studies have shown similar efficacy of combined acetaminophen and ibuprofen when compared with acetaminophen and narcotic combinations. IV acetaminophen is also available for patients unable to take oral medications. Nonsteroidal anti-inflammatory drugs can be used to reduce narcotic dosages and side effects postoperatively. Use of epinephrine may be added to traditional local anesthetics such as lidocaine and marcaine to prolong the anesthetic effects. Table 21-5 provides dosages for commonly used analgesics.

Emotional Support

Even the most routine operation is often a major traumatic event for patients and their families. Children between the ages of 1 and 4 years are aware enough to be afraid, although they cannot understand the bewildering events going on around them. Older children and adolescents are particularly fearful of physical injury and mutilation. Parents are often devastated at the prospect of their child having to undergo an operation, with the dread of general anesthesia often superseding that of the operative procedure itself.

Much can be done to alleviate the anxiety of both children and parents. The approach must be individualized, depending on the age of the child and the temperament of the patient and family. Honest and open explanations are best. The child should be included in the discussions and

TABLE 21-5. Dosages of Local Anesthetics and Analgesics in Children

Bupivacaine (0.5% or 0.25%) with or without 1% epinephrine	Maximum of 3 mg/kg injected intraoperatively (or 0.5 mL/kg of the 0.5% solution)
Lidocaine without epinephrine	Maximum of 5 mg/kg without epinephrine (or 1 mL/kg of the 0.5% solution)
Lidocaine with epinephrine	Maximum of 10 mg/kg with epinephrine (or 2 mL/kg of the 0.5% solution)
Morphine	0.1 mg/kg intravenously every 1-2 h
Fentanyl	1-2 μg/kg intravenously every 1-2 h
Acetaminophen	10-15 mg/kg orally or rectally every 4 h

provided with ample opportunity for questions. With the assistance of a child life specialist, videos, booklets, and a facility tour can transform an alien, hostile setting into a familiar, friendly one. Even when procedures are unpleasant or painful, children fare better when they know what to expect. Separation from parents should be minimized. In some hospitals, parental presence at anesthesia induction has been shown to reduce both patient and parental anxiety and improve overall satisfaction with care. For the parent, an excellent relationship with the surgeon and a clear understanding of the events is important because parents often transmit their own feelings to their children. Informed parents can do much to prepare children at home. Special use of in-person or video language interpretation is often necessary.

Premedication, including versed, is often given to allay anxiety and should be administered orally because an injection would defeat its purpose. In the OR, anesthesia induction in younger patients is performed with a face mask, which can be flavored. Older children can choose between mask and IV induction.

NEONATAL SURGICAL CONDITIONS

Birth defects are the most common cause of perinatal mortality and a major source of morbidity in the United States. In most instances, the etiology of these malformations is unknown and likely results from a combination of genetic and environmental factors. Many of these defects require surgical intervention for either cure or palliation. With the increasing use of antenatal screening modalities, particularly ultrasonography, more anomalies are being discovered in utero. For a limited number of conditions (eg, hydronephrosis, hydrocephalus, space-occupying lesions of the chest), intrauterine operations may be beneficial, but these are still experimental procedures and are performed in only specialized centers. Myelomeningocele has been shown to have improved outcomes with fetal intervention, and fetal closure has become a standard-of-care option. Nevertheless, prenatal diagnosis allows for family counseling regarding the management of the pregnancy and planning of the timing, mode, and location of delivery. Most importantly, personal relationships can be established between the parents and the health care team at an early stage.

Congenital Diaphragmatic Hernia

A congenital diaphragmatic hernia (CDH) is a condition in which the absence of a portion of the diaphragm can lead to life-threatening respiratory compromise. It occurs in about 1:3,300 live births and serves as a prototype for surgical causes of neonatal respiratory distress. As a result of recent advances in management, the survival rate has steadily improved. The opening in the diaphragm can vary in location and size. By far the most common type is the Bochdalek hernia, which is a defect of the posterolateral diaphragm, usually on the left. Morgagni hernias, which are retrosternal defects, rarely present as emergencies in the newborn period.

Embryology

The etiology of CDH is unknown. Embryologically, the extruded midgut normally returns to the abdominal cavity between the 9th and 10th weeks of gestation. If the pleuroperitoneal canal through the posterolateral portion of the diaphragm remains open, the viscera will pass into the chest and compress the developing lungs. The resulting pulmonary hypoplasia and abnormalities of the pulmonary vasculature affect both lungs but are more severe when ipsilateral. The timing and severity of the pulmonary compression determine the physiologic consequences.

Pathophysiology

CDH causes respiratory distress by a combination of physical compression of the lungs by the herniated viscera, pulmonary hypoplasia, and resultant pulmonary hypertension. Although the mechanical lung compression is relieved by surgery, pulmonary hypoplasia can be fatal if severe. Pulmonary hypertension results from the abnormally high pulmonary vascular resistance caused by the paucity of pulmonary arterioles and the abnormal vascular reactivity of the vessels that are present. This increased pulmonary vascular resistance causes right-to-left shunting of desaturated blood across the foramen ovale and ductus arteriosus, exacerbating the hypoxemia.

Clinical Presentation and Evaluation

A newborn with CDH has a variable degree of dyspnea and cyanosis. There are diminished breath sounds on the side of the hernia and a shift of the heart to the opposite side. The abdomen is characteristically scaphoid. The diagnosis is confirmed by a CXR that shows air-filled loops of bowel in the chest (or opacity in the right chest if the liver is involved), loss of the diaphragmatic contour, and mediastinal deviation (Figure 21-2).

Treatment

Initial resuscitation of a newborn with a CDH includes immediate endotracheal intubation with mechanical ventilation and supplemental oxygenation. Positive pressure ventilation through a face mask is contraindicated because gas will enter the GI tract and further compress the lungs. A nasogastric tube is placed to minimize gastric distention.

The ventilatory management of babies with CDH both preoperatively and postoperatively is most critical, as

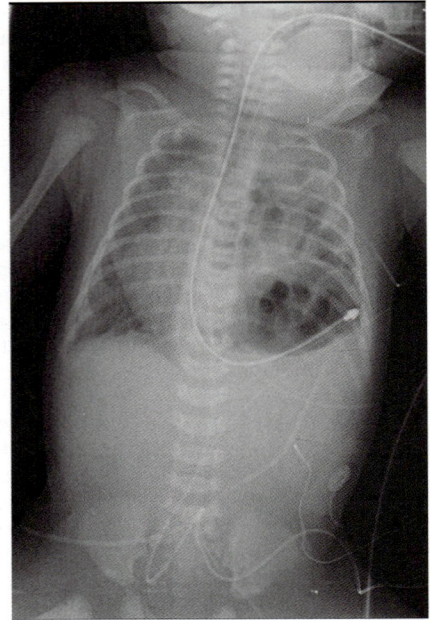

Figure 21-2. Congenital diaphragmatic hernia in a neonate. Intestinal loops and an orogastric tube are seen on the left side of the chest, with mediastinal displacement to the right.

too-high ventilator settings will irreversibly damage hypoplastic lungs. A strategy of "permissive hypercapnia" and "gentle ventilation" consists of strictly limiting the ventilatory pressures and oxygen concentrations while counterintuitively accepting some degree of hypercarbia and hypoxemia; this method has significantly improved survival. Adjuncts may include the administration of inhaled nitric oxide (a pulmonary vasodilator) and the use of high-frequency ventilation. Finally, if all else fails, ECMO can provide complete respiratory support, allowing time for pulmonary hypertension to improve while avoiding further lung damage by high ventilator settings.

The timing of the surgical repair of the CDH itself is no longer considered emergent, and there is value in a delay of several days to stabilize the baby and improve the elevated pulmonary artery pressures. The operative approach is usually through the abdomen, although it may also be through the chest cavity. Minimally invasive techniques are increasingly favored. The viscera are reduced, and the diaphragmatic defect is closed primarily or, if it is large, with a prosthetic patch.

CDH is often diagnosed by antenatal ultrasound. Delivery is then planned to take place in a specialized center. Although antenatal repair of the defect has not been successful technically, inducing lung growth by fetoscopic tracheal occlusion or by the administration of pulmonary growth factors is being evaluated in clinical trials. Antenatal measurement of lung-to-head ratio of less than 1.4 portends a worse outcome.

Prognosis

The overall survival of babies with CDH is about 70% to 80%, with a combination of permissive hypercapnia, delayed surgery, and the judicious use of ECMO having led to these improved survival rates. Most survivors have had little disability because the lungs continue to grow postnatally. Yet, as more severely affected babies with CDH survive, more are showing evidence of long-term problems with pulmonary function, poor growth, and developmental delay. It is paramount that these children undergo long-term follow-up and screening for these potential complications, as well as for recurrence.

Neonatal Thoracic Mass Lesions

Mass lesions in the chest cavity of newborns are infrequent but not rare and may be life threatening. These conditions include congenital lobar emphysema, congenital pulmonary airway malformation (CPAM), pulmonary sequestration, bronchogenic cysts, and foregut duplication cysts. The lesions may be asymptomatic, or they may cause symptoms as a result of a primary compressive effect or secondary infection, including chest pain, wheezing, dyspnea, and fever. These malformations are increasingly detected prenatally on ultrasound and then confirmed by postnatal imaging. A computed tomography (CT) scan should be obtained to help delineate the anatomy, but delaying this to 3 to 6 months of age helps with imaging unless the child is symptomatic.

Patients with congenital lobar emphysema (which represents hyperinflation of normal lung tissue) who are not significantly symptomatic may be observed. Other lesions such as extra-lobar sequestrations have also been safely observed, and there is ongoing debate as to which lesions should be resected in the asymptomatic child.

Unborn infants with CPAMs can be risk-stratified on the basis of the size of the lesion. A CPAM volume ratio is calculated on the basis of the volume of the lesion in comparison with head circumference. A value greater than 1.6 portends a worse prognosis, and maternal steroid administration as well as fetal interventions such as thoracoamniotic shunts are potentially beneficial interventions. Fetal resection is performed at specialized centers but is reserved only for cases in which hydrops is present and the gestational age prohibits earlier delivery.

For intralobar lesions, lobectomy is the standard operation, and it can be performed with minimally invasive thoracoscopic techniques. Lobectomy is very well tolerated by neonates, and their remaining lung is able to compensate over time such that their future pulmonary function is not compromised.

Esophageal Atresia and Tracheoesophageal Fistula

Esophageal atresia (EA) is a congenital interruption in the continuity of the upper and lower portions of the esophagus (Figure 21-3A). A tracheoesophageal fistula (TEF) is an abnormal communication between the trachea and esophagus (Figure 21-3E). Either condition may occur alone, but they usually appear in some combination (Figure 21-3B–D). The most common pattern is type C, in which the upper esophagus ends blindly and the lower portion communicates with the trachea. Overall, these anomalies are found in 1:4,000 live births.

Pathophysiology

The etiology of EA and TEF is unknown, but it is believed that the septation process that normally divides the foregut into the trachea and esophagus by the seventh week of gestation is incomplete. In addition, the more rapidly growing trachea may partition the upper and lower esophagus into discontinuous segments. Neonates with EA and TEF often have certain other abnormalities, known as the VACTERL (**vertebral, anal, cardiac, tracheal, esophageal, radial or renal, limb**) association. The presence of an anomaly of any of these structures should prompt a search for others through additional midline workup with ultrasound.

Clinical Presentation and Evaluation

An infant with EA, with or without a TEF, immediately chokes and regurgitates with feeding, as the blind-ending upper esophageal pouch rapidly fills. An alert nurse usually notes excessive drooling even earlier because the infant cannot swallow saliva. An attempt should be made to pass an OG tube. Resistance is encountered, and an x-ray confirms that the tip is in the upper mediastinum. Air visualized in the abdomen confirms the presence of a TEF. An isolated EA is associated with no gas in the GI tract. A provider may inject 1 to 2 mL of air through the OG tube immediately prior to CXR to delineate the upper pouch. A contrast study of the upper pouch should not be attempted.

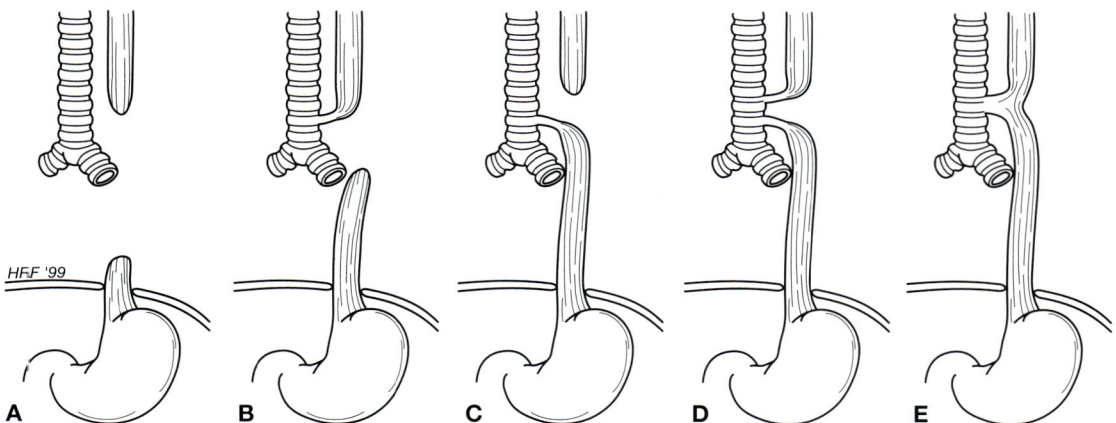

HFF '99

A   **B**   **C**   **D**   **E**

Figure 21-3. Anatomic patterns and approximate percentages of occurrence of esophageal atresia and tracheoesophageal fistula. A. Isolated esophageal atresia (8%). B. Proximal tracheoesophageal fistula (<1%). C. Distal tracheoesophageal fistula (85%). D. Double fistula (<1%). E. "H" type fistula (5%). (From Lawrence PF. *Essentials of Surgical Specialties.* 3rd ed. Lippincott Williams & Wilkins; 2007.)

An isolated TEF, the H-type fistula (Figure 21-3E), is more insidious because the esophagus is patent. These individuals have recurrent aspiration pneumonia, and the diagnosis is established by endoscopy or pull-back esophagram.

Treatment

Immediate measures are taken to prevent aspiration. The baby is kept with the head elevated to minimize reflux of gastric contents through the fistula into the trachea. To avoid the accumulation of oral secretions, a double-lumen tube is placed in the upper pouch for suctioning. IV fluids and broad-spectrum antibiotics are administered. Echocardiogram should be performed to evaluate for significant intracardiac lesions as well as document the side of the descending aorta.

Most neonates with EA and TEF undergo primary repair within the first few days of life, with division of the fistula and anastomosis of the upper and lower esophageal segments through a right thoracotomy, although some surgeons prefer to approach this with thoracoscopic techniques. If the infant is extremely premature, has other major illnesses and cannot tolerate a lengthy procedure, or has a long gap between esophageal segments, a staged repair is preferable. In that case, a gastrostomy is performed initially to keep the stomach empty and prevent aspiration. It is subsequently used for feeding after the TEF is ligated. Upper and lower esophageal segments may require several months to grow close enough to permit approximation. Only in rare instances is a colon interposition, gastric interposition, or reversed gastric tube necessary to bridge the gap.

Common Complications

Postoperative complications include anastomotic leak, stricture, recurrent TEF, GER, and tracheomalacia. Esophageal anastomosis dilations are generally required but should be reserved for patients at least 1 month out from surgery. Tracheomalacia is caused by the underdevelopment of the cartilaginous tracheal rings and may be manifested by noisy respirations, a barking cough, and apneic spells. When severe, this can require operative correction with aortopexy performed through a left anterolateral thoracotomy. Reflux is especially common and may require subsequent fundoplication.

Prognosis

Most neonates with EA and TEF have excellent results. Mortality is usually limited to those who are extremely premature or have other major anomalies. Long-term follow-up is mandatory because these children can develop anastomotic strictures, chest wall anomalies, and other complications that can be addressed to improve the quality of life for these patients.

Congenital Gastrointestinal Obstruction

Congenital GI obstruction refers to an obstruction that is present at birth. The site of the obstruction may be anywhere from the stomach to the anus, and it can result from a wide variety of causes. These disorders should be managed with some urgency because the obstructed neonate can rapidly develop fluid and electrolyte derangements, may aspirate vomitus, and can acquire sepsis from perforation of the distended bowel or necrosis from an underlying volvulus.

Clinical Presentation and Evaluation

The clinical manifestations of congenital intestinal obstruction will vary depending on the site of obstruction. The four key signs are listed herewith:

1. Polyhydramnios. The fetus swallows 50% of the amniotic fluid daily, which is largely absorbed in the upper intestinal tract. A high obstruction allows this fluid to back up and accumulate in excessive quantities as may be noted on routine maternal ultrasound.
2. Bilious vomiting. Nonbilious vomiting is common in infants. Bilious vomiting is often pathologic.
3. Abdominal distention. Distention develops within 24 hours of birth in distal obstructions because swallowed air accumulates above the blockage.
4. Failure to pass meconium. Within 24 hours of birth, 95% of term babies pass meconium. A delay may signify obstruction.

If obstruction is suspected, plain x-rays are performed because swallowed air is an excellent contrast material. If a few dilated loops of the bowel with air-fluid levels and no distal air can be seen (Figure 21-4), complete, proximal obstruction is diagnosed and no further imaging studies are needed. If the obstruction appears to be partial or is questionable, with some distal air visualized, an upper GI (UGI) contrast study can be helpful. If many distended loops of the bowel are seen, suggesting a distal obstruction, a contrast enema is indicated. Tables 21-6 and 21-7 compare features of the common causes of neonatal upper and lower GI obstruction, respectively.

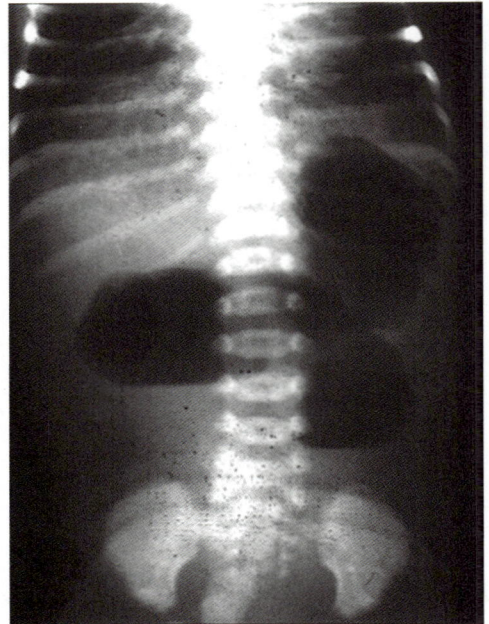

Figure 21-4. Congenital intestinal obstruction. Proximal obstruction ("triple bubble") from jejunal atresia. Air is visualized in the stomach and proximal jejunum only.

TABLE 21-6. Neonatal Upper Intestinal Obstruction: Differential Diagnosis

	Pyloric Stenosis	Duodenal Atresia	Midgut Volvulus
Onset of symptoms	2-8 wks	Birth	Any time
Overall appearance	Hungry, dehydrated	Well	Well initially, then acutely ill
Abdominal pain	None	None	+++ (May be none early)
Vomiting	Nonbilious projectile	Bilious	Bilious
Abdominal distention	None	None	+++ (May be none early)
Abdominal x-ray	Large gastric bubble	"Double-bubble" sign	Variable
Upper gastrointestinal study	Narrowed pyloric channel	Complete or partial duodenal obstruction	Duodenal obstruction; "corkscrew" appearance
Ultrasound	Enlarged pylorus	Dilated stomach	Twisted mesentery
Treatment	Pyloromyotomy	Duodenoduodenostomy	Ladd procedure with or without bowel resection
Urgency of surgery	Minimal	+	+++
Prognosis	Excellent	Good	May lead to short bowel syndrome or death

Treatment

Initial management should always include OG tube decompression, IV hydration, and prophylactic antibiotics. The need for and timing of surgery then depends on the nature of the obstruction and the overall condition of the baby.

Duodenal Obstruction

Duodenal obstruction is commonly caused by (1) atresia and (2) malrotation. Most obstructions of this type are distal to the ampulla of Vater, so the vomiting is bilious. Atresia may take several forms, including complete separation of the proximal and distal duodenal segments, stenosis, or a web across the lumen. During fetal development, the duodenal epithelium overgrows and transiently occludes the lumen. Failure of subsequent complete recanalization is believed to account for the various forms of atresia. There is a strong association of atresia with trisomy 21. An annular pancreas is frequently encountered, in which the ventral pancreatic bud fails to rotate around and becomes incorporated into the dorsal buds. The two instead fuse around the duodenum, creating a ring effect.

Rotation of the intestine normally occurs in the fetus after the midgut (ie, the bowel from the duodenum to the transverse colon) has returned to the abdominal cavity from the yolk sac. The vertical midgut rotates 270° in a counterclockwise direction, placing the cecum in the right lower

TABLE 21-7. Neonatal Lower Intestinal Obstruction: Differential Diagnosis

	Intestinal Atresia	Meconium Ileus	Meconium Plug	Hirschsprung Disease
Onset of symptoms	Birth	Birth	Birth	Any time (usually infancy)
Association	None	Cystic fibrosis	Prematurity	Trisomy 21
Abdomen	Distended if distal, soft	Distended, doughy feel, visible loops	Distended, soft	Distended, soft
Abdominal x-ray	Dilated bowel loops, air-fluid levels	Dilated bowel without air-fluid levels, "soap-bubble" appearance in the right lower quadrant	Moderately dilated bowel loops, air-fluid levels	Dilated bowel loops, air-fluid levels
Contrast enema	Narrow colon, proximal obstruction, and anastomosis	Narrow colon, meconium pellets in the distal ileum	Normal colon with meconium plugs	Transition zone usually in rectosigmoid
Treatment	Bowel resection	Contrast enema; laparotomy if unsuccessful	Contrast enema usually therapeutic	Neonatal pull-through procedure
Prognosis	Excellent	Poor (cystic fibrosis)	Excellent	Good

quadrant and the duodenojejunal junction in the left upper quadrant. Subsequently, the ascending and descending colon are fixed retroperitoneally by fibrous attachments that arise from the lateral abdominal wall. In malrotation, this process is incomplete. The cecum is located in the right upper quadrant or remains completely in the left abdomen, and the duodenojejunal junction is located to the right of the midline. This configuration allows the intestine, which is suspended between these closely fixed points, to twist as a midgut volvulus (Figure 21-5A and B) around the superior mesenteric artery. Midgut volvulus may occur at any age in the presence of malrotation but is most common in the first month of life. It is the most dangerous form of intestinal obstruction, potentially progressing to necrosis of the entire midgut if not urgently recognized and corrected.

In infants with malrotation, the peritoneal attachments to the lateral abdominal wall, which normally fix the cecum retroperitoneally, now cross over the duodenum to reach the high, malrotated cecum. These attachments are called Ladd bands and may be another cause of partial or complete obstruction by compression of the duodenum (Figure 21-5C). A UGI x-ray will reveal an obstructed duodenum and the presence of distal intestinal gas (Figure 21-5D).

The diagnosis of complete duodenal obstruction can often be seen prenatally with ultrasound and at birth is established by visualizing a "double bubble" on x-ray, because air is present in the stomach and in the proximal, dilated duodenum, but none is seen distally (Figure 21-6). If the obstruction is incomplete, some air will be noted below. This should prompt emergent evaluation with UGI contrast evaluation to rule out malrotation, or if radiology is unavailable, proceed to laparotomy, because the consequences of a missed volvulus can be disastrous.

If there is no concern for malrotation, true duodenal atresia is an elective operation generally scheduled within a few days following the required echocardiogram. For

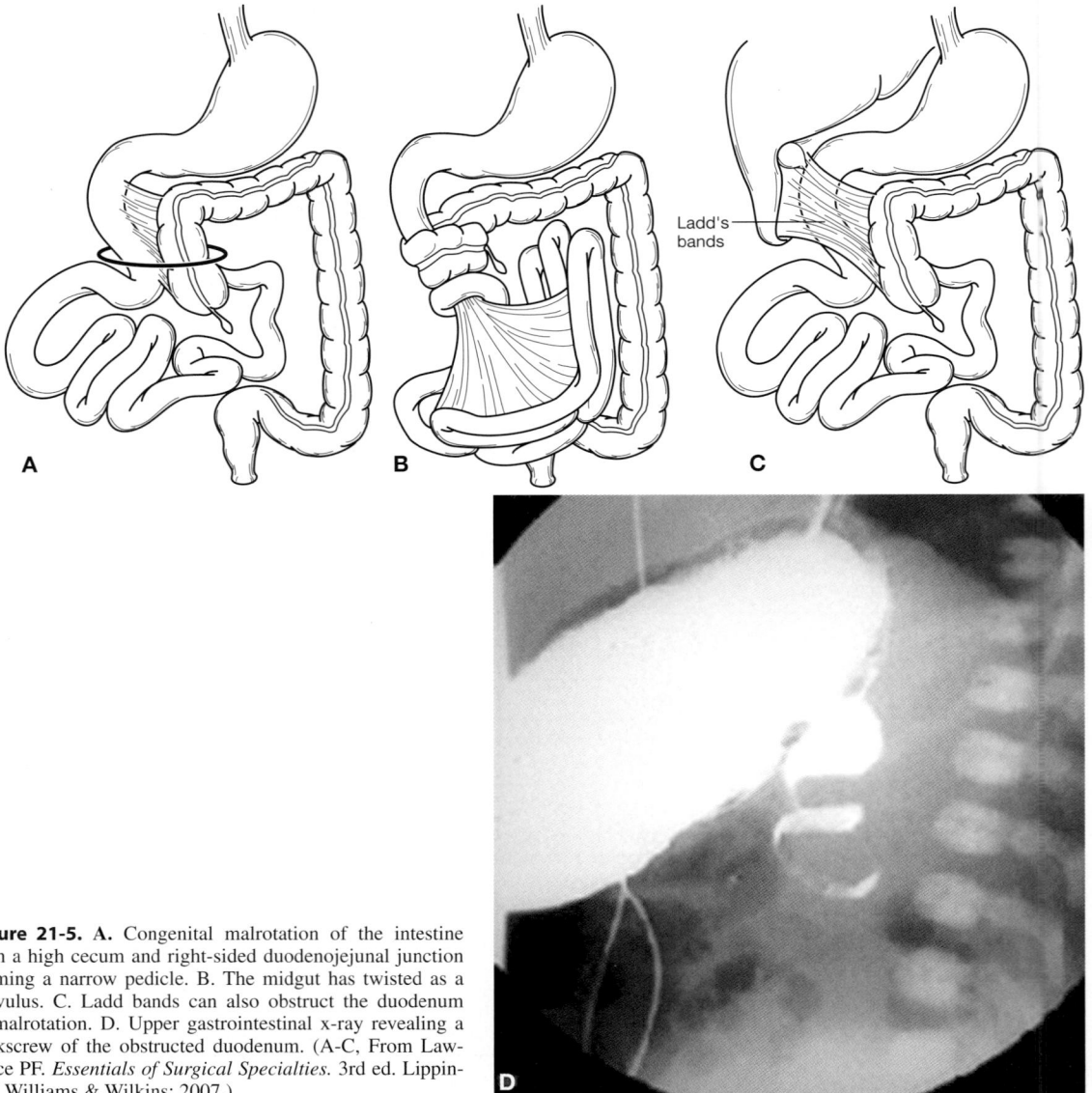

Figure 21-5. A. Congenital malrotation of the intestine with a high cecum and right-sided duodenojejunal junction forming a narrow pedicle. **B.** The midgut has twisted as a volvulus. **C.** Ladd bands can also obstruct the duodenum in malrotation. **D.** Upper gastrointestinal x-ray revealing a corkscrew of the obstructed duodenum. (A-C, From Lawrence PF. *Essentials of Surgical Specialties.* 3rd ed. Lippincott Williams & Wilkins; 2007.)

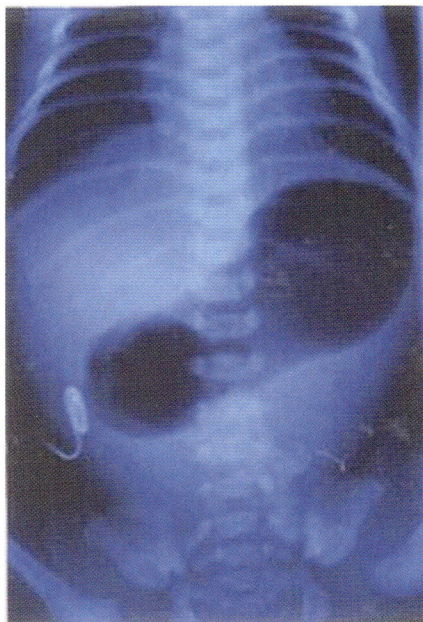

Figure 21-6. "Double-bubble" sign in a neonate with duodenal atresia. Air is visualized in the stomach and proximal dilated duodenum only.

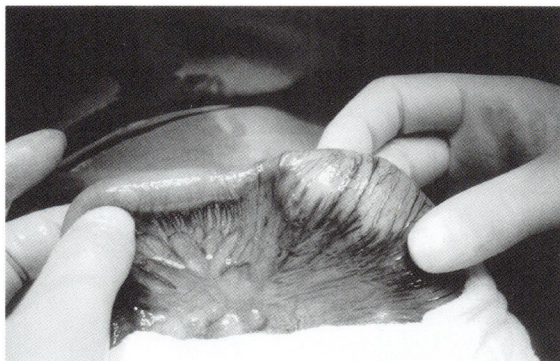

Figure 21-7. Atresia of the small intestine caused by an intraluminal web. A size discrepancy between the dilated proximal and decompressed distal bowel is seen. (From Lawrence PF. *Essentials of Surgical Specialties.* 3rd ed. Lippincott Williams & Wilkins; 2007.)

atresia with or without an annular pancreas, the obstruction is bypassed through an anastomosis between the proximal duodenal segment and the distal duodenum or a loop of the jejunum (a gastrojejunostomy is poorly tolerated in infants). In malrotation, the volvulus (if present) is untwisted, Ladd bands are divided, and the base of the small bowel mesentery is widened. Because the bowel must be returned to the abdomen in the nonrotated position, an appendectomy is also performed to avoid misleading presentations of appendicitis. The entire operation (termed a Ladd procedure) can now be performed laparoscopically.

Small Intestinal Obstruction

Congenital obstruction of the small intestine is usually caused by atresia, meconium ileus, and intestinal duplication. Like its duodenal counterpart, atresia of the small intestine may range from a web across the lumen (Figure 21-7) to complete separation of the intestinal segments. The defects may be multiple. Unlike duodenal atresia, the proposed etiology is an in utero vascular accident, such as a localized twist or intussusception.

Meconium ileus is caused by the impaction of sticky, thick meconium in the distal ileum, the narrowest portion of the intestinal tract. It occurs in 15% of infants with cystic fibrosis, from the abnormally viscid enzymes secreted by the pancreatic and intestinal glands. Of note, almost 100% of babies presenting with meconium ileus will have cystic fibrosis. One in 30 Americans are noted to be carriers of this gene that produces a faulty CFTR protein. A family history of cystic fibrosis, an autosomal recessive disorder, is suggestive, but is positive in only 25% of patients. X-rays often demonstrate a peculiar foamy appearance of the dilated meconium-filled bowel loops and a lack of air-fluid levels, as the thick meconium is mixed with

air and fails to layer out. Calcification on abdominal x-ray indicates that an antenatal perforation has occurred.

Duplications are endothelial-lined cystic or tubular structures adjacent to any portion of the alimentary tract. They are found on the mesenteric side of the normal bowel, usually sharing a common wall and may or may not communicate with the primary lumen. Mucous secretions or stool may accumulate in the duplication, causing it to distend. Obstructive symptoms from pressure on neighboring bowel or localized volvulus may appear during or after the neonatal period.

Atresias and duplications are managed surgically by resection and primary anastomosis. Meconium ileus can frequently be treated nonoperatively with diatrizoate (Gastrografin) enemas. Gastrografin is a radiopaque fluid with a very high osmolarity that causes fluid to be drawn into the bowel lumen. The sticky meconium is hydrated and may be spontaneously evacuated. IV fluids must be infused during the procedure to avoid systemic hypovolemia. If the obstruction persists or if there is evidence of perforation, surgery is mandatory.

Colon Obstruction

Congenital colorectal obstruction may be caused by (1) Hirschsprung disease, (2) a meconium plug, (3) neonatal small left colon syndrome, and, rarely, (4) atresia.

Hirschsprung disease is a disorder in which ganglion cells of the parasympathetic nervous system are absent from the wall of the distal intestinal tract. Embryologically, these cells migrate from the esophagus to the anus. In Hirschsprung disease, ganglion cells are arrested in their descent or development. The transition zone between the narrow aganglionic distal bowel and the dilated normal proximal bowel is usually in the rectosigmoid colon but can occur anywhere, with the entire colon or even the small intestine being aganglionic. The aganglionic bowel is not capable of normal peristalsis, producing a functional obstruction at the transition zone. The condition may first present in the newborn as a lower bowel obstruction or later in childhood as severe chronic constipation. A contrast enema usually demonstrates the transition zone (Figure 21-8), and anorectal manometry will show the absence of the internal sphincter relaxation reflex. A suction

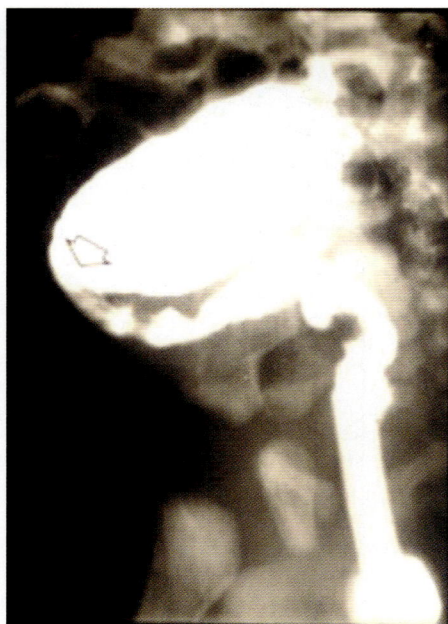

Figure 21-8. Infant with Hirschsprung disease. Barium enema shows the transition zone (arrow) between the distal aganglionic rectum and the dilated proximal colon.

rectal biopsy will confirm the absence of ganglion cells and can be augmented by staining for acetylcholinesterase, which is increased with hypertrophied nerves as well as for calretinin, which in the context of Hirschsprung will show the absence of staining. This can be performed at the bedside of neonates, typically up to about 6 months of age.

The treatment for Hirschsprung disease is resection of the diseased segment of aganglionic colon, which can be performed with laparoscopic assistance or completely transanally with endorectal techniques. Historically, a colostomy was performed after confirming the level of aganglionosis, and a staged pull-through procedure was performed; however, this is rarely necessary. Initial management with antibiotics and rectal irrigations helps avoid the complication of Hirschsprung disease–associated enterocolitis. Single-staged definitive surgery is possible within the first few months of life as long as the child is nutritionally optimized.

Children with Hirschsprung disease may develop severe enterocolitis, with dehydration, peritonitis, and sepsis. This may be the first manifestation of the disease, or it may even occur after surgery. Treatment of Hirschsprung enterocolitis must be prompt with IV fluids, antibiotics, and colonic irrigations.

Meconium plug and small left colon syndrome are functional causes of large bowel obstruction, likely caused by transient motility disturbances of the immature colon. Meconium plugs frequently occur in premature babies, whereas small left colon syndrome is most common in infants of mothers with diabetes. A contrast enema is generally both diagnostic and therapeutic. Babies are usually normal after treatment, but subsequent testing for Hirschsprung disease or cystic fibrosis may be indicated because both are diagnoses of exclusion.

Anorectal Malformations

Anorectal malformations (imperforate anus) represent a spectrum of disorders in which the rectum fails to reach its normal perineal termination. When the rectum ends above the levator muscles, the malformations are classified as high, and when it passes through these muscles, the malformations are low. High lesions are more frequent in males and low ones in females.

Pathophysiology

Although the rectum may end blindly in both types of defects, it usually terminates in an anterior fistulous tract. In high anomalies, the fistula communicates with the urethra or bladder in males (Figure 21-9A) and with the vestibule of the vagina in females. A true rectovaginal fistula in a female is rare and potentially represents a cloaca (Figure 21-9C). In low malformations, the fistula drains externally in both genders, anterior to the normal anal site (Figure 21-9B and D). Imperforate anus is part of the VACTERL association (see section "Esophageal Atresia and Tracheoesophageal Fistula"), and associated abnormalities, particularly genitourinary, frequently occur.

Clinical Presentation and Evaluation

The diagnosis of an imperforate anus is usually obvious on inspection. Either no perineal opening exists (Figure 21-10) or a fistula may be visible. In males, the external fistula is usually a small opening in the anterior perineum or as far forward as the scrotal raphe. Females may also have an external fistula draining into the anterior perineum or else into the posterior vulva (vestibular fistula). A single perineal orifice in a female signifies a cloaca, where the rectum, vagina, and urethra all open into one common chamber. Common cloacal channel lengths greater than 3 cm represent a severe malformation and should be referred to specialty centers.

The management of babies with high and low anorectal malformations differs considerably, and it is therefore essential to distinguish between them. The presence of an external fistula *usually* signifies a low lesion. In the absence of a visible fistula, most lesions are intermediate or high. If the level of the rectal termination is not clear, an "invertogram" is traditionally performed. The baby is held prone and head-down, and if on lateral x-ray air in the rectum rises to within 1 cm of the perineal skin, the lesion is low; if not, it is likely high. The invertogram is being replaced by ultrasound, CT, and magnetic resonance imaging (MRI) to identify the level of the rectum more precisely.

Treatment

Continence normally depends on the coordinated actions of the external sphincter, internal sphincter, and levator muscles. Because the levators are the most important, infants with low lesions in which the bowel descends normally within the levator sling have an excellent functional outlook. A fistula only slightly anterior to the normal anal location (anterior anus) can often function normally and may therefore be left alone. Otherwise, a perineal anoplasty can be performed to establish adequate communication between the rectum and the perineum, at the center of the external sphincter. This operation may be done in the newborn period or later, if the external fistula can be dilated sufficiently to permit the passage of stool.

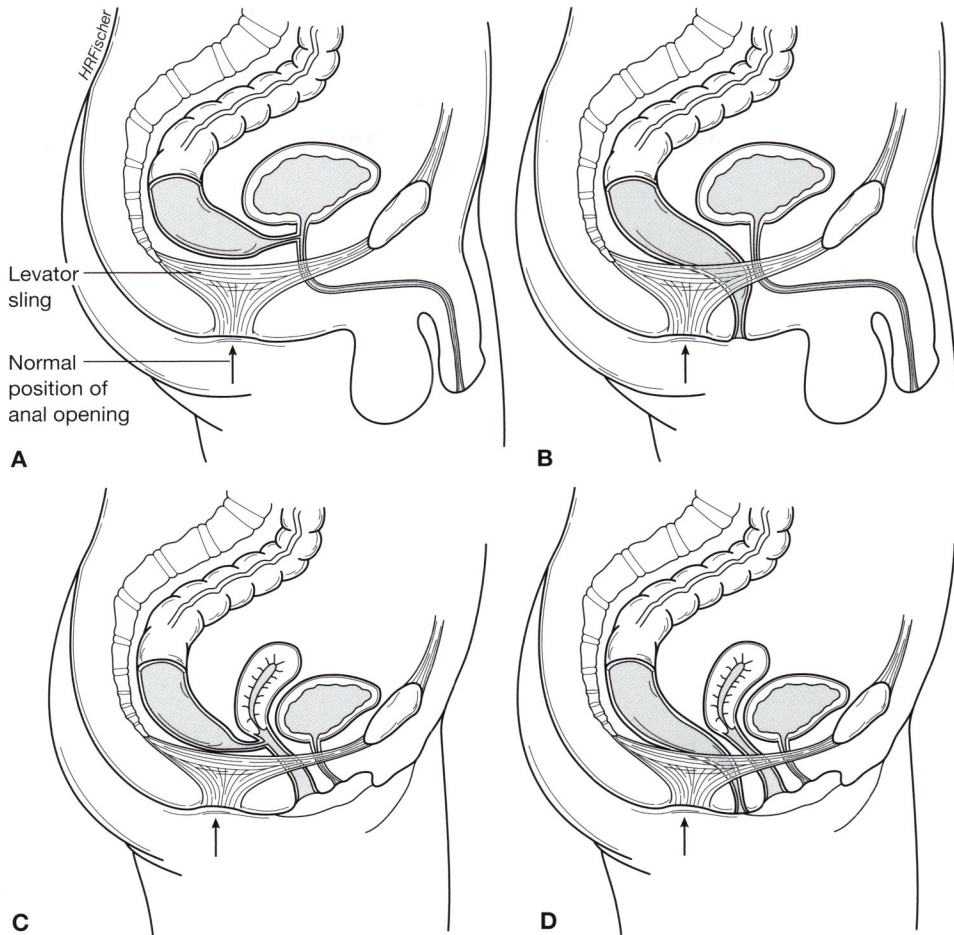

Figure 21-9. **Congenital anorectal malformations.** A. A boy with a high defect and a rectourethral fistula. B. A boy with a low defect and an anoperineal fistula. C. A girl with a high rectovaginal fistula. D. A girl with a rectovestibular fistula. The normal location of the anal opening should be at the external sphincter (arrows). (From Lawrence PF. *Essentials of Surgical Specialties.* 3rd ed. Lippincott Williams & Wilkins; 2007.)

Infants with intermediate and high malformations traditionally require an initial colostomy. Over the next several months, a pull-through procedure is performed, in which the rectum is mobilized, brought through the center of the levator sling, and anastomosed to the perineum. Although various types of pull-throughs have been described, the Peña operation, in which all the muscles are divided posteriorly in the midline from a prone approach, has become the standard because of the excellent visualization that is obtained. More recently, a laparoscopic-assisted approach has been advocated, with or without the use of a protective colostomy. The laparoscopic approach is especially helpful in high malformations because this allows better visualization of the fistula and complete mobilization of the rectum.

Prognosis

The functional prognosis for these children is mixed. Those with low lesions achieve excellent continence, although they often suffer from constipation and may require daily laxatives. Children with high anomalies often have difficulty toilet training, and the majority have at least occasional soiling. These patients often require a structured bowel management program, including daily retrograde enemas to achieve "functional continence." Additionally, the Malone antegrade continence enema (MACE) procedure offers affected children and families improved hygiene through a surgically created appendicostomy that allows daily enema therapy.

Necrotizing Enterocolitis

Necrotizing enterocolitis (NEC) is an acquired ischemic necrosis of the intestine in neonates. It is primarily a disease of premature infants but occasionally occurs in full-term babies. It is the most common indication for emergency surgery in neonates and is a major cause of death in premature infants who survive the first week of life.

Pathophysiology

NEC initially affects the mucosa but can extend to full-thickness injury and perforation. The precise

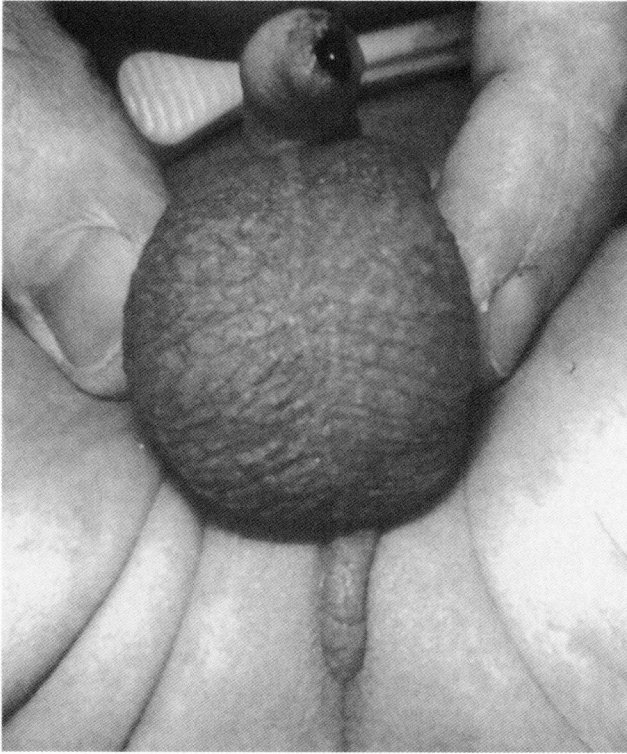

Figure 21-10. A newborn boy with a high anorectal malformation and a rectourethral fistula. The perineal opening is absent, and meconium is seen at the urethral meatus. (From Lawrence PF. *Essentials of Surgical Specialties.* 3rd ed. Lippincott Williams & Wilkins; 2007.)

pathogenesis of NEC is not clear but almost certainly involves an interaction between environmental stressors and unique responses of the GI tract of premature infants. A number of conditions have been shown to increase the incidence of NEC, and all are related to a reduction in the perfusion of the GI tract. Many types of bacteria are associated with NEC, including gram-positive and gram-negative aerobes and anaerobes. NEC is most common in babies who have already been fed because feedings act as a substrate for bacterial proliferation in the intestinal tract. The ileocecal region is most often affected, but any portion of the GI tract may be involved.

Clinical Presentation and Evaluation

Clinical signs of NEC are initially nonspecific and may consist of lethargy, feeding intolerance, temperature instability, and apnea. GI manifestations follow and include vomiting, bloody stools, abdominal distention, and tenderness. Full-blown sepsis may supervene.

Abdominal x-rays may be nonspecific and show only dilated, air-filled loops of the bowel. Pneumatosis intestinalis, the radiographic appearance of intramural gas produced by enteric organisms, is pathognomonic for this disease. Portal venous air may be seen when the intraluminal gas enters the venous drainage system of the GI tract. Laboratory findings are consistent with a systemic infection and include positive blood cultures, leukocytosis or leukopenia, thrombocytopenia, and acidosis.

Metabolic derangements, including positive blood culture, acidosis, bandemia, thrombocytopenia, hyponatremia, hypotension, and neutropenia, should be followed,

and the presence of three of these factors predicts a clinical trajectory that could necessitate surgery.

Treatment

Most babies with NEC recover with medical management and do not need surgery. The goals of treatment are to maximize perfusion of the intestine and treat the infection. Fluid resuscitation is undertaken to restore intravascular volume, an OG tube is inserted to decompress the intestinal tract, broad-spectrum antibiotics are administered, and the infant is observed closely. Indications for surgery are intestinal perforation and full-thickness necrosis. Perforation is usually identified by the presence of pneumoperitoneum (free air) on x-ray (Figure 21-11A and B). Full-thickness necrosis without perforation and perforation without free air on x-ray are difficult to diagnose but are suggested by systemic signs of progressive sepsis (eg, worsening cardiorespiratory function, increased fluid needs, thrombocytopenia) or physical findings of peritonitis (tenderness, guarding, erythema, or edema of the abdominal wall). In equivocal cases, paracentesis that yields peritoneal fluid containing intestinal contents or bacteria strongly suggests bowel necrosis. Surgical therapy usually consists of a laparotomy in which the entire intestine is inspected (Figure 21-11C), and all areas of necrosis are resected. The ends of the viable bowel are usually exteriorized as stomas, but a primary anastomosis may be performed if the disease is limited and the patient is otherwise stable. Alternatively, extremely small (<1,000 g), critically ill infants have been treated initially by the insertion of Penrose drains through a mini-laparotomy, which can be performed at the patient's bedside (Figure 21-11D). The patient is followed closely, and laparotomy is undertaken if the clinical condition fails to improve.

Prognosis

The overall survival rate of babies with NEC is 80%. In those who require emergency surgery, the survival rate is 50% to 80%. Of those who are initially treated successfully nonoperatively, 10% later have a stricture and require an operation for intestinal obstruction.

Short Bowel Syndrome

Short bowel syndrome (SBS) occurs when there is insufficient small intestine to digest and absorb essential nutrients for growth and development. The incidence is increasing because more infants and children are surviving following

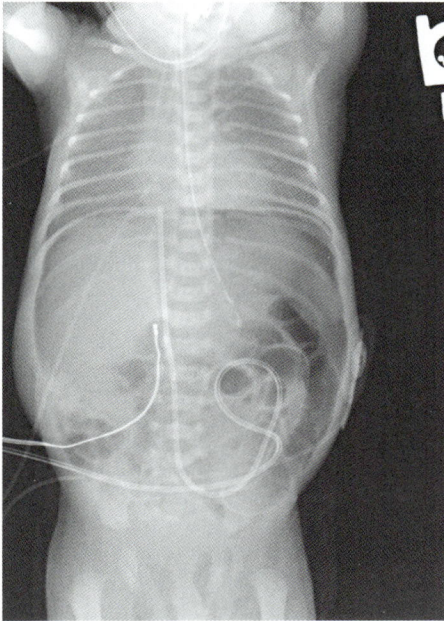

A

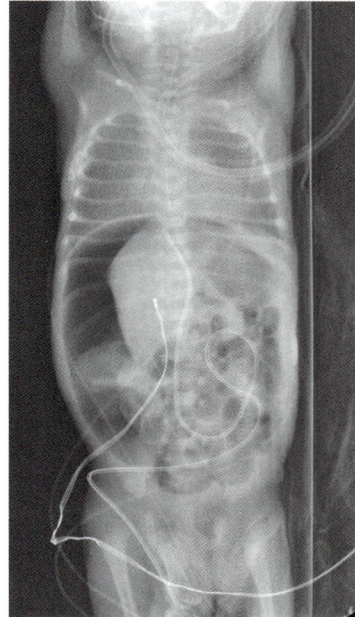

B

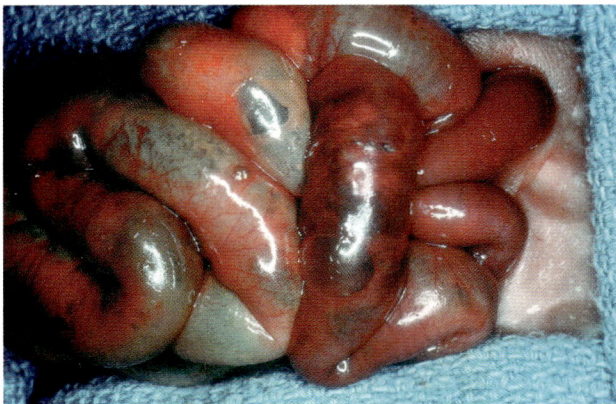

C

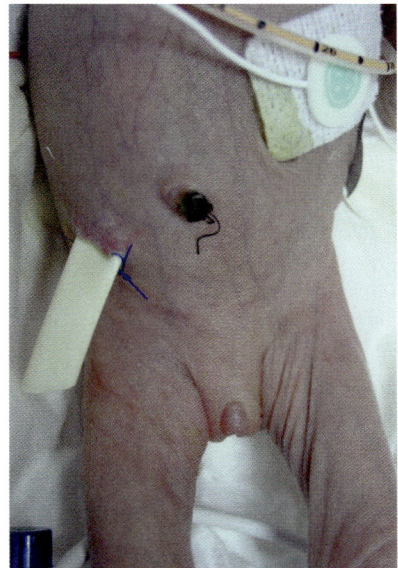

D

Figure 21-11. A premature infant with necrotizing enterocolitis and pneumatosis intestinalis. A. The "football sign" of massive pneumoperitoneum. B. Left lateral decubitus in the same patient. C. Intraoperative photograph revealing patchy ischemia. D. A premature infant treated with bedside Penrose drain.

the loss of massive lengths of small intestine from conditions such as NEC, midgut volvulus, and long-segment Hirschsprung disease. The severity depends not only on the absolute length of the remaining small intestine but also on the age of the child, the particular portion of small bowel remaining, the presence of an ileocecal valve and colon, and the degree of adaptation that has occurred. Although the term infant normally has 200 to 250 cm of small intestine, survival without IV nutrition has eventually been attained with as little as 15 to 20 cm with an ileocecal valve and 40 cm without one.

Malabsorption, along with the malnutrition and diarrhea that result, is primarily caused by the loss of mucosal absorptive surface and a decrease in transit time through the foreshortened GI tract. These problems may be compounded by osmotic and secretory diarrhea that can be produced by insufficient absorption of digestive enzymes, fermentation of undigested sugars by colonic bacteria, the irritative effect of unabsorbed bile salts, and acid hypersecretion by the stomach due to elevated gastrin levels. Other major complications of SBS are sepsis from translocation of intestinal bacteria and liver failure. Fortunately, adaptation occurs over time as the intestine lengthens and dilates, villi undergo hypertrophy, and transit time decreases. The ileum is more capable of undergoing adaptation than is the jejunum. In addition, the use of newer formulations of parenteral nutrition not metabolized by the liver has resulted in a significant decrease in liver failure, allowing children to receive sufficient parenteral calories for lengthy periods of time.

Treatment of SBS is primarily a delicate balancing act between IV and enteral feedings. Elemental formulas are employed initially and are often better absorbed when administered continuously than by bolus. These enteral feeds are gradually increased as adaptation occurs and are slowly transitioned to more complex formulas. Medications may also be beneficial and can include drugs to reduce intestinal motility (eg, loperamide, diphenoxylate); drugs to decrease gastric secretion (histamine-2 blocking agents such as ranitidine or proton pump inhibitors such as omeprazole); cholestyramine to bind bile salts; somatostatin to decrease biliary, pancreatic, and intestinal secretions; and antibiotics to inhibit bacterial overgrowth.

The goals of surgical therapy, employed when medical management and intestinal adaptation fail, are as follows: reestablish intestinal continuity, eliminate stasis, and increase effective absorptive surface. Serial transverse enteroplasty procedure (STEP) produces an elongated bowel and will allow many children to be weaned from IV nutrition. Finally, if all other measures prove unsuccessful in managing SBS, particularly when accompanied by liver failure, intestinal transplantation or multivisceral transplantation should be considered.

Neonatal Jaundice: Biliary Atresia and Choledochal Cyst

Neonatal jaundice is usually caused by physiologic indirect hyperbilirubinemia and is self-limited. A direct bilirubinemia of more than 2 mg/dL that persists for more than 2 weeks warrants further investigation.

Pathophysiology

Biliary atresia is a progressive inflammatory obliteration of unknown etiology that may affect part or all of the biliary ductal system. Infantile choledochal cysts, which usually consist of rounded, cystic dilatations of the common bile duct with distal narrowing, producing biliary obstruction, may be another manifestation of the same disease. The incidence of these disease processes is significantly increased in individuals of Asian descent.

Clinical Presentation and Evaluation

An infant with biliary atresia has progressive jaundice during the first several weeks of life. The stools are pale, the liver is usually enlarged, and levels of serum conjugated bilirubin, alkaline phosphatase, and other liver enzymes are elevated. Choledochal cysts may present in a similar fashion, although the typical presentation would be later in life with pancreatitis. Also, these lesions are increasingly identified on prenatal imaging. Other causes of neonatal jaundice include TORCH (toxoplasmosis, rubella, cytomegalovirus, and herpes) infections, α_1-antitrypsin deficiency, galactosemia, and TPN or hypoxic injury to the liver. The usual evaluation includes ultrasound and hepatic scintiscan. Ultrasonography and magnetic resonance cholangiopancreatography can identify a choledochal cyst, and the demonstration of bile flow into the duodenum or the scintiscan excludes the diagnosis of biliary atresia. A percutaneous liver biopsy may also be helpful.

Treatment

If biliary atresia is not excluded in the evaluation of persistent direct hyperbilirubinemia, a laparotomy is performed, the hilum of the liver is inspected, and a cholangiogram is performed. The finding of a patent biliary system excludes the diagnosis of biliary atresia. If biliary atresia is confirmed, a Kasai portoenterostomy is performed. This procedure involves the excision of the atretic extrahepatic biliary system with the creation of a jejunal conduit for bile drainage from the fibrous-appearing tissue in the hilum of the liver that contains microscopic biliary ductules. Success after this procedure is greatest if it is performed before the child is 60 days of age. In cases of choledochal cyst, the cyst is excised and the biliary system is reconstructed either by anastomosing a defunctionalized Roux-en-Y bowel loop to the proximal hepatic ducts or by direct connection of the hepatic duct to the duodenum.

Prognosis

The success of the Kasai operation depends on the age of the patient, the diameter of the microscopic hepatic ductules, and the severity of hepatic fibrosis. Recurrent postoperative cholangitis is common and results in a progressive deterioration of hepatic function. Portal hypertension with esophageal varices may develop even with the restoration of bile flow.

Approximately 30% of infants ultimately do well after portoenterostomy and do not require additional surgery. Liver transplantation is the other available therapy and is generally reserved for patients with severe hepatic fibrosis at presentation or progressive liver disease. Infant livers are rarely available, so segments from adult donors are used. In contrast to the prognosis for patients with biliary atresia, the prognosis for patients who undergo excision of choledochal cysts is excellent. Unresected choledochal cysts have significant potential for cholangiocarcinoma.

Abdominal Wall Defects: Omphalocele and Gastroschisis

Omphalocele and gastroschisis are congenital defects of the abdominal wall through which the abdominal contents variably protrude externally. The incidence of gastroschisis is reported to be between 1:2,000 and 1:3,000 live births, with increasing frequency. Omphalocele occurs in approximately 1:5,000 live births. Although these conditions are in many ways similar, there are important differences.

Embryology

The abdominal wall is formed by four folds, the cephalic, the caudal, and two lateral folds, which converge ventrally to form a large umbilical ring surrounding the umbilical cord vessels and yolk sac. During development, the ring contracts to close the abdominal wall. Between the fifth and tenth weeks of gestation, the rapidly growing intestine is extruded out of the umbilical ring and into the yolk sac. It then returns to the abdominal cavity, where it undergoes rotation.

Pathophysiology

An omphalocele results when the lateral folds do not close and the extruded viscera remain in the yolk sac. Gastroschisis may be caused by an in utero perforation of the developing abdominal wall at the point where one of the paired umbilical veins undergoes atrophy, an area of relative weakness; alternatively, there is evidence that gastroschisis may be produced by the antenatal perforation of a small omphalocele sac.

Clinical Presentation

Babies with an omphalocele have an opening in the center of the abdominal wall, and the protruding viscera are covered by a translucent membrane (Figure 21-12). The umbilical cord inserts into the center of the omphalocele sac. In babies with gastroschisis, the opening is lateral to the umbilical cord, usually to the right (Figure 21-13A). The exteriorized viscera are not covered by a membrane and often become thickened and edematous. In both conditions, the size of the defect and the amount of protruding viscera are variable.

Babies with an omphalocele have a high incidence of associated congenital anomalies, including chromosomal defects. In contrast, the only associated disorder noted with increased frequency in babies with gastroschisis is intestinal atresia. These atresias are probably caused by in utero compression and vascular compromise of the bowel against the rim of the abdominal defect.

Treatment

Immediately after birth, infants with abdominal wall defects are at risk for fluid and heat loss from the exposed viscera. The viscera should be kept moist with saline, and the abdomen should be wrapped in plastic. IV fluids and broad-spectrum antibiotics are given, and nasogastric decompression is instituted. In babies with gastroschisis, the viscera should remain on top of the baby or the baby turned on their side to avoid kinking the vascular supply of the protruding bowel. Cyanosis of the viscera mandates immediate enlargement of the fascial defect at the bedside.

Babies with gastroschisis require emergency surgery to replace the viscera in the abdomen and close the defect. If the abdominal cavity is too small to allow primary closure without undue tension, a prefabricated silo is used to protect the bowel because a provider gradually reduces the bowel over the next week (Figure 21-13B). A preformed spring-loaded silo is also available for this purpose. The silo is manually compressed daily over the course of a week to gradually reduce the viscera and expand the abdominal cavity. Increasingly, babies are being treated with immediate reduction with coverage of the defect with the umbilical cord. The umbilical cord is then secured in place with Steri-strips, and a dressing is applied. No sutures are applied, and this can be accomplished at the bedside without the baby ever requiring anesthesia. The defect can completely close with this technique.

An omphalocele is treated in a similar fashion, except that surgery is not so emergent and time can be taken to evaluate associated anomalies. In cases of severe associated malformations or prohibitive operative risks, the omphalocele sac can be painted with an antiseptic (eg, silver sulfadiazine [Silvadene] or povidone-iodine). The sac eventually epithelializes and contracts, leaving a ventral hernia that can be repaired electively. Large omphaloceles present a particular challenge, given the underdevelopment of the abdominal cavity and poor tolerance of reductions.

Atresias associated with gastroschisis are best repaired after the swelling and inflammation subside (Figure 21-14). Recovery and enteral autonomy may be prolonged.

Prognosis

Infants with gastroschisis may have prolonged intestinal dysfunction after surgery as a result of chronic inflammation of the exposed bowel. However, the long-term outlook is generally good. The ultimate prognosis for babies with omphaloceles is usually related to any associated anomalies that may be present.

Circumcision

Circumcision, among the oldest surgical procedures known, is the most frequently performed operation on males in the United States. Although approximately 90% of boys in the United States undergo neonatal circumcision, routine circumcision is performed in only 32% of boys in Canada, 15% in Australia, and rarely in Europe. Circumcision remains a controversial topic, even within the medical profession. The American Academy of Pediatrics Task

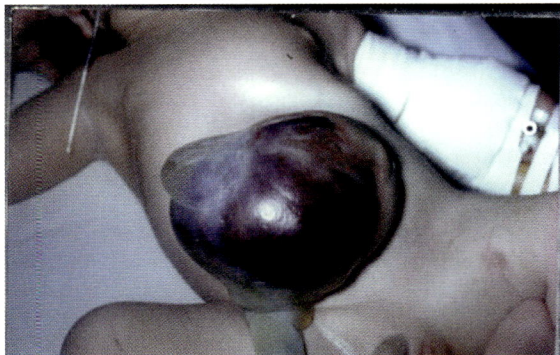

Figure 21-12. A large omphalocele that contains visible loops of the intestine. The umbilical cord arises from the intact sac.

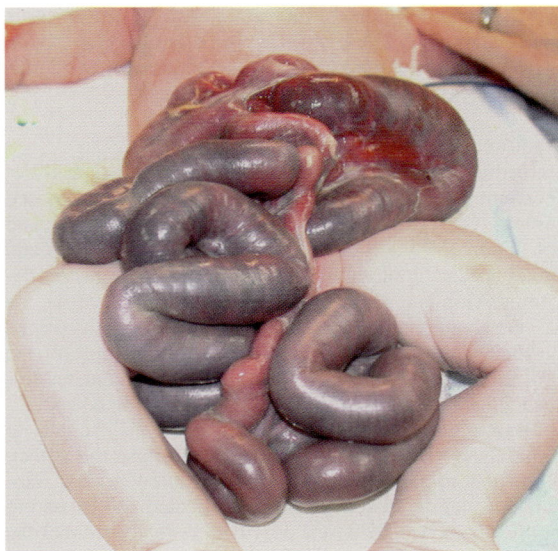 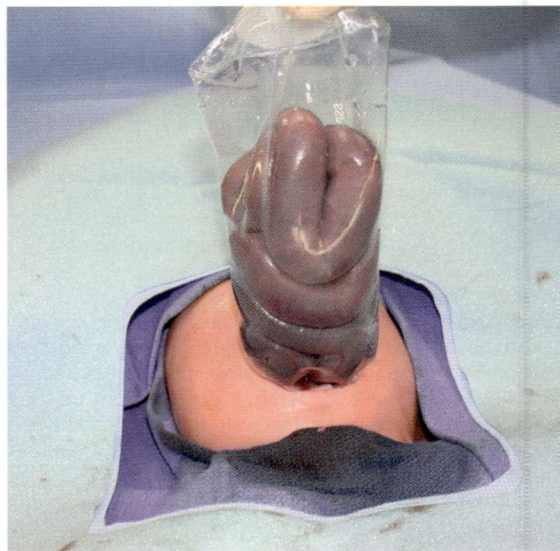

A   B

Figure 21-13. **A.** Gastroschisis, with exteriorized intestine that is not covered by a sac. B. Bowel secured in prefashioned silo placed at the bedside.

Force on Circumcision, in its updated 2012 policy statement, endorsed neonatal circumcision, stating that the risks were outweighed by the benefits, including prevention of urinary tract infections, reduced risk of penile cancer, and reduced transmission of some sexually transmitted infections without adversely affecting penile sexual function or sensitivity. Other notable organizations have warned that the risks outweigh the benefits in routine neonatal circumcision. Effective analgesia, such as a penile nerve block, is strongly recommended for the procedure.

The prepuce, or foreskin, completely covers the glans, except for a small opening at the urethral meatus. The undersurface of the foreskin is fused with the glans at birth with congenital adhesions, and it is not until later in childhood that the foreskin is fully retractable. In uncircumcised boys, attempts at retraction should be avoided until 2 to 3 years of age. True phimosis is the inability to pull back the foreskin because of fibrotic narrowing at the preputial orifice, not these physiologic adhesions.

SURGICAL CONDITIONS IN THE OLDER CHILD

Inguinal Hernia and Hydrocele

Inguinal hernias and hydroceles are extremely common in children. Their repair is the most common operation performed by pediatric surgeons. Hernias occur in 3% to 5% of children overall. The incidence rises to 30% in very premature infants. Conditions that may increase intra-abdominal pressure or weaken connective tissues (eg, ascites, connective tissue disorders) may also predispose children to hernias. Boys are affected 6 times as often as girls. Inguinal hernias in children are virtually all indirect, with the hernia sac emerging through the internal inguinal ring. Direct and femoral hernias are rare.

Embryology

At 3 months' gestation, the processus vaginalis forms as an outpouching of the peritoneum and passes through the internal inguinal ring. This structure then migrates down the inguinal canal, out of the external ring, and into the scrotum, preceding the testicle, and comes to lie within the spermatic cord. The processus usually becomes obliterated around the time of birth, except for the most distal portion, which remains surrounding the testicle as the tunica vaginalis (Figure 21-15A).

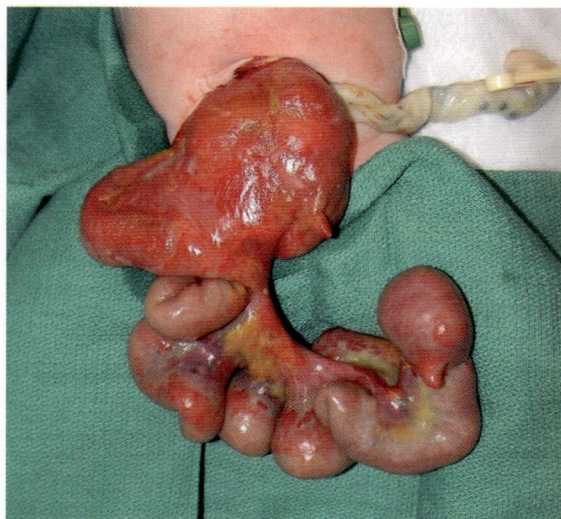

Figure 21-14. Complicated gastroschisis with intestinal atresia and short bowel syndrome. Note that the defect is to the right of the umbilical cord.

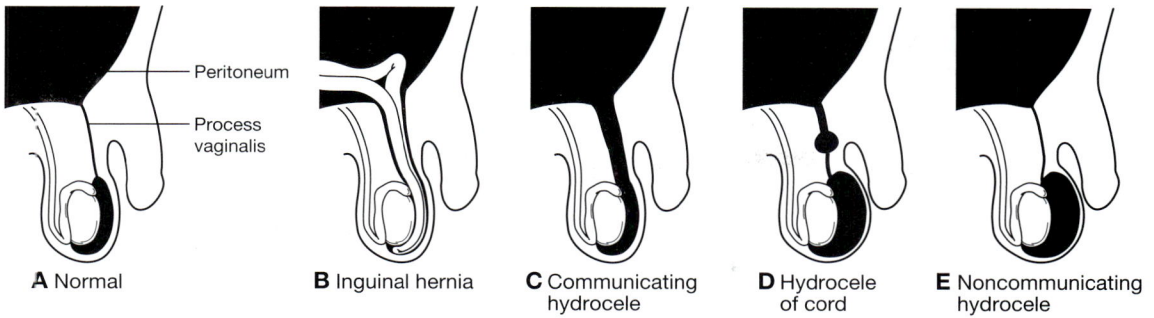

Figure 21-15. A. Normal anatomy. B. Inguinal hernia. C. Communicating hydrocele. D. Hydrocele of cord. E. Noncommunicating hydrocele. (From Lawrence PF. *Essentials of Surgical Specialties*. 3rd ed. Lippincott Williams & Wilkins; 2007.)

Pathophysiology

Continued patency of part or all of the processus vaginalis accounts for the development of hernias and hydroceles. If the processus remains widely open proximally, in continuity with the peritoneal cavity, the intra-abdominal contents may variably protrude into it, forming an inguinal hernia (Figure 21-15B). If the processus remains open but is too narrow to admit any viscera, only peritoneal fluid may enter. Usually, this fluid surrounds the testicle within the widened tunica vaginalis, forming a communicating hydrocele (Figure 21-15C). Less often, if the distal processus is obliterated, the fluid accumulates above the testicle as a hydrocele of the spermatic cord (Figure 21-15D). Finally, with obliteration of the proximal processus, fluid may remain trapped distally in the tunica vaginalis, producing a noncommunicating hydrocele (Figure 21-15E).

In girls, the round ligament is a vestigial structure analogous to the spermatic cord and has the same relation to the processus vaginalis. In addition to the bowel, the ovary or Fallopian tube may enter a patent processus. Of note, sliding hernias are more common in girls.

Clinical Presentation and Evaluation

Approximately half of all inguinal hernias appear during the first year of life. They occur twice as often on the right side as on the left because the right testicle descends later embryologically, and its processus is therefore less likely to have closed. Ten percent of inguinal hernias are bilateral. The hernia usually causes an intermittent bulge in the groin or scrotum, brought on by crying or straining. On examination, it is palpable as a firm mass that completely disappears with digital pressure (Figure 21-16). If not apparent, a hernia may be brought out by applying suprapubic pressure in infants or by asking older children to jump or strain. Suggestive evidence of an inguinal hernia consists of a palpable thickening of the spermatic cord where it crosses the pubic tubercle (ie, "silk glove" sign). A hydrocele usually causes diffuse swelling of the hemiscrotum. If it communicates with the peritoneal cavity, it fluctuates in size throughout the day as it fills and empties. Noncommunicating hydroceles remain fairly constant in size but may gradually regress as fluid is absorbed.

Hernias can almost always be differentiated from hydroceles on physical examination. A hydrocele is more mobile, is not reducible, and does not extend upward into the internal ring. A hydrocele of the cord may be more difficult to distinguish from an incarcerated hernia because both are manifested as an irreducible mass above the testis. Hydroceles, however, produce no symptoms, whereas incarcerated hernias are quite painful and may produce intestinal obstruction. Transillumination is not particularly reliable, especially in infants in whom the thin bowel wall may transmit light readily. Table 21-8 summarizes the differences between hernias and hydroceles.

Treatment

Inguinal hernias in children never resolve and are at risk for incarceration and strangulation. The incarceration rate of inguinal hernia is approximately 10%, with the highest incidence occurring in the first 6 months of life. Therefore, all inguinal hernias should be repaired by high ligation of the hernia sac at the internal ring. Repair of the floor of the inguinal canal, as is performed in adults, is unnecessary. The operation is usually carried out on an outpatient basis soon after diagnosis and can be performed via a small groin incision. Recently, some surgeons have adopted a laparoscopic approach. A dilemma is presented in the treatment of the very young and especially the premature infant because of the predisposition to postanesthesia apnea. If surgery is performed less than 52 weeks from conception, overnight monitoring in the hospital is necessary,

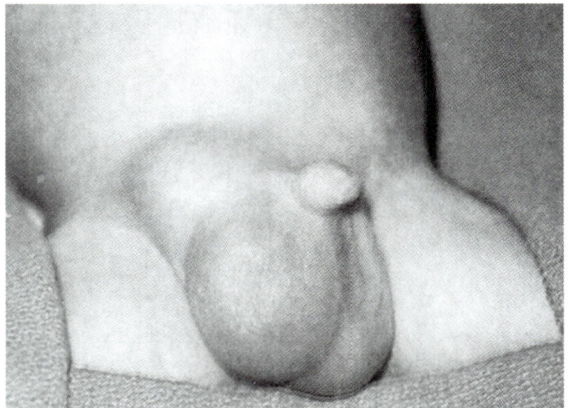

Figure 21-16. A right inguinal hernia in a 5-month-old boy. (From Lawrence PF. *Essentials of Surgical Specialties*. 3rd ed. Lippincott Williams & Wilkins; 2007.)

TABLE 21-8. Differential Diagnosis of Groin Masses in Children

	Hydrocele	Reducible Inguinal Hernia	Incarcerated Inguinal Hernia
Age	Most <1 y	Any age	Any age
Overall state	Well	Well	Ill, anorexic, vomiting
Pain and tenderness	None	None	Severe
Diurnal changes	None or evening fluctuation	Protrudes on straining	Always protruded
Site of swelling	Usually scrotum	Groin with or without scrotum	Usually groin and scrotum
Physical findings	Round, smooth, mobile	Firm, elongated, disappears completely with pressure	Firm, fixed; cannot feel superior edge
Transillumination	++	None (except in infants)	±
Reducible	No	Yes	Possible
Abdominal x-ray	Normal	With or without air in the groin	All in the groin; bowel obstruction
Treatment	Repair at 1 y	Elective repair	Immediate attention

including routine use of an apnea monitor. Postoperative recovery is rapid in children, and complications (eg, damage to the vas deferens or testicular vessels) and recurrence are uncommon.

An incarcerated hernia is an emergency, not only because of the risk of strangulation of the hernia contents but also because the testicle may become ischemic. An incarcerated hernia in a child can almost always be reduced. Slow, persistent pressure is applied bimanually on the mass. Sedation is not uniformly required. Following successful reduction, hernia repair is delayed for 24 to 48 hours until the edema of the sac subsides. If reduction fails, surgery is performed without delay.

A child with one inguinal hernia has an increased risk of having another one on the contralateral side. Although opinions vary, historically, surgeons recommend routine exploration of the opposite side in children with a greater likelihood of bilaterality, such as in premature boys, as well as in young girls. Currently, most surgeons simply observe the contralateral side or perform diagnostic laparoscopy by inserting a small-angled laparoscope into the peritoneal cavity through the hernia sac to visualize the opposite internal ring. Both internal rings are routinely examined in a primary umbilical laparoscopic approach.

Unlike hernias, most neonatal noncommunicating hydroceles resolve within the first or second year of life. Hydroceles that persist after that time or develop later are unlikely to resolve and should be electively repaired.

Umbilical Hernia

Pathophysiology

Umbilical hernias are caused by the failure of the umbilical ring to contract completely. They are especially common in African American infants or children, in whom the incidence approaches 50%. Unlike inguinal hernias, most umbilical hernias resolve spontaneously during childhood. The risk of incarceration in infants is extremely low.

Clinical Presentation and Evaluation

The diagnosis is apparent by the presence of a bulge within the umbilicus. The fascial defect is readily palpable after the mass is reduced. Diastasis recti, which does not require operative intervention, may occasionally be confused with an abdominal wall hernia.

Treatment

Surgery is usually recommended when the hernia persists beyond 4 years of age. Parents are often anxious about these very visible protrusions. If the fascial defect remains larger than 1.5 cm by the time the child is 2 years old, spontaneous closure is unlikely and early repair may be considered. Girls especially should have an umbilical hernia corrected before pregnancy, a time when increased intra-abdominal pressure could lead to complications. Skin excoriation over the hernia and pain from incarcerated fat are other rare indications for early operation. Occasionally, a proboscis skin deformity will necessitate tissue rearrangement through umbilicoplasty at the time of primary fascial repair.

Cryptorchidism

A cryptorchid testis is one that has not descended into the scrotum, an event that normally takes place between the seventh and ninth months of gestation. The incidence of cryptorchidism at the time of birth is 3% in term infants and up to 30% in preterm infants. Most testes that are cryptorchid at birth spontaneously descend within the first year.

Pathophysiology

Ultrastructural studies show that by the second year of a child's life, undescended testes already have histologic abnormalities. The fertility potential of an undescended testis is never 100%, but its repositioning in the cooler scrotal environment maximizes the potential for sperm production and function. Evidence suggests that if a testis is left undescended, it may adversely affect spermatogenesis in the opposite, normally descended testicle.

The incidence of subsequent testicular malignancy in children with undescended testes is 10 to 40 times that of the general population. This risk begins to increase in young adulthood. Recent evidence, based on longitudinal studies of adults who had orchidopexy performed as young children, suggests that successful orchidopexy in young childhood reduces the risk of subsequent testicular cancer to that of normal controls. Orchidopexy performed in older children and adolescents does not reduce the risk of testicular malignancy, but it facilitates the early detection of testicular tumors on physical examination. Other problems encountered in boys with cryptorchidism include an increased risk of testicular torsion, more vulnerability to trauma, and psychological concerns.

Clinical Presentation and Evaluation

A cryptorchid testicle is absent from the scrotum and may be palpable in the groin. It must be differentiated from the much more common retractile testis that is pulled up transiently by an active cremasteric reflex. If the testicle can be manipulated into the scrotum without tension, even if it does not remain there, the parents can be assured that no abnormality is present and that observation alone is indicated. A daily family journal of testicular position might also help differentiate retractile testicle from cryptorchid testicle. A cryptorchid testis may also be present ectopically. Therefore, examination should include careful palpation of the suprapubic, perineal, and upper inner thigh areas.

A testicle that is not palpable may be absent or located above the internal ring. Although ultrasound, CT, and MRI scanning have been advocated as imaging modalities, failure to visualize a testicle is not sufficient proof of its absence. Laparoscopy has become the procedure of choice because in many instances it allows both accurate diagnosis and treatment (Figure 21-17). In infants with bilateral nonpalpable testes, a human chorionic gonadotropin (hCG) stimulation test may be performed. If the serum testosterone level does not rise markedly in response to hCG administration, no testicular tissue exists.

Treatment

Hormonal treatment with hCG and, more recently, luteinizing hormone–releasing hormone has been advocated as an initial treatment of cryptorchidism. However, the results are conflicting. Hormonal therapy may be rationally attempted in boys with bilateral cryptorchidism, in whom it is more plausible that an underlying hormonal deficiency is responsible for the undescended testes.

Orchidopexy is recommended for all boys whose testes remain undescended. It is usually performed between 6 and 12 months of life. After appropriate dissection and closure of the patent processus vaginalis, the testicle is secured to a dartos pouch in the lower hemiscrotum (Figure 21-18). A two-stage Fowler-Stephens approach may be required for intra-abdominal testis. Orchiectomy, either laparoscopic or open, is indicated for atrophic testes and those first encountered in late puberty. Testicular prosthesis can be considered.

Prognosis

After early successful orchidopexy for unilateral cryptorchidism, 80% to 90% of boys are subsequently fertile. Only 50% of boys with bilateral cryptorchidism are fertile after bilateral orchidopexy. In contrast, testosterone production by the testes is unaffected by their location, and secondary sexual characteristics develop normally in all of these boys. Young men whose orchidopexy was performed in older childhood should be advised to do regular testicular self-examinations.

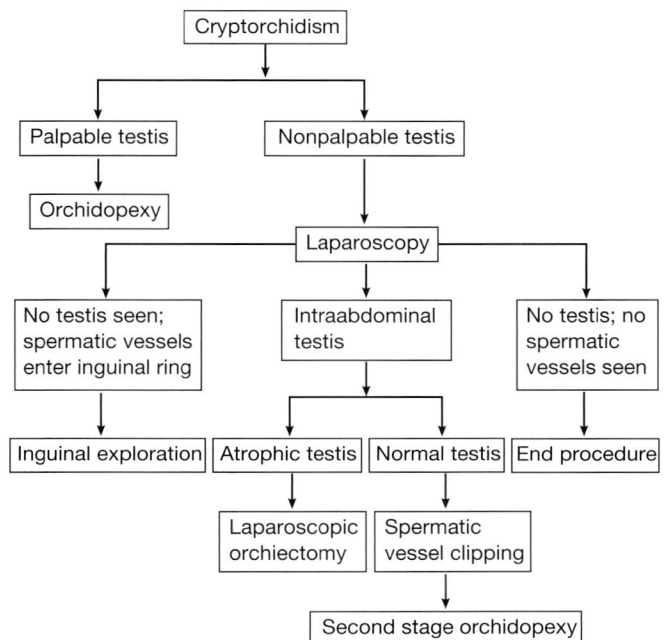

Figure 21-17. Algorithm for the management of a cryptorchid testis. (From Lawrence PF. *Essentials of Surgical Specialties*. 3rd ed. Lippincott Williams & Wilkins; 2007.)

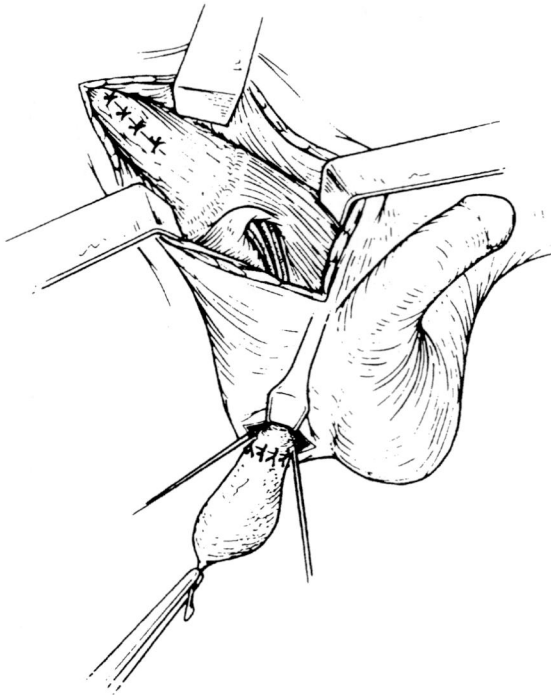

Figure 21-18. Orchiopexy for cryptorchidism. The undescended testicle is brought down and implanted into the scrotum between the dartos layer and the skin. (From Lawrence PF. *Essentials of Surgical Specialties.* 3rd ed. Lippincott Williams & Wilkins; 2007.)

Pyloric Stenosis

Pyloric stenosis is a progressive hypertrophy of the musculature of the pylorus in infancy, leading to gastric outlet obstruction. It is a common disorder, occurring in 1:500 infants. It affects males 4 times as often as females, and it has a strong familial component.

Pathophysiology

The etiology of pyloric stenosis is not known. One hypothesis suggests abnormal development of the ganglion cells in the wall of the pylorus. Another proposal is that milk curds propelled against the pylorus produce submucosal edema that initially blocks the gastric outlet, leading to subsequent work hypertrophy of the muscular pylorus.

Clinical Presentation and Evaluation

An infant with pyloric stenosis typically presents at 2 to 8 weeks of age with nonbilious vomiting after feeds. The vomiting, which may be projectile, becomes progressively worse until little is kept down. The infant remains hungry between vomiting episodes and sucks vigorously. Stool frequency and urinary output may diminish.

On examination, the infant may appear irritable and dehydrated to a variable degree. Peristaltic waves are sometimes seen moving across the abdomen. The hallmark of pyloric stenosis is the palpable "olive," a hard, round, movable mass in the epigastrium. Success in palpating the pyloric mass depends on the examiner's experience and

patience. The infant can be given an electrolyte and mineral supplement (Pedialyte) or a pacifier coated with sugar to promote relaxation. Then the stomach can be emptied with a nasogastric tube. When an olive is identified, no imaging studies are necessary.

If no palpable olive is found, ultrasonography is highly accurate in diagnosing pyloric stenosis because the length, diameter, and wall thickness of the pylorus are all increased (Figure 21-19). If this study is equivocal, an UGI is obtained. It shows a narrowed, elongated pyloric channel with shouldering.

Treatment

Appropriate preoperative rehydration is essential. Pyloric stenosis is a medical, not surgical, emergency. These infants have been vomiting gastric contents and often have hypochloremic, hypokalemic, metabolic alkalosis. Depending on the extent of dehydration and alkalosis, D5% in ½ normal saline or D5% in normal saline with 20 to 40 mEq/L KCl is administered at 1½ to 2 times the maintenance rate. When urine output is 1 to 2 mL/kg/h and serum electrolytes are normal, operative correction may proceed with a pyloromyotomy, either open or laparoscopically. This procedure involves a longitudinal split of the hypertrophic pyloric muscle that extends down to the mucosa but does not enter it (Figure 21-20). Surgeon knowledge of the precise ultrasound measurements is helpful during the pyloromyotomy. Feeding is initiated 2 to 4 hours postoperatively and increased gradually until a regular schedule is tolerated. Most infants are discharged within 24 to 48 hours postoperatively.

Prognosis

Infants may have transient vomiting postoperatively, either as a result of a chronically overdistended stomach or from mucosal irritation. Significant complications are rare.

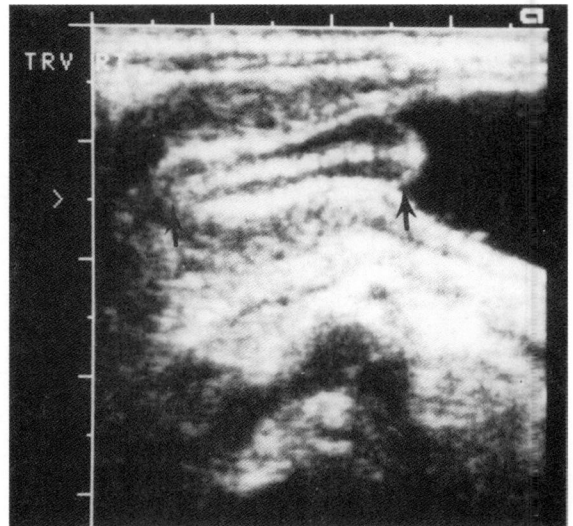

Figure 21-19. Ultrasound appearance of pyloric stenosis. The narrowed, elongated pyloric channel (between arrows) has thickened walls. (Reprinted from Lesions of the stomach. In Ashcraft K, ed. *Atlas of Pediatric Surgery.* WB Saunders; 1994:292. Copyright © 1994 Elsevier, with permission.)

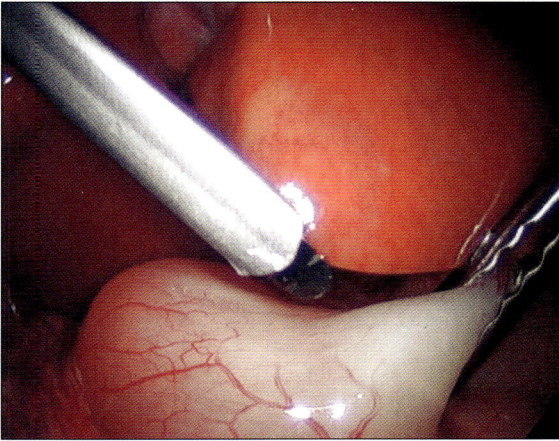
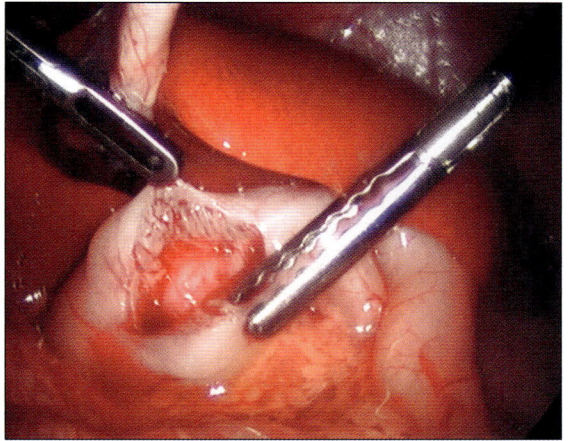

A **B**

Figure 21-20. Laparoscopic pyloromyotomy. A. The hypertrophic pylorus is secured. B. Longitudinal incision that extends down to, but not through, the mucosa.

Acute Abdomen

Children who have acute abdominal pain present a challenge for all physicians involved in their care. The diagnostic dilemma involves differentiating children who need immediate surgery from the many others who may be managed conservatively. Several factors contribute to the diagnostic challenge:

1. Young children tend to have a uniform response to infection. Whether they have streptococcal pharyngitis, pneumonia, viral gastroenteritis, or appendicitis, they often have fever, vomiting, and a stomachache.
2. Most surgical diseases in children are age dependent. The relative risks for various conditions vary significantly with age.
3. Children have a limited ability to express their symptoms. The younger they are, the less likely they are to have classic manifestations of various abdominal conditions.
4. A child who is in pain is not a cooperative patient, and even a simple abdominal examination can be a challenge. A child who is asleep or lying in their parent's arms should be first examined in that position. Waking the child or placing them in the supine position causes crying and voluntary guarding and significantly reduces the effectiveness of the examination. Building trust through patient interaction with the child and very gentle initial palpation is crucial.
5. Parental anxiety adds to the stress of the situation.

Despite these factors, in most cases, a diagnostic decision can be made chiefly on the basis of a thorough clinical assessment and a few simple added investigations. Although a pathologic diagnosis must be sought, the key decision in acute abdominal pain is whether the child warrants observation or requires immediate surgery. The index of suspicion must be high. In cases of uncertainty, overnight observation with serial examinations by the same observer is warranted.

Appendicitis

Acute appendicitis is the most common condition that requires emergency surgery in childhood. It is rare in infancy, but after that, its incidence increases progressively, peaking in adolescents and young adults. Appendicitis is caused by obstruction at the base of the appendiceal lumen by a fecalith or lymphoid hyperplasia. Mucosal secretions distend the appendix and increase intraluminal pressure, leading to bacterial overgrowth and impairment of perfusion. Without prompt treatment, perforation occurs in 24 to 48 hours. Delayed presentation is much more likely in young children and thus perforation rates are higher.

Clinical Presentation and Evaluation

The initial symptom is almost always pain, although the classic migratory progression from the periumbilical area to the right lower quadrant may not be elicited. Anorexia, nausea, and vomiting are common. The temperature is typically mildly elevated. An early, high fever suggests another diagnosis. Later, it may signify a ruptured appendix. The cheeks are often flushed, and the child is unusually quiet, lying with the knees pulled up. Abdominal examination usually shows diminished bowel sounds and signs of localized peritonitis, with involuntary guarding, tenderness, and rebound in the right lower quadrant. Children with a ruptured appendix are often septic, have abdominal distention from the ileus, and have frank peritonitis. They may also have a right lower quadrant or rectal mass.

Laboratory studies should include a CBC and urinalysis. The white blood cell count is usually elevated or shifted to the left. β-hCG levels should always be obtained in adolescent girls to exclude ectopic pregnancy. Abdominal x-ray films are obtained only in patients in whom the diagnosis of appendicitis is questionable and in the very young in whom the diagnosis is always difficult. The only pathognomonic sign of appendicitis is a calcified fecalith that can be visualized in 5% to 15% of cases (Figure 21-21). Ruptured appendicitis in children may lead to an intra-abdominal

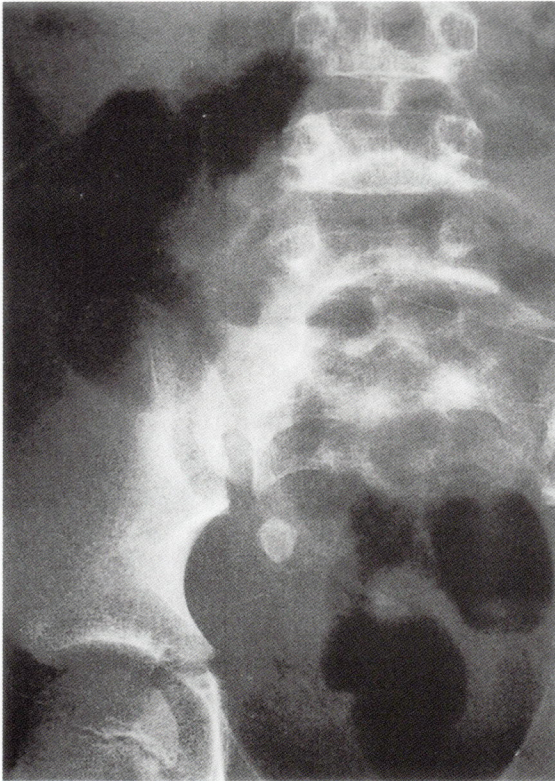

Figure 21-21. Calcified fecalith. (Reprinted from Liebert PS, ed. *Color Atlas of Pediatric Surgery*. 2nd ed. WB Saunders; 1996:188. Copyright © 1996 Elsevier, with permission.)

abscess or incomplete small bowel obstruction. CT scans are reported to be 95% accurate in identifying an acutely inflamed appendix but are associated with significant exposure to ionizing radiation. Of increasingly recognized importance, data suggest that 1 in 1,000 children who receive an abdominal CT scan will develop a life-threatening malignancy later in life. Unlike the adult population, CT scan should not be routinely performed when investigating appendicitis. In children in whom there is doubt about the diagnosis of appendicitis, ultrasonography is preferred, and in expert hands, it is more than 90% accurate.

Treatment

The standard treatment for acute appendicitis is appendectomy performed after IV hydration and the administration of broad-spectrum antibiotics. Timing of appendectomy has evolved from a true surgical emergency to a more accepted practice of performing the procedure within 8 hours of arrival. This case can be done laparoscopically, but the advantages in children are less pronounced compared with the adult population. Single-incision laparoscopic surgery is a technique gaining increasing popularity for the treatment of appendicitis. If the appendix is not ruptured, postoperative antibiotics are unnecessary. For perforated appendicitis, antibiotics are usually given for a minimum of 4 days postoperatively and discontinued when the child is afebrile and has a normal white blood cell count. Recovery from nonruptured appendicitis is rapid, and children

are usually discharged within 24 hours. Children who present with perforated appendicitis and an established intra-abdominal abscess are referred to interventional radiology for percutaneous image-guided drain. An "interval" appendectomy is then performed electively in 6 to 8 weeks, although recent evidence questions whether this operation is necessary.

Common Complications

Perforated appendicitis has a significant incidence of complications, particularly intra-abdominal abscesses and wound infections. Abscesses are often drained percutaneously or transrectally under ultrasound guidance. Wound infections are opened and drained. Trocar complications including bladder and bowel injuries are rare.

Intussusception

Intussusception is the telescoping of one portion of the intestine into another. It is usually ileocolic, and the distal ileum invaginates and advances for a variable distance into the colon. Intussusception is an emergency condition because the involved intestine can become strangulated.

Pathophysiology

Intussusception typically affects children between 6 and 18 months of age. Viral hypertrophy of Peyer patches in the intestinal submucosa accounts for most cases. Less often, a pathologic lead point is found (eg, Meckel diverticulum, polyp, lymphoma, hematoma). These conditions are more prevalent in children who have intussusception at a later age.

Clinical Presentation and Evaluation

Intussusception often follows a viral illness and is seasonal. It is characterized by intermittent bouts of colicky abdominal pain during which the child cries and draws the knees to the chest. Between episodes, the child is initially well but becomes increasingly lethargic. Vomiting is common and eventually becomes bilious as intestinal obstruction develops. Blood and mucus may be passed rectally as "currant jelly" stools as a result of congestion and ischemia of the intestinal mucosa.

On examination, these children may be irritable or somnolent, as well as dehydrated. A tender, sausage-shaped mass can sometimes be palpated in the right upper abdomen. Digital rectal examination may yield blood and mucus. Abdominal x-rays may appear normal or show a paucity of air in the right lower quadrant. Eventually, dilated small intestinal loops consistent with obstruction develop.

Unfortunately, the diagnosis can be difficult because intermittent crying spells are very nonspecific in children and many more suggestive findings may be absent. If intussusception is suspected, the standard investigation is barium or air-contrast enema. Ileocolic intussusception appears as a filling defect in the colon, at which point the flow of contrast material stops (Figure 21-22). Ultrasound can also be diagnostic by showing the intussuscepted mass in the right flank, with obstructed flow across the ileocecal valve.

Treatment

The pressure of contrast or air (favored) during administration of the enema is used to reduce the intussusception and is successful in over 90% of cases. Repeat enema, several hours following the initial attempt, is appropriate for a partially reduced intussusception. After successful reduction,

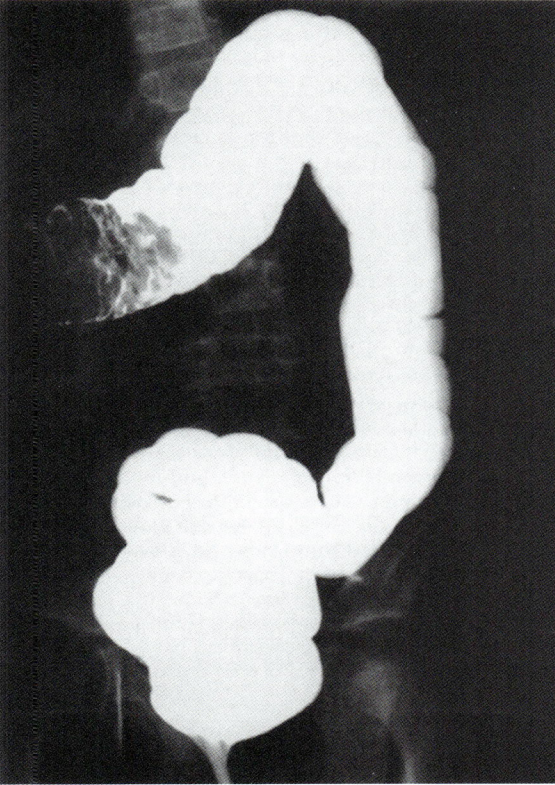

Figure 21-22. Ileocolic intussusception. Barium enema outlines a filling defect in the transverse colon. (From Lawrence PF. *Essentials of Surgical Specialties*. 3rd ed. Lippincott Williams & Wilkins; 2007.)

the child is admitted overnight for observation. Surgery must be performed promptly if nonoperative reduction fails. After expeditious hydration and antibiotics, the intussusception is manually reduced, either laparoscopically or via an open procedure, and the surgeon investigates for a lead point.

Prognosis

Recurrent intussusception occurs in 5% to 8% of children, regardless of the method of reduction.

Meckel Diverticulum

A Meckel diverticulum occurs in 2% of the population. It is located in the ileum, within 2 ft (100 cm) of the ileocecal valve.

Pathophysiology

A Meckel diverticulum contains heterotopic tissue in 50% of symptomatic patients. It is most often lined with gastric mucosa. Embryologically, the yolk sac communicates with the intestine through the vitelline (omphalomesenteric) duct. If this structure does not involute and remains completely open, intestinal contents drain from the umbilicus after cord separation, and a vitelline fistula forms. Much more commonly, only the intestinal side of the vitelline duct remains patent and creates a Meckel diverticulum. The distal end may lie freely or may be attached to the undersurface of the umbilicus by a fibrous band.

Clinical Presentation and Evaluation

Although most Meckel diverticula are clinically silent, they may be complicated by bleeding, obstruction, and inflammation. Bleeding results from peptic ulceration of the normal bowel adjacent to the ectopic gastric mucosa of the diverticulum. It usually occurs in children younger than 5 years of age. The bleeding is typically dark red and painless, and it may be massive. Contrast x-rays rarely visualize the diverticulum. Technetium-99m pertechnetate isotope scan is preferred because the isotope is taken up by the ectopic gastric mucosa.

A Meckel diverticulum can cause intestinal obstruction by acting as the lead point of an intussusception or by allowing the intestine to twist around it as a volvulus when the diverticulum is fixed to the anterior abdominal wall.

Meckel diverticulitis occurs in somewhat older children and is almost always misdiagnosed preoperatively because its manifestations are so similar to those of appendicitis. Whenever a normal appendix is found at laparotomy for presumptive appendicitis, the distal ileum must be inspected for the possibility of Meckel diverticulitis.

Treatment

A symptomatic Meckel diverticulum is resected by laparotomy or laparoscopic surgery. Asymptomatic diverticula found incidentally at the surgery are usually resected if the child is young, if the diverticulum has a narrow neck, if it is attached to the abdominal wall, or if heterotopic tissue is palpable within its lumen.

Gastrointestinal Bleeding

GI bleeding may be frightening to parents, but it is usually mild and readily managed. The most likely sources of bleeding in a child may be suspected by the patient's age, the level of the bleeding (upper or lower), the color and amount of blood, and the associated findings. If the bleeding is massive and the child is hemodynamically unstable, rapid resuscitation is required, with insertion of large-bore IV catheters, fluid administration, blood transfusions, and prompt investigation of the cause. For smaller amounts of bleeding, which is much more common, outpatient evaluation is appropriate. Common causes include anal fissure, gastroenteritis, polyps, and inflammatory bowel disease.

Gastroesophageal Reflux

The reflux of stomach contents into the esophagus is known as GER. GER is particularly common in infants and children who have neurologic impairments. Although most children with GER are managed successfully with medical measures alone, surgical procedures to combat reflux are now among the most common major operations performed in children.

Pathophysiology

GER is common in normal babies because the lower esophageal sphincter is relatively incompetent for the first few months of life. This type of GER is usually self-limited because its incidence and severity decrease with normal growth and development. Patients with neurologic disorders may have motor and reflex abnormalities of the entire foregut, including disordered swallowing, reduced esophageal clearance, an incompetent lower esophageal sphincter, and delayed gastric emptying. All of these conditions predispose patients to GER and its complications at all ages.

Clinical Presentation and Evaluation

In most infants, GER is of minor consequence. It is responsible for the occasional regurgitations and "wet burps" seen. In some cases, vomiting is more severe and may even mimic pyloric stenosis. Clinically significant complications of GER include (1) failure to thrive (inadequate growth and weight gain because of chronic regurgitation); (2) aspiration of gastric contents into the lungs, causing recurrent pneumonia or reactive airway disease; (3) apnea, probably because of reflux-induced laryngospasm or a vagal reflex (may be one cause of sudden infant death syndrome); and (4) peptic esophagitis, which can lead to GI bleeding, stricture formation, and Barrett esophagus (more common in older children). Patients who have certain underlying disorders, including chronic neurologic impairment, EA, and diaphragmatic hernias, are more likely to have severe GER.

Evaluation of a child with significant GER is initiated with a barium swallow to rule out obstructive lesions and to define the anatomy. If massive GER is observed, no further diagnostic studies may be necessary. If GER is suspected clinically but not documented radiographically, more sensitive tests such as a pH probe study are indicated. Endoscopy is useful to demonstrate esophagitis and its complications, but it is used much less often in children than in adults. Manometry is rarely useful in children outside of cases of suspected achalasia.

Treatment

GER is so common in babies that the diagnosis and initial treatment are often based on the clinical impression alone. Medical management, including upright positioning, thickening of feeds, and agents to promote gastric emptying (eg, metoclopramide), is usually effective for uncomplicated reflux. H_2 blockers or proton pump inhibitors are used to prevent or treat esophagitis.

Surgery is indicated if medical management does not control the complications of GER or sooner for life-threatening complications (eg, apnea or aspiration pneumonia). Surgery is more likely to be necessary if the child has an underlying condition that predisposes to GER. Many operative procedures have been devised, but the Nissen fundoplication, in which the gastric fundus is wrapped 360° around the lower esophagus, is most commonly performed and may be done laparoscopically. If long-term access for enteral feeding is anticipated, a gastrostomy tube is placed at the time of the procedure.

Common Complications

Possible complications of antireflux procedures include the inability to vomit and the gas-bloat syndrome, in which patients become distended after feeding because they cannot burp. Children usually outgrow these problems. Recurrence of GER after antireflux surgery is much more common in neurologically impaired children who routinely and sometimes violently retch than in the general population.

Chest Wall Deformities

A variety of skeletal malformations of the chest wall may present at birth or in early childhood. The most common of these are pectus excavatum, pectus carinatum, and mixed defects.

Pathophysiology

Pectus excavatum, or "funnel chest," is characterized by a depression of the sternum and sharp angulation of the lower costal cartilages where they bow out over the upper abdomen (Figure 21-23). It occurs in up to 1 in 400 births and has a strong familial component. Several theories exist to explain the pathogenesis of pectus excavatum, but none has been proven. The involved costal cartilages are abnormal, on both gross and microscopic inspection. Pectus carinatum, or "pigeon breast," is characterized by protrusion of the anterior chest wall. It is believed to be caused by an overgrowth of the costal cartilages and is much less common than pectus excavatum.

Clinical Presentation and Evaluation

Young children with chest wall deformities are usually brought for evaluation by parents who are concerned about the obvious cosmetic problem. Boys may be unwilling to expose their chests while swimming or engaging in sports. Symptoms caused by restrictive pulmonary changes are more common in older children and adolescents, and include easy fatigability, reduced stamina and endurance, and an increased incidence of respiratory illness. In severe forms of pectus excavatum, the heart is displaced into the left side of the chest, and inspiratory expansion of the lungs is inhibited. Thoracic CT scans

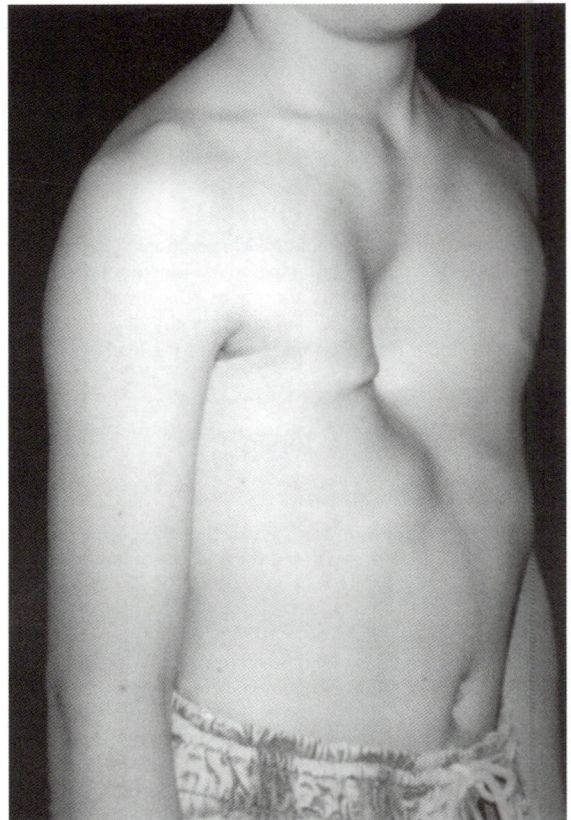

Figure 21-23. A 15-year-old boy with pectus excavatum. (From Lawrence PF. *Essentials of Surgical Specialties.* 3rd ed. Lippincott Williams & Wilkins; 2007.)

are usually reserved for young teens and may provide information regarding displacement of the heart and assessment of lung volumes. Additionally, the Haller index, representing a ratio of the greatest transverse diameter of the chest compared with the maximal depression of the sternum, is calculated. Pulmonary function tests can be used to determine the physiologic abnormalities when symptoms are present. Most children with pectus carinatum do not have cardiopulmonary impairment, and consideration for operative correction is based on the cosmetic severity of the deformity.

Treatment

The traditional operation for pectus excavatum involves resection of the involved costal cartilages for the entire length of the deformity and elevation of the sternum to a neutral position via a wedge osteotomy anteriorly. The sternum is then stabilized in this position using a supporting substernal stainless steel bar that is removed within a year as healing in the new position is complete. A similar procedure is performed for pectus carinatum. Of note, custom bracing is a viable nonoperative option for pectus carinatum, especially in young patients. The Nuss procedure is now favored and involves the insertion of a semicircular bar under the sternum and anterior ribs via small incisions on either side of the chest under thoracoscopic vision. The bar is left in place for 2 years when permanent remolding of the sternum and costal cartilages has occurred. Liberal use of cryoablation of multiple rib segments has revolutionized pain control for this procedure.

Common Complications

Early postoperative complications of the traditional procedure for pectus excavatum and carinatum include pneumothorax; fluid accumulation in the pleural cavity, mediastinum, or subcutaneous space; and wound infection, dehiscence, and hematoma. Late complications include migration of the stabilizing bar, and a 5% to 10% rate of recurrence after the bar is removed. Impaired chest wall growth has been noted in adolescents whose corrective surgery was done during young childhood. This has been attributed to intraoperative injury to the costochondral junctions, which are the longitudinal growth centers for the ribs. Surgery is now delayed until after the pubertal growth spurt.

Neck Masses

Neck masses are often found in children and seldom carry the same ominous import as they do in adults, although certain malignancies do occur. In most cases, neck masses are accurately diagnosed by history and physical examination alone. Surgical excision may be required for definitive treatment and occasionally for diagnosis. Neck masses are classified according to their location. Table 21-9 lists the most common types of neck masses in children.

Midline Neck Masses

Among the midline neck masses found in the older child are thyroglossal duct cysts, ectopic thyroid, dermoid or epidermoid cysts, enlarged lymph nodes, and thyroid masses. Some surgeons recommend thyroid scan prior to the excision of thyroglossal ducts; however, others argue that the tissue is dysgenetic and should be removed regardless.

TABLE 21-9. Neck Masses in Children	
Location	**Type**
Midline	Thyroglossal duct cyst
	Ectopic thyroid
	Thyroid masses
	Dermoid and epidermoid cysts
	Lymphadenopathy
Lateral	Lymphadenopathy
	Cystic hygroma
	Branchial cleft cysts
	Torticollis

Embryologically, the thyroid gland descends from the base of the tongue. If the thyroglossal duct, along the path of descent, does not obliterate, a thyroglossal duct cyst can result. This cyst usually appears between 2 and 10 years of age as a firm, round, midline neck mass (Figure 21-24). It rises with swallowing and protrusion of the tongue. Infection often occurs. A thyroglossal duct cyst must be removed with its tract and the center of the hyoid bone, or recurrence can be expected.

In an ectopic thyroid, the gland is arrested in its antenatal descent. It may present as a midline neck mass and is the patient's only thyroid tissue. An ectopic thyroid gland

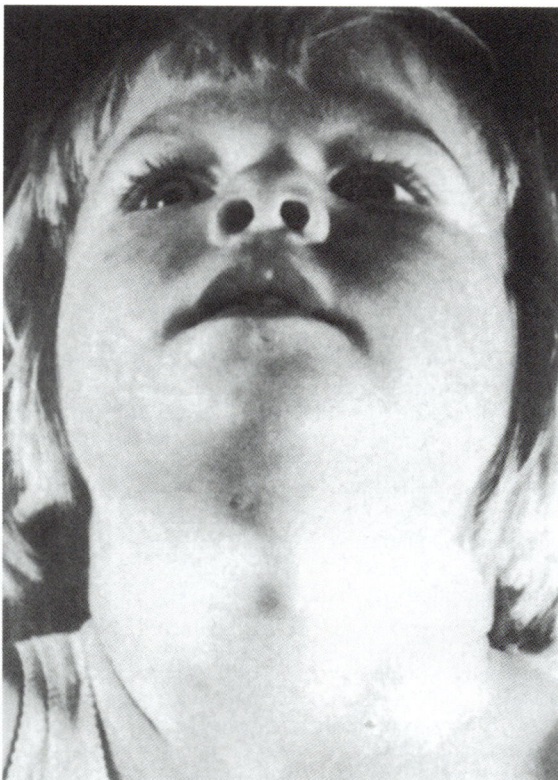

Figure 21-24. A thyroglossal duct cyst in a 5-year-old girl. (From Lawrence PF. *Essentials of Surgical Specialties*. 3rd ed. Lippincott Williams & Wilkins; 2007.)

may be divided and moved bilaterally or excised. The patient then receives thyroid replacement therapy.

A dermoid or epidermoid cyst arises from trapped epithelial elements and may present as a midline neck mass. It is usually more superficial than a thyroglossal duct cyst. Enlarged lymph nodes (lymphadenopathy) may also appear in the midline of the neck.

Thyroid masses are usually recognized by their location. Although uncommon in children, they may be caused by the same abnormalities as in adults. A thyroid nodule in a child is more likely to be malignant. Either lobectomy with biopsy or needle aspiration biopsy and an attempt at suppression with thyroid hormone (if the patient does not have hyperthyroidism) is recommended.

Lateral Neck Masses

Lateral neck masses in older children may involve the lymph glands, lymphatic vessels, branchial cleft cysts and sinuses, or the sternomastoid muscle.

Acute cervical lymphadenitis occurs predominantly in young children as a result of staphylococcal or streptococcal infection, usually after an upper respiratory infection. The child is febrile, and the swelling shows signs of inflammation, including erythema and tenderness. Antibiotics may be curative, but if the mass becomes fluctuant, incision and drainage are necessary.

Chronic lymphadenopathy is extremely common in the cervical region. It usually represents nonspecific benign hyperplasia. Other causes of chronically enlarged cervical lymph nodes are infections with mycobacteria (usually nontuberculous), cat scratch disease, and, rarely, lymphoma. Lymphoma is more likely if the nodes are hard or fixed, if the nodes continue to grow, and if the patient has systemic symptoms of fever, malaise, and weight loss. An open biopsy of enlarged cervical lymph nodes is indicated if they are larger than 2 cm and persist for 6 weeks, or sooner if malignancy is suspected on the basis of physical findings.

Cystic hygromas, or lymphangiomas, are congenital malformations of the lymphatic vessels characterized by multiloculated cysts filled with lymph. They may occur anywhere but are most common in the posterior triangle of the neck, followed by the axilla. Many are present at birth and almost always appear by 2 years of age. A multimodal approach, including a liberal use of sclerosing agents such as doxycycline and/or surgical excision, offers the best opportunity for permanent cure. Infants with large airway-compromising hygromas may require ex utero intrapartum treatment procedures for safe delivery.

Branchial cleft cysts and sinuses arise when the various branchial clefts and arches do not completely resorb. Sinuses usually present in early childhood as small cutaneous openings that drain clear fluid. Cysts are noted as subcutaneous masses in older children because fluid gradually accumulates within them. They are less complete abnormalities than sinuses, in that external closure has occurred. Skin tags and collections of cartilage may also occur. Remnants of the second branchial cleft are the most common and are located along the anterior border of the sternomastoid muscle. Remnants of the first cleft are found near the ear or the angle of the mandible. These cysts and sinuses may become infected, and resection is indicated as soon as infection is controlled.

Neonatal torticollis, or wry neck, is caused by fibrosis and shortening of the sternomastoid muscle. A traumatic cause is hypothesized, with hematoma formation and organization within the muscle. The infant has a firm neck mass. The face is rotated away from the affected side, and the head is tilted toward the ipsilateral shoulder. Ultrasound confirms that the mass is within the muscle. Passive rotational exercises by the parents are usually curative. Surgical division of the sternomastoid muscle is reserved for rare treatment failures. Untreated torticollis may lead to permanent facial asymmetry.

Vascular Tumors

Vascular tumors are common in childhood and are found in 10% of children during the first year. The terminology used to describe them is variable and confusing. Biologic classification is the most useful. Hemangiomas are biologically active benign vascular tumors characterized initially by cellular proliferation and followed in most cases by involution. In contrast, vascular malformations are biologically inert errors of morphogenesis of vessels. They are not proliferative and grow only with the child. Many leading children's hospitals have instituted a vascular anomalies program to foster a multidisciplinary approach, including surgery, interventional radiology, and oncology, when treating these children.

Hemangiomas

Most hemangiomas appear within the first few weeks after birth as a small red spot that grows rapidly during the first year and then slowly regresses over the next several years. They are commonly located on the head and neck but may be found anywhere. Hemangiomas may be superficial or deep and may involve the viscera. Superficial lesions, or capillary hemangiomas, are firm, bright red, and raised. They are the most likely to regress (Figure 21-25). Deep or cavernous lesions are softer and may have a blue discoloration. They may be less likely to resolve.

Most hemangiomas should be left alone because the overwhelming majority resolve spontaneously in early childhood. Indications for treatment include significant facial distortion, interference with function (eg, as occurs with lesions of the eyelid or airway), thrombocytopenia from platelet trapping, and congestive heart failure. Management includes steroids (by intralesional injection or systemically), cyclophosphamide, α-interferon, embolization, and surgical excision, depending on the location and characteristics of the hemangioma.

Vascular Malformations

Vascular malformations are much less common than hemangiomas and tend to remain stable over time. One such malformation, the port wine stain, is seen at birth as a red or purple nonraised lesion, usually on the face. Another vascular malformation is a congenital arteriovenous fistula. These anomalies are most common in the extremities and central nervous system (CNS). In the extremities, they are usually multiple and may cause heart failure and hypertrophy of the involved limb.

A port wine stain never regresses and is best treated with laser photocoagulation. The treatment of a congenital arteriovenous fistula, although not completely satisfactory, consists of elastic compression, ligation of the involved vessels, embolization, or surgical excision.

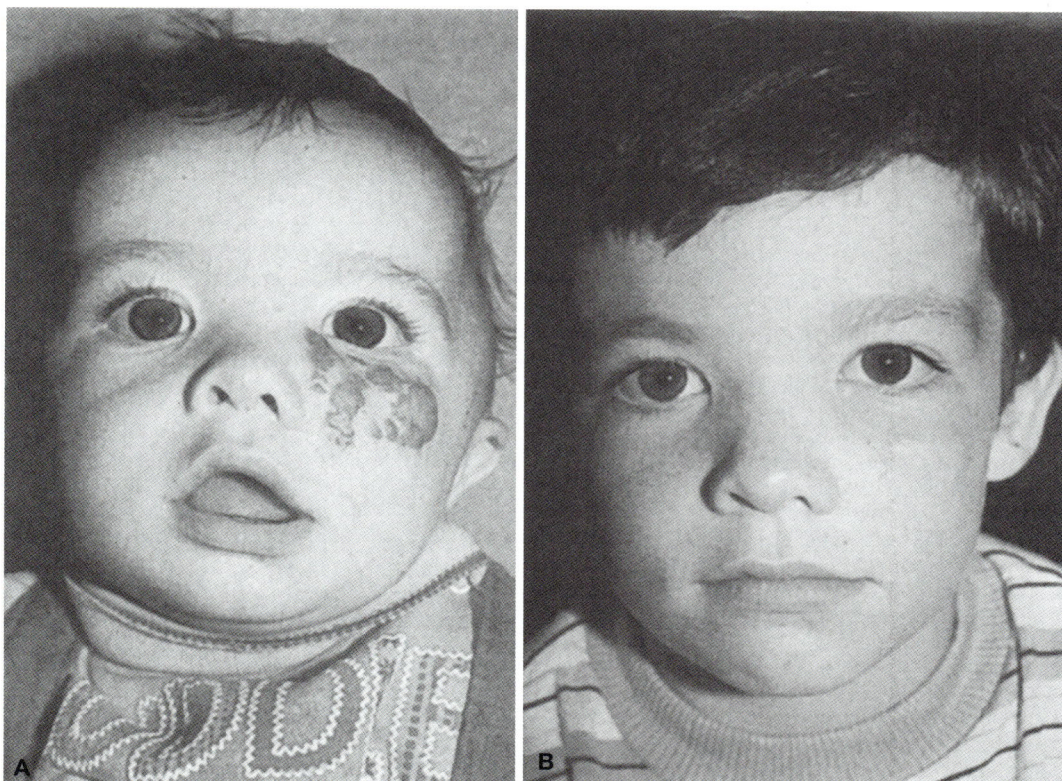

Figure 21-25. **A.** A superficial hemangioma in an infant boy. B. Regression by 5 years of age. (From Lawrence PF. *Essentials of Surgical Specialties*. 3rd ed. Lippincott Williams & Wilkins; 2007.)

TUMORS

Few ordeals are more devastating for young people and their families than childhood cancer. Cancer accounts for 11% of all childhood deaths. The frequency and distribution of malignant neoplasms in children differs markedly from that in adults. Leukemia (25%), CNS tumors (20%), and lymphoma (12%) predominate. Neuroblastoma and Wilms tumors each account for 5% to 10% of pediatric cancers, followed by malignancies of the liver, bone, and other soft tissues.

Fortunately, the outlook for children with malignancies has improved markedly in the last two decades, largely as a result of multicenter clinical trials. Individual hospital data and outcomes collected through the Children's Oncology Group have generated uniform treatments for uncommon diseases. The pediatric surgeon almost always treats children with solid malignancies as a part of a multidisciplinary team that combines the use of surgery, chemotherapy, radiation therapy, and sophisticated diagnostic imaging. Peer discussion at tumor board is recommended to fully vet treatment options and optimize results. Each of these modalities of therapy has side effects that affect surgical therapy. For example, chemotherapy may cause renal dysfunction that affects fluid and electrolyte therapy in the perioperative period. Radiation has an effect on wound healing that must be considered in surgical planning. Secondary malignancies can occur as a consequence

of therapy, and pediatric surgeons are often involved in the management of these problems.

Vascular access devices offer a substantial advantage in children with many types of cancer. These catheters are used to administer chemotherapy, IV nutrition, and blood products, as well as to sample blood. Some catheters (eg, Hickman, Broviac) have a subcutaneous cuff and external tubing. Others (eg, Port-A-Cath) are completely internalized and have implanted subcutaneous reservoirs that are easily accessed percutaneously with a special needle. These implanted devices are associated with a lower infection rate and are less limiting to patient activities when not in use.

Neuroblastoma

Neuroblastoma is the most common extracranial solid tumor of childhood. It has the unique ability to undergo maturation to a benign form, ganglioneuroma, or to spontaneously regress altogether.

Pathophysiology

The tumor is derived from embryonal neural crest tissue. It arises anywhere in the sympathetic nervous system. Three-quarters of neuroblastomas are intra-abdominal. Of these, most arise from the adrenal medulla. Other sites include the posterior mediastinum, neck, and brain. Most children with neuroblastoma excrete catecholamines, and their breakdown products can be found in the urine.

Clinical Presentation and Evaluation

One-half of neuroblastomas occur in the first 2 years of life, and 90% are found by the time a child is 8 years old. An abdominal mass is the presenting feature in most patients. Tumors of the mediastinum may produce respiratory distress, may cause Horner syndrome because of involvement of the stellate ganglion, or may be noted incidentally on CXR. Paraplegia can occur if there is an extension through the intervertebral foramina with compression of the spinal cord. Systemic symptoms are common and include fever, weight loss, failure to thrive, anemia, and hypertension. Most children have metastases at diagnosis, with the most common sites of spread being bone, bone marrow, lymph nodes, liver, and subcutaneous tissue.

A child with a suspected neuroblastoma undergoes studies that include ultrasonography, CT or MRI scan, bone scan, bone marrow aspiration, and measurement of urinary catecholamines. An MRI is performed preoperatively if intraspinal extension is suspected. Several staging systems have been proposed to specify the extent of disease and the completeness of surgical resection. Tumor specimens are examined for histology, karyotype, and genetic analysis. Prognostically positive features include favorable nuclear and stromal histologic characteristics (Shimada classification), DNA aneuploidy, and lack of amplification of the N-*myc* oncogene.

Treatment

Therapeutic protocols are based on the child's age, tumor location and characteristics, and extent of disease. Surgical resection remains the mainstay of treatment and is currently the only method of cure. In cases in which tumor recurrence is likely or there is residual cancer, postoperative radiation and multiple-agent chemotherapy are usually indicated. For advanced disease with an unresectable tumor, chemotherapy may be given initially to shrink the lesion and permit subsequent resection. Bone marrow transplantation rescue has been used after massive chemotherapy and total body irradiation, with prolonged relapse-free survival. Immunotherapy is being evaluated as well.

Prognosis

The overall survival rate is 40% to 50%, but it depends greatly on the age of the patient and the site and characteristics of the tumor. The survival rate for infants less than 1 year of age is 84%, but it is only 42% for children older than 1 year. Children with localized, completely resected disease have a 90% survival rate. However, for those with metastatic disease, the survival rate is less than 20%. An unusual form of this disease occurs in infants younger than 1 year of age who have metastases limited to the liver, bone marrow, and skin. The survival rate for these children is approximately 80%, even with little or no treatment.

Nephroblastoma (Wilms Tumor)

Pathophysiology

Nephroblastoma, or Wilms tumor, is an embryonal neoplasm of the kidney. It is often associated with other anomalies (eg, hypospadias, hemihypertrophy, and aniridia [congenital absence of the iris]). The tumor occurs bilaterally in approximately 10% of patients, is often familial, and is associated with a deletion at the 11p13 and 11p15 chromosome sites.

Clinical Presentation and Evaluation

Most children with Wilms tumors are 1 to 5 years old. They usually have an asymptomatic abdominal mass. Occasionally, they have abdominal pain, hematuria, or hypertension, but systemic manifestations (eg, fever, anorexia, weight loss) are much less frequent than in children with neuroblastoma. Metastases are also less common and tend to occur in regional lymph nodes and in the lungs. Wilms tumors may also invade the renal vein and extend into the inferior vena cava. Investigations include ultrasonography and CT scans of the abdomen and chest (Figure 21-26).

Treatment

Resection of the tumor as a total or partial nephrectomy is the mainstay of treatment. Preoperative chemotherapy is given initially for unresectable tumors. Most children receive chemotherapy postoperatively. Radiation therapy is added for those with unfavorable histology, residual tumor, or metastatic disease. Children with bilateral Wilms tumors usually undergo partial nephrectomies and chemotherapy in an effort to preserve renal tissue.

Prognosis

Survival depends on the stage, size, and histologic type of the tumor, and on the patient's age. Younger children fare better, and the long-term survival rate for patients with localized tumors is more than 90%. Even for those with extensive disease and unfavorable histology, it is more than 50%.

Teratomas

Teratomas are neoplasms that originate early in embryonic cell division, yet they can manifest at any age. It is unclear whether they arise from germ cells or from other totipotential embryonic cells. Teratomas often occur in the gonads or near the midline of the body, where undifferentiated cells might be found. They contain a wide spectrum of tissue types of varying degrees of differentiation, and they may be benign or malignant. Benign teratomas produce symptoms by compressing adjacent organs or by torsion. Malignant teratomas may invade and metastasize.

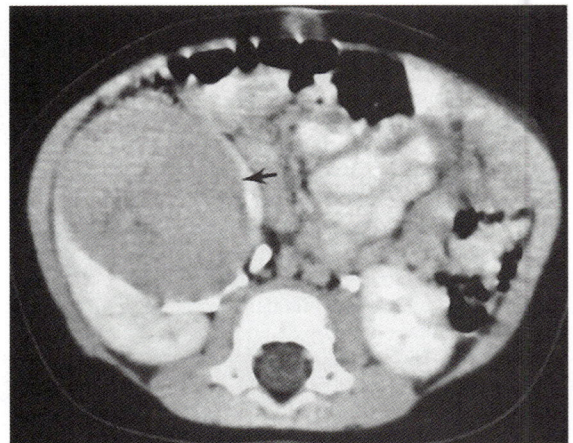

Figure 21-26. Large Wilms tumor of the right kidney (arrow) seen on computed tomography. (From Lawrence PF. *Essentials of Surgical Specialties*. 3rd ed. Lippincott Williams & Wilkins; 2007.)

The most common locations for teratomas in children are the sacrococcygeal region and the ovary. Other sites are the neck, anterior mediastinum, retroperitoneum, testes, and CNS. Operative resection is curative for benign teratomas. Patients with malignant teratomas usually undergo resection followed by chemotherapy, but recurrences and metastases are common.

Sacrococcygeal teratoma is the most common tumor found in neonates. It occurs predominantly in girls and can be massive (Figure 21-27A and B). It arises from the coccyx and usually has an external component that is covered with skin. It may also have a significant internal portion that extends in front of the sacrum and enters the pelvis. Rarely, the entire tumor is internal, with no visible abnormality. Initial treatment involves surgical resection, which is curative in benign sacrococcygeal teratomas. The outlook for cure and for normal function in these patients is excellent. However, survival after malignant transformation is unlikely. Sacrococcygeal teratomas are increasingly diagnosed in utero. Delivery by cesarean birth is recommended for large tumors because rupture with exsanguination can occur during vaginal delivery.

Hepatic Tumors

Tumors of the liver are the third most common abdominal malignancy in childhood, after neuroblastomas and Wilms tumors. Approximately three-fourths of hepatic neoplasms in children are malignant.

Malignant Tumors

The most common malignant tumors are hepatoblastoma and hepatocellular carcinoma. Hepatoblastoma is more common and is typically found in children younger than 3 years of age and particularly in children with a history of prematurity.

Patients with liver tumors usually have an abdominal mass that is often associated with discomfort, anorexia, weight loss, and occasionally jaundice. Serum α-fetoprotein levels are usually elevated. Hepatocellular carcinoma usually occurs in older children, is more invasive, and is more often multicentric. Resection is the treatment of choice and may follow a course of chemotherapy if the tumor is initially unresectable. Liver transplantation should be considered for unresectable hepatoblastomas without metastases. The survival rate for patients with hepatoblastoma is more than 50%. It is substantially lower for those with hepatocellular carcinoma.

Benign Tumors

Hemangiomas are the most common benign tumors of the liver in children. Other benign liver lesions in children are adenomas and focal nodular hyperplasia. Hemangiomas appear as dilated vascular spaces and may be solitary or multiple. They are sometimes accompanied by cutaneous hemangiomas and may produce congestive heart failure and platelet trapping. Asymptomatic hepatic hemangiomas are best left alone; many spontaneously regress. Symptomatic lesions are treated with propranolol, which induces regression, although embolization, ligation of the hepatic arteries, or surgical resection are sometimes required. Digitalis and diuretics may be beneficial for heart failure.

Rhabdomyosarcoma

Rhabdomyosarcoma is the most common soft-tissue sarcoma in children, accounting for approximately 4%

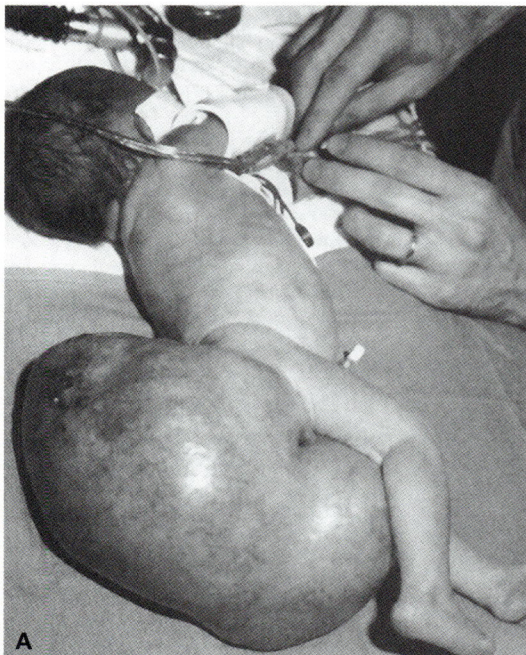

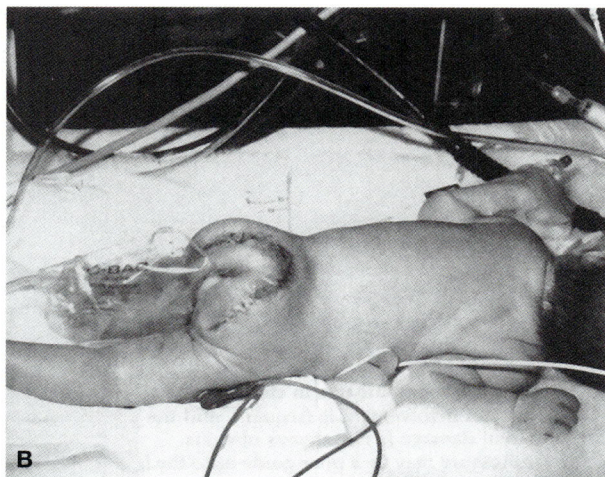

Figure 21-27. **A.** A sacrococcygeal teratoma in a newborn infant displacing the anus anteriorly. **B.** The same infant postoperatively. (From Lawrence PF. *Essentials of Surgical Specialties*. 3rd ed. Lippincott Williams & Wilkins; 2007.)

of pediatric malignancies. Rhabdomyosarcomas are a diverse group of tumors derived from primitive mesenchymal cells that may occur anywhere in the body. The embryonal type, found mostly in infants and young children, tends to occur in the genitourinary tract, head and neck, and orbit. The alveolar type occurs in older children and usually involves the trunk and extremities. These tumors invade locally and metastasize by lymphatic and hematogenous spread. The clinical presentation depends on the site of the disease, but often consists of an asymptomatic mass. Careful planning, including imaging studies, must be done before the biopsy to allow for subsequent excision. Multimodal therapy now allows for much less radical therapy than was advocated in the past. DNA fusion status, anatomic location, nodal status, and size are the important prognostic features of this tumor, with overall survival rates ranging from 90% for orbital lesions to 65% for extremity lesions.

TRAUMA

Trauma is the leading cause of childhood mortality, potential years lost, and medical cost in developed countries. In fact, trauma accounts for more fatalities than all other causes combined. Every year, there are 12,000 children killed in the United States by injuries, over 50,000 are permanently disabled, and 9.2 million are temporarily incapacitated and require emergency department evaluation. According to the Centers for Disease Control, the lifetime medical cost (treatment and rehabilitation) of unintentional injury of children is over $77 million and the total work loss cost (wages, benefits, etc) is approximately $12 billion. Differences in leading causes of death exist between infants (suffocation), children 1 to 4 years of age (drowning), and those over 5 years of age (motor vehicle collisions). Racial and ethnic disparities exist in injury-related mortality. It is estimated that 90% of injuries are predictable and preventable, and thus the term "accident" may no longer be appropriate. Firearm injuries rate as the second most common cause of traumatic death in children. National organizations such as the American Pediatric Surgical Association (APSA) and the Pediatric Trauma Society (PTS) have recently produced position papers, promoted gun safety protocols, and advocated for public health initiatives to decrease pediatric firearm injuries. Both organizations aim to create a safer America for our children regardless of political beliefs.

Since 1992, the National Center for Injury Prevention and Control has funded research for injury prevention and developed strategies for control of these preventable harms. Focused efforts to reduce injuries include decreasing water heater temperatures, adding trigger locks to prevent accidental gun discharge, using bike helmets and safety glasses, the softening of playground services, and constructing sidewalks for safety while walking. The treatment that young trauma victims receive determines whether they survive and if they will have permanent disabilities. To ensure the best outcome, children with serious injuries should be transported to specialized trauma centers. The most effective means for reducing deaths and disability from childhood trauma is prevention through education and legislation.

Differences in Trauma Care Between Adults and Children

Many of the basic principles of trauma care are the same in children and adults, but there are important differences, as follows:

1. Blunt trauma predominates in children, where there are often multiple injuries, and the extent of internal damage is not always obvious on initial evaluation.
2. Hypoxia is the most common cause of cardiac arrest in the injured child. Prompt management of the airway and breathing are of the highest priorities.
3. Hypotension is not a sensitive sign for shock. Children can compensate very effectively for hypovolemia by increasing their peripheral vascular resistance and heart rate. Hypotension develops only after a loss of 30% to 40% of the total blood volume.
4. Children are more vulnerable to head injury because the head is relatively large and poorly stabilized. The subarachnoid space is relatively smaller and less protective of the brain.
5. Children are at greater risk for hypothermia because of their proportionately larger body surface areas.
6. The young skeleton is quite flexible and more readily transmits applied forces. Children may therefore sustain major internal damage without overlying fractures.
7. Injury to the epiphyseal growth plate can result in growth inhibition and deformity.
8. Gastric distention is more common in children because they tend to swallow air. This may compromise respiration, promote aspiration, or mimic significant intra-abdominal injuries.

Evaluation of the Injured Child

The first priority of management involves the primary survey and ABC (airway, breathing, and circulation) of resuscitation, focusing on life-threatening conditions of ABC. The secondary survey, which is a more complete evaluation, then follows.

Primary Survey
The initial ABCs include the following principles:

1. Airway evaluation and maintenance are the top priority. The airway is cleared of blood, vomitus, and debris and positioned in such a way that the tongue and soft tissues do not obstruct. An endotracheal tube may be required. Techniques in video laryngoscopy are increasingly used. In the rare instance in which an airway is needed and orotracheal intubation is not possible, surgical cricothyroidotomy is recommended in children over 10 years of age and needle cricothyroidotomy in those under 10.
2. The neck must be immobilized until a cervical spine injury is ruled out.
3. Supplemental oxygen is provided, and breathing is supported by positive pressure ventilation if necessary. A tension pneumothorax should be decompressed immediately by needle aspiration, after which a chest tube is placed.
4. The circulation must be supported. External bleeding is controlled by direct pressure. Large-bore IV catheters

are inserted. For children younger than 3 to 5 years of age in whom emergency IV access cannot be obtained, an intraosseous route below the tibial tuberosity or through the upper femur using a bone marrow or spinal needle is temporarily acceptable for fluid infusion. Blood samples are sent for type and crossmatching, a CBC, and an amylase level. Lactated Ringer solution may be administered rapidly in 20 mL/kg boluses. If the patient does not improve with three such infusions, blood transfusion is indicated, MTP is ordered, and surgical intervention must be considered.

Further resuscitation at this time includes the placement of monitoring devices (ECG, pulse oximeter, temperature probe), a nasogastric tube to decompress the stomach (if there is a risk of cribriform plate injury, the tube may be placed through the mouth), and a Foley catheter to obtain urine for analysis and to monitor the output as a guide to further resuscitation. A contraindication to the insertion of a Foley is an injury to the urethra, as evidenced by blood at the urethral meatus or a hematoma at the prostate on rectal examination. Unstable fractures are splinted, and open wounds are covered. Focused assessment with sonography in trauma (FAST) scanning is routinely performed at the bedside to assess cardiac function and hemoperitoneum.

Secondary Survey

Following the primary survey and general resuscitation, a more detailed, head-to-toe physical examination (the secondary survey) is completed. X-rays of the chest and pelvis are usually taken early in the resuscitation phase. Later, films of the remainder of the spine and extremities may be obtained, as indicated by the mechanism of injury and findings on physical examination. CT scans are obtained if needed. A decision must be made as to whether an urgent operation is needed or if the child should be transported to a suitable facility for further support and monitoring.

Head Injuries

Head injury is a major cause of death of injured children. A CT scan provides excellent anatomic definition and should be obtained promptly for any suspected injury. Localized intracranial hematomas require immediate surgical drainage. More commonly, a cerebral contusion occurs, possibly resulting in diffuse edema that can raise intracranial pressure and impair brain perfusion. Oxygen delivery to the brain is optimized by maintaining good blood pressure and oxygen saturation and controlling intracranial hypertension. Intracranial pressure is minimized by mild hyperventilation to produce hypocapnia (which limits cerebral vasodilation), liberal use of sedation and 3% normal saline, upright posture, and drainage ventriculostomy. Continuous intracranial pressure monitoring is helpful in children with unreliable exams. Compared with adults, children have an enhanced ability to recover from severe head trauma. Inpatient rehabilitation stays maximize functional outcomes.

Chest Injuries

Although thoracic trauma occasionally requires immediate, dramatic intervention, most injuries to the chest can be managed nonoperatively with chest tube drainage and supportive care. Indications for surgery are massive, continued blood loss, uncontrolled air leaks through chest tubes,

pericardial tamponade, and suspected injury to the esophagus, diaphragm, and great vessels. Pericardiocentesis can be lifesaving for tamponade but should always be followed by operative repair of the underlying cardiac injury. Pulmonary contusions are very common in children following blunt trauma and appear as focal or diffuse infiltrates on CXR, often in the absence of rib fractures. Treatment consists of respiratory support as needed. Recently, rib plating has been recommended in older children, with multiple rib fractures causing a flail chest.

Abdominal Injuries

Abdominal surgery following trauma is required for a child with a distended, tense abdomen or free intraperitoneal air on x-ray because these findings indicate either massive intra-abdominal bleeding or a perforated viscus. In other stable-injured patients, if abdominal injury is suspected, a contrast scan is indicated (Figure 21-28). CT scans can reliably identify intraperitoneal blood, intraperitoneal free air, and solid organ injuries that may be the source of bleeding. A laparotomy is usually not necessary for intra-abdominal bleeding. If the child can be stabilized with IV fluids and transfusions, close observation is prudent. Diagnostic peritoneal lavage has been replaced with FAST scanning. Every effort should be made to salvage a ruptured spleen, whether surgery is required or not, because children are particularly susceptible to overwhelming postsplenectomy sepsis (OPSI). Intravascular embolization through interventional radiology remains an important adjunct in cases of active splenic, hepatic, and pelvic hemorrhage, as noted with contrast extravasation on CT scan. Previously, children managed nonoperatively required obligatory days of bedrest on the basis of the grade of injury; however, current evidence has shifted attention to physiologic performance as a better guide.

Urinary Tract Injuries

Trauma to the urinary tract usually produces hematuria, which is an indication to perform a CT scan. Most injuries are minor and resolve with observation. Surgical repair is necessary if there is any extravasation of urine from the kidneys or intraperitoneal bladder and for injuries of the

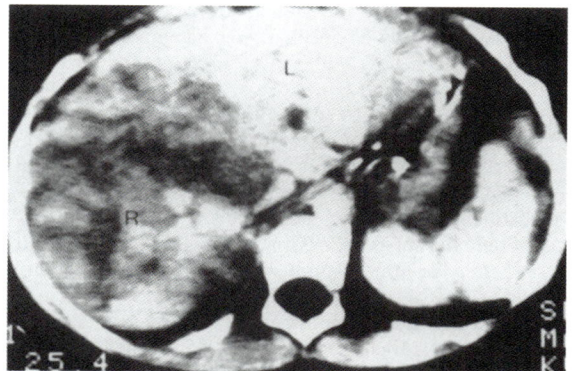

Figure 21-28. Computed tomography from a 7-year-old girl with intrahepatic hemorrhage from an automobile accident. (From Lawrence PF. *Essentials of Surgical Specialties*. 3rd ed. Lippincott Williams & Wilkins; 2007.)

major renal vessels. The presence of gross blood at the urethral meatus requires the performance of a urethrogram to rule out a urethral injury before inserting a Foley catheter.

Burns

After the automobile, burns are the second most common cause of accidental death in children. One-third of burn injuries are caused by child abuse. Major burns produce a profound physiologic insult to the child. The burned individual rapidly develops severe hypovolemia from evaporative loss through the damaged skin barrier and from the seepage of plasma into the tissues through leaky capillaries. There is a marked hypermetabolic state, and multiple organ failure frequently supervenes. Infection is a constant threat. Children with significant burns should be cared for in a specialized burn center.

Clinical Findings

Burns are classified according to their depth, as follows:

1. First degree: Involves epidermis only and produces erythema, as in sunburn.
2. Second degree: Involves partial thickness of dermis while sparing enough epidermal appendages to allow spontaneous healing. Wounds are characterized by painful blistering.
3. Third degree: Necrosis of full-thickness dermis, including the epidermal appendages. Skin is leathery with no sensation.

When calculating the percentage of body surface area burns in young children, the Rule of Nines used for adults does not apply. The Lund and Browder chart (Figure 21-29) may be used to estimate burn size according to the age of the child and should include all second- and third-degree burns. Most patients will have a mixed burn pattern. Hospital admission is advised if a second-degree burn involves more than 10% of the body surface area or a third-degree burn covers more than 2%. Inpatient care is also recommended for significant burns of the hands, feet, face, or perineum and in children under 2 years of age.

Treatment

Minor burns are treated by debridement of devitalized tissue, antimicrobial cream, and occlusive dressings. Intact blisters are generally left alone. The wound should then be washed and dressed once or twice a day at home. Scrupulous care is necessary because infection can convert a partial-thickness injury into full-thickness necrosis.

Major burns are treated with full-scale resuscitative efforts. Burns are cleansed and dressed. Silver-containing products are the norm for the prevention of infection. Bronchoscopy and pulmonary support may be needed for inhalational injuries. Analgesia should be provided. Circumferential third-degree burns impair distal perfusion to an extremity or limit respiration. Emergency escharotomy is necessary.

Fluid resuscitation should always be adjusted to the responses of the patient. However, several formulas provide initial guidelines. The Parkland formula is as follows:

- Lactated Ringer solution is administered at 4 mL/kg per % burn for 24 hours, with half being given in the first 8 hours.

- Colloid is usually started after 24 hours when capillary integrity is improved.
- Enteral fluids and nutrition are administered as soon as the ileus resolves.

Full-thickness burns are surgically excised and covered within several days of injury, to restore normal physiology and prevent infection. Coverage may be provided with partial-thickness autografts or temporarily with pigskin or cadaveric grafts. For large burns, multiple staged excisions are necessary.

Rehabilitation may be prolonged and often includes a compressive, elastic garment that is worn for months in order to limit hypertrophy of the burn scar. Graft contracture is common, especially in burns crossing joints, and may require revision as the child grows. Psychological problems are common and must be fully addressed.

Child Abuse

Overall, the incidence of child abuse is unknown but likely increasing. During the recent COVID-19 pandemic, children had less exposure to child health advocates such as teachers, school nurses, coaches, and religious leaders. Thus, many cases of child abuse were underreported. Certain elements of the history and clinical examination should raise the suspicion of intentional injury. These features are itemized in Table 21-10. The physician must treat the injuries medically, admit the child to the hospital for protection, consult the forensics team, and contact the proper authorities. Difficult discussions with family members should be expected. A high index of suspicion with a constant focus on the welfare of the child is paramount.

Foreign Body Aspiration and Ingestion

Young children put all manner of objects into their mouths, some of which are aspirated or ingested. Among children under the age of 4 years, aspirated and ingested foreign bodies are among the top four causes of accidental death.

Aspiration

An aspirated object that completely obstructs the larynx will rapidly lead to suffocation unless it is coughed out or promptly removed. A smaller object that passes through the larynx usually lodges in a main bronchus, usually the right. Complete obstruction will cause atelectasis as air is absorbed distally, and pneumonia often results. In contrast, partial obstruction of a bronchus produces hyperinflation distally through a ball valve effect, as the airway collapses around the object during expiration and excessive air is trapped.

Clinical Manifestations

Choking and coughing may or may not occur. Once these symptoms subside, the patient frequently produces unilateral wheezing or decreased air entry on the affected side. A CXR will rarely reveal a radiopaque foreign body but often demonstrates hyperaeration of the involved lung or lobe. Expiratory films and fluoroscopy are very helpful because expiration exaggerates the hyperinflation and produces a mediastinal shift in the opposite direction (Figure 21-30).

Estimation of Size of Burn by Percent

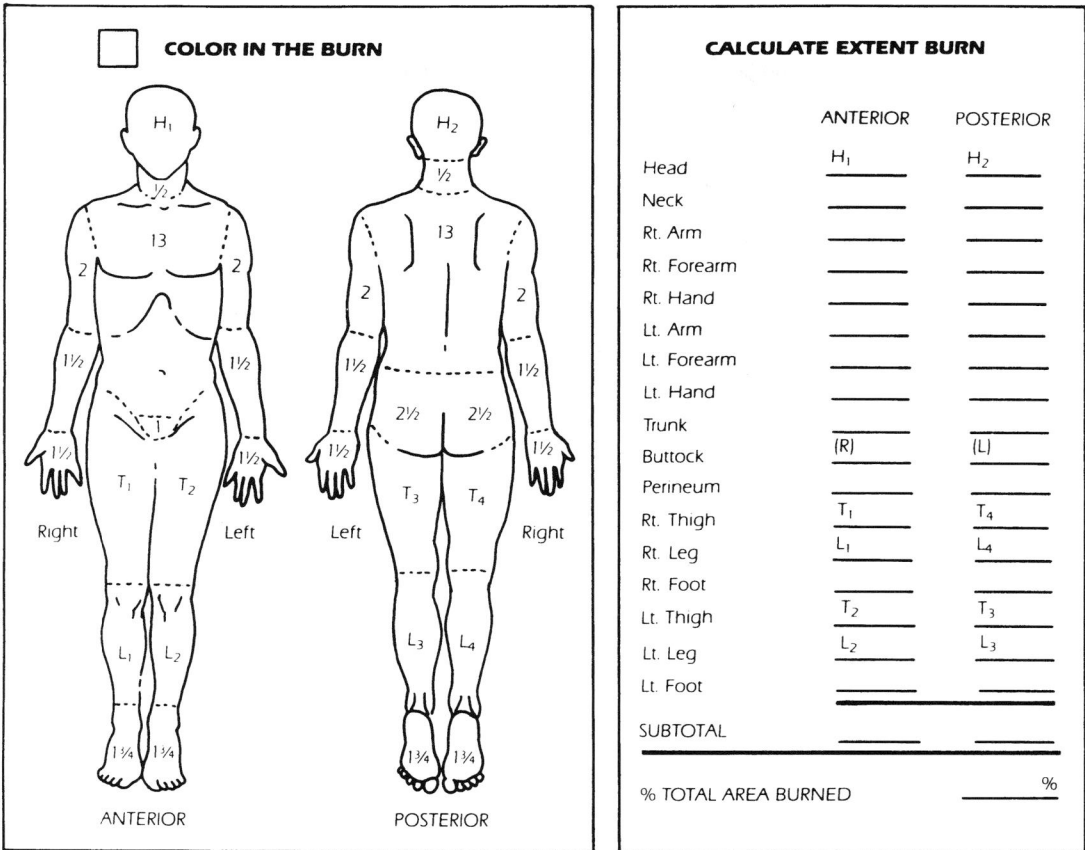

COLOR IN THE BURN

ANTERIOR   POSTERIOR

Right   Left   Left   Right

ANTERIOR   POSTERIOR

CALCULATE EXTENT BURN

	ANTERIOR	POSTERIOR
Head	H_1 _____	H_2 _____
Neck	_____	_____
Rt. Arm	_____	_____
Rt. Forearm	_____	_____
Rt. Hand	_____	_____
Lt. Arm	_____	_____
Lt. Forearm	_____	_____
Lt. Hand	_____	_____
Trunk	_____	_____
Buttock	(R) _____	(L) _____
Perineum	_____	_____
Rt. Thigh	T_1 _____	T_4 _____
Rt. Leg	L_1 _____	L_4 _____
Rt. Foot	_____	_____
Lt. Thigh	T_2 _____	T_3 _____
Lt. Leg	L_2 _____	L_3 _____
Lt. Foot	_____	_____
SUBTOTAL	_____	_____
% TOTAL AREA BURNED	_____ %	

CIRCLE AGE FACTOR	PERCENT OF AREAS AFFECTED BY GROWTH AGE					
	0-1	1-4	5-9	10-14	15	Adult
H (1 or 2) = ½ of the Head	9½	8½	6½	5½	4½	3½
T (1, 2, 3, or 4) = ½ of a Thigh	2¾	3¼	4	4¼	4½	4¾
L (1, 2, 3, or 4) = ½ of a Leg	2½	2½	2¾	3	3¼	3½

Figure 21-29. Modified Lund and Browder chart. Only second- and third-degree burns should be used in the calculation. (From Lawrence PF. *Essentials of Surgical Specialties*. 3rd ed. Lippincott Williams & Wilkins; 2007.)

Treatment

If there is any suspicion of foreign body aspiration, rigid bronchoscopy is performed under general anesthesia and any object identified is removed. Close communication with pediatric anesthesia and liberal use of bronchodilators is critical for minimizing laryngospasm and bronchospasm while optimizing outcomes.

Ingestion

Most foreign objects, even sharp ones, which are swallowed, will reach the stomach and pass unimpeded through the GI tract (Figure 21-31). More commonly, a coin (or other smooth object) is swallowed that can become lodged along the esophagus, particularly at the cricopharyngeus (Figure 21-32A). Drooling and mild chest pain are

TABLE 21-10. Child Abuse: Suspicious Clinical Features
History
Discrepancy between history and physical findings
Prolonged delay before seeking medical care
Recurrent trauma
Inappropriate parental response to child or medical advice
Examination
Child is overly fearful or withdrawn.
Sharply demarcated burns in unusual areas
Long bone fractures in children <3 y
Trauma in genital or perianal areas
Multiple old scars or healed fractures
Bizarre injuries (eg, bites, cigarette burns, rope marks)

common. Timely flexible or rigid esophagoscopy is recommended and is curative. Foley balloon extraction is a secondary option.

An exception to the above-mentioned recommendations concerns swallowed alkaline disk batteries, which can leak and cause local necrosis. To avoid complications, including esophageal perforation, tracheal fistula, or erosion through great vessels, emergent removal is required. Children may be given honey at diagnosis to limit the caustic nature of the injury as the OR is prepared. Although similar in appearance to a less-harmful coin, a seasoned practitioner will note the double ring or halo appearance of a disk battery on plain film (Figure 21-32B). If the battery passes beyond the esophagus, expectant observation is still warranted, but if it fails to advance beyond the stomach for 24 hours, or the same area of the

intestine for a week in spite of purgatives and enemas, removal is indicated.

Caustic substances may be ingested accidentally by young exploring children or purposely by adolescents in a suicide attempt. Strong alkalis (such as lye), which penetrate tissues deeply and produce liquefaction necrosis, predominantly injure the esophagus. Acid causes a surface coagulation necrosis that tends to limit deeper penetration of the esophagus and more frequently damages the stomach. All patients who potentially have ingested corrosive substances require prompt evaluation. For severe injuries, airway control and fluid resuscitation may be necessary. Rarely, emergency surgery is required for peritonitis or mediastinitis, which are indicative of full-thickness necrosis. Otherwise, endoscopy is indicated to assess the degree of injury. Although the approach is controversial, significant esophageal burns are usually treated with steroids and antibiotics. A feeding tube is passed for enteral nutrition and to maintain access through the length of the esophagus if subsequent stricture dilatation is necessary. The rare stricture that is resistant to dilatation is treated surgically by esophageal replacement with either a gastric or colon interposition. Patients who have sustained caustic strictures to the esophagus are at an increased risk for later development of esophageal carcinoma.

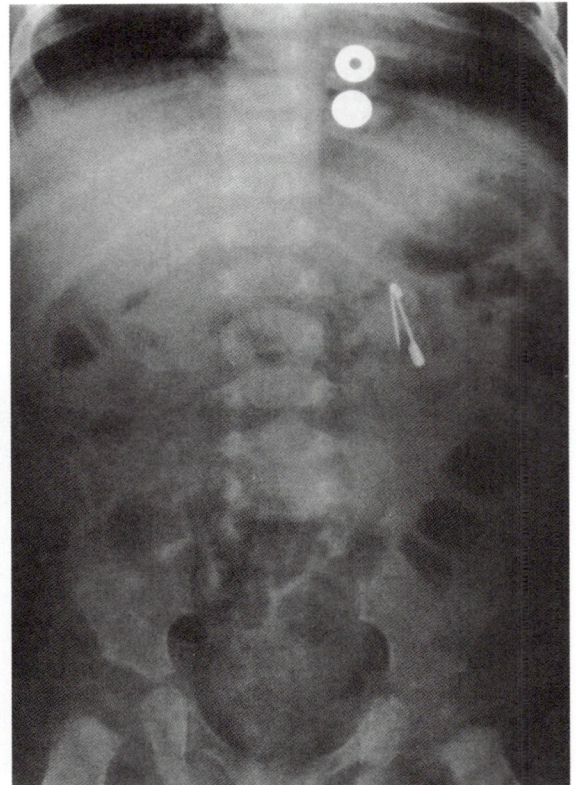

Figure 21-31. Abdominal radiograph of an infant with a swallowed sharp foreign object that passed uneventfully. (From Lawrence PF. *Essentials of Surgical Specialties.* 3rd ed. Lippincott Williams & Wilkins; 2007.)

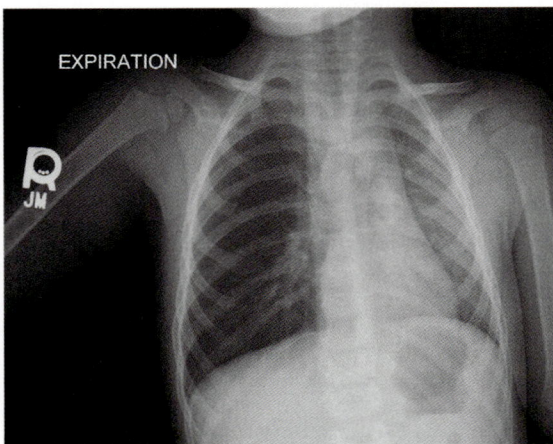

Figure 21-30. Expiratory film of a child with peanut aspiration. Film reveals hyperexpansion of the right chest and mediastinal shift to the left.

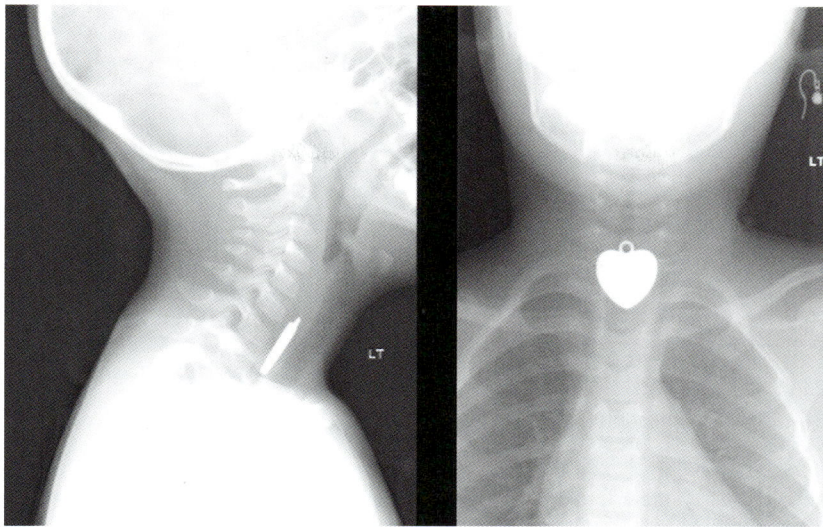

A

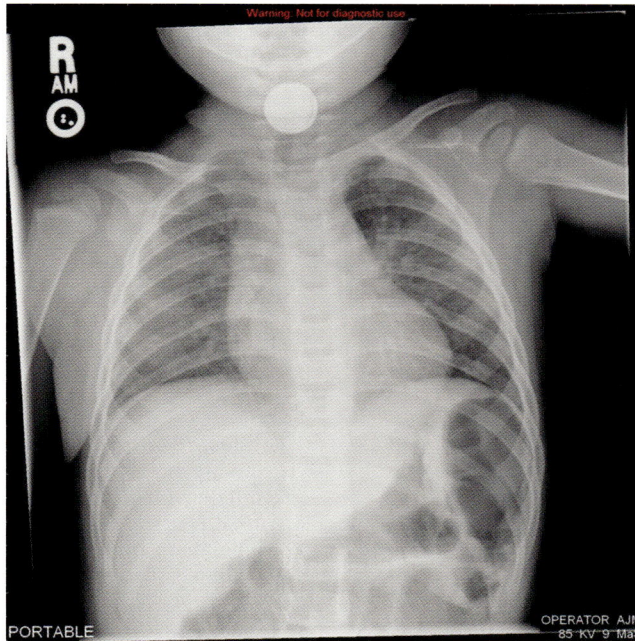

B

Figure 21-32. A. A preschooler who ingested a heart-shaped pendant. **B.** A toddler with watch button battery ingestion. Note "double-ring" lucency.

Regulatory Consideration and Resource Allocation

In 2015, the american college of surgeons (ACS) introduced the *Optimal Resources for Children's Surgical Care,* which has established standards required to improve the surgical care of children 17 years of age or younger. Similar to trauma verification, children's hospitals undergo a formal on-site, extensive chart and facility review and will receive appropriate designation (levels 1 to 3). Ongoing commitment to improving surgical access and care, appropriate physician staffing, data surveillance, quality improvement, and education are key factors in designation. Additionally, many state legislatures across the United States have passed laws defining designation for NICUs, maternal services, and stroke services. On-site review has historically been the gold standard; however, changes related to the COVID-19 pandemic have increased the virtual format for surveys.

SUGGESTED READINGS

Bhakta N, Liu Q, Ness KK, et al. The cumulative burden of surviving childhood cancer: an initial report from the St Jude Lifetime Cohort Study (SJLIFE). *Lancet.* 2017;390:2569-2582.

Calder BW, Vogel AM, Zhang J. Focused assessment with sonography for trauma in children with blunt abdominal trauma: a multi-institutional analysis. *J Trauma Acute Care Surg.* 2017;83:218-224.

Harbaugh CM, Lee JS, Hu HM, et al. Persistent opioid use among pediatric patients after surgery. *Pediatrics.* 2018;141(1):e20172439. doi:10.1542/peds.2017-2439

Rotondo MF, Cribari C, Smith RS, eds. *Resources for the Optimal Care of the Injured Patient.* American College of Surgeons; 2014.

Task Force for Children's Surgical Care. Optimal resources for children's surgical care in the United States. *J Am Coll Surg.* 2014;218:479-487, 487.e1-e4.

SAMPLE QUESTIONS

QUESTIONS

Choose the best answer for each question.

1. Concerning pediatric nutrition, which is false?
   A. Both adults and infants require approximately 25 to 30 kcal/kg to meet nutritional demands.
   B. TPN can be expensive and requires the placement of a PICC line or central line.
   C. Enteral nutrition need not reach goal rates to be beneficial.
   D. Long-term enteral nutrition is best facilitated through a surgically placed gastrostomy.
   E. Enteral nutrition promotes intestinal microvilli and is associated with decreased cost compared to TPN.

2. A referring NICU calls about a term newborn with a CDH that they would like to transfer to your institution. The child is on room air and has an OG tube in place. All of the following are true, except:
   A. Statistically speaking, this child most likely has a left-sided Bochdalek hernia.
   B. Morgagni hernias are central defects and often do not present in the newborn period.
   C. An OR should be available within 2 hours for emergent repair via a left subcostal incision.
   D. Pulmonary hypertension and pulmonary hypoplasia are responsible for the respiratory distress seen in these neonates. ECMO may be required.
   E. Many CDHs are diagnosed prenatally, and therefore, delivery can be planned to take place in a highly specialized center.

3. The most common type of EA is:
   A. type A, pure EA with no fistula.
   B. type B, EA with a proximal TEF.
   C. type C, EA with a distal TEF.
   D. type D, EA with both a proximal and distal TEF.
   E. type E, "H-type" fistula; TEF without EA.

4. You are managing a term child with suspected EA. Midline workup reveals a left-sided aortic arch and mild hydronephrosis. Which of the following is true about this newborn with EA?

A. An esophagram with contrast is required to make the diagnosis.
B. Intubation and mechanical ventilation are preferred in order to protect the airway of a child with EA/TEF.
C. Most neonates with type C EA/TEF require a gastrostomy tube and delayed repair.
D. Postoperative complications include GER, anastomotic leak, tracheomalacia, and anastomotic stricture.
E. "H-type" fistulas are always discovered in the newborn period because of severe respiratory failure and inability to swallow.

5. You are making rounds in the NICU with your attending surgeon. She asks you to define expected findings in newborns with congenital intestinal obstruction. All of the following are true, except:
   A. polyhydramnios.
   B. bilious emesis.
   C. abdominal distention.
   D. failure to pass meconium.
   E. renal failure.

6. You are called to the emergency department to evaluate a 4-week-old, previously healthy term child who presents with abdominal distention and bilious vomiting. Child is lethargic. Pertinent labs include pH of 7.2, WBC of 3.5, and Hgb of 17. Parents report last wet diaper 8 hours ago. If malrotation with midgut volvulus is suspected, clinicians should:
   A. refer the child to an outpatient pediatric surgery clinic to be seen within the next 2 weeks.
   B. discuss the case with radiology and await a formal UGI contrast study to confirm the diagnosis.
   C. proceed immediately to the OR to perform an exploratory laparotomy and possible Ladd procedure which includes lysing Ladd bands, widening of the small bowel mesentery, and appendectomy.
   D. begin IV fluid resuscitation, OG tube decompression, serial exams, and admission to the med/surg ward.
   E. obtain a suction rectal biopsy to rule out Hirschsprung disease.

7. A 7-year-old presents to the emergency department following a football helmet strike in the abdomen. He is tender in the left upper quadrant. Successful management of pediatric solid organ injury includes the following principles, except:

   A. Children are more susceptible to postsplenectomy sepsis and therefore attempts at splenic salvage are recommended.
   B. MTPs offer a balanced resuscitation approach and should be considered early in the trauma evaluation.
   C. Traditional diagnostic peritoneal lavage (DPL) remains favored over FAST in the preteen population.
   D. Stable children with contrast extravasation on CT can be referred to interventional radiology for selective embolization.
   E. Splenic and/or hepatic injuries can generally be managed with fluid resuscitation and close observation. Surgery is rarely required.

8. Possible signs of child abuse include the following, except:

   A. history discrepancy between caregivers.
   B. delay in obtaining health care.
   C. long bone fractures in infants.
   D. an interactive child who is not withdrawn.
   E. multiple injuries in various stages of healing.

9. A 2-year-old presents to the emergency department with excessive salivation and refusing to take a bottle. There are no respiratory symptoms. You are concerned with possible ingested foreign body. He last ate 4 hours ago. Which of the following is not correct:

   A. Obtain a portable CXR to diagnose an esophageal foreign body, such as a coin. If the coin has passed into the stomach, there is no additional immediate action.
   B. Immediately give the child honey if a watch battery is seen in the esophagus as noted by a halo sign on plain film.
   C. If the child is stable, preoperative consultation with pediatric anesthesia is recommended to determine the appropriate NPO period before proceeding to the OR for flexible esophagoscopy for a lodged esophageal coin in the proximal esophagus.
   D. If a coin is lodged in the distal esophagus, the child should be taken to the OR for endoscopic removal.
   E. Watch battery ingestions in the esophagus are relatively benign, and these cases should be added onto the OR schedule in the morning.

ANSWERS AND EXPLANATIONS

1. Answer: A

Understanding of pediatric nutrition is required when managing pediatric surgical patients. Overall, enteral nutrition is preferred as it promotes intestinal microvilli, is more physiologic, is cheaper, and is easier to administer. In certain conditions, such as obstruction to the GI tract, TPN will be required.

Of note, the nutritional demands of children far outweigh those of their adult counterparts. Most infants require 100 kcal/kg of nutrition in order to grow. For more information on this topic, please see section "Nutrition."

2. Answer: C

Surgical repair of a CDH is not emergent. In fact, emergent repair increases the stress on the newborn and results in increased morbidity and mortality. Repair should be delayed until signs of pulmonary hypertension have improved. Bochdalek hernias are 4 times more common than Morgagni hernias, and because of their location, Morgagni hernias often present later in life and sometimes can be relatively asymptomatic. Many birth defects can be identified on prenatal ultrasound, and a CDH is one of them. For more information on this topic, please see section "Congenital Diaphragmatic Hernia."

3. Answer: C

A type C proximal atresia with a distal TEF is by far the most common type (85%). Pure atresia (type A) occurs in approximately 8% of cases, type B occurs in less than 1% of cases, type D occurs in less than 1% of cases, and type E occurs in 5% of cases. For more information on this topic, please see section "Esophageal Atresia and Tracheoesophageal Fistula."

4. Answer: D

GER is common after the repair of EA. Other complications include anastomotic leak, anastomotic stricture, and tracheomalacia. Diagnosis can often be made by an attempt at OG tube placement combined with a CXR. Intubation and mechanical ventilation can make for an unstable situation because of positive pressure forcing air through the fistula and away from the lungs. H-type fistulas are often not discovered in the newborn period because the esophagus is in continuity. For more information on this answer, please see section "Esophageal Atresia and Tracheoesophageal Fistula."

5. Answer: E

Not every child with GI obstruction will have these findings, but polyhydramnios, bilious emesis, abdominal distention, and failure to pass meconium are all common symptoms. Renal failure is unrelated to intestinal obstruction. For more information on this answer, please see section "Congenital Gastrointestinal Obstruction."

6. Answer: C

Malrotation with midgut volvulus is the one diagnosis that is a true surgical emergency. Any delay can result in complete ischemia of all bowels supplied by the superior mesenteric artery (duodenum through mid-transverse colon). Confirmatory upper contrast study is helpful but not required. If suspicion is high, surgeons should proceed directly to the OR without confirmatory imaging. After counterclockwise rotation of the twisted bowel, a Ladd procedure, which includes removal of the appendix, is performed because it no longer sits in the right lower quadrant. For more information on this answer, please see section "Congenital Gastrointestinal Obstruction."

7. **Answer: C**

Key characteristics of successful management of pediatric trauma include increasing nonoperative management, aggressive burn resuscitation and subsequent enteral nutrition for burn patients, and early deployment of the MTP. Historically, DPL has been used as a window into the peritoneal cavity to diagnose intra-abdominal hemorrhage or bowel injury. DPL has largely been replaced by FAST which aims to detect free fluid in the abdomen as an indicator of hemorrhage. For more information on this topic, please see section "Evaluation of the Injured Child."

8. **Answer: D**

Nonaccidental injury to a child, otherwise known as child abuse, remains a public health crisis. High index of suspicion is required. Work with pediatric forensics team, child protective services, and close follow-up are recommended. Clinicians may find family discussions concerning possible child abuse to be difficult; however, a frank and honest discussion with a singular focus on the child's health should be the goal. Most children who are abused tend to be fearful and withdrawn. For more information on this topic, please see section "Child Abuse."

9. **Answer: E**

Children are curious creatures. Through exploring their environments, they will often put things in their mouths, such as coins, sharp objects, pins, and even watch batteries. Many objects will pass naturally. Occasionally, objects will become lodged in the proximal esophagus at the cricopharyngeus or in the distal esophagus at the lower esophageal sphincter. Watch battery ingestions present a unique, potentially life-threatening problem and require immediate endoscopic removal. Honey can help neutralize the harsh alkaline levels and thus protect the delicate esophageal tissue. During the COVID-19 pandemic, the prevalence of watch battery ingestions rose dramatically since children were spending more time at home. For more information on this topic, please see section "Foreign Body Aspiration and Ingestion."

22

Plastic Surgery: Diseases of the Skin and Soft Tissue, Face, and Hand

Seung Ah Lee, Gregory R. D. Evans, and Gregory A. Greco

The field of plastic and reconstructive surgery is concerned with the reconstruction or improvement of the form and function of many areas of the body. Rarely can either form or function be sacrificed for the other, but one is often of greater concern. This chapter concentrates on reconstructive surgery that is required because of abnormalities of the skin and soft tissues. These abnormalities may be caused by trauma, malignancies, congenital deformities, or other diseases.

Because plastic surgery almost always involves the skin, this chapter begins with a review of the structure of the skin, the process of wound healing, and the reconstruction of large defects (see Chapter 5). These discussions are followed by sections on benign skin lesions, facial trauma, hand surgery, congenital deformities, acquired deformities, and, finally, aesthetic surgery. This type of surgery differs from reconstructive surgery because it is directed at the cosmetic improvement of normal structures.

SKIN STRUCTURE

The skin, or integument, is the largest organ of the body and completely envelops its surface. The skin is both the primary defense against the environment and the principal means of communicating with it. The skin also serves important functions in terms of homeostasis and thermoregulation. The integument is an indispensable organ: Total destruction of the skin is incompatible with life.

The skin is divided into two embryologically distinct layers: the epidermis and the underlying dermis (Figure 22-1). The epidermis has five distinct strata, the cells of which all derive from the innermost of these strata, the stratum germinativum, or basal layer. Mitosis of this layer, with transformation of these cells as they migrate outward, forms the other strata of the epidermis. Located within the basal layer are the pigment-containing melanocytes. The epidermis is devoid of vasculature and receives its nourishment from the underlying dermis. Epidermal projections known as "rete pegs" extend down into the underlying dermis.

The dermis is 15 to 40 times thicker than the epidermis. It is divided into the thin papillary dermis, located beneath the epidermal rete pegs, and the thicker subjacent reticular dermis. The papillary dermis contains reticular and elastic fibers intermingled with a rich capillary network. The reticular dermis contains dense bundles of collagen parallel to the surface of the skin. This layer provides much of the tensile strength of the skin. Also contained within the dermis are pilosebaceous apparatus, eccrine and apocrine units, and important nerve end organs (eg, Pacinian and Meissner corpuscles).

WOUND HEALING

Wound healing has three phases. The inflammatory or substrate phase is characterized by inflammation around the edges of the wound, a nonspecific reaction to any injury. Leukocytes remove debris and bacteria. Toward the end of this relatively brief phase, activated macrophages appear and direct the next phase. The inflammatory phase lasts approximately 3 days in wounds with little contamination but may be significantly prolonged in contaminated wounds. The second phase, the proliferative phase, is characterized by collagen production by fibroblasts. Tissue fibroblasts synthesize collagen at an increased rate for approximately 6 weeks in normal wound healing. This synthesis causes a rapid gain in wound tensile strength that peaks at the end of this phase (Figure 22-2). The third phase, the maturation phase, consists of the remodeling of collagen by the formation of intermolecular cross-links. This phase, which lasts 6 to 12 months, leads to a flatter, paler scar, with little increase in tensile strength through a dynamic balance of collagenolysis and collagen synthesis.

Wound healing is classified as healing by primary, secondary, or tertiary (delayed primary) intention. Healing by primary intention involves recent, clean wounds that are managed by suture repair. These wounds are first gently irrigated and debrided to minimize the inflammatory process. Debridement consists of removing foreign material and devitalized tissue. After debridement, the tissue planes are approximated accurately to provide optimal healing. At the peak of collagen synthesis, the scar is mildly inflamed. It is raised, red, and often pruritic. Over time, the scar flattens, thins, and becomes much lighter. The process takes at least 9 to 12 months in an adult and somewhat longer in a child. The final appearance of a scar depends on the initial injury, the amount of contamination and ischemia, and the method and accuracy with which the wound was closed. Wound healing is delayed by multiple factors, including impaired circulation, immunosuppression, infection, or inadequate nutrition. Absorbable sutures are usually used below the skin surface. Nonabsorbable sutures are used for the outer closure because they are less reactive (Figure 22-3).

Wounds that are left open to heal without surgical intervention heal by secondary intention. This secondary closure is characterized by a prolonged inflammatory phase that persists until the wound is covered with epithelium. Wounds treated in this manner eventually heal, unless factors such as infection and foreign bodies are present. Epithelialization from the wound margins proceeds at approximately 1 mm/d in a concentric pattern. Wound

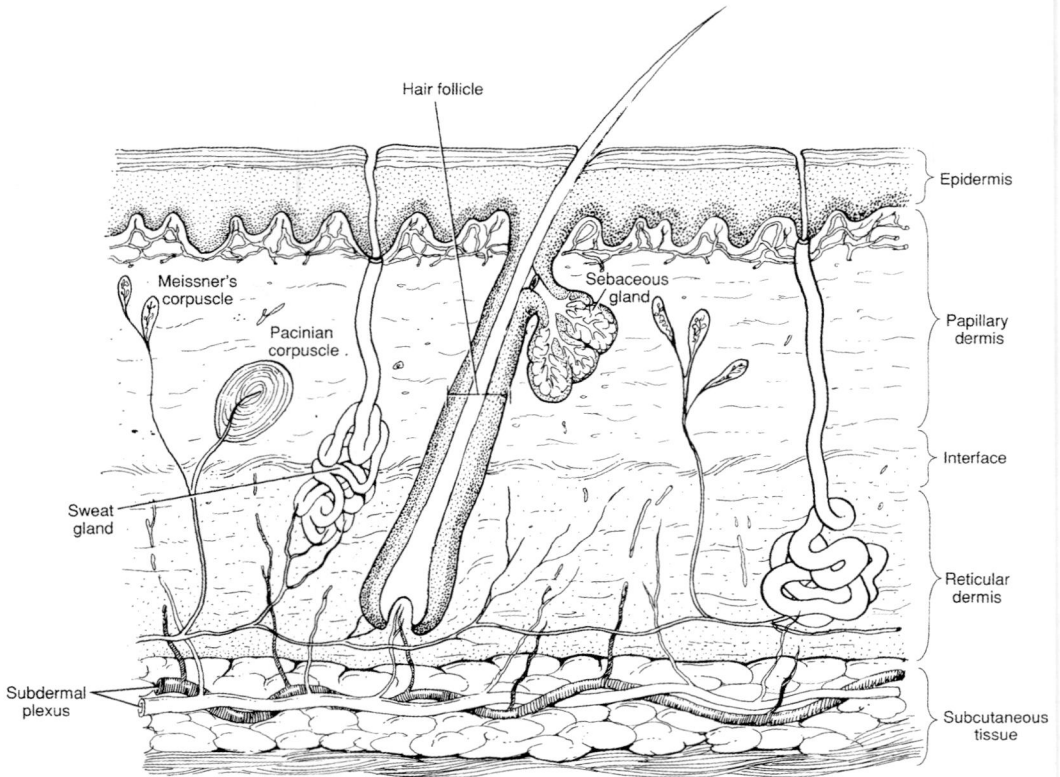

Figure 22-1. Cross section anatomy of the skin. (From Lawrence PF. *Essentials of Surgical Specialties*. 3rd ed. Lippincott Williams & Wilkins; 2007.)

contraction greatly reduces the size of the wound, although it never approaches the final appearance of a primarily closed wound. Healing by secondary intention is indicated in infected or severely contaminated wounds because abscess or wound infection rarely develops in an open wound.

Delayed primary closure, or healing by tertiary intention, involves the subsequent repair of a wound that was initially left open or was not repaired. This method is indicated for

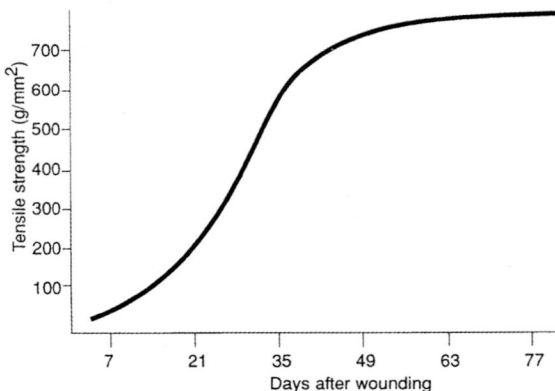

Figure 22-2. Wound tensile strength as a function of days. (From Lawrence PF. *Essentials of Surgical Specialties*. 3rd ed. Lippincott Williams & Wilkins; 2007.)

wounds with a high ($>10^5$) bacterial content (eg, human bite), a long time lapse since the initial injury, or a severe crush component with significant tissue devitalization. Successful closure depends on the cleanliness of the wound, the preparedness of the wound edges, and the absence of significant bacterial colonization ($<10^5$ bacteria/g tissue).

Abnormal healing may take the form of **hypertrophic scars** or **keloids.** Hypertrophic scars are raised, widened, and red. They may be pruritic, with tissue remaining within the boundaries of the scar (Figure 22-4A). Keloids have an abnormal growth of tissue that usually mushrooms over the edges of the wound and extends outside the boundaries of the scar (Figure 22-4B). Keloids are more common in African Americans and Asians. Differentiating between the two scars is important because their treatment differs. A hypertrophic scar often improves with time or may be improved by surgical revision. A keloid may be made worse by revision and is treated with intralesional steroids, external pressure, radiation, or a combination of modalities (see Chapter 5).

Suture Material

Suture material, suture placement, and knot-tying are fundamental elements to a successful surgical outcome. Understanding the properties of suture material and becoming proficient in knot-tying are critical skills for most physicians, not just surgeons. Properly tying sutures requires a great deal of practice.

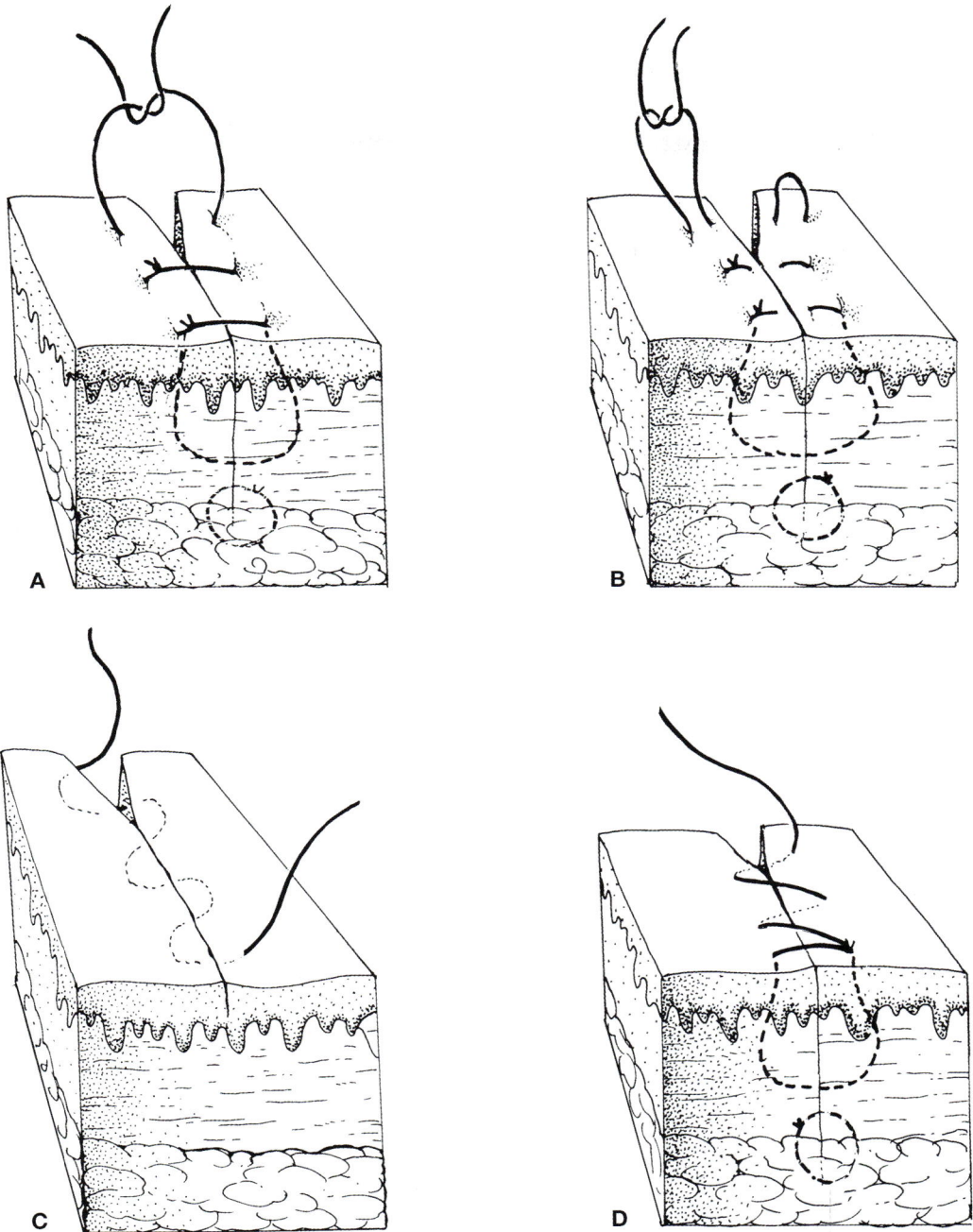

Figure 22-3. Techniques of skin closure. A. Simple interrupted sutures. B. Vertical mattress sutures. C. Running intracuticular (subcuticular) sutures. D. Continuous simple sutures. (From Lawrence PF. *Essentials of Surgical Specialties*. 3rd ed. Lippincott Williams & Wilkins; 2007.)

Types of Wounds and Their Treatment

Different wounds have specific causes and treatment guidelines.

Lacerations

Lacerations consist of cut or torn tissue. Care includes gentle handling of tissues. In addition, the wound should be cleansed of clots, foreign material, or necrotic tissue and irrigated with a physiologic solution (eg, saline, lactated Ringer solution). Administering a local anesthetic before the final cleansing is helpful. Once cleansed, lacerations are closed with an atraumatic technique, with care taken to avoid further crushing or injuring the tissues. Careful closure of wound margins gives the best chance for ideal healing with minimal scarring (Figure 22-5). Dressings should

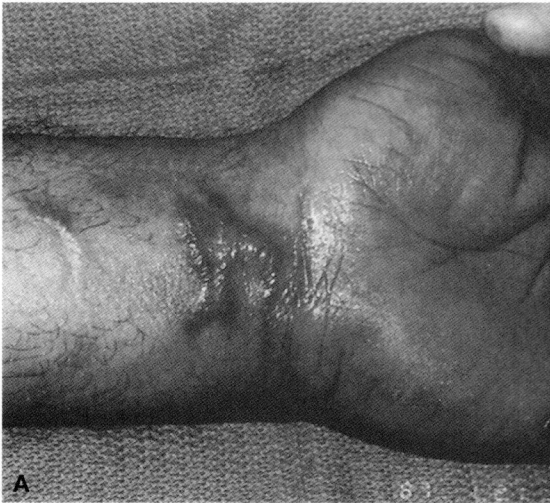

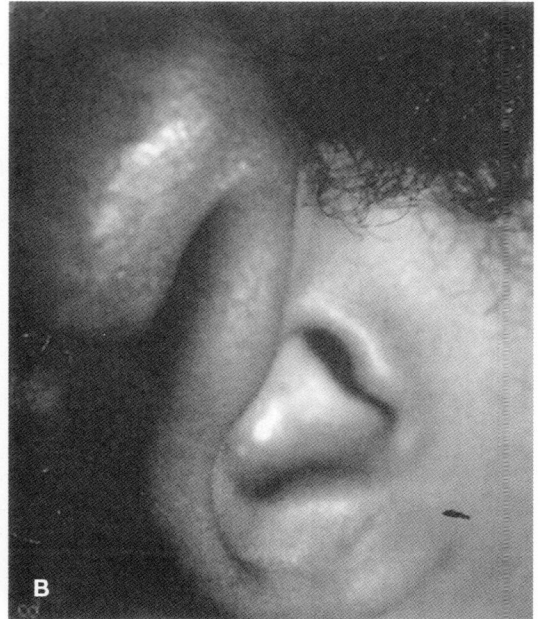

Figure 22-4. A. Hypertrophy of a scar on the volar wrist. The scar does not extend beyond the boundaries of the original scar. B. Keloid of a scar of the helical rim. The scar tissue mushrooms out beyond the boundaries of the original scar. (From Lawrence PF. *Essentials of Surgical Specialties*. 3rd ed. Lippincott Williams & Wilkins; 2007.)

consist of sterile material that will protect the wound and absorb some wound drainage. Immobilization is helpful in complex extremity wounds.

Abrasions

Abrasions are injuries in which the superficial skin layer is removed. They may be of variable depth. Abrasions should be gently cleansed of any foreign material. Occasionally, more vigorous rubbing with a scrub brush is appropriate. A local anesthetic can facilitate cleansing. Dirt and gravel are removed to prevent permanent discoloration (traumatic tattooing). The wound must be cleansed within the first day after injury. After this cleansing, an abrasion can be cared for by any method that keeps it clean and moist. The use of topical antibiotic ointment or protective dressings is appropriate.

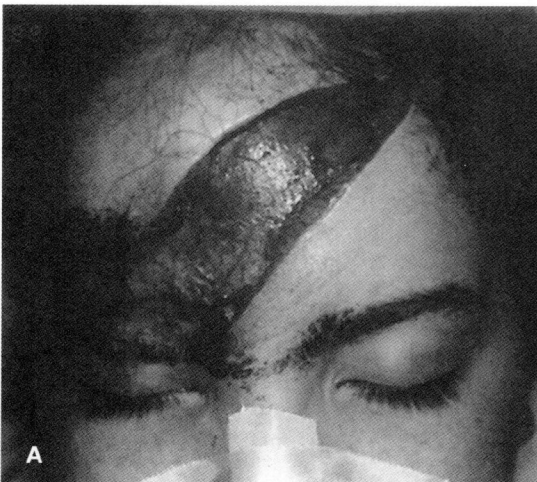

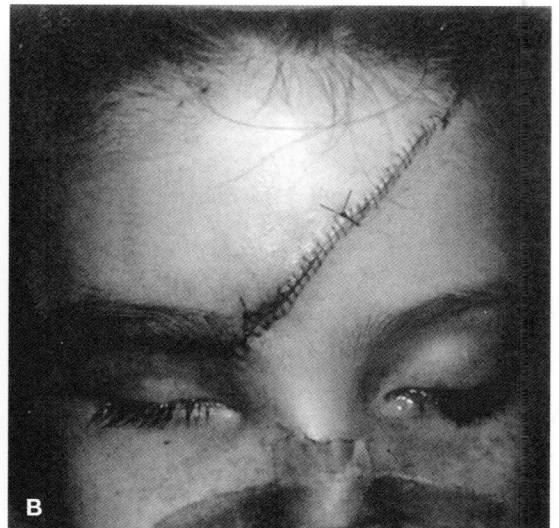

Figure 22-5. Complex laceration of the forehead and eyelid. A. Before debridement and closure. B. After debridement and closure. (From Lawrence PF. *Essentials of Surgical Specialties*. 3rd ed. Lippincott Williams & Wilkins; 2007.)

Contusions

A contusion is an injury that is caused by a forceful blow to the skin and soft tissues. The entire outer layer of skin is intact, although it is injured. Contusions require minimal early care. They should be evaluated early to diagnose a possible deep hematoma or tissue injury. Large or expanding hematomas may require evacuation, particularly if, through pressure, they threaten the viability of the overlying skin, cause vascular or neurologic compromise, or cause airway obstruction.

Avulsions

Avulsions are injuries in which the tissue is torn off, either partially or totally. In partial avulsions, the tissue is elevated but still attached to the body. If this raised portion of the tissue is adequately vascularized and appears viable, it is gently cleansed, irrigated, replaced into its anatomic location and anchored with a few sutures. If the tissue is not viable but is still attached, the best approach is usually to excise the tissue and use an alternate method of closure (eg, skin graft, local flap; discussed later). Completely avulsed tissue usually cannot be directly replaced as a graft because it is too thick to permit reliable healing. In some cases, the skin is debulked, defatted, and used as a skin graft.

Major avulsions (eg, amputation of extremities, fingers, ears, nose, scalp, eyelids) require specialty evaluation and care. Because replantation of some avulsed tissue is possible if it is handled appropriately, a replant team should be consulted promptly. For appropriate tissue preservation techniques, see the discussion of amputations.

Bites

Bites from animals and humans are a major problem because they are heavily contaminated by bacteria. Although dog bites may be appropriately left open for wound care, most, if handled appropriately, can be closed and heal without infection. Because of their much heavier bacterial contamination, however, human bites should be irrigated, debrided, and left open. In sensitive areas such as the face, thorough debridement and attempted closure may be appropriate. Broad-spectrum antibiotics should also be administered. Human bites to the hand are a special topic and are discussed later. Immobilization and elevation of extremity wounds aid in the healing of these heavily contaminated wounds.

Contaminated Wounds

A contaminated wound is one that has been exposed to bacteria from the body or local environment. The management of acute, significantly contaminated wounds consists of debridement, irrigation, and healing by secondary or tertiary intention. The use of antibiotics is reserved for severely contaminated wounds, wounds in immunocompromised patients, contaminated wounds that involve deeper structures (eg, joints, fractures), and obvious infection. The choice of antibiotic depends on the most likely organisms, given the cause of the injury. Broad-spectrum antibiotics with coverage of *Staphylococcus aureus* are usually recommended. Contaminated wounds are closed cautiously, depending on the degree of contamination and the location of the wound. Deep sutures should be kept to a minimum and should be monofilament. Patients with contaminated wounds are reevaluated within 24 to 48 hours. If any signs of deep infection are seen on reevaluation, at least a portion of the wound is opened by removing the sutures.

Contaminated Chronic Wounds

Lacerations and open injuries that are older than 24 hours require debridement and irrigation. With few exceptions, systemic antibiotics are not helpful in controlling bacterial colonization within a contaminated chronic wound. Antibiotic penetration into a chronic wound, with its granulating fibrous bed, is poor and unpredictable. Topical antibiotic cream (eg, silver sulfadiazine [Silvadene], bacitracin, Neosporin) may be helpful in areas of partial-thickness skin loss. However, some of these topical agents inhibit epithelialization and the initial aspects of wound healing. Highly toxic solutions (eg, alcohol, hydrogen peroxide) may adversely affect wound healing by destroying normal tissue. Contaminated wounds should be closed only after bacterial contamination is controlled. Chronic wounds that show no evidence of epithelialization or contraction or that are any color but the beefy red of a granulating bed usually have significant bacterial contamination and may be clinically infected. Although the type of organism is important, the principal determinant of wound sepsis seems to be the total bacterial load per gram of tissue ($>10^5$ bacteria/g tissue). Proteinaceous and necrotic debris may also be treated with enzymatic (eg, collagenase and urea) as well as surgical debridement.

Wound Management

The initial care of the wound is a major determinant in healing. Methodical assessment of the injury, followed by meticulous closure, minimizes deformity and maximizes the functional result. Evaluation includes an assessment of tissue injury, the amount of tissue lost, and the degree of injury to deeper structures. Treatment of a wound begins after the patient is evaluated and stabilized. After careful debridement and hemostasis, the injury pattern and tissue deficit are defined before the appropriate reconstructive technique is selected. Bleeding within the wound is controlled by direct pressure. Random clamping of tissue with hemostats should be avoided because it can crush normal tissue or injure other structures (eg, nerves). Because a tourniquet can increase venous bleeding or cause limb ischemia, it is used only to control life-threatening hemorrhage that cannot be controlled by other means. After bleeding is controlled, the wound is gently irrigated with a physiologic solution (eg, normal saline).

After the wound is cleaned, the viability of the wound margins is assessed. Clean lacerations have minimal surrounding tissue injury. Contused, contaminated wounds have a crush component of surrounding ischemic tissue. In general, recent, clean wounds without tissue loss can be gently irrigated and closed. However, crushed, contaminated wounds have areas of tissue injury and devitalization that may require debridement and closure, delayed closure, or even the use of skin grafts or flaps to resurface injured areas that have inadequate overlying tissue. Specialized tissues (eg, eyebrows, eyelids, ears, lips) and other tissues that are difficult to replace precisely should be debrided only by a physician experienced in complicated wound care. Some areas of the body (eg, face) have a rich vascular supply and tend to heal well. However, the viability of portions of these wounds initially may be in question. As

TABLE 22-1. Immunization Recommendations

| History of Immunization | Tetanus Prone | | Nontetanus Prone | |
	Tetanus Toxoid	Tetanus Immune Globulin	Tetanus Toxoid	Tetanus Immune Globulin
Unknown or incomplete	0.5 mL[a]	Yes	0.5 mL[a]	No
Complete, last booster >5 y ago	0.5 mL	No	No[b]	No
Complete, last booster <5 y ago	No	No	No	No

[a]In unimmunized children, diphtheria, tetanus or diphtheria, pertussis, or tetanus is used. Completion of immunizations is necessary.
[b]Yes, if booster >10 years ago.

a rule, any questionable tissue should be gently irrigated and reexamined 24 to 48 hours later. Although contused, crushed injuries predictably have a less favorable outcome, precise reconstruction can optimize the results.

A recent adjunct to wound management has been a negative pressure wound dressing, such as the vacuum assisted closure (VAC, Kinetic Concepts, Inc., San Antonio, TX). This device consists of a sponge that is placed in the wound bed, which is then sealed with a dressing and connected to suction. The ability to prescribe negative pressure wound therapy provides multiple benefits for wound management and closure. The VAC system will assist in the promotion of granulation tissue formation, aid in the removal of interstitial fluid, and uniformly draw wound edges closer together through the use of the controlled, localized negative pressure.

For all penetrating injuries and many nonpenetrating injuries (eg, abrasions, burns, frostbite), the patient's tetanus immunization status must be determined. Guidelines for wounds that may be tetanus prone should be followed (Table 22-1).

RECONSTRUCTION OF LARGE WOUNDS AND TISSUE DEFECTS

Wounds that cannot be repaired by simple approximation of the wound margins often require an alternate method of reconstruction (eg, graft, flap). When choosing the appropriate method of reconstruction, the concept of a "reconstructive ladder" must be kept in mind (Figure 22-6). This ladder is a classification of the methods of wound reconstruction in order of increasing complexity. Simpler methods are often best, but they do not always suffice. The different "rungs" of the ladder are discussed in this section (direct closure, where appropriate, was discussed previously under "Types of Wounds and Their Treatment").

Skin Grafts

A skin graft is a portion of the skin (including the epidermis and a variable amount of dermis) that is completely removed from its original location (donor site) and transferred to another area of the body (recipient site). No underlying tissue is included. Because of its separation, a skin graft derives all of its nutritional supply from its recipient bed. It carries neither vasculature nor any lymphatic or nerve structures. Skin grafts are categorized according to species and thickness.

Species Classification

An autograft is a graft taken from one place on an individual and transplanted to another place on the same individual. Immunologic compatibility is ensured, and the graft is considered permanent. An **allograft** (homograft) is a graft taken from one individual (usually a cadaver) and transplanted to another individual of the same species. These grafts are useful for temporarily resurfacing defects. Rejection eventually occurs, except in cases of transplantation between identical twins or, potentially, in people who are permanently immunosuppressed. The third type of species graft, a xenograft (heterograft), is a graft from a donor of one species to a recipient of a different species. This type of graft, commonly used in clinical practice, entails

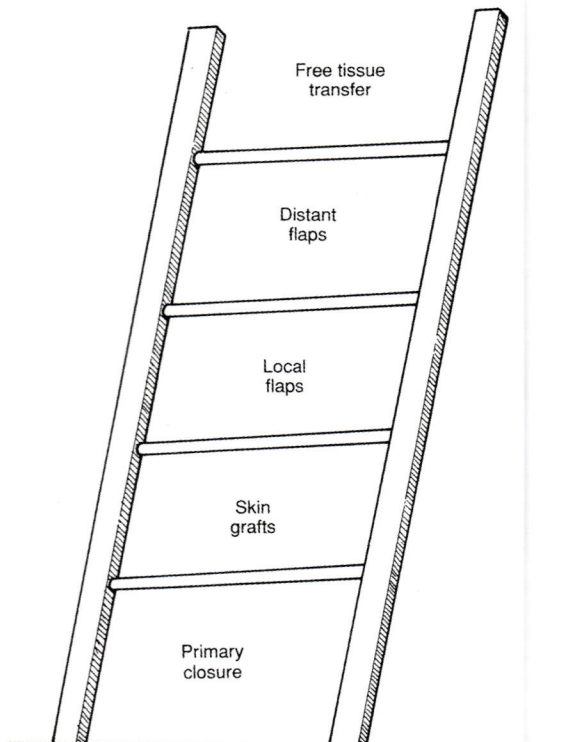

Figure 22-6. The reconstructive ladder. (From Lawrence PF. *Essentials of Surgical Specialties.* 3rd ed. Lippincott Williams & Wilkins; 2007.)

the use of porcine skin to cover large skin and soft tissue defects on a temporary basis.

Recently, various types of dermal substitutes have been developed and widely used for wound care and soft tissue reconstruction. One such dermal substitute product, acellular dermal matrix (ADM), is different from classic allografts or xenografts in that it is prepared by decellularizing donor dermis and leaving only extracellular matrix components. Alloderm (LifeCell, Branchburg, NJ) is a type of ADM made from human cadaver dermis. Thus, Alloderm promotes revascularization and dermal regeneration. It was initially used in burn reconstruction but is now also used for other large soft tissue defect reconstructions as well as chest and abdominal wall repair. Other commercially available allogeneic ADM products are DermaMatrix (MTF, Edison, NJ), FlexHD (MTF, Edison, NJ), GraftJacket (Wright Medical Technology, Arlington, TN), DermACELL (Arthrex, Naples, FL), Repriza (Specialty Surgical Products, Victor, MT), DermaSpan (Biomet, Warsaw, IN), and AlloMax (CR Bard, Warwick, RI). Xenogeneic ADM, on the contrary, is created by using porcine or bovine dermal sources, which require extra processing to reduce immunogenicity. The examples of xenogenic ADM include Surgisis Biodesign (Cook Surgical, Bloomington, IN), Oasis (Cook Biotech, Lafayette, IN), Tutopatch (RTI Biologics, Alachua, FL), and Strattice (LifeCell, Branchburg, NJ) and TELA bio (Malverne, PA). Some skin substitutes are available in a bilayer form in which one layer emulates the epidermis, whereas the other layer functions as the dermis. For example, Integra (Integra LifeSciences, Plainsboro, NJ), widely used for various types of wounds, consists of a porous layer of bovine collagen and glycosaminoglycan (GAG) matrix attached to a silicone membrane layer. The collagen-GAG matrix serves as a dermal replacement, whereas the silicone layer provides a barrier against moisture loss. In contrast to acellular dermal substitutes, the cellular dermal matrix contains living fibroblasts. Apligraf (Organogenesis, Canton, MA), a type of cellular dermal matrix, was initially approved by the Food and Drug Administration (FDA) for the treatment of venous ulcers that have failed to heal with conventional wound care. It is created by culturing fibroblasts derived from neonatal foreskin in a bovine type I collagen matrix. Although the long-term stability of these skin substitutes is less than that of autografts, they can play a significant role in early wound coverage.

Thickness Classification

A **split-thickness skin graft** includes the epidermis and a portion of the dermis (Figure 22-7). The graft includes a variable number of dermal appendages, depending on the thickness of the dermis taken with the graft. The success of the skin graft increases with thinner grafts because less vascular ingrowth is required to maintain their viability. Thinner grafts can also be expanded to a greater degree than thicker grafts. They are used in areas of large skin loss (Figure 22-8), over areas of granulating tissue, and in areas of marginal vascularity or potential contamination. These grafts are harvested with an air- or electric-powered dermatome or a specialized freehand knife. The donor site, which represents a partial-thickness loss, heals by reepithelialization from

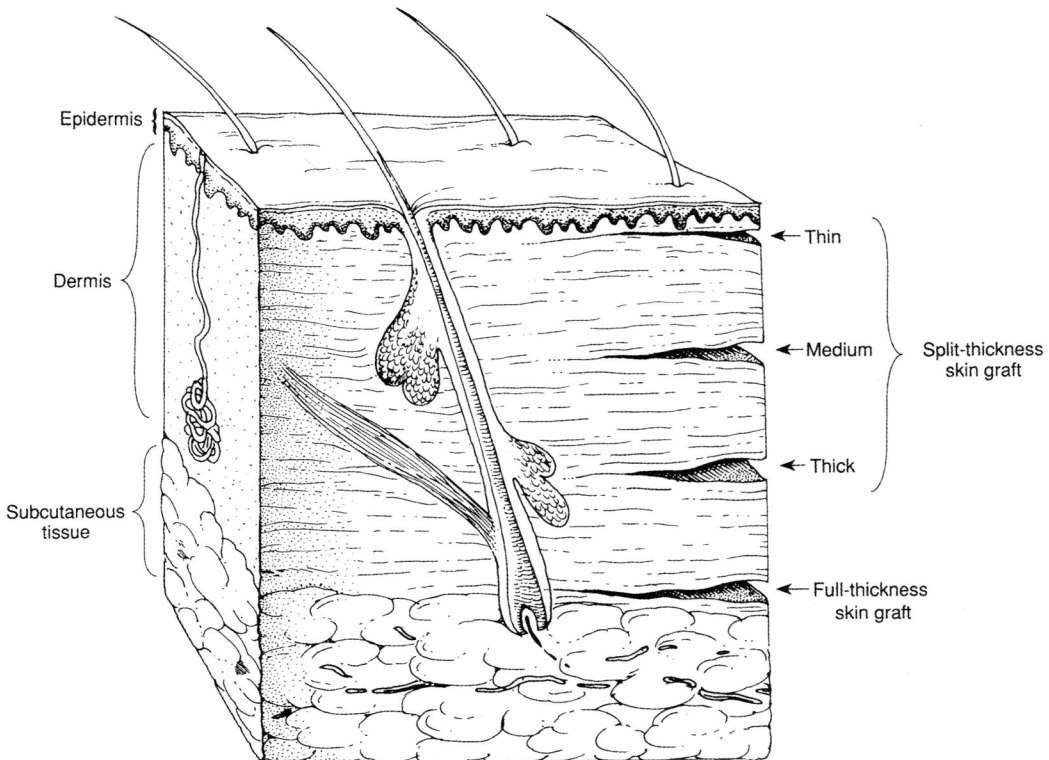

Figure 22-7. Different levels of thickness of skin grafts. (From Lawrence PF. *Essentials of Surgical Specialties*. 3rd ed. Lippincott Williams & Wilkins; 2007.)

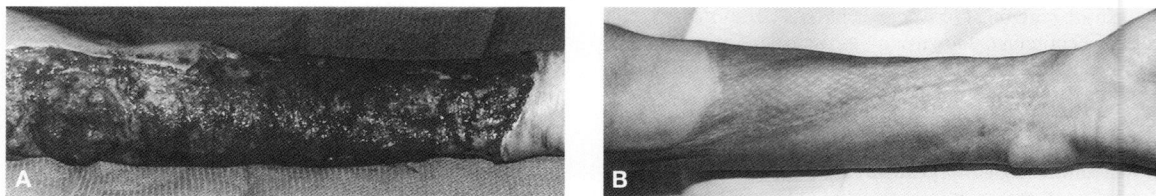

Figure 22-8. Open wound of the forearm. A. Before split-thickness skin grafting. B. After successful healing of a meshed graft. (From Lawrence PF. *Essentials of Surgical Specialties*. 3rd ed. Lippincott Williams & Wilkins; 2007.)

wound edges and from residual deeper skin dermal appendages scattered throughout the wound base. The donor site requires ongoing care to prevent secondary infection, which can create full-thickness loss. This care consists of keeping the wound moist while minimizing contamination, pressure, and desiccation. Split-thickness skin grafts are usually taken from the buttock or high thigh area because of the large amount of surface area available and the relatively inconspicuous location. Split-thickness skin grafts have an added benefit in that they can easily be "meshed" with an operative device at various ratios (eg, 2:1, 3:1, 4:1). This allows for gentle separation of the meshed tissue for greater surface area coverage.

A **full-thickness skin graft** consists of the epidermal layer and the entire thickness of the dermis (see Figure 22-7). In contrast to a split-thickness graft, it provides a more durable form of coverage, its appearance is more normal, and it carries an increased number of dermal appendages. However, because of its greater thickness and slower revascularization, it may be less likely to succeed than a split-thickness skin graft. The absolute thickness may vary according to the thickness of the dermis at the donor site. A thin full-thickness skin graft may be obtained from the eyelid or postauricular areas. Thicker full-thickness skin grafts can be obtained from the cervical and groin areas. Full-thickness grafts are usually used on the face because of their better color match, on the fingers to avoid joint contractures, and at any site where thicker skin or less secondary contraction is desired. Because the donor site is a full-thickness defect, it is managed by either primary closure or split-thickness skin grafting. This factor limits the size of full-thickness skin grafts. These grafts are usually taken from the groin, postauricular area, upper eyelid, supraclavicular area, or scalp. The last four locations are useful for reconstruction in the head and neck because of proper color match, but a limited amount of skin is available (Figure 22-9).

When a graft is harvested, it contracts immediately after it is freed from the surrounding tissue. This primary skin graft contraction is related to the number of elastin fibers in the graft. Thus, the thicker the graft (because of the greater number of elastin fibers it contains), the greater the primary contraction.

Secondary contraction occurs during the healing phase (Figure 22-9). As healing occurs, the graft contracts to leave a smaller surface area. The thicker the graft, the less secondary contraction occurs. This phenomenon is more closely related to the percentage of the dermis in the graft than to the actual thickness. Consequently, a graft that includes 50% of the dermis would be predicted to contract less than a graft that contains 30%. Secondary contraction is mediated by myofibroblasts (specialized fibroblast-like cells that contain smooth muscle contractile elements)

within the wound. The dermis suppresses the myofibroblast population. Greater suppression is seen with greater thickness of the dermis.

Contraction must be taken into account when planning reconstruction. Thus, reconstruction of defects or scar contractures may need more graft placed than initially predicted. On the contrary, secondary graft contraction may be used to provide an advantage. A large defect can be surfaced with a thin split-thickness skin graft with the expectation that the total surface area will shrink with the skin graft contraction. A secondary procedure can be performed to excise a portion of the defect and leave a much smaller defect.

Skin Graft Healing

Because the skin graft is completely isolated from its original nutrient source when it is harvested, it must survive initially by diffusion of oxygen and nutrients from the recipient bed. The diffusion of nutritional elements and fluid from the recipient site and the subsequent diffusion back to the host bed of metabolic waste products is called "plasmatic imbibition." This process allows the skin graft to survive for the first 48 to 72 hours after placement. Vascular ingrowth begins shortly after the skin graft is placed on the host bed. However, adequate nutritional exchange to maintain tissue viability does not occur until 48 to 72 hours after graft placement. The new ingrowth of capillary tissue into the graft (neovascularization) is known as "inosculation." The recipient bed is prepared by minimizing the bacterial concentration and removing poorly vascularized tissue. Wounds may require debridement at grafting or even several days before grafting. An adequate vascular supply must be ensured, particularly in the compromised extremity. Physical examination is usually sufficient, but Doppler examination or arteriography may be necessary. If local blood flow is inadequate, vascular bypass or another

Split-thickness graft	Full-thickness graft
Success higher (more reliable)	Success lower
Less first degree contraction	Greater first degree contraction
Greater second degree contraction	Less second degree contraction
Donor site heals by reepithelialization	Donor site must be closed
May be used in most wounds	Used in specialized situations

Figure 22-9. Comparison of split-thickness and full-thickness skin grafts. (From Lawrence PF. *Essentials of Surgical Specialties*. 3rd ed. Lippincott Williams & Wilkins; 2007.)

procedure may be necessary. A well-vascularized recipient site, if kept clean, shows signs of local capillary proliferation. The mixture of capillary buds and connective tissue (granulation tissue) is usually beefy red and bleeds easily to touch. In most cases, it forms a good recipient bed for skin grafting, but because it is a chronic open wound, it also supports bacterial growth.

The graft should be immobilized on the recipient site to prevent shear forces from dislodging the tenuous ingrowth of new capillaries. Separation of the graft from its bed prevents both the diffusion of nutrients and the ingrowth of new vascular tissue, resulting in the loss of the skin graft. Because skin grafts require a well-vascularized recipient bed, they do not take on relatively avascular structures (eg, bone, tendon, heavily irradiated areas, infected wounds). However, skin grafts take well on periosteum, peritenon, and perichondrium. Immobilization can occur by wrapping and splinting on an extremity or placement of a bolster dressing on the scalp, trunk, or extremity. Occasionally, a negative pressure wound dressing can also apply the immobilization that is required.

Graft failure is usually caused by a mechanical blockage of diffusion (eg, hematoma or seroma under the graft), shearing forces that dislodge the graft from its recipient bed, or an inadequate recipient site (because of contamination or poor blood supply). Systemic factors (eg, malnutrition, sepsis, medications) may also play a role in the success of the skin graft. Systemic steroids, antineoplastic agents, and vasoconstrictors (eg, nicotine) may adversely affect skin graft survival and wound healing in general.

Flaps

Tissues that are transferred from one location to another and are supported by an intact blood supply are commonly known as "flaps." They are typically used to replace tissue that is lost because of trauma or surgical excision. Flaps provide temporary or permanent skin coverage in critical areas that require good soft tissue bulk for underlying structures (eg, tendons, joints). They may also provide increased padding over bony prominences (eg, pressure sore reconstruction). They bring a better blood supply to relatively poorly vascularized areas and are occasionally used to improve sensation to an area by bringing in an accompanying nerve supply. In addition, they are used to carry specialized reconstructive tissue (eg, bone, cartilage). Flaps may consist of skin, subcutaneous tissue, muscle, bone, cartilage, nerve, and specialized tissues such as jejunum, omentum, or fascia. Skin flaps are classified according to their vascular anatomy as random or axial and according to their anatomic location as local, regional, or distant.

A **random-pattern skin flap** is an area of skin and subcutaneous tissue that has no specifically defined vascular distribution (Figure 22-10). For viability, the flap depends mostly on the random dermal and subdermal plexus of vascular structures. It has a limited length-to-width ratio to ensure that enough blood vessels are included to provide nutrition throughout its length. Random flaps may be raised in any location, assuming normal vascularity of the skin.

A **Z-plasty** is a specific use of random-pattern skin flaps. It involves raising two random flaps in a Z-shape. The flaps are interpolated and then interdigitated with one another (Figure 22-11). In so doing, two things are accomplished. First, the scar is lengthened at the expense of width. Second, the direction of the scar is reoriented. Z-plasties are often used when scar contractures have developed. Varying the angle of the Z will vary the amount of lengthening of the skin. The normal angles are usually 60 and 120°.

Axial-pattern, or arterialized, flaps differ from random-pattern flaps because they are based on a named blood supply (Figure 22-12). The underlying vasculature must be well mapped, and the flap outline must be designed to maximize the vascular supply. The vascular supply must include a direct artery and accompanying veins. Specific axial-pattern skin flaps in different anatomic locations take advantage of known cutaneous arteries. Because of this known arterial supply, a greater length-to-width ratio (up to 5:1 or 6:1) is usually possible than with the random flap. Some axial flaps may be used as free flaps (see later discussion).

Tissue expansion uses the ability of the skin to relax and expand as a result of tension applied to it. When local tissue directly adjacent to the wound is the best option for reconstruction (eg, scalp defects), the two-stage process of tissue expansion is used. An inflatable prosthesis is placed beneath the skin or other tissue to be expanded. After initial healing occurs, the expander is serially inflated through a valve or injection port, usually weekly. When full expansion is achieved, the expander is removed at a second operation. The expanded tissue is used as a local flap to reconstruct the wound (Figure 22-13).

Composite Flaps

Composite flaps offer another technique for reconstruction. In this technique, multiple tissue types such as skin, fascia, and bone are transferred to allow closure of critical defects with materials similar to those that were lost.

Myocutaneous flaps are the next most complex type of flaps used for reconstruction (Figure 22-14). The skin overlying many muscles of the body is supported by vessels that course directly from the muscle to the skin (musculocutaneous perforators). Large amounts of skin left attached to the underlying muscle can be transferred from one location to another as long as the blood supply to the underlying muscle is preserved. Knowledge of the blood supply to these muscles allows rotation or transposition of the tissue from the donor site to the reconstructed wound. The location of the dominant vasculature is used as the pivot point for the arc of rotation. In some cases, a muscle alone is transferred and subsequent skin grafting is performed.

Fasciocutaneous flaps can also be used for coverage. These flaps are similar to myocutaneous flaps, except that the blood supply to the skin does not course through muscle. Consequently, these flaps provide thin and well-vascularized coverage from a named artery to assist in covering defects.

Vascularized composite allotransplant is a continuously evolving technique with significant potential for complex wound care. It comprises the transplantation of a vascularized human body part that includes different tissue types such as skin, muscle, cartilage, bone, nerves, lymph nodes, and blood vessels. With this technique, body parts like the hand, abdominal wall, larynx, trachea, penis, and knee have been transplanted. The first face transplantation on a living human using a vascularized composite flap was carried out in 2005 in France.

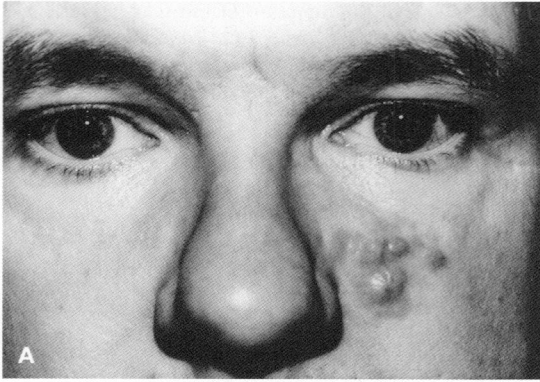

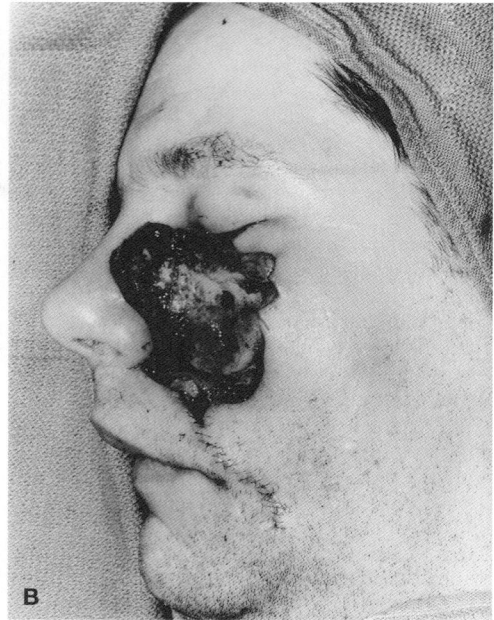

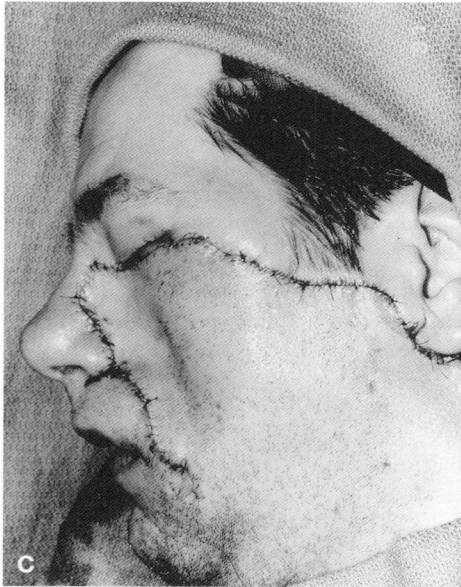

Figure 22-10. A. Patient with a dermatofibrosarcoma protuber-ans of the left lower eyelid and cheek. B. After radical resection. C. After coverage with a random-pattern skin flap of adjacent cheek and neck skin. The length-to-width ratio of the flap is ap-proximately 1:1. (From Lawrence PF. *Essentials of Surgical Spe-cialties*. 3rd ed. Lippincott Williams & Wilkins; 2007.)

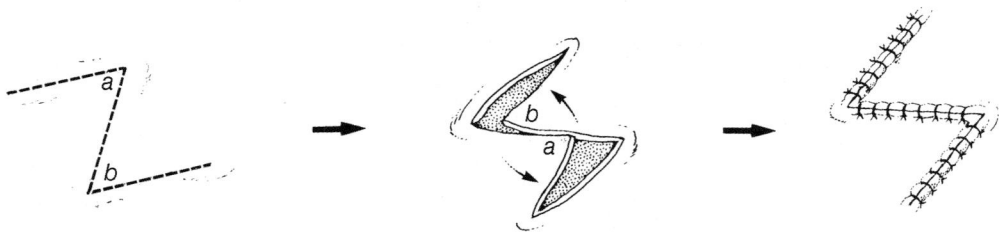

Figure 22-11. A Z-plasty is used to reorient and lengthen a scar (distance *a* to b) at the expense of width. (From Lawrence PF. *Essentials of Surgical Specialties*. 3rd ed. Lippincott Williams & Wilkins; 2007.)

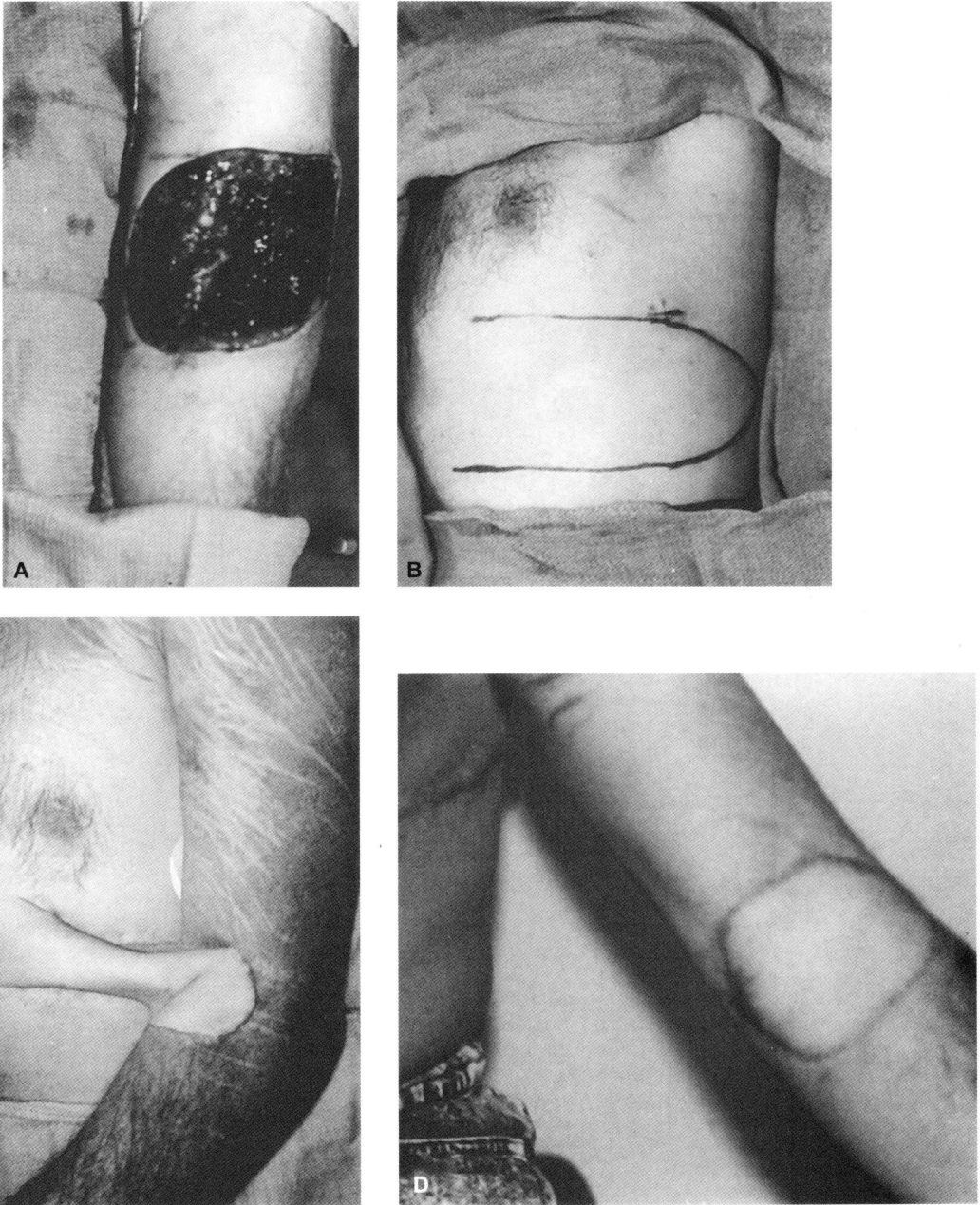

Figure 22-12. A. Open wound of the antecubital fossa. B. A thoracoepigastric axial-pattern skin flap is designed. Its length greatly exceeds its width. C. The flap is attached as a pedicled flap and left for several weeks before the pedicle is divided. D. After the pedicle is divided, is inset, and has healed. (From Lawrence PF. *Essentials of Surgical Specialties*. 3rd ed. Lippincott Williams & Wilkins; 2007.)

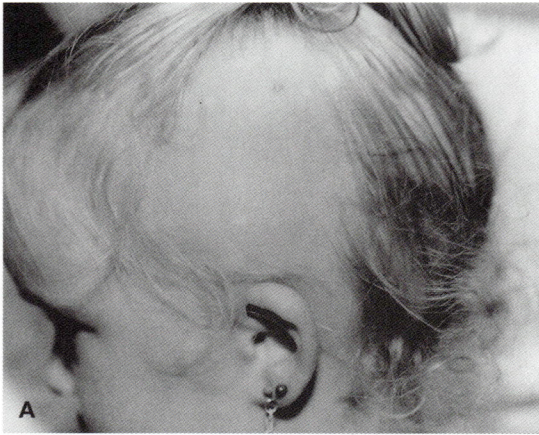

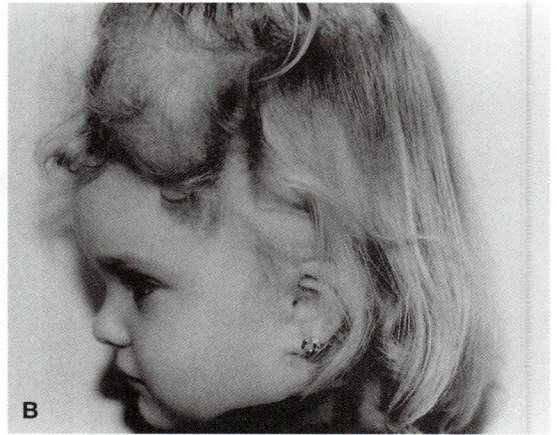

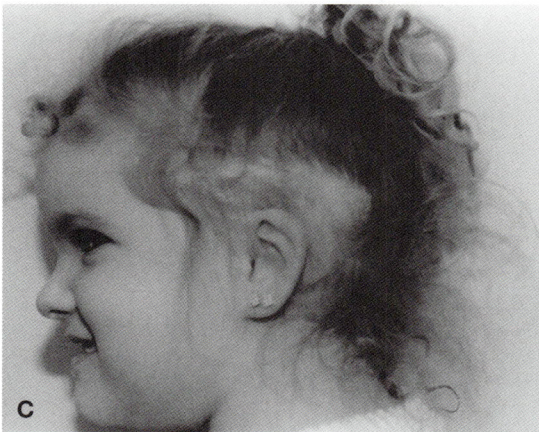

Figure 22-13. A. A young patient with a large sebaceous nevus of the scalp. B. A tissue expander is placed anteriorly and fully inflated. C. Result after resection of the lesion and coverage with the expanded scalp skin. (From Lawrence PF. *Essentials of Surgical Specialties*. 3rd ed. Lippincott Williams & Wilkins; 2007.)

Flaps Used in Microvascular Surgery

Free flaps raised from a distant site may be used if local skin flaps or regional myocutaneous flaps are not available for wound reconstruction. These flaps are transplanted from one site of the body to another by isolating the dominant artery and veins to a flap and performing a microscopic anastomosis between these and the vessels in or near the recipient wound. Muscle and skin are most commonly used, although bone, nerves, tendons, jejunum, and omentum may also be transferred. Although these flaps may be used in almost any reconstruction situation, they are predominantly used in lower extremity, breast, and head and neck reconstructions (Figure 22-15).

MANAGEMENT OF BENIGN SKIN LESIONS

Types of Lesions

Skin lesions are either benign or malignant. Differentiation is important in providing appropriate care. Common benign lesions include the **nevus**, keratosis, verruca, fibroma, and **hemangioma and vascular malformation**. Common malignant lesions include basal cell carcinoma, squamous cell carcinoma, and malignant melanoma (see Chapter 25).

The nevus is the most common lesion in the adult. It is usually brown and slightly raised, and it may have hair (Figure 22-16). Nevi are subclassified according to the appearance and depth of active proliferating cells. Dysplastic nevi have the potential for malignant transformation. They have irregular borders and varying shades of pigmentation. It is impractical to excise all nevi, but suspicious pigmented lesions that have had a recent change in size, elevation, color (brown to black or gray), or irregular borders (notching) should be excised. In addition, lesions that have a surface discharge, a tingling sensation, bleeding, or itching and those that are constantly irritated (eg, those under a belt line or bra) should be excised. All significant nevi should be carefully observed.

The second most common type of benign lesion is keratosis. It is subclassified into seborrheic keratoses, actinic keratoses, and **keratoacanthomas**. A seborrheic keratosis is elevated and brown and has a greasy feeling. It usually has a "stuck-on" appearance and can be treated by freezing, scraping, cauterizing, or excision. If the diagnosis is

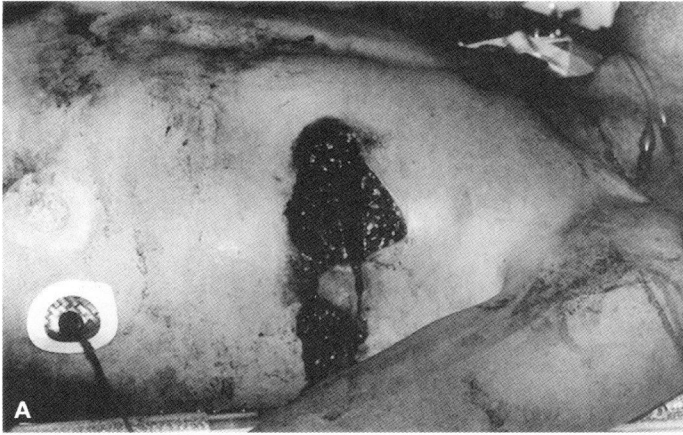

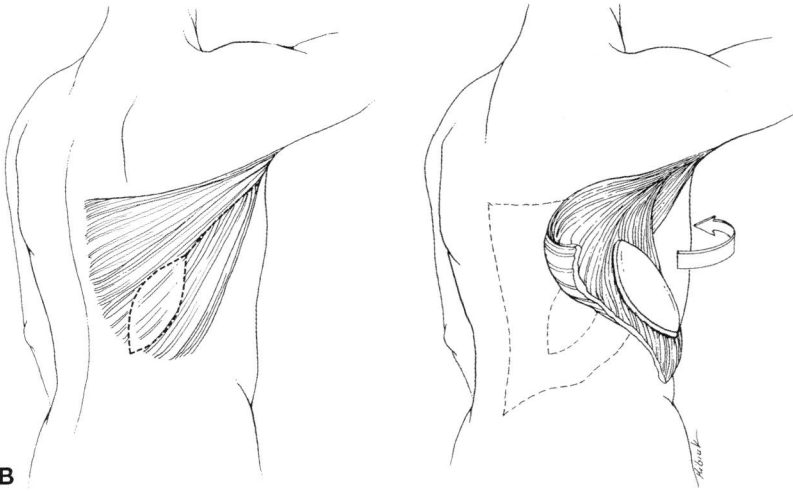

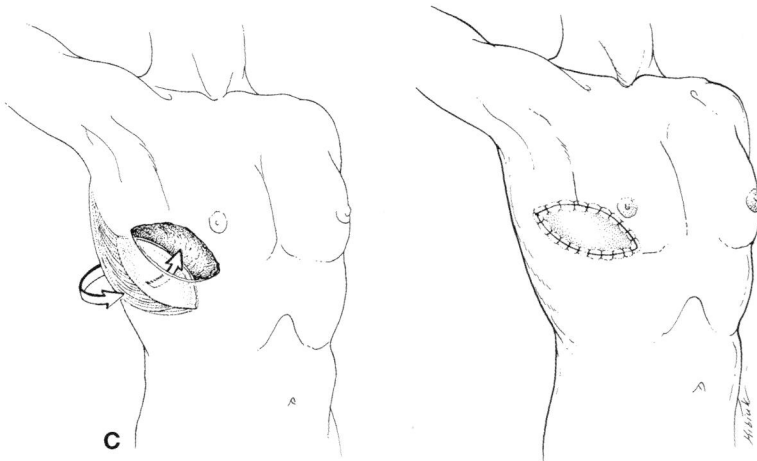

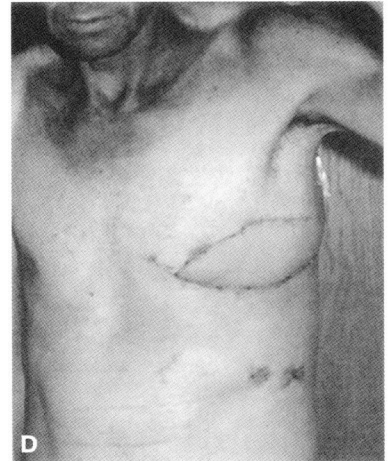

Figure 22-14. A. A patient who had a point-blank shotgun blast to the chest. B. The defect is closed with a latissimus dorsi myocutaneous flap. C. Once the flap is elevated, it is tunneled into the defect on the chest. D. The patient after successful reconstruction. (From Lawrence PF. *Essentials of Surgical Specialties*. 3rd ed. Lippincott Williams & Wilkins; 2007.)

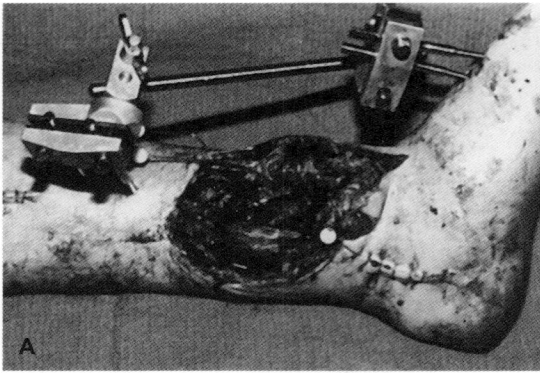

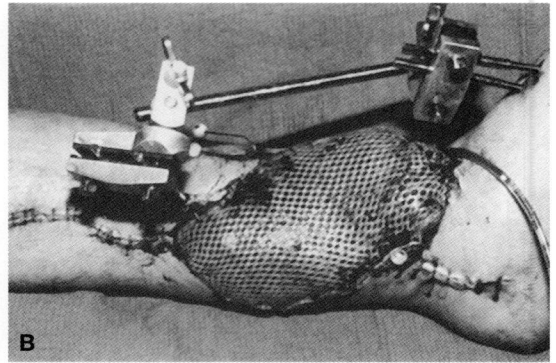

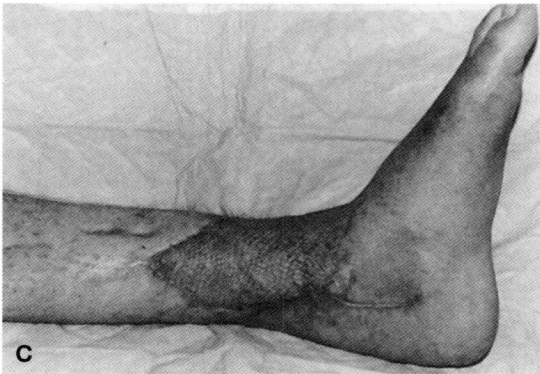

Figure 22-15. A. A close-range shotgun blast to the ankle required external fixation of the ankle and vascular reconstruction. B. The ankle immediately after reconstruction with a free muscle flap and a skin graft. C. Long-term result showing satisfactory reconstruction. (From Lawrence PF. *Essentials of Surgical Specialties*. 3rd ed. Lippincott Williams & Wilkins; 2007.)

uncertain, it should be excised. An actinic keratosis is a rough, irregularly shaped, brownish patch, most commonly seen in the older adult. Because these keratoses may be premalignant, some may be removed at the discretion of the surgeon and patient. A keratoacanthoma is a rapidly growing, elevated lesion that may have a central crater or ulceration (Figure 22-17). It usually resolves spontaneously in 4 to 6 months; however, concern over its growth and appearance often justifies excision for diagnosis.

A verruca (wart) usually has a viral etiology. It is characteristically self-limiting. Spontaneous disappearance after several years is the rule. Surgical excision is occasionally indicated, especially if the lesion occurs on pressure points

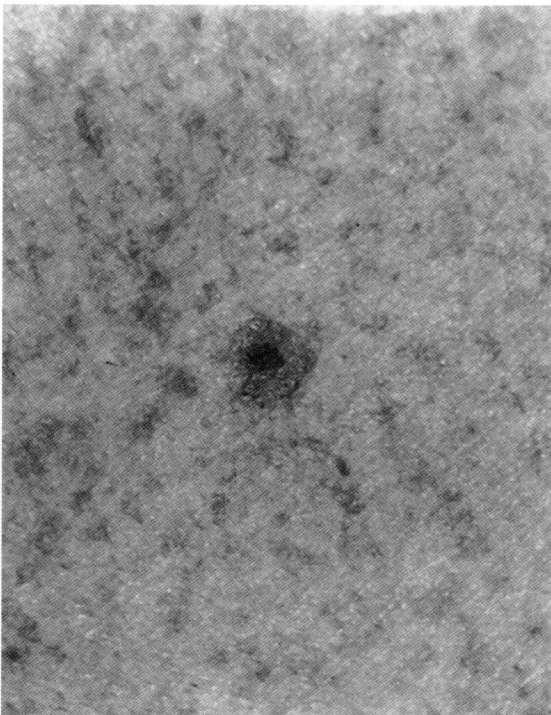

Figure 22-16. Benign nevus. (From Lawrence PF. *Essentials of Surgical Specialties*. 3rd ed. Lippincott Williams & Wilkins; 2007.)

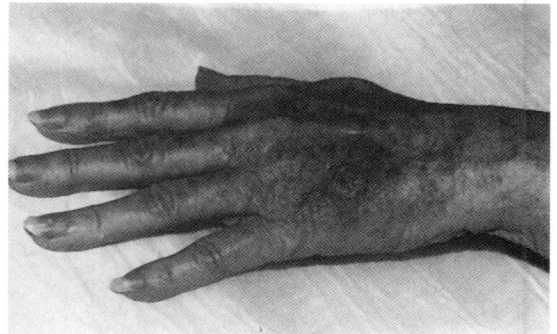

Figure 22-17. Keratoacanthoma of the hand, with a central crater or ulcer. (From Lawrence PF. *Essentials of Surgical Specialties*. 3rd ed. Lippincott Williams & Wilkins; 2007.)

and is symptomatic (eg, soles of feet, palms of hands). However, these lesions are usually removed with cryosurgery or laser vaporization. Persistently enlarging lesions may suggest verrucous carcinoma, a type of squamous cell carcinoma, and require surgical excision.

Fibromas are solid lesions. They occur just below the skin surface and may involve skin structures. They are subclassified into fibromas, neurofibromas, and dermatofibromas. Large or symptomatic fibromas should be removed.

Hemangioma is the most common benign tumor of infancy. It consists of an abnormal collection of blood vessels. Several classifications exist on the basis of the likelihood of proliferation or regression. Hemangiomas tend to involute more than 90% by 9 years of age. Therefore, they are often managed conservatively. However, either medical or surgical treatment is required if proliferation of the lesion causes functional impairment or significant disfigurements. Propranolol, a nonselective β-blocker, induces involution of infantile hemangiomas and is now considered first-line medical treatment for problematic lesions. Steroids, either oral or intralesional, can also prevent further growth of the hemangioma. Pulsed dye and Nd:YAG lasers can also be utilized for both proliferating and residual vessels from hemangiomas. Surgical excision is often delayed until school age and when the child starts to experience psychological distress because of the hemangioma. Surgery can be urgently performed when the lesion is causing visual, airway, or auditory canal obstruction.

Vascular malformations are the other classification of pigmented congenital lesions. They are classified into capillary, lymphatic, venous, and arteriovenous malformations. They present at birth and tend to grow with the child, with no regression being seen. A variety of options exist for these lesions, including laser therapy, embolization, and surgical excision.

Techniques for Excision

In excising small skin lesions or subcutaneous lesions, the goal is to completely remove the lesion while leaving as inconspicuous a scar as possible. Although the surgical technique significantly affects the final appearance of the scar, other factors (eg, location, size, and orientation of the lesion; overall health; age) also influence the result. A spindle-shaped, or lenticular, incision is made. The total length of the spindle is approximately twice the diameter of the lesion. The long axis of the incision should parallel lines of relaxed skin tension. The incision is made distinctly into the subcutaneous tissue but should not penetrate into the fascia or deeper structures. Gentle undermining can help reduce tension on the closure. Careful layered closure provides the best result. The specimen should always be sent to the pathologist, even when it appears to be benign.

FACIAL TRAUMA

The patient with facial injuries requires early wound care; accurate diagnosis by history, physical examination, and radiographic studies; and appropriate wound repair and fracture stabilization. Facial fractures should be reduced and stabilized within the first 5 to 7 days. If the patient's condition allows it and evaluation of the facial injuries is complete, early repair is preferable.

If the patient has other significant injuries (eg, closed head, intrathoracic, cervical spine, or intra-abdominal injuries), medical attention to these injuries takes priority over repair of the facial fractures. However, fixation of a facial fracture can be combined with neurosurgical, orthopedic, or other procedures without increased morbidity. This approach allows early or immediate repair of the facial injuries, diminishing the effects of soft tissue contraction, potential infection, and scarring. Secondary revision of facial injuries may be required but should be delayed until scars mature and fractures heal (6-12 months). Occasionally, skin grafts and flaps are required for large soft tissue defects.

Emergency Care

The initial care of the patient with facial injuries focuses on managing the airway, immobilizing the cervical spine, and controlling bleeding. Foreign material and blood are removed from the airway either by hand or by suction. Tracheostomy is seldom indicated when the injury involves only the facial soft tissues. However, for facial fractures, bleeding, and potential cervical spine injuries, cricothyroidotomy or early tracheostomy may be appropriate. After the airway is clear and adequate ventilation is established, bleeding should be controlled. Direct pressure is usually adequate. Dressings wrapped around the face rarely ensure prolonged control of bleeding. Vessels should not be clamped until the injury is adequately visualized because blind clamping can injure important structures (eg, facial nerve).

After the extent of injury is assessed, the wound is carefully cleansed. All foreign material should be carefully removed. The wound is also palpated or gently explored to detect underlying injury to bony structures. Manual physical examination is the most sensitive means of detecting facial fractures. After initial wound care and hemostasis, the underlying structures can be repaired.

Soft Tissue Defects

As soon as the patient's general condition allows, soft tissue injuries are treated. Ideally, treatment occurs within the first several hours after injury. If the patient's general condition is not good, primary wound closure may be delayed. Because of the excellent vascular supply of the face, facial wounds can be closed up to 24 hours after injury if necessary. Soft tissue repair of the face requires gentle cleansing, minimal debridement, and restoration of all available parts. Most injuries cause little or no tissue loss once they are evaluated. The illusion of skin loss is the result of skin elasticity and retraction. Although nonviable tissue should be removed, questionable areas of skin should be replaced gently.

Early, skillful repair of soft tissue injuries provides the best result. Local anesthetics that contain epinephrine are used to allow adequate wound cleansing and hemostasis. After the wound is irrigated and debrided, it is carefully closed. The possibility of injury to deeper structures (eg, facial nerve, lacrimal apparatus, parotid duct) is considered next (Figure 22-18). Although a rapid assessment of facial nerve function is possible in the awake, cooperative patient, it can be extremely difficult in the multiply injured or comatose patient. Ideally, facial nerve injuries should be identified on initial physical examination so that repair may be planned. Parotid duct injuries should be suspected when a cheek laceration crosses a line from the tragus of the ear to the base of the nose.

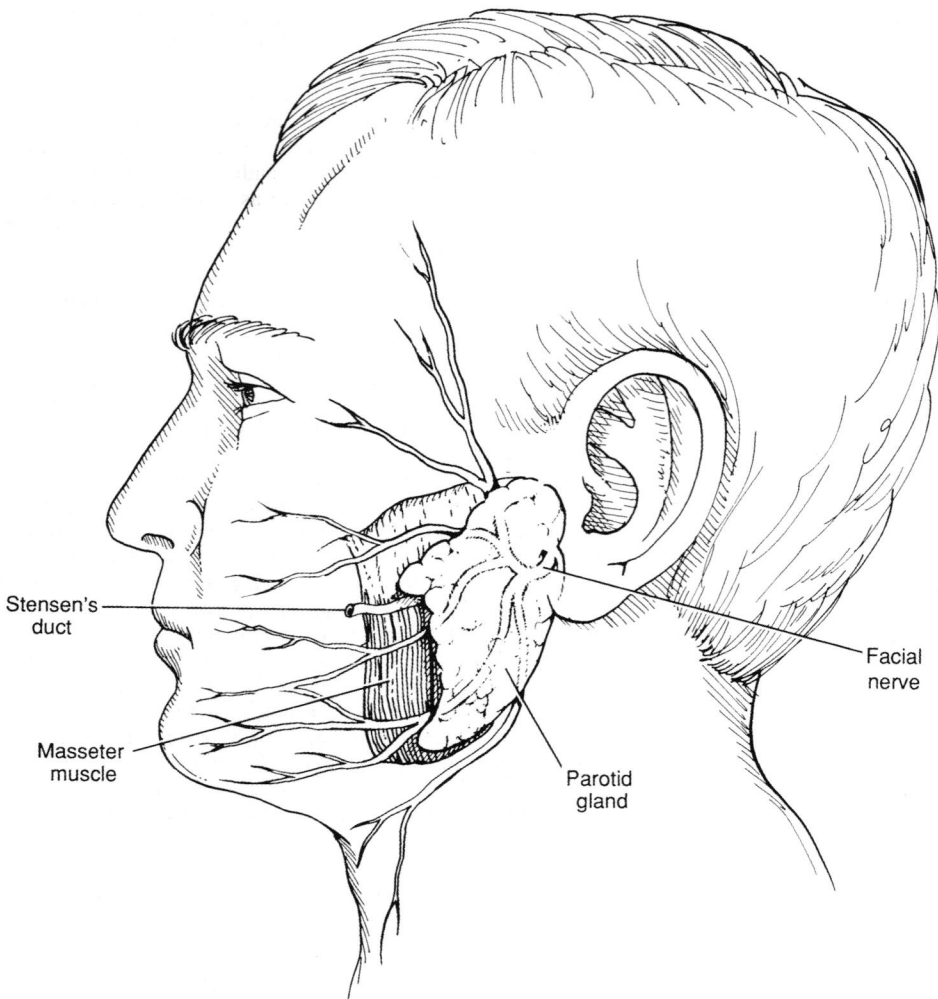

Figure 22-18. Anatomy of the parotid gland showing Stensen duct and the relation of the facial nerve to the parotid gland and the face. (From Lawrence PF. *Essentials of Surgical Specialties*. 3rd ed. Lippincott Williams & Wilkins; 2007.)

Injuries around the eyelids should be carefully evaluated because of the precision of repair required and the possibility of injury to the lacrimal apparatus. Debridement must be conservative in areas such as the eyebrows, eyelids, nose, ears, and lips. Because these areas are extremely difficult to reconstruct, it is better to repair questionably ischemic areas, even if a minor revision is required later, than to sacrifice large portions of usable tissue. However, obviously nonviable tissue must be debrided.

Treatment of specific injuries (eg, abrasions, lacerations) is similar to that in other parts of the body. Lacerations around the lip and other such areas require independent reconstruction of the muscle layers. For most injuries, topical antibiotic ointments are adequate to keep the wound clean and moist. Their antimicrobial component has minimal effect. Systemic antibiotics are not routinely required in facial injuries unless there is massive gross contamination or open injury to deeper structures (eg, cartilage, bone). Tetanus prophylaxis should always be considered. Sutures are left in place for 5 to 6 days.

In significantly contused and crushed tissue, sutures may be left a few days longer. Although the initial injury and the patient's genetic makeup are the main determinants in the outcome of healing, appropriate initial handling of the wound is also an important factor.

Simple lacerations are appropriately repaired by a generalist who uses careful technique. More complex injuries that involve stellate lacerations, crush injuries, or devitalized or avulsed tissue should be referred to a specialist. Likewise, significant injuries to the eyelids and injuries that involve deeper structures (eg, nerve injury, parotid duct injury, fractures) require prompt referral.

Facial Fractures

General Principles

Facial fractures are common in patients who have traumatic injuries. Common causes include motor vehicle accidents, assaults, falls, and athletic injuries. These fractures may be open or closed. The overlying tissue may be significantly injured or contused in closed injuries. A history of the injury often indicates the facial area involved. The nasal bone and the zygomatic-malar area are the most commonly injured areas, followed by the mandible and the maxilla. Many patients have multiple facial fractures.

Most facial fractures can be diagnosed on the basis of physical examination, which should include gentle examination and palpation of the facial bones. A fracture is suspected if there is any mobility of facial bones, asymmetry, palpable bony step-offs, extraocular muscle irregularities, sensory loss, localized pain or tenderness, or malocclusion of the teeth. This examination should be followed by radiographic evaluation after the cervical spine is cleared. Of patients with significant facial injuries, 15% to 25% have concomitant cervical spine injuries. The possibility of skull fracture and intracranial injury is also evaluated.

X-ray evaluation consists of a complete facial bone series, which includes the Water, anterior-posterior, Caldwell, and lateral views. When computed tomographic (CT) scan is not available or the index of suspicion for any bony injury is low, these plain radiographs can be used as screening examination.

The Water view, an oblique anterior-posterior projection or occipitomental view, shows most clearly the entire facial complex, thus rendering it the most helpful. Lateral skull films can show the anteroposterior position of the globe. Currently, however, CT scans in both the axial and coronal planes are the most accurate method of visualizing complex fractures. Three-dimensional (3D) CT scans or reconstructions are available in many centers. However, they add little to the acute management of facial fractures over what can be learned from routine CT scans. Mandibular x-ray evaluation is best obtained with the panorex (panoramic x-ray) view. This specialized x-ray is superior to plain films of the mandible. However, in most facilities, the patient must be upright, a difficult position for the patient with multiple injuries.

After facial fractures are identified, the urgency of their treatment is assessed. Urgency depends on the likelihood of continued bleeding, cerebrospinal fluid (CSF) leak, or loss of airway because of shifting oropharyngeal structures. Early consultation with all services that treat facial fractures should be made. If the patient is stable and treatment is not urgent, repair of the facial fractures may be appropriately delayed for up to 5 to 7 days without adverse effects. This interval allows adequate time for evaluation and treatment of other injuries and for reduction of facial edema. CT scan examination can also evaluate mandibular injury.

The principal goal of facial fracture reconstruction is the restoration of normal (premorbid) function and appearance. This goal is achieved by precise, anatomic reconstruction of all fractured bone segments, usually by open reduction and internal fixation. Although closed reduction may be adequate for simple fractures, internal fixation with interosseous wires or with plates or screws is usually performed. The bony pieces should be replaced if possible into the defect. If these bony fragments are unusable, immediate bone grafts should be considered, providing there is adequate soft tissue surrounding the structures. Recently, 3D CT reconstruction and computer-generated models of the facial skeleton have become useful tools for fracture analysis and surgical planning because it enables surgeons to see the extent of fracture lines and the spatial displacement more clearly. These modalities, however, are much less useful in minor facial trauma.

Mandibular Fractures

Mandibular fractures often occur in facial trauma. They are rarely isolated to one location. Because of the ring structure of the mandible, 94% of patients with mandibular fractures have associated fractures in a second area of the mandible. When sufficient force is applied at one point to produce a fracture, a second fracture site is likely because the force is transmitted to the entire ring. Some regions are more commonly associated with multiple fractures (Figure 22-19). Fractures of the mandibular condyle are often associated with fractures of the symphysis and the corresponding condyle on the contralateral side. Mandibular body fractures are associated with fractures of the contralateral mandibular angle.

The classification of mandibular fractures is similar to that of long bone fractures. Closed fractures show no break in the overlying skin or mucosa. Open fractures, extremely common in the mandible, involve an external or internal (intraoral) wound associated with the fracture site. Although the overlying skin may not be broken, fractures into the tooth-bearing area are essentially open and should be treated as such. Antibiotic prophylaxis is recommended for any patient with an open fracture. Penicillin covers most oral bacteria, and clindamycin can be used for patients with a penicillin allergy. Alveolar or dentoalveolar fractures involve the alveolar process, but no other portions of the main body of the bone. These fractures are more common in the maxillary than in the mandibular area. Multiple fractures are common. (Anatomically, most adult mandibular fractures occur in the condylar area. The mandibular body in the molar region is the next most common location, followed by the angle of the mandible.)

Dislocation of the mandibular condyle is occasionally seen and may be unilateral or bilateral. Signs are the inability to close the jaw, malocclusion, and pain. The dislocation is reduced by pressing downward on the mandible and sliding it posteriorly into position. Because the muscles of mastication (primarily the masseter and temporalis) quickly go into spasm, reduction may require sedation and occasionally general anesthesia. Recurrence is common.

Evaluation

The first priority in evaluating the patient with a mandibular fracture is assessment of the airway. Manual displacement of the mandible forward usually relieves obstruction by the tongue. In some cases, emergent definitive airway management is needed. Routine complaints include alteration of normal **dental occlusion**, abnormal position of the teeth, and abnormal mobility of the mandible. This may present itself by a cross or overbite with the teeth. Manual palpation shows disjointed movement of the mandible and some separation between mandibular fragments. Patients almost uniformly have pain. The presence of crepitus because of the fracture is unusual in mandibular fractures but is virtually pathognomonic of a fracture. Patients may also have lacerated gingiva or mucosal ecchymosis. Occasionally, patients have anesthesia in the lower teeth secondary to injury or contusion of the inferior alveolar nerve.

Fractured mandibles are usually displaced. Appreciation of the normal pull of the muscle of mastication can

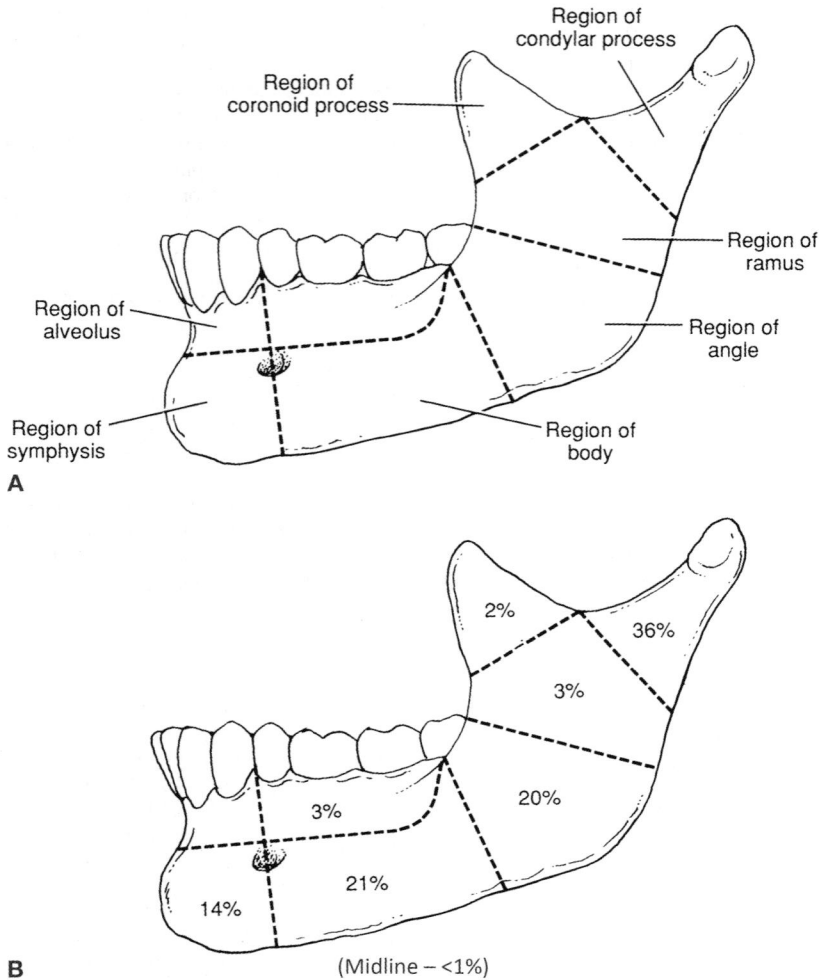

Figure 22-19. A. Anatomy of the mandibular regions. B. Frequency of fractures by mandibular region. (From Lawrence PF. *Essentials of Surgical Specialties*. 3rd ed. Lippincott Williams & Wilkins; 2007.)

be used to predict motion of the mandibular fragments. By evaluating the location of the mandible fracture and the angle of the fracture, and taking into account the location of muscle insertion and the vector of pull, it is possible to accurately predict the direction of displacement and estimate the ultimate stability of the fracture. If the normal muscle pull tends to reduce the mandibular fracture, the fracture is favorable. If the normal muscle pull tends to distract the bony fragments, the fracture is unfavorable. This distinction can be helpful in determining whether a closed reduction is adequate or an open reduction is needed.

Treatment

Treatment methods include closed reduction (maxillomandibular fixation), open reduction with internal fixation, and external fixation (primarily used for infected wounds or for significant loss of bony segments). A minimally displaced fracture can be treated by closed reduction (wiring the teeth together into normal occlusion). Good dentition, with reliable and stable occlusion, is necessary for this type of treatment. This method involves the placement of maxillary and mandibular arch bars that are wired or banded together in interdental fixation. In adults, 4 to 6 weeks of fixation is necessary; 2 to 4 weeks is necessary in children. Open reduction, with direct visualization of the fractures and wiring or plating in some configuration, is often necessary. This method provides better approximation of the fracture site. In addition, internal fixation prevents displacement and movement of the fracture, which provides a more precise restoration of occlusion. Open reduction is accomplished either extraorally (through a neck incision) or intraorally. Interdental fixation is almost always used with internal fixation methods to help with fracture alignment. The concept is to align the fractured bone with stable, unfractured bone. This allows a stable platform to build on for fixation of the fractured segments. The open technique has a higher incidence of infection (4%-5%) than the closed technique. However, it allows earlier mandibular movement, with reduced morbidity from immobilization because of tightening of the muscles of mastication. External fixation with an external appliance may be used in complicated fractures, severely infected fractures, or fractures with significant bone loss.

During the period of interdental fixation, attention to oral hygiene is necessary. Although it is difficult to brush the teeth normally, frequent cleansing with a pulsatile water hygiene device and the use of mouthwash can be very helpful.

Complications

Mandibular fractures may have multiple complications. Delayed healing occurs in the presence of inadequate or loosened fixation, an infection, or a fault in the reduction and fixation technique. Loosened fixation is associated with initially poor technique, poor patient compliance, or secondary infection. Malunion is caused by a lack of adequate treatment or a lack of patient compliance with proper oral hygiene and wound care. Malunion essentially allows healing to take place in a nonanatomic position. It causes significant functional difficulty because of the resultant malocclusion. Malunion may require further surgery. Nonunion is caused by delayed healing, which often occurs secondary to inadequate fixation or infection. Nonunion may require secondary bone grafting, external fixation, or bone transport.

Special Cases

Mandibular condyle fractures deserve separate consideration. Patients routinely have tenderness and pain in the preauricular area. The mandible may deviate toward the fractured side on opening because of pterygoid muscle function. Mandibular movement is limited, and there may be malocclusion and preauricular swelling. On examination, there is pain on palpation of the anterior wall of the external auditory canal. Occasionally, hemotympanum or external auditory canal laceration is noted. (Radiographically, a panorex view is the best diagnostic tool. CT scan is rarely helpful in evaluating a difficult mandibular fracture.)

Treatment of mandibular condyle fractures is usually by closed reduction, which is accomplished by interdental fixation with the patient in correct occlusion. When adequate occlusion cannot be obtained by closed reduction, open reduction of the condylar fracture is indicated. Complications of mandibular condyle fractures include ankylosis, temporomandibular joint dysfunction, limited postoperative motion, malocclusion, occasional sequestration of a dislocated fragment, and chorda tympani nerve damage (especially with dislocation). In children, aseptic necrosis, with disruption of mandibular growth, may occur. Rarely, seventh nerve paralysis occurs in association with open reduction.

Edentulous patients with mandibular fractures present a therapeutic problem. Signs and symptoms are the same as for patients with dentition. However, bilateral body fractures are more common because of the atrophy of the mandibular segment in that area. Edentulous patients also have a much higher incidence of nonunion because of poor bone stock and reduced strength of the small atrophic mandible.

Zygomatic Maxillary Complex Fractures

The anatomy of the zygomatic and orbital regions has several important features. The orbit is composed of the maxilla, lacrimal, frontal, sphenoid, palatine, zygoma, and ethmoid bones. The orbital rims are composed of a confluence of bones that is relatively strong. By comparison, the floor and walls of the orbit are composed of bone that is thin and easily fractured. The eyelids are attached by ligaments at the medial and lateral canthi. The lateral canthal ligament is attached to the zygoma, and the medial canthal ligament is attached to the lacrimal bone. Each canthus may be displaced by certain fractures. The orbit also contains (and protects) many important structures. Cushioned within a layer of periorbital fat are the globe, optic nerve, ophthalmic artery, extraocular muscles, and their accompanying nerves. Injury to these structures in specific fractures is not uncommon.

Evaluation

Periorbital injuries and fractures are extremely common (Figure 22-20). Patients routinely have chemosis (subconjunctival hematoma), which causes a ballooning effect of the conjunctiva and swelling over the cheek area. Palpation, however, shows flatness of the cheekbones (malar eminence) on that side. The injury may be missed if the examiner is unaware that overlying edema tends to mask this depression. Patients may have limited mandibular opening because the depressed zygomatic arch impinges on the temporalis muscle as it inserts on the coronoid process of the mandible. These patients may have anesthesia in the distribution of the infraorbital nerve, which traverses the floor of the orbit. Oblique canting of the eye may be caused by a depression of the lateral palpebral fissure because of displacement of the lateral canthus (Figure 22-21). Periorbital edema and ecchymosis are also present. Careful evaluation may show **enophthalmos**, diplopia (secondary to entrapment of periorbita), and step-offs at the inferior and lateral rims. The patient should be examined for intraoral buccal ecchymosis. Limitation of gaze in multiple planes is associated with corresponding entrapment of orbital contents. Loss of integrity of the orbital floor may allow herniation of orbital contents into the maxillary antrum, with downward displacement of the globe.

The patient should be evaluated with routine facial x-rays, which often show separation of the frontozygomatic suture, fractures or fragments of the lateral maxilla, orbital rim discrepancies, and opacification of a maxillary sinus. Unilateral opacification of a maxillary sinus is considered a presumptive sign of a facial fracture until proven otherwise. A submental vertex view is important because it may show depression of the zygomatic arch. CT scans in the axial and coronal planes most clearly define the location of fractures.

Treatment

Treatment of zygomaticomaxillary complex fractures usually requires open reduction with internal fixation of the fracture segments at several locations. Orbital floor exploration may be necessary to rule out floor fracture. The infraorbital nerve is commonly contused. Consequently, there is some anesthesia in the area of its distribution. Return of sensation may take several weeks or months, although, in some cases, anesthesia of varying degrees may persist. However, this nerve is rarely lacerated.

Complications

Because of the possibility of ocular injury in any significant facial injury, ophthalmologic evaluation and consultation

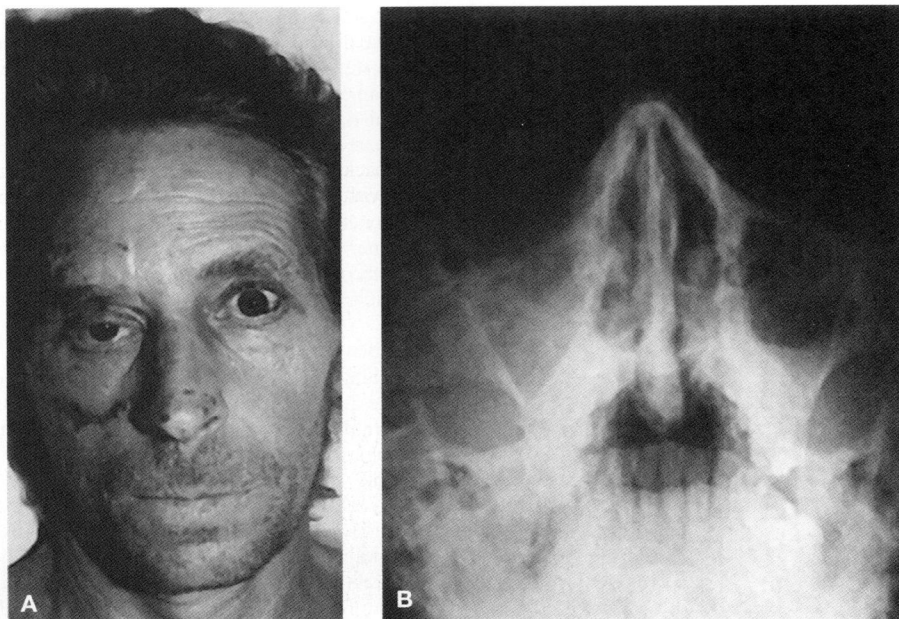

Figure 22-20. A. Grossly displaced right zygomatic maxillary complex fracture. B. X-ray showing the fracture lines and clouding of the right maxillary sinus. (From Lawrence PF. *Essentials of Surgical Specialties*. 3rd ed. Lippincott Williams & Wilkins; 2007.)

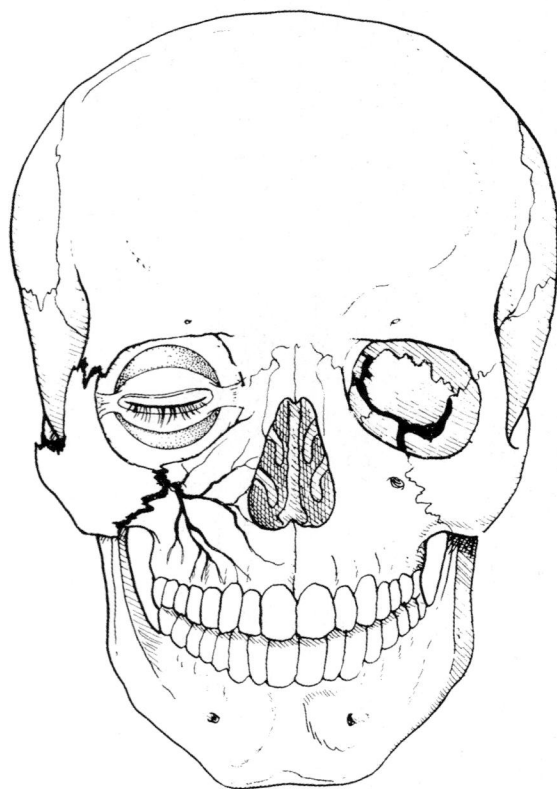

Figure 22-21. Zygomaticomaxillary complex fracture. The fracture through the infraorbital rim extends through the infraorbital foramen, where it can injure this sensory nerve. (From Lawrence PF. *Essentials of Surgical Specialties*. 3rd ed. Lippincott Williams & Wilkins; 2007.)

should be sought if an injury is suspected. Blood observed in the anterior chamber or retrobulbar hematoma, usually diagnosed by pain, periorbital ecchymosis, and/or proptosis of the globe, occasionally occurs and should be treated immediately. In addition, the optic nerve may be involved, and loss of vision may occur. The presence of any of these symptoms requires immediate ophthalmologic consultation. Residual entrapment of orbital contents may occur after treatment. If residual entrapment occurs, reexploration is required. Late **enophthalmos** can occur and may be secondary to atrophy of periorbital fat with protrusion of the intraorbital structures. Surgical correction depends on the symptoms. It is critical to assess vision before any type of reduction. Visual changes following surgery can occur because of bone fixation. Immediate evaluation is critical in order to prevent permanent injury.

Orbital Blow-Out Fractures

A **blow-out fracture** of the orbit is a relatively common fracture complex. It is an isolated fracture of the orbital floor. A segment of the orbital floor and a portion of the periorbital contents are displaced downward into the maxillary sinus, with or without extraocular muscle entrapment. In a pure blow-out fracture, there is no infraorbital rim fracture. However, a blow to the globe may transmit force to the orbital floor, causing the thin bone to break. Alternatively, a blow to the orbital rim may momentarily deform the rim, causing the floor to buckle and break without fracturing the rim. Either mechanism causes the floor to fracture into the maxillary antrum, creating a blow-out of the orbital region.

Evaluation

The patient may present with reduced extraocular muscle function and some diplopia. Evaluation may be difficult because of surrounding swelling, edema, and ecchymosis. There may be some evidence of enophthalmos, and anesthesia of the infraorbital nerve and some inequality in pupil height may be noted. Because these findings are relatively mild in most cases, radiographic confirmation is usually indicated. Plain radiographs rarely show any findings other than clouding of the maxillary sinus. CT scans more accurately show fractures (Figure 22-22).

Treatment

Operative treatment of orbital floor fractures depends on the associated symptoms. Patients with minimal orbital floor fractures and who are asymptomatic or who report transient diplopia require no treatment. However, persistent diplopia, enophthalmos, displacement of the globe into the maxillary sinus, and a large fracture seen on CT scan are indications for operative repair. This repair involves exploration of the orbital floor, reduction of periorbital contents back into the orbit, and reconstruction of the orbital floor with bone grafts (usually autogenous cranial bone, rib, or allogeneic rib) or prosthetic materials (eg, vitallium, titanium mesh, or resorbable plates). Long-term complications are usually post-traumatic enophthalmos or diplopia, especially if the fracture was inadequately treated.

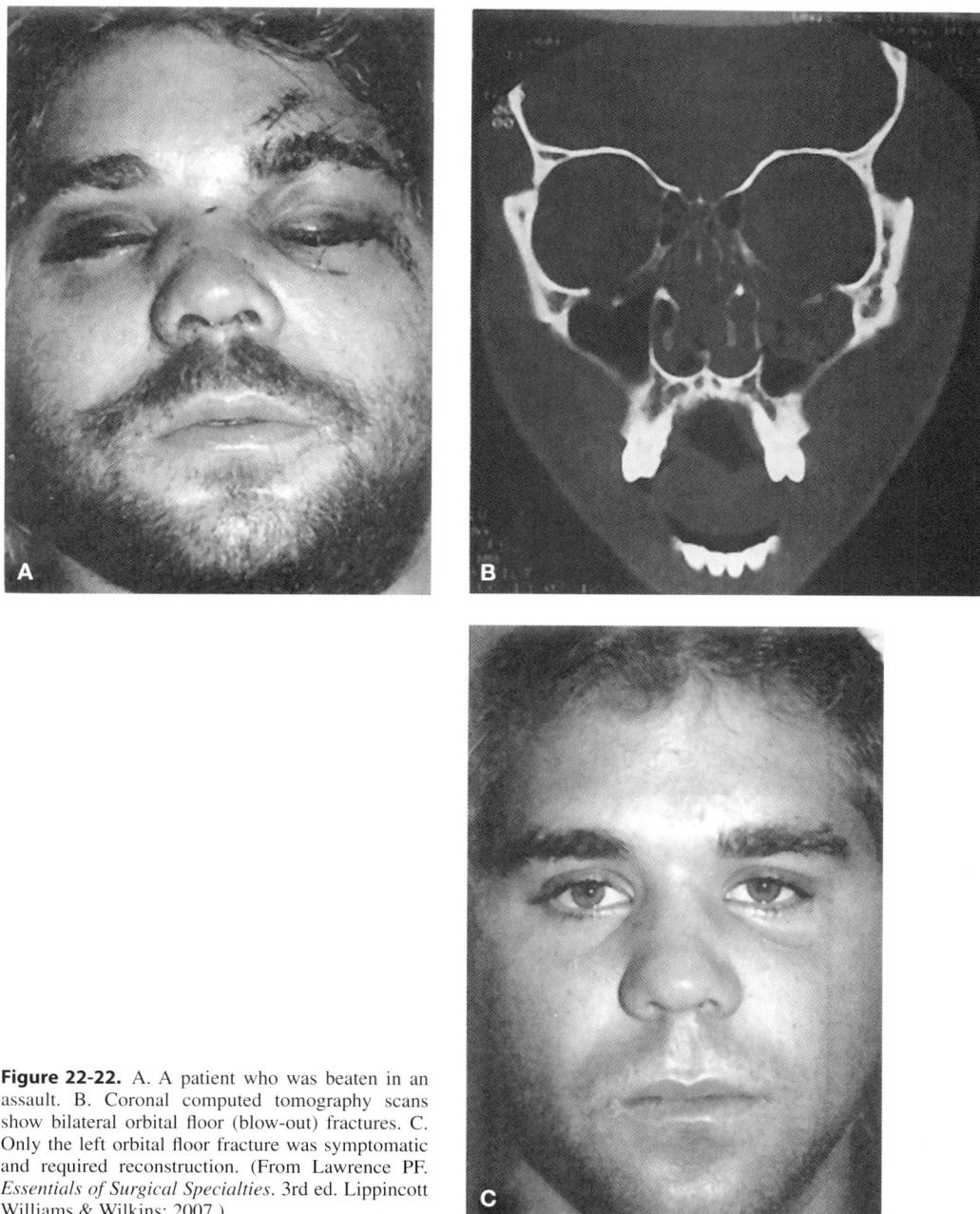

Figure 22-22. A. A patient who was beaten in an assault. B. Coronal computed tomography scans show bilateral orbital floor (blow-out) fractures. C. Only the left orbital floor fracture was symptomatic and required reconstruction. (From Lawrence PF. *Essentials of Surgical Specialties*. 3rd ed. Lippincott Williams & Wilkins; 2007.)

Nasal and Nasoethmoidal Fractures

The nasal bone is the most commonly fractured bone of the face because of its relative weakness and prominent position. The thin nasal bones fuse laterally with the frontal process of the maxilla and superiorly with the frontal bone. Internally, the perpendicular plate of the ethmoid articulates posteriorly with the sphenoid and the vomer. In addition, the cartilaginous skeletal anatomy consists of upper lateral, lower lateral, septal, and accessory cartilages.

Evaluation

The mechanism of injury affects the nature of the fracture. Anterior blows usually produce a comminuted fracture, with flattening of the bridge or telescoping (shortening) of the nose. Lateral blows depress the affected side and cause a convex deformity on the other side. Patients always have significant swelling, which may make precise examination of nasal deformities difficult. **Epistaxis**, facial asymmetry, nasal airway obstruction, and periorbital ecchymosis are usually signs. However, crepitus over the nasal bones and septal hematomas are not uncommon.

Nasoethmoidal fractures cause all of the abovementioned symptoms as well as telecanthus (increase in the inner canthal distance) and severe depression of the nasal bridge, usually with telescoping of the nasal bones and fractures of the inferior orbital rims. CSF rhinorrhea, pneumocephalus, or anosmia may also be present. Simple nasal fractures are best evaluated by physical examination alone. Nasoethmoidal fractures require visualization by CT scans. Comparison of the patient's appearance with previous photographs is helpful in determining the extent of deformity.

Treatment

Treatment of nasal fractures can rarely be achieved early because of the amount of edema that rapidly develops. After the edema resolves (usually 3-4 days), operative repositioning of the nasal bones, or closed reduction, may be achieved. Delays of longer than 10 days make closed reduction difficult. Septal hematomas should be drained immediately, because undrained hematomas may produce pressure necrosis of the septum or secondary problems such as saddle nose deformity. Further description of septal hematoma can be found in Chapter 25. Repositioning of the nasal septum may be required. The nasal bones are usually stabilized with external splints and internal packs. Patients who have obvious nasal deformities and minimal or no acute swelling may have old nasal fractures that cannot be treated with closed reduction.

Nasoethmoidal fractures usually require open reduction and internal fixation. Although a number of approaches are used, the best is through a bicoronal incision that allows exposure of the glabellar, medial canthal, and superior orbital regions. Significant lacerations may also be used as an approach to the fractures. The goal of fixation is to reestablish or repair the nasal pyramid, medial canthal region, medial orbits, and normal restoration of the intercanthal distance. Interosseous wiring, plate-and-screw fixation, transnasal wiring of the medial canthal ligaments, and immediate bone grafting may be used.

Complications

Postoperatively, nasal and nasoethmoidal fractures may be complicated by residual nasal and septal deformities, with resultant nasal airway obstruction. Deformities of the medial canthi are common. They are usually caused by inadequate treatment and produce telecanthus, which requires secondary correction. CSF rhinorrhea may complicate more significant fractures. This rhinorrhea usually ceases after adequate fracture fixation, but complex neurosurgical procedures are occasionally needed. Damage to the lacrimal apparatus is common and is repaired secondarily.

Maxillary Fractures

Maxillary fractures may be subdivided according to the **LeFort classification.** Although not all fractures fit this classification, it remains useful.

LeFort I Fractures

A LeFort I fracture is a transverse fracture that extends through the maxilla and pterygoid plates above the floor of the maxillary sinus (Figure 22-23A). The etiology is usually traumatic and most commonly involves a central midline blow. The patient has consistent findings of malocclusion and mobility of the maxilla. On examination, patients have ecchymosis in the buccal vestibule, some crepitus in the maxillary area, and false motion of the lower maxilla, with stability of the upper nose and orbits. Patients occasionally have airway obstruction, noticeable lengthening of the face, nasal septal deformities, and paresthesia in the distribution of the infraorbital nerve. Such patients should be evaluated by routine facial x-rays and CT scans if appropriate.

Treatment of LeFort I facial fractures involves establishing the mandible as a foundation on which to base other repairs. Therefore, mandibular injuries are usually repaired before maxillary injuries. In most cases, intermaxillary fixation, with or without internal plate fixation, provides sufficient reduction and stabilization. Bone grafts may also be needed if severe comminution is present. Complications of LeFort I facial fractures often include malocclusion, paresthesia, nasal septal deformities, and facial asymmetry.

LeFort II Fractures

A LeFort II fracture is a zygomatic midfacial fracture with a floating, pyramid-shaped fragment (Figure 22-23B), from which the term *pyramidal fracture* is derived. The central portion of the face is free floating, but the lateral orbits and cranium are stable. The patient has flattening of the naso-orbital region and mobility across the nasal bridge. **Epistaxis** is common. The maxilla is mobile and moves with the nasal bridge and the medial component of the inferior rim. The lateral orbital rim and forehead remain stable. Open-bite deformities and malocclusion are also common. Palpation along the orbital rims and nasofrontal areas usually shows step deformities. CSF leaks are relatively common. The patient may also have some lengthening of the midface and paresthesia of the infraorbital nerve. Diplopia and reduced intraocular muscle function may occur when there is significant disruption of the orbital floor. Although most fractures are diagnosed on physical examination, a CT scan is usually indicated.

Treatment involves restoration of the anatomic configuration and structure. Intermaxillary fixation is performed after stabilization of mandibular fractures. Direct fixation in the areas of the lateral maxilla, infraorbital rim, and nasofrontal angle is achieved with plate-and-screw fixation,

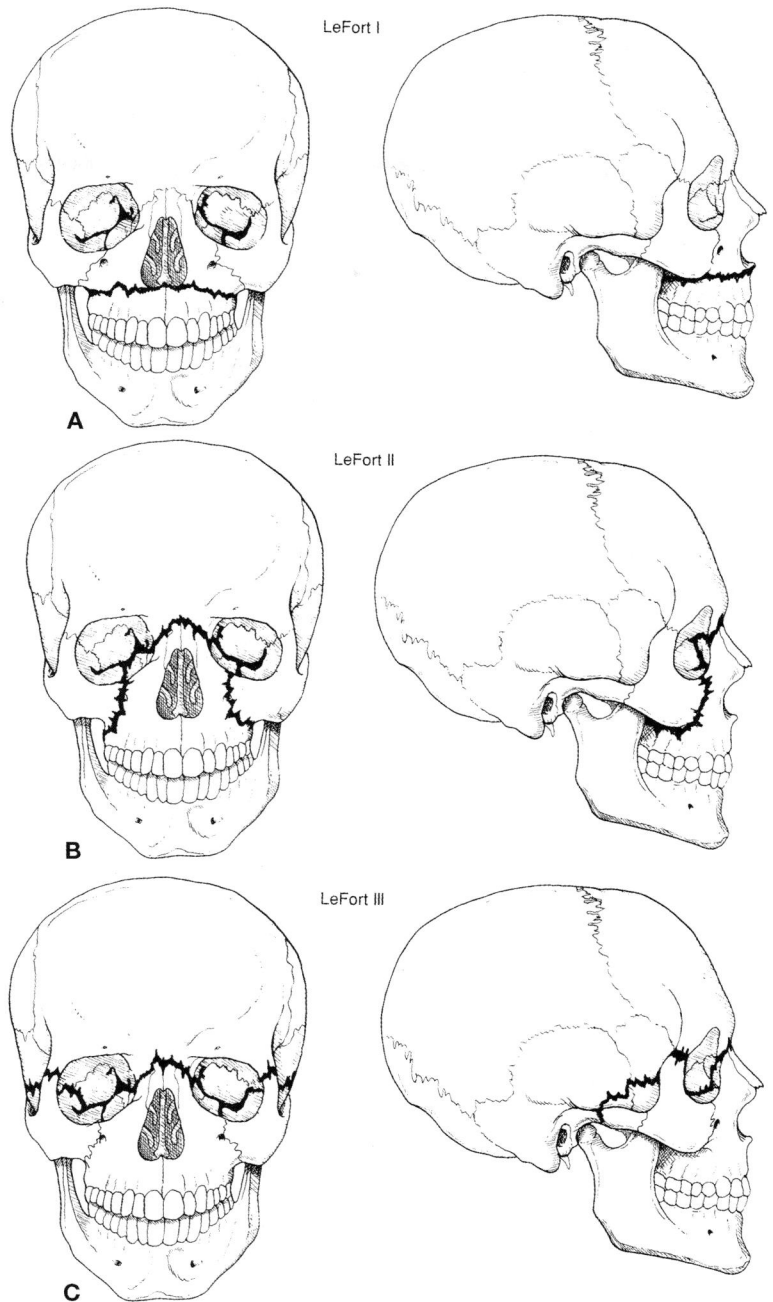

Figure 22-23. The LeFort classification of maxillary fractures. A. LeFort I fracture. B. LeFort II fracture. C. LeFort III fracture. (From Lawrence PF. *Essentials of Surgical Specialties*. 3rd ed. Lippincott Williams & Wilkins; 2007.)

which allows early motion and release of intermaxillary fixation. Bone grafts are used, if necessary, in cases of severe comminution or bone loss.

Basic complications of the LeFort II facial fracture are the same as those of the LeFort I fracture. If the fracture is incorrectly or inadequately corrected, the midface might be lengthened. There is a higher incidence of orbital injuries, CSF leaks, nasal deformities, and midface abnormalities involving the lacrimal system.

LeFort III Fractures

A LeFort III fracture is a severe fracture that completely separates the midface from the upper face (craniofacial disjunction) (Figure 22-23C). The signs and symptoms of LeFort III fractures are similar to those of LeFort II fractures, with additional signs associated with basilar skull fractures. Depressed zygomatic arches are often found, with the inferior orbital rims intact. Relatively common findings are **Battle sign** (ecchymosis in the mastoid region),

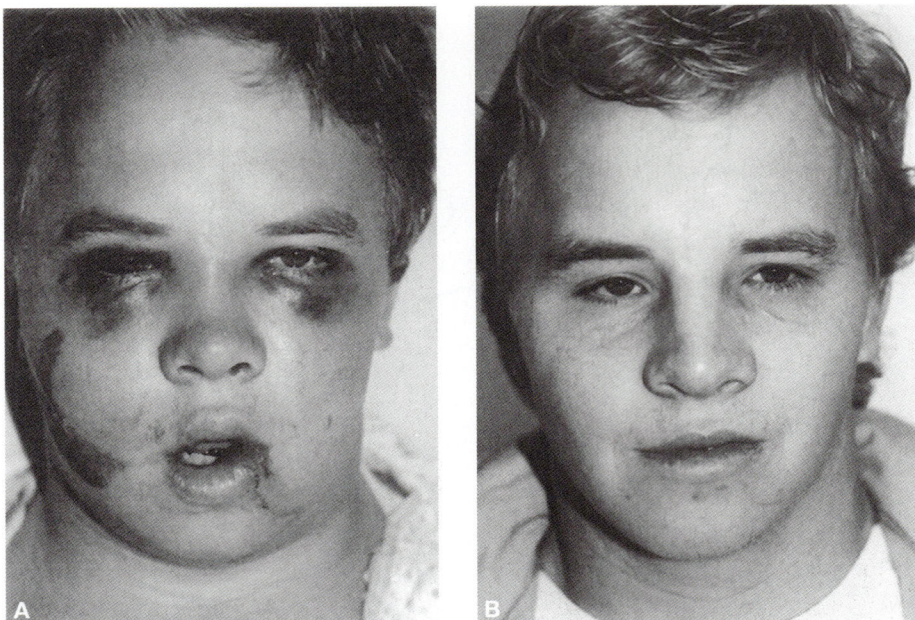

Figure 22-24. A. A patient with multiple facial fractures, including a LeFort III fracture. Note the raccoon eyes. B. After fracture fixation and facial reconstruction. (From Lawrence PF. *Essentials of Surgical Specialties*. 3rd ed. Lippincott Williams & Wilkins; 2007.)

bilateral orbital ecchymosis (raccoon eyes) (Figure 22-24), CSF otorrhea, and hemotympanum.

Diagnosis depends on the facial examination. On manipulation of the maxilla, movement is felt at the frontonasal angle and frontozygomatic sutures. However, the entire midface remains intact. Zygomatic arch fractures are also palpated. Radiographic diagnosis is usually made by CT scans, which also evaluate cranial vault fractures and intracranial injuries.

As in other facial fractures, the goal is anatomic restoration of the fracture complex. The general treatment protocol is the same as that for LeFort II fractures, except that the inferior orbital rims are no longer available for superior stabilization. Thus, stabilization must be achieved at the frontozygomatic sutures and zygomatic arches. Complications of LeFort III facial fractures are the same as those of LeFort II facial fractures, with the possible addition of injuries to the cranial base, with neurologic damage.

Panfacial Fractures

Patients who have facial trauma because of high levels of kinetic energy (eg, high-speed motor vehicle crashes) often have multiple fracture complexes (Figure 22-25). When they involve all areas of the face, they are known as panfacial fractures. The same principles of diagnosis and treatment that are used in isolated fracture complexes are applied to these complex injuries. To avoid serious soft tissue contraction of the overlying facial skin, early fixation is usually indicated. Sequencing of fracture repair varies from physician to physician, but the concept of stable fixation to those structures that are not fractured is critical.

Cerebrospinal Fluid Rhinorrhea

CSF rhinorrhea occurs in as many as 25% of high-level midface injuries that involve the paranasal sinuses. Most of these cause leakage within the first 48 hours after injury.

Less commonly, rhinorrhea occurs 5 to 7 days later. Clinically, CSF rhinorrhea is associated with a fracture of the cribriform plate and a dural tear in association with midface fractures. After this injury, the clear, watery CSF begins to leak out slowly. If the patient remains supine, fluid drains down the posterior pharynx and the patient may not be aware of any leakage. Nasal packing should be avoided, and any attempt at passing a nasogastric or nasotracheal tube is contraindicated.

Early reduction of facial fractures usually stops CSF leakage within a few days. Prophylactic antibiotics are used *only* perioperatively. If CSF rhinorrhea persists after fracture fixation, intracranial repair of the dural tear may be required. Accordingly, neurosurgical consultation is needed.

HAND SURGERY

The hand and upper extremity form a unique functional organ system that allows complex interaction between an individual and the environment. The hand both manipulates the external environment and receives sensations from it.

Because hand injuries are often seen in clinical practice, all physicians should have a basic knowledge of hand anatomy and injuries to assess the need for primary treatment or referral. Because definitive treatment of the hand is usually performed by a specialist, emphasis is given to diagnosis and early treatment of the injured or diseased hand. Second only to back injuries, injuries to the hand and upper extremity are the most common reason for loss of work days in the United States.

Functional Anatomy and Examination

The hand is composed of multiple finely balanced units. Its intricate anatomy allows specialized and refined functions.

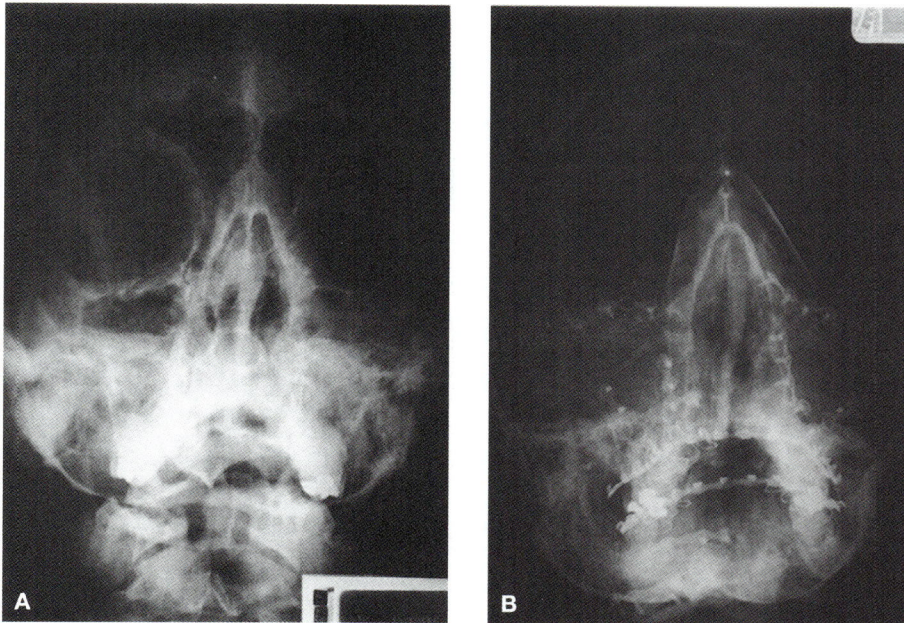

Figure 22-25. X-rays of a patient with panfacial fractures. A. Before fixation. B. After fixation with both intermaxillary fixation and rigid internal fixation. (From Lawrence PF. *Essentials of Surgical Specialties*. 3rd ed. Lippincott Williams & Wilkins; 2007.)

Disturbance of these units, their interaction, or their innervation causes dysfunction and ultimate disability. To properly treat diseases and injuries of the hand, an understanding of its anatomy is essential. Hand anatomy is quite complex but can be greatly simplified when broken down into its components. Therefore, hand anatomy is discussed in terms of its subsystems: nerves, muscles, tendons, bones, and blood vessels.

Terminology

In discussing hand anatomy, standard terminology should be used to avoid confusion. In addition, when describing hand injuries to a specialist, it is important to use a consistent, precise, and uniformly accepted vocabulary. In this way, injuries can be clearly delineated and safe treatment plans implemented.

The fingers should be named rather than numbered (ie, thumb; index, long or middle, ring, and small fingers). The hand and digits have a dorsal and a volar, or palmar, surface. Each has a radial and an ulnar border (Figure 22-26). The volar surface of the hand has a thenar and a hypothenar eminence and a midpalmar area between the two. The thenar eminence is the muscle mass overlying the thumb metacarpal. The hypothenar eminence is the muscle mass overlying the small finger metacarpal. Each finger has a proximal, middle, and distal phalanx. Each finger has a metacarpophalangeal (MCP) joint, proximal interphalangeal (PIP) joint, and distal interphalangeal (DIP) joint. The thumb has only a proximal and distal phalanx, an MCP joint, and a single interphalangeal (IP) joint (Figure 22-27).

Nerve Anatomy and Evaluation

The hand is innervated by the median, ulnar, and radial nerves. The median nerve enters the hand at the wrist through the carpal tunnel accompanied by the nine extrinsic flexor

tendons of the digits (Figure 22-28). The median nerve motor branch to the thenar musculature arises within the carpal tunnel or just distal to it. The common digital branches innervate the lumbrical muscles to the index and long fingers. The median nerve divides into sensory branches that serve the volar aspect of the thumb, the index and long fingers, and the radial half of the ring finger (Figure 22-29A). The ulnar nerve enters the hand at the wrist accompanied by the ulnar artery through Guyon canal. Within the hand, motor

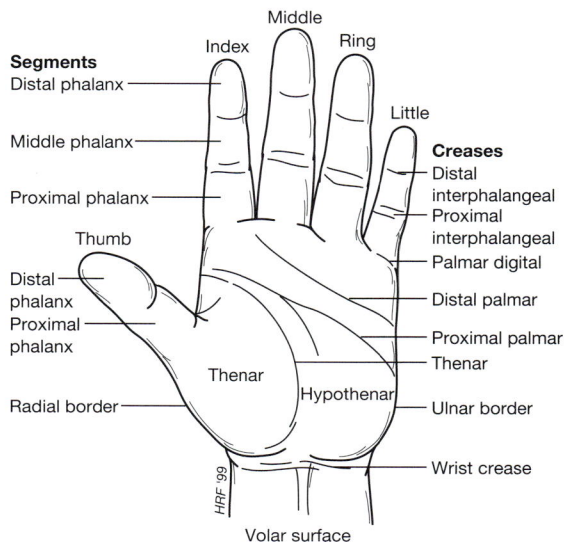

Figure 22-26. Surface anatomy of the hand. (From Lawrence PF. *Essentials of Surgical Specialties*. 3rd ed. Lippincott Williams & Wilkins; 2007.)

Bones
Distal phalanges
Middle phalanges
Proximal phalanges
Distal phalanx
Proximal phalanx
Metacarpals
Trapezoid
Trapezium
Capitate
Scaphoid
Hamate
Triquetrum
Pisiform
Lunate

Joints
Distal interphalangeal (DIP)
Proximal interphalangeal (PIP)
Metacarpophalangeal (MCP)
Interphalangeal
MCP
Carpometacarpal ("saddle joint")

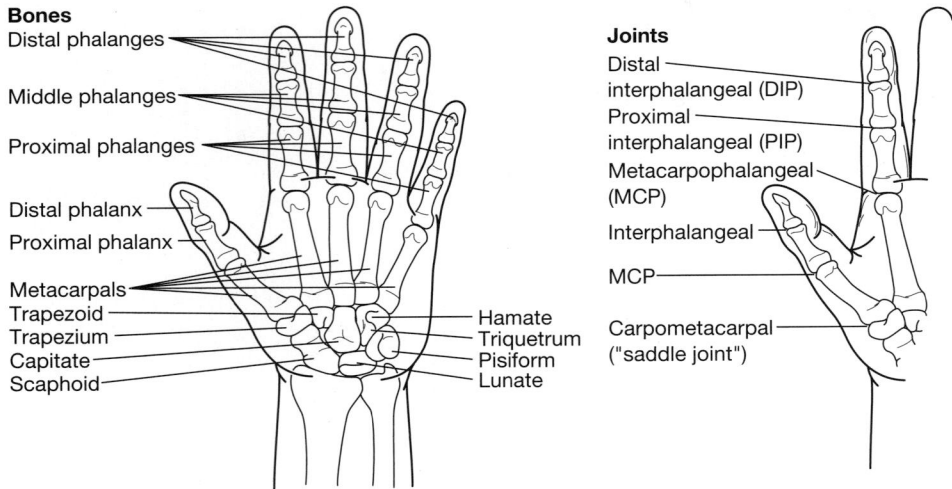

Figure 22-27. Skeletal structure of the hand and wrist. (From Lawrence PF. *Essentials of Surgical Specialties*. 3rd ed. Lippincott Williams & Wilkins; 2007.)

branches to the intrinsic muscles arise from the ulnar nerve. Digital branches provide sensation to the volar and dorsal aspects of the ulnar half of the ring finger and to the entire small finger (Figure 22-29B). The radial nerve (Figure 22-29C) lies dorsally. It provides sensation to the dorsal aspects of the thumb, the index and long fingers, and half of the ring finger. The motor component of the radial nerve innervates the muscles that extend the wrist and MCP joints and abduct and extend the thumb. Significant anatomic variation may occur in these innervation patterns.

When examining the hand, tests of motor and sensory function of the nerves can be performed. Sensory function is usually tested by light touch from a wisp of cotton or fine filament, as well as by two-point discrimination. The patient is asked to look away from the hand during the examination. If it is not clear whether there is sensory loss, the examination is repeated later. Median nerve motor function is tested by assessing the ability to flex the fingers and to oppose the thumb and small finger. Because the thenar muscles are innervated by the median nerve, asking the patient to touch the thumb to the small finger tests distal median motor function. The interosseous muscles, which abduct and adduct the fingers, are innervated by the ulnar nerve. The motor function of the ulnar nerve is tested by asking the patient to spread the fingers against resistance or to hold a piece of paper between opposing surfaces of adjacent fingers while the examiner attempts to withdraw it. The motor function of the radial nerve is tested by asking the patient to extend the wrist against resistance.

Motor Unit Anatomy

The muscles of the hand can be divided into extrinsic and intrinsic muscle groups. Extrinsic muscles, both flexors and extensors, have their origins in the forearm and their tendon insertions in the hand. Extrinsic flexors are located on the volar aspect of the forearm and are responsible for flexion of the digits and the wrist. Extrinsic extensors are located on the dorsal aspect of the forearm and produce extension of the wrist and digits. The intrinsic muscles have their origins and insertions completely within the hand.

Flexor Anatomy and Examination

Flexion of the MCP, PIP, and DIP joints is served by separate musculotendinous units. The lumbricals, which are intrinsic muscles, arise within the hand and insert into the proximal phalanges, crossing the MCP joint (Figure 22-30). These, along with the interossei, are responsible for MCP joint flexion and for DIP and PIP joint extension. The extrinsic flexors, the flexor digitorum superficialis and the flexor digitorum profundus, are responsible for flexion at the PIP and DIP joints, respectively.

The flexor digitorum profundus muscle originates in the forearm and gives rise to four tendons that run through the wrist within the carpal tunnel to insert at the base of the distal phalanges of the fingers. Its function is tested by blocking flexion at the PIP joint of the involved finger and observing flexion at the DIP joint (Figure 22-31). Because a single muscle gives rise to all four deep flexor tendons, the flexor digitorum profundus acts as a unit, and independent DIP flexion is not observed. PIP flexion is achieved through the action of the flexor digitorum superficialis. This muscle is also located in the forearm and sends four flexor tendons through the carpal tunnel to ultimately insert on the base of the middle phalanges of the fingers. Separate muscle fibers give rise to each of the tendons, allowing independent flexion. To test the function of the flexor digitorum superficialis, passive extension of adjacent fingers is maintained (to block the deep flexor unit). Flexion of the PIP joint of the affected finger is observed (Figure 22-32). The flexor pollicis longus muscle has its origin in the forearm, and it inserts on the volar base of the distal phalanx of the thumb. Flexor pollicis longus function is tested by asking the patient to flex the IP joint of the thumb against resistance.

Extensor Anatomy and Examination

Finger extension is achieved through the action of both intrinsic and extrinsic muscles that insert into a complex tendinous system on the dorsum of the fingers (extensor apparatus) (Figure 22-33). The extensor digitorum communis is a common extrinsic extensor muscle that inserts

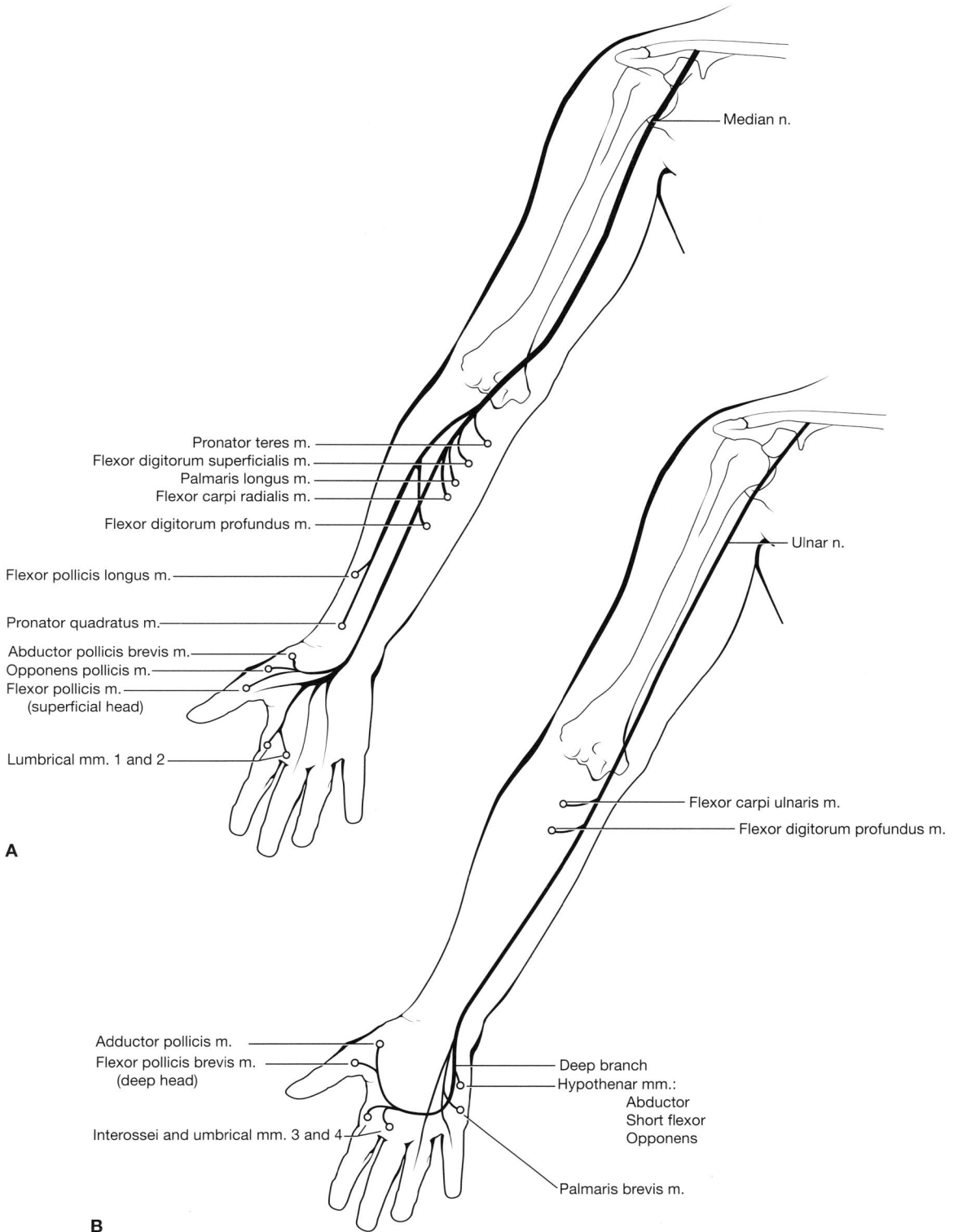

Figure 22-28. A. Muscles innervated by the median nerve in the forearm and hand. **B.** Muscles innervated by the ulnar nerve in the forearm and hand.

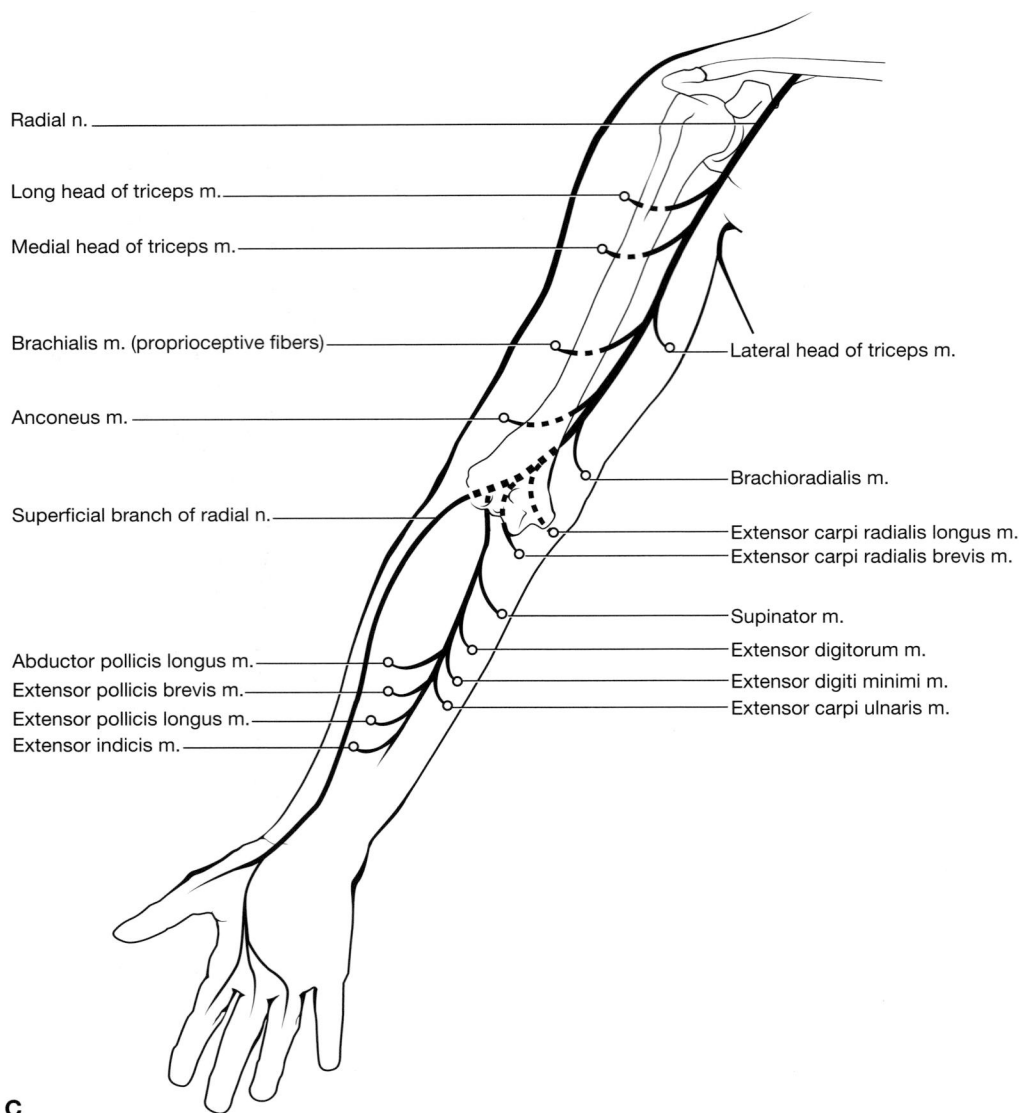

Figure 22-28. (*continued*) C. Muscles innervated by the radial nerve in the forearm and hand. (From Lawrence PF. *Essentials of Surgical Specialties*. 3rd ed. Lippincott Williams & Wilkins; 2007.)

onto the extensor apparatus and provides MCP extension, as a unit, of the index, long, ring, and small fingers. Independent extension of the index and small fingers is provided by two independent extensors (extensor indicis proprius and extensor digiti quinti minimi, respectively). PIP and DIP joint extension is achieved through an interplay of the common extensors and the intrinsic muscles of the hand (lumbricals and interossei). The intrinsic muscles travel volar to the axis of rotation of the MCP joint to insert into the lateral bands of the extensor apparatus (see Figure 22-30). This unique position allows the intrinsic muscles to act as flexors at the MCP joint and as extensors at the PIP and DIP joints.

Examination of the extensor function of the hand involves observation of extension, with or without resistance, of each of these elements. Because independent extension of the index and small fingers is provided, these digits must be evaluated both separately and as a unit with the long and ring fingers.

Thumb extension is also provided by extrinsic and intrinsic muscles. The extensor pollicis brevis and extensor pollicis longus are extrinsic muscles located within the forearm. They give rise to tendons that insert on the bases of the proximal and distal phalanges, respectively. These muscles provide extension at the MCP and IP joints of the thumb. The abductor pollicis, an intrinsic muscle of the hand, is innervated by the ulnar nerve and has tendinous insertions onto the extensor apparatus of the thumb. In this way, thumb IP extension is assisted by the intrinsic muscles. Thumb extension is also assisted by abduction of

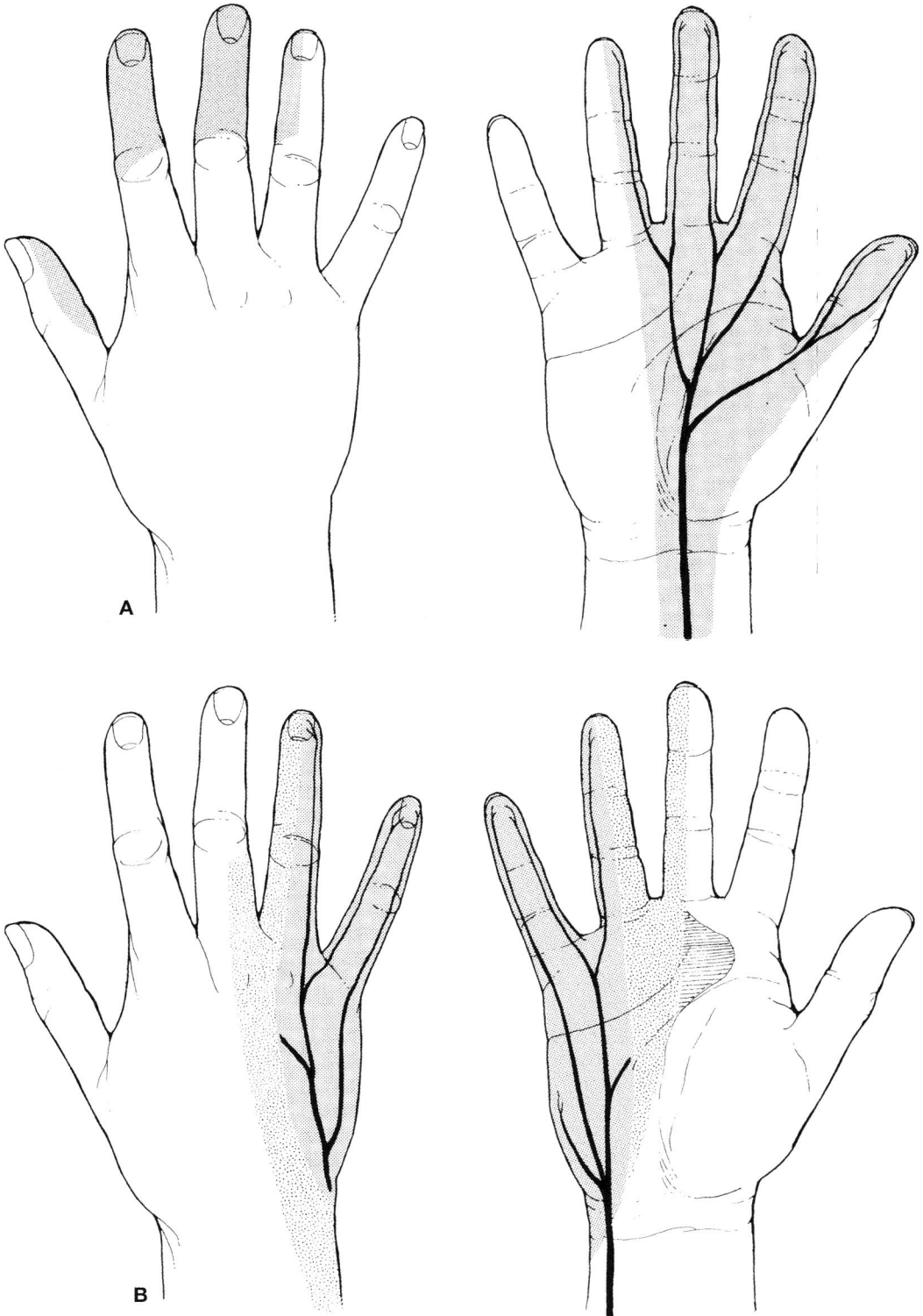

Figure 22-29. Sensory innervation of the hand. A. Median nerve. B. Ulnar nerve.

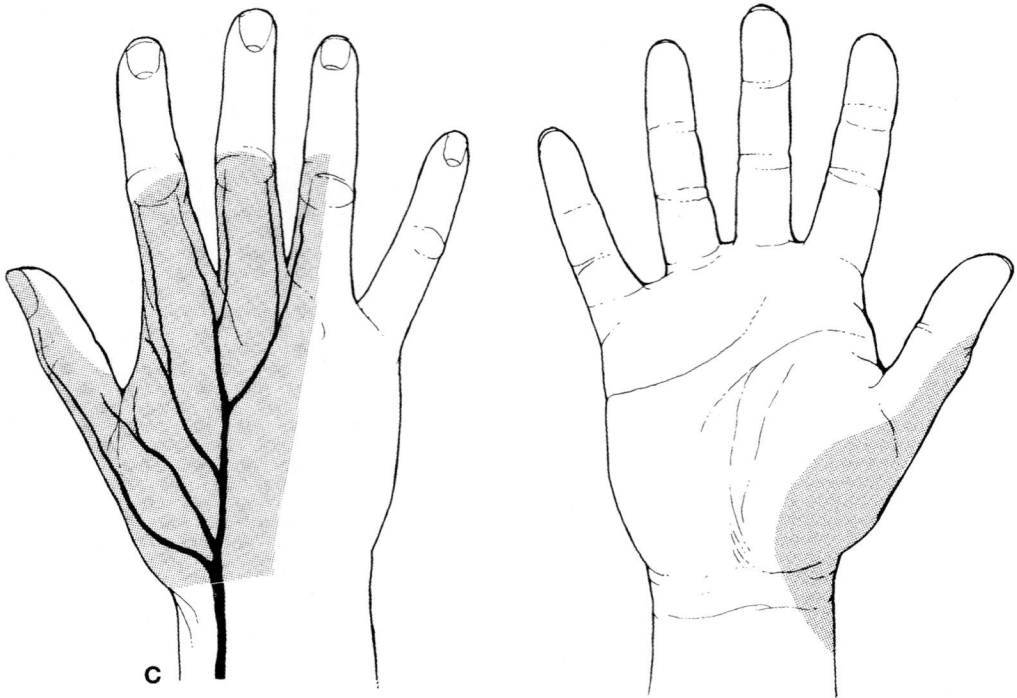

Figure 22-29. (*continued*) C. Radial nerve. (From Lawrence PF. *Essentials of Surgical Specialties*. 3rd ed. Lippincott Williams & Wilkins; 2007.)

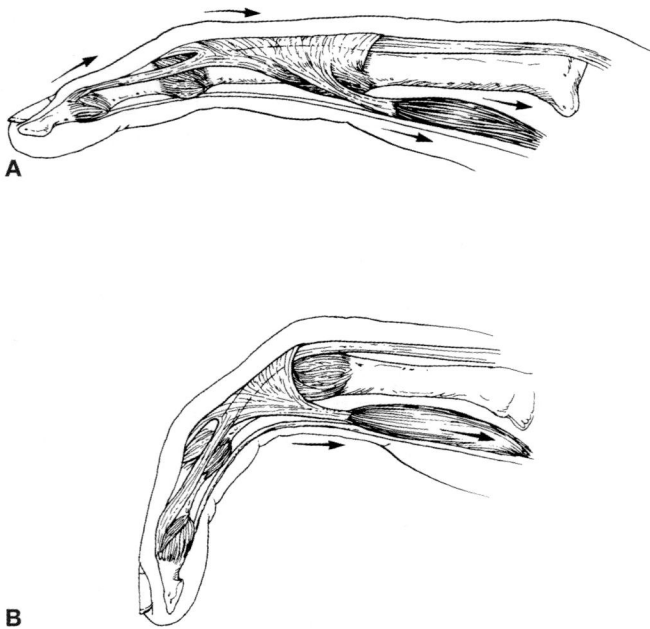

Figure 22-30. Anatomy and function of the lumbrical muscle. A. The insertion of the lumbrical muscle onto the extensor apparatus allows extension of the distal interphalangeal and proximal interphalangeal joints on contraction of the lumbrical muscle. B. Because the lumbrical tendon passes on the volar surface of the metacarpophalangeal joint, flexion of the metacarpophalangeal joint is achieved by contraction of the lumbrical muscle. (From Lawrence PF. *Essentials of Surgical Specialties*. 3rd ed. Lippincott Williams & Wilkins; 2007.)

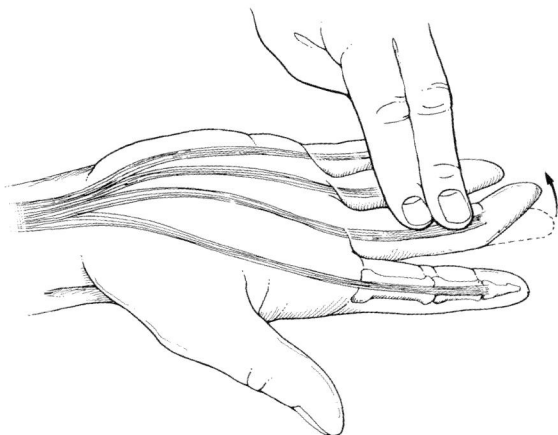

Figure 22-31. Examination of the flexor digitorum profundus. The integrity of the flexor digitorum profundus musculotendinous unit is examined by blocking flexion at the proximal interphalangeal joint and observing flexion at the distal interphalangeal joint of the finger. (From Lawrence PF. *Essentials of Surgical Specialties*. 3rd ed. Lippincott Williams & Wilkins; 2007.)

the thumb by the abductor pollicis longus, which crosses the wrist to insert on the thumb metacarpal. The area between the tendons of the extensor pollicis longus and the abductor pollicis longus on the radial aspect of the wrist is known as the "anatomic snuff box."

The extensor tendons of the wrist and fingers are arranged in specific anatomic compartments on the dorsal surface of the wrist (Figure 22-33B). Each compartment is a separate tunnel enclosed in a tough fibrous capsule through which the extensor tendons travel.

Thumb Opposition

Opposition of the thumb is the movement that allows the thumb to be approximated successively to the tip of each of the fingers. Specifically, the movement is described by radial extension, palmar abduction, and IP joint flexion. Thumb opposition, a unique ability of the hands, is provided by the muscles of the thenar eminence (opponens pollicis, flexor pollicis brevis, and abductor pollicis brevis). Opposition is assisted by flexion of the thumb IP joint, which is provided by the flexor pollicis longus, an extrinsic flexor whose tendon travels through the carpal tunnel and inserts on the base of the distal phalanx.

Bony Anatomy

The skeleton of the hand consists of 27 bones. It can be divided into three segments: phalanges, metacarpals, and carpal bones (Figure 22-34). The fingers each have three phalanges; the thumb has two. The five proximal phalanges all articulate with their respective metacarpals. The metacarpals articulate with the carpal bones, which as a unit form the wrist joint. This joint articulates with the radial head. The carpal bones are arranged in two rows. The proximal row includes the scaphoid, lunate, triquetrum, and pisiform. The distal row includes the trapezium, trapezoid, capitate, and hamate. The wrist bones are interconnected through a complex of ligaments that also reinforce the articulations with the radius and ulna.

Vascular Anatomy

Both the radial and ulnar arteries contribute to the blood supply of the hand (Figure 22-35A). Usually, the ulnar artery is dominant. Together, these arteries form two arches, or arcades, within the hand. The common digital arteries arise from these arcades. Each common digital artery gives off "proper" digital arteries. The proper digital vessels travel along the radial and ulnar sides of the digits, and their respective digital nerves form neurovascular bundles. The integrity of the digital vessels may be checked by observing capillary refill in the fingers. The radial and ulnar arteries and their vascular arcades are examined with **Allen test** (Figure 22-35B). In this test,

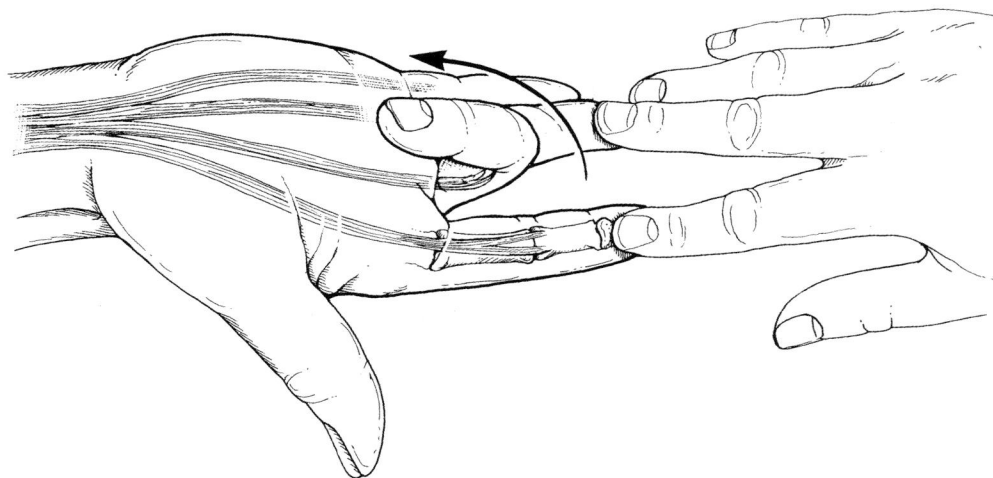

Figure 22-32. Examination of the flexor digitorum superficialis. Because the tendons of the flexor digitorum profundus have a common muscular origin, the action of this musculotendinous unit is blocked by maintaining adjacent fingers in extension. Flexion of the finger is then a function of only the flexor digitorum superficialis. (From Lawrence PF. *Essentials of Surgical Specialties*. 3rd ed. Lippincott Williams & Wilkins; 2007.)

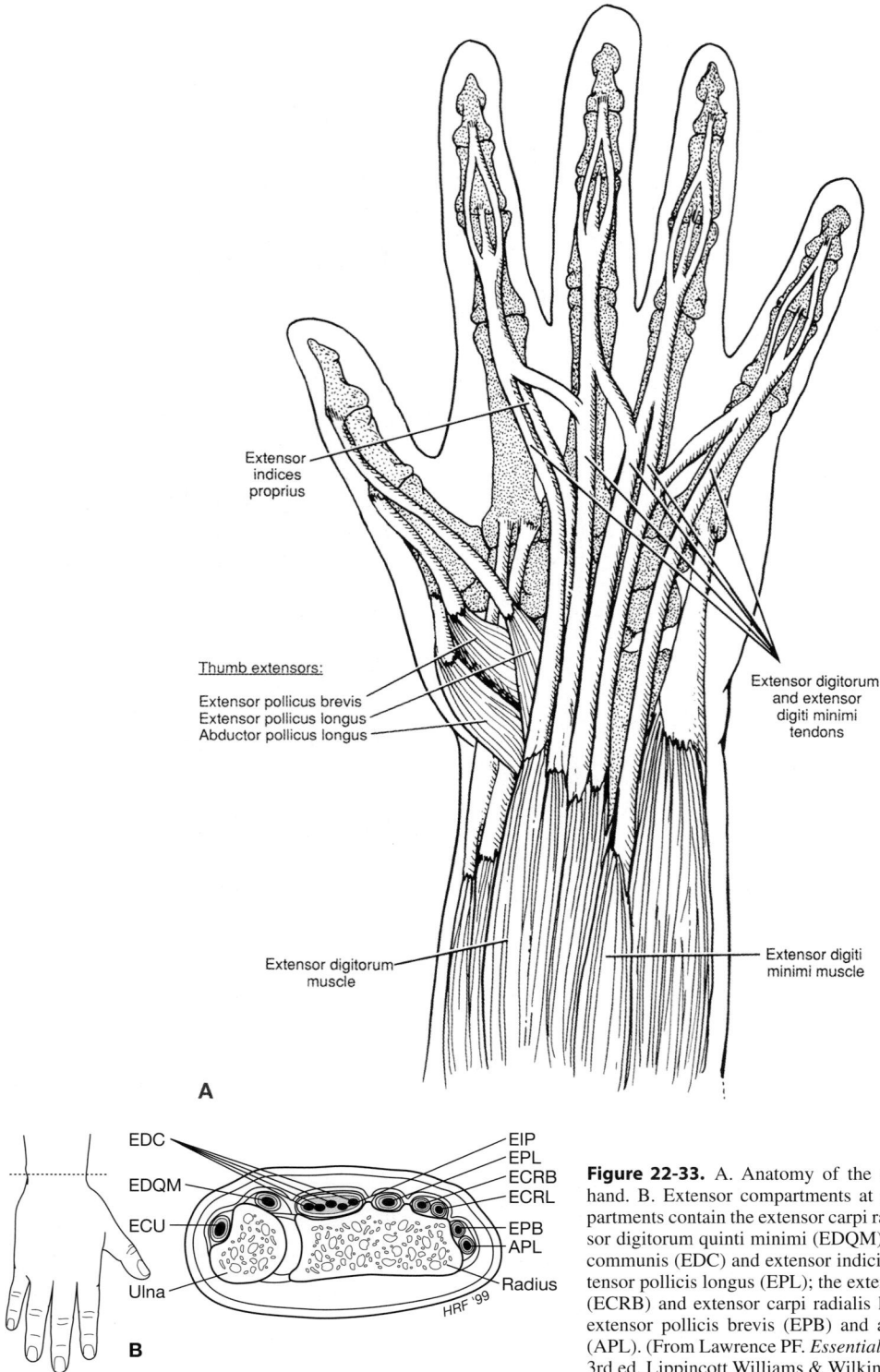

A

B

EDC

EDQM

ECU

Ulna

EIP
EPL
ECRB
ECRL
EPB
APL
Radius

Extensor
indices
proprius

Thumb extensors:

Extensor pollicus brevis
Extensor pollicus longus
Abductor pollicus longus

Extensor digitorum
and extensor
digiti minimi
tendons

Extensor digitorum
muscle

Extensor digiti
minimi muscle

HRF '99

Figure 22-33. A. Anatomy of the extensor tendons to the hand. B. Extensor compartments at the wrist. The six compartments contain the extensor carpi radialis (ECU); the extensor digitorum quinti minimi (EDQM); the extensor digitorum communis (EDC) and extensor indicis proprius (EIP); the extensor pollicis longus (EPL); the extensor carpi radialis brevis (ECRB) and extensor carpi radialis longus (ECRL); and the extensor pollicis brevis (EPB) and abductor pollicis longus (APL). (From Lawrence PF. *Essentials of Surgical Specialties.* 3rd ed. Lippincott Williams & Wilkins; 2007.)

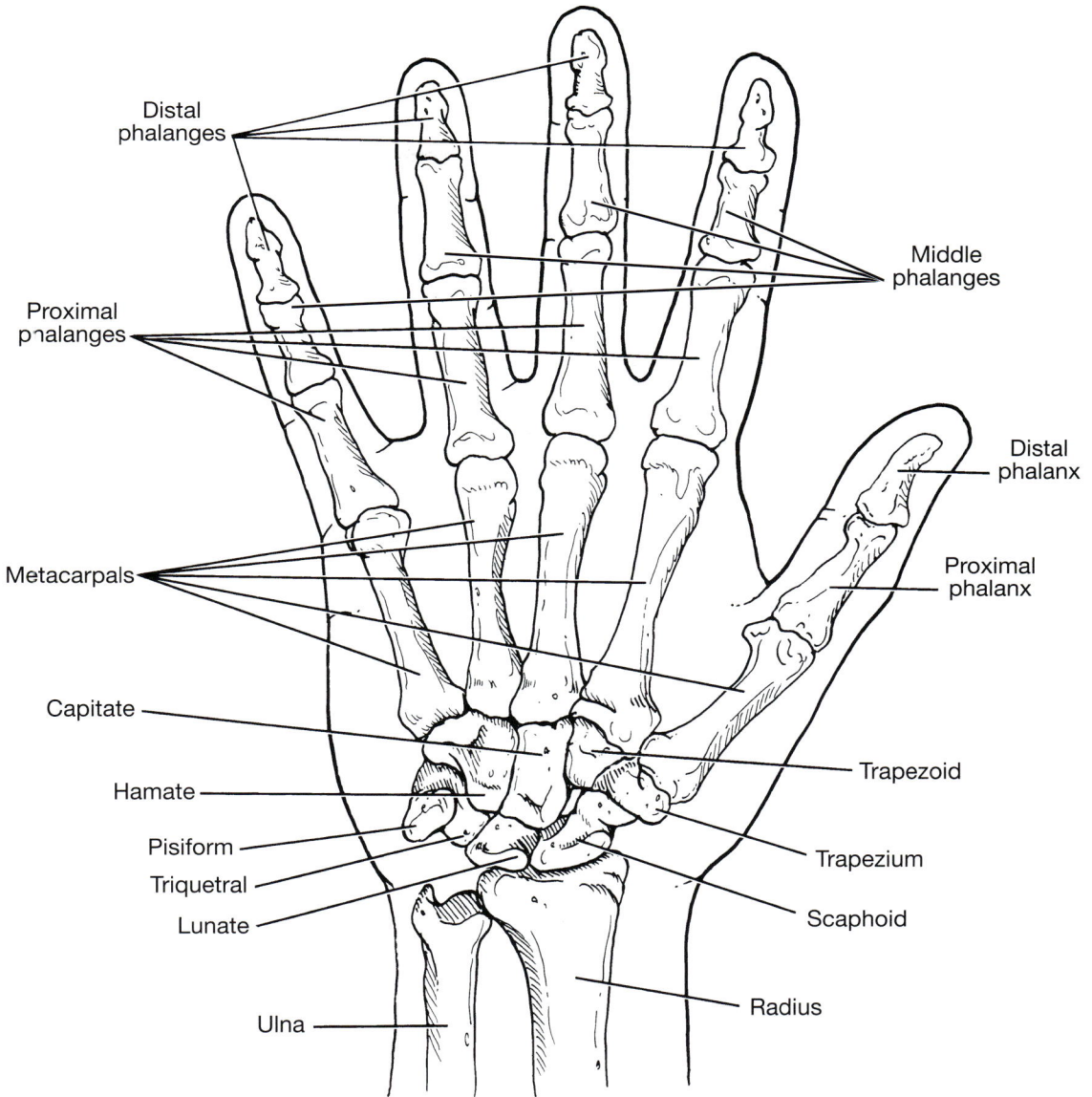

Figure 22-34. Skeletal anatomy of the hand. (From Lawrence PF. *Essentials of Surgical Specialties*. 3rd ed. Lippincott Williams & Wilkins; 2007.)

the radial and ulnar arteries are compressed at the wrist. The patient is asked to open and close the first several times, thus exsanguinating the hand and leaving the skin blanched. The fingers are held extended while the radial artery is released from compression. If the radial artery is patent, with good collateral flow to the ulnar artery, the palm and all five digits turn pink. Arterial compression and exsanguination are repeated, but this time, the ulnar artery is released. If the ulnar artery is patent, with good collateral flow into the radial artery, the hand and all five digits turn pink. If vascular integrity is still uncertain, a Doppler examination may be helpful.

Diagnosis of Hand Injuries

Because of the complex anatomy and function of the hand and the potentially severe consequences of hand injuries, most significant injuries should be treated by a hand specialist. However, the nonspecialist may be the first person to encounter these injuries and thus must be able to evaluate, initially treat, and, if appropriate, refer these patients for specialty consultation.

Evaluation of the hand begins with a proper history. The time and mechanism of injury and the environment in which the injury occurred are of paramount importance,

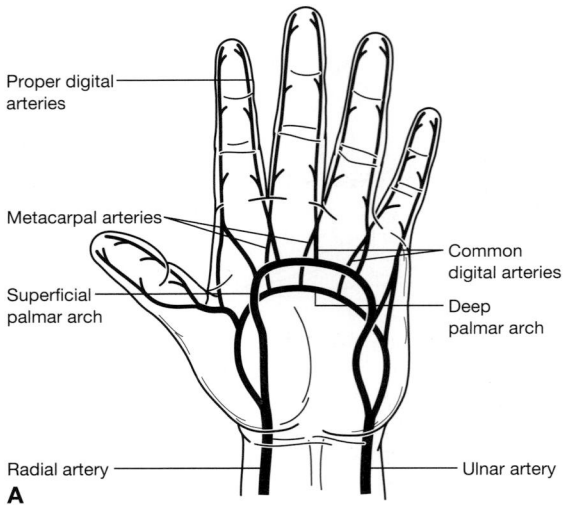

Figure 22-35. A. Vascular anatomy of the hand. B. Allen test for vascular patency. (From Lawrence PF. *Essentials of Surgical Specialties*. 3rd ed. Lippincott Williams & Wilkins; 2007.)

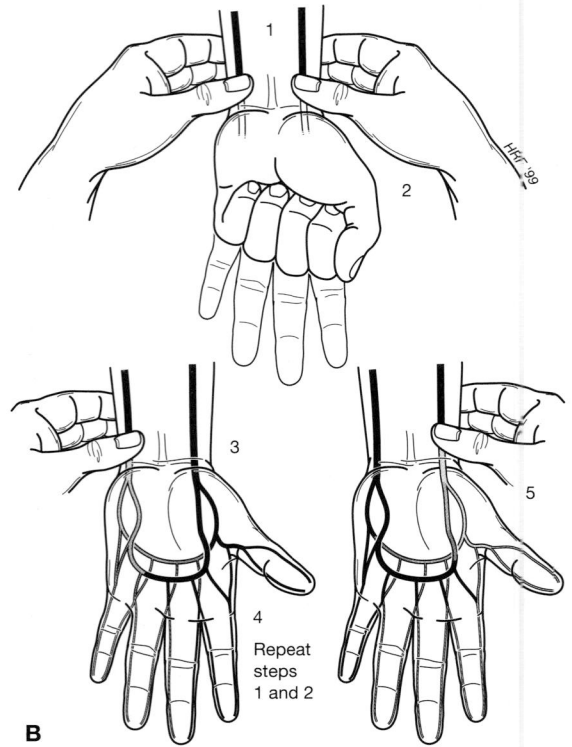

particularly with open wounds. The patient's overall medical condition, allergies, medications, tetanus immunization status, and previous injuries are also documented. The patient's hand dominance, occupation, and avocations play an important role in therapeutic decision-making. They should be noted and communicated to the hand specialist.

Before the hand is examined in detail, its vascular integrity is evaluated, so that if revascularization is needed, the patient can be referred immediately. Bleeding is controlled with direct pressure alone. Bleeding vessels are not clamped because of the risk of damaging accompanying nerves or further damaging reparable vessels. A pneumatic tourniquet is used only in extreme cases. The nail bed of each digit is examined for capillary refill, and the wrist and forearm are checked for pulse. Doppler examination can be used to confirm the patency of the ulnar and radial arteries, palmar arch, and digital arteries. If major portions of the hand appear ischemic, plans are made to transfer the patient to a replantation center with microvascular capabilities or to the operating room.

A careful examination of all motor and sensory units is performed. The distribution of each major sensory nerve should be tested and recorded. Each flexor and extensor tendon should be individually examined, as previously outlined. When fractures are suspected, appropriate radiographs are obtained. Complex injuries that involve multiple tendons and nerves can be simply and well delineated with a thorough examination. Careful documentation of these injuries is required.

During the initial evaluation of the hand, fractures should be suspected and diagnosed. Inspection of the hand is often diagnostic when localized swelling, angulation, or rotational deformity is seen. Tenderness to palpation over the fracture site is the rule. In addition, there may be limitation of motion of the involved finger. A survey x-ray of the entire hand should be obtained, followed by anterior-posterior and lateral x-rays of the affected part. If suspected fractures are not well visualized, oblique views may be obtained.

Treatment of Hand Injuries

Soft Tissue Injuries

Open wounds of the hand should be copiously irrigated with a physiologic solution. For highly contaminated wounds, multiple liters of saline irrigation may be required. If no sensory or motor injuries are present, these wounds are simply closed in a sterile manner. Antibiotics are recommended for contaminated wounds or for open wounds with underlying bone, joint, or tendon injuries. Tetanus immunization status must be ascertained.

A lacerated nerve requires microscopic repair in the operating room. This type of injury does not require immediate repair if it is not convenient; it can be delayed for several days.

Flexor tendon injuries must also be repaired in the operating room. These injuries can be classified according to zone (Figure 22-36). Injuries within zone II (no man's land) can be the most difficult to manage. The deep and superficial flexor tendons run within the flexor sheath in this location. Once they are repaired, adhesions may form and restrict normal motion. A flexor tendon laceration can be repaired immediately or within several days. Simple skin closure and referral for repair within a few days are acceptable management of these injuries.

Many extensor tendon injuries can be repaired in the emergency department at the discretion of the hand

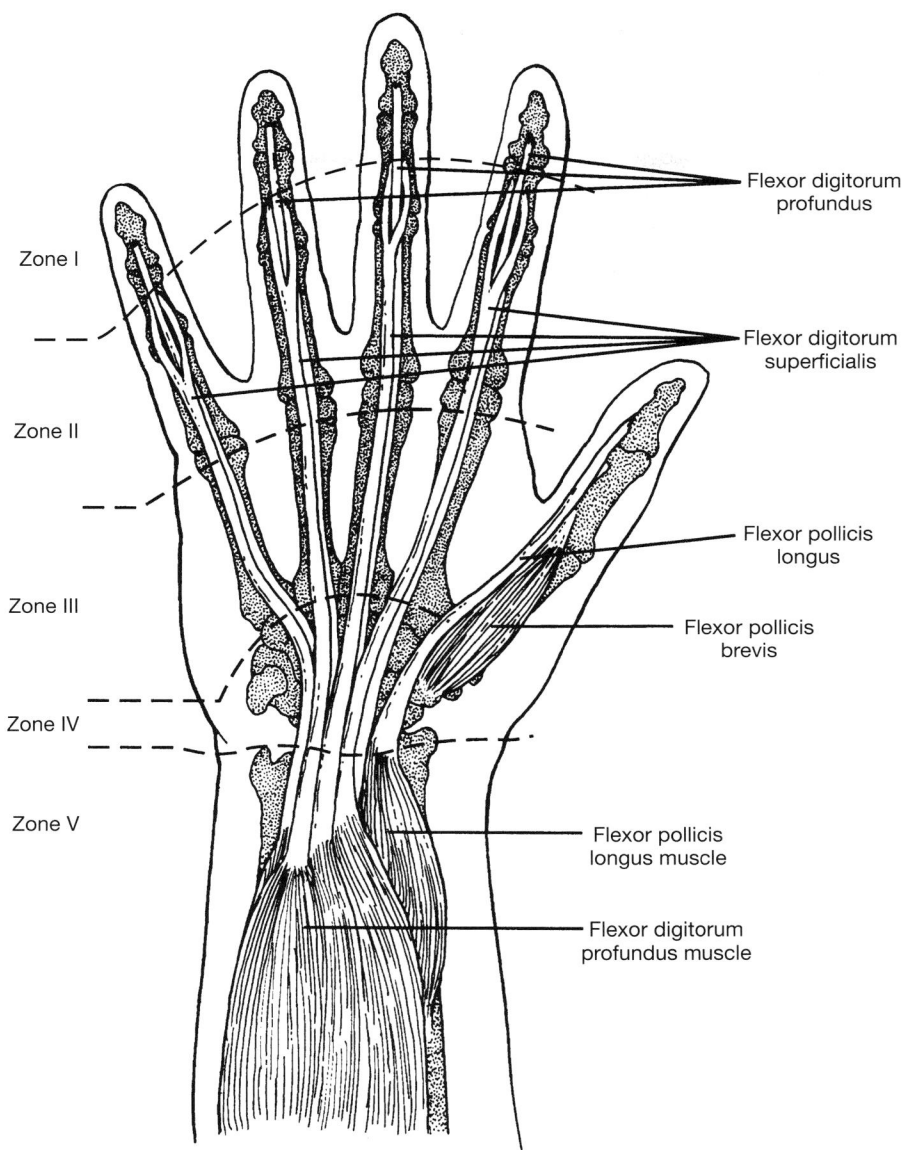

Figure 22-36. Zones of flexor tendon injuries. (From Lawrence PF: *Essentials of Surgical Specialties*. 3rd ed. Lippincott Williams & Wilkins; 2007.)

surgeon. Injuries to the extensor tendon overlying the DIP joint cause **mallet finger** (loss of active extension through the DIP; Figure 22-37A). Injuries to the central portion of the extensor mechanism at the PIP joint produce a boutonnière deformity (PIP flexion with DIP hyperextension; Figure 22-37B). Laceration of the extensor tendon in the hand prevents extension of the finger (Figure 22-37C).

Fractures of the Hand

Fractures of the hand are a common component of injury. The goal of treatment is proper reduction of the fracture and maintenance of the reduction with splinting, casting, or fixation (either internal or external). To achieve as near-normal function as possible, anatomic reduction of all fractures is ideal. In some fractures, minor discrepancy in final bone alignment can be tolerated. Because of the complexity of the hand and its fractures, nearly all fractures require the consultation of a hand surgeon.

Closed fractures are usually treated electively as the localized swelling allows. Proper splinting until fixation reduces patient discomfort and swelling. All open fractures should be treated acutely as the patient's overall condition allows. With the exception of very minor fractures and those treated with casting alone, all definitive reduction and fixation should be done in the operating room. Although an in-depth discussion of specific hand fractures is beyond the scope of this chapter, a few types are discussed here.

Probably the most common fracture is that of the end of the distal phalanx, or distal tuft. Because the fracture occurs distal to the insertion of the extensor and flexor a result of a blow to another object (eg, an opponent's chin) (Figure 22-38). Angulation or rotational deformity is often seen. Although 20 to 30° of volar angulation of the fourth and fifth metacarpals may be acceptable, little or no angulation of the other metacarpals is acceptable. Likewise, rotational deformity is unacceptable because it interferes with normal motion. Boxer fractures and other stable, nondisplaced metacarpal fractures may be treated with casting alone, but most others require additional methods of fixation.

Fractures of the scaphoid usually occur after a fall on the outstretched hand. This history and tenderness over the anatomic snuff box are key to making the diagnosis. Although initial radiographs may not show a fracture, repeat films in 1 to 3 weeks may. Because of the problems with nonunion in improperly treated scaphoid fractures, patients who are suspected of having such injuries, but whose initial x-rays are negative, should be casted and treated as though they have this fracture. Repeat x-rays are obtained 2 weeks later. Avascular necrosis is a common complication of the fractured scaphoid. This issue is further addressed in Chapter 26.

Splinting of the injured hand is important and deserves special note. Prolonged splinting in an inappropriate position may cause joint stiffness, shortening of musculotendinous and ligamentous units, and ultimate loss of some function. Although certain fractures or tendon injuries may require splinting in different positions, most injured hands should be splinted in the "safe" position to preserve function (Figure 22-39). In this position, the wrist is in 20 to 30° of extension, the MCP joints are flexed at 80 to 90°, and the IP joints are straight or nearly so. The thumb is held in palmar abduction. Splints to maintain this position are usually placed on the volar surface of the hand, wrist, and forearm.

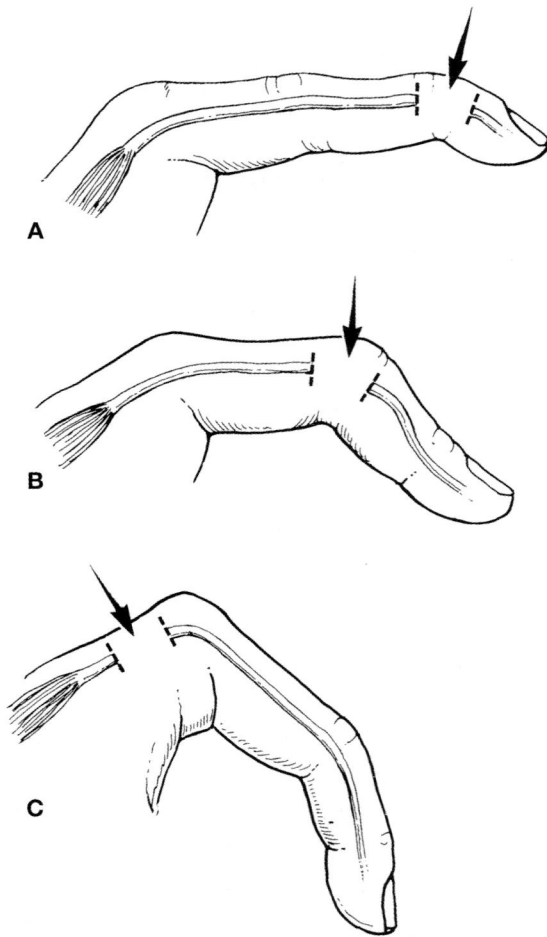

Figure 22-37. Extensor tendon injuries. A. Mallet finger deformity caused by a laceration of the extensor tendon at or just proximal to the distal interphalangeal joint. B. Boutonnière deformity caused by a laceration of the central slip of the extensor apparatus at or just proximal to the proximal interphalangeal joint. C. Extensor tendon laceration proximal to the metacarpophalangeal joint. (From Lawrence PF. *Essentials of Surgical Specialties.* 3rd ed. Lippincott Williams & Wilkins; 2007.)

tendons, precise anatomic reduction is not required. These fractures can be easily treated with splints for 2 to 3 weeks, usually without complications. Seriously crushed tips may require some molding during splinting to achieve the best result, and associated nail bed injuries require careful repair under loupe magnification. If the fracture involves the DIP joint space or any tendinous insertion, referral should be sought.

Fractures of the middle and proximal phalanges are also common. Stable fractures can be treated with splints or "buddy taping," whereby the injured finger is taped to an adjacent finger that functions as a splint. Unstable, comminuted, or spiral fractures and those that involve the joint space may require more complex fixation.

Fractures through the head or neck of the metacarpals often result from altercations. A **boxer fracture** is a fracture through the fourth or fifth metacarpal neck, usually as

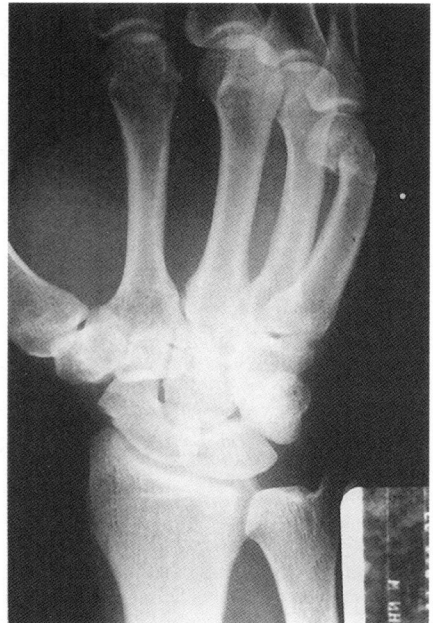

Figure 22-38. Boxer fracture. (From Lawrence PF. *Essentials of Surgical Specialties.* 3rd ed. Lippincott Williams & Wilkins; 2007.)

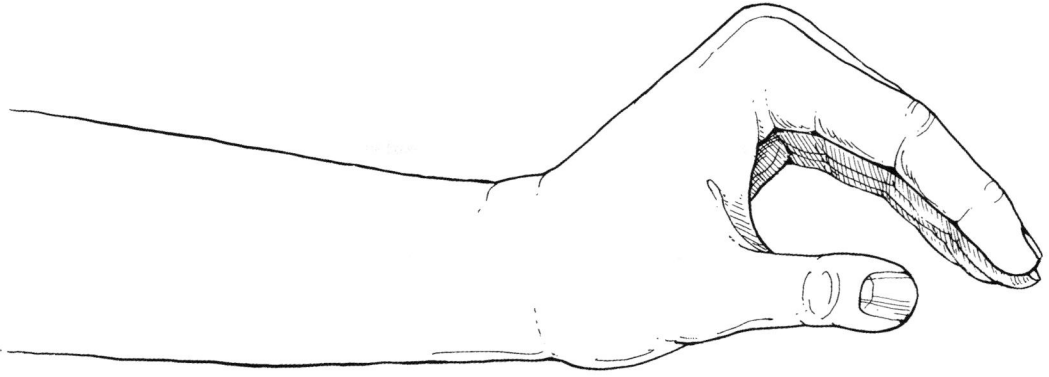

Figure 22-39. Safe position for immobilization of the hand. (From Lawrence PF. *Essentials of Surgical Specialties.* 3rd ed. Lippincott Williams & Wilkins; 2007.)

Special Injuries
Fingertip Injuries

Although fingertip injuries are common, their care can be very complex because of the structure and function of the fingertip. The goals of treatment are to maintain adequate length and normal sensibility. Simple distal skin losses can be treated with dressings alone and allowed to heal by contraction. However, injuries that involve the distal phalanx or nail bed require complex repairs. If the distal amputated part is available, it should be handled gently and cared for properly (see section "Amputations").

Amputations

Particular care is given to amputated parts. Digits or significant portions of digits are often amputated in industrial accidents that occur in unsanitary settings. The amputated part should be rinsed with saline to remove debris and gross contamination. The amputated part is then wrapped in moist gauze and placed in a watertight plastic bag. The bag is sealed and placed in a container filled with iced saline. The amputated part should not be allowed to become waterlogged by being placed directly in saline or frozen by being placed directly on ice. X-ray films of the amputated part should be obtained before it is transferred.

Although not all amputated parts can or should be replanted, the ultimate decision regarding replantation should be made by the replant surgeon. Replantation is always considered in thumb amputations, amputations distal to the PIP joint, multiple-digit amputations, bilateral amputations, hand or hemihand amputation, and in children. Replantation of severely crushed or avulsed parts is usually not indicated, nor is replantation of parts that have undergone warm ischemia for more than 6 to 12 hours.

Thermal Injuries

The thermally injured hand offers a challenge to the initial treating physician. Correct early treatment significantly improves outcome. The burned hand should be cleansed gently with physiologic solution and, if necessary, with mild soap. All foreign material (eg, burned clothing) should be removed. Blisters should be left intact because they signify a second-degree burn and protect the underlying tissue. When these blisters eventually break on their own, they should be gently debrided. Capillary refill of all burned digits should be checked because circumferential burns can interfere with distal circulation. This interference may take several hours to develop; if it does, escharotomy may be required.

After the hand is cleaned, an antibiotic ointment (eg, Silvadene) is applied. The hand is placed in a bulky dressing and splinted in the safe position. Therapy consists of daily whirlpool baths, dressing changes, and aggressive range-of-motion exercises to prevent joint contracture. Patients who have significant partial-thickness burns or full-thickness burns that require skin grafting should be referred.

Burns represent a unique form of trauma. The role of the surgeon may involve patient care only for burn reconstruction or from the initial trauma all the way through reconstruction. The burned patient should be approached in the same logical and orderly manner as any other trauma patient at the onset, but a quality understanding of the unique characteristics of burn patients and burn care is critical to the near- and long-term successful treatment of that patient. An excellent review of trauma and burns can be found in Chapters 7 and 8.

Frostbite is a unique form of thermal injury classified as a local injury and, therefore, separated from systemic hypothermia. The overall pathophysiology consists of the formation of ice crystals in the tissue fluid, leading to cellular injury. This injury must be recognized early and treated aggressively. Successful treatment is based on rapid tissue rewarming in a 40 °F water bath. After this, the normal components of monitoring a burn patient (eg, airway, breathing and circulation [ABCs], urine output, monitoring for infection), wound management, and evaluation of tetanus status can be applied. As the pathophysiology of frostbite is associated with vascular thrombosis, tissue plasminogen activator and intravenous (IV) heparin can be administered. Prophylactic oral antibiotic use is controversial. Topical antibiotic should be avoided because it can cause maceration. Depending on the location of the injury and total areas involved, therapy for range of motion and strength exercises might be necessary.

Hand Infections

The complex structure of the hand offers multiple sites for infection. Although superficial cellulitis and subcutaneous abscesses can occur in the hand as in other locations, some infections are peculiar to the hand. Such infections can occur within the lateral nail bed (**paronychia**), at the finger pulp (**felon**), in the tendon sheaths (**tenosynovitis**), and in the deeper structures of the hand (deep-space infections). Human bites to the hand are a common infectious problem. The successful management of hand infections depends on knowledge of both hand anatomy and the specific treatment of each infection.

In the hand, infection usually progresses rapidly. Without prompt diagnosis and treatment, the infection can spread quickly along fascial planes, causing damage to adjacent structures. In addition, this rapid spread can lead to massive tissue necrosis, which may require amputation of the extremity. At a minimum, it can result in a stiff, nonfunctional extremity. The treatment of suppurative infections of the hand is based on adequate surgical drainage. Although systemic symptoms may be present, signs and symptoms are usually localized to the hand. Serious infections of the hand are usually treated in the operating room under regional or general anesthesia, with tourniquet control. Appropriate aerobic and anaerobic cultures are taken. After adequate surgical drainage, the hand is immobilized in the protective splinted position and elevated. Antibiotics are routinely administered (usually a first-generation cephalosporin or a penicillinase-resistant antibiotic). After surgical drainage, the hand is reevaluated frequently, and antibiotics are adjusted according to intraoperative culture results. Further extension of the infection is possible, and adequate drainage should be verified by progressive resolution of pain and swelling.

Paronychia

Paronychia, an infection of the lateral nail fold, usually presents as a small collection of purulent material at the side of the nail. If seen early, it is properly treated by elevating the skin over the nail or excising a small lateral, longitudinal portion of the nail to drain the purulent material (Figure 22-40). More advanced infection may require incision within the nail fold for drainage. This procedure is followed by soaking the finger in warm water several times a day. Chronic paronychia suggests secondary colonization with more complex organisms. Antibiotic treatment for chronic paronychia should await results of cultures. Fungal nail infections or herpetic infection (herpetic whitlow) may be confused with chronic paronychia. Proper diagnosis is vital, because operating on a fungal or herpetic infection

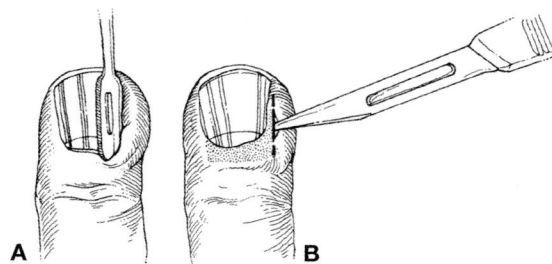

Figure 22-40. Treatment of paronychia. A. Elevation of the nail fold. B. Placement of an incision. (From Lawrence PF. *Essentials of Surgical Specialties.* 3rd ed. Lippincott Williams & Wilkins; 2007.)

may worsen the condition by allowing secondary bacterial infection and delayed wound healing.

Felon

A felon, a purulent infection of the pad of the finger, is usually extremely painful. Fibrous septa within the tip of the finger allow a significant amount of pressure when only a minimal amount of purulent material is present. This condition also increases local tissue pressure to the point of interrupting capillary flow, which can produce ischemia and necrosis. The felon can be drained by various methods (Figure 22-41). If skin necrosis is present, the incision can be made over it, or the incision can be made at a point of maximum tenderness. Alternatively, it is drained through a small stab incision laterally on the noncontact side of digit pad (eg, radial side of the thumb, ulnar side of the fingers). In draining a felon, it is important to adequately disrupt the fibrous septa to provide enough drainage.

Tenosynovitis

Tenosynovitis is a painful inflammation of the tendon sheath. Suppurative tenosynovitis is usually caused by a puncture wound over the volar aspect of the hand. It can also develop from the extension of a felon (Figure 22-42). Diagnosis is usually made by observing four signs (**Kanavel signs**): (a) finger held in slight flexion, (b) fusiform swelling of the finger, (c) tenderness over the tendon sheath, and (d) pain on passive extension. The fourth sign is usually the key to diagnosis.

Prompt and appropriate treatment is required to prevent complications. Some very early infections can be treated with IV antibiotics, elevation, and immobilization. However, for more advanced infections or when the initial symptoms fail to improve after 24 hours with the above-mentioned treatment, surgical drainage of the tendon sheath is carried out in the operating room by a hand surgeon.

Deep-Space Infections

Infection of the deep spaces of the hand or thenar eminence can also occur. Patients usually have pain and swelling. Although the primary problem may be in a volar location, more dorsal swelling is almost always present. Treatment is surgical drainage of the affected spaces. The complexity of the anatomy of the deep spaces of the hand complicates their drainage. Referral to a hand surgeon is usually necessary. Deep-space infections of the hand initially involve specific sites (eg, thenar, hypothenar, midpalmar, parona's space). Infections are typically caused by a penetrating injury, but the actual presence of a foreign body on radiographs is rare. Clinical examination is considered the hallmark of diagnosis. The space involved will generally show signs such as a loss of palmar concavity (midpalmar space) or a wide abduction of the thumb and difficulty with opposition (thenar space). Urgent surgical intervention is required to provide adequate treatment of the infection, and frequently, postoperative therapy is necessary to maintain range of motion and strength.

Human Bites

Human bites to the hand can produce devastating complications because of the degree of wound contamination from human saliva. The diagnosis is often complicated by an inaccurate or misleading history given by the patient.

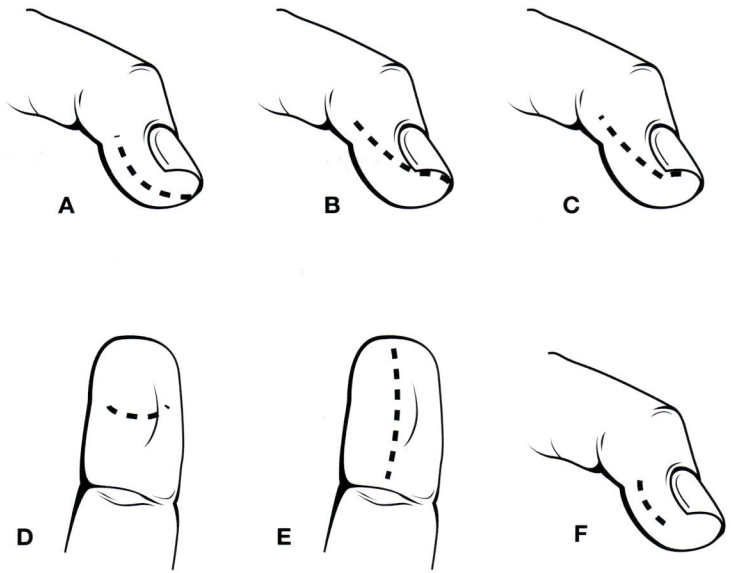

Figure 22-41. Drainage approaches for a felon. A–C. "Hockey stick" or J incision around the tip of the finger. D. Transverse incision across the pulp of the finger. E. Longitudinal incision down the center of the finger pad. F. Incision on the lateral aspect of the finger. (From Lawrence PF. *Essentials of Surgical Specialties.* 3rd ed. Lippincott Williams & Wilkins; 2007.)

Lacerations overlying the dorsal MCP joint (knuckle) should always be suspected of being a "fight bite" (Figure 22-43). The patient's hand must be examined in a clenched position to avoid missing deeper wounds. Lacerations from human bites should never be closed but must be left open to drain. Patients are admitted for 24 to 48 hours of IV antibiotics, with the hand elevated and immobilized. Bites that are not treated within 24 hours require longer hospitalization and more complex treatment. Those that are properly treated within 24 hours virtually always have a favorable outcome.

Tumors of the Hand

Benign Tumors

Ganglion Cyst

The most common soft tissue mass of the hand is a **ganglion cyst**. These cysts occur in several anatomic locations. The ganglion is an outpouching of the synovium, usually of a joint or tendinous structure. The most common location is on the dorsal radial aspect of the wrist, where the cyst originates from the ligament joining the scaphoid and lunate bones. These cysts may also occur on the volar radial area of the wrist or along the palmar surface of the hand or finger overlying the flexor tendon sheath. A ganglion cyst presents as a mobile mass that transilluminates. Symptomatic ganglion cysts are surgically removed. Untreated, they tend to increase in size slowly but progressively. Other methods of treatment (eg, digital rupture, aspiration, injection with steroids or sclerosing materials) are usually ineffective.

Mucous Cyst

A mucous cyst is not a true cyst, but a ganglion arising from the dorsum of the finger overlying the DIP joint. These often present in older females and are usually associated with degenerative changes in the DIP joint. Surgical

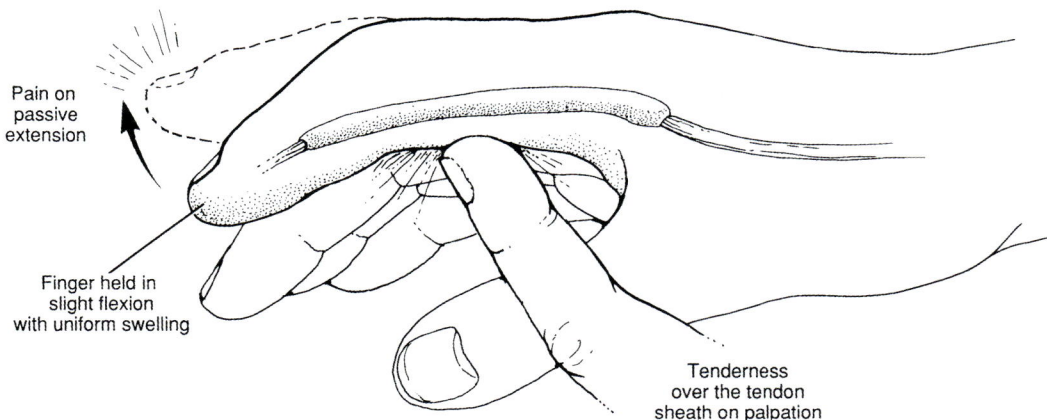

Figure 22-42. Flexor tenosynovitis. The diagnosis is made by Kanavel four signs: the finger held in slight flexion, fusiform swelling of the finger, tenderness over the tendon sheath, and pain on passive extension. (From Lawrence PF. *Essentials of Surgical Specialties.* 3rd ed. Lippincott Williams & Wilkins; 2007.)

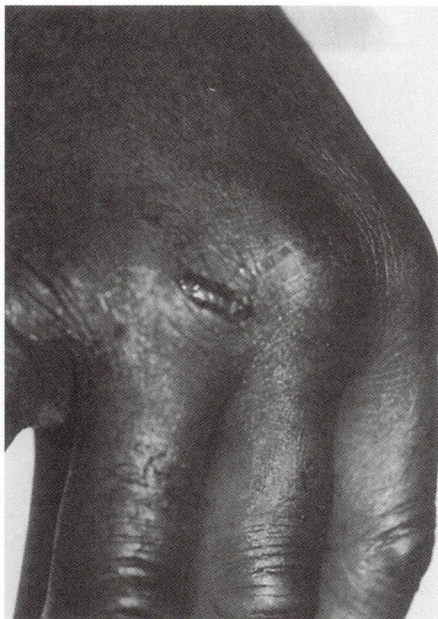

Figure 22-43. Human bite to the metacarpophalangeal joint.
This is the typical appearance of a "fight bite." (From Lawrence
PF. *Essentials of Surgical Specialties.* 3rd ed. Lippincott Wil-
liams & Wilkins; 2007.)

resection is complicated by the need to excise the cyst, usually with some overlying skin and underlying osteophytes.
Small skin grafts or skin flaps may be required for closure.

Giant Cell Tumor

Another soft tissue tumor that occurs in the wrist or finger
is the giant cell tumor (xanthoma). This slowly growing,
yellow-brown tumor invades surrounding structures. It has
a high recurrence rate after resection because of satellite
lesions. Surgical excision is carefully performed under
low-power magnification.

Malignant Tumors

Squamous and basal cell carcinomas of the skin are relatively common in the hands. They are usually caused by
aging and sun exposure. As in other parts of the body, treatment is with wide local excision followed by soft tissue
reconstruction. Malignant melanoma may be present under
the nail bed, and the nails should be carefully examined.
Melanomas in the hand are managed with wide local excision or amputation.

Other Conditions That Require Surgery

Arthritis

Some common problems with the hands involve either
degenerative or rheumatoid arthritis. These conditions are
extremely debilitating and may cause permanent disability.
The primary treatment of both diseases is medical. Surgical treatment is reserved for maintaining or restoring functional ability. In many patients, improvement is provided
by early surgical intervention for joint reconstruction,
muscle and tendon rebalancing, and synovectomy.

Dupuytren Disease

Dupuytren disease is progressive fibrosis of the palmar
fascia of the hand. The etiology of the disease is unclear,
but it has a definite hereditary pattern. It usually occurs after
40 years of age, is more common in men (7:1 ratio), and occurs bilaterally in more than 50% of cases. It causes increasing contraction of the fibrous palmar fascia that presents as
nodules, cords, and contractures in the hand because of disorganized type III collagen. The natural course is progressive contracture of the hand and the inability to fully extend
the digits. There is no known medical treatment. However,
steroid or collagenase injections have gained popularity because of convenience and patient tolerance. Indications for
surgery include limited finger extension (eg, any PIP joint
contracture, >30° MP joint contracture), rapid progression
of the disease, and painful nodules. The best surgical results
occur when the patient is evaluated early and when surgical resection is performed before the formation of joint abnormalities or fixed joints. At surgery, the involved palmar
fascia is removed, and the skin is repaired to alleviate scar
contractures. Care must be taken because the neurovascular
bundles may be encased in the diseased tissue.

Compression Neuropathy

Although compression neuropathy occurs in many locations of the upper extremity, the most common location
is the carpal tunnel. The median nerve is compressed as
it passes through the wrist within the carpal tunnel, which
is bounded dorsally by the carpal bones and volarly by a
tough ligament, the volar carpal ligament. Nine flexor tendons accompany the median nerve through the carpal tunnel (the four tendons of the flexor digitorum superficialis,
the four tendons of the flexor digitorum profundus, and the
tendon of the flexor pollicis longus). Patients usually have
numbness and tingling, particularly at night, within the median nerve sensory distribution of the hand. They may also
have difficulty grasping objects. These patients often have
occupations that require a large amount of repetitive manual work. Usually, pain and tingling can be reproduced by
percussing the median nerve within the carpal tunnel (**Tinel
sign**). In advanced cases, atrophy of the thenar musculature
can occur. Nerve conduction studies usually show delays.

Treatment is directed at relieving the compression and
resultant inflammation of the median nerve. In early cases,
splinting or alteration of work habits may be helpful. However, these measures usually provide only transient help.
Definitive operative treatment involves division of the volar
carpal ligament and, occasionally, internal neurolysis of the
median nerve. Surgery should not be delayed until thenar
atrophy develops because this condition can be permanent.

CONGENITAL DEFECTS

Congenital Defects of the Hand

Congenital defects of the hand can occur either alone or
in association with multiple other medical syndromes.
Early diagnosis allows planned treatment. Common defects include webbed fingers (**syndactyly**) (Figure 22-44)
and extra digits (polydactyly). Syndactyly is routinely repaired before the infant is 6 to 12 months of age. Repair
should not be delayed past 12 months of age unless other

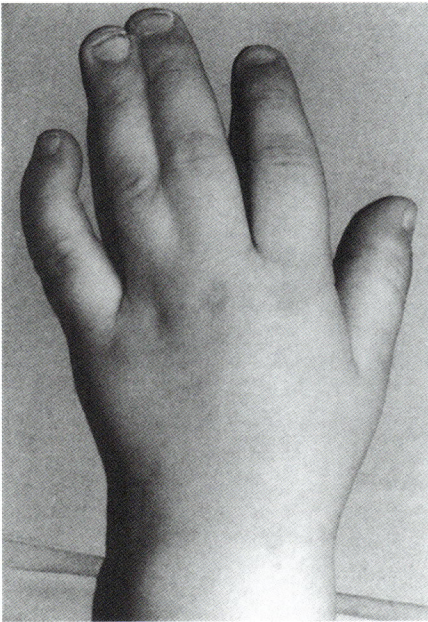

Figure 22-44. Simple syndactyly. (From Lawrence PF. *Essentials of Surgical Specialties*. 3rd ed. Lippincott Williams & Wilkins; 2007.)

associated medical problems are present. If the two digits fused together are of unequal length (eg, ring and small fingers, thumb and index finger), progressive contracture and bony angulation will occur as the child grows. Another reason to proceed early with separation is the presence of complex syndactyly in which fusion of adjacent phalanges occurs. This fusion causes significant growth abnormalities if the phalanges are not divided early.

Surgical care of polydactyly usually involves amputation of the extra digits. Amputation should be done only after complete evaluation is made of the functional status and potential of all of the digits. Such an evaluation may require waiting for several months, or even more than a year, until it is evident which digit will be the most functional. Occasionally, combining some elements of one digit with those of the other is indicated.

Two congenital hand problems require early treatment. One is a constriction ring deformity, in which a band of amniotic tissue forms a tourniquet around a finger or another part of the body (eg, wrist, leg, toe). The constriction must be at least partially relieved early because it tends to limit circulation. A second defect that benefits from early treatment is the significantly deviated hand (eg, radial club hand). Very early splinting prevents increasing angulation and deformity.

Cleft Lip and Palate

The most common developmental anomalies of the face are cleft lip and cleft palate. The incidence of clefts is between 1:600 and 1:1,000 live births. A cleft of the left lip and palate is more common in boys and has a hereditary component. A cleft palate alone is seen more often in girls and does not have a hereditary component. The etiology of clefts is not completely understood, but because heredity plays a significant role, many patients are concerned about the risk of clefts in their offspring. If one parent has had a cleft, a child has a 7% chance of having a cleft. This figure increases to 14% if there is already a sibling with a cleft. When two normal parents already have a child with a cleft, a second boy has a 4.5% chance of being born with a cleft.

The lip and palate structures are divided anatomically into prepalatal (primary palate) and palatal (secondary palate) structures. The incisive foramen, located in the midline on the hard palate, just behind the alveolus, divides prepalatal and palatal clefts. The embryology of these clefts is different.

The prepalatal structures form between the fourth and seventh weeks of fetal life and arise from three mesenchymal islands (one central and two lateral). Incomplete migration of these elements can lead to clefts. Prepalatal clefts involve the lip, alveolus, nose, and nasal cartilage. Cleft lips may be unilateral or bilateral, and complete or incomplete. At 7 weeks of gestation, the palatal structures are composed of two palatal shelves that are vertically oriented along the sides of the tongue. As the neck of the fetus straightens, the tongue drops, and the palatal shelves rotate upward to become horizontal by the 12th week. Palatal clefts are caused by an incomplete fusion of the palatal shelves. They involve the hard palate, soft palate, and uvula. Various combinations of clefts of the prepalatal and palatal structures are seen.

Treatment of the cleft lip is directed at returning the different lip elements to their normal position to improve appearance and correct minor functional problems, such as lisping (Figure 22-45). The timing of cleft lip repair is controversial. Repair is usually begun when the infant is 6 to 12 weeks of age and completed by 6 to 9 months of age. The ideal lip repair will establish symmetrical nostrils, alar bases, natural philtral columns and central dimple, as well as the Cupid bow and vermilion tubercle. Functionally, the muscular repair will provide normal activity and lip competence. Although multiple cleft lip repairs have been described in the past (eg, Le Mesurier, Randall-Tennison), the most common unilateral cleft lip reconstruction is the Millard rotation-advancement. This repair advances a mucocutaneous flap from the lateral lip element into the cleft gap to approximate the rotated (inferiorly and into the cleft gap) medial segment.

Recent utilization of artificial intelligence can help in planning and developing options for lip closures. This may be most useful virtually to allow surgeons in other countries to perform the surgery with guidance through virtual technology.

Treatment of the nasal deformity is much more difficult because of the underdevelopment and malposition of the nasal cartilage. The cleft lip nasal deformity may require several revisions that extend into the teenage years. However, primary treatment of the nose at the time of lip repair is now commonly performed and provides either complete correction or significant improvement.

Although cleft lip is repaired primarily for the sake of appearance, cleft palate is repaired to ensure function, specifically, speech. The competent palate (or velum) elevates and meets the posterior pharyngeal wall (creating velopharyngeal closure) during speech and swallowing. The inability to elevate the palate produces abnormal speech, which can range from hypernasal to nearly unintelligible. The

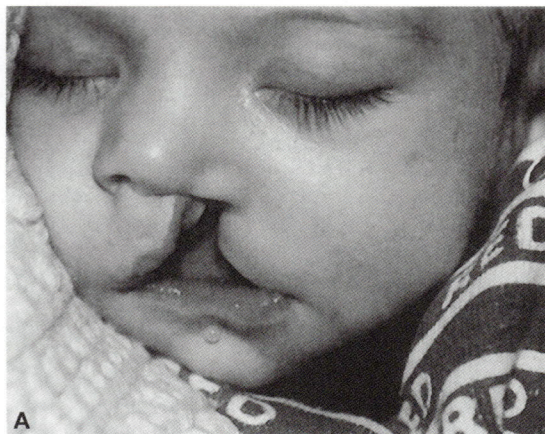

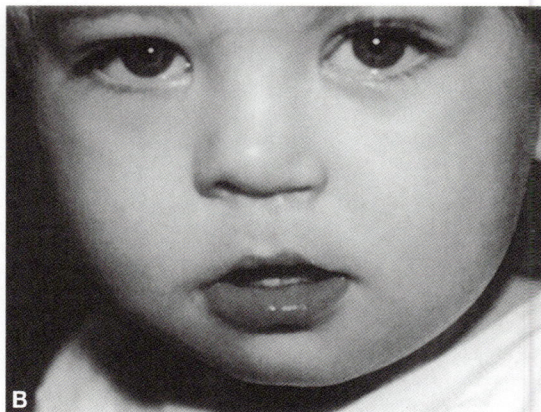

Figure 22-45. A. A 4-week-old child with a complete cleft of the left lip. B. The same child at 2 years of age, after lip repair with a rotation advancement method. (From Lawrence PF. *Essentials of Surgical Specialties.* 3rd ed. Lippincott Williams & Wilkins; 2007.)

various cleft palate repairs are designed to reorient the musculature of the palate, close the cleft, and lengthen the palate. As with the lip, the timing of cleft palate repair varies. Many surgeons now prefer earlier closure (by 6-12 months of age) to allow for more normal speech development.

The cleft palate repair options are based primarily on the anatomic defect to be corrected. Because no two cleft palates are exactly alike, the goal of the cleft palate repair must be the correction of a functional defect. These repairs generally are accepted to include palatal closure alone, palatal closure in concert with palatal lengthening, or either of these with direct palatal muscle reapproximation. The techniques include a V-Y pushback, the von Langenbeck procedure, intravelar veloplasty, or even the double-opposing Z-plasty technique. Future procedures may be indicated to correct speech abnormalities, such as a pharyngoplasty or pharyngeal flap.

Because of the abnormal orientation of the palatal musculature around the pharyngeal opening of the eustachian tube, middle ear infections are very common in these patients. Almost all of these children require myringotomy tubes to avoid long-term hearing problems. Another relatively uncommon cleft disorder is Pierre-Robin sequence, in which the palatal cleft is associated with a small or retropositioned mandible and a posteriorly displaced tongue. Emergency treatment may be required to maintain the airway.

A child with a cleft palate may have numerous developmental problems. Therefore, treatment should be conducted by a team of specialists under the direction of the plastic surgeon. The treating specialists should work efficiently to coordinate the integrated protocol of the Parameters of Care Guidelines, as established by the American Cleft Palate Craniofacial Association.

Other Congenital Head and Neck Anomalies

Branchial Cleft Cysts

Many other anomalies are possible within the head and neck area. The most common are variations of the **branchial cleft cyst** or sinus. This anomaly involves an epithelial tract along the *lateral* neck, which is seen along the anterior border of the sternocleidomastoid muscle. The cyst or sinus tract can range from a small blind pouch to

a tract that extends completely into the oral cavity. Treatment consists of surgical resection. The timing may vary according to the symptoms.

Thyroglossal Duct Cyst

A **thyroglossal duct cyst** or sinus is an opening or defect in the absolute *midline* of the neck around the hyoid bone. The defect may be either a small blind pouch or a sinus tract that extends into the base of the tongue at the foramen cecum and is noted to move with protrusion of the tongue or deglutition. Occasionally, as in the branchial cleft cyst, infection occurs, and a brief course of antibiotics may be required. However, the definitive treatment is surgical excision. Because a thyroglossal duct cyst routinely goes through the middle of the hyoid bone, adequate resection requires the removal of the central portion of the hyoid bone as well as the complete sinus, usually all the way to the base of the tongue.

Congenital Ear Deformities

Another type of congenital deformity is an ear deformity. Although complete absence of the ear (**anotia**) is rare, abnormally forming cartilage (eg, protruding or prominent ears) and deficient cartilage (**microtia**) are relatively common. Anotia or microtia requires reconstruction of the cartilaginous framework of the ear. A large piece of cartilage is harvested, usually from the patient's rib, and carved to resemble the scaffolding of the ear. The cartilage is implanted and covered with adequate skin. Although the technique is difficult and demanding, in expert hands, it can produce excellent results. The amount of reconstruction depends on the severity of the defect. Routinely, three to four surgical procedures are required. Microtia repairs can be performed after a child is 6 years old because the ear is almost adult size and adequate rib cartilage is available.

Congenital protruding ears can be treated with molding techniques initiated within the first 72 hours after birth, or are repaired by removing some of the conchal cartilage and plicating the remaining cartilage to the mastoid fascia. Acquired ear deformities, as in partial amputation, can be repaired with techniques similar to those used to reconstruct congenital defects.

ACQUIRED DEFORMITIES

Treatment of acquired soft tissue deformities often requires reconstructive surgery. Several factors are important to a successful reconstruction, beginning with a careful consideration of the etiology of the deformity and the natural history of the disease that produces it. Next, the deformity itself is considered. The amount and type of missing tissue and the function of the tissue are important. Through this evaluation, the patient's reconstructive needs can be understood. Finally, the reconstructive surgeon must choose the most appropriate method of reconstruction, keeping in mind the reconstructive ladder.

In many cases, several reconstructive options are appropriate, or at least possible. A careful, comprehensive discussion of these options with the patient is important because the patient is an important part of the decision-making process. Further, because each patient has different needs, desires, and expectations, it is difficult to follow a "cookbook" approach that always treats certain wounds with specific operations. Each patient must be considered individually to appreciate their unique differences and needs.

Postmastectomy Breast Reconstruction

During the past 45 years, major advances have occurred in postmastectomy breast reconstruction. Technical advances include the development of tissue expanders, improvement in breast prostheses, and new methods of flap reconstruction. Psychological considerations have also come to be appreciated. The patient's psychological well-being and recovery may be significantly affected by proper breast reconstruction. As general surgeons have come to understand the methods of breast reconstruction, better collaboration with the reconstructive surgeon has resulted. Surgeons now understand that breast reconstruction can often be begun or completed at the time of mastectomy and that the method chosen must take into account the patient's body habitus, lifestyle, healing capabilities, adjuvant therapy (chemotherapy and radiation), and desires. The skin-sparing mastectomy, which preserves all or most of the breast skin (except the nipple-areola complex and the biopsy site), provides dramatic reconstructive results without compromising on cancer cure. Recently, nipple-sparing mastectomy has been gaining popularity as a breast cancer treatment or prophylactic procedure. In this method, all the glandular breast tissues are removed through inframammary, lateral, or periareolar incision approaches, but the nipple-areolar complex is preserved. This method eliminates the need for nipple reconstruction and is associated with a more natural look following reconstruction. Another recent advancement in breast surgery is the development of oncoplastic reconstruction. Oncoplastic technique involves complete resection of cancer with better margin control while preserving normal breast parenchyma as much as possible. This aims to improve aesthetic outcomes and to reduce patient morbidity. Techniques such as partial mastectomy, local tissue rearrangement, reconstruction by reduction mammoplasty, mastopexy, and local or regional flaps allow patients who otherwise would have to undergo traditional mastectomy to become eligible for breast-conserving therapy.

Psychological Considerations

Because many options for breast reconstruction are available, adequate time must be spent with the patient to determine how to best suit their needs. All options must be discussed with the patient, and the patient's preference must be elicited. When two options are equally appropriate or nearly so, the patient may choose the operation they prefer. The patient should also be counseled about what to expect regarding the operation, recovery, and ultimate aesthetic results. The reconstructed breast often looks as good as or better than the contralateral breast. In other cases, the reconstruction may appear only adequate (especially when the patient is fully clothed) but is superior to an external prosthesis.

Before undertaking breast reconstruction, the surgeon must determine whether the procedure should be performed, what the timing should be, will postoperative radiation and or chemotherapy be necessary, and what method should be used. Although some form of reconstruction is possible for most patients, other patients, because of advanced disease, associated illness, or unrealistic expectations, should be counseled instead about external prostheses. Reconstruction can be immediate, starting with the mastectomy, or delayed, beginning after the mastectomy wound heals. Although a number of factors must be considered, the patient's desires are often the most important.

Reconstruction

Reconstruction of the breast can be divided into reconstruction of the breast mound and reconstruction of the nipple-areola complex. For the breast mound, local tissue with an implant or distant tissue, with or without an implant, may be used. A small or medium implant placed beneath the chest wall skin and the muscles of the chest wall (pectoralis major and serratus anterior) often gives an acceptable breast mound. Recent techniques allow placement of direct implants or tissue expanders placed prepectorally, providing mastectomy flaps are viable and not too thin. This helps prevent "animation deformity" occasionally seen following reconstructive surgery. If enough local tissue is not available to cover the implant chosen, a tissue expander may first be placed. The tissue expander is serially inflated during office visits to create enough soft tissue coverage to accommodate the appropriate permanent implant, which is placed at a second operation.

When local tissue is not available or not preferred, distant tissue can be used. In the past, the most common source of soft tissue was the lower abdominal wall, or transverse rectus abdominis myocutaneous **(TRAM) flap** (Figure 22-46). A transverse paddle of skin and fat from just above the umbilicus down to the pubic hairline can be elevated and supported by the deep superior epigastric vessels that lie within the rectus abdominis muscle. By maintaining the attachment to one or both rectus abdominis muscles, the tissue can be transferred to the chest to create a breast mound. This procedure not only provides the best breast reconstruction aesthetically but also improves the donor site by providing an abdominal lipectomy. Back skin and fat transferred with the underlying latissimus dorsi, supported by the thoracodorsal vessels, may also be used. This flap is exceedingly reliable and can be used when other

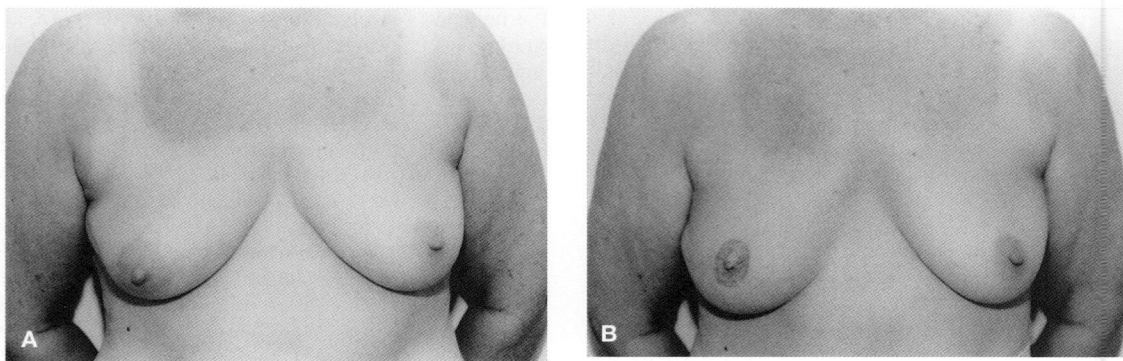

Figure 22-46. A. A woman with biopsy-proven carcinoma of the right breast before mastectomy. B. The result after skin-sparing mastectomy and immediate breast reconstruction with a transverse rectus abdominis myocutaneous flap, followed by nipple and areolar reconstruction. (From Lawrence PF. *Essentials of Surgical Specialties*. 3rd ed. Lippincott Williams & Wilkins; 2007.)

options are unavailable. It is also used to salvage reconstructions by other methods when difficulties occur. A small breast implant can be placed beneath these flaps to provide the necessary breast mound projection. Free flaps are also used. A TRAM flap can be based on the deep or superficial inferior epigastric vessels and transferred as a free flap with only a small amount of underlying muscle. Newer complex microsurgical techniques allow transfer of this abdominal skin with no sacrifice of muscle. The deep inferior epigastric perforator (DIEP) flap has now become the most popular option for breast reconstruction. Unlike in TRAM flaps, the abdominal skin and subcutaneous fat are taken without sacrificing the rectus abdominis muscles or rectus sheath fascia. Therefore, the DIEP flap is associated with less postsurgical abdominal wall weakness and a lower chance of abdominal wall hernia development compared with the TRAM flap. Other popular alternative microsurgical flaps include transverse upper gracilis (TUG), superior gluteal artery perforator (SGAP), and superficial inferior epigastric artery (SIEA).

When the abovementioned reconstruction options are not available, such as in a patient with a thin abdomen, a history of previous abdominal surgeries, or a plan for future pregnancy, other donor sites can be used. These include the back, the buttocks, and the thigh. For example, the latissimus dorsi myocutaneous flap is commonly used because of its consistent pedicle anatomy and large vessel diameters. Transposition of this flap to the chest provides excellent coverage of mastectomy defects. A tissue expander or an implant can be used with the flap to add more volume. Free flaps with gluteal arteries are also reliable alternatives to soft tissue from the abdomen. Either the SGAP or the inferior gluteal artery perforator can provide a thick fasciocutaneous flap that is adequate for breast reconstruction. The medial thigh region can also be used as a soft tissue donor site. For example, the TUG, diagonal upper gracilis, and transverse musculocutaneous gracilis have been demonstrated as reliable breast reconstruction options.

Reconstruction of the nipple and areola, which completes breast reconstruction, is chosen by many patients. The nipple is created by a flap of local tissue folded on itself to give adequate projection or by a free graft from the contralateral nipple, if it is quite large. The areola can then be mimicked by intradermal tattooing to match the color of the normal areola or by a full-thickness graft of the contralateral areola if a breast lift (**mastopexy**) is being performed. The risk of transferring potential cancer cell should be considered with this technique, however. Full-thickness skin grafts from the groin or upper inner thigh can also be used for areolar reconstruction.

Lower Extremity Reconstruction

The soft tissues of the leg often require reconstruction of defects caused by trauma, vascular disease, or diabetes. Trauma is the most common cause for reconstruction. High-energy blunt trauma (eg, motor vehicle accident, crush injury, fall) is the most complex to repair. Wounds can involve the skin, bone, and vasculature of the leg. Loss of soft tissue causes exposure of fracture sites, orthopedic hardware, or vascular reconstruction, allowing infection. The infection can cause loss of fixation, disruption of vascular anastomoses, or osteomyelitis. Compartment syndrome can occur as a complication from lower extremity trauma. This typically presents with the six Ps (pain out of proportion, pressure, paresthesia, paralysis, pallor, and pulselessness). Any of these complications may cause loss of the extremity.

Trauma

Because of the complex nature of traumatic wounds, a team approach that involves trauma, vascular, orthopedic, and plastic surgeons is used. The first priority is survival of the patient. Next, the viability of the leg must be ensured, with vascular reconstruction undertaken as necessary. Bony fixation or stabilization is achieved to ensure adequate limb length, proper orientation, and a stable skeletal platform for soft tissue reconstruction. Afterward, all efforts are directed at achieving adequate soft tissue coverage of open wounds and exposed fracture sites. Open fractures of the leg present the most challenging reconstruction problems. Some wounds can be managed with skin grafts, skin flaps, or fasciocutaneous flaps, but muscle flaps are usually required. These flaps can cover large areas of exposed bone, obliterate dead space, and provide a rich vascular coverage of exposed fracture sites to aid in bone healing.

In terms of available muscle coverage, the leg is divided into proximal, middle, and distal thirds. Wounds of the proximal third are usually reconstructed with the medial or lateral gastrocnemius muscles, usually covered by a skin graft. Likewise, the middle third of the leg is the domain of the soleus muscle flap. Because of the lack of local muscle flaps in the distal third of the leg, free muscle transfers are usually required (see Figure 22-15). Free flaps may also be required for more proximal reconstruction when local muscles are unusable because of trauma.

Systemic Disease

When systemic disease causes defects (usually ulcers) in the soft tissues of the leg, the underlying disease must first be treated. Ischemic limbs should be revascularized. When venous or lymphatic insufficiency is the underlying cause, patients should be put to bed with their extremities elevated. In addition to treatment of the underlying disease, infection should be treated and appropriate wound care administered. Wounds that result from these diseases can usually be reconstructed with skin grafts. Prolonged bed rest, elevation, and, occasionally, adjuncts (eg, hyperbaric oxygen, pharmacologic agents, growth factors) are necessary. In other cases, more complex reconstructive methods are needed.

Pressure Sore Reconstruction

Pressure sores are caused by irreversible tissue damage that occurs if a patient—because of paralysis and insensitivity, debilitation, or disease—lies in a given position for more than 2 hours. Traditionally, the pressure required to induce these changes over this time frame is 30 mm Hg. Patients with spinal cord injuries are the most susceptible because of their insensibility in areas of pressure. These patients cannot feel pain caused by the evolving pressure-related wound or injury. Pressure sores can develop in any location, but they usually develop over a bony prominence. They are most commonly located in the regions of the ischial tuberosities, sacrum, and trochanter. Less commonly, they are found at the elbows, heels, and occiput. The muscle and subcutaneous tissues are most susceptible to pressure damage and are closest to the bony prominences. Most sores are larger at their base than at their visible surface, assuming the shape of an inverted cone.

Pressure sores are graded by severity: Grade 1 has skin redness only; grade 2 involves the skin and subcutaneous tissue; grade 3 involves the skin, subcutaneous tissue, and muscle; and grade 4 involves the skin, subcutaneous tissue, muscle, and bone.

Pressure sores add significant cost and complexity to patient care. Obviously, prevention is the best treatment. Patients who cannot turn themselves require frequent repositioning. Alternatively, patients at risk can be placed on a fluidized air bed, which distributes pressure evenly throughout the body.

Once a pressure sore forms, treatment is directed at caring for the wound and placing the patient on a fluidized air bed to prevent further pressure-related damage. After the wound is debrided and is sufficiently clean, reconstruction is considered. The best candidates for reconstruction are those who are alert and cooperative enough to prevent the recurrence of pressure sores, as well as having a support and rehabilitation system in place following surgery, along with nutritional maximization preoperatively. Patients who are likely to have pressure sores immediately after treatment should be managed with wound care alone. Likewise, patients who have malnutrition or other major systemic illnesses should have these problems addressed before they are considered for reconstruction. Operative treatment is directed at total excision of the ulcer, removal of the underlying bony prominence, and coverage with healthy tissue. Although many sores can be covered with local skin flaps, muscle flaps are of great benefit and are most often used (Figure 22-47).

In patients with spinal cord injuries, virtually any muscle or myocutaneous flap may be used for soft tissue coverage. Commonly used muscles include the gluteus maximus, gracilis, tensor fasciae latae, and hamstrings. However, in ambulatory patients, many of these muscles are needed for ambulation and their function cannot be sacrificed. In addition, because pressure sores may be a chronic problem, when possible, flaps should be designed to allow their reuse if another pressure sore develops.

Abdominal Wall Reconstruction

Goals of abdominal wall reconstruction should be stable and secure protection of the abdominal viscera and prevention of recurrent herniation. When planning reconstruction, the size, location, and nature of the defects and other

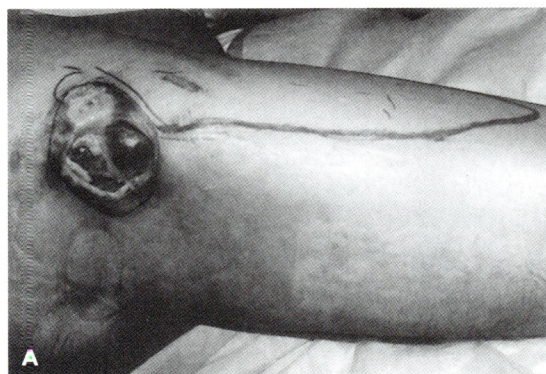

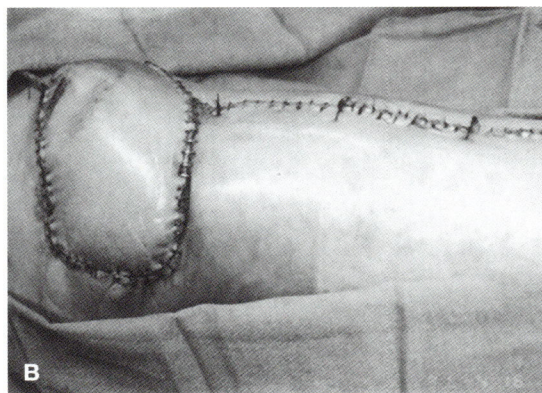

Figure 22-47. A. A paraplegic patient with a trochanteric pressure sore. B. The sore is closed with a tensor fasciae latae myocutaneous flap. (From Lawrence PF. *Essentials of Surgical Specialties*. 3rd ed. Lippincott Williams & Wilkins; 2007.)

conditions such as fistulas, adhesion, intra-abdominal sepsis, or hemorrhage should be considered. Reconstruction after tumor resection or uncomplicated hernia repair can be performed immediately. However, delayed reconstruction is warranted with patient instability or any active intra-abdominal issue, such as infection.

Partial abdominal wall defects, in which there is loss of skin and subcutaneous tissue with an intact myofascia, can be corrected with skin grafts or local tissue mobilization and advancement. For fascial defects, prosthetic mesh (eg, polypropylene, expanded polytetrafluoroethylene), fascia lata, or ADM (eg, Alloderm, Strattice, FlexHD, SurgiMend) can be used to securely cover the defects. ADM mesh has become a popular option because it is readily available, covers large defects, and can be placed in contaminated wounds. Mesh can be placed in different layers of the abdominal wall. The onlay technique places the mesh between the subcutaneous tissue and the anterior rectus sheath. The inlay technique places the mesh between the fascial edges of the rectus muscles. These two techniques have been reported with higher recurrence rates. On the contrary, the underlay technique, in which the mesh is placed below the fascial layers, has been reported with lower recurrence rates.

When direct closure of midline abdominal defect with minimal tension is not feasible, component separation with or without mesh can be performed. Ramirez first popularized component separation in the 1990s. In this method, the external oblique aponeurosis is incised vertically, lateral to the linea semilunaris. The plane between the internal and external oblique muscles is dissected, leading to the separation of the two muscles. This also allows medialization of the rectus abdominis muscle, and up to 10 cm of medial advancement of each flap becomes possible.

Perineal Reconstruction

Deformities of the perineal regions often result from malignancy and its resection. Resection often involves vulva, vagina, penis, anus, rectum, and surrounding soft tissues. The majority of these patients with cancer are also treated with adjuvant radiation therapy, which makes reconstruction even more challenging. However, multiple pedicled flaps from the region can be utilized for effective reconstruction. Commonly used flaps are the vertical rectus abdominis myocutaneous flap, the gracilis muscle flap, the pudendal flap (or Singapore flap), and the thigh flap. Perineal reconstruction faces unique postoperative issues. First, infection and wound breakdown are common because of the high bacterial count in the area. The reconstructed areas are also subject to significant pressure in both recumbent and sitting positions, which may lead to pressure ischemia and subsequent flap necrosis.

Head and Neck Reconstruction

Malignancy involving the head and neck, often intraoral squamous cell carcinoma, is by far the most common disease for which tissue reconstruction in that area may be needed. Trauma and other diseases also produce defects that require reconstruction of the skin of the head and neck, of the intraoral mucosal lining, or of the bone (usually the mandible). In cancer resection, reconstruction is usually performed at the time of tumor ablation. A number of axial-pattern skin flaps and myocutaneous flaps are useful in reconstructing some defects. The most common is the pectoralis major myocutaneous flap (Figure 22-48). Because it is based on the thoracoacromial vessels, the flap can be elevated and tunneled through the neck for use in many areas of the head. Other myocutaneous flaps are

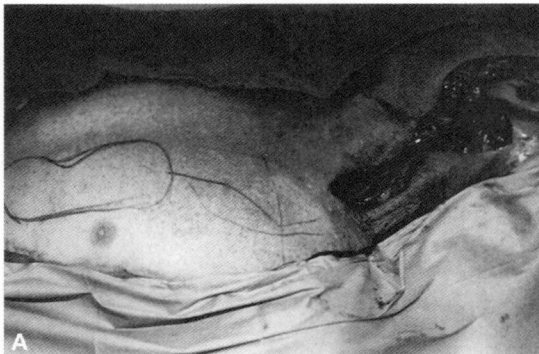

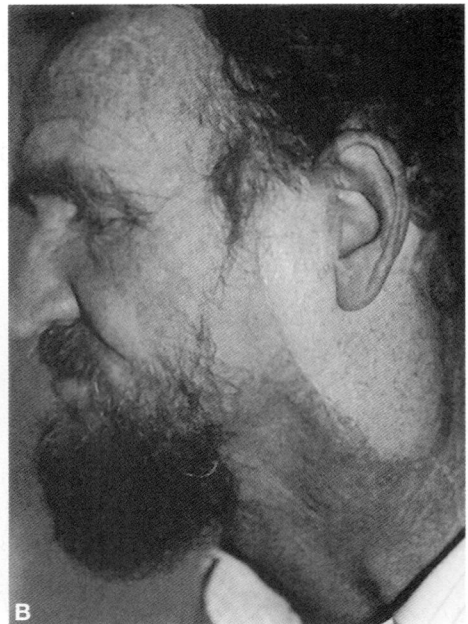

Figure 22-48. A. Radical resection for recurrent squamous cell carcinoma of the cheek and underlying parotid gland. B. After reconstruction with a pectoralis major myocutaneous flap. (From Lawrence PF. *Essentials of Surgical Specialties*. 3rd ed. Lippincott Williams & Wilkins; 2007.)

also used (eg, latissimus dorsi, trapezius). Free flaps can also provide excellent reconstruction. Osteocutaneous free flaps, or free flaps that include bone (eg, radial forearm flap with a portion of the underlying radius, iliac flap with a portion of the underlying iliac crest), may be used when mandibular reconstruction is desired.

AESTHETIC SURGERY

Aesthetic surgery involves improving the form of a normal structure. All aesthetic surgery is considered elective and should be undertaken only under optimal conditions and with the patient's clear understanding of all aspects of the surgery and recovery. Because these operations are directed at correcting perceived abnormalities, extensive preoperative consultation is required to understand such perceptions and how surgery will affect them. Aesthetic surgery is broadly divided into body-contouring surgery and surgery of the aging face. Some operations are performed for either aesthetic or reconstructive purposes (eg, **rhinoplasty** can be performed to improve the nasal profile or to correct a nasal deformity caused by trauma).

Body-Contouring Surgery

Surgery of the Breast

Surgery of the breast involves changing both the shape and size of the breast. It includes **reduction mammaplasty**, **augmentation mammaplasty**, and **mastopexy**.

Operations aimed primarily at reducing the size of the breast (reduction mammaplasty) are reconstructive. Excessively large breasts create both physical and psychological problems. Physical problems include neck and back pain, posture-related problems, grooves in the shoulders created by bra straps, numbness of the arms, and skin problems within the inframammary fold. Psychological problems occur in adolescents who are teased by their peers for having ample breasts at a young age. The goal of reduction mammaplasty is to reduce the size of the breast, elevate the nipple position, and preserve the blood supply to the nipple-areola complex (Figure 22-49). Most of these operations leave the nipple-areola complex attached to a pedicle of underlying breast tissue from which it receives its blood supply. These procedures are described by the orientation of the pedicle (eg, inferior pedicle, superior pedicle,

central pedicle). The correct nipple location must be chosen immediately preoperatively with the patient upright. At this time, all skin markings for the reduction are made.

Breasts that are considered too small can be enlarged through breast augmentation (augmentation mammaplasty). Breast implants are placed either directly beneath the breast tissue (subglandular) or beneath the pectoralis major (subpectoral or submuscular) by various approaches in skin incisions. Implants that are currently in use are constructed of an outer silicone shell filled with either silicone or saline. A round shape implant is most commonly used in the United States. The most recent generation of silicone implant is made of cohesive silicone gel and is form-stable, which offers a more natural breast shape. Implant leak or rupture is rare but is best evaluated by magnetic resonance imaging (MRI) or high-resolution ultrasound. The most common problem with implants is breast firmness, which can result from excessive scar tissue or from a capsule that normally forms around all implants. Capsular contractures cause symptoms in 15% to 20% of patients, and a few may require reoperation.

When breast size is adequate but shape is inadequate because of ptosis or sagging caused by pregnancy, aging, or weight loss, then a mastopexy, or breast lift, may be done. The nipple position is elevated by an appropriate skin excision. In some patients, breast augmentation is combined with mastopexy.

Breast implant–associated (BIA) capsular malignancies such as anaplastic large cell lymphoma (ALCL) and squamous cell carcinoma have been diagnosed with increasing incidence. BIA-ALCL is a rare type of CD30-positive peripheral T-cell lymphoma that develops around breast implants. The most common symptom of BIA-ALCL is a late-onset seroma. Therefore, patients who present with periprosthetic seromas at least 1 year after implantation should be screened for BIA-ALCL using CD30 immunohistochemistry and flow cytometry. The pathophysiology of this disease is largely unknown. However, recent studies have found that the incidence of BIA-ALCL is higher in patients with textured implants as opposed to those with smooth implants. BIA-ALCL follows an indolent course, and its prognosis is excellent, especially in patients who are diagnosed in the early stages of the disease. A rare form of squamous cell carcinoma has also been associated with the breast implant capsules.

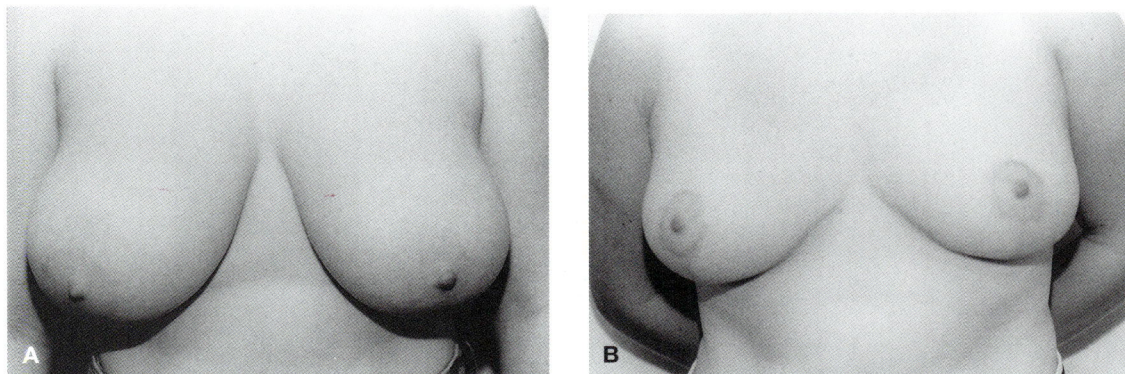

Figure 22-49. A. Mammary hyperplasia. B. After bilateral reduction mammaplasty. (From Lawrence PF. Essen*tials of Surgical Specialties*. 3rd ed. Lippincott Williams & Wilkins; 2007.)

Abdominoplasty

Reshaping the abdominal wall usually involves the excision of abdominal skin and fat (abdominoplasty) and the repair or tightening of the rectus abdominis muscle (repair of rectus diastasis). The latter is considered reconstructive in women because it addresses abnormalities of the abdominal wall that result from pregnancy and childbearing and the resultant symptoms of back pain and inadequate abdominal support. Although a low abdominal incision is most commonly used, a vertical orientation or another orientation may be required if previous surgical scars are present. In general, the goal of skin excision is to remove the skin between the umbilicus and the pubic hair region. The abdominal skin and fat are elevated from the underlying musculature (from the pubic region up to the costal margin), the abdominal wall muscles are invaginated, the laxity is removed by sutures, and the excess skin is removed. The umbilicus is left attached to the underlying abdominal wall and is repositioned after skin excision (Figure 22-50).

Suction-Assisted Lipectomy

Suction-assisted lipectomy is directed at the removal of fat collections that are out of proportion to the patient's normal subcutaneous fat distribution. These procedures are not for patients who are obese, nor are they designed for weight reduction. Rather, they are performed on patients who are close to their ideal weight. In women, the lateral hips, thighs (saddlebags), legs, and abdomen are most commonly treated. In men, the hip rolls (love handles) and abdomen are often suctioned.

Through small incisions, suction cannulae are introduced. When connected to two atmospheres of suction, the normally solid fat can be aspirated as a semisolid material. Ultrasound, power, or water assistance can be used to aid in the removal of the adipose tissue and to aid in suction lipectomy. Important technical considerations include appropriate fat removal, preservation of a normal subcutaneous fat layer, and prolonged postoperative compression (6-8 weeks).

Surgery of the Aging Face

The effects of aging are often seen in the skin and underlying tissue of the face, including the eyelids, forehead, and neck. These changes are produced by a combination of factors, including gravity, atrophy or thinning of the skin, and sun damage. Although these processes are most evident in the skin, the underlying fat and musculature of the skin and neck are also affected. The signs of aging are predominantly sagging (ptotic) skin, wrinkles, and herniation of the underlying fat. The age at which these changes appear is variable. Some individuals in their 30s benefit from surgical correction of the aging process, particularly if they have a hereditary predisposition to early signs of aging or if they have had excessive sun damage. Most patients seek such surgery in the fifth, sixth, or seventh decade of life.

Facelift

A facelift, or **cervicofacial rhytidectomy**, is directed at correcting the effects of aging, generally below the level of the eyes and including the neck. Areas that are most affected include the nasolabial folds, jawline (jowls), and neck. In this procedure, the skin of the face and neck is lifted from the underlying skin and facial musculature to a variable degree through an incision placed in front of, beneath, and behind the ear, and within the hairline. A small submental incision is also used. Usually, a deeper layer of facial muscle and platysma is also dissected. During the operation, this deeper layer (the superficial musculoaponeurotic system) is tightened, excess fat from the neck is removed, and the excessive skin is resected (Figure 22-51). The most feared complication is injury to the branches of the facial nerve that run beneath the superficial musculoaponeurotic system. Other complications include bleeding and skin slough, seen mostly in cigarette smokers.

Blepharoplasty

Recontouring of the eyelids is achieved with **blepharoplasty** because these structures are changed very little by

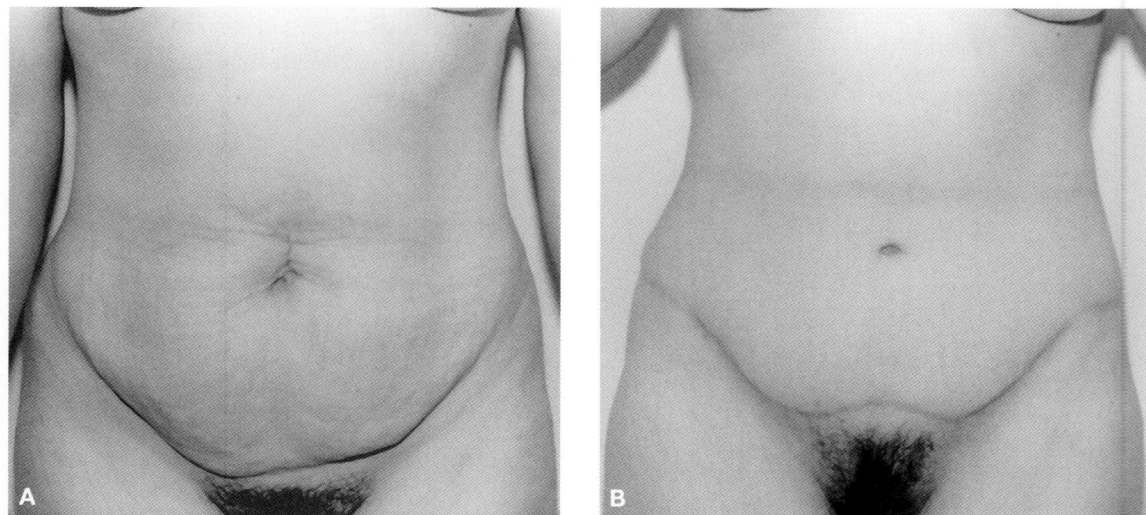

Figure 22-50. A. After her childbearing years, this patient underwent abdominoplasty. B. Six months after surgery. (From Lawrence PF. *Essentials of Surgical Specialties.* 3rd ed. Lippincott Williams & Wilkins; 2007.)

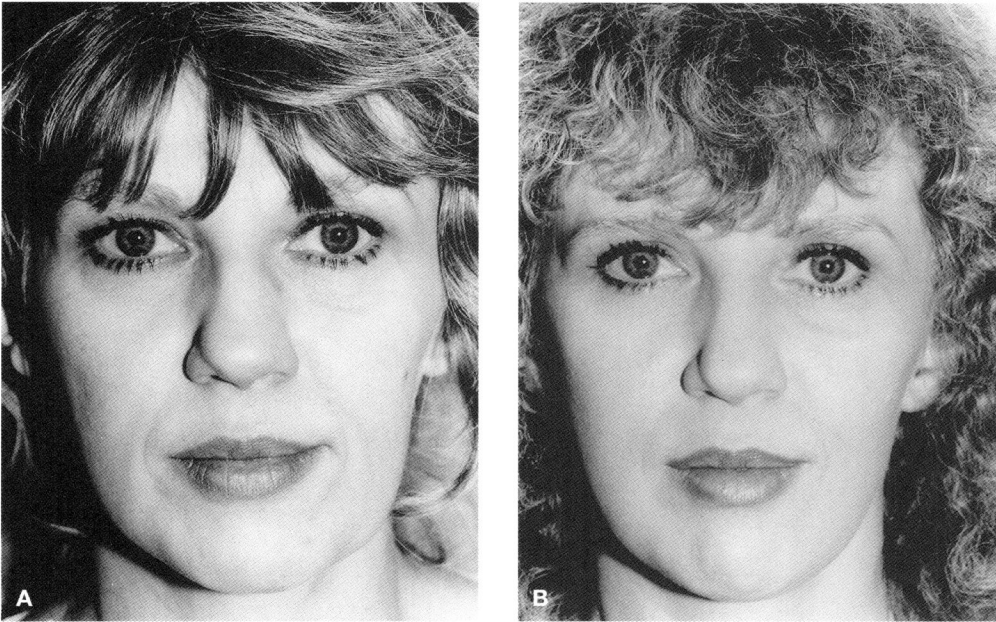

Figure 22-51. A. Before upper and lower lid blepharoplasty. B. After surgery. (From Lawrence PF. *Essentials of Surgical Specialties.* 3rd ed. Lippincott Williams & Wilkins; 2007.)

a facelift (Figure 22-51). This procedure removes excess skin from both the upper and lower eyelids. Fat pockets within the eyelids tend to become much more pronounced with age. Fat pockets in the lower eyelids give the impression of "bags" beneath the eyes. Some patients have a strong family predisposition to lower lid fat pockets and benefit from a lower lid blepharoplasty at a young age.

For an upper lid blepharoplasty, the incision is placed within the normal eyelid crease above the eye. In the lower eyelids, the incision is placed just beneath the eyelashes. Through these incisions, fat from the pockets is appropriately resected, and excess skin and muscle (orbicularis oculi) are removed. Newer concepts allow fat repositioning to obtain a more youthful appearance. Major complications result from bleeding or excess skin removal.

Laser-Assisted Skin Resurfacing

Laser resurfacing was first introduced in the 1980s. Since then, a variety of lasers have been developed to achieve the desired outcome while minimizing side effects. They range from ablative and nonablative laser technology to light-based devices. What laser is used depends on the indication, which includes skin resurfacing, treatment of hyperpigmentation, scars, and vascular lesions. Some contraindications include a history of scleroderma, systemic lupus erythematosus (SLE), keloids, skin hypersensitivity, or hypertrophic scarring. As with all devices, there are risks/complications associated with lasers, including hypertrophic scarring, hypopigmentation, and skin infections. All in all, most laser devices have a good safety profile and when used correctly can achieve desirable outcomes in a noninvasive manner.

The carbon dioxide laser has been an important tool for the removal of fine lines and wrinkles from the face, with or without incisions to remove excess skin. The target of this laser is water within the skin. As the laser is applied to an area of skin, the superficial layers are vaporized because the water molecules absorb the energy from the laser beam. As these areas heal, the skin appears tauter and has fewer wrinkles. The development of a computed pattern generator attached to the handpiece of a CO_2 laser allows a grid of laser points to be set down in a single burst and allows the use of this technology for resurfacing of the entire face, segmental resurfacing of specific areas of the face, and blepharoplasty. Other ablative (surface-removing) lasers, such as the erbium YAG and nonablative (surface-retaining) techniques can be used to tighten skin and treat other skin lesions. Intense pulsed light (IPL) and broadband light (BBL) are wavelengths of light ranging from 500 to 1,200 nm and treat a variety of vascular and pigmented lesions of the skin. These are not lasers (single coherent wavelength). Nonablative laser techniques such as a diode laser do not induce epidermal vaporization; therefore, recovery is faster. Lasers are also used for tattoo and vascular lesion removal.

Rhinoplasty

Patients seek changes in the shape of the nose because of trauma or a desire to improve the normal nasal profile. In cases of trauma, the operation is considered reconstructive (Figure 22-52). In other cases, the correction is considered aesthetic. In both cases, the rhinoplasty is performed in much the same way. Although this complex operation is being performed, attention must be given to the nasal airway. When this airway is obstructed, surgery on the nasal septum, nasal value, or turbinates may be needed.

Through incisions that are usually placed within the nose, the nasal cartilage and bones are exposed. They are reshaped to give a better profile. Common areas of patient concern are a broad nasal bridge, a dorsal hump, or a bulbous nasal

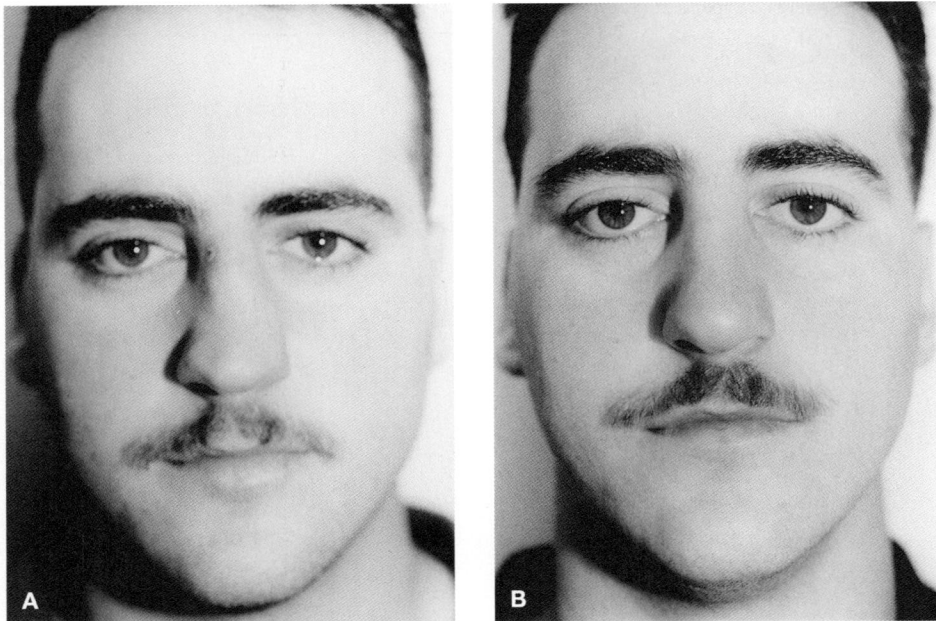

Figure 22-52. A. A young man with a posttraumatic nasal deformity. B. After reconstructive rhinoplasty. (From Lawrence PF. *Essentials of Surgical Specialties*. 3rd ed. Lippincott Williams & Wilkins; 2007.)

tip. Because the nasal bones are usually cut, postoperative support is required with a splint and nasal packs.

Chemical Peels

Chemical peels induce regeneration of skin by the controlled creation of a partial-thickness injury. Superficial peels penetrate into the epidermal-dermal junction and help correct mild dyschromia, melasma, and keratosis. Jessner solution (a mix of resorcinol, salicylic acid, and lactic acid in 95% ethanol), salicylic acid, and α hydroxy acid are commonly used. Twenty percent to thirty percent trichloroacetic acid (TCA) peels are commonly utilized for medium-depth peels. TCA penetrates the papillary and upper reticular dermis and thus corrects superficial rhytids. Phenol (carbolic acid)-croton oil peels penetrate into the upper to mid-reticular dermis and treat both fine and coarse rhytids and irregular pigmentation. Both hypo- and hyperpigmentation can occur as side effects from chemical peels.

Neurotoxin

Botulinum toxin injection is the most commonly performed cosmetic procedure in the United States. Botulinum toxin A is an exotoxin derived from the bacterium *Clostridium botulinum*. This toxin targets the SNAP/SNARE docking protein in the presynaptic nerve and inhibits the release of acetylcholine. Consequently, this weakens the action of postsynaptic musculature and thus smooths wrinkles. Its effect lasts for 3 to 6 months with minimal complications. Botox (Allergan, Irvine, CA) was the first agent approved by the FDA for forehead lines, crow's feet lines, and glabellar lines. Dysport® (Medicis Aesthetics, Scottsdale, AZ), Xeomin (Merz Pharmaceuticals, Greensboro, NC), Jeaveau (Evolus, Newport Beach, CA), and Daxxify (Revance Therapeutics, Nashville, TN) are also approved by the FDA for glabellar rhytids. Their

uses, however, expanded beyond FDA-approved purposes. Botulinum toxin injection is contraindicated for patients with neuromuscular disorders, such as myasthenia gravis or Lambert-Eaton syndrome.

Soft Tissue Fillers

Injectable fillers are a popular method for soft tissue volume restoration. Both biologic and synthetic fillers and autologous fat are widely used. In fact, injection of soft tissue filler is currently ranked as the second most frequently performed rejuvenation procedure following botulinum toxin injection. Autologous fat injection is commonly used to restore subcutaneous volume in the various parts of the body, including areas of depressed scars, radiation damage, chronic ulcers, congenital deformities such as pectus excavatum, and other soft tissue defects. In autologous fat injection, immunogenicity, allergic response, and toxicity are not concerns. Achieving satisfying results, however, depends on several variables, such as harvest methods, the types of fat, and the skills of injectors. The longevity of results can also be unpredictable. Synthetic biodegradable materials, such as hyaluronic acid, calcium hydroxyapatite, and poly-L-lactic acid, are widely used as filler agents. Hyaluronic acid fillers (eg, Juvederm Voluma, Restylane, Belotero Balance) have become the most popular filler materials because of ease of use, natural results, and relatively low complication rates. Hyaluronic acid is a type of GAG that naturally exists in human tissue and, therefore, has no immunogenicity. It will create volume for 4 to 12 months before eventually degrading.

Calcium hydroxyapatite is synthetically created with calcium and phosphate ions and is identical to the mineral portion of the bone. This was initially used for oral maxillary defects and vocal cord insufficiency. Radiesse (Merz Aesthetics, Raleigh, NC) is made of calcium hydroxyapatite microspheres suspended in an aqueous carrier gel. The FDA approved its use for the correction of moderate-to-severe facial folds and rhytids and for the correction of human immunodeficiency virus (HIV)-associated lipoatrophy in 2006. The volume typically lasts from 9 to 18 months as the microspheres are slowly degraded into calcium and phosphate ions and cleared from the body. Poly-L-lactic acid (Sculptra, Galderma, SA) is a synthetic, biodegradable polymer derived from the α-hydroxy acid family. It is currently approved by the FDA for mid-to-deep facial rhytids and folds and for volume augmentation for HIV lipoatrophy. Microparticles of poly-L-lactic acid are degraded by hydrolysis and replaced by collagen. The effect typically lasts for 2 years.

SUGGESTED READINGS

Althubaiti G, Butler CE. Abdominal wall and chest wall reconstruction. *Plast Reconstr Surg*. 2014;133(5):688e-701e.

Carruthers J, Carruthers A, Humphrey S. Introduction to fillers. *Plast Reconstr Surg*. 2015;136(5 Suppl):120S-131S.

Curtis W, Horswell BB. Panfacial fractures: an approach to management. *Oral Maxillofac Surg Clin North Am*. 2013;25(4):649-660.

Silverstein MJ, Mai T, Savalia N, Vaince F, Guerra L. Oncoplastic breast conservation surgery: the new paradigm. *J Surg Oncol*. 2014;110(1):82-89.

Sosin M, Devulapalli C, Fehring C, et al. Breast cancer following augmentation mammaplasty: a case-control study. *Plast Reconstr Surg*. 2018;141(4):833-840.

SAMPLE QUESTIONS

QUESTIONS

Choose the best answer for each question.

1. The skin is the largest organ of the body and serves as the primary defense against the environment. The skin serves important functions in both homeostasis and thermoregulation. Several distinct layers make up the human skin. Which of the following statements best describes the structure of the human skin?

   A. Skin is divided into two embryologically distinct layers: the epidermis and the subcutaneous fatty layer.
   B. The pigment-containing melanocytes are located in the epidermis.
   C. The dermis contains the pilosebaceous apparatus and the eccrine and apocrine units.
   D. The dermis is 2 times thicker than the epidermis.
   E. The epidermis contains a rich vascular network and epidermal projections known as rete pegs that extend down into the underlying dermis.

2. A patient presents to the emergency department 10 days after an open appendectomy. The patient has mild pain, redness, and irritation at the operative site. The chief resident performs an incision and drainage of the wound. The abdominal wall fascia is noted to be completely intact. The wound is gently cleansed and sterile dressing applied. The attending surgeon and chief resident decide not to reclose the wound. Which statement regarding this type of wound healing is most accurate?

   A. Epithelialization from the wound margins proceeds at approximately 1 cm/d in a concentric pattern.
   B. Wound healing by secondary intention is characterized by a prolonged inflammatory phase that persists until the wound is covered with epithelium.
   C. Wound contraction rarely occurs in wounds that heal by secondary intention.
   D. Delayed primary closure or healing by tertiary intention involves resection of the previously healed scar.
   E. Open contaminated wounds are more likely to develop infections and, therefore, should be closed whenever possible.

3. A 79-year-old woman has a large squamous cell carcinoma of the right lower extremity. She will require a wide skin resection that will be approximately 6 × 6 cm in diameter. You are quite certain you will not be able to close this defect primarily. At your preoperative visit, you have informed the patient that you feel that a skin graft would be best to close the defect. Which of the following is the most appropriate statement about a skin graft?

   A. A split-thickness skin graft has greater primary contraction and less secondary contraction.
   B. A full-thickness skin graft has greater primary contraction and more secondary contraction because of the full complement of dermal appendages.
   C. Unlike a xenograft, an allograft is harvested from the same person it will be used on to repair the wound.
   D. An allograft (homograft) is typically harvested from one individual and transplanted to another individual of the same species.
   E. A split-thickness skin graft is typically harvested with a special instrument and contains only epidermis that may be "meshed" for greater surface area coverage.

4. A 56-year-old female comes into your office for evaluation of a raised brown lesion on the right cheek. The lesion has been present for several years;

however, she feels that the lesion is starting to increase in size. Which of the following is the most accurate statement about such a skin lesion?

A. Dysplastic nevi have the potential for malignant transformation and may have irregular borders and varying shades of pigmentation.

B. All nevi should be excised to rule out malignant transformation, regardless of size, shape, or color.

C. Actinic keratoses are usually "stuck on" in appearance, elevated, brown, and greasy feeling.

D. Hemangioma is the most common benign tumor of infancy and consists of an abnormal collection of blood vessels that rarely resolves on its own.

E. When excising a skin lesion, the incision should be oriented so that the long axis of the incision runs perpendicular to the lines of relaxed skin tension.

5. A 31-year-old male presents to your office stating that the side of his nail has been painful for several days. There is no drainage, and he denies fever or chills. Which of the following statements is most accurate?

A. This condition may be diagnosed by observing Kanavel four signs.

B. Lacerations of the hand from human bites should be closed tightly and often do not require antibiotics.

C. A paronychia is an infection of the lateral nail fold and usually presents as a small collection of purulent material at the side of the nail.

D. A felon is a purulent infection of the thenar eminence that is usually painful and may be drained by various methods.

E. Hand infections are usually self-limited and rarely need to result in functional deficits of the extremity.

ANSWERS AND EXPLANATIONS

1. Answer: C

The skin is the largest organ of the body. The epidermis is devoid of vasculature. The dermis is 15 to 40 times thicker than the epidermis. The dermis contains the pilosebaceous apparatus, eccrine and apocrine units, nerves, and organs such as Pacinian and Meissner corpuscles. For more information on this topic, see section "Skin Structure."

2. Answer: B

Healing by primary intention involves the suture closure of a clean wound. Healing by secondary intention is marked by a prolonged inflammatory phase; these wounds will heal as long as there is no marked infection or foreign body. Wound contraction greatly reduces the size of these wounds, and healing by secondary intention is indicated for severely contaminated or infected wounds. For more information on this topic, see section "Wound Healing."

3. Answer: D

Split-thickness skin grafts include the epidermis and a portion of the dermis. Full-thickness skin grafts typically have greater primary contraction because of their higher elastin fiber content but less secondary contracture, whereas split-thickness skin grafts undergo less primary contracture and greater secondary contracture. An allograft is harvested from one individual (usually a cadaver) and transplanted to another individual; it will eventually be rejected. For more information on this topic, see section "Skin Grafts."

4. Answer: A

The nevus is the most common lesion in the adult. Not all nevi need to be excised. Lesions should be excised if they have had a recent change in shape, elevation, or color. Seborrheic keratoses are benign, raised, waxy, "stuck-on" lesions. Actinic keratosis is typically rough and irregularly shaped and may be brown. Ninety percent of all hemangiomas involute by age 9. Skin excisions should run parallel to the lines of relaxed skin tension. For more information on this topic, see section "Types of Lesions" under the heading "Management of Benign Skin Lesions."

5. Answer: C

Tenosynovitis is a painful inflammation of the tendon sheath. Diagnosis is made by observing Kanavel four signs: the finger held in slight flexion, fusiform swelling, tenderness of the tendon sheath, and pain on passive extension. Human bites should never be closed. Patients are typically admitted and treated with IV antibiotics. A felon is a purulent infection of pad of the finger. Hand infections can be devastating if not treated promptly and can result in restricted motion. For more information on this topic, see section "Hand Surgery."

23

Cardiothoracic Surgery: Diseases of the Heart, Great Vessels, and Thoracic Cavity

Peyman Benharash, Constantine Poulos, and Kwame S. Amankwah

Cardiovascular diseases are the most common causes of significant morbidity and mortality in all sectors of the population. Enormous resources are consumed in treating these diseases, and it remains a major concern to patients, physicians, and policymakers alike. This chapter discusses cardiovascular system pathology, including ischemic heart disease, valvular diseases, acquired traumatic lesions, and aneurysmal degenerations.

DISEASES OF THE HEART

ANATOMY

The heart is a hollow, muscular organ that provides the physical force necessary to deliver oxygen-rich blood to the body and to return oxygen-poor blood to the lungs. The anatomy of the normal heart is well suited for this task because blood destined for the lungs is kept separate from blood destined for the periphery. The atria receive blood from the peripheral or central circulation and send it through one-way atrioventricular valves (tricuspid on the right; mitral on the left) into the primary pumping chambers or ventricles. The left ventricle, which delivers blood against systemic vascular resistance, is more muscular than the right ventricle, which delivers blood against the less-resistant pulmonary circuit. The heart is an end organ that receives its circulation from the epicardial coronary arteries that arise from the left and right sinuses of Valsalva, distal to the aortic valve. The left main coronary artery branches into the left anterior descending (LAD) coronary artery and the circumflex coronary artery. Each of these in turn may give off additional branches. The right coronary artery usually supplies the posterior descending coronary artery distally and a posterolateral branch (Figure 23-1). The blood supply to the sinus and atrioventricular nodes usually arises from the right coronary artery and often explains the occurrence of heart block in the presence of a right coronary occlusion or infarct.

As an end organ, the heart is affected by the same physiologic disturbances that affect peripheral organs. The ability of the heart to provide blood to the periphery may be adversely affected by any alteration in the normal anatomy of the heart (eg, defects of the atrial or ventricular septum, valvular incompetence or stenosis, and coronary artery obstruction).

PHYSIOLOGY: CARDIAC FUNCTION AND ITS ASSESSMENT

Physiologic manipulation of the circulation is essential for treating patients with cardiovascular disease. It should always be recognized that cardiac function can be clinically assessed with simple parameters (blood pressure, urine output, skin color and texture, mental status, and heart rate). Unfortunately, these measurements do not always reflect changes in cardiac function until deterioration has occurred, sometimes irreversibly. Earlier detection of myocardial dysfunction is possible with both noninvasive and invasive techniques that permit pharmacologic and mechanical intervention to halt deterioration.

A catheter can be placed via a central vein so that its tip lies within the thoracic cavity to monitor **central venous pressure** (CVP). The limitation of the CVP is that it does not directly measure the function of the left side of the heart. It measures the ability of the right side of the heart to deal with the volume load delivered by systemic veins and can be useful in detecting compromised left ventricular function (in patients who do not otherwise have heart disease). When there is intrinsic cardiac disease, the response of the left side of the heart will likely differ from that of the right side. Further, any clinical derangement that affects both the systemic volume and, indirectly, pulmonary vascular resistance may alter CVP without altering cardiac function. A single CVP measurement will probably overassess or underassess the dysfunction. A record of changes in CVP over time is more useful than an isolated measurement.

A flow-directed pulmonary artery catheter may be inserted into a large central vein and "floated" through the right heart and out into the pulmonary artery (Figures 23-2 and 23-3). This is usually done with a Swan-Ganz catheter, which can be used to measure CVP, pulmonary artery pressure, pulmonary capillary wedge pressure (PCWP), and cardiac output. When the balloon on the end of the catheter is inflated, the catheter can be wedged into a small pulmonary artery. The pressure measured in this position is called the PCWP. By the laws of hydraulics, this will reflect left atrial pressure, which, in the absence of mitral valve disease, reflects pressure in the left ventricle at the end of diastole when the mitral valve is open (left ventricular end-diastolic pressure [LVEDP]).

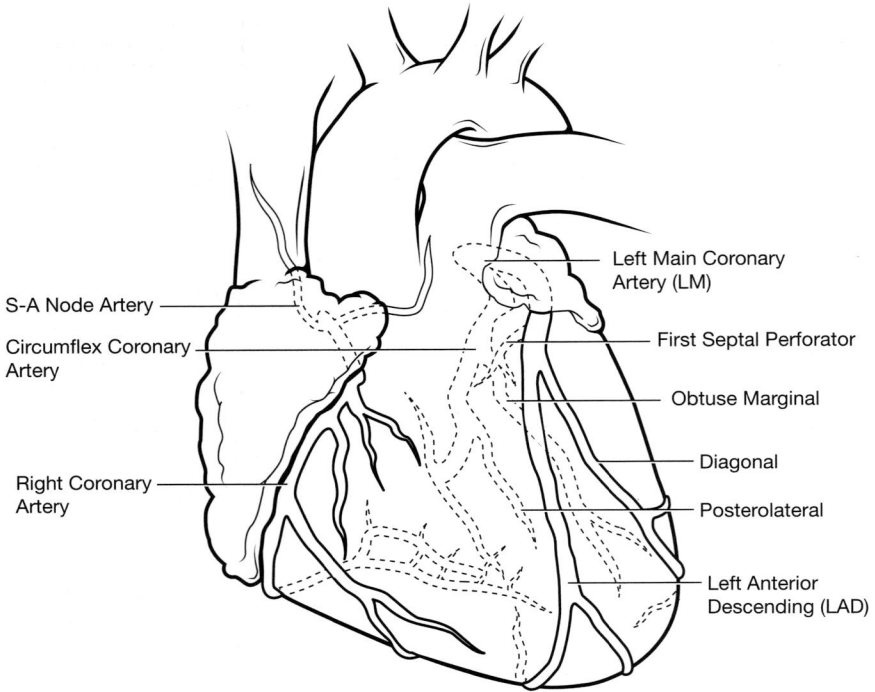

Figure 23-1. Diagram of heart and coronary arteries. S-A node, sinoatrial node. (From Lawrence PF. *Essentials of Surgical Specialties.* 3rd ed. Lippincott Williams & Wilkins; 2007.)

In turn, this pressure reflects the left ventricular end-diastolic volume component of cardiac output. According to Starling law, left ventricular muscle contractile force is proportional to myocardial fiber stretch: The greater the volume of blood within the ventricle is at the end of diastole, the greater the force of contraction and therefore of cardiac output. Because rapid and accurate bedside methods to measure end-diastolic volume are not readily available, measurements of LVEDP are used instead. LVEDP is used as a guide to the volume status, or filling pressure, of the heart. The translation of left ventricular end-diastolic volume into a clinically useful pressure measurement (LVEDP) assumes that compliance of the ventricle remains constant. However, that is not always the case. Certain clinical conditions that acutely alter left ventricular compliance (eg, left ventricular hypertrophy,

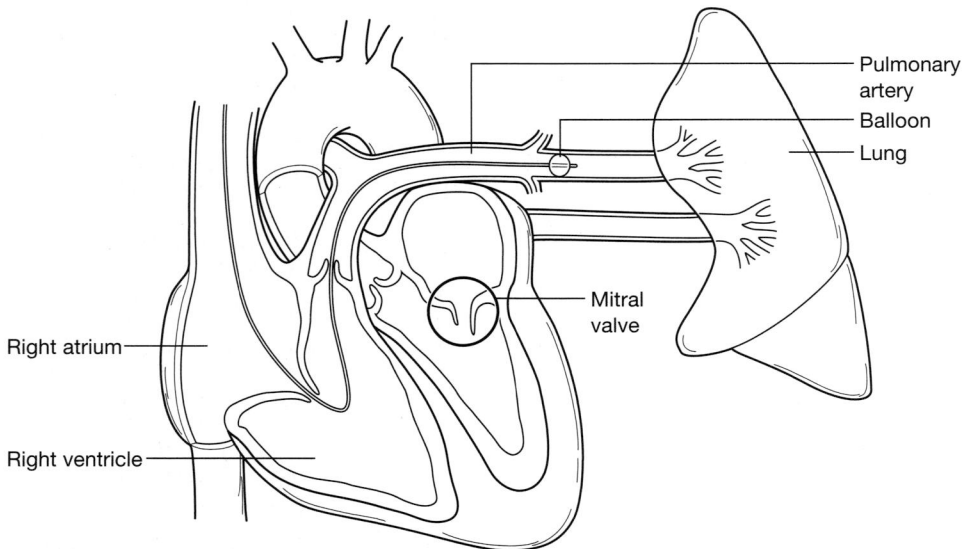

Figure 23-2. A flow-directed pulmonary artery catheter in place. (From Lawrence PF. *Essentials of Surgical Specialties.* 3rd ed. Lippincott Williams & Wilkins; 2007.)

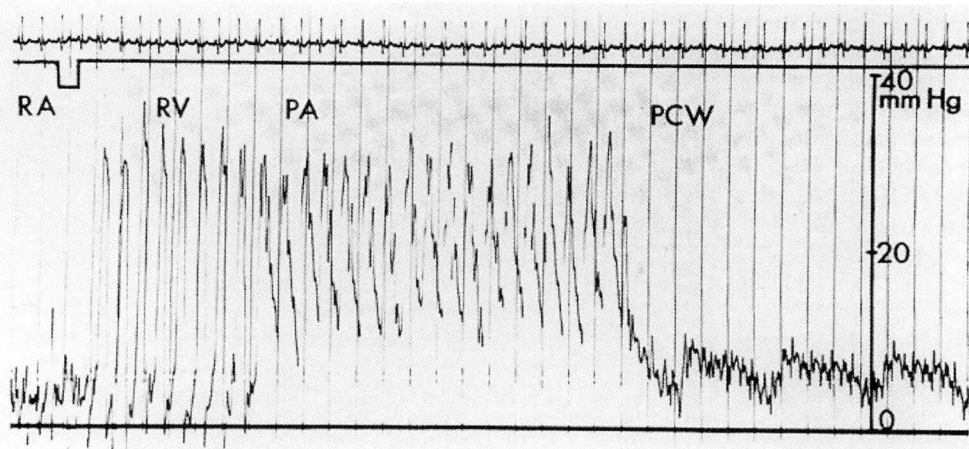

Figure 23-3. Tracing from a flow-directed pulmonary artery catheter. PA, pulmonary artery; PCW, pulmonary capillary wedge; RA, right atrium; RV, right ventricle. (From Lawrence PF. *Essentials of Surgical Specialties.* 3rd ed. Lippincott Williams & Wilkins; 2007.)

acute myocardial infarction) can change the relation between left ventricular end-diastolic volume and pressure.

Cardiac output can be measured using the Swan-Ganz catheter by means of thermodilution techniques that use a thermistor at the tip of the catheter. This calculation is combined with blood pressure, CVP, and PCWP to calculate resistance and assess cardiac function. Adding a fiberoptic system that can provide real time, online measurement of oxygen saturation in the pulmonary artery allows further discrimination in such assessment. The mixed venous oxygen saturation (SvO$_2$) reflects cardiac index and systemic oxygen delivery as long as hemoglobin levels and oxygen extraction (metabolic activity and work) are accounted for. A decrease in SvO$_2$ can be caused by a decrease in cardiac output, a decrease in hemoglobin levels, or an increase in the amount of oxygen extracted at the cellular level. Careful assessment is necessary to decide which variable is operational in any given patient. The mixed SvO$_2$, although affected by hemoglobin concentration, is a clinically useful tool for moment-to-moment assessment of cardiac function. Table 23-1 shows the basic formulas used to assess myocardial function based on measurements available in an intensive care unit.

When these types of invasive monitoring are available, it is easy to distinguish the etiology of hypotension and shock. A patient who is in hypovolemic shock may be diagnosed by clinical signs (trauma, hemorrhage, vomiting, diarrhea, and dehydration) and simple bedside measurements (assessment of mucous membranes, skin turgor, urine output, blood pressure, and pulse rate). However, when clinical indicators are equivocal, invasive measurements that show low pulmonary artery wedge pressure (PAWP), CVP, and cardiac index usually confirm a low circulating volume. Appropriate therapy is transfusion with blood products or balanced electrolyte solutions. Both clinical and invasive measurements are used to gauge patient response.

Usually, patients who have heart failure because of chronic conditions (eg, valvular heart disease) or acute problems (eg, acute myocardial infarction) have elevated PAWP because of inadequate myocardial pump function

and diminished cardiac index. However, the caution about the integration of myocardial compliance, wedge pressure, and cardiac index is often forgotten in the setting of acute cardiac dysfunction. For example, a patient who has an acute myocardial infarction, a cardiac index of 1.8 L/min/m^2, and a wedge pressure of 6 mm Hg is hypovolemic. The patient's edematous infarcted myocardium may require filling pressures greater than the "normal" wedge pressure of 12 to 15 mm Hg to stretch the myocardium sufficiently to generate adequate cardiac output. Conversely, another patient who has an acute myocardial infarction may have a cardiac index of 1.8 L/min/m^2 but a wedge pressure of 25 mm Hg. This patient is clearly in pulmonary edema and will benefit from a reduction in the filling pressures of the left ventricle to allow improved coronary perfusion of the critical areas of subendocardial myocardial muscle mass. According to Laplace law, wall tension is directly proportional to the radius of the heart chamber and the pressure within it. Therefore, a dilated left ventricle will have subendocardial perfusion deficits based on transmyocardial pressure gradients within the coronary circulation (especially during diastole, when most coronary perfusion occurs). Reducing the radius of the left ventricle with pulmonary vasodilators (eg, morphine, nitroglycerin), diuretics (eg, furosemide), or phlebotomy (actual or rotating tourniquets) will decrease wall tension and increase subendocardial perfusion and therefore improve overall cardiac function. When hypertension is present, afterload reduction is likewise helpful. Continued low cardiac output may require the use of inotropes, intra-aortic balloon, or emergency invasive intervention.

Vasodilatory shock can be associated with early sepsis or other causes leading to the lowering of systemic resistance. In this situation, hypotension may in fact be associated with a high cardiac output and normal or elevated filling pressures. Vasoconstrictive agents are indicated in this situation to maintain adequate pressure to perfuse the end organs.

The shock associated with cardiac tamponade can be very difficult to assess and can lead to a delay in treatment that may be fatal. In this situation, low blood pressure is

TABLE 23-1. Assessment of Myocardial Function

Function	Normal Values
Arterial blood pressure	120/80 mm Hg
Mean arterial pressure (MAP) $\dfrac{\text{Pulse pressure}}{3} + \text{Diastolic blood pressure}$	70-90 mm Hg
Heart rate	60-100 beats/min
Central venous pressure (CVP)	2-8 mm Hg
Pulmonary artery pressure (PAP)	10-25 mm Hg
Pulmonary wedge pressure (PWP)	6-12 mm Hg
Cardiac index (CI)	2.5-3.0 L/min/m^2
Systemic vascular resistance (SVR) $\dfrac{\text{MAP} - \text{CVP} \times 80}{\text{CO (cardiac output)}} + \text{Diastolic blood pressure}$	900-1,200 dyn/s/cm^{-5}
Peripheral vascular resistance (PVR) $\dfrac{\text{PAP(mean)} - \text{PWP} \times 80}{\text{CO}} + \text{Diastolic blood pressure}$	150-250 dyn/s/cm^{-5}
Stroke volume (SV) $\dfrac{\text{CO}}{\text{Heart rate}}$	60-70 mL/beat
Stroke index (SI) $\dfrac{\text{SV}}{\text{BSA (body surface area)}}$	35-45 mL/beat/m^2
Left ventricular stroke work index (LVSWI) SI × MAP × 0.014	51-61 g/min/m^2
Arterial O$_2$ content (CaO$_2$) = % saturation (hemoglobin) × 1.39 + 0.003 (PaO$_2$ [partial pressure of oxygen, arterial])	18-20 mol/dL
Arterial O$_2$ delivery (DO$_2$) = CI × CaO$_2$	550-600 mol/min/m^2
Mixed venous O$_2$ saturation (SvO$_2$)	55%-70%

associated with a low cardiac output, elevated filling pressure, and, usually, elevated systemic resistance. One of the hallmarks of tamponade is "equalization of pressures," that is, filling pressures on both sides of the heart tend to equalize, systemic pressure drops, pulmonary pressure rises, and pulse pressure may narrow. Treatment requires immediate relief of the tamponade by mechanical interventions such as pericardiocentesis or surgical drainage of the pericardium.

Although invasive monitoring devices provide valuable information, they can cause complications. Depending on the site of insertion, any central venous cannulation can cause hemorrhage and pneumothorax. In a critically ill patient whose condition is acutely deteriorating, proper insertion techniques must be used. The safest approach to introducing a pulmonary artery flotation catheter is a posterior-superior approach to the right internal jugular vein. In this approach, the introducer needle is never in contact with the lung. Lower jugular or subclavian approaches are more likely to cause pneumothorax. They are used especially cautiously in patients with blood dyscrasias and clotting abnormalities because direct pressure cannot be applied to the subclavian vein or the internal jugular vein beneath the clavicle. In these patients, a high cervical approach to the central veins or the temporary use of the femoral vein is recommended. Perforation of the pulmonary artery with massive **hemoptysis** may occur after the insertion of a pulmonary artery catheter. In addition, cardiac arrhythmias can occur when the catheter is passed through the right ventricle. Infectious endocarditis is also a potential problem, especially when the catheter is in place for more than 3 days.

Additional noninvasive means of assessing cardiac function include radionuclide scanning, echocardiography, and cardiac magnetic resonance imaging (MRI). Multiple gated acquisition (MUGA) scans show ejection fractions quite accurately and can therefore categorize cardiac function, but they are not easily performed at the bedside. Echocardiography and transesophageal echocardiography (TEE) can be performed at the bedside but must be interpreted by an experienced echocardiographer. Cardiac MRI is a newer method of cardiac evaluation and can be very accurate in the assessment of cardiac function but, again, is not available at the bedside. During surgical procedures, TEE can be used to continuously monitor cardiac volume, function, and wall motion.

CARDIOPULMONARY BYPASS AND MYOCARDIAL PROTECTION

The ability to perform surgery on the heart and great vessels depended on the development of a method to artificially support the circulation and respiration while, at the same time, preventing significant damage to the heart. This method of support is the heart-lung machine, which consists of multiple components, as shown in Figure 23-4. Either a roller pump or a centrifugal pump can substitute for the pump function of the heart to provide circulation of blood. Membrane oxygenators exchange

blood gases to take the place of pulmonary function. Temperature regulation is maintained by a heater-cooler, and blood lost in the operative field is returned to the machine by suction catheters. Filtering devices, sensors, and traps are present to prevent air and particulate embolization as debris infused into the arterial circulation may lead to stroke and other end-organ damage. Because blood comes into contact with the thrombogenic "foreign" surfaces of the heart-lung machine, systemic anticoagulation with heparin is used to prevent thrombosis. During cardiopulmonary bypass, blood is withdrawn from the venous circulation from the right atrium or the venae cavae. The venous blood collects in a reservoir, is pressurized via the pump, and subsequently passes through an oxygenator, where oxygen levels are replenished, and carbon dioxide is removed. The oxygenated blood is then reintroduced into the circulation through either the ascending aorta or a peripheral large artery. Varying degrees of hypothermia are used to decrease the metabolic demand of the body.

Most cardiac surgical procedures require temporarily stopping the heart using cardiopulmonary bypass. The goal is to provide a motionless and bloodless field for performing the operative procedure while preventing permanent damage to the heart muscle. The myocardial cells are protected by minimizing the metabolic demand of the heart while it is deprived of its normal circulation and oxygen supply. Recalling the determinants of oxygen demand (wall tension, heart rate, and contractility), this is

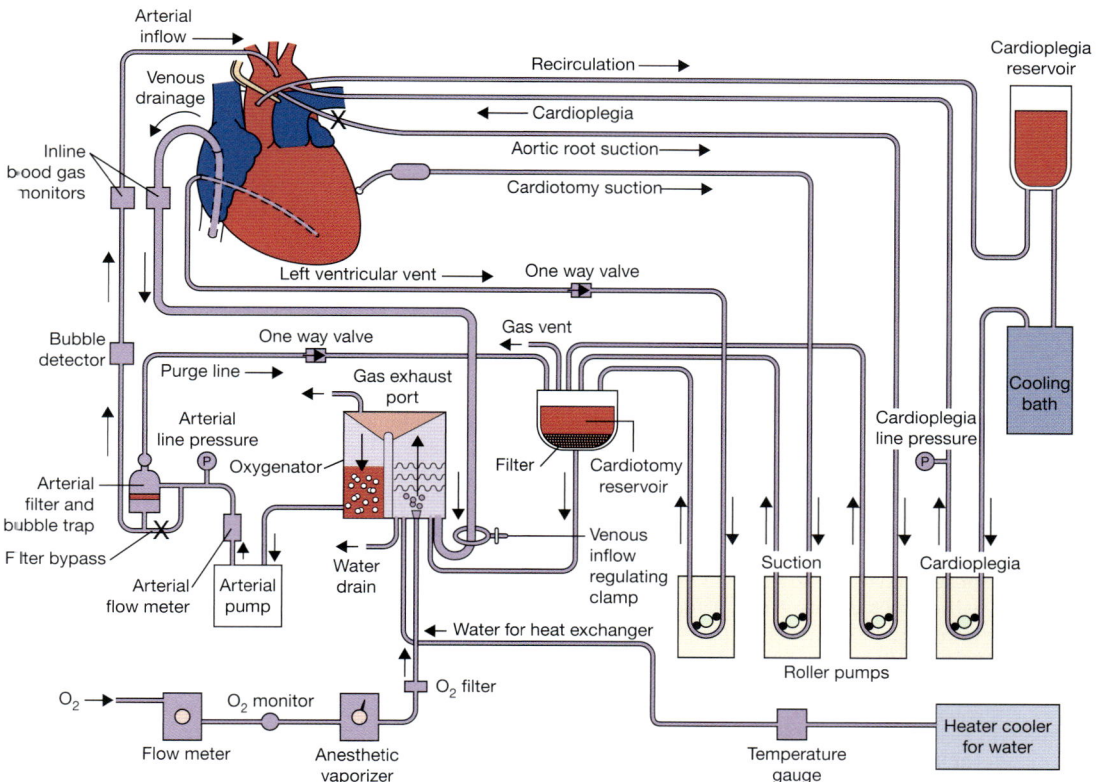

Figure 23-4. Extracorporeal cardiopulmonary bypass circuit. (Reprinted with permission from Morrison WE, McMillan KLN, Shaffner DH. *Rogers' Handbook of Pediatric Intensive Care.* 5th ed. Wolters Kluwer; 2017; Figure 56-1.)

achieved by emptying the heart, stopping it, and eliminating any work it must do (taking over its pumping function). This form of myocardial protection requires the use of a solution called cardioplegia, which provides cardiac arrest along with a chemical milieu that preserves myocardial viability. The heart is stopped after initiating cardiopulmonary bypass by applying a cross-clamp to the aorta and delivering cardioplegia into the aortic root and down the coronary arteries. Cardioplegia solutions typically contain high concentrations of potassium (20-25 mEq/L) and eliminate the potassium concentration gradient across the cell membrane, inducing electrochemical quiescence of the myocardium. The composition of the cardioplegic solution varies among institutions, but it usually consists of a crystalloid or a blood carrier, a buffer to reverse acidosis that results from anaerobic metabolism, and a hyperosmotic agent (eg, mannitol) to reduce intracellular edema. To overcome the heterogeneous distribution of antegrade cardioplegia that may result from coronary artery stenosis, some surgeons infuse cardioplegic solution in a retrograde fashion through the coronary sinus. Periods of ischemic cardioplegic arrest lasting 1 to 3 hours are well tolerated. Cardiac activity resumes after normal perfusion is restored with the removal of the aortic cross-clamp.

ISCHEMIC HEART DISEASE

Pathophysiology

Ischemic heart disease results from the occlusion or severe stenosis of large epicardial vessels in the heart by diseases such as atherosclerosis of the coronary arterial wall. Other less common etiologies include vasculitis, congenital coronary anomalies, embolic events, and dissection of the thoracic aorta if the ostia of the coronary arteries are involved. In each of these disorders, the underlying pathophysiology is the mismatch of myocardial oxygen supply and demand. Conventionally, a narrowing of more than 50% of the cross-sectional diameter of a coronary artery is considered a flow-limiting lesion. The usual manifestation of ischemia is angina pectoris, characterized by substernal chest pain or pressure that may radiate down the arm. Other "anginal equivalents," however, may be present (eg, jaw pain, throat pain, arm pain, or dyspnea on exertion). Individuals with diabetes and women may not exhibit the typical symptoms of angina and may instead present with vague symptoms such as gastrointestinal (GI) upset, generalized malaise, and dyspnea.

The physiology of oxygen supply to the heart is unique compared with that of other end organs. Although other organs are perfused mainly during systole, the heart receives most (~80%) of its blood flow during diastole, when intracavitary pressure of the heart and the resulting transmural pressure gradient are low. The heart extracts 70% or more of the oxygen carried by capillary blood before the blood is returned to the venous system. Consequently, the heart cannot meet increased metabolic demands by increasing the extraction of oxygen from the blood, as most other organs do. Instead, it must rely on increased blood flow to the myocardium to meet these needs.

The supply of oxygen to the heart is determined by the duration of the diastolic interval (which decreases as heart rate increases or obstruction to left ventricular outflow occurs); the oxygen-carrying capacity of the blood

(hemoglobin level and oxygen saturation); and the unimpeded flow of blood through the coronary arteries. Stenosis that narrows the cross-sectional area of a large epicardial coronary artery by more than 75% (50% of cross-sectional diameter) impedes the required increase in blood flow to the bed supplied by that coronary artery when metabolic demand increases.

Demand of the heart for oxygen has three major determinants: (a) wall tension as measured by Laplace law (tension = [pressure × radius]/2 × wall thickness), (b) heart rate, and (c) the level of contractility of the heart (Starling law). Laplace law summarizes the effects of preload (radius of the chamber and pressure in the chamber during diastole), afterload (pressure during systole), and wall thickness (compensatory changes to chronic increases in afterload).

The etiology of atherosclerotic cardiovascular disease is multifactorial. It is a progressive disease that can appear microscopically, even in adolescents. The lesions develop over time as a complex interaction of lipid deposition within the intima of the vessel wall, along with blood and blood products, fibrous tissue, and calcification. After significant stenosis occurs, symptoms may ensue. In addition, dynamic plaques (intermittent closure), rupture of plaques with hemorrhage into the wall, or acute thrombosis superimposed on these plaques can contribute to episodes of ischemia or to the development of myocardial infarction, even if oxygen demand on the heart is not increased. More recently, factors associated with inflammation and the inflammatory response have been implicated in these changes.

Many factors are recognized as contributing to the development of atherosclerotic cardiovascular disease. These include genetic factors, hypertension, diabetes, obesity, hypercholesterolemia, stress, inactivity, and smoking. Many of these factors can be modified to alter the progressive course of the disease.

Clinical Presentation and Evaluation

History and Physical Examination

Patients may present emergently with acute onset of severe chest pressure or pain (often radiating down the arm), diaphoresis, nausea, and vomiting. Alternatively, patients may acutely develop heart failure manifested by pulmonary edema or hypotension. Such patients are likely to be evolving an acute myocardial infarction or having severe unstable angina. These patients require hospitalization for further emergency diagnosis and treatment.

Other patients have more chronic forms of ischemic heart disease. They often have angina associated with different levels of physical activity. A complete, careful history and physical examination often raise the suspicion of ischemic heart disease. The history should focus on defining the nature and location of the discomfort while identifying factors that bring on the symptoms (eg, exercise, physical exertion, and emotional stress). Angina must be differentiated from other causes of chest pain, such as the epigastric discomfort of heartburn, the chest pain of pericarditis or pleuritis, or the discomfort of bursitis or inflammatory problems in the chest wall. Additional inquiries should be made regarding family history of heart disease, hypertension, diabetes, or connective tissue disorders. Questions should be asked about smoking, exercise, dietary habits, and the use of medications.

The examiner should attempt to elicit signs of coronary artery disease or other diseases that may be associated with atherosclerotic disease of the heart. Peripheral signs of atherosclerosis include carotid bruits, abdominal aortic aneurysms, loss of peripheral pulses, and symptoms of leg ischemia and cerebral ischemia. Signs of heart failure include rales, peripheral edema, and hepatic enlargement. On cardiac examination, the patient may show signs of increased cardiac size and abnormal heart sounds or an irregular rhythm that suggests heart failure. The presence of any cardiac murmurs should prompt a search for valvular lesions, usually by transthoracic echocardiography.

Diagnostic Evaluation

In the emergency setting, acute changes are often noted on an electrocardiogram (ECG), especially when there is ongoing pain. These changes may include Q waves that indicate myocardial cellular necrosis because of the inability of dead cells to become electrically excitable; ST-segment elevations caused by the inability of the affected myocyte to repolarize normally; and T wave inversions and QT prolongations that reflect ongoing cardiac ischemia because of delayed repolarization. Creatine phosphokinase isoenzymes and troponin levels are elevated when myocardial cellular damage has occurred.

In the more chronic situation, if the index of suspicion for ischemic heart disease is high, further diagnostic studies are often needed. The usual process is to proceed to stress testing. Stress is induced to increase the metabolic demands of the heart and can be accomplished by physical exercise or by medications causing coronary vasodilation and steal from territories with significant stenosis. The patient who is physically able exercises progressively to gradually increase the heart rate and myocardial O_2 consumption, usually by walking and running on a treadmill

at increasing rates and levels of inclination while blood pressure and ECG are monitored. The patient is questioned about any symptoms of angina. The onset of symptoms, especially when associated with significant ECG changes, is considered positive for ischemia. The development of hypotension associated with a stress test is an ominous sign that strongly suggests left main vessel or critical triple-vessel disease. The accuracy of a stress test alone is approximately 70%. The accuracy can be increased to approximately 90% with the addition of thallium or technetium. A stress thallium examination shows electrocardiographic changes of ischemia if they are present and graphically locates the ischemic myocardium by reduced tracer uptake in ischemic areas. In this test, the radioisotope is injected intravenously (IV), and the heart is scanned before and after stress is induced. Ischemic areas show diminished radiolabeled tracer activity (Figure 23-5). Resting echocardiography easily shows regional wall motion abnormalities consistent with ischemia or infarction, and allows estimates of valvular dysfunction, pulmonary artery pressures, and chamber size. In patients with normal resting values, an inotropic challenge with dobutamine may unmask an ischemic myocardium.

The decision to proceed with more invasive testing depends on the index of clinical suspicion (even in the absence of a positive stress test), the severity of the disease, and the concern for impending cardiac events (eg, myocardial infarction). Invasive testing with cardiac catheterization must fall into 1 of 166 indications for appropriate use of this diagnostic tool. Catheterization remains the gold standard in the diagnosis of ischemic heart disease although magnetic resonance (MR) angiography and computed tomography angiography (CTA) may someday replace diagnostic coronary angiograms. The procedure requires that a catheter be placed through a peripheral artery (either radial or femoral)

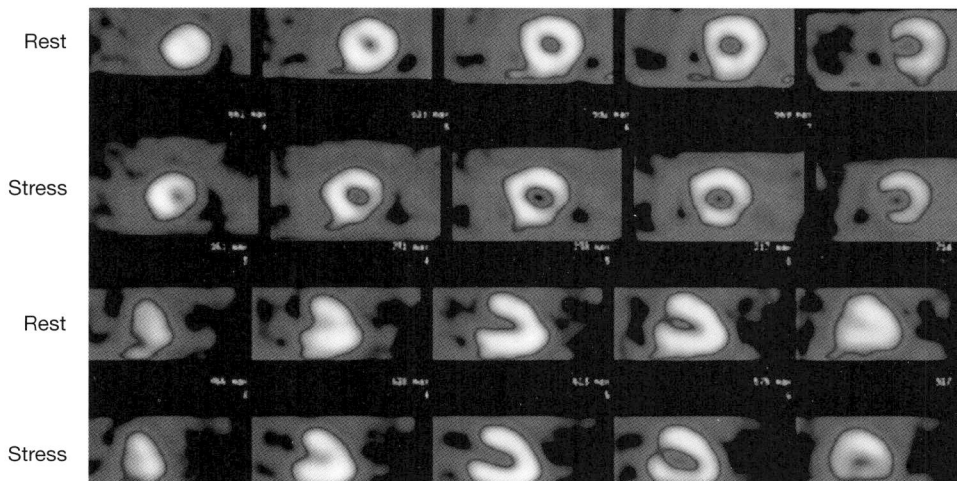

Figure 23-5. Myocardial perfusion imaging. Myocardial perfusion scan from a 61-year-old woman presenting with recurrent typical exertional chest pain (CP). The test was stopped because of typical chest discomfort (CD); electrocardiography shows 1-mm ST depression. Findings: no rest perfusion abnormalities. During stress, moderate-severe ischemia in the lateral wall from apex to base (6 of 25 segments, typical left circumflex coronary artery [LCx] territory). Subsequent coronary angiogram: left anterior descending (LAD) 40% stenosis, LCx totally occluded distally, obtuse marginal branch 95% stenosis, and right coronary artery small and totally occluded. Thus, LCx and right coronary artery (RCA) are both occluded. Both the lateral and inferior walls still show normal perfusion at rest. This appearance can be explained by sufficient collateral flow at rest, but insufficiency of the collateral flow during stress is first manifested in the lateral wall. (Reprinted by permission from Lee RT. Current science. In: Lee RT, Braunwald E, eds. *Atlas of Cardiac Imaging*. 1st ed. Current Medicine; 1998.)

and passed retrograde to the aortic root and coronary ostia, where injected contrast reveals angiographically significant lesions (Figure 23-6). Fractional flow reserve and instant wave-free ratio are techniques performed at the time of coronary catheterization that permit physiologic assessment of restricted flow by detecting a pressure drop across a lesion. Catheterization may also include measurements of pressure in the aorta and left ventricle. Left ventriculography (in which dye is injected into the left ventricular cavity to evaluate left ventricular function) is sometimes performed, and the results are reported as a global ejection fraction with additional description of regional wall motion abnormalities. If valvular lesions are suspected, more extensive pressure measurements may be required.

Coronary anatomy is commonly discussed in terms of the two major coronary arterial systems: the left and the right coronary arteries (see Figure 23-1). The left main coronary artery divides into the LAD coronary artery and the circumflex coronary artery. The right coronary artery usually supplies a branch to the atrioventricular node and is the origin of the posterior descending coronary artery 80% to 85% of the time (right dominant system). Branches of the LAD are referred to as diagonal arteries and septal perforators. Obtuse marginal arteries are branches of the circumflex coronary artery. Obstruction of the left main coronary artery carries a significantly worse prognosis because both the circumflex and the anterior descending systems are included within its watershed. A 50% stenosis of a coronary artery visualized in two planes at angiography qualifies as a hemodynamically significant lesion. Studies of the natural history of coronary artery disease show that the prognosis worsens as the disease increases from one to three vessels, as would be expected when larger amounts of myocardium are placed in jeopardy. It is not enough, however, to denote single-, double-,

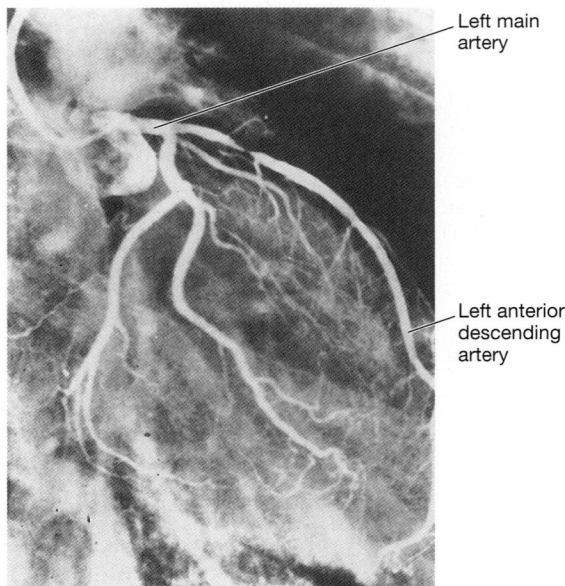

Figure 23-6. Coronary angiography showing a lesion in the proximal left anterior descending artery. (From Lawrence PF. *Essentials of Surgical Specialties.* 3rd ed. Lippincott Williams & Wilkins; 2007.)

or triple-vessel disease without allowing for variations in the amount of myocardium served by each vessel (ie, myocardium at risk). For example, high-grade stenosis of a nondominant right coronary artery is not an indication for coronary revascularization, whereas high-grade stenosis of a large, dominant right coronary artery would be likely to require revascularization of some kind.

The presence of left ventricular dysfunction is significant in terms of prognosis, with and without further therapy, and may dictate treatment. When ventricular dysfunction is associated with large areas of scarred myocardium, revascularization may be of no value. However, "hibernating" myocardium that is nonfunctional because of chronic ischemia or "stunned" myocardium that is nonfunctional because of an acute ischemic episode from which it has not recovered may benefit from revascularization and may have improved long-term outcomes. Current strategies allow safe coronary revascularization for patients with a very low (20%) ejection fraction when ischemic myocardium is present.

Treatment

Three types of therapy are available to patients with ischemic heart disease: medical, percutaneous interventions, and surgery. Treatment decisions must be individualized and are based on the symptoms, the anatomy, and the risks of the selected therapy. In all patients, however, risk factor modification of lifestyle and dietary habits may be of considerable benefit, especially when coordinated with smoking cessation, cholesterol-lowering strategies, and medical regimens selected on an individual basis.

Medical Management

When the risk of impending myocardial infarction is low, medical therapy to control symptoms may be appropriate. Medical therapy includes treatment with β-blockers to minimize increases in heart rate in response to physical and emotional demands, calcium channel blockers to decrease afterload and prevent coronary spasm, and nitrates to decrease preload and dilate the vessels that supply ischemic coronary beds. In theory, only after all three modes of medical therapy have been used simultaneously and at maximally tolerated doses is a patient considered to have "failed medical therapy" and to be a candidate for another more invasive mode of treatment.

Percutaneous Interventions

Percutaneous transluminal coronary angioplasty (PTCA) is performed in a cardiac catheterization laboratory to open partially and even totally occluded coronary vessels percutaneously. In addition to PTCA, these procedures may include laser angioplasty, directed atherectomy, and the placement of intracoronary stents. With techniques similar to cardiac catheterization, a guidewire is directed across the coronary lesion under fluoroscopic control. A PTCA balloon is passed over the guidewire and across the lesion. After the balloon is inflated, it compresses the lesion against the walls of the vessel (Figure 23-7). Similarly, placement of an intracoronary stent requires that a tubelike scaffold often impregnated with anti-inflammatory medication be compressed around a PTCA balloon. Following balloon inflation, the stent remains in place to hold open the artery.

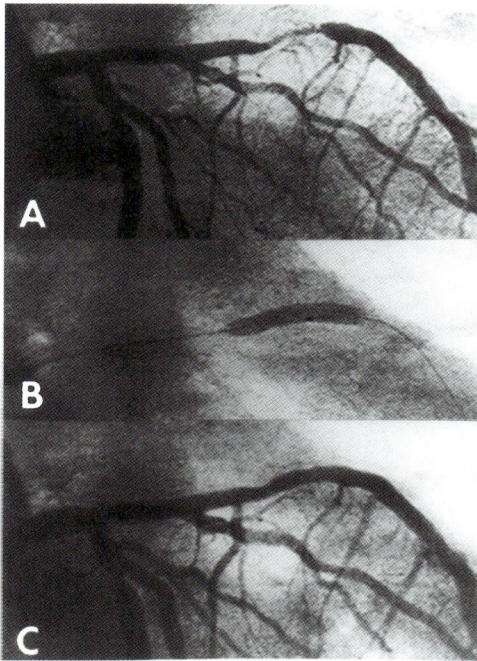

Figure 23-7. A. Narrowing of the coronary artery. B. Balloon inflated across the obstruction. C. The end result is near-normal diameter at the site of the previously obstructing lesion. (Reprinted with permission from Vogel JHK, King SB III. *Practice of Interventional Cardiology*. 2nd ed. Mosby-Year Book; 1993:84. Copyright © 1998 Elsevier, with permission.)

Surgical Treatment

The decision to use coronary artery bypass grafting (CABG) to treat patients with ischemic heart disease is based on the anatomy, the symptoms, and the potential risks to the patient, as well as the long-term benefits of the operation. The American Heart Association (AHA) and the American College of Cardiology (ACC) have developed specific guidelines for the selection of patients being considered for CABG. Certain anatomic situations alone (eg, left main artery disease, left main equivalent, proximal LAD, and circumflex occlusions) may warrant surgery, even in the absence of symptoms because of the large amount of myocardium in jeopardy and the recognized high mortality rate without surgical treatment (especially sudden death). Patients with stable angina that is unresponsive to medical therapy, unstable angina (eg, pain at rest, preinfarction angina, or postinfarction angina), or double- or triple-vessel disease with diminished left ventricular function are likewise candidates for surgical intervention. In these patients, surgery usually relieves symptoms, prevents myocardial infarction, and prolongs life. In addition, concomitant CABG may be indicated for patients who undergo surgery for complications of myocardial infarction (eg, acute mitral regurgitation, ventricular septal defect, free rupture of the heart) or those who undergo elective valve replacement procedures when critical vessel occlusions are identified preoperatively.

CABG can be performed with or without the use of the heart-lung machine. Traditionally, cardiopulmonary bypass has been used to provide a stable, bloodless field in which to perform the precise distal anastomoses to the coronary arteries required for successful long-term results. Off-pump coronary artery bypass surgery (OPCAB) has been introduced as a method of performing CABG without the use of cardiopulmonary bypass in the hope of reducing some of the complications (especially neurologic) and the need for transfusion associated with its use. OPCAB is performed through a standard median sternotomy or, in certain circumstances, via a limited thoracotomy. Once the technique has been mastered and the "learning curve" has been passed, many centers report excellent results. Long-term results, however, reveal few benefits of OPCAB when compared to CABG performed using cardiopulmonary bypass.

For some patients, the risks of surgery far outweigh its benefits. For example, patients with limited life expectancy from other diseases, the very old, and the physically impaired might not be surgical candidates because of associated conditions. In these cases, further medical treatment or attempts at partial revascularization with PTCA and stenting may be more appropriate. Although the benefits of CABG to patients with decreased ventricular function and double- or triple-vessel disease are well recognized, poor ventricular function adds to the mortality of patients who undergo the operation. The Society of Thoracic Surgeons Adult Cardiac Surgery Risk Calculator can be used to provide an individual assessment of CABG risk (http://riskcalc.sts.org/stswebriskcalc).

On the day of surgery, the patient receives preoperative medications, including prophylactic antibiotics, to minimize the risk of perioperative infection. In many cases, the morning dose of cardiac drugs is given, including aspirin and a β-blocker. Monitoring devices (Swan-Ganz catheter, CVP, and arterial line) are inserted and the patient is anesthetized. Once the patient has been prepped and draped, the incision used to expose the heart (usually a median sternotomy) is performed. For almost all CABG procedures, one or both of the internal mammary arteries are harvested from beneath the chest wall. The other conduits to be used for bypasses (saphenous veins from the leg or radial artery from the forearm) are harvested simultaneously under direct vision or using endoscopic techniques to minimize the extent of the skin incisions. The patient is heparinized, and cardiopulmonary bypass is initiated with the heart-lung machine. The aorta is cross-clamped, and the heart is arrested with cardioplegia to provide a stable, bloodless field in which to perform the distal microsurgery and to protect the heart during these periods of global ischemia. Bypasses are then performed. While using surgical loupes to magnify the operative field, the surgeon makes a small opening in the native coronary artery. The size of the opening is approximately twice the diameter of the artery. The conduit used to bypass the obstruction in the coronary artery is then sutured to it. The bypass is completed by suturing the proximal end of the conduit to the aorta. The proximal end of the mammary artery, where it branches from the subclavian artery, is left intact (Figure 23-8). After the patient is weaned from the heart-lung machine, the heparin is reversed with protamine, hemostasis is obtained, and the incisions are closed. Temporary pacing wires are usually placed on the atrium and ventricle, should they be needed. Chest tubes are placed to drain blood from around the heart and from the pleural space.

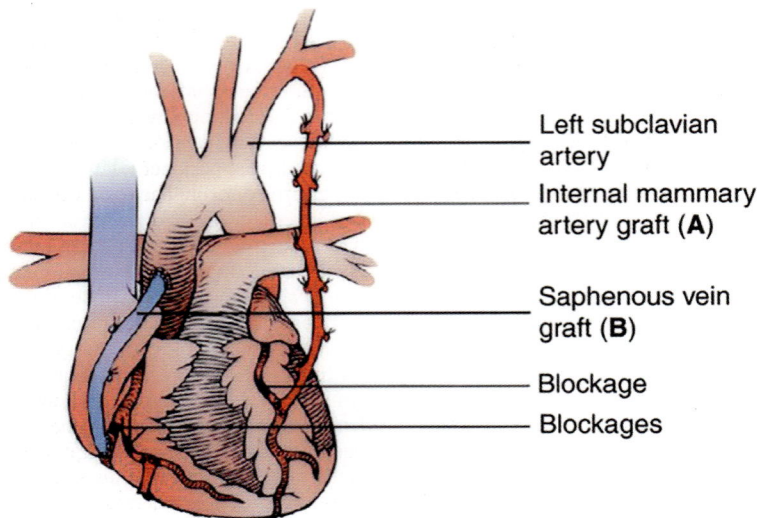

Left subclavian
artery

Internal mammary
artery graft (**A**)

Saphenous vein
graft (**B**)

Blockage

Blockages

Figure 23-8. Illustration of two-vessel coronary artery bypass grafting using the left internal mammary artery (A) to the left anterior descending coronary artery and a segment of reversed greater saphenous vein (B) to the right coronary artery. (Reproduced with permission from Rosdahl CB, Kowalski MT. *Textbook of Basic Nursing.* 12th ed. Wolters Kluwer Health and Pharma; 2022.)

Preoperative and Postoperative Care

Most elective CABG and valve procedures are now performed with the patient admitted to the hospital on the morning of surgery. Anticipated discharge home for low-risk patients is on the fourth or fifth postoperative day. Consequently, almost all preparations are made on an outpatient basis. Other patients with acute symptoms or unstable coronary syndrome (as many as 50% in some institutions) will require surgery while in the hospital following catheterization. Regardless of their status, a complete history and physical examination are required. In addition, attention is directed to documenting the absence of associated carotid disease, which could increase the risk of stroke at the time of CABG. The finding of significant carotid stenosis may prompt pre-CABG carotid endarterectomy or a simultaneous approach to decrease the risk of perioperative stroke. The presence of suitable conduits for the procedure must be verified, especially in patients with varicose veins, a history of deep vein thrombophlebitis, a previous operation, or severe peripheral vascular disease. The patient and the family are provided extensive education about the short- and long-term risks and benefits of the procedure, about the hospitalization itself, and about the postoperative recuperation.

Years of experience and attention to detail in the preoperative, intraoperative, and postoperative care of patients who undergo CABG have resulted in almost routine care of these patients. Many patients are extubated within hours of return to the intensive care unit. They are often transferred to a step-down unit in less than 24 hours. Early mobilization is emphasized, as are the prevention of pulmonary problems and the prophylactic treatment of atrial fibrillation (incidences of up to 40% are reported) with β-blockers or other drugs. Aspirin is prescribed to increase long-term bypass graft patency unless contraindicated. Because of the fluid weight gained during the surgery, aggressive diuresis to return patients to their preoperative weight is emphasized. Discharge from the hospital on the fourth

or fifth postoperative day is not uncommon, especially for patients younger than 65 years who do not have associated diseases.

At discharge, patients are likely to feel easily fatigued and have some minor sternal discomfort. Recovery over 4 to 6 weeks is one of gradually increasing ambulation and activity. After 6 weeks, most patients undergo a repeat stress test. If the stress test documents the absence of ongoing ischemia, most patients are enrolled in an exercise rehabilitation program for rapid reconditioning. Patients can often return to work within 6 to 8 weeks of discharge from the hospital, especially if their work is primarily sedentary. Patients whose work requires heavy physical activity may need to wait 3 to 6 months after discharge to permit the sternum to heal completely.

Postoperative Complications

Patient survival following complications that may occur after CABG is based on early recognition of problems as they develop and rapid and appropriate responses to them. Close monitoring with invasive devices (eg, arterial line, Swan-Ganz catheter) and appropriate therapeutic interventions can prevent many complications. Monitoring of systemic blood pressure, pulmonary artery pressures, and cardiac index has made it easier to differentiate among the several major early postoperative complications. Hypotension caused by volume loss, cardiac tamponade, low peripheral resistance, or cardiac failure can be diagnosed and treated. Hypovolemia requires rapid replacement of blood volume. Signs of tamponade necessitate early return to the operating room or emergency opening of the median sternotomy incision in the intensive care unit to relieve the tamponade and to correct the source of bleeding. Low peripheral arterial resistance may require α-adrenergic agents to improve vascular tone. Myocardial failure requires treatment with inotropic agents. Inotropic agents with direct β-adrenergic effects on the heart are most appropriate and include dopamine, dobutamine, epinephrine, and norepinephrine. Phosphodiesterase inhibitors (eg, milrinone) are also helpful agents to increase cardiac contractility while decreasing pulmonary artery resistance.

If these interventions do not reverse a low-output state caused by cardiac failure, the use of mechanical cardiovascular support may be indicated. The first tier of such support includes the intra-aortic balloon pump (IABP) and the Impella catheter (Figure 23-9). These devices reduce the cardiac work of providing adequate systemic blood flow. An IABP is normally inserted percutaneously through the femoral artery to lie in the descending thoracic aorta. A cylindrical balloon mounted on the end of the catheter is positioned just distal to the left subclavian artery. It inflates and deflates synchronously with the ECG. Inflation occurs during diastole and results in high augmented diastolic pressure that causes increased coronary blood flow. Deflation occurs just before systole, causing significant afterload reduction resulting in decreased myocardial oxygen requirements. Alternatively, the Impella catheter assists the heart by pumping blood out of the heart. The device is placed percutaneously across the aortic valve with a blood inlet portion of the catheter in the left ventricle and a blood outlet area in the ascending aorta. The device then pumps oxygenated blood from the left ventricle into the ascending aorta, where the closed aortic valve causes distal systemic perfusion.

When first-tier measures of mechanical support fail, complete support of the failing myocardium is required with a ventricular assist device. These devices assume 100% of the pumping function of the left, the right, or both sides of the heart. The heart may recover function over time when extensive myocardial stunning occurs and sufficient time for recovery is provided. Failure to recover function within 1 week usually requires implantation of a more permanent assist device as a "bridge" to heart transplantation, if the patient meets the criteria for transplantation.

There are many potential complications in the early postoperative period. Essentially, any organ system can be affected by complications of CABG and the physiologic disruptions associated with the use of the heart-lung machine. Heart failure is only one of these complications. As in all surgical patients, infections such as pneumonia, urinary sepsis, or superficial or deep infection in surgical wounds may occur. The most catastrophic complication is mediastinitis with true infection of the mediastinum and associated osteomyelitis of the sternum. This complication requires a major revision of the incision, with extensive debridement and either a repeat closure or, more likely, closure with vascularized muscle flaps or omentum.

Although there is controversy about the significance of perioperative microembolization, clinically evident stroke occurs in 1% of all patients undergoing CABG. Stroke is usually related to unrecognized carotid stenosis, intravascular air, or particulate embolization from the aorta. Manipulation of the ascending aorta by a cross-clamp or side-biting clamp is increasingly recognized as the major source of gross neurologic damage at the time of any heart surgery. Respiratory failure may occur, especially in patients with underlying pulmonary disease, those who have received large amounts of blood products, and those who have undergone bypass for prolonged periods. Renal insufficiency or failure can occur, especially in patients with preexisting renal problems or diabetes. These patients may require temporary or permanent dialysis.

The desire to minimize the possibility of certain complications was a major motivation to explore less invasive methods of coronary revascularization, such as OPCAB, by eliminating the use of cardiopulmonary bypass. The results have been mixed but seem to demonstrate a decreased incidence of stroke (but only when aortic clamps are avoided), decreased renal insufficiency, and a decreased

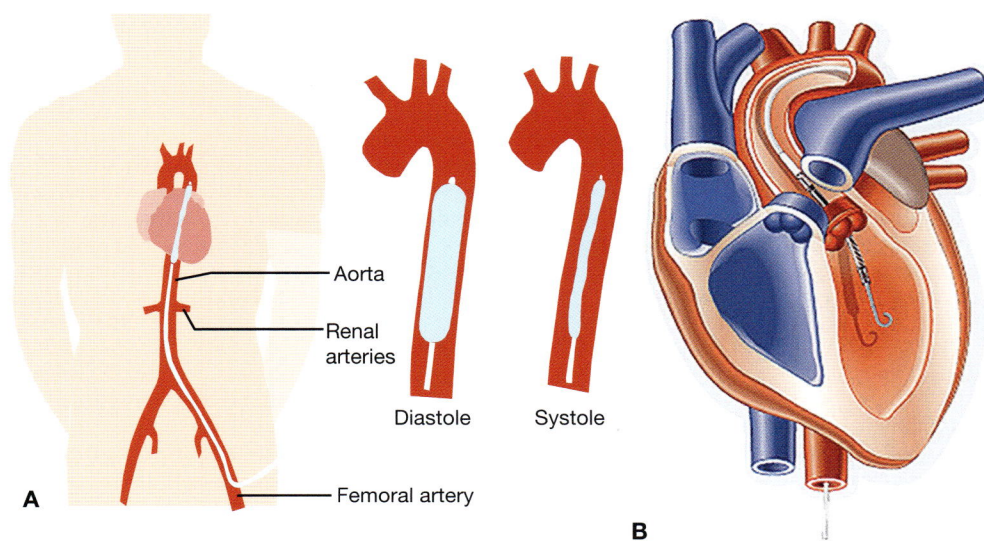

Figure 23-9. A. The intra-aortic balloon pump (IABP) is placed in the descending thoracic aorta. In diastole, the balloon inflates to augment coronary perfusion pressure. In systole, the balloon actively deflates to decrease afterload. B. The Impella (Abiomed, Inc.) uses a novel catheter-based pump motor to actively pump blood from the left ventricular inlet portion of the cannula to the aortic outlet site to augment native cardiac pump function. (A. Reproduced with permission from Nettina SM, *The Lippincott Manual of Nursing Practice*. 7th ed. Lippincott Williams & Wilkins; 2001. B. Reproduced with permission from Moscucci M. *Grossman & Baim's Cardiac Catheterization, Angiography, and Intervention*. 8th ed. Wolters and Kluwer Health and Pharma; 2013.)

use of blood and blood products. Minimally invasive approaches have been applied to CABG and valve replacement to limit incision size while using standard techniques of bypass and cardioplegia. Robotic techniques and the use of other specially developed instruments have seen increasing use to potentially provide decreased pain, less bleeding, shorter recovery time, and decreased incidence of wound infection.

Prognosis

Although CABG produces excellent results, many factors contribute to operative mortality and morbidity. At most major centers, the mortality rate for all patients who undergo CABG is 2% to 4%. Survival rates of 95%, 88%, 75%, and 60% at 1, 5, 10, and 15 years, respectively, are reported. Freedom from angina is reported as 95%, 83%, 63%, and 37% at 1, 5, 10, and 15 years, respectively. Freedom from myocardial infarction approaches 99%, 96%, 85%, and 64% at 1, 5, 10, and 15 years, respectively.

The importance of the conduit used for revascularization appears to be of crucial importance for the long-term benefits of surgery. The most common conduit used is the greater saphenous vein. The patency of this vein varies from 50% to 70% at 10 years. The internal thoracic artery (internal mammary) has a much better patency (>90% at 10 years) and has resulted in improved survival. In addition, the reoperation rate is halved (from 10%-15% to 5%-10%) within the first 10 postoperative years when at least one mammary artery is used. Because of the apparent benefit of using an arterial conduit, many investigators have attempted to use other arteries, including both internal mammary arteries and the radial artery. Early results appear favorable, but no long-term studies have been completed to verify their benefit and long-term patency.

VALVULAR HEART DISEASE

Because there is no ideal valve replacement prosthesis, all decisions about surgical intervention in patients with valvular heart disease must be made carefully. As such, the inherent advantages and disadvantages of each particular type of prosthetic device must play a role in this decision. The natural history of the disease and the risks associated with the surgical procedure must also be carefully considered. In some cases, methods of valvular repair rather than replacement have excellent long-term results, and as a result, earlier intervention may be indicated.

AORTIC VALVE DISEASE

The etiology of aortic valvular disease is varied. Isolated aortic stenosis usually occurs because of progressive degeneration and calcification of a normal trileaflet valve resulting in reduced valve area. Congenitally bicuspid aortic valves, however, are particularly prone to develop early stenosis caused by calcification. The disease is progressive and frequently clinically silent until symptoms begin to develop as the degree of obstruction to left ventricular outflow increases. The left ventricle concentrically hypertrophies to overcome outflow obstruction. Eventually, however, the ventricle begins to dilate, and signs of

congestive heart failure develop. The onset of symptoms (ie, angina, heart failure, and syncope) portends a poor prognosis without surgical intervention. The mortality rate approaches 100% within 3 to 5 years of the onset of symptoms. Congestive heart failure is the poorest prognostic sign, and the presence of all three symptoms should lead to prompt evaluation and surgery.

Aortic regurgitation can be an even more indolent disease, without the development of significant symptoms, even in the presence of massive cardiac enlargement. Volume overload of the ventricle associated with regurgitation causes dilation of the ventricle and significant cardiomegaly. Causes of aortic regurgitation include aortic annular dilation and valvular damage from bacterial endocarditis. Acute regurgitation related to aortic dissection or acute bacterial endocarditis is poorly tolerated and can lead to fulminant heart failure and death without early or even emergent treatment. Symptomatic patients with severe aortic regurgitation should be offered surgical treatment. Likewise, surgery should be offered to asymptomatic patients with cardiomegaly, especially if there is progression with medical management. The mortality rate associated with aortic valve replacement is closely related to the degree of ventricular dysfunction present at the time of surgery. ECG is the ideal noninvasive measurement tool used to follow patients with aortic disease and to pinpoint timely surgical intervention.

Transcatheter aortic valve replacement (TAVR) is an alternative, catheter-based procedure for treating aortic valve stenosis (Figure 23-10). Performed as a percutaneous or minimally invasive surgical procedure, a catheter is advanced through a peripheral artery to the ascending aorta and placed across the diseased aortic valve. The device includes a bioprosthetic aortic valve in a stent that is collapsed against the catheter. The valve is deployed into the native stenotic aortic valve by actively expanding a balloon or by releasing a self-expanding type of valve. Once deployed, the native aortic valve is opened against the wall of the aortic root with a fully functional valve in the center. Originally designed for nonoperative patients, the procedure has gained widespread and rapid adoption and now appears safe and effective for even moderate-risk candidates. Long-term studies of structural valve deterioration and residual aortic insufficiency will ultimately define the appropriate application for this technology.

MITRAL VALVE DISEASE

Chronic mitral regurgitation is caused predominantly by myxomatous degeneration of the mitral leaflets, previous myocardial infarction, or endocarditis. Acute fulminant mitral regurgitation can be related to myocardial infarction, rupture of the papillary muscle, or acute bacterial endocarditis with valve disruption. These conditions may require lifesaving emergency valve surgery. Mitral regurgitation can lead to signs of pulmonary hypertension, atrial arrhythmia, and left and right heart failure. In mitral regurgitation, the left ventricle may sustain damage because of associated volume overload. This regurgitant fraction of left ventricular ejection into the low resistance left atrium may lead to gross underestimation of left ventricle systolic function when using ejection fraction. Patients with severe

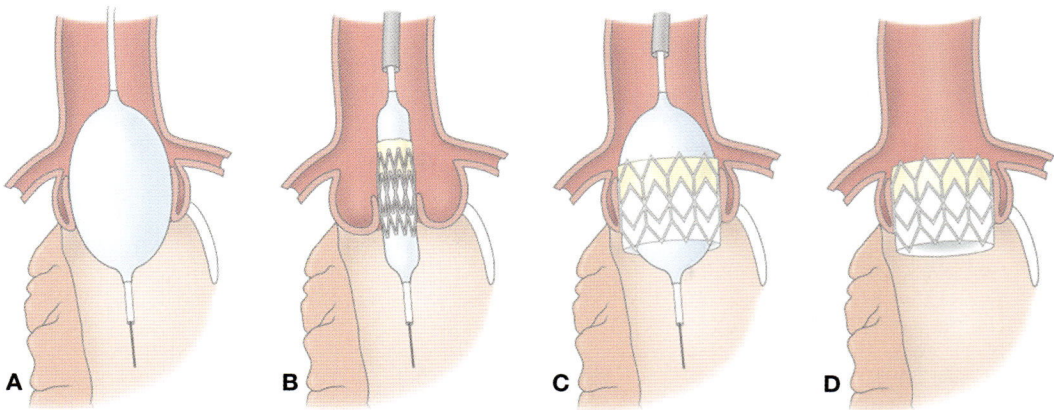

Figure 23-10. **Procedure for transcatheter aortic valve replacement (TAVR).** A. Balloon aortic valvuloplasty. B. TAVR catheter positioned across the native stenotic aortic valve. C. The fully inflated TAVR balloon and stent expanded within the aortic valve orifice. D. The completed deployment of the TAVR valve. (Reproduced with permission from Timby BK, Smith NE. *Introductory Medical-Surgical Nursing*. 12th ed. Wolters and Kluwer Health and Pharma; 2017.)

dysfunction of the left ventricle face a very high operative mortality rate and a poor prognosis, even when the operation is successful.

All patients with mitral valve disease (except perhaps those with end-stage mitral regurgitation) should be offered surgical intervention once symptoms of heart failure develop or the left ventricle shows signs of decompensation. When repair of the mitral valve (mitral annuloplasty, leaflet resection, chordal repair, etc) is believed to be technically possible, earlier intervention may be indicated. Currently, catheter-based mitral valve repair and replacement devices are under clinical investigation to provide percutaneous or minimally invasive solutions for mitral valve disease.

TRICUSPID VALVE DISEASE

Until recently, isolated disease of the tricuspid valve was uncommon; however, endocarditis of the tricuspid valve as a result of IV drug misuse has recently reached epidemic proportions. In early or less destructive forms of infection, these valves can be repaired but often require bioprosthetic replacement. Formerly, most patients developed tricuspid regurgitation secondary to pulmonary hypertension associated with left heart failure or left-sided valve dysfunction, which results in dilatation of the tricuspid annulus. Annuloplasty of the tricuspid valve, a procedure in which the dilated annulus is reduced to a normal circumference, in conjunction with repair or replacement of the left-sided valves, remains the procedure of choice in such circumstances.

VALVE REPLACEMENT PROSTHESES

Mechanical prostheses are made of pyrolytic carbon, metal, and cloth. Bileaflet valves dominate the market because of their low profile and relatively low thrombogenicity (Figure 23-11A). The leaflets of these valves are made of pyrolytic carbon, and the housings are made of titanium.

They may not be visible on chest x-rays unless they are made lucent by metallic rings or other material added to the pyrolytic carbon. These foreign and thrombogenic valve constituents necessitate lifelong anticoagulation.

Bioprostheses are either xenografts or homografts. Xenografts are made from the aortic valve of a pig or the pericardium of a pig or cow (Figure 23-11B). They are either mounted on a metal stent for suturing or inserted freehand into the aortic root. All xenografts are treated with chemicals such as glutaraldehyde to render the tissue nonimmunogenic and to sterilize the tissue before packaging. Homografts are harvested from cadavers within 24 hours of death. The ascending aorta and aortic valve are removed as a unit. They are then sterilized and frozen for storage (cryopreserved). They are thawed later for an isolated valve or root replacement of the aorta. Autografting an autologous pulmonary valve into the aortic position (Ross procedure) with homograft replacement of the pulmonic valve is an option, especially in younger adults and children. Insertion of homografts and autografts is technically more challenging than that of mechanical valves or stent-mounted xenografts.

Each type of valve has advantages and disadvantages (Table 23-2). Mechanical prostheses are the most durable and rarely require replacement for structural dysfunction. However, valve closure may be audible and thus disturbing to the patient. They uniformly require anticoagulation, usually with warfarin (Coumadin). Lower levels of anticoagulation have been used in recent years without an increase in the risks of thromboembolism to decrease the rate of anticoagulant-associated hemorrhage. These patients currently suffer bleeding complications in the range of 1.5% to 7%/patient-year and thromboembolic rates of 2% to 3.5%/patient-year.

Xenografts normally do not require anticoagulation in the aortic position, but their durability is lower, especially in younger patients and those with renal failure. Autografts and homografts have somewhat intermediate durability. They offer low thrombogenicity and have the lowest incidence of prosthetic endocarditis. Historically, patients under 60 years of age were counseled to have a

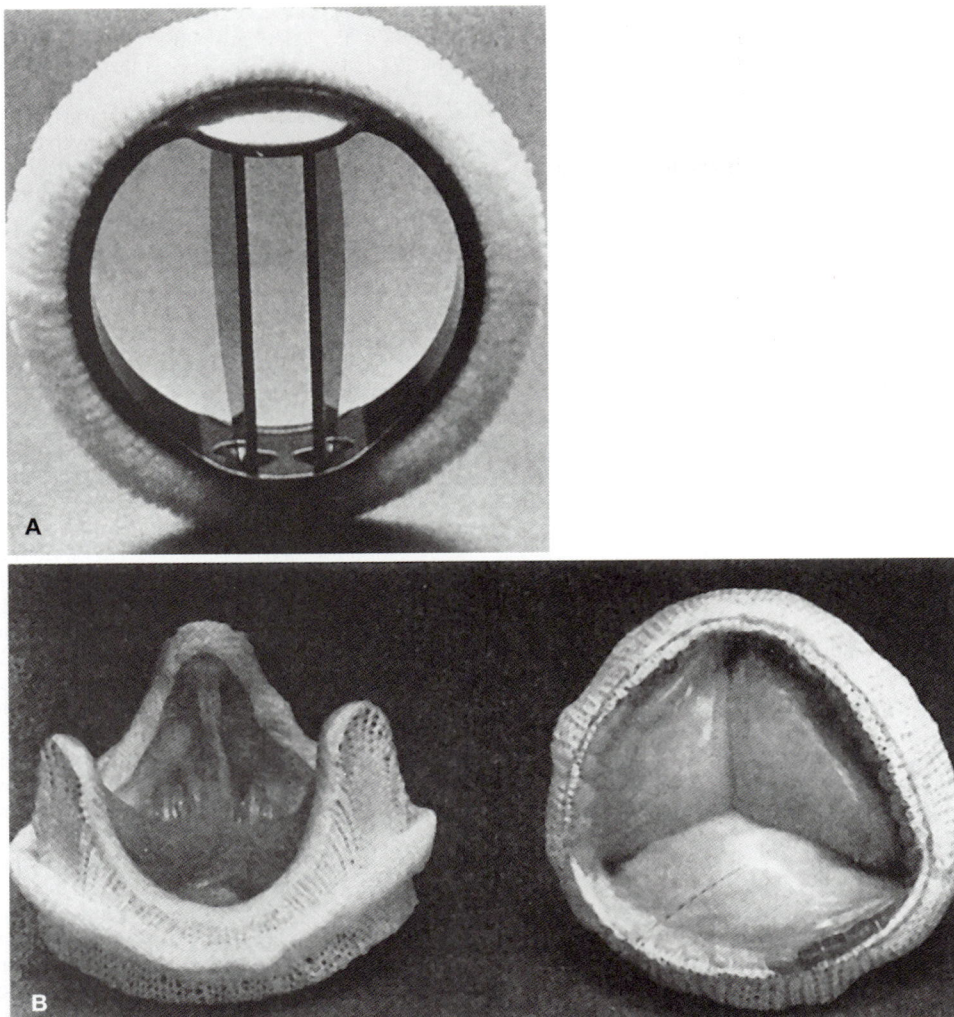

Figure 23-11. Valve prostheses. A. Mechanical bileaflet valve. B. Porcine bioprosthetic valve. (From Lawrence PF. *Essentials of Surgical Specialties.* 3rd ed. Lippincott Williams & Wilkins; 2007.)

mechanical prosthesis implanted unless anticoagulants were contraindicated. Older patients, especially those with a life expectancy of 20 years or less, were offered a xenograft or homograft. Since the advent of TAVR, however, bioprosthetic valves have been more frequently chosen even in younger patients. Early results show that a TAVR valve can be safely and effectively deployed into a failing bioprosthetic aortic or mitral valve. This strategy allows younger patients to avoid the anticoagulation required of a mechanical valve in exchange for a second procedure (TAVR) in the future when the biologic valve begins to structurally deteriorate.

Valve replacement is not curative; it merely substitutes one disease (the problems associated with the prosthesis) for another (the diseased valve itself and the secondary physiologic derangement of the heart). Common sequelae of valve replacement are thromboembolism (2%-6%),

TABLE 23-2. Comparison of Prosthetic Heart Valves

	Mechanical Valves	Bioprosthetic Valves
Durability	++	±
Thromboembolism	−	+
Obstruction in small sizes	+	−
Calcification with age	+	−
Calcification with dialysis	+	−

+, valve compares favorably; −, valve compares unfavorably.

mechanical failure (including valve thrombosis if inadequately anticoagulated), prosthetic endocarditis (1%-2%), and bioprosthetic deterioration (30% at 10 years). The newest generation of bioprostheses seems to last longer before deterioration. In contrast to valve replacement, valve repair (when properly performed) is safe, effective, and durable, especially for mitral stenosis and regurgitation.

ANTIBIOTIC PROPHYLAXIS FOR THE PREVENTION OF BACTERIAL ENDOCARDITIS

Deciding on antibiotic prophylaxis for patients with heart disease is complex, and the decision is tailored to individual patient risk factors. It is unclear whether antibiotic prophylaxis is completely effective in preventing endocarditis. It is also unclear how many patients are at risk for endocarditis with bacteremia and which regimens are most effective. Theoretically, transient bacteremia can occur after tooth extraction, periodontal surgery, tooth brushing, urologic manipulation, endoscopic procedures on the bronchial and GI systems, and normal obstetric delivery.

Because of the complexity of this problem, the AHA has published guidelines for the prevention of bacterial endocarditis. In 2017, the AHA and ACC published a focused update to their previous guidelines. These guidelines support infective endocarditis premedication for a relatively small subset of patients (Table 23-3). This recommendation is based on a review of scientific evidence, which showed that the risk of adverse reactions to antibiotics generally outweighs the benefits of prophylaxis for many patients who would have been considered eligible for prophylaxis in previous versions of the guidelines.

DISEASES OF THE GREAT VESSELS

ANATOMY

The aorta is the main conduit and reservoir of oxygenated blood. As a muscular artery, it is composed of three layers: the intima or the innermost layer composed of a single endothelial cell layer; the media or middle layer composed of elastin, collagen, and smooth muscle cells (the thickest layer); the adventitia or the outermost layer composed of loose connective tissue and vasa vasorum. Although the

TABLE 23-3. Patients at Increased Risk for Developing Endocarditis
Prosthetic valve
History of endocarditis
Congenital heart or heart valve defects
Hypertrophic cardiomyopathy
Heart transplant

elasticity of the aorta is attributed to the media, the tensile strength of the vessel arises from the adventitia. The vasa vasorum is the arcade of vessels that supply blood to the aortic wall.

The thoracic aorta comprises the aortic root, aortic arch, and the descending aorta. The aorta traverses the mediastinum from the aortic valve cephalad, arches posterolaterally, and descends through the thorax along the vertebral column outside the pleura. It passes through the diaphragm and enters the abdominal cavity. The vessels that originate from the arch are designated as the great vessels. The vessels are the innominate artery (also known as the brachiocephalic artery), which bifurcates into the right subclavian artery and right common carotid artery (CCA) at the base of the neck. The other branches are the left CCA and the left subclavian artery.

PATHOPHYSIOLOGY

The origins of the vessels as well as the arch can demonstrate anatomic variability, which can be both congenital and acquired. As stated above, the innominate artery bifurcates into the right CCA and the right subclavian artery. When the left CCA originates from the innominate as well, it is termed a bovine origin of the left CCA, or a bovine arch. This is seen in 7% to 20% of the population. Another variation encountered is a separate origin of the left vertebral artery off the aortic arch. The left vertebral artery is typically identified between the origins of the left CCA and the left subclavian artery. This is noted in approximately 0.5% to 6% of individuals. Another rare congenital anomaly is a separate origin of the right subclavian artery. The aberrant right subclavian artery usually arises just distal to the left subclavian artery and crosses in the posterior portion of the mediastinum on its way to the right upper extremity. Occasionally leading to dysphagia, a course of the artery behind the esophagus is seen in 80% of these cases, between the esophagus and the trachea in 15%, and anterior to the trachea or main stem bronchus in 5%.

Atherosclerosis

Atherosclerosis contributes to diseases of the thoracic aorta. It can affect the ascending aorta, the arch, the descending aorta, or the great vessels. Atherosclerosis affects the intima and media layers of the aorta, which can cause aneurysm formation or dissection. Progression of aortic atherosclerotic disease is associated with conventional cardiac risk factors of hypertension, hyperlipidemia, smoking, and hyperglycemia. The development of complex atherosclerotic plaque can lead to embolization (portions of the plaque breaking off) or occlusion, resulting in cerebrovascular (eg, stroke) or peripheral arterial occlusive events (eg, mesenteric ischemia or extremity ischemia).

Aortitis

Aortitis is an inclusive term ascribed to inflammation of the aorta. The cause of this inflammation may be the result of infectious or noninfectious causes. The noninfectious causes often encountered are giant cell arteritis (GCA) and Takayasu arteritis (TA).

Giant Cell Arteritis

GCA is the most common of the systemic vasculitides. The diagnosis of GCA should be considered in a patient over the age of 50 years who complains of or is found to have one of the following symptoms or signs: (1) new headaches; (2) abrupt onset of visual disturbances (eg, transient monocular visual loss); (3) jaw claudication; (4) unexplained fever, anemia, or other constitutional symptoms and signs; and (5) a high erythrocyte sedimentation rate and/or high serum C-reactive protein (CRP). Temporal artery biopsy remains the traditional gold standard for the diagnosis of GCA, although the use of ultrasound color Doppler has shown to be a reasonable alternative to the diagnosis of GCA in place of biopsy. In patients with GCA not complicated by symptoms or signs of ischemic organ damage (eg, visual loss), prednisone is recommended, along with the addition of low-dose aspirin (81-100 mg/d). The prednisone may require adjustment over time to achieve control of symptoms. Once achieved, the medication can be gradually reduced over time. An association has been found between a history of GCA and the development of aortic aneurysm, particularly thoracic aortic aneurysm, as a manifestation of extracranial involvement. Patients treated for GCA have a 17-fold increase in the incidence of thoracic aortic aneurysm compared with age- and sex-matched control patients. About 18% of patients with GCA and aortic aneurysm are diagnosed with thoracic aortic aneurysm at the time of diagnosis in this population, whereas most develop aneurysms during follow-up at a median of 5.8 years after the initial diagnosis.

Takayasu Arteritis

TA is a large-vessel vasculitis that primarily affects the aorta and its primary branches. The pathogenesis of TA is poorly understood. TA is an inflammatory disorder of the aorta that typically affects women younger than 40 years. Its prevalence is higher in Asian and African populations than in those of European or North American descent. A subacute inflammatory phase of the illness is demonstrated by constitutional symptoms. The signs and symptoms associated with TA are claudication of the extremities, decreased pulsation of one or both brachial arteries, difference of at least 10 mm Hg in systolic blood pressure between arms, bruit over one or both subclavian arteries or the abdominal aorta, and evidence on arteriography or CTA of narrowing or occlusion of the entire aorta, its primary branches, or large arteries in the proximal upper or lower extremities, not due to arteriosclerosis, fibromuscular dysplasia, or other causes. Treatment is corticosteroids. Patients may develop occlusive disease that becomes symptomatic. Surgical bypass or endovascular stent may be used for treatment only after the inflammatory phase has subsided.

Connective Tissue Disorders

Marfan syndrome (MFS) is one of the most common inherited disorders of connective tissue disease. It is an autosomal dominant condition with a reported incidence of 1 in 3,000 to 5,000 individuals. There is a comprehensive variety of clinical severity associated with MFS, which is beyond the scope of this chapter; however, many clinicians view MFS in terms of classical findings of ocular, cardiovascular, and musculoskeletal abnormalities, but manifestations also include involvement of the lung, skin, and central nervous system. Most patients with the typical Marfan phenotype harbor mutations involving the gene (*FBN1*) encoding the connective tissue protein fibrillin-1. The mutation affects the microfibrils in the aortic wall, which are weakened and are associated with defects in the collagen microarchitecture. This change in structure can eventually cause progression to aneurysm formation and dissection.

Aneurysms occurring in the ascending aorta, involving at least the sinuses of Valsalva, aortic regurgitation, and dissection are the major contributors to morbidity and mortality in the population with MFS. Dissection generally begins just above the coronary ostia and can extend the entire length of the aorta. About 10% of dissections begin distal to the left subclavian.

An important question has been the timing of aortic root surgery to prevent expansion leading to dissection and aortic regurgitation. An aortic dilatation beyond 40 mm is now the indication for surgery. Often the entire aortic root must be replaced, and the coronary arteries reimplanted. In cases of mitral valve insufficiency, a mechanical prosthesis is often placed given the young age of these patients at presentation. The use of β-blockers and angiotensin-converting enzyme inhibitors has been suggested in the literature to delay aortic dilatation.

Aortic dissection is the most common cause of premature death; however, the prognosis of individuals with MFS has improved significantly over the years. Early diagnosis and use of aortic imaging, β-blockers, and elective aortic root repair have all contributed to prolong survival with average life expectancy into the seventies.

Ehlers-Danlos syndrome (EDS) is another genetic disorder affecting collagen formation and function. It can affect every organ system which can result in significant morbidity and mortality. There are 13 subtypes described in the classification system; however, vascular EDS (vEDS) is a rare form of EDS and is considered the most serious. Patients with vEDS may have skin that easily bruises, thin skin with visible vessels on the upper chest and legs, hypermobile fingers and toes, varicose veins at an unusually early age, unusual facial features (thin nose, small earlobes, large eyes, and thin lips) and fragile blood vessels and organs that may tear or rupture causing internal catastrophes. vEDS involves an autosomal dominant inheritance pattern. Its mutation is the result of decreased amount of type III collagen, which is caused by the genetic mutation in the COL3A1 gene resulting in connective tissue fragility causing arterial rupture, organ rupture (uterine, intestinal), and untimely mortality. Sudden onset of pain in a patient with known vEDS should result in rapid medical evaluation in the presence or absence of trauma. Any surgical intervention in vEDS, including emergent lifesaving measures, poses a risk of complications due to the fragility of the blood vessels and organs. Postoperatively, these individuals are at risk for further complications due to prolonged healing times and risk of bleeding.

Blunt Aortic Injury

Blunt aortic injury (BAI) from trauma usually occurs because of deceleration injuries, most often as a result of motor vehicle accidents. Many patients die at the scene because of rapid exsanguination. However, 20%

of individuals who suffer BAI survive long enough to be treated. The most common site of thoracic aortic injury occurs at the isthmus just distal to the left subclavian artery at the insertion of the ligamentum arteriosum. Tears just above the aortic valve are almost uniformly fatal. Other sites that can be involved are the transverse arch, proximal ascending aorta, and descending aorta just proximal to the diaphragm. The shearing force of sudden deceleration leads to transection of intimal and medial layers, and the aorta is often held together by a thin layer of adventitia and mediastinal tissues.

Approximately 5% of patients develop chronic false aneurysms, also known as pseudoaneurysms. Chronic pseudoaneurysms may be identified months to years later, as they expand. Although pseudoaneurysms may not have immediate physiologic consequences, a heightened awareness of the possibility of aortic disruption is needed when treating patients with a history of traumatic injury. Knowledge of the mechanism of injury is important. History of a decelerating injury or a fall from a great height should prompt a search for the injury as soon as possible. (Traumatic aortic rupture is also covered in Chapter 7.)

Clinical Presentation and Evaluation

Many patients with BAI have multiple system injuries. There are no symptoms or clinical signs of sufficient sensitivity to accurately clinically diagnose BAI. Therefore, a high index of suspicion is necessary when treating this population. Failure to recognize BAI and manage it nonoperatively places patients at increased risk for mortality.

Physical examination of a patient with BAI may include signs of significant chest wall trauma such as a seat belt or steering wheel imprint. Other clinical findings may be cardiac or interscapular murmur or left subclavicular hematoma. Upper extremity hypertension, also known as pseudocoarctation, or bilateral femoral pulse deficit (as a result of intimal or luminal obstruction), can also be a sign of aortic injury or rupture.

Chest x-ray remains an important initial screening tool. Radiologic findings on a supine anterior-posterior portable chest x-ray include widening of the mediastinum to more than 8 cm (upright >6 cm) at the level of the aortic knob, a left apical pleural cap (indicating the presence of an extrapleural mediastinal hematoma at the apex of the left hemithorax), loss of the contour of the aortic knob and aortopulmonary window, depression of the left mainstem bronchus, rightward deviation of a nasogastric tube (indicating displacement of the esophagus), and wide left paravertebral stripe.

All of these findings on chest x-ray indicate the presence of a mediastinal hematoma and are not specific for great vessel injury. The trauma surgeon must distinguish between great vessel injury, which requires immediate treatment, and mediastinal hematoma of another cause. Mediastinal hematoma is largely the result of injury to small arteries and veins in the mediastinum. When BAI is suspected, further imaging is needed to definitively identify or exclude BAI.

Angiography for many years was considered the gold standard for the diagnosis of BAI. However, computed tomography (CT) of the chest has supplanted it to become the diagnostic test of choice. Chest CT is a highly sensitive and specific test for BAI. Thoracic aortography is no longer routinely used to identify BAI because it is invasive and can be associated with delays.

Findings on chest CT indicative of BAI are intimal flap, luminal filling defect, aortic contour abnormality, periaortic hematoma, pseudoaneurysm, contained rupture, vessel wall disruption, and active extravasation of IV contrast from the aorta. As a result of high-resolution imaging offered by multidetector CT, subtle arterial injuries that may have been previously undetected are being identified more frequently. This has led to aortic injury grading to aid in managing patients on the basis of the grade of injury. There are four types of aortic injury: type I, which is an intimal tear; type II, which is an intramural hematoma; type III, which is a pseudoaneurysm; and type IV, which is aortic rupture (eg, periaortic hematoma, free rupture).

Management

The approach to management of the patients with BAI has changed significantly over the past several years. The decision on how to treat patients with BAI depends on the hemodynamic status of the patient, grade of aortic injury, and the presence of other injuries and medical comorbidities.

Before the advent of high-resolution multidetector CT scans of the chest, all patients with BAI were consistently taken to the operating room for open surgical repair when the injury was identified. With improved imaging, a grading system for BAI has been designated, and it accurately identifies a subgroup of lower-grade injuries that do not require intervention. Contemporary studies, consisting primarily of retrospective reviews, support conservative management of minor BAI, delayed repair of contained thoracic aortic injury in the face of multiple other injuries, and preference for thoracic aortic stent grafting rather than open surgical repair, when anatomically feasible.

The following represents recommendations for the type of BAI identified. Type I injuries with limited aortic injury can be managed nonoperatively with heart rate and blood pressure control and serial imaging. Types II, III, and IV injuries warrant repair, whether immediate or delayed. Outcomes of untreated thoracic aortic rupture are poor. Before intervention, appropriate management of blood pressure and heart rate is needed. Delayed repair may be appropriate for patients who are hemodynamically stable, particularly if the patient has severe concomitant injuries.

Repair of BAI injury can be performed using open or most commonly endovascular techniques. Open repair involves primary repair of the aorta or replacement of the diseased aortic segment with a tube prosthetic graft through a thoracotomy incision. Endovascular thoracic aortic repair involves the placement of modular covered stent graft components that are delivered via the iliac or femoral arteries to line the thoracic aorta and exclude the injury from the circulation.

Degenerative Disease: Aortic Dissection

Pathophysiology

Acute aortic dissection is a catastrophic event, and without appropriate recognition and prompt treatment, it carries greater than 90% mortality. The primary etiology is the separation of the layers of the aortic wall that originates at a site known as the entry tear. The dissection occurs into the media, functionally separating the intima from the adventitia. The "false lumen" forms between the intima and the adventitia and becomes pressurized. As the adventitia is stronger than the intima, the "true lumen" becomes compressed. This compression may result in antegrade and/or retrograde propagation and compromise perfusion, leading to end-organ ischemia. Intimal rupture may occur into the aortic lumen or externally into the pericardium or mediastinum. External rupture often results in fatal cardiac tamponade.

Diseases that weaken the aortic wall predispose patients to dissection. The underlying pathogenesis is an abnormal aortic intima caused either by hemorrhage into atherosclerotic plaques or by cystic medial degeneration of the vessel caused by a connective tissue disorder (eg, MFS and EDS).

Anatomy and Classification

Classically, there are two common classifications that are used worldwide: Stanford and DeBakey. Both classification systems depend on the anatomic location of the dissection with the takeoff of the left subclavian artery used as the distal extent of the aortic arch. According to the Stanford University classification, all dissections that involve the ascending aorta, regardless of origin, are considered type A. Dissections that are confined to the descending thoracic aorta, distal to the left subclavian artery, are classified as type B. The DeBakey system categorizes dissections based on the origin of the intimal tear and the extent of dissection. Aortic dissections involving the ascending and descending aorta and the arch are type I. Dissections confined only to the ascending aorta are type II. Aortic dissections that originate and propagate distal to the left subclavian artery are type III (IIIa is limited to the descending thoracic aorta and IIIb extends below the diaphragm) (Figure 23-12).

More recently, this system has been expanded upon and standardized through a collaborative effort of both the Society for Vascular Surgeons and the Society for Thoracic Surgeons. The new system divides the aorta into 12 discrete zones numbered zone 0 to zone 11. Zone 0 is the most proximal zone encompassing the ascending aorta and brachiocephalic takeoff, while zone 11 is the most distal zone representing the external iliac arteries with the remaining zones contained between these two limits. These level designations are combined with the classic Stanford Classification to yield a composite designation that allows clinicians to rely on information about the location and

extent of dissection. For example, in this system, an A_9 dissection refers to a dissection that extends from the ascending aorta to the infrarenal aorta, while a $B_{3,10}$ refers to a dissection that extends from the aorta just distal to the left subclavian to the iliac bifurcation (Figure 23-13).

Previous classification of dissections defined "acute" dissections are those that present within 14 days or less, whereas "chronic" dissections describe those present for more than 2 weeks. Contemporary classification now defines the time from onset of symptoms as *hyperacute* as less than 24 hours, *acute* as 1 to 14 days, subacute as 15 to 90 days, and *chronic* as greater than 90 days. Acute Stanford A dissections account for more than 60% and are considered surgical emergencies requiring immediate operation.

Clinical Presentation and Evaluation

The classic presentation is acute, severe, and "tearing or ripping" chest pain radiating to the back and flanks. This pain may be described as the "worst pain imaginable" and is often confused with coronary ischemia. Careful history can help to differentiate between the chest pressure of angina and the tearing pain of aortic dissection. Dissection may be accompanied by symptoms of end-organ ischemia such as syncope, stroke, coronary ischemia, abdominal pain, oligo-anuria, lower extremity ischemia, paresis, or paraplegia.

Physical examination findings of hypotension, muffled heart sounds, and jugular vein distension are known as the Beck triad and are pathognomonic of cardiac tamponade. Pulse differentials between the arms and/or the legs, bloody diarrhea, hemiparesis, and abdominal tenderness are other diagnostic clues that are observable on physical examination.

While a normal ECG and abnormal chest x-ray that shows widened mediastinum may help in differentiating dissection from myocardial infarction, the diagnosis is most commonly made by CTA or TEE. TEE, when readily available, can identify the proximal entry tear and its origin. It is also effective in differentiating type A and type B dissections and can assess cardiac function without the use of contrast or ionizing radiation (Figure 23-14). CTA, however, has the advantage of being readily available in most emergency rooms and is less operator dependent.

DeBakey Classification   Stanford Classification

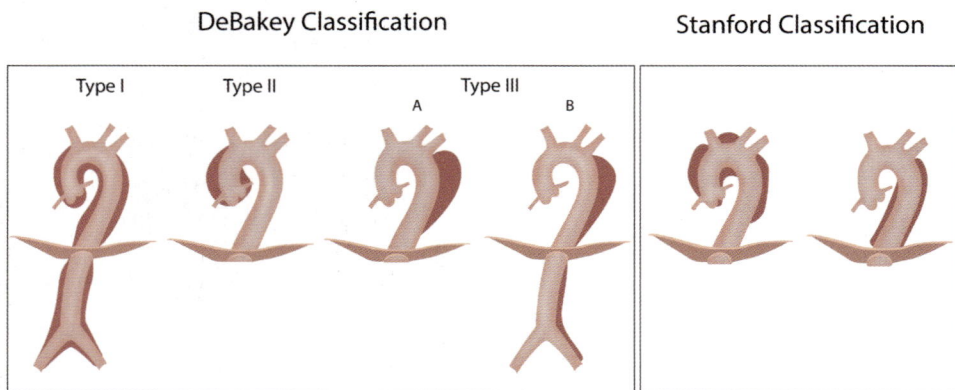

| Type I | Type II | Type III |
| | | A | B |

Figure 23-12. Schematic illustration comparing the Stanford classification and DeBakey classification. (Illustration by Alexandra Wedro.)

administered initially to reduce the rate of change of blood pressure ($\delta P/\delta t$) and the shear forces on the aortic wall. Target heart rate should be maintained around 60 to 80 beats/min, with a target systolic blood pressure of 100 to 120 mm Hg. These targets may be lowered if the patient's symptoms persist, as long as adequate perfusion is maintained, judged by urine output and mentation.

Aortic dissection involving the ascending aorta is a lethal condition if surgical intervention is not performed early. The current best practice guidelines for type A dissection repair involve ascending aortic replacement and open distal anastomosis (hemiarch) under circulatory arrest with varying degrees of hypothermia and selection of cerebral protection techniques, including antegrade or retrograde cerebral perfusion, or deep hypothermia alone. The goals of surgical management are to prevent or treat rupture and/or ischemia from vessel malperfusion. The operative mortality rate is 5% to 20% and is highest when the tear originates in the aortic arch. Hybrid endovascular techniques involving ascending aortic replacement, arch debranching, and antegrade endovascular stent deployment are showing some promising results that may reduce mortality and improve morbidity.

Medical management of uncomplicated type B dissection with antihypertensive therapy remains the preferred treatment. Surgical repair is reserved for uncomplicated type B dissection that fails control with antihypertensive medication or continues to have pain despite appropriate pain medication and for those who develop complications such as rupture or malperfusion. Thoracic endovascular aortic repair (TEVAR) has largely replaced open surgery. The endovascular graft seals the entry tear and most likely causes false lumen thrombosis, restoring distal perfusion through the true lumen. TEVAR has improved early mortality and morbidity rates for patients presenting with complicated type B dissection. The role of TEVAR in patients presenting with acute and subacute uncomplicated type B continues to be discussed, but several studies (INSTEAD, INSTEAD XL, ADSORB, VIRTUE) have shown there may be a benefit for early intervention (Figure 23-16).

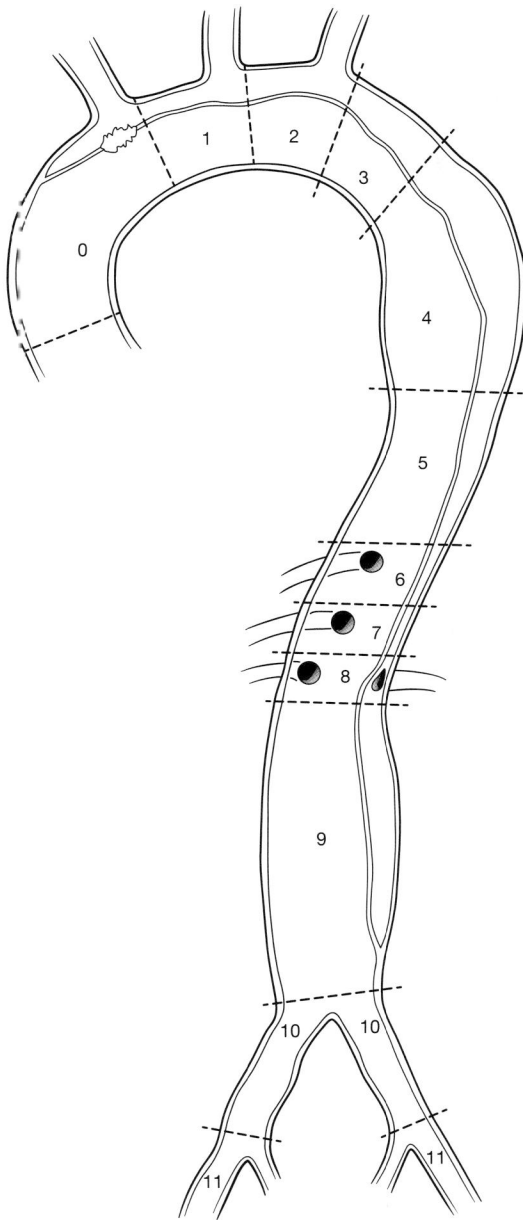

Figure 23-13. Schematic illustration of the new classification system created by the Society for Vascular Surgeons and the Society for Thoracic Surgeons. The illustration demonstrates what an A_9 dissection looks like. https://www.sts.org/sites/default/files/documents/STS-SVS-ReportingStandardsTypeBAorticDissections.pdf

It can also identify rupture, end-organ ischemia, the extent of distal dissection, and the relative size of the true and false lumens. For this reason, CTA has become the most expeditious and useful modality to diagnose aortic dissection (Figure 23-15).

Treatment

Medical management is critical for all patients with acute aortic dissection, whether or not surgery is performed. Initial management is focused on strict blood pressure and heart rate control. β-Adrenergic antagonists should be

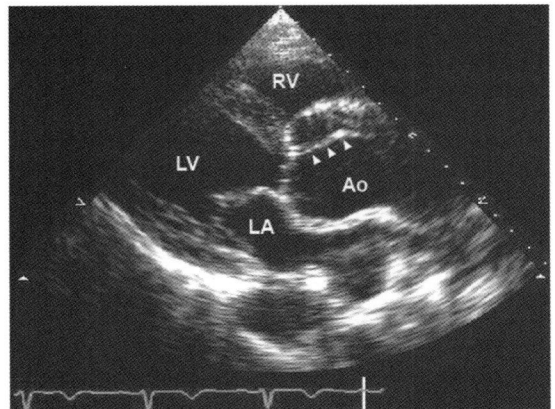

Figure 23-14. Transesophageal echo evidence of ascending aortic dissection (ASC AO). Arrowheads denote intimal flap. Ao, Aorta; LA, left atrium; LV, left ventricle; RV, right ventricle. (Reprinted with permission from Eidem BW, O'Leary PW, Cetta F. *Echocardiography in Pediatric and Adult Congenital Heart Disease.* 2nd ed. Wolters Kluwer Health; 2015.)

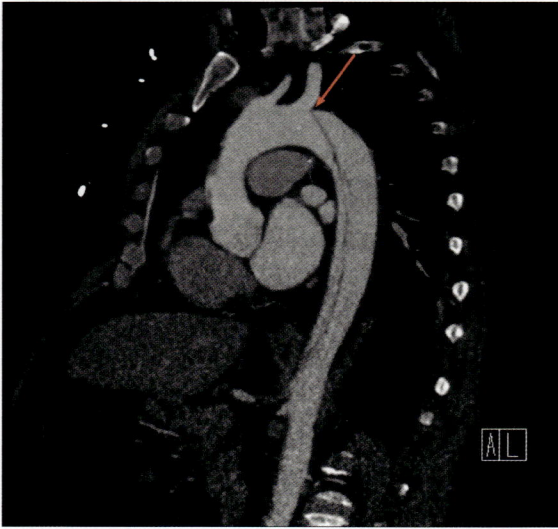

Figure 23-15. Computed tomography scan with intravenous contrast showing dissection in the descending thoracic aorta extending to the iliac bifurcation (not shown in the image). The red arrow denotes proximal extent of intimal flap just distal to the left subclavian artery.

Atherosclerotic Disease: Aneurysm

Atherosclerotic, posttraumatic, and chronic dissections with dilatation and infectious aneurysms may affect the thoracic aorta. Recognizable symptoms (eg, chest and back pain caused by enlargement of the aneurysm against the vertebral column) and discovery on routine chest x-rays are common presentations. Indications for treatment include symptomatic

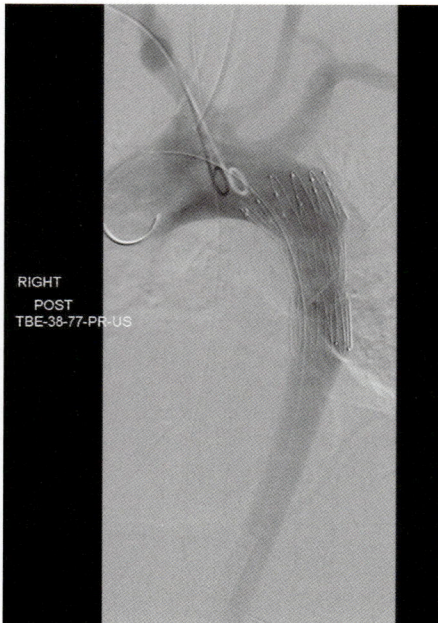

Figure 23-16. Thoracic aortic angiogram showing the placement of thoracic endovascular aortic repair graft over the left subclavian artery, resulting in the exclusion of antegrade flow in the entry tear proximally.

aneurysms, enlarging aneurysms, and aneurysms larger than 5.5 cm in diameter in the ascending or 6.5 cm in the descending thoracic aorta. Aneurysms in the ascending aorta and aortic arch are approached through a median sternotomy and usually necessitate axillary artery perfusion in order to provide selective brain perfusion while the body is under a no-flow condition known as circulatory arrest. The patient is often placed in hypothermic (18-22 °C) total circulatory arrest to protect the brain and viscera. Numerous grafting and repair techniques are used; most include resection and grafting of the aneurysmal tissue with Dacron grafts.

An alternative approach to open surgery is TEVAR, which involves the placement of an endovascular stent to exclude the aneurysmal segment of the diseased aorta. Results have been successful in a selected group of patients when the aneurysm is confined to the descending thoracic (or abdominal above the celiac artery) aorta. Multiple studies, which include registries, randomized control, and retrospective studies, have demonstrated the safety and efficacy of this technique. Cardiovascular and pulmonary complications and spinal cord ischemia occur less often in the TEVAR group when compared to the open group (Figure 23-17). In the last 5 years, there has been considerable advancement in the endovascular treatment of the ascending aortic and transverse aortic disease. Certain sites within the United States have been involved in treating aneurysmal and dissection within the ascending and transverse aorta with fenestrated grafts. These grafts, with similarities to fenestrated grafts for abdominal aneurysmal disease, have allowed vascular and cardiac surgeons to provide less invasive treatment. Within the graft, there are openings (fenestrations) which are meant to be aligned with the flow channels of the innominate, left common carotid, and left subclavian. Once aligned, short stents are placed into each fenestration and then the graft can be fully deployed. Once deployed, the aortic graft and stents within the fenestrations create a seal for blood flow to travel only through the graft and not within the areas of disease. Several studies have demonstrated the safety and efficacy of this treatment modality. Further investigations being conducted are on long-term morbidity and mortality and aneurysmal/dissection remodeling. These grafts are still investigational and are not currently approved by the U.S. Food and Drug Administration (FDA).

DISEASES OF THE THORACIC CAVITY: CHEST WALL, MEDIASTINUM, AND LUNGS

Thoracic surgeons treat many patients with both benign and malignant disease processes (eg, lung and esophageal cancer, pleuropulmonary infection, and chest trauma). An understanding of the anatomic structures of the thoracic cavity and familiarity with respiratory physiology are crucial elements for a thorough understanding of this field.

ANATOMY

The thorax is a flexible cage whose framework is made up of the ribs, sternum, vertebrae, scapula, and clavicles. Its main function is to facilitate the mechanics of ventilation. These structures also protect the heart, lungs, and great vessels from trauma. The inner pleural cavity is lined by a layer of parietal

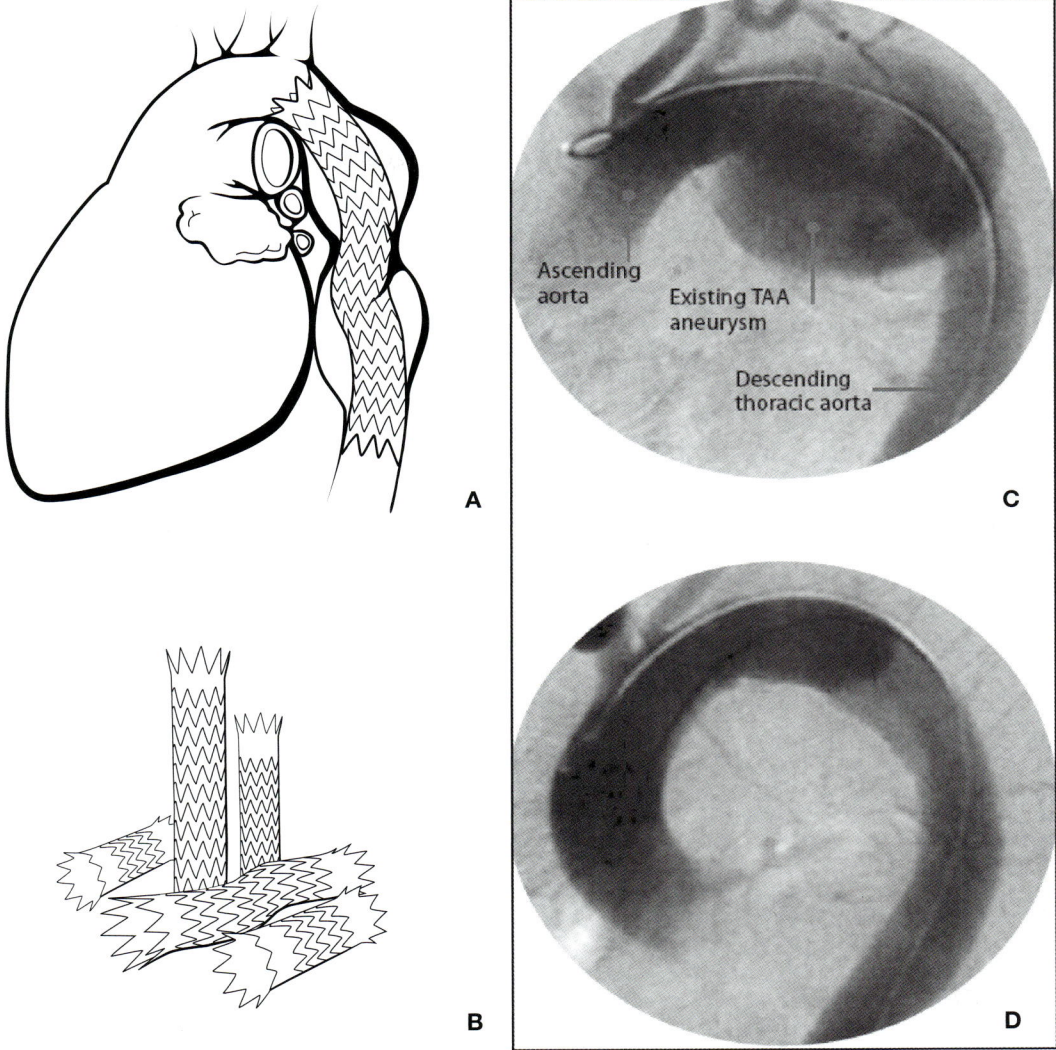

Figure 23-17. Thoracic aortic graft (TAG) endovascular graft. A. Artist's rendition of the delivery of a TAG thoracic endoprosthesis, allowing for endovascular repair of a thoracic aortic aneurysm (TAA). B. TAG thoracic endoprosthesis. C. Preoperative TAA. D. Postoperative TAA. No blood flow to the aneurysm. All blood flows through the TAG thoracic endoprosthesis. (Adapted with permission from W.L. Gore & Associates, Inc., Medical Products Division. *An Endovascular Treatment for Thoracic Aortic Aneurysm.* 2005.)

pleura whereas the lungs are covered by visceral pleura. These linings allow frictionless movement of the lungs with normal respiration and normal flow of lymphatics.

The trachea bifurcates into the right and left mainstem bronchi; subsequent branching results in a total of 23 generations of airways. The right lung is made of three lobes: upper, middle, and lower; the left has two lobes: upper and lower. Each lobe is further subdivided into bronchopulmonary segments. These are the anatomic units of the lung with an individual blood supply and bronchus. There are generally 10 segments on the right and 8 on the left.

The last generation of the airway is the terminal bronchiole, which ends in alveolar ducts and sacs. This is where gas exchange occurs between the sacs and the capillaries, which are the terminal destinations of the pulmonary arterial system.

PHYSIOLOGY

Inspiration is an active process caused by coordinated muscular contraction (mainly the intercostal muscles and diaphragm, and, to a lesser extent, the sternocleidomastoid and serratus posterior muscles). This process decreases the intrathoracic pressure and leads to the inflow of air. At the end of inspiration, elastic recoil of the chest wall and of the lungs increases the intrathoracic pressure and forces air out. Thus, expiration is a passive process.

The alveoli are held open by a balance between the outward elastic recoil of the chest and the inward collapse of the lung. Pulmonary surfactant, which is secreted by type II pneumocytes, helps keep alveoli open by decreasing the surface tension within the alveoli.

PATHOPHYSIOLOGY

Pathology of the thoracic cavity includes anything that disrupts the normal respiratory function and includes a variety of inflammatory, infectious, and neoplastic processes. Details are discussed under specific disease processes.

CLINICAL PRESENTATION AND EVALUATION

Thoracic pathology presents in a number of ways, from an asymptomatic abnormality detected on chest x-rays to life-threatening hemoptysis. The workup is influenced by the presentation.

History

A thorough history is part of the workup of any thoracic problem. The history emphasizes the following elements:

1. Past illnesses (episodes of pneumonia, bronchitis, asthma, or other related illness)
2. Allergies that affect the respiratory system
3. Exposure (occupational or other, including ionizing radiation, asbestosis, or other chemical exposure)
4. Habits (smoking or exposure to secondhand smoke)
5. Previous chest x-rays or their interpretation

Physical Examination

A thorough, complete physical examination is an essential part of the thoracic workup. The examination should focus on the integrity of the chest wall, auscultation and percussion of the lungs, and drainage of the lymph nodes in the axilla, neck, and scalene area.

Laboratory and Diagnostic Evaluation

Initial tests include posteroanterior and lateral chest x-rays and laboratory tests (eg, complete blood count, blood chemistry). More specialized tests include sputum culture and sensitivity, cytology, arterial blood gases, and pulmonary function tests. Further radiologic evaluation is done most often by CT scans, positron emission tomography scans, MRI, and radionuclide studies. Direct evaluation of the airways is performed with bronchoscopy.

TREATMENT

After a thorough workup that includes diagnostic tests, a tentative diagnosis can usually be made. Some pathology, especially infectious and inflammatory diseases, may be managed nonoperatively. The details of the treatment of these medical diseases are beyond the scope of this chapter, but some of the basic principles are discussed later. Other types of pathology (eg, neoplasm) are managed primarily with surgery. This treatment is more fully described.

Hemoptysis

The principal causes of hemoptysis have changed, over the last two decades, from tuberculosis and bronchiectasis to bronchitis and cancer. Bronchitis and other inflammatory and infectious processes now account for approximately

50% of cases of hemoptysis. Tumors account for almost 20%. Most hemoptysis is treated with bed rest, humidification, antitussives, antibiotics, and sedation.

Any patient who has persistent, recurrent, or massive hemoptysis should undergo a thorough workup. If the hemoptysis is not massive (<400 mL/24 h), the workup can be done electively. If it is massive, the patient requires immediate diagnostic and therapeutic intervention. In approximately 90% of cases, posteroanterior and lateral chest x-rays followed by bronchoscopy show the cause of hemoptysis. Bronchoscopy is necessary to identify the site of bleeding. The patient is positioned with the side of the bleeding dependent, to minimize aspiration of blood into the other lung. Endobronchial occlusion of the appropriate bronchus is then performed. If bleeding is massive, an aortogram with bronchial arteriography facilitates management because bronchial artery embolization temporarily controls hemoptysis in some patients. Determining the site of bleeding can be difficult because blood may collect throughout the endobronchial tree. Diligent bronchoscopy with occluding catheters and angiography may be necessary.

Surgical treatment is based on the etiology of the hemoptysis. In benign disease, as little lung as possible is resected. For any potentially curable malignancy, more extensive anatomic resection is necessary. The photocoagulating yttrium-argon-garnet (YAG) laser is used with some success to control hemoptysis from proximal endobronchial tumors.

Solitary Pulmonary Nodule

Some pulmonary masses are first noted as incidental findings on chest x-rays. If the radiograph shows a solitary pulmonary nodule or coin lesion, a workup is required to formulate a management plan (Figure 23-18). The importance of previous chest radiographs cannot be overstated. Management decisions are greatly affected by knowledge of previous lesions and estimates of growth rates. Stable lesions or those that double in size in less than 6 months are usually benign. New or enlarged masses must be presumed malignant until proved benign.

Pleural Effusion

For diagnostic and therapeutic reasons, pleural effusions (fluid in the pleural space) are divided into two types: transudates and exudates. Transudates originate from some external cause that upsets the normal balance of fluid secretion and absorption in the pleural space, allowing fluid to accumulate. Common causes include congestive heart failure, cirrhosis, and atelectasis. Exudates are caused by primary disease processes of the pleural cavity (eg, malignancies that exude fluid or block lymphatic channels).

Symptoms of pleural effusions include shortness of breath, pleuritic pain, and a sense of fullness in the chest. Decreased breath sounds and dullness to percussion are noted on physical examination. Thoracentesis is the primary diagnostic procedure. The fluid is analyzed to determine whether it is a transudate or an exudate (Table 23-4). Gram stain and culture are also routinely performed. Usually, the removal of as much fluid as possible allows subsequent chest x-rays to detect otherwise hidden lesions.

Treatment of pleural effusion depends on its cause (Table 23-5). Transudates rarely require chest tube

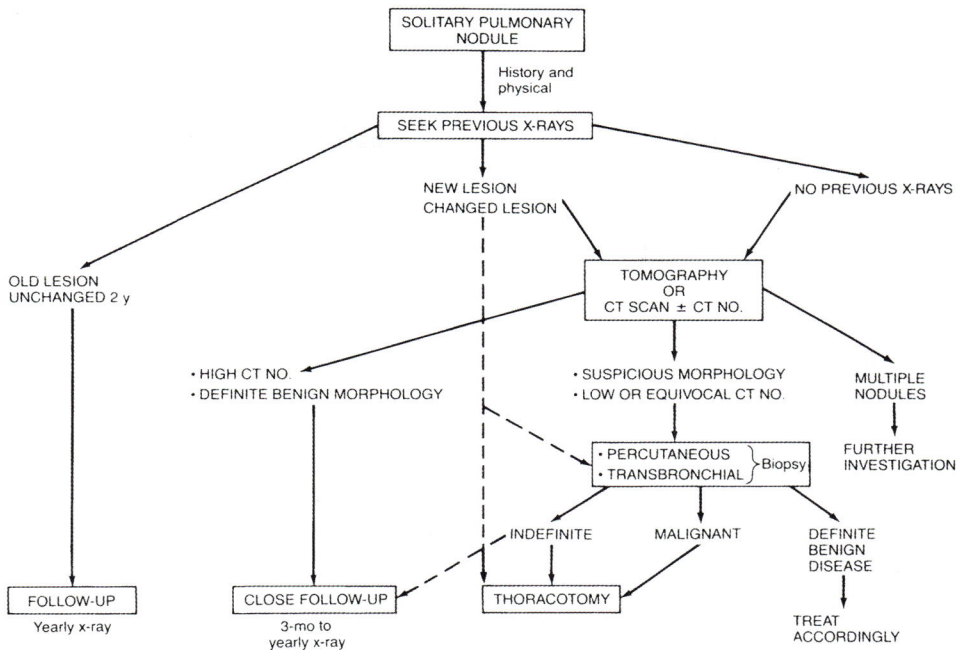

Figure 23-18. Management plan for the assessment of patients with an asymptomatic solitary pulmonary nodule. CT, computed tomography. (From Lawrence PF. *Essentials of Surgical Specialties.* 3rd ed. Lippincott Williams & Wilkins; 2007.)

drainage. They are treated by addressing the underlying cause (eg, congestive heart failure). Exudates usually require chest tube drainage. Malignant effusions often recur after thoracentesis alone. They also require chest tube drainage. Drainage of the pleural space with a chest tube until the space is dry and instillation of a chemical sclerosing agent (eg, tetracycline, bleomycin, and talc) prevents reaccumulating in 60% to 80% of cases. For sclerosis to be effective, the underlying lung must reexpand and allow apposition of the visceral and parietal pleura. Occasionally, mechanical abrasion (pleurodesis) or excision of the pleura (pleurectomy) is indicated.

Lung Abscess

A lung abscess is suspected in any patient who has a fever and an air-fluid level seen within the lung parenchyma on chest x-ray. CT scan usually permits differentiation between a lung abscess (parenchymal process) and an empyema (extraparenchymal process). The most common cause of lung abscess is aspiration pneumonia. Persistent pneumonia can evolve into a lung abscess, as can pulmonary infarction. A bronchial neoplasm or an aspirated foreign body may also be the cause and can be excluded by bronchoscopy.

Treatment of a lung abscess consists of prolonged antibiotic therapy and vigorous respiratory physiotherapy. Until the pathogen is identified, broad-spectrum antibiotics are indicated. An abscess caused by aspiration may include *Staphylococcus* species, fusiform bacilli, α-hemolytic streptococcus, and *Bacteroides fragilis*. Patients who are immunocompromised because of acquired immune deficiency syndrome (AIDS), chemotherapy, or malignancy may harbor gram-negative organisms, such as *Proteus*, *Pseudomonas*, *Escherichia coli*, and *Klebsiella*.

In most patients with a lung abscess, bronchoscopy is indicated to obtain cultures, promote drainage, and rule out an endobronchial tumor or foreign body. Surgery is indicated only if the patient continues to be septic, has an enlarging cavity, or has a resectable endobronchial lesion. Resection and tube drainage of the abscess are the principal surgical treatment techniques.

TABLE 23-4. Tests to Differentiate Transudative From Exudative Pleural Fluid

Test	Exudate	Transudate
Protein (g/dL)	>0.3	<0.3
Pleural fluid/serum protein (g/dL)	>0.5	<0.5
Lactate dehydrogenase (IU/L)	>200	<200
Pleural fluid/serum lactate dehydrogenase (g/dL)	>0.6	<0.5

TABLE 23-5. Common Causes of Pleural Effusion

Transudates	Exudates
Congestive heart failure	Infection
Cirrhosis	Malignancy
Hypoalbuminemia	Chylothorax
Nephrotic syndrome	Tuberculosis

Pneumothorax

Pneumothorax is the partial or total collapse of the lung caused by air collecting in the pleural space. It eliminates the normal negative intrapleural pressure that counteracts the elastic recoil of the lung and prevents lung collapse. Spontaneous pneumothorax may be caused by rupture of subpleural blebs. Sometimes, it occurs for no apparent reason (primary) or is caused by lung pathology (secondary). The diagnosis is made by history (chest pain or pressure) and physical examination (decreased breath sounds on auscultation and tympany on percussion). The diagnosis is confirmed by chest x-ray. Care is taken to differentiate a pneumothorax from hyperinflated bullae, which also appear with no lung markings (eg, giant bulla) on chest x-ray.

A significant or symptomatic pneumothorax usually requires a chest tube. The tube is placed in the fourth or fifth interspace in the midaxillary line unless the pneumothorax is loculated. In this case, the tube may be more appropriately directed using ultrasound or CT guidance. The tube should reach the apex of the thoracic cavity, where most blebs are located. After anesthetizing the area, a 2- to 4-cm incision is made, and blunt dissection with a surgical clamp (Peon) through the muscles, over the top of the rib, and into the pleural cavity allows easy placement of the tube. For spontaneous pneumothorax, a 28F tube is adequate. The tube is placed to -20 cm H_2O suction. A lung that reinflates too rapidly may cause significant transient pain that requires analgesia. The chest tube usually can be removed after the air leak stops. Occasionally, patients who have prolonged air leaks are discharged with chest tubes in place, connected to a one-way valve.

Surgical intervention should be considered for patients who have an air leak that persists for more than 7 to 10 days, recurrent pneumothorax, or bilateral simultaneous pneumothoraces. Surgery is considered for an initial pneumothorax in certain patients whose occupations put them at risk, such as deep-sea divers or airline pilots. Surgery consists of closure and exclusion of the ruptured bleb or any other large blebs with surgical staplers and mechanical pleurodesis. Pleurodesis, the creation of a fibrous adhesion between the visceral and the parietal layers of the pleura, is accomplished by abrading the parietal pleura with dry gauze to create an inflammatory reaction. This reaction, when coupled with complete lung expansion, ensures obliteration of the pleural space and prevents recurrence of pneumothorax. Mechanical pleurodesis is preferred over pleurectomy (removal of the pleura) because it has a much lower complication rate. A newer surgical approach is video-assisted thoracoscopic surgery (VATS). VATS allows the resection of blebs, lysis of adhesions, and sclerosis through multiple, small (~1 cm) incisions on the chest. The thoracoscopic approach permits earlier mobilization, discharge, and return to normal activity.

Empyema

Empyema is an abscess of the pleural space and typically occurs in conjunction with an underlying bronchopulmonary infection such as pneumonia. Initially thin, the fluid changes to a thick fibrin-laden collection after a few days and must be drained with a large chest tube. Indications for drainage include organisms seen on Gram stain, pH less than 7.1, glucose less than 40 mg/dL, and lactate dehydrogenase greater than 1,000 IU/L (Light criteria), all of which are indicative of a cellular exudate. The chest tube can be removed once the space is evacuated, the lung has reexpanded, and the fluid is no longer purulent. The tube may be left in place for several weeks and may be allowed to extrude over several more weeks. If treatment is delayed, tube drainage will not suffice because the thick fluid in the later stages of empyema will not be completely evacuated with a chest tube alone. In these cases, more invasive methods may be needed. In a procedure called decortication, VATS can be used to drain loculations and remove the encasing fibrin peel. Complex empyemas may require further procedures (eg, additional chest tubes, rib resection and drainage, decortication) (Figure 23-19). Obliteration of the pleural space is the single most important principle that guides therapy for empyema. Once adherence between the parietal and the visceral pleural surfaces occurs, resolution is all but ensured. If the lung cannot expand adequately to fill the space, the space must be obliterated by other means. One method includes transposing thoracic muscles into the pleural cavity (commonly used muscles are the serratus anterior or latissimus dorsi). Another old method used for tuberculosis is to collapse the chest wall by excising ribs (called a *thoracoplasty*). This latter option is quite disfiguring and is rarely used in modern surgery.

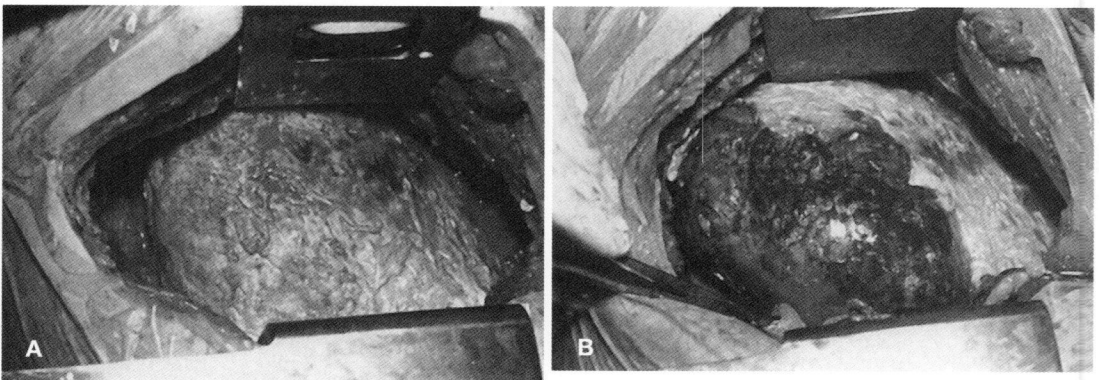

Figure 23-19. A. Lung trapped by exudative rind. Note the space between the lung and the chest wall. B. Partial decortication The lung is released from entrapment and is beginning to expand. (From Lawrence PF. *Essentials of Surgical Specialties.* 3rd ed. Lippincott Williams & Wilkins; 2007.)

Trauma

Although chest trauma accounts for 25% of all trauma deaths, fewer than 15% of patients who have chest trauma require thoracic surgery. It is important for all physicians to understand thoracic trauma. Chest trauma causes a wide variety of conditions, the most common of which are discussed in the succeeding text.

Open Pneumothorax

In open pneumothorax, the integrity of the chest wall is disrupted by an opening into the thorax. This opening interferes with respiration because it disrupts the negative pressure that is normally present for lung expansion. It is corrected with an occlusive dressing over the hole and a chest tube or, conversely, by endotracheal intubation with positive pressure breathing, which obviates the need for an intact chest wall. Definitive treatment requires operative debridement and wound closure, often with muscle flaps.

Tension Pneumothorax

A tension pneumothorax develops when a pneumothorax causes pressure to build within the thorax, as with a one-way valve effect. A tension pneumothorax is often an emergency, with acute, severe shortness of breath. Decompression with a chest tube or a large-bore needle (inserted over the second or third rib in the midclavicular line) is followed by a confirmatory chest x-ray. The tension is the result of positive pressure in the chest, which causes the lung to deflate and mediastinal structures to shift. This shifting of structures can kink the superior and inferior venae cavae, leading to a relative obstruction of venous return to the heart. Symptoms include shortness of breath and lightheadedness. Signs include absent breath sounds, hypotension, and often jugular venous distension. Cardiovascular collapse may occur. Placement of a chest tube rapidly alleviates this condition.

Massive Hemothorax

Significant bleeding into the thoracic cavity can interfere with respirations by limiting the volume available for lung expansion. Most cases are treated with chest tube drainage. Operation is indicated for a continued blood drainage rate of greater than 200 mL/h for 4 hours or more or an initial drainage of greater than 1.5 L.

Flail Chest

Fracture of a rib or ribs in more than one location may cause a portion of the chest wall to move paradoxically to the rest of the chest. On inspiration, as the rest of the chest expands, this segment is pulled in by the intrathoracic negative pressure. On expiration, as the normal chest wall collapses inward, this segment bulges outward because of the positive intrathoracic pressure. If physiologically severe compromise is demonstrated, the patient may require mechanical ventilation until the chest wall is stabilized by surgery or fracture healing. The most significant pathology is usually not the flail segment of chest wall, but damage to the underlying lung.

Neoplasms

Chest Wall Tumors

Half of all chest wall tumors are primary tumors. Of these, 60% are malignant. The rest are metastatic, arising mainly from lung, thyroid, GI, or genitourinary tumors. Both types

TABLE 23-6. Chest Wall Tumors

Benign	Malignant
Fibrous dysplasia	Chondrosarcoma
Chondroma	Osteogenic sarcoma
Osteochondroma	Plasmacytoma
Eosinophilic granuloma	Ewing sarcoma

usually cause enlarging chest wall masses. Malignant lesions are more often painful, perhaps because of rapid expansion. The most common primary malignant tumor is chondrosarcoma. The most common benign tumor is fibrous dysplasia (Table 23-6).

All chest wall tumors should be considered malignant until they are proven benign. A careful history and physical examination may show a source of metastatic disease. Posteroanterior and lateral chest x-rays and CT scan of the chest are performed to further define the tumor. CT scan details whether the mass is solitary and provides an assessment of the underlying lung parenchyma and mediastinal structures. A bone scan helps to determine other sites of osseous involvement.

With the exception of plasmacytoma, which is treated as systemic myeloma, most solitary primary malignant tumors are removed with a wide excision that encompasses the involved soft tissues, ribs, sternum, and underlying lung or pericardium. Margins of 2 to 4 cm are recommended, and a variety of muscle pedicle flaps are used for reconstruction. Patients who have Ewing sarcoma, osteogenic sarcoma, or other soft tissue sarcomas are candidates for postoperative adjuvant therapy with radiation therapy, chemotherapy, or both.

Mediastinal Tumors

Several benign and malignant tumors, both primary and metastatic, occur in the mediastinum. Although most tumors are first found on standard posteroanterior or lateral chest x-rays, CT scanning is essential to localize the tumor accurately. MRI offers no significant advantages over CT scanning, except in posterior paraspinal tumors.

Mediastinal tumors are divided according to their location (Figure 23-20). The anterior mediastinum is defined by an imaginary line that extends along the anterior wall of the trachea and down over the anterior pericardium. The posterior mediastinum is defined by an imaginary line that extends from the anterior border of the vertebral bodies to the costovertebral sulci. The middle mediastinum is the space in between. Tumors occur most often in the anterior mediastinum and least often in the middle mediastinum.

The most common tumors of the anterior mediastinum are thymoma, substernal thyroid tumor, teratoma (germ cell tumor), and lymphoma. Symptoms in patients with malignant lesions include chest pain, dyspnea, fever, chills, and cough. Patients who have benign lesions are usually asymptomatic, and the lesions are found only on routine chest x-ray. A careful history and physical examination can give clues as to the type of tumor present.

Lymphoma can cause night sweats, weight loss, and peripheral adenopathy. Lymphomas are best treated with chemotherapy and radiation. A mediastinal germ cell

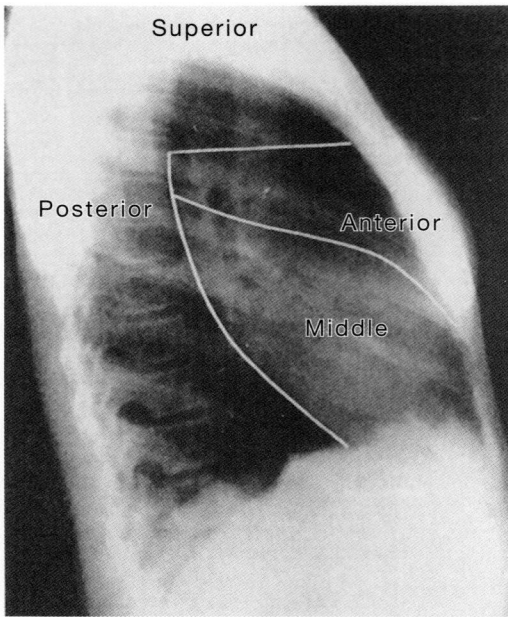

Figure 23-20. Lateral film of the chest showing the anatomic divisions into four subdivisions of the mediastinum. (Reprinted with permission from Sabiston DC, Spencer FC, eds. *Surgery of the Chest.* 5th ed. WB Saunders; 1990:872. Copyright © 1998 Elsevier, with permission.)

metastasis can appear as a testicular mass. A thymoma can cause symptoms of myasthenia gravis. A substernal thyroid tumor often partially compresses the trachea, one of the few tumors to do so. Excision is the best treatment, except for lymphoma, which usually requires anterior mediastinotomy and biopsy to make the diagnosis if no extramediastinal adenopathy exists. Almost all substernal thyroids can be removed through a cervical incision. Resection of all other anterior mediastinal tumors is best approached with a median sternotomy.

The most common masses in the middle mediastinum are enterogenous cysts and metastatic lymph nodes from lung cancer. Asymptomatic mediastinal adenopathy can be a manifestation of sarcoidosis and can be diagnosed by mediastinoscopy. Middle mediastinal cysts (bronchogenic, esophageal, and pleuropericardial) are removed by lateral thoracotomy to rule out a malignancy that has similar radiographic findings.

The most common tumors of the paravertebral sulci are of neurogenic origin: neurilemoma, neurofibroma, ganglioneuroma, and neuroblastoma. Tumors in this location must be evaluated by MRI to determine whether there is extension into the spinal canal. If they extend into the canal, a combined neurosurgical-thoracosurgical approach is essential to ensure complete removal. Failure to remove the spinal canal component can cause paralysis years later, as the residual tumor slowly grows and presses against the spinal cord.

Lung Cancers

Lung cancer is the most common nondermatologic cancer in North America. It accounts for 14% of all new cancers and 30% of cancer deaths and is now the leading cause of

cancer death in both men and women. More than 85% of patients with lung cancer have a significant smoking history. Other reported causative exposures are to radioactive materials, including asbestos dust and fluorspar, and secondary cigarette smoke.

The pathology of lung cancer may be either primary or secondary. Primary lung cancer progresses from dysplastic changes to in situ changes to frankly invasive carcinoma. It develops from two distinct cell lines, large cell lines (eg, squamous cell, adenocarcinoma, and mixed cell type) and small cell lines (eg, oat cell, intermediate cell type, and mixed cell type). Information about cell type is obtained from a variety of diagnostic procedures. These include cytologic evaluation of sputum and bronchial washings, and histologic and cytologic evaluation of tumor tissue obtained by direct or transpulmonary biopsy. The biopsy is performed through the bronchus or the chest wall by fine needle aspiration. Identification of the originating cell line is important in determining treatment. Because tumors from the small cell line tend to metastasize earlier, they are often managed systemically with a combination of chemotherapy and radiation therapy rather than with a primary surgical approach. However, surgery may play a role in selected early lesions that have no evidence of metastasis. Patients with neoplasms of large cell origin are always evaluated with resection in mind because surgical removal offers the best chance for cure.

Secondary lung cancers are caused by metastasis of lesions elsewhere in the body. These lesions usually originate in the breast, GI system, genitourinary tract, or soft tissue. Surgery is an option when there is no evidence of other distant metastatic lesions. In some cases, surgical removal of solitary or well-localized metastatic lesions in the lung is justified by improvement in the survival rate. The development of metastatic lesions to the lung carries a generally poor prognosis. However, aggressive combination therapy can produce long, disease-free intervals and, in some cases, improve survival rates.

The clinical presentation of lung cancer is highly variable. Approximately 5% of patients are asymptomatic, and a lesion is discovered incidentally by chest x-rays performed for some other reason. Because the yield is low, especially in nonsmokers, routine screening chest x-rays are usually not recommended, although screening of selected populations may be revisited. If radiographs show a solitary pulmonary nodule (coin lesion), a workup is required to formulate a management plan (see Figure 23-18). Stable lesions are usually benign. New masses and those that show enlargement are presumed malignant until proven benign.

The other 95% of patients are symptomatic, with signs and symptoms that can be categorized as bronchopulmonary, extrapulmonary, metastatic, nonspecific, or nonmetastatic (Table 23-7). Extrapulmonary signs and symptoms suggest advanced disease. Paratracheal lymph node metastases may produce hoarseness because of the involvement of the recurrent laryngeal nerve. Superior vena cava obstruction may occur with right-sided nodal enlargement or direct invasion. Pleural effusion may be caused by metastatic disease in the pleura, obstructive pneumonia, or lymphatic obstruction. Neurologic changes, abnormal liver function test results, and bone pain suggest metastases. A thorough search for metastases must be undertaken with CT scans of the brain and abdomen and bone scans. Nonmetastatic symptoms (paraneoplastic syndromes) occur in

TABLE 23-7. Signs and Symptoms in Patients With Lung Cancer

Type	Signs and Symptoms
Bronchopulmonary	Cough (most common symptom) Chest pain (may indicate involvement of chest wall) Dyspnea (because of airway obstruction or pleural effusion) Hemoptysis
Extrapulmonary	Superior vena caval obstruction Hoarseness (recurrent laryngeal nerve invasion) Pleural effusion
Metastatic	Neurologic (headache, change in mental status) Skeletal (bone pain) Visceral (Liver or adrenal metastases are often asymptomatic.)
Nonspecific (usually occurs late in the course of the disease)	Weight loss Anemia Fatigue
Nonmetastatic	Dermatologic (hyperpigmentation, dermatomyositis)
Encocrine (Some tumors secrete hormonelike substances causing hypercalcemia or syndrome of inappropriate antidiuretic hormone secretion.)	Vascular (Patients with lung cancer may become hypercoagulable.) Neurogenic (Eaton-Lambert syndrome, autonomic neuropathy, etc) Metabolic (hypercalcemia, Cushing syndrome, carcinoid syndrome, etc) Hematologic (anemia, thrombocytosis, etc) Skeletal (pulmonary osteoarthropathy, clubbing)

a small percentage of patients and may be very early signs of primary lung cancer. These include hypercalcemia and inappropriate secretion of the antidiuretic hormone.

Once the possibility of bronchogenic cancer is raised, the physician must formulate a management plan. The plan depends on a precise diagnosis, the stage of the disease, and the ability of the patient to undergo operative treatment. The following three questions must be answered:

1. What is the diagnosis?
2. Can the patient undergo an operation?
3. Can the patient tolerate the maximally anticipated lung resection?

Diagnosis

The diagnosis of bronchogenic carcinoma is confirmed by bronchoscopy or percutaneous needle biopsy. Flexible or rigid bronchoscopy is used to visualize proximal tumors. Direct biopsy (or the use of washings and brushings) provides a precise diagnosis in more than 90% of patients. Even patients with peripheral lesions that are not directly visible endoscopically can undergo biopsy with fluoroscopic guidance into the appropriate bronchopulmonary segment. Lesions that are not amenable to bronchoscopic biopsy are evaluated with percutaneous needle biopsy guided by either fluoroscopy or CT scan. Cytologic analysis is also performed, although some needles yield only a small histologic specimen. In most cases, clinical management is properly guided by the findings of needle biopsy.

The stage of the tumor determines the treatment. The size and spread of the tumor are important elements of staging. The most widely used classification is the TNM system of the American Joint Committee on Cancer Staging:

T = Size and location of the tumor
N = Presence and location of lymph node metastases
M = Presence of distant metastases

The TNM classification allows the surgeon to provide a stage grouping for the patient. Based on the stage, statistical prognostication can be made for most patients. Generally, tumors with extensive contralateral lymph node involvement or metastatic disease require systemic chemotherapy and local radiation whereas limited tumors of lower stage can be treated with surgical excision and lymph node dissection.

After the tumor is localized by bronchoscopy and radiologic evaluation, its resectability is determined. With rare exceptions, tumors at or near the carina are not considered resectable. The proximity of the tumor to vital structures can be determined with bronchoscopy and CT scanning with contrast.

In a patient who has lung cancer, the search for metastatic disease must be as complete as possible before a pulmonary resection. A resection that leaves malignancy behind is both fruitless and dangerous. As such, it is imperative to obtain an adequate assessment of mediastinal and hilar lymph nodes as their involvement may suggest advanced disease. In addition to traditional high-resolution CT imaging, fludeoxyglucose-positron emission tomography (FDG-PET) scans can provide an accurate assessment of both the size and metabolic activity of draining lymph node basins. Any suspicious lymph nodes should be biopsied so that they may undergo microscopic and histochemical evaluation. Traditionally, biopsy was completed via mediastinoscopy; however, minimally invasive techniques including endobronchial ultrasound or navigational bronchoscopy are becoming increasingly utilized. The presence of metastases in these nodes reduces the surgical cure rate to a level at which few centers attempt surgical resection. With rare exceptions, patients with a tumor limited to the ipsilateral hemithorax, with no evidence of mediastinal lymph node metastases and no involvement of other vital structures, are considered surgical candidates (Figure 23-21).

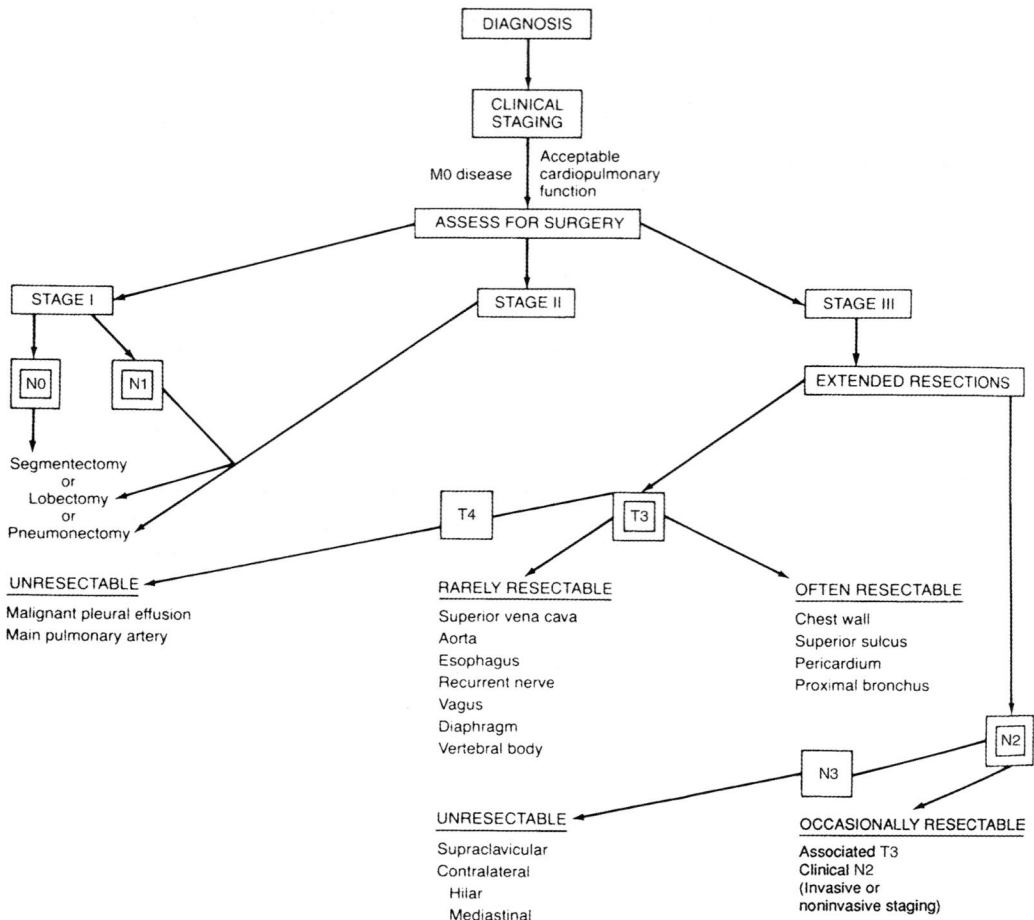

Figure 23-21. Staging of lung cancer to assess resectability. (From Lawrence PF. *Essentials of Surgical Specialties.* 3rd ed. Lippincott Williams & Wilkins; 2007.)

Preoperative Evaluation

The decision to perform elective thoracotomy with resection is based on the patient's ability to tolerate a thoracic operation. This judgment is based on an assessment of comorbid conditions (eg, age; cardiac, renal, hepatic, or neurologic conditions that may adversely affect operative risk). Cardiac reserve is evaluated by history, physical examination, ECG, and, occasionally, stress testing (Figure 23-22). Pulmonary reserve is estimated by history, physical examination, and exercise testing. Evaluation is best carried out with pulmonary function tests, measurement of arterial blood gases, and sometimes selective ventilation-perfusion scanning. Spirometry evaluates a number of components of respiration and allows for the quantification of a patient's lung function. In general, when assessing a patient's operative candidacy, the forced expiratory volume during 1 second (FEV_1) and the diffusion capacity of carbon monoxide (DLCO) are most important. FEV_1 represents the volume of air a patient can maximally exhale in 1 second after full inhalation. DLCO helps to evaluate the alveolar-capillary membrane and its function. A predicted postoperative value of less than 40% of either the FEV_1 or DLCO is considered high risk and

typically prohibitive of surgical lobectomy. Preoperative assessment of respiratory risk is outlined in Figure 23-23.

Measurement of arterial blood gases is also useful in predicting pulmonary reserve. The concentration of carbon dioxide in the blood (PCO_2) indicates the adequacy of alveolar ventilation. Carbon dioxide retention, particularly after exercise, may preclude pulmonary resection. Usually, PCO_2 greater than 50 mm Hg contraindicates resection. Interpretation of the oxygen concentration in the blood (PO_2) is more difficult. Many believe that a PO_2 of less than 50 mm Hg, or less than 90% saturation, is usually associated with such severe dysfunction that pulmonary resection is not advisable.

Aggressive perioperative management of patients who undergo thoracotomy plays a crucial role in their recovery. In addition to careful patient selection, as outlined earlier, this management involves pulmonary physiotherapy and pain control. Factors that seem to favorably influence perioperative outcomes are smoking cessation, bronchodilators, pulmonary physiotherapy, and short-term corticosteroids in patients with asthma or bronchitis. Epidural anesthesia and long-acting regional blocks like intercostal blocks greatly facilitate pain management and

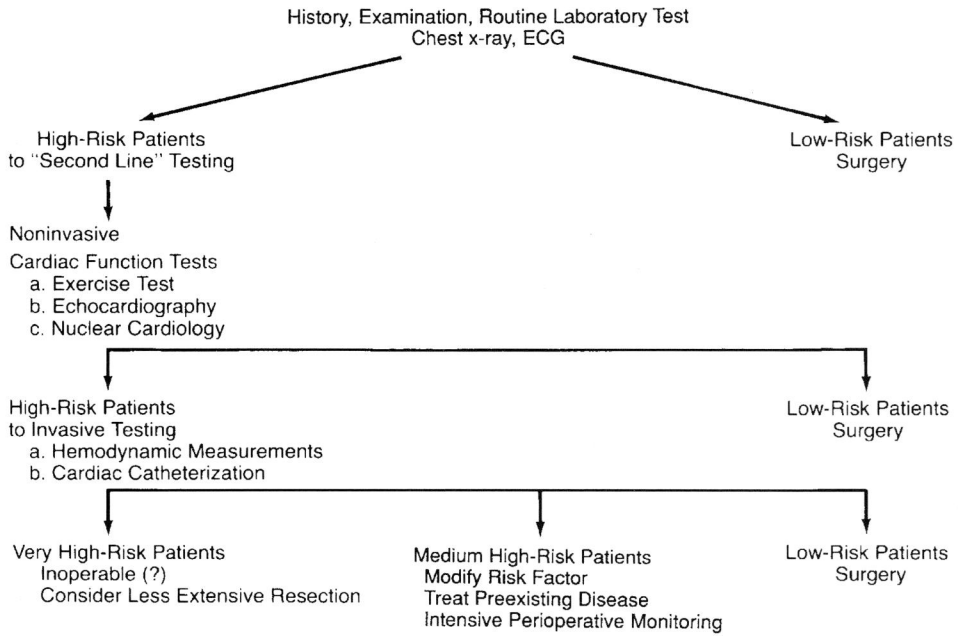

Figure 23-22. Preoperative assessment of cardiac risk. ECG, electrocardiogram. (From Lawrence PF. *Essentials of Surgical Specialties.* 3rd ed. Lippincott Williams & Wilkins; 2007.)

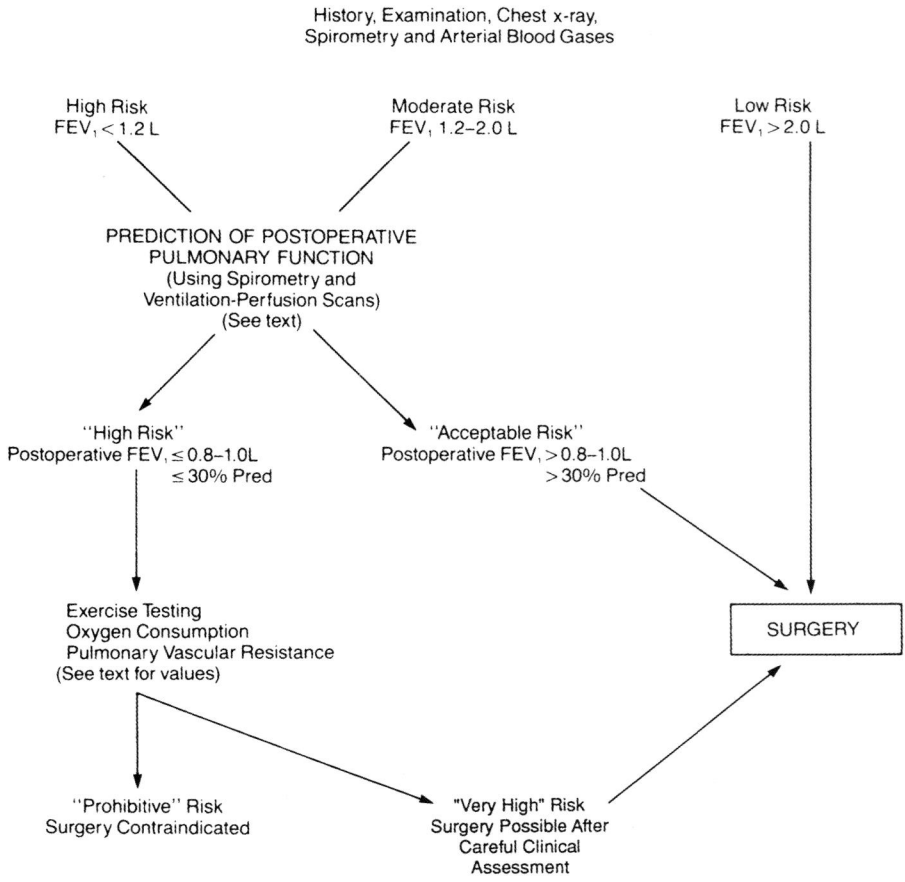

Figure 23-23. Preoperative assessment of respiratory risk. FEV_1, forced expiratory volume in 1 second. (From Lawrence PF. *Essentials of Surgical Specialties.* 3rd ed. Lippincott Williams & Wilkins; 2007.)

postoperative respiratory function in patients with thoracic conditions. These techniques are now used routinely.

Treatment

Upfront surgery is indicated after a patient is deemed operable and the tumor is deemed resectable. The vast majority of these patients have small, localized tumors less than three centimeters but upfront surgery can sometimes be indicated for tumors as large as 7 cm if they do not involve major structures. The ideal goal of surgery is the complete removal of the tumor by anatomic resection while preserving enough lung tissue to permit satisfactory respiration. Anatomic resection allows for the removal of the tumor and lung parenchyma along with its draining lymph node basins. Depending on the size and location of the tumor, this can be accomplished by removing a segment (segmentectomy), a lobe (lobectomy), or the whole lung (pneumonectomy). In some cases, it may be necessary to perform more complex operations that involve bronchoplastic reconstruction of the tracheobronchial tree.

Resection is the best treatment for patients who have localized non-small cell primary lung cancer. The risk of death at resection is 2% to 5%, depending on the extent of the resection and the age and underlying condition of the patient (Table 23-8). The long-term survival of patients who undergo pulmonary resection depends on the stage of the tumor and its cell type. In patients who have a well-differentiated squamous cell carcinoma that is completely resected, the 5-year survival rate is 60% to 70%. Patients who have more advanced or less well-differentiated tumors carry different prognoses (Table 23-9). A small number of patients have totally resectable small cell lung cancer. Accepted primary treatment for most patients with small cell carcinoma is a combination of chemotherapy and local radiation.

For patients who cannot tolerate anatomic resection, there are a number of alternative treatment options. Nonanatomic resection, or wedge resection, can be used in patients with lung function prohibitive of extensive resection. For exceptionally high-risk patients for which surgery is not an option, stereotactic beam radiation therapy (SBRT) delivers focused radiation to targeted lesions causing tumor necrosis. While this treatment modality avoids surgery altogether, it does not allow for mediastinal node dissection that typically accompanies surgical resection. Lastly,

TABLE 23-9. Analysis of Survival According to State and Histology From the Lung Cancer Study Group

Stage	Subset	Cell Type	4-y Survival Stage Subset (%)
I	T_1N_0	Squamous cell	85
		Adenocarcinoma	72
	T_1N_1	Squamous cell	80
		Adenocarcinoma	63
	T_2N_0	Squamous cell	65
		Adenocarcinoma	60
II, III		Squamous cell	37
		Adenocarcinoma	25

Postoperative mortality is excluded.
T, tumor size; N, lymph node.

immunotherapy, specifically modern tyrosine kinase inhibitors, has played an increasing role in both the neoadjuvant and adjuvant settings for advanced disease.

Common Complications After Pulmonary Resection

Postoperatively, early mobilization and full expansion of the lungs appear to favorably influence recovery. Patients require a variety of types of perioperative analgesia. Modalities that appear to help include enhanced recovery pathways, local intercostal blocks, epidural analgesia, and multimodal pain regimens. Postoperative bleeding, pneumonia, wound infection, and cardiac events are rarely seen. The most common complication after lung surgery is atelectasis. Adequate analgesia and incentive spirometry can be helpful in its prevention. About 30% of patients may develop atrial fibrillation in the postoperative period.

Newer Surgical Procedures and Techniques

Lung Reduction Surgery

Lung reduction surgery is an innovative procedure that involves the excision of a bullous portion of the lung in patients with severe emphysema. After this procedure, it is anticipated that the remaining, more normal lung will expand and that lung mechanics, including chest wall compliance, will improve, thereby palliating the severe symptoms of dyspnea. Some reported results are quite promising, but the exact indications and long-term results are still under investigation. For selected patients, lung reduction surgery is considered an alternative to lung transplantation.

Minimally Invasive Surgery

With the increasing use of minimally invasive surgery, there has been renewed interest in thoracoscopic surgery. This technique was first described in 1910. Endoscopic surgery is performed through several small incisions and transthoracic ports as a video-assisted procedure similar to laparoscopic (Figure 23-24) methods. There is markedly decreased postoperative pain and interference with respiratory mechanics. This technique has the benefit of small incisions which cause less pain and less disruption in the mechanics of respiration. Even more so, robotic-assisted

TABLE 23-8. Postoperative Mortality Rate After 2,220 Pulmonary Resections for Lung Cancer

Type of Resection and Age of Patient	Number of Resections	30-d Mortality Rate
All resections	2,220	3.7
Pneumonectomy	569	6.2
Lobectomy	1,508	2.9
Segmentectomy or wedge resection	143	1.4
60 y	847	1.3
60-69 y	920	4.1
70 y	443	7.2

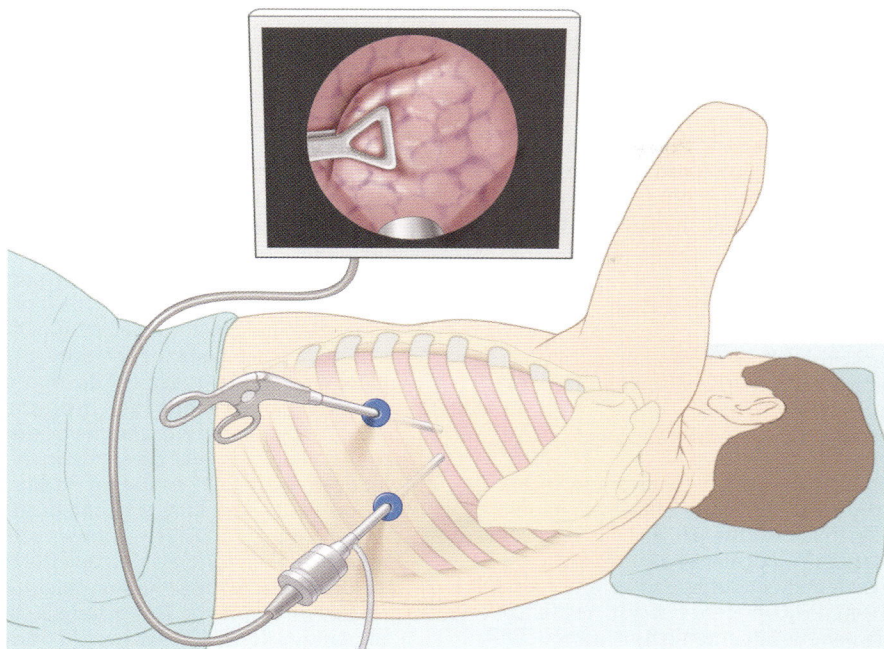

Figure 23-24. Video-assisted thoracic (thoracoscopic) biopsy of the lung.

techniques provide minimally invasive advantages similar to thoracoscopic approaches while maintaining the dexterity and accuracy of open thoracotomies. With that said, conversion to thoracotomy may still be necessary if the surgeon encounters bleeding or cannot accomplish the surgical objectives. Thoracoscopic and robotic techniques are becoming increasingly common for procedures such as:

1. Pleural diseases: Video-assisted debridement and decortication, pleurodesis, and pleural biopsy
2. Parenchymal diseases: Lung biopsy, management of spontaneous pneumothorax, and management of bullous disease
3. Pulmonary nodules: Investigation of the indeterminate solitary pulmonary nodule (if it is accessible). Definitive treatment for lung cancer is also by performing VATS lobectomies.
4. Mediastinal procedures: Investigation of primary lesions of the mediastinum (thymectomy, biopsy of mediastinal masses, excision of bronchogenic or esophageal cysts)
5. Thoracic sympathectomy for hyperhidrosis

SUGGESTED READINGS

Altorki N, Wang X, Kozono D, et al. Lobar or sublobar resection for peripheral stage IA non-small-cell lung cancer. *N Engl J Med.* 2023;388(6):489-498.

Lawton JS, Tamis-Holland JE, Bangalore S, et al. 2021 ACC/AHA/SCAI guideline for coronary artery revascularization: a report of the American College of Cardiology/American Heart Association Joint Committee on Clinical Practice guidelines. *Circulation.* 2022;145(3):e18-e114.

Lombardi JV, Hughes GC, Appoo JJ, et al. Society for Vascular Surgery (SVS) and Society of Thoracic Surgeons (STS) reporting standards for type B aortic dissections. *J Vasc Surg.* 2020;71(3):723-747.

Mack MJ, Leon MB, Thourani VH, et al. Transcatheter aortic-valve replacement with a balloon-expandable valve in low-risk patients. *N Engl J Med.* 2019;380(18):1695-1705.

Otto CM, Nishimura RA, Bonow RO, et al. 2020 ACC/AHA guideline for the management of patients with valvular heart disease: a report of the American College of Cardiology/American Heart Association joint committee on clinical practice guidelines. *Circulation.* 2021;143(5):e72-e227.

SAMPLE QUESTIONS

QUESTIONS

Choose the best answer for each question.

1. A 70-year-old woman in the critical care unit develops hypotension 2 days after being hospitalized for acute myocardial infarction. Regarding cardiac function assessment to correct her hypotension, which of the following statements is true?

A. She requires fluid bolus because her CVP is low.
B. She requires fluid bolus because her cardiac index is low and wedge pressure is low.
C. She requires fluid bolus because her cardiac index is normal and wedge pressure is high.
D. She requires fluid bolus because her cardiac index is low and wedge pressure is high.
E. She requires fluid bolus because her CVP is high.

2. A 20-year-old man involved in a motor vehicle accident presents to the emergency department having been intubated in the field. His blood pressure is 100/70 mm Hg with a heart rate of 80 beats/min. He has a right femur fracture and bruising of the left thorax. A CT scan of the thorax demonstrates a grade 1 aortic tear and pulmonary contusion and no hemothorax or pneumothorax. What would be your expected management?

A. Emergent thoracotomy and open repair of the aorta
B. Placement of a left-sided chest tube
C. Pericardiocentesis
D. Anti-impulse therapy with blood pressure and heart rate control with interval imaging to confirm no change in grade
E. Placement of a thoracic aortic endograft

3. A 38-year-old woman with no significant medical or surgical history presents to your office with general malaise and anemia over the last 2 weeks. Your examination reveals a normal-appearing woman and her general examination is unremarkable; however, you note a 20-mm Hg difference in systolic blood pressure between the left and the right arms. A CRP is sent and is found to be elevated. You plan to do more testing, but what is your presumed diagnosis at this time?

A. GCA
B. Fibromuscular dysplasia
C. Atherosclerosis
D. Aortic dissection
E. TA

4. A 40-year-old man is referred to your office after his primary care physician noted a bulge in the upper portion of the esophagus along the posterior wall on a GI report. The patient states he has been having some mild problems associated with swallowing. You suspect a vascular anomaly. Which of the following anatomic variability do you suspect?

A. A separate origin of the left vertebral of the aorta
B. The right subclavian arising distal to the left subclavian artery
C. The left common carotid originating off the innominate artery
D. The right vertebral originating off the right subclavian
E. The left subclavian originating off the aortic arch

5. Insertion of a pulmonary artery catheter can help to measure cardiac output and provide valuable information. However, complications of pulmonary artery catheters include:

A. Hemoptysis, pneumothorax, and infective endocarditis
B. Acute mitral regurgitation
C. Pyogenic pericarditis
D. Respiratory insufficiency and cardiac arrhythmias
E. Congestive heart failure

ANSWERS AND EXPLANATIONS

1. **Answer: B**

CVP measurement is not reliable in a patient with heart disease. Usually, patients who have heart failure because of chronic conditions (eg, valvular heart disease) or acute problems (eg, acute myocardial infarction) have elevated PAWP because of inadequate myocardial pump function and diminished cardiac index. However, the caution about the integration of myocardial compliance, wedge pressure, and cardiac index is often forgotten in the setting of acute cardiac dysfunction. For example, a patient who has an acute myocardial infarction, a cardiac index of 1.8 L/min/m², and a wedge pressure of 6 mm Hg is hypovolemic. This patient's edematous infarcted myocardium may require filling pressures greater than the "normal" wedge pressure of 12 to 15 mm Hg to stretch the myocardium sufficiently to generate adequate cardiac output. Conversely, another patient who has an acute myocardial infarction may have a cardiac index of 1.8 L/min/m², but a wedge pressure of 25 mm Hg. This patient is clearly in pulmonary edema and will benefit from a reduction in the filling pressures of the left ventricle to allow improved coronary perfusion of the critical areas of subendocardial myocardial muscle mass. For more information on this topic, please see section "Physiology: Cardiac Function and Its Assessment."

2. **Answer: D**

The patient has suffered from BAI. He has a type 1 tear, which is an intimal tear. This type of injury can be managed nonoperatively with heart rate and blood pressure control and serial imaging. Both an emergent thoracotomy and repair of the aorta and placement of a thoracic endograft would be inappropriate for this injury. The patient has no evidence of cardiac injury or lung injury; therefore, placement of a chest tube and pericardiocentesis would also be unnecessary. For more information on this topic, please see section "Blunt Aortic Injury."

3. **Answer: E**

This woman is suffering from TA. It is an inflammatory disorder of the aorta that typically affects women younger than 40 years. Signs and symptoms that can be associated with Takayasu are claudication of the extremities, decreased pulsation of one or both brachial arteries, and a difference of at least 10 mm Hg in systolic blood pressure between arms. CRP can be elevated in both giant cells and TA. The difference is that GCA typically occurs in women older than 50 and has signs and symptoms dissimilar to TA. Fibromuscular dysplasia can affect young women; however, it usually affects the renal arteries or carotids. This is a young woman who has no medical or surgical conditions; therefore, atherosclerosis would be unlikely to be a cause. Aortic dissection would not be a likely choice because the woman has no history or suggestion of being at high risk for a dissection. For more information on this topic, please see section "Aortitis."

4. **Answer: B**

This patient has an aberrant right subclavian artery. It is a congenital anomaly in which the aberrant right subclavian artery usually arises just distal to the left subclavian artery and crosses in the posterior portion of the mediastinum on its way to the right upper extremity. Occasionally leading to dysphagia, the course of the artery behind the esophagus is seen in 80% of these cases, between the esophagus and the trachea in 15%, and anterior to the trachea or main stem bronchus in 5%. This is not seen with the other choices described. A separate origin of the left vertebral artery off the aortic arch is incorrect. The left vertebral artery is typically identified between the origins of the left CCA and the left subclavian artery. This is noted in approximately 0.5% to 6% of individuals. A bovine arch is described as the left common carotid originating off the innominate artery. This is seen in 7% to 20% of the population. The right vertebral off the right subclavian and the left subclavian off the aortic arch represent normal anatomy. For more information on this topic, please see section "Anatomy" under the heading "Diseases of the Great Vessels."

5. **Answer: A**

The safest approach to introducing a pulmonary artery catheter is using the right internal jugular vein. The introducer can be placed under ultrasound guidance, lessening the risk of pneumothorax. Perforation of the pulmonary artery with massive hemoptysis can occur and should be used especially carefully in patients with clotting abnormalities. If the catheter is in place for more than 3 days, the risk for infectious endocarditis increases. Cardiac arrhythmias can be caused by the catheter passing through the right ventricle, but this should not increase the risk of respiratory insufficiency or cause congestive heart failure. Pyogenic myocarditis is rare and usually seen in infants or young children with sepsis. For more information on this topic, please see section "Physiology: Cardiac Function and Its Assessment."

24

Diseases of the Vascular System

James B. Alexander, Jessica Beth O'Connell, Roman Nowygrod, Matthew R. Smeds, and Peter F. Lawrence

ARTERIAL DISEASE

Anatomy

The vascular system consists of a network of branching, interconnected blood vessels that conduct the blood flow to and from the heart and throughout the body. The components of the vascular system are divided into arteries, veins, and lymphatics. These are not passive conduits but dynamic and responsive tissues that continuously interact with the blood elements and are under endocrine and neural influences. The three layers of the arterial wall are the intima, media, and adventitia (Figure 24-1). The internal elastic lamina separates the intima from the media, and the external elastic lamina separates the media from the adventitia. There are similar layers of the venous wall, although the ratio of the intima, media, and adventitia is different, so a vein wall acts more passively than the more vasoactive arterial wall.

The endothelium, which is derived from hemangioblasts, lines the inner aspect of the intima of both arteries and veins. Given the large number of blood vessels, the collective mass of endothelial cells in arteries is greater than that of the liver. The endothelial layer interacts with both cellular and soluble blood components and the dynamics of blood flow. The endothelium functions as an antithrombotic surface that expresses proteins C and S, antithrombin III, prostacyclin, thrombomodulin, heparin, and tissue plasminogen activator (tPA). Conversely, it also modulates hemostasis by contributing von Willebrand factor, thromboxane, coagulation factor V, and platelet-activating factor. Endothelial cells also generate vasoactive agents such as nitric oxide, which results in vasodilation and angiotensin converting enzyme, facilitating vasoconstriction. They also have low-density lipoprotein receptors on their surface and produce lipoprotein lipase. In addition, they are an important source of growth factors such as the so-called platelet-derived growth factor, which modulates their interactions with the cellular elements of the blood.

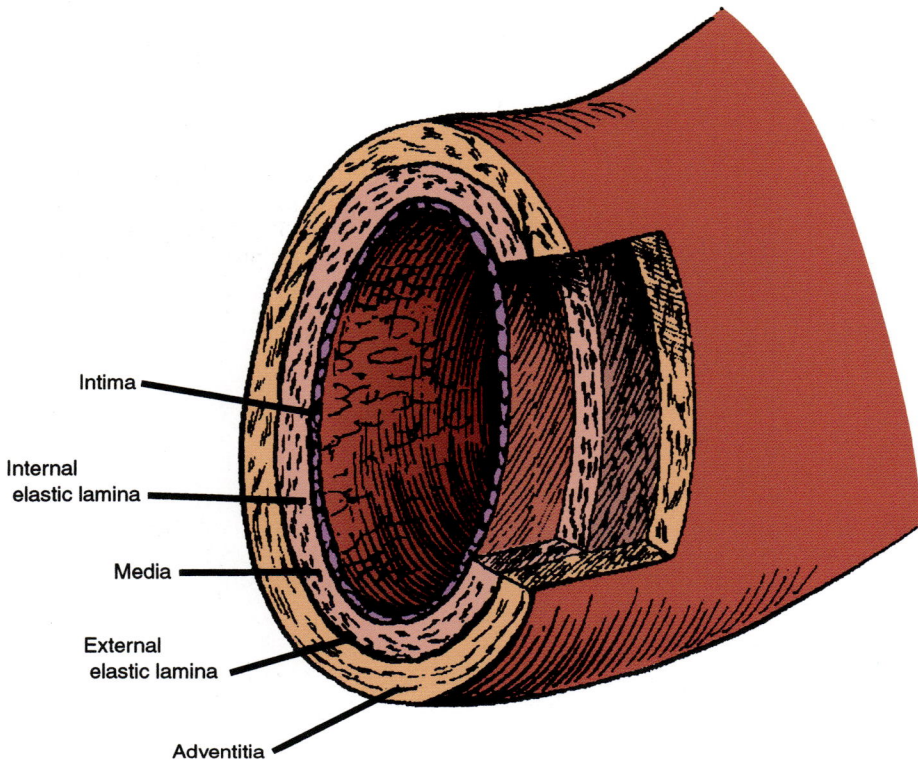

Figure 24-1. Layers of the arterial wall.

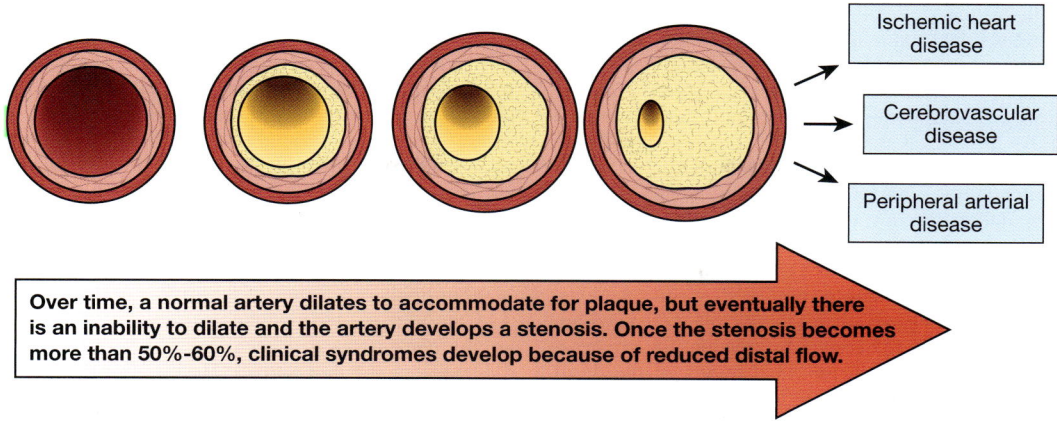

Over time, a normal artery dilates to accommodate for plaque, but eventually there is an inability to dilate and the artery develops a stenosis. Once the stenosis becomes more than 50%-60%, clinical syndromes develop because of reduced distal flow.

Figure 24-2. Time course of human atherosclerosis.

The media is the thickest layer of the arterial wall. It is composed chiefly of smooth muscle cells, along with a connective tissue matrix that includes elastin, collagen, and proteoglycans. The smooth muscle cells are predominantly aligned circumferentially around the lumen such that contraction will produce vasoconstriction and relaxation will yield dilation. The smooth muscle cells and surrounding matrix are organized into discrete bundles or lamellae. Larger vessels, which have more lamellar units stacked in cross section, have their own blood supply, from the vasa vasorum, which penetrates from the adventitia in the outer portion of the arterial wall. Arteries with fewer lamellar units, however, are oxygenated directly by diffusion of blood-borne oxygen from within the lumen.

The adventitia is the outermost layer. It extends beyond the external elastic lamina and is composed of connective tissue, fibroblasts, capillaries, and neural fibers. The adventitia is also rich in collagen. It is the site of vessel nutrition and neural innervation. Despite its thin and fragile appearance, it is important in containing hemorrhage after trauma or arterial dissection.

Atherosclerosis

The most common cause of arterial stenosis and occlusion is atherosclerosis, a degenerative disease that is characterized by endothelial cell dysfunction, inflammatory cell adhesion and infiltration, and the accumulation of cellular and matrix elements. These processes lead to the formation of fibrocellular plaques. In the end stages of the disease, advanced plaques impede blood flow (Figure 24-2) and lead to chronic ischemic syndromes of angina pectoris in the heart, intermittent claudication in the legs, and organ-specific syndromes such as renovascular hypertension (HTN). More sudden events (eg, myocardial infarction [MI], stroke, atheroembolism) are usually caused by unstable plaques that may rupture into the arterial lumen, like a volcano, causing acute thrombosis of the vessel wall at the plaque, or the material embolizing distally.

Risk factors for the development of atherosclerosis include cigarette smoking, HTN, abnormalities in cholesterol metabolism (elevated levels of low-density lipoprotein and depressed levels of high-density lipoprotein), diabetes mellitus, obesity, coagulation disorders, and regions of turbulence within the arterial circulation. It appears that smoking is a greater risk factor for peripheral atherosclerosis than for coronary atherosclerosis. The common thread is that all these factors cause inflammation and injury to the arterial wall. The Framingham Study has shown that the presence of multiple risk factors compounds the risk (Figure 24-3).

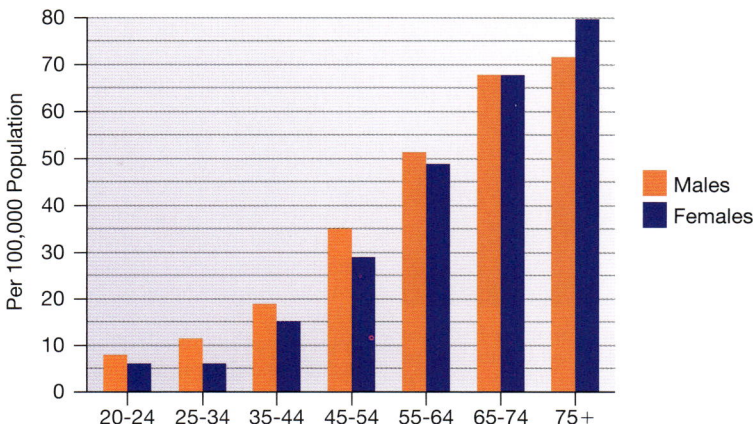

Figure 24-3. Risk factors and age. Risk factors are both modifiable and nonmodifiable. Smoking, hypertension, diabetes, lipid disorders, obesity, and a sedentary lifestyle are cumulative risk factors that increase with age.

The first signs of atherosclerosis may appear early in adolescence as lipid- and macrophage-laden fatty streaks on the endothelial surface. Although they may regress early in their development, they often progress to fibrous plaques, consisting of macrophages encapsulated by collagen and elastin. As the fibrous plaque matures, regions within the plaque become necrotic and eventually rupture, leading to plaque ulceration. Within these complex plaques, regions of microcalcification develop and can progress to significant calcium deposits.

Although atherosclerosis is usually considered a systemic disease, plaques tend to localize in specific regions. The most common sites of atherosclerotic plaques are within the coronary arteries, the carotid bifurcation, the proximal iliac arteries, and the adductor canal region of the distal superficial femoral arteries. Arterial bifurcations are also predisposed to the development of atherosclerotic plaques because of turbulence at the flow divider that results in regions of low shear stress and flow stagnation (Figure 24-4). This stasis allows greater contact time between the vessel wall and lipids and other atherogenic factors in the blood.

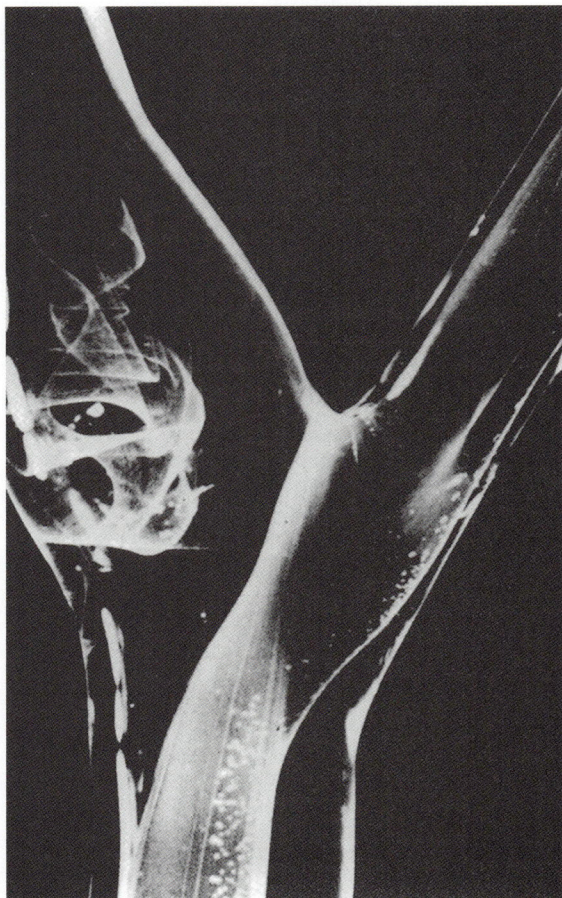

Figure 24-4. Glass model of the carotid bifurcation. Hydrogen gas bubbles show the streamlining of flow fields at the carotid flow divider and the complex counterrotating helical pattern at the arterial wall opposite the flow divider. (Reprinted from Zarins CK, Glagov S. Arterial wall pathology in atherosclerosis. In: Rutherford RB, ed. *Vascular Surgery*. 4th ed. Vol 1. WB Saunders; 1996:214. Copyright © 1996 Elsevier, with permission.)

Atherosclerosis is a progressive disease manifested by the development of symptomatic ischemic syndromes. The best way to retard its progression is to modify atherosclerotic risk factors. Programs that use a combination of risk factor modification and specific pharmacologic agents that slow the progression of atherosclerosis, such as antiplatelet agents, statins, β-blockers, antihypertensives, and nutritional modification, have been shown to dramatically reduce the frequency of cardiovascular events. Exercise has a protective effect by increasing the level of high-density lipoproteins, which enhance the transport and metabolism of other lipids.

Common sequelae of atherosclerosis are (1) MI or angina pectoris as a result of coronary atherosclerosis; (2) transient ischemic attack (TIA) or stroke as a result of carotid bifurcation atherosclerosis; and (3) lower-extremity ischemia that can cause difficulty in walking (claudication), ischemic rest pain, or gangrene. Less common clinical presentations are renal hypoperfusion caused by renal artery stenosis, small bowel ischemia due to mesenteric stenosis or occlusion, and upper extremity ischemia. The symptoms of arterial stenosis are caused by either gradual, progressive occlusion from an enlarging plaque that limits distal flow or by sudden thrombosis of the artery superimposed on an underlying plaque. Gradual stenosis of the artery may allow for the development of arterial collaterals to maintain distal perfusion, but sudden arterial occlusion does not allow for the development of collateral arterial channels and often leads to acute and severe ischemia. Plaque ulcerations often become a nidus for platelet deposition and thrombus formation, and distal embolization of this material may produce an acute occlusive event with a sudden onset of symptoms.

Aneurysms

An aneurysm is a focal dilation of an artery to more than one-and-a-half times its normal diameter. Aneurysms may be either "true" aneurysms, which include all three layers of the arterial wall, or "false" aneurysms (pseudoaneurysms), which do not include all three layers of the arterial wall. Secondary aneurysms occur due to trauma, infection, or disruption of an arterial bypass anastomosis. Many times, the outer wall or the capsule of a pseudoaneurysm is only composed of a thickened fibrous membrane. Aneurysms are also classified by their shape. A fusiform aneurysm is diffusely dilated, whereas a saccular aneurysm is an eccentric outpouching of an otherwise normal-appearing artery (Figure 24-5).

Aneurysms may occur in any location within the arterial tree but are most common in the infrarenal aorta, iliac arteries, and popliteal arteries (Table 24-1). Aneurysms also have a predilection to form at arterial branch points. It is estimated that 3% of all men older than 70 years have an aortic aneurysm, but patients with high-risk factors may have a lifetime incidence of up to 10%. Aneurysms are also a systemic disease, so a patient with one popliteal aneurysm has more than a 50% chance of having an aneurysm in the contralateral popliteal artery and a 50% chance of harboring an abdominal aortic artery (AAA). Aneurysmal formation is also often a familial disease. Approximately 20% of patients with AAA have a first-degree relative with the same disease.

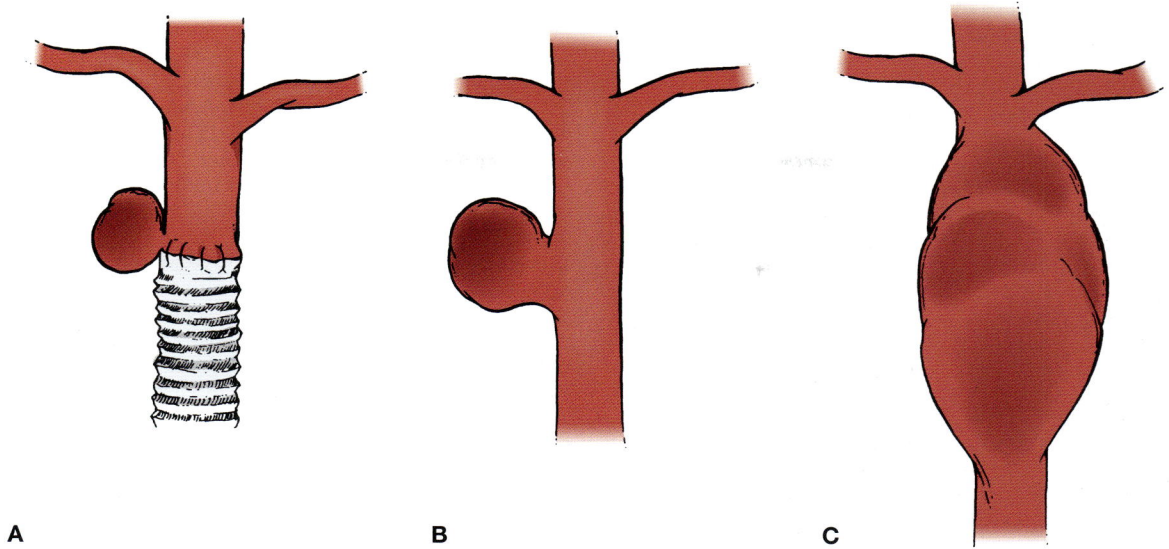

A **B** **C**

Figure 24-5. Classification of aneurysms. A. Pseudoaneurysm. B. Saccular atherosclerotic aneurysm. C. Fusiform atherosclerotic aneurysm.

The majority of aneurysms are associated with atherosclerosis. Although the precise etiology is not known, atherosclerosis may impair the diffusion of nutrients and predisposes to metalloproteinase-mediated arterial wall degeneration. Recent studies have demonstrated increased levels of matrix-metalloproteinase-2 (MMP-2) and MMP-9 in early AAA, and an abundance of MMP-9 levels in patients with larger AAA. Less common causes of aneurysm formation include connective tissue disease (Marfan syndrome, Ehlers-Danlos syndrome), infection (mycotic aneurysm), cystic medial degeneration, disruption of anastomotic connections (anastomotic pseudoaneurysm), and trauma (traumatic pseudoaneurysm) (Table 24-2).

The most serious complication of aneurysms is their propensity for enlargement and rupture. The growth rate of aneurysms is variable; although most AAAs enlarge at an average rate of approximately 0.3 cm/year, the range of expansion rates is great; some aneurysms double in size over a few years. The size of an aneurysm is important because the risk of rupture is diameter dependent. According to a modification of the law of Laplace, the larger an aneurysm grows and the thinner its wall becomes, the higher its tangential wall stress (J):

$$J = P \times r/t,$$

where P is the pressure, r is the radius, and t is the tension.

As the diameter increases at the aneurysmal portion of the artery, the velocity of the blood flow decreases, which can also result in thrombus formation along the wall. Such thrombi can embolize to the more distant arterial circulation, especially when they occur in peripheral aneurysms.

Clinical Presentation of Aneurysms

Aneurysms are often discovered as asymptomatic pulsatile masses on routine physical examination or during diagnostic tests, such as ultrasound, computed tomography (CT) scan, or MRI performed for other conditions. Approximately 20% of aneurysms cause symptoms, including pain, thrombosis, distal embolization, or rupture, which is the most life-threatening occurrence (Figure 24-6). The clinical presentation reflects the location of the aneurysm. When abdominal and thoracoabdominal aortic aneurysms rupture, they present as a clinical catastrophe with acute back pain and hemodynamic collapse. Popliteal and femoral aneurysms rarely rupture, but laminated thrombus along the wall can dislodge and embolize into the arteries of the calf and foot, causing acute arterial ischemia. This is likely due to the constant motion of the vessel during movement of the associated joint. Extracranial carotid artery aneurysms, which are relatively rare, may cause cerebrovascular ischemia, including TIA or stroke, when they embolize.

TABLE 24-1. Localization and Incidence of Abdominal Aneurysms	
Location of Aneurysm	**Incidence**
Abdominal aorta	1.5%-3.0%
Common iliac artery	20%-40% present with AAA 0.03% isolated, without AAA
Splenic artery	0.8% 60% of all splanchnic artery aneurysms
Renal artery	0.1%
Hepatic artery	0.1%
Superior mesenteric artery	0.07%
Celiac axis	0.05%

AAA, abdominal aortic aneurysm.

TABLE 24-2. Etiology of Aneurysmal Disease

Congenital
  Idiopathic
  Tuberous sclerosis
  Turner syndrome
  Poststenotic dilation (eg, aortic coarctation)

Inherited abnormalities of connective tissue
  Marfan syndrome
  Ehlers-Danlos syndrome
  Cystic medial necrosis

Dissection

Infection
  Mycotic
  Posttraumatic
  Infection of existing aneurysm

Inflammatory

Aneurysms that enlarge/rupture during pregnancy
  Splenic artery
  Mesenteric vessels
  Renal artery

Aneurysms associated with arteritis
  Takayasu disease
  Giant cell arteritis
  Polyarteritis nodosa
  Systemic lupus erythematosus

Pseudoaneurysm

Nonspecific aortic aneurysms: "atherosclerotic"

If an aneurysm is suspected, the patient should undergo a diagnostic evaluation. The best and most cost-effective screening test for most aneurysms (except for aneurysms in the thorax) is ultrasonography. A well-performed ultrasound assesses the size and general location of the aneurysm with more than 95% accuracy. If the diagnosis of AAA of significant size is established, the patient should undergo CT angiography (CTA) to evaluate the full extent of the aneurysm, its precise location (infrarenal or suprarenal), and better assess the need for intervention. In the past, most AAAs were further evaluated with invasive contrast angiography, but because of improvements in the performance and interpretation of CTAs, most patients proceed to operation without angiography. CTA is also advised for peripheral artery aneurysms to plan the arterial reconstruction.

Treatment of Aortic Aneurysms

The natural history of AAA is to enlarge and rupture; as a consequence, patients with large AAA have a greatly decreased life expectancy compared with age-matched controls. The risk of rupture is directly related to the diameter of the aneurysm; most clinical studies show that a 4-cm AAA has an annual risk of rupture of less than 1% (5-year risk of rupture is 5%-6%), but the annual rate increases to more than 10% when the AAA reaches 6 cm (Figure 24-7).

The treatment of smaller aneurysms is being carefully studied. Two studies, the United Kingdom Small Aneurysm

Trial and the VA Cooperative Small Aneurysm study, demonstrated equivalent "all-cause" mortality in patients with asymptomatic AAA between 4 and 5.5 cm, whether they were treated medically or surgically. This would indicate that men may be followed if their AAAs are asymptomatic and 5.0 to 5.5 cm. In contrast to this recommendation, women, who start with a smaller aorta, have a 4-fold increased risk of rupture in aneurysms from 5 to 5.5 cm.

Treatment of AAAs

Currently, approximately 80% of AAAs are treated with an endovascular repair, whether the procedure is elective or emergent, due to a lower periprocedural morbidity and mortality. The procedure involves placing a bifurcated prosthetic graft with wire supports that attach to the uninvolved aorta above the aneurysm and to the iliac vessels distal to the aneurysm. The graft is initially loaded into a delivery catheter and introduced from a remote access site in the common femoral artery into the infrarenal aorta and iliac arteries (Figure 24-8). The attachment to the aorta and the iliac vessels is accomplished through the outward radial force of self-expanding stents or hooks that embed in the aortic wall.

Endovascular repair of AAAs has been shown to be associated with decreased perioperative mortality, decreased blood loss, shortened hospital stays, and a more rapid return to normal activity. Recent studies have also shown decreased short-term mortality with endovascular repair (~1.5%) compared to conventional open aortic repair (~3%). Endografts with branches to the internal iliac, renal, and mesenteric arteries are used when the aneurysm involves these vessels, and they have also significantly reduced the procedural mortality.

The disadvantages of endovascular repair include the need for regular follow-up requiring annual abdominal ultrasound or CT scans, an increased rate of secondary interventions to correct problems with the fixation of the aortic graft, leakage of blood into the aortic aneurysm sac, and the risk of renal dysfunction secondary to the contrast agents used for visualization of the graft.

Elective open surgical treatment of AAAs is the traditional approach and is usually accomplished with a midline abdominal or left flank retroperitoneal incision. Although most surgeons use the anterior approach, the advantages of the retroperitoneal incision are decreased postoperative pulmonary dysfunction and ease of access to the perirenal and suprarenal aorta. It is also particularly useful for those patients who have a "hostile abdomen" secondary to previous intraperitoneal operations or inflammatory aneurysms.

During the operative approach, the normal aorta proximal to the AAA and arteries distal to the aneurysmal disease are dissected and isolated. After heparinization, the aorta is clamped, and the aneurysm is incised. A prosthetic graft is sewn in place and covered with the residual aneurysm sac (Figure 24-9). Aneurysms that involve the more proximal (suprarenal) portions of the abdominal or thoracic aorta are technically more challenging, requiring suprarenal or supraceliac clamping and reimplanting of the renal and intestinal arteries, but good results are consistently reported in modern series. The operative mortality for elective repair of an infrarenal AAA is less than 3% in good-risk patients, but a thoracoabdominal aneurysm repair has a slightly higher operative mortality.

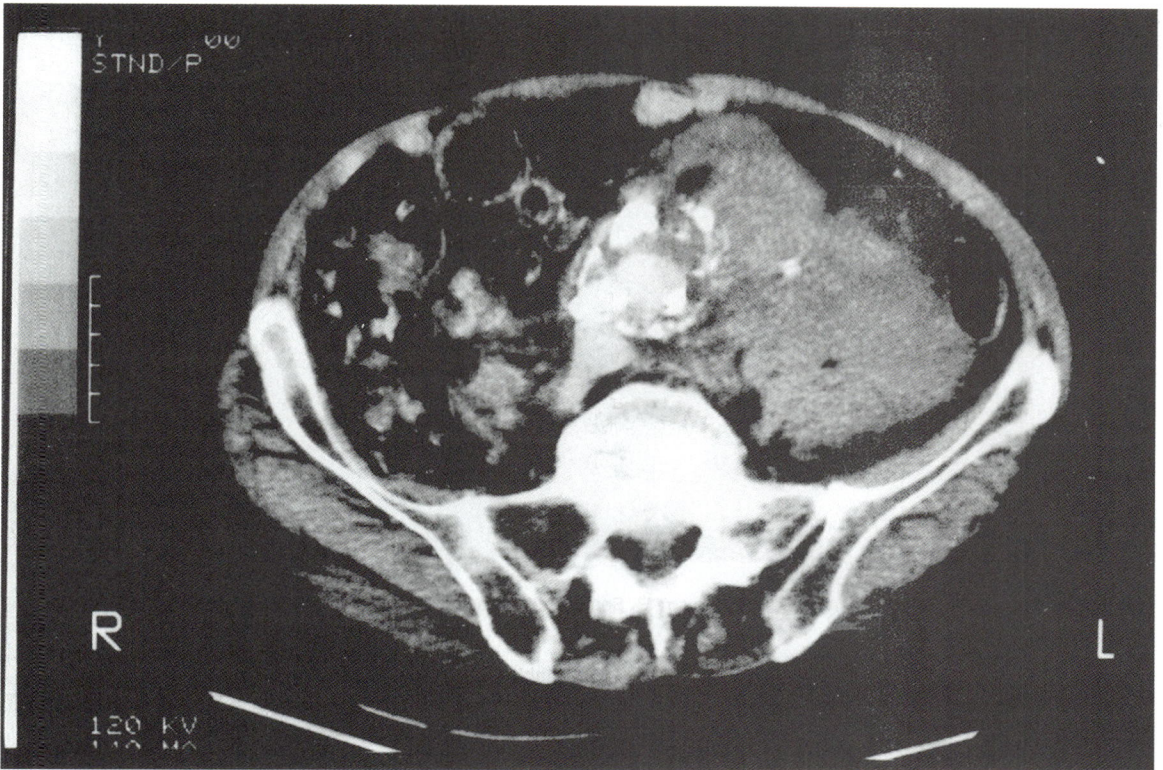

Figure 24-6. Computed tomography scan of a calcific abdominal aortic artery with a contained rupture into the left retroperitoneum.

Patients who have a rupture of an aneurysm will succumb unless they are immediately treated. Those patients with the classic triad of back pain, hypotension, and a pulsatile abdominal mass should be taken to the operating room immediately for repair. These patients should be resuscitated with blood products while being prepared for operation. The best survival is achieved with a technique of

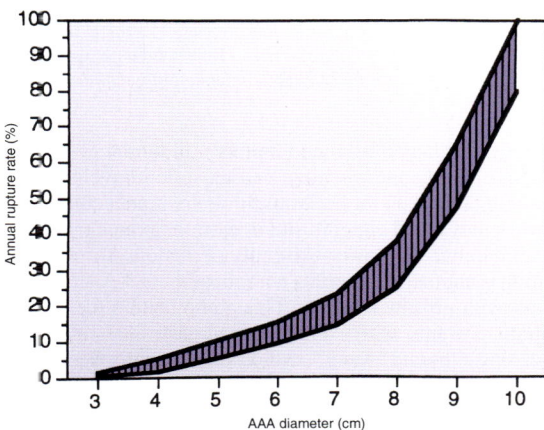

Figure 24-7. **The annual risk of aneurysm rupture according to size.** AAA, abdominal aortic artery. (Reprinted with permission from Zarins CK, Gewertz BL. Aneurysms. In: *Atlas of Vascular Surgery*. Churchill Livingstone; 1989:51.)

"permissive hypotension," with a restriction of volume resuscitation such that the blood pressure is titrated to maintain a systolic blood pressure between 70 and 80 mm Hg with monitoring of mental status and organ perfusion. This technique strives to minimize ongoing blood loss through the aortic defect. Despite advances in surgical critical care, the 30-day mortality of open ruptured aneurysm repair remains as high as 40% to 70%. Many survivors have major complications, including renal dysfunction, MI, bowel ischemia, cerebrovascular accident (CVA), and hernias. Endografts are now being used routinely to repair ruptured AAAs with a reduction in mortality to 20% to 30%, especially in those centers that perform a large number of elective AAA endografts.

Complications of Aortic Aneurysm Repair

Immediate complications after elective repair of aortic aneurysms include MI, renal failure, colonic ischemia, distal emboli, and hemorrhage. Long-term complications include aortic graft infection, aortoenteric fistula, and graft thrombosis. After aortic repair, colonic ischemia can result from the disruption of pelvic arterial collateral flow, occlusion of the inferior mesenteric artery, or perioperative hypotension. The patient with postoperative colonic ischemia usually presents with colonic emptying, bloody diarrhea, or abdominal pain. Patients who experience diarrhea immediately postoperatively, with or without blood, should undergo sigmoidoscopy to evaluate the sigmoid colon and rectum. If the colon is frankly infarcted, the affected colonic

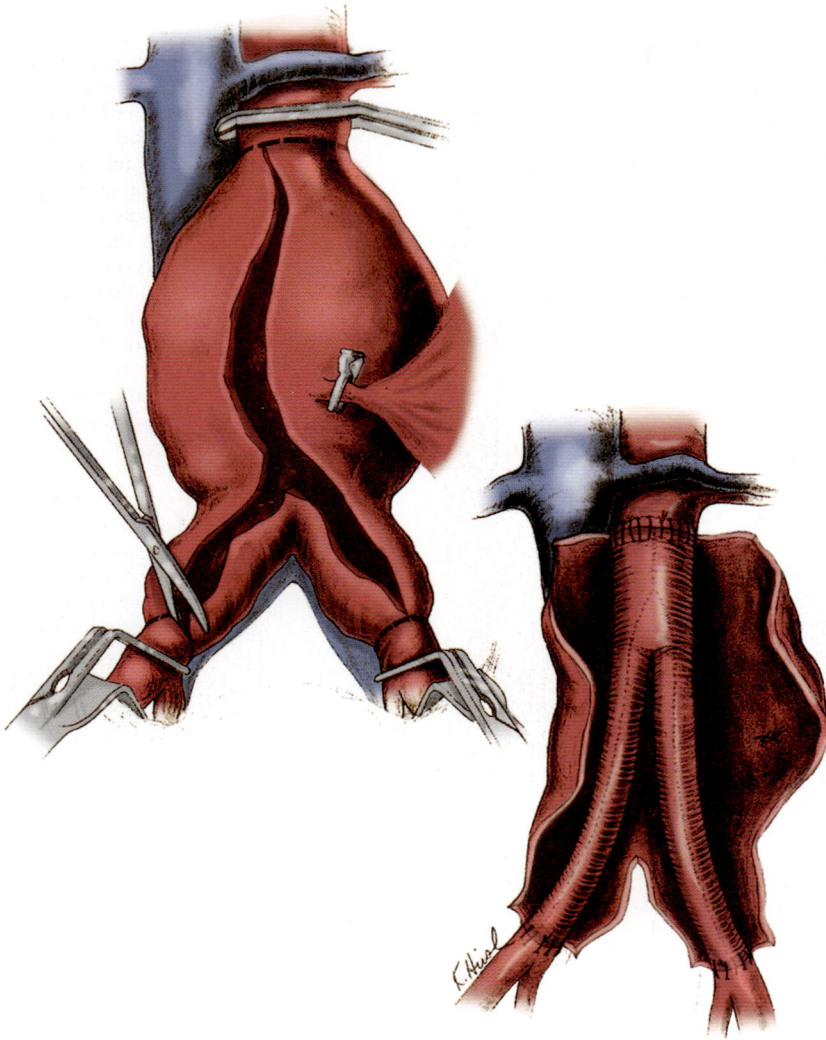

Figure 24-8. Example of an endovascular aortic stent graft. There is a main body of the graft that is implanted in the aorta just below the renal arteries and then limb extensions that are intussuscepted into the gates for extension into the iliac arteries. The distal aspect of the extension limbs comes in multiple diameter sizes to allow for the treatment of different-sized iliac arteries. (Reprinted with permission from Porrett PM, Atluri P, Karakousis GC, et al. *The Surgical Review: An Integrated Basic and Clinical Science Study Guide.* 4th ed. Wolters Kluwer; 2016.)

portion must be resected and a colostomy performed. If the colonic inner lumen appears ischemic but without frank necrosis, the patient is treated with blood pressure support and broad-spectrum antibiotics. Frequent repeat sigmoidoscopy is used to ensure that the ischemia has not progressed to frank necrosis. As with all complications, prevention is far more desirable than treatment after the fact. Colonic ischemia can be prevented by ensuring the maintenance of adequate collateral flow through patent superior mesenteric and internal iliac arteries or reimplanting a patent inferior mesenteric artery into the prosthetic graft in patients anatomically predisposed to poor colonic blood flow.

Graft infection following open repair and prosthetic graft replacement is a devastating complication with a mortality exceeding 40%. Any patient with a history of aortic graft implantation presenting with sepsis should be urgently evaluated by blood cultures, indium-111-labeled whole blood count scanning, and most definitively by CT scanning to search for perigraft fluid. Treatment consists of graft removal and either in situ or extra-anatomic bypass to restore pelvic and lower-extremity perfusion. Aortoenteric fistula is another serious late complication of AAA replacement with prosthetic grafts. This complication most commonly presents with sudden upper gastrointestinal (GI) bleeding ("herald bleed"), which may initially be limited in quantity. CT scans or bleeding scans are often inconclusive. The best diagnostic procedure is direct evaluation with upper endoscopy, using an orally placed colonoscope. Since communication generally occurs between the third portion of the duodenum and the proximal aortograft anastomosis, it is important that the endoscopist fully evaluate the entire duodenum. Endoscopic findings can vary from

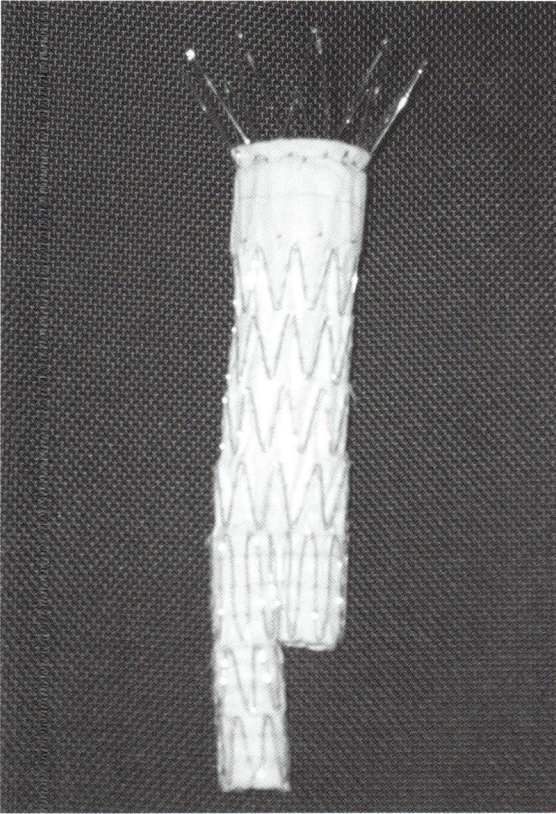

Figure 24-9. Repair of an abdominal aortic artery and a bilateral iliac artery aneurysm with an aortoiliac bypass graft. (Reprinted from Zarins CK, Gewertz BL. Aneurysms. In: Zarins CK, Gewertz BL, eds. *Atlas of Vascular Surgery*. 1st ed. Churchill Livingstone; 1989:51. Copyright © 1989 Elsevier, with permission.)

an irregular erythematous region in the third portion of the duodenum to the observation of the aortic graft through an erosion in the duodenal wall.

Prompt surgery is the procedure of choice. Treatment entails graft removal, extra-anatomic or in situ aortic graft replacement, and duodenal repair.

Endoleak is a complication associated with the endovascular repair of aortic and iliac aneurysms. An endoleak represents leakage of blood into the aneurysm sac and is classified as types I to IV. A type I endoleak represents a leak at either the proximal or distal attachment site. This is associated with a high rate of aneurysm sac expansion and rupture and should be repaired with either placement of an additional stent graft or replacement of the endovascular graft with an open repair. A type II endoleak represents persistent flow into and out of the aneurysm sac from lumbar or inferior mesenteric arteries. Generally, type II endoleaks are not treated unless there is an expansion of the aneurysm sac. Type III endoleaks occur from a disconnection between components of the stent graft or a tear in the fabric of the graft. They should be repaired when identified. A type IV endoleak is due to the diffusion of blood and serum through the graft; it generally will resolve once anticoagulation is reversed at the conclusion of the surgical procedure.

Peripheral Aneurysms

Popliteal artery aneurysms cause either distal emboli or thrombosis. Complete thrombosis of a popliteal artery aneurysm has a poor prognosis and a 50% amputation rate. The morbidity is high because a popliteal artery aneurysm often thromboses after it has showered multiple emboli to the lower extremity, thrombosing the outflow vessels. To treat this sequence, angiography and thrombolytic therapy of the outflow vessels are required before arterial reconstruction. Because of the risk of embolization and thrombosis, popliteal aneurysms should be repaired if they exceed 2 cm in diameter, if there is evidence of thrombus formation in the aneurysm, if there is distal embolization, or if there is compression of the nearby structures causing deep vein thrombosis or nerve pain. Preoperative CTA or magnetic resonance arteriography [MRA]) is essential for planning the reconstruction and/or delivery of thrombolytic (clot-dissolving) therapy to recanalize thrombosed distal vessels.

Popliteal aneurysm repair can be accomplished with either open surgery or a covered stent graft. The preferred surgical conduit is the saphenous vein graft because of its superior patency record for below-the-knee (BK) revascularization. Popliteal aneurysms can also be treated with covered stent grafts, especially in high-risk patients or in patients whose popliteal aneurysm only involves the region of the popliteal artery proximal to the knee joint. This less-invasive approach can often have excellent initial technical results, but endografts do not have long-term patency rates comparable to open repair.

Femoral artery aneurysms are less morbid than popliteal aneurysms because they embolize and thrombose less frequently. Treatment involves open interposition bypass grafting since endovascular stent grafts cover the critical profunda femoris artery and have a high risk of stent fracture and thrombosis since they cross the hip joint.

Aortic Dissection

Aortic dissection is one of the most common aortic diseases; it results from a tear in the intima, which results in pulsatile blood in the media of the aortic wall. This dissection may be due to trauma from HTN, structural changes from atherosclerosis, or other diseases such as Marfan and Ehlers-Danlos syndromes that predispose to medial degeneration and disruption. Once the tear in the aortic wall is created, the dissection can extend (or "propagate") proximally or distally as a pulsatile blood column traveling through the media of the thoracic and abdominal aorta in the "false" lumen. This creates a "double-barreled" aorta, with the false lumen often occupying 50% or more of the aortic circumference. In some cases, the origins of critical arterial branches can be compressed, with ischemia of the spinal cord, intestines, kidneys, or extremities. Preservation of flow to these critical branches must be maintained while the flow to the false lumen is closed with flow restoration to the true lumen. Dissections classically begin in the thoracic aorta and are classified as A or B by their site of origin. Stanford type A dissections involve the ascending thoracic aorta and may or may not extend into the descending thoracic aorta, whereas Stanford type B dissections begin in the descending aorta distal to the left subclavian artery and often extend into the abdominal aorta.

Most dissections present with severe acute chest pain, described by patients as "tearing." The pain is differentiated from other cardiac problems by its location, radiation, severity, and timing. Complications from an ascending aortic dissection relate to retrograde or antegrade propagation of the dissection. With retrograde dissection toward the aortic valve, the origins of the coronary arteries can be obstructed, resulting in acute myocardial ischemia. The dissection can also extend into the aortic valve leaflets and result in acute aortic valve insufficiency. The most devastating complication is the proximal extension of the dissection into the aortic root and free rupture into the pericardial sac, causing cardiac tamponade. Dissection can also extend into the brachiocephalic vessels and cause stroke. The diagnosis of aortic dissection is confirmed by transesophageal echocardiography, CT scan, or angiography. Dissections can also lead to free rupture into the thoracic or abdominal cavities.

Type A dissections are managed by emergent surgery. In contrast, many type B dissections are treated successfully by lowering blood pressure and heart rate and decreasing the velocity of left ventricular contraction (dp/dt) to reduce the stress on the arterial wall. Aortic stent grafting for type B dissection is indicated for those dissections that fail to be controlled with pharmacologic management or that compromise flow in the mesenteric, renal, or iliac arteries, producing ischemia of the respective organs. Surgery is indicated for type B lesions that form large enough aneurysms that threaten to rupture. Indeed, enlargement of a chronic dissection with aneurysm formation is the main indication for elective repair.

Peripheral Arterial Occlusive Disease

Peripheral arterial disease (PAD) is characterized by occlusions or stenoses (partial occlusions) of the arteries of the lower extremities. Specific symptoms are dictated by the number and severity of occlusions, the degree of collateralization, and the patient's tolerance to limitations in walking distance.

Stenosis or occlusion of the aorta and iliac arteries (aortoiliac occlusive disease) is more common in adults between 45 and 65 years. The predilection to aortoiliac disease is increased by cigarette smoking, HTN, and hyperlipidemia. Disease confined below the inguinal ligament is known as femoropopliteal occlusive disease. The most common site of disease is the distal superficial femoral artery (SFA) within the adductor (Hunter) canal. Femoropopliteal occlusive disease may be asymptomatic unless a patient participates in extensive exercise because collateral blood flow from the profunda femoris artery can usually provide sufficient foot and calf blood flow at rest. Involvement of the arteries below the popliteal trifurcation is called "tibial occlusive disease." Tibial occlusive disease is common in patients with diabetes, end-stage renal failure, and advanced age.

Physiology

Large atherosclerotic plaques occlude the arterial lumen, impede blood flow, and diminish blood pressure distal to the stenosis. The loss of pressure caused by a reduction in a vessel's diameter is described by Poiseuille law. While it was originally formulated for a cell-free "Newtonian" liquid and not a cellular fluid like blood in a pulsatile system, it does provide a reasonable description of the flow dynamics:

$$\Delta P = 8QL\eta/\pi r^4$$

where ΔP is change in pressure, Q is volume of blood flow, L is arterial length, η is density, and r is arterial radius.

The loss in pressure is directly proportional to the volume of blood flow and the arterial length but inversely proportional to the fourth power of the radius. Hence, a reduction in radius has the most profound effect on ΔP. In general, ΔP is small until the reduction in diameter or "stenosis" is reduced by 50% in diameter or 75% in cross-sectional area (Figure 24-10). At that point, pressure and flow past the point of narrowing decrease exponentially with greater narrowing.

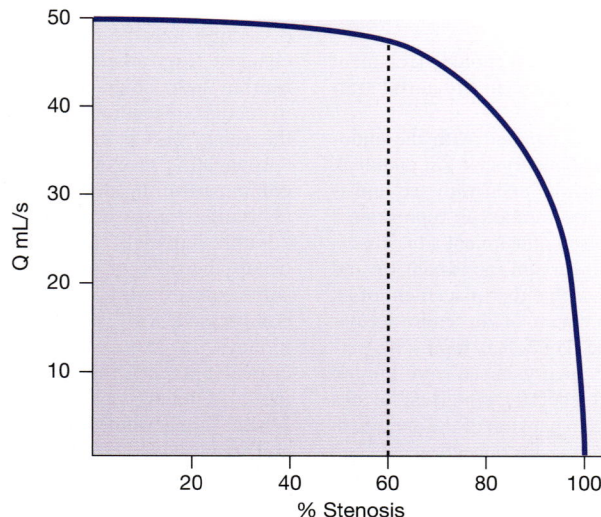

Figure 24-10. Relationship between degree of stenosis and flow. Focal accumulation of plaque occurs at sites of turbulence and reduced shear stress. When plaque forms, reduction in flow occurs only when 60% to 70% of the artery diameter is narrowed.

Enlargement of an atherosclerotic plaque is the leading cause of the development of symptoms of peripheral vascular arterial occlusive disease. Studies have shown that as a plaque grows, the vessel initially adapts and enlarges its overall diameter. Once maximal enlargement is attained, this compensation is exhausted, and the luminal area is progressively decreased by the atherosclerotic process (Figure 24-11). Other less common causes of arterial occlusive disease include Buerger disease (thromboarteritis obliterans), cystic adventitial disease, iliac endofibrosis, and compression of arteries by aberrant muscular bands (eg, popliteal artery entrapment syndrome and cervical rib).

Clinical Presentation

Ischemia of the lower extremity can progressively cause intermittent claudication, ischemic rest pain, skin ulceration, and gangrene. The degree of ischemia determines the presentation. Claudication, from the Latin *claudatio* (to limp), is characterized by reproducible pain in a major muscle group that is precipitated by exercise and relieved by rest. The joints and foot are spared because they have little muscle mass. The mechanism is straightforward; these patients maintain adequate arterial perfusion at rest, but their arterial occlusions prevent the augmentation of blood flow necessary to meet the metabolic demands of active muscles during exercise. The result is conversion to anaerobic metabolism and painful local metabolic acidosis. The muscle groups that are affected by claudication are always one level "downstream" from the level of arterial obstruction. Hence, aortoiliac occlusion classically causes Leriche syndrome, defined by impotence, lower-extremity claudication, and muscle wasting of the buttocks. Occlusion of the SFA causes calf, but not thigh,

claudication because the thigh blood supply comes from the profunda femoris artery.

The natural history of untreated claudication is frequently benign. In one landmark population study (Framingham), the risk of major amputation was only 5% within 5 years if claudication was treated conservatively. With cessation of cigarette smoking and an organized exercise program, as many as 50% of patients with claudication improve or completely resolve their symptoms. The most common cause of death in patients with claudication is the systemic manifestation of atherosclerosis, such as cardiac or cerebral events.

More profound ischemia is categorized as chronic limb-threatening ischemia (CLTI) and includes ischemic rest pain and/or tissue loss/ulceration. Patients with ischemic rest pain have pain in the toes and metatarsal heads while lying down at night. Temporary relief is achieved by dangling the legs over the side of the bed or walking. By making the feet more dependent, gravitational hydrostatic pressure increases arterial pressure and temporarily enhances oxygen delivery. Rest pain is caused by nerve ischemia of tissues that are most sensitive to hypoxia.

Ulceration of the skin of the toes, heel, or dorsum of the foot can occur as a result of advanced arterial insufficiency. Even minor trauma such as friction from an ill-fitting shoe, poor nail care, or a small break in the skin can lead to progressive ulceration in the setting of insufficient arterial flow. Ulcers caused by arterial insufficiency are usually painful, except in patients with diabetes who often have associated peripheral neuropathy. Ischemic ulcers may have a punched-out appearance and a pale or necrotic base. By comparison, ulcerations caused by venous insufficiency usually occur at the level of the medial or lateral malleolus ("gaiter zone").

Diabetic ulcerations are painless and are located on the plantar or lateral aspect of the foot, in areas of pressure. They are a direct result of the neuropathy of diabetes. Because of the injury to the autonomic, motor, and sensory nerves, the skin becomes dry, and the foot can become deformed (Charcot foot) and insensate.

The outlook for patients with rest pain or ulceration is far worse than that for patients with claudication. If untreated, nearly 50% of patients with CLTI come to amputation for intractable pain or gangrene within a short time period. Dry and wet gangrene are differentiated clinically. Dry gangrene is the mummification of the digits of the foot without associated purulent drainage or cellulitis. Wet gangrene is associated with ongoing infection. The severely ischemic foot is a nidus for the colonization and growth of bacteria and is generally malodorous with copious purulent drainage. The outlook is ominous with likely sepsis and immediate limb loss unless the necrotic tissue is removed, and the limb is revascularized. The most common cause of a major limb amputation is diabetes, and a person with diabetes with a limb amputation has a 2-year survival rate of 50%. The WiFi classification system evaluates the three components of a foot ulcer that predict healing—perfusion, infection, and ulcer depth—to determine the extent of treatment needed to avoid an amputation.

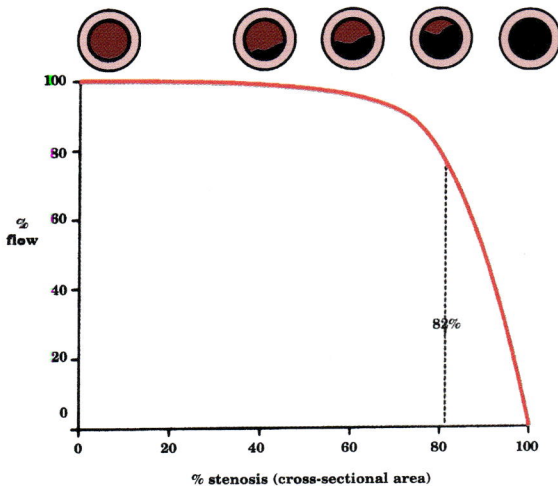

Figure 24-11. Proposed arterial adaptation to enlarging atherosclerotic plaques. Initially, the artery enlarges to maintain the luminal diameter despite the enlarging plaque. After the plaques create a stenosis of more than 40%, the artery can no longer adapt, and a luminal stenosis develops. (Rasmussen T, Clouse WD, Tonnessen BH. *Handbook of Patient Care in Vascular Diseases*. Wolters Kluwer; 2019.)

Evaluation

Routine evaluation of patients with PAD includes a thorough physical examination and noninvasive vascular testing. Inspection of the legs and feet may show loss of

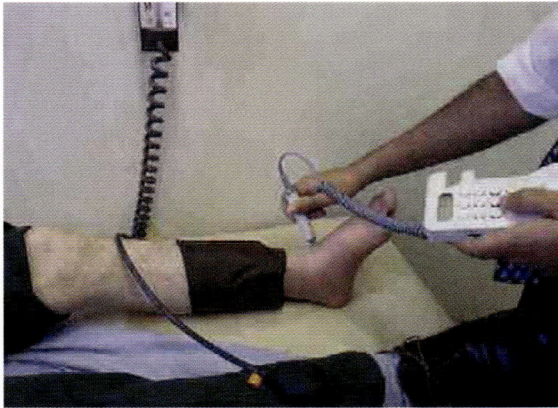

Figure 24-12. A continuous-wave handheld Doppler is an inexpensive instrument that can be used at the bedside to both grade the quality of arterial signals and measure ankle or arm arterial pressures.

hair on the distal aspect of the leg, muscle atrophy, color changes in the leg, ulcers, or gangrene. Patients with severe PAD often have dependent rubor. When the foot is dangled, pooling of oxygenated blood in the maximally dilated arteriolar bed distal to an arterial occlusion causes the foot to appear red. When the extremity is elevated, hydrostatic pressure decreases, pooled blood drains, and the foot becomes white, hence the description of dependent rubor and pallor on elevation. Intermittent claudication can be differentiated from musculoskeletal or neurogenic pain by a careful history, physical examination, and noninvasive vascular evaluation. Neurogenic lower-extremity pain is usually not located in major muscle groups and is rarely precipitated by exercise. Straight-leg raised lifts and findings of sensory examinations may be abnormal. Musculoskeletal pain is often present at rest. Pain secondary to spinal stenosis is relieved by bending forward while walking. It often radiates down the limb and is not relieved immediately by resting.

Physical examination should include an investigation of the presence and character of the arterial pulse in the groin (femoral artery), in the popliteal fossa (popliteal artery), in the dorsum of the foot (dorsalis pedis artery), and posterior to the medial malleolus (posterior tibial artery).

Patients with extremity ischemia may also be examined with continuous-wave Doppler ultrasound (Figure 24-12), which provides a qualitative assessment of the degree of stenosis (Figure 24-13).

In addition to the qualitative assessment of arteries, the systolic pressure within the arteries of the foot can be determined. A blood pressure cuff is inflated in the calf and then slowly deflated while the Doppler signal is monitored. The pressure at which a signal "reappears" is the systolic pressure within the artery. The pressure is normalized for all patients by dividing the ankle pressure by the systolic blood pressure in the arm and calculating the ankle-brachial index (ABI). The calculated ABI is a physiologic test that correlates with the extent of ischemia; an ABI greater than 0.9 is normal, an ABI less than 0.8 is consistent with claudication, and an ABI less than 0.4 is usually associated with CLTI. Patients may also be observed while walking on a treadmill; the ABI of claudicators will drop when symptoms occur, whereas patients with other causes of leg pain will not show any change in pressure measurements. Advances in ultrasound technology have also led to anatomic correlation using arterial duplex scanning. Duplex scanners can calculate the velocity of flowing blood in regions of significant stenosis, and high-velocity jets are seen as blood travels through the narrow lumen. Duplex scanning is a technique for imaging arteries and not a physiologic study.

Diagnostic Imaging in Vascular Disorders

Patients with severe lifestyle-limiting claudication, rest pain, or gangrene may undergo diagnostic MRA or CTA. Contrast arteriography, performed with a percutaneous femoral artery puncture, is only used when diagnosis is combined with a planned therapeutic procedure.

MRA and CTA do not require a puncture of an artery to obtain images. In these studies, the dye is injected into a peripheral vein, and the timing of the images is critical to obtain quality studies of the area under investigation. The contrast complications exist, though small. Gadolinium (an MRA contrast agent) may rarely cause subcutaneous fibrosis in patients with renal failure, and most CTA contrast agents may exacerbate renal insufficiency. Newer iron imaging techniques are sometimes used for patients with renal insufficiency.

Angiography involves the puncture of a peripheral artery, with the passage of an intravascular catheter for selective injection of arteries (Seldinger technique)

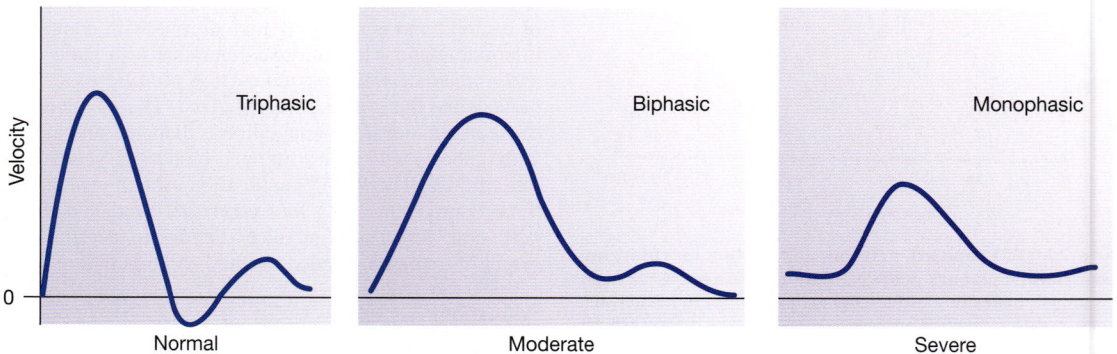

Figure 24-13. A Doppler ultrasound instrument provides an analog display of blood flow velocity (waveform). With progressive occlusion, the waveform changes from triphasic to biphasic to monophasic.

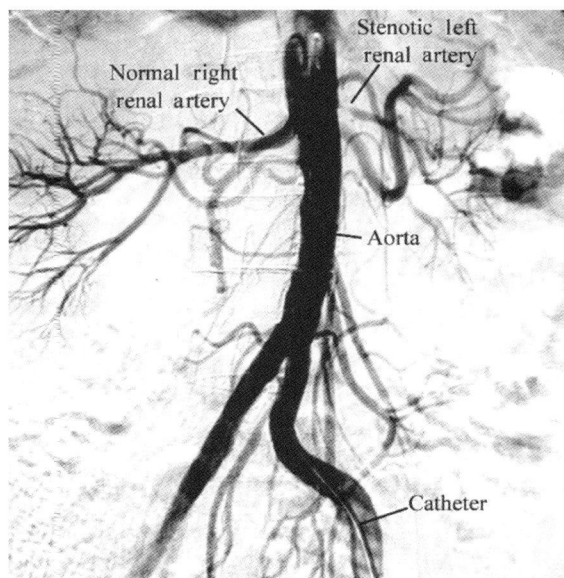

Figure 24-14. Example of an angiogram of the abdominal aorta. A proximal left renal artery stenosis is visualized.

(Figure 24-14). A needle and then a guide wire are percutaneously inserted into the femoral artery and advanced into the aorta under x-ray guidance. A catheter is then inserted over the wire into the aorta. After the removal of the wire, a liquid contrast agent is injected into the catheter. When the catheter is removed, the puncture site is either compressed manually or closed with a permanent or absorbable mechanical device.

In patients with known hypersensitivity to iodinated contrast material, steroids and antihistamines can be administered before the procedure to reduce the incidence and severity of reactions. All patients should be questioned about previous allergic reactions before CT, MR, catheter angiography, or venography is performed. Hydration before and after angiography is important in all patients, particularly in those with renal insufficiency.

Treatment of Peripheral Arterial Occlusive Disease
Medical Management
All patients with PAD require medical therapy. The leading cause of death for patients with PAD is MI; proper risk factor modification is associated with decreased cardiovascular event rates. Medical therapy includes diet modification, exercise, tobacco cessation, antiplatelet therapy, a statin (irrespective of the lipid profile), and cardiovascular risk modification including treatment of HTN, dyslipidemia, and diabetes mellitus. For patients with diabetes, a regular program of foot care (such as nail trimming, orthotic shoes, and shaving of calluses) helps prevent foot ulceration.

Endovascular Therapy
Endovascular therapy involves revascularization of stenotic or occluded lesions via a minimally invasive procedure performed inside the blood vessel with techniques such as balloon angioplasty, stenting, or atherectomy. Percutaneous transluminal angioplasty (PTA) has been used to treat short-segment stenosis of peripheral arteries since 1979 (Figure 24-15). PTA entails the passage of a small caliber wire through the region of stenosis or occlusion from a remote percutaneous puncture site. In the simplest of cases, a balloon catheter is then passed over the wire and inflated in the region of narrowing, thereby dilating the vessel and restoring its luminal diameter. This may be all that is needed, provided there is no significant dissection created at the site and no recoil of plaque resulting in residual stenosis. This approach can address short and complex long-segment stenoses and even total occlusions. Passage of the wire in between the layers of the wall, called "subintimal recanalization," can also be performed to create a new channel that can then be balloon-dilated to restore flow through the vessel without a surgical bypass.

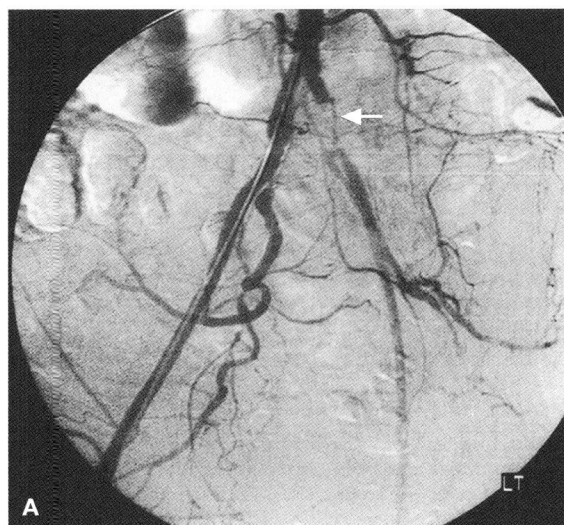

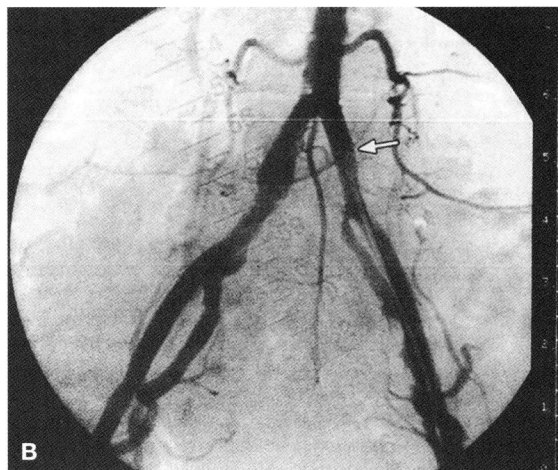

Figure 24-15. A. Angiogram showing a short-segment occlusion of the proximal left common iliac artery (arrow). **B.** Successful percutaneous balloon angioplasty of the iliac lesion (arrow).

PTA can be complicated by acute vessel occlusion, usually the result of plaque rupture or intimal disruption and dissection, restenosis caused by elastic recoil, and vessel disruption. These events generally require stenting or, less commonly, need immediate surgical intervention.

Several adjunctive techniques have improved the overall technical success of PTA. Balloon-expandable stainless-steel stents, which create high radial force, are well suited for focal calcified lesions, which often occur at major vessel origins (common iliac, renal). Self-expanding nickel-titanium (nitinol) stents offer more flexibility and range in diameter and length to accommodate lesions in long or tortuous arteries (external iliac, superficial femoral), but they provide less radial force. Most recently, drug-eluting balloons and stents coated with antineoplastic, cytotoxic, or immunosuppressant drugs have been approved, and initial studies have shown promising patency results, although systemic effects of the drugs are still being investigated. All stents are at risk for fracture, so caution must be used in placing them in areas of high flexion, such as hip or knee joints.

Atherectomy, or removal of the plaque, is an alternative to angioplasty or displacement of plaque (Figure 24-16). This debulking approach, using rotational or orbital blades or laser energy, is appealing because of its potential to re-establish maximal luminal area and limit or avoid foreign body application. Finally, covered stent grafts have begun

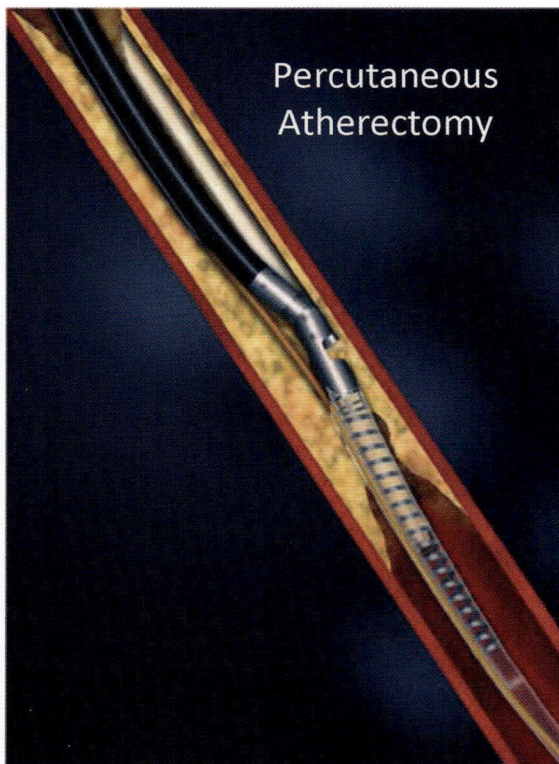

Figure 24-16. Atherectomy refers to the mechanical removal of plaque by debulking it, as opposed to compressing it against the arterial wall, which occurs with balloon angioplasty. However, atherectomy exposes the arterial flow surface to debris and has a high incidence of restenosis.

to emerge with favorable results over uncovered bare metal stents, especially in regions of previous stent placement or when the arterial lumen has renarrowed after angioplasty.

Irrespective of the approach used to open a stenotic or occluded limb artery, studies demonstrate the significant potential for restenosis. This complication of luminal diameter reduction begins at 6 months to 1 year postprocedure and is best explained as a remodeling of the artery in reaction to the trauma of the initial intervention and the development of neointimal hyperplasia. This is a complex inflammatory mechanism involving cellular proliferation, monocytic invasion, and ultimately smooth muscle cell migration and collagen deposition. Neointimal hyperplasia continues to limit the long-term efficacy of minimally invasive interventions. Multiple approaches are being studied in an attempt to inhibit neointimal hyperplasia and reduce the incidence of restenosis. These include systemic anti-inflammatory regimens, continued development and evaluation of other drug-eluting stents, bioabsorbable stents, biologic adjuncts, and brachytherapy.

Iliac interventions, which usually involve stenting as well as angioplasty, demonstrate 70% to 90% primary patency at 1 year. This success has reduced the use of open aortofemoral reconstructions in favor of this less-invasive interventional approach.

In contrast, infrainguinal interventions still remain a therapeutic challenge. SFA stenoses or occlusions can typically be treated with high initial technical success rates, but neointimal hyperplasia can occur anywhere along the vessel and lead to failure. Several approaches are utilized, including PTA/stenting, subintimal angioplasty, atherectomy, drug-eluting balloons and stents, and covered stent grafting to reduce restenosis. These interventional approaches to SFA disease may be most applicable to patients with critical limb ischemia, in whom bypass surgery may not be desirable because of other risk factors. Overall, the incidence of interval restenosis and intervention failure is between 20% and 50% at 1 year. Antiplatelet agents and statins are routinely used following any endovascular intervention to prevent acute thrombosis.

The extent of atherosclerotic disease impacts the long-term results of endovascular procedures. Longer, more extensive arterial stenoses and occlusions have been shown to reduce the long-term patency. Angioplasty of the infrapopliteal and tibial vessels is generally reserved for patients who have poor surgical risks or who have limited bypass conduit and need to heal an ischemic foot ulcer.

Surgical Management of PAD

Surgical management of PAD may include endarterectomy, bypass, or hybrid procedures that utilize these surgical procedures with endovascular components. Endarterectomy (excision of the diseased arterial wall, including the endothelium, the occluding plaque, and a portion of the media) is the standard operative treatment for carotid bifurcation atherosclerosis, but endarterectomy has more limited usefulness in the treatment of lower-extremity occlusive diseases because lower-extremity atherosclerotic disease is often extensive with no discrete starting or ending points. Few patients with aortoiliac disease are candidates for aortoiliac endarterectomy, but many surgeons use local endarterectomy of the common femoral artery and profunda femoral arteries to improve outflow for an aortcfemoral bypass graft or inflow for an infrainguinal bypass. Common femoral endarterectomy is becoming an increasingly important technique in combined approaches, when used with either iliac or SFA stenting. This hybrid approach makes the overall procedure far less invasive.

Bypass procedures are the "gold standard" treatment for PAD. Aortoiliac occlusive disease may be treated with aortcbifemoral bypass although endovascular approaches are the current method of choice for many patients. When the aortic disease is extensive and the aorta is occluded and must be bypassed, using a combination of abdominal and groin incisions, a prosthetic graft is sutured to the infrarenal aorta and tunneled through the retroperitoneum to both femoral arteries (Figure 24-17). In patients with concomitant SFA occlusion, the profunda femoris artery is the primary outflow bed. Aortofemoral bypass grafting is a durable procedure with a 5-year patency rate of greater than 90%. When aortofemoral bypass graft limb occlusion occurs, it is usually caused by the progression of distal outflow disease, which limits blood flow through the graft.

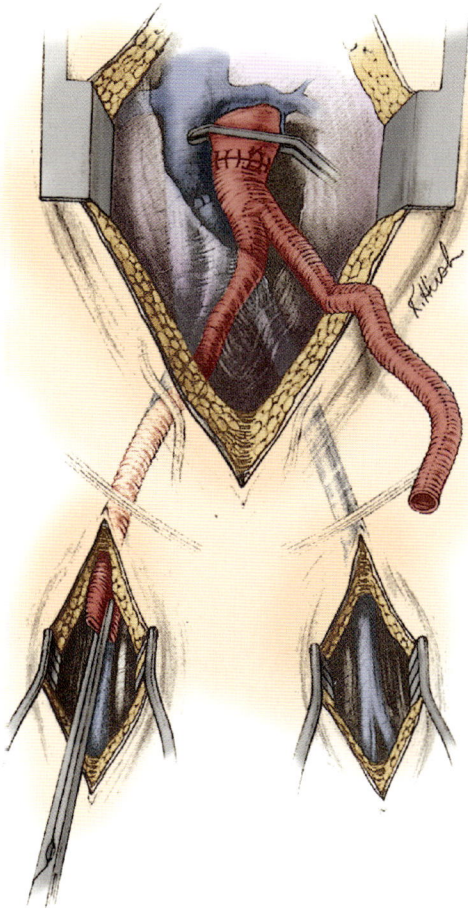

Figure 24-17. Aortobifemoral bypass graft showing the creation of the retroperitoneal tunnels to the groins. (Reprinted from Zarins CK, Gewertz BL. Aneurysms. In: Zarins CK, Gewertz BL, eds. *Atlas of Vascular Surgery*. 1st ed. Churchill Livingstone; 1989:51. Copyright © 1989 Elsevier, with permission.)

If the patient has an occluded aorta and is a prohibitive surgical risk for an intra-abdominal procedure or has had multiple intra-abdominal procedures or infections ("hostile" abdomen), extra-anatomic bypasses are considered. Extra-anatomic bypasses include axillary artery-to-femoral artery bypass grafts and femoral artery-to-femoral artery bypass grafts. These grafts typically use prosthetic conduits tunneled from one artery to the other in the subcutaneous tissue. In critically ill patients, this procedure may actually be performed with local anesthesia and intravenous (IV) sedation. The patency rates for extra-anatomic bypasses are lower than those for aortofemoral bypass grafts, but still acceptable. Occlusions typically occur because of neointimal hyperplasia at the anastomoses or because of progression of distal disease, but can also occur secondary to the longer length of the bypass graft and/or graft compression or kinking within the subcutaneous tunnels. Systemic anticoagulation is often used to improve patency.

In patients with ischemic rest pain and occluded superficial femoral arteries with proximal profunda femoral artery stenoses, opening the stenoses by profundaplasty, combined with femoral endarterectomy, can increase lower leg perfusion through collaterals and relieve most symptoms. However, if the ischemia has progressed to tissue loss or gangrene, it is unlikely that profundaplasty alone can adequately increase arterial inflow into the leg to heal the ulcerative lesions. In this case, an arterial bypass must be performed.

Patients who have infrainguinal occlusive disease can often be treated with a bypass of the occluded segment. Bypass to the popliteal artery above the knee is performed with either the patient's own (autologous) vein or a prosthetic graft; both have comparable initial results, although the autologous vein is more durable. In contrast, prosthetic bypasses to arteries below the knee function poorly, so these distal bypass procedures are best accomplished with an autologous vein (Table 24-3). Bypass grafts to the vessels in the foot are now routinely used for limb salvage.

Saphenous vein bypass grafts are harvested and either reversed, so that the venous valves are in the same direction

TABLE 24-3. Outcomes of Infrainguinal Arterial Bypasses

Graft Type	2-y Patency (%) Primary/ Secondary	4-y Patency (%) Primary/ Secondary
Above-knee femoropopliteal, PTFE	75	60
Above-knee femoropopliteal, vein	80	70
Below-knee femoropopliteal, PTFE	60	40
Below-knee femoropopliteal, vein	75-80/90	70-75/80
Femoral-tibial bypass, PTFE	30	20
Femoral-tibial bypass, vein	70-75/80-90	60-70/75-80

PTFE, polytetrafluoroethylene.

as that of arterial flow, or alternatively, in situ bypasses can be performed in which the saphenous vein is left in its normal anatomic position and the vein valves are disrupted with a valvulotome. This approach allows a better size match between the artery and the vein and can often be performed with minimal incisions. Disadvantages of in situ bypass include endothelial injury during passage of the valvulotome and the possibility of missing a valve cusp (retained valve).

In situations where an ipsilateral saphenous vein is not available, an alternative conduit must be used. The contralateral saphenous may be used if available, but caution must be taken to consider the circulation in the other leg and the potential need for its own bypass. Upper extremity veins can also be a valuable source of conduit. Cephalic and basilic veins can often be harvested and combined to create a composite or "spliced" graft long enough to accomplish a leg bypass. If no adequate venous conduit is available, a prosthetic bypass to the tibial level can still be used. Outcomes can be improved with the use of a vein patch or cuff at the distal anastomosis in an effort to improve the hemodynamics of this critical connection. In instances of toe or foot gangrene and no available autologous conduit, "CryoVein" (cryopreserved human vascular allografts or cadaver vein) or human umbilical vein can be used as alternative conduits. Patency rates are much poorer than with autologous vein, but they may remain patent long enough to heal an ulcer or amputation wound.

Immediate complications of arterial bypass graft procedures include postoperative bleeding from the anastomotic sites, graft thrombosis, wound infection, and lymphatic leakage that results in a lymphocele (lymphatic fluid collection). Because many patients with peripheral arterial occlusive disease have concomitant coronary artery disease, renal insufficiency, or pulmonary obstructive disease, other serious postoperative cardiopulmonary complications are always a concern in the postoperative period.

Postoperative duplex ultrasound surveillance of vein bypass grafts is useful in identifying anastomotic and midgraft stenoses that, if uncorrected, could lead to graft failure. The combination of duplex graft surveillance and either balloon angioplasty or surgical repair of stenotic lesions results in higher long-term patency of the saphenous vein bypass graft. The "assisted" patency rates of these vein grafts approach 90% at 2 years post bypass. In contrast, if a stenosis of a saphenous vein graft is allowed to progress to occlusion before it is revised, the patency rate at 2 years is only 30%.

In summary, lower-extremity revascularization must be individualized to each patient. Claudication can be adequately treated by risk factor modification, especially smoking cessation and structured exercise. Interventions in this setting should be justified by advanced, debilitating symptoms or critical limb ischemia that restricts daily activities or threatens an individual's livelihood. A percutaneous approach for intervention using any of the techniques described may be the most appropriate first line of treatment in this setting, reserving more invasive approaches for more advanced disease. For limb-threatening diseases such as rest pain, tissue loss, or gangrene, a bypass is often the best option. Interventional techniques in this setting should be used for patients with high surgical risk. In either case, the best long-term results require the appropriate

use of antiplatelet or anticoagulant therapy, ideal medical management of other risk factors, and vigilant surveillance with reintervention if needed.

Amputation may be the only option in some patients with severe rest pain or gangrene who are not candidates for revascularization. In general, the more distal the amputation is, the better the rehabilitation potential is, although the level of amputation depends on the extent of tissue loss and arterial inflow. Distal amputations include toe, transmetatarsal, and Syme (ankle) amputations. If arterial inflow is inadequate and an arterial bypass cannot be performed, then a below-the-knee amputation (BKA) or above-the-knee amputation (AKA) may be required.

It is important to choose the appropriate site for amputation to ensure adequate wound healing. A BKA is often the lowest level that will heal; it is important to attempt to preserve the knee joint because significantly more energy is required to ambulate with an AKA prosthesis.

AKA is required when profound ischemia and gangrene extend to the knee. At this higher amputation level, healing is likely, even in advanced ischemia. AKA amputation is also indicated in patients who are bedridden or represent a high surgical risk because of other medical conditions.

Chronic Intestinal Ischemia

The visceral arterial supply includes the celiac axis, superior mesenteric artery (SMA), and inferior mesenteric artery. If one of these visceral vessels becomes stenotic or occluded, the other two vessels, through the gastroduodenal artery and marginal artery, can supply significant collateral flow (Figure 24-18). If the gastroduodenal artery is not well developed or there is occlusion of two of the three major arterial pathways to the visceral organs, patients may experience visceral ischemic symptoms. Once two vessels are occluded, symptoms become very common.

Clinical Manifestations and Diagnosis

The clinical manifestations of chronic intestinal ischemia include postprandial abdominal pain and weight loss. Postprandial pain usually occurs within an hour after meals and ranges from a persistent epigastric ache to severe,

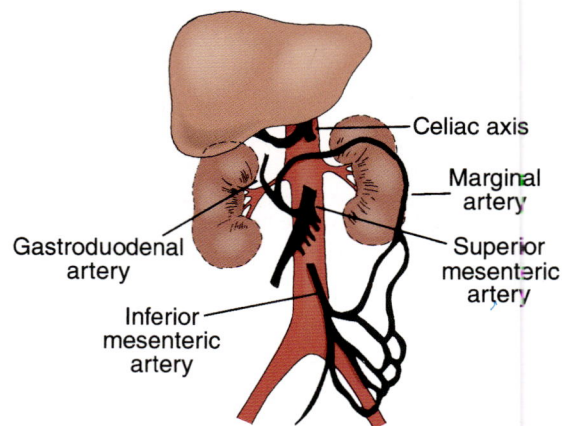

Figure 24-18. The intestinal circulation is characterized by three main vessels: the celiac axis, superior mesenteric artery, and inferior mesenteric artery. Collaterals connect these vessels so that chronic occlusion of one vessel is well compensated.

disabling, cramping pain. Many patients have a fear of food because of the intimidation of postprandial pain and limit their oral intake. This factor accounts for the significant weight loss seen in many patients. The malnutrition associated with chronic visceral ischemia can be severe and is frequently mistaken for carcinomatosis or primary visceral malignancies. Associated symptoms of systemic atherosclerotic disease are often present (eg, coronary artery disease, claudication, CVA).

The diagnosis is based on an accurate history and physical examination as well as duplex ultrasound studies, CTA, and mesenteric angiography of the visceral vessels. Noninvasive duplex scans assess the flow within the visceral vessels as well as the presence of a proximal arterial stenosis. The limitation of the duplex scan is its inability to evaluate the visceral vessels if a significant amount of bowel gas is present or if there is significant calcification in the visceral vessels. Therefore, CT or MR angiograms are the best diagnostic study. They are used to show hemodynamically significant lesions of at least two of the three major visceral vessels and evidence of collateral flow circumventing the stenotic mesenteric vessel. Catheter angiograms are used for interventions.

Treatment

Mesenteric revascularization usually provides symptomatic improvement and prevents catastrophic mesenteric infarction and should be considered in patients who have symptoms consistent with mesenteric ischemia as well as angiographic evidence of significant visceral occlusive disease.

Proximal mesenteric artery balloon angioplasty and stenting are being used much more frequently in the treatment of chronic mesenteric ischemia, for both thrombotic occlusions and pre-occlusive stenoses. Although the long-term durability of angioplasty/stenting is not quite as good as a surgical bypass (~70% PTA vs 90% surgical over 3 years), the immediate morbidity is much less, favoring the use of these techniques in older and nutritionally depleted patients.

Surgical revascularization options include endarterectomy of the proximal visceral vessels or bypass with synthetic grafts. An autogenous vein is used only when infection is a significant risk. Many experienced surgeons routinely revascularize at least two of the visceral vessels to maximize the durability of the repair. Bypass routes are either retrograde or antegrade bypass to the SMA and celiac axis. The antegrade bypass from the supraceliac aorta is preferable because of the direct course of the bypass graft and a reduced risk of kinking, but this procedure is more stressful because of the need to temporarily occlude the aorta above the celiac artery. Retrograde bypasses can originate from either the infrarenal aorta or an iliac artery but are more prone to kink when the mesentery is returned to its normal position.

Renovascular Hypertension

Renovascular HTN accounts for approximately 5% of the causes of HTN, but this disease is responsible for a disproportionately high proportion of cases of curable HTN, especially in children and young adults. Atherosclerosis is the most common cause of renal artery stenosis, but it occurs in older patients. Fibromuscular dysplasia and posttraumatic

dissections are less common causes but are, in fact, more amenable to treatment. Although most patients with renal artery stenoses are asymptomatic, these obstructive lesions may be associated with poorly controlled blood pressure (renovascular HTN) or renal insufficiency (ischemic nephropathy). Other causes of surgically correctable HTN include pheochromocytoma, aldosterone-secreting tumors, and descending thoracic aortic coarctation.

Atherosclerotic renal artery lesions usually occur in the proximal portion of the renal artery and often represent an extension of an aortic plaque into the renal artery ostium. In contrast, fibromuscular dysplasia most commonly involves the middle to distal portion of the renal artery, with sparing of the proximal aspect of the renal artery (Figure 24-19). Fibromuscular dysplasia is a hyperplastic, fibrosing process of the intima, media, or adventitia. It occurs in children (equal sex distribution) or in the second to fourth decade (more common in women). Bilateral involvement is seen in as many as 50% of cases.

Critical stenosis of the renal artery causes decreased blood pressure and flow to the kidney as well as decreased glomerular filtration. This change stimulates the renal juxtaglomerular apparatus to produce renin, which catalyzes the conversion of angiotensinogen to angiotensin I. Angiotensin converting enzyme then converts angiotensin I to angiotensin II, a potent vasoconstrictor. Angiotensin II also stimulates the production of aldosterone, causing sodium retention and increased plasma volume. This combination of vasoconstriction and sodium retention causes a hypertensive state. With the progression of bilateral renal artery stenoses, patients may have inadequate blood flow to support renal function and may develop ischemic nephropathy.

Most untreated patients have profound diastolic HTN, with diastolic pressures occasionally exceeding 120 mm Hg. An epigastric or flank bruit may be noted on auscultation of the abdomen and suggests turbulent flow within the renal artery.

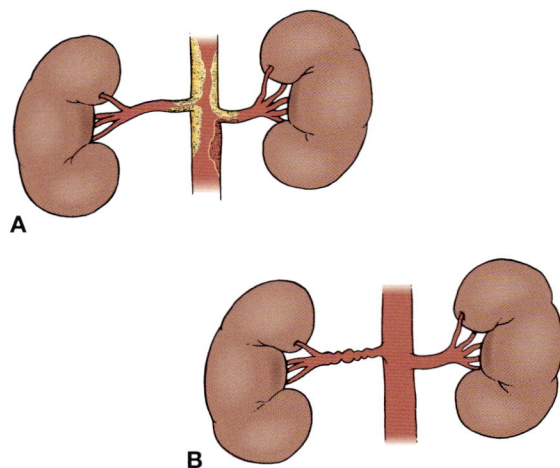

Figure 24-19. A. Stenotic lesions of the renal artery cause hypoperfusion of the kidney and activation of the renin-angiotensin system. As a result, significant hypertension occurs. Atherosclerotic lesions usually involve the origin to the middle portion of the renal artery. B. Fibromuscular hyperplasia involves the middle to distal portion of the renal artery.

Diagnosis

Renal artery stenosis should be suspected with the onset of HTN in patients younger than 35, worsening of previously well-controlled blood pressure, uncontrolled HTN despite three or more antihypertensive medications, flash pulmonary edema, or severe HTN with a rapid decline in renal function. For patients with suspected renal artery stenosis, screening studies include renal duplex scan, renal function studies, and CT or MR angiography.

Renal duplex ultrasonography can assess the flow velocity profile in both renal arteries and the juxtarenal aorta. A significant difference in renal artery velocities (renal artery-to-aorta ratio >3.5) suggests the presence of a hemodynamically significant renal artery stenosis. The duplex scan can also determine the renal parenchymal size and assess whether one of the kidneys is atrophying as a result of ischemia. With an experienced technologist, the sensitivity and specificity of renal artery duplex ultrasonography for detecting significant renal artery stenosis are greater than 90%.

A functional test for renovascular HTN is the captopril challenge test. Captopril, an angiotensin II–converting enzyme inhibitor, prevents the conversion of angiotensin I to angiotensin II. Because of the blockage of synthesis of angiotensin II, more renin is produced, and plasma renin levels are elevated after captopril administration. A positive captopril test also leads to a decrease in the glomerular filtration rate because of the blockage of the effect of angiotensin II on the efferent arteriole of the renal glomeruli. Without the vasoconstriction of the efferent renal arteriolar bed, there is decreased outflow resistance and less of a pressure gradient to allow for renal filtration.

CT or MR angiography can reliably detect renal artery stenosis. Unfortunately, a CT scan is associated with the use of potentially nephrotoxic IV contrast agents that can worsen renal function, and MR angiography does not identify calcium and may overestimate the severity of stenosis. Also, these studies are expensive to use as screening tools. Catheter renal arteriography not only detects renal artery stenoses but also assists in determining kidney size by evaluating the postinjection nephrogram. At the time of renal angiography, a pressure gradient can be measured using a pressure sensing wire or a small catheter that is attached to a pressure monitor and withdrawn across the region of suspected stenosis. A pressure gradient greater than 10 mm Hg is consistent with a significant renal artery stenosis.

Treatment

In young patients with fibromuscular dysplasia, antihypertensive medications are often ineffective in controlling severe renovascular HTN. For example, angiotensin II–converting enzyme inhibitors, usually very effective drugs for HTN, should be avoided in cases of bilateral renal artery stenoses because these drugs decrease glomerular filtration by altering postglomerular capillary tone. In the worst circumstances, they may cause acute renal failure.

In patients with severe HTN and hemodynamically significant renal artery stenoses, renal revascularization should be considered. Fibromuscular dysplasia responds exceptionally well to percutaneous transluminal balloon angioplasty without stenting in all age groups. Current experience with fibromuscular disease in pediatric patients and young adults suggests that more than 95% of patients are cured or significantly improved with renal artery angioplasty. Atherosclerotic lesions of the proximal renal artery are most frequently treated with both angioplasty and stenting because angioplasty alone is associated with a high rate of restenosis. Unfortunately, few patients are cured of their HTN after angioplasty/stenting for atherosclerotic renal artery stenosis, although a significant portion may have improved blood pressure control. The procedure may be complicated by worsening renal function from contrast nephrotoxicity or atheroembolism. Many vascular specialists recommend angioplasty/stenting as the initial method of treatment for renal artery stenosis. Open surgical revascularization is reserved for those patients who fail endovascular intervention. A recent study comparing revascularization to medical therapy suggested limiting revascularization to a very selective group of patients.

Surgical treatment for renal vascular HTN is performed in patients who have recurrent stenosis after angioplasty. It is also performed when lesions are not correctable with angioplasty. Surgical interventions include endarterectomy of the atherosclerotic lesions and bypass to the renal artery from the aorta, iliac, hepatic, or splenic arteries.

Acute Arterial Occlusion

Acute occlusion of an extremity or visceral vessel can cause limb, intestinal, or life-threatening ischemia. Etiologies of acute arterial occlusion include in situ thrombosis of preexisting atherosclerotic occlusive disease, arterial emboli from another site, penetrating and blunt trauma, and thrombosis of a preexisting arterial aneurysm. Patients with preexisting arterial occlusive disease may have a history of claudication or intestinal angina before arterial thrombosis occurs. These patients may already have a well-developed collateral bed and may therefore develop less acute symptoms. In contrast, patients with arterial emboli, vascular trauma, or thrombosis of a preexisting aneurysm are usually asymptomatic before the arterial occlusion occurs and may have more profound ischemic symptoms.

Clinical Manifestations and Diagnosis

The classic presentation of limb-threatening acute arterial occlusion includes the "six Ps": *p*allor, *p*ain, *p*aresthesia, *p*aralysis, *p*ulselessness, and *p*oikilothermia (change in temperature). These changes are limited to the area distal to the region of acute arterial occlusion. For example, with femoral artery occlusion, the ischemic changes occur in the distal ipsilateral limb. The great majority (80%) of arterial emboli originate in the left side of the heart. Thrombi form in the left atrium in patients with atrial fibrillation and in hypokinetic regions of previous MI. Mural thrombi within thoracic, abdominal aortic, and popliteal aneurysms can also cause distal embolization. These thrombi can dislodge and embolize to the peripheral circulation, often lodging at sites of abrupt reduction of luminal caliber, such as arterial bifurcations or branches. Nonthrombotic emboli can also occur from detached fragments of atherosclerotic lesions of the aorta and aortic valve. The most common site of embolic occlusion is the femoral artery. Other common sites are the axillary, popliteal, and iliac arteries, the aortic bifurcation, and the mesenteric vessels.

Acute mesenteric ischemia results from arterial occlusion (embolus or thrombosis), mesenteric venous occlusion, or nonocclusive mesenteric ischemia (especially vasospasm). Presenting symptoms may include abdominal pain out of proportion to the examination, diarrhea, and bloody stools. Embolization to the SMA accounts for approximately 50% of all cases of acute mesenteric ischemia; 25% of cases occur secondary to the thrombosis of a preexisting atherosclerotic lesion. Most emboli to the SMA lodge just distal to the origin of the middle colic artery, approximately 5 to 10 cm from the origin of the SMA (Figure 24-20). Nonocclusive mesenteric ischemia accounts for an additional 25% of cases of acute mesenteric ischemia. The etiology of nonocclusive mesenteric ischemia is multifactorial but usually involves moderate to severe mesenteric atherosclerotic lesions in association with a low cardiac output state or the administration of vasoconstricting medications, such as digitalis.

Acute mesenteric venous occlusion usually involves the superior mesenteric vein and its branches. It is an infrequent but life-threatening condition generally in patients with portal HTN or hypercoagulability, and in older patients with a history of poor oral intake and dehydration. It presents as acute abdominal pain, with early lab values pointing toward intestinal ischemia. Diagnosis is aided by a CT scan with IV contrast, which shows the thrombus within the mesenteric veins, as well as a thickened bowel wall.

Treatment

Treatment of acute mesenteric venous thrombosis is anticoagulation; prompt surgery with venous thrombectomy is performed only for an acute abdomen; if the bowel is viable, continued systemic anticoagulation with heparin and a second-look surgery within 24 hours to assess bowel viability is recommended.

Irrespective of the arterial bed involved, patients with acute arterial occlusion require rapid evaluation and diagnosis to prevent limb-, bowel-, or life-threatening ischemia. Immediate anticoagulation with IV heparin is administered

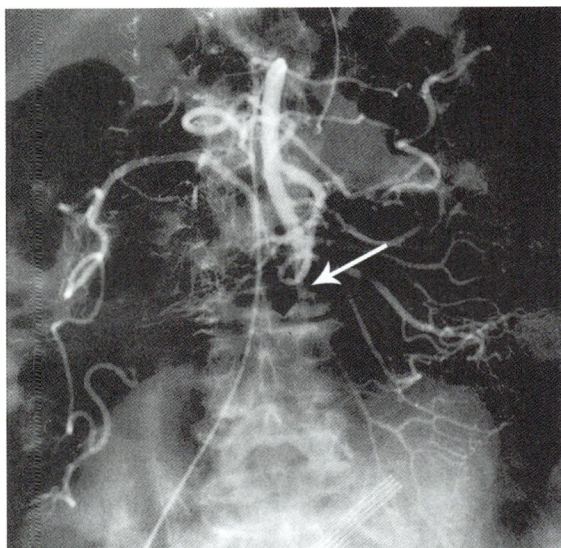

Figure 24-20. Acute embolus of the proximal superior mesenteric artery (arrow).

to prevent further propagation of the thrombus, but heparin does not lyse existing clots. Contraindications to anticoagulation include a history of GI bleeding, a new neurologic deficit, head injury, ongoing sites of active bleeding, and antibodies to heparin. Aggressive fluid resuscitation and correction of ongoing systemic acidosis should be performed. Patients who are in critical condition may require inotropic cardiac support. Interventions should not be significantly delayed, allowing for correction of the acidosis because the ongoing ischemia is usually the primary contributor to the acid-base disturbance.

In cases of limb-threatening ischemia (with motor deficits), immediate surgical thrombectomy or embolectomy is performed. Preoperative arteriography may be of benefit in patients who have a history of arterial occlusive disease to determine the sites of potential bypass. In contrast, in previously normal patients with sudden acute ischemia, arteriograms should be avoided, and immediate surgical revascularization performed, with the exploration based on the level at which pulses are absent. More recently, some have advocated thrombolysis as first-line therapy. Patients with acute mesenteric ischemia should likewise undergo emergent revascularization of the occluded vessel to prevent intestinal necrosis. There is less evidence for thrombolysis in these patients.

The surgical approach is directed toward rapidly reperfusing the threatened extremity or organ. Reperfusion can be accomplished by embolectomy, endarterectomy, or surgical bypass depending on the extent/etiology of the disease, limb or organ ischemia, and success or failure of the techniques used. The results of revascularization are variable and depend on the extent of the occlusive disease and the duration of ischemia. In embolic occlusion, embolectomy is performed through peripheral vessels with specialized balloon-tipped catheters. Complete thrombectomy is performed both proximally and distally. Distal thrombectomy is essential because nearly one-third of patients with arterial occlusions have additional thrombus past the point of occlusion. Pathologic evaluation should be performed of all emboli, especially in the absence of atrial fibrillation, to ensure that the embolus is not of malignant origin.

After extremity or organ revascularization, the reperfused organ is examined to determine the extent of tissue damage and the potential for edema. If there is lengthy extremity ischemia (>4-6 hours), fasciotomy is often required to decompress the muscular compartments and prevent compression of the arteries, nerves, and veins (ie, compartment syndrome).

Unfortunately, the mortality rate from acute arterial occlusion is relatively high. This high rate is related to the advanced age of the patient population as well as to comorbid factors such as severe myocardial disease. In the case of embolic arterial occlusion, postoperative long-term anticoagulation must be considered because one-third of patients have recurrent emboli within 30 days if not anticoagulated.

In patients who have acute arterial occlusion but present prior to profound ischemia, thrombolytic therapy has become a first-line treatment if possible. The goal of thrombolysis is to reperfuse the limb or organ gradually, causing fewer systemic effects. It also spares the patient a surgical procedure with the attendant complications. This approach requires arterial cannulation of the area proximal to the area of occlusion and the administration of a thrombolytic agent such as tPA. If therapy is unsuccessful or if there are signs of progressive critical ischemia, thrombolytic therapy is aborted and surgical revascularization is performed.

In any acute arterial occlusion involving the extremities, systemic ischemia-reperfusion syndrome may be expected. It is characterized by compartment syndrome, hyperkalemia, metabolic acidosis, myoglobinuria, and renal and pulmonary insufficiency. Vigorous hydration, alkalinization of the urine by IV route, and fascial decompression are all important treatments in this setting. Regardless of the surgical or endovascular treatment used, all patients with acute limb or mesenteric ischemia should be anticoagulated postoperatively unless contraindicated.

Cerebrovascular Insufficiency

Arterial cerebrovascular insufficiency can result from occlusive, ulcerative, or aneurysmal disease of the carotid or vertebral arteries. The most devastating complication of cerebrovascular insufficiency is stroke. Stroke is the fifth leading cause of death in North America and the leading cause of long-term disability. Every year, more than 795,000 new strokes and 129,000 stroke-related deaths occur. The medical cost of managing patients after stroke is estimated at $40 billion per year.

Strokes are caused by infarction or hemorrhage within the cerebral hemispheres. Approximately one-third of strokes are caused by embolism from atherosclerotic plaques in the carotid arteries of the neck. Although medical management, including antihypertensive, hypocholesterolemic, and antiplatelet agents, may help prevent carotid atheroembolism, the most effective strategy is either removal of the plaque through carotid endarterectomy (CEA) or carotid stenting.

Blood reaches the brain through the paired carotid and vertebral arteries (Figure 24-21). The right and left carotid arteries originate from the innominate artery and the aortic arch, respectively. The vertebral arteries arise from the proximal portions of the subclavian arteries. The common carotid arteries in the neck bifurcate into the external carotid arteries (which supply the muscles of the face) and the internal carotid arteries. The internal carotid arteries have no branches in the neck, but they enter the petrous portion of the skull and give rise to the ophthalmic artery of the eye and the anterior and middle cerebral arteries that serve the cerebral cortex. The paired vertebral arteries form a single blood vessel within the brainstem (basilar artery) and then give rise to the posterior cerebral arteries and the arteries of the cerebellum. The arteries of the anterior and posterior circulation are part of a rich collateral network of vessels (circle of Willis) that is composed of the P1 segments of the posterior cerebral arteries, the posterior communicating arteries, the A1 segments of the anterior cerebral arteries, and the anterior communicating artery. Theoretically, an intact circle of Willis allows cerebral perfusion to be maintained in the face of occlusion or stenosis of one or more of the main branches. Unfortunately, this collateral network is complete in less than 25% of people.

Approximately 15% of the cardiac output is directed to maintain cerebral perfusion. The resting total cerebral blood flow is 100 mL/min/100 g brain matter, with as much as 50 to 60 mL/min/100 g directed to the more cellular gray matter and 20 mL/min/100 g to the less cellular white matter. Cerebral ischemia can result once the

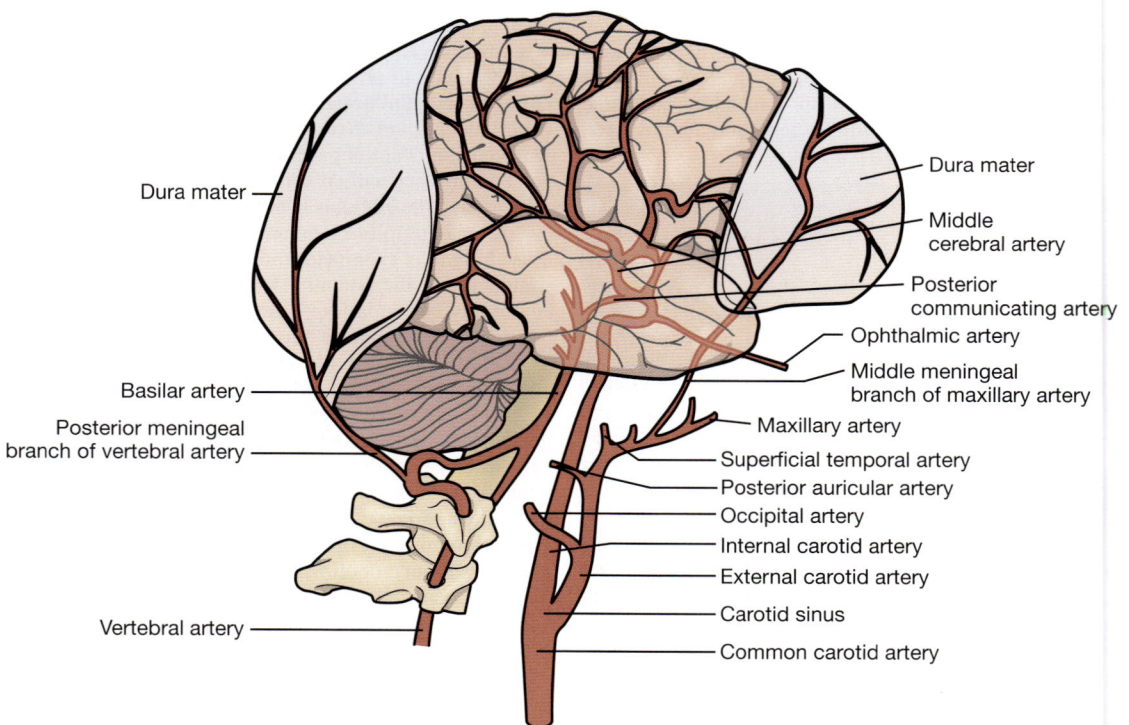

Figure 24-21. The cerebrovascular anatomy has multiple interconnecting arteries, although the circle of Willis is complete in only 25% of patients. Occlusion of one vessel may not lead to cerebral ischemia if the other vessels are patent.

total perfusion is less than 18 mL/min/100 g brain matter. Cerebral infarction can occur after the cerebral perfusion decreases to less than 8 mL/min/100 g.

A number of mechanisms maintain cerebral blood flow in the face of systemic hypotension or fixed lesions in the carotid and vertebral arteries and intracerebral branches. Baroreceptors located at the carotid sinus sample and regulate blood pressure and heart rate. Further, cerebral vessels dilate in response to decreased perfusion pressure (autoregulation). This change is probably mediated by local receptors in the vascular smooth muscle and by autoregulatory autacoids (eg, nitric oxide).

Although cerebral ischemia occasionally results from systemically induced decreased blood flow, atheroembolism is by far the most common cause of cerebral infarction. Cerebral embolism may originate from any source between the left atrium and cerebral arteries, including the atrial appendage, left ventricle, aortic valve, aortic arch, carotid bifurcation, carotid siphon, or small vessel intracranial disease. The most common source of emboli is an atherosclerotic lesion at the carotid bifurcation. Experimental models show that the carotid bifurcation contains areas of low and oscillatory shear stress. This finding may account for the transfer of circulating lipids to predisposed segments of the carotid bifurcation and the development of occlusive plaques. Like any lesion in the body, most plaques are eventually covered with a fibrous cap, or scar, and separated from the circulation. Occasionally, however, the fibrous cap is disrupted, allowing embolism of exposed plaque elements or laminated thrombus. Less common causes of carotid arterial occlusive disease include fibromuscular dysplasia, Takayasu arteritis, arterial dissection, and trauma.

Hypoperfusion can cause neurologic deficits in the watershed areas between the perfused territories of the main cerebral arteries, where collateral flow is marginal. Sudden thrombosis of the carotid artery can cause massive cerebral infarction or may be asymptomatic if there is adequate collateral circulation from the contralateral carotid artery and the basilar artery (silent occlusion).

Clinical Presentation

Symptoms of cerebral vascular insufficiency are classified according to the location of the deficit, its duration, and the presence of cerebral infarction. These symptoms can be either transient or permanent. Amaurosis fugax (fleeting blindness) is a transient monocular blindness ipsilateral to the carotid stenosis that is caused by emboli to the ophthalmic artery. Classically, amaurosis fugax is described as a curtain of blindness being pulled down from superior to inferior and involving the eye ipsilateral to the carotid lesion. TIAs are short lived, with often repetitive changes in mentation, vision, or sensorimotor function that are completely reversed within 24 hours. Most TIAs last only a few minutes before they resolve completely. Because TIAs often involve the middle cerebral artery distribution, patients often have arm, leg, and facial weakness contralateral to the carotid stenosis. Patients may also have expressive or receptive aphasias (difficulty speaking or understanding others). A stroke in evolution is a rapid progressive worsening of a neurologic deficit. A cerebral infarction, or CVA, is a permanent neurologic deficit, or stroke. Cerebral CT scan or MRI of a patient who had a stroke shows a region of nonviable cerebral tissue. MRI diffusion–weighted imaging is generally the most sensitive in detecting cerebral infarction. Atherosclerotic carotid artery disease is not the only etiology of these clinical presentations. TIAs are also caused by migraines, seizure disorders, brain tumors, intracranial aneurysms, and arteriovenous malformations (AVMs).

The severity of the neurologic deficit is determined by the volume and location of the ischemic area of the brain. The most commonly involved area is the perfused territory of the middle cerebral artery (parietal lobe), which is the main outflow vessel of the carotid artery. Hypoperfusion of the middle cerebral artery causes contralateral hemiparesis or hemiplegia and, occasionally, paralysis of the contralateral lower part of the face (central seventh nerve paralysis). Difficulty with speech (aphasia) is noted if the dominant hemisphere is involved. The left hemisphere is dominant in nearly all right-handed people and most left-handed people.

Patients with ischemia of the brain tissue that is supplied by the anterior cerebral artery have contralateral monoplegia that is usually more severe in the lower extremity. Posterior cerebral artery ischemia is usually related to the obstruction of both vertebral arteries or the basilar artery. Dizziness or syncope may be accompanied by visual field defects, palsy of the ipsilateral third cranial nerve, and contralateral sensory losses.

As with most syndromes of vascular insufficiency, the diagnosis is usually suggested by the history alone. Patients may also be asymptomatic with incidental findings found on imaging. A carefully elicited history may also localize the neuroanatomic deficit and the offending arterial lesion. Physical examination should include a thorough neurologic examination as well as a search for evidence of arterial occlusive disease in other vascular beds. The classic finding in a patient with carotid stenosis is a cervical bruit (high-frequency systolic murmur) heard during auscultation with a stethoscope placed at the angle of the jaw. Unfortunately, there is little correlation between the degree of stenosis and the pitch, duration, or intensity of the bruit. A minimal stenosis can produce a loud bruit, but a near-total occlusion may not produce a bruit at all. A bruit can also be produced from other cervical blood vessels or transmitted from the aortic valve. Because of the close proximity of the carotid artery to the ear, some patients actually note a buzzing or heartbeat in their ear referred to as carotid stenosis. During ophthalmologic examination, small, yellow refractile particles (Hollenhorst plaques) may be seen at the branch point of the retinal vessels. These plaques are cholesterol emboli from a carotid artery, aortic arch, or aortic valve plaque. Fisher plugs are caused by platelet emboli and are not refractile.

Noninvasive tests can determine the extent of carotid artery stenosis without the use of arteriography. Candidates for noninvasive testing include patients with cerebrovascular symptoms, those with cervical bruits, and, in some cases, those who are undergoing major vascular procedures (eg, coronary artery bypass grafting). Noninvasive, yet direct, evaluation of the extracranial carotid arterial vessels is obtained with Doppler ultrasound. The nature of the plaque (soft, calcific, or ulcerated) and its precise location (common vs external vs internal carotid artery) can be determined with duplex ultrasound. The accuracy of imaging is enhanced by combining B-mode ultrasound with Doppler-derived assessments of blood flow velocity (duplex scan). In more than 90% of patients with carotid bifurcation plaque, no further diagnostic test is needed to institute therapy. A limitation of duplex scanning is the inability to assess the intracranial circulation and the origins of the common carotid arteries from the aortic arch. Occasionally, visualization of the carotid bifurcation is impaired by calcification of the vessels.

The definitive study of the extracranial carotid arterial system is arteriography. Arterial injections offer the clearest definition of carotid plaques and potential ulcerations (Figure 24-22). Arteriography is indicated in patients who have a potential aortic arch or intracranial lesion, those with uncertain symptoms, and those in whom the carotid stenosis cannot be clearly visualized on duplex ultrasonography. Complications are rare but can be devastating. They include CVA (~0.5% of cases). As a consequence, most diagnostic angiograms today employ CT technology, which does not require arterial catheterization. These CT angiograms nearly match catheter-based studies in detail and diagnostic quality but have lower risks involved.

Recent improvements in CTA, cerebral MRI, and MRA have led to increased application in patients with carotid occlusive disease. CTA with 3-D reconstruction is as accurate as catheter angiography for carotid and intracerebral vascular evaluation. MRI is useful for the evaluation of the brain tissue for infarction, tumor, AVM, and hemorrhage. MRA also provides detailed visualization of the carotid arterial system without requiring arterial puncture and injection (Figure 24-23).

Treatment

Medical therapy for cerebrovascular disease is directed at the control of risk factors (HTN, smoking, diabetes, and hyperlipidemia) and anticoagulation (vitamin K antagonists, direct oral anticoagulants) or administration of antiplatelet drugs (aspirin, clopidogrel). Anticoagulation and antiplatelet therapies are most commonly used in patients with ulcerative nonstenotic lesions or severe intracranial disease because surgical therapy would not change the natural history of the disease process as well as for patients who have asymptomatic mild or moderate carotid stenosis. Patients with symptomatic moderate or severe carotid stenosis and those with severe stenosis may benefit from CEA. In this procedure, an incision in the neck is used to isolate the common, internal, and external carotid arteries. After control is obtained proximally and distally, an arteriotomy is performed with the removal of the atherosclerotic plaque, intima, and a portion of the media via endarterectomy. The arteriotomy is closed with a patch. A prospective randomized study (North American Symptomatic Carotid Endarterectomy Trial [NASCET]) evaluated the treatment of patients with internal carotid artery stenosis and cerebrovascular symptoms. After 2 years of follow-up, researchers found that in symptomatic patients who had more than 70% ipsilateral stenosis and were managed with antiplatelet therapy alone, the risk of CVA or death was approximately 26% compared with 9% in patients who were treated with operative repair of the carotid through CEA. The risk in symptomatic patients with 50% to 69% stenosis was also reduced with CEA.

Asymptomatic patients with documented 60% or greater carotid stenosis were studied in the Asymptomatic Carotid Atherosclerosis Study (ACAS). The risk of stroke in the medically managed group was calculated at 11% in 5 years. CEA reduced the risk to 5%. Although not as dramatic as the reduction in symptomatic patients, these findings firmly established the role of CEA in the prevention of stroke in properly selected patients with significant carotid stenosis. However, aggressive risk factor management, which was not used during ACAS, makes surgical and medical treatment of asymptomatic carotid stenosis comparable.

In experienced hands, the morbidity and mortality rates for CEA are less than 2%. Recurrent lesions may occur in as many as 10% of endarterectomized arteries, so long-term follow-up with serial ultrasonography is advised. Restenosis within 2 years usually represents intimal hyperplasia, whereas late recurrence is usually a manifestation of recurrent atherosclerosis.

Carotid angioplasty with placement of a metallic stent from a transfemoral access (transfemoral carotid stenting) has been evaluated and has been used to treat symptomatic carotid stenosis. The Carotid Revascularization Endarterectomy versus Stenting Trial (CREST) showed comparable overall results: patients with carotid angioplasty had more postprocedure strokes but fewer MIs, and patients

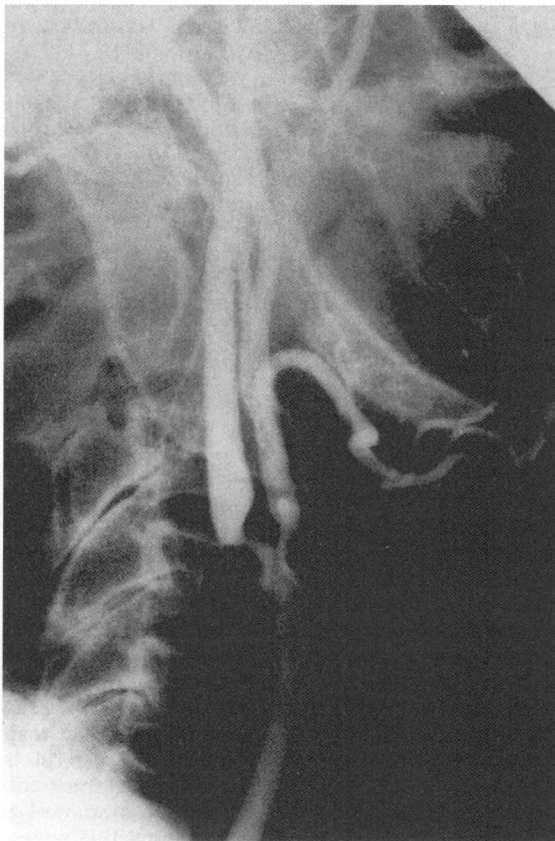

Figure 24-22. Angiogram of an internal carotid stenosis showing an ulcerative and stenotic atherosclerotic lesion at the carotid bifurcation in a patient who has transient ischemic attacks.

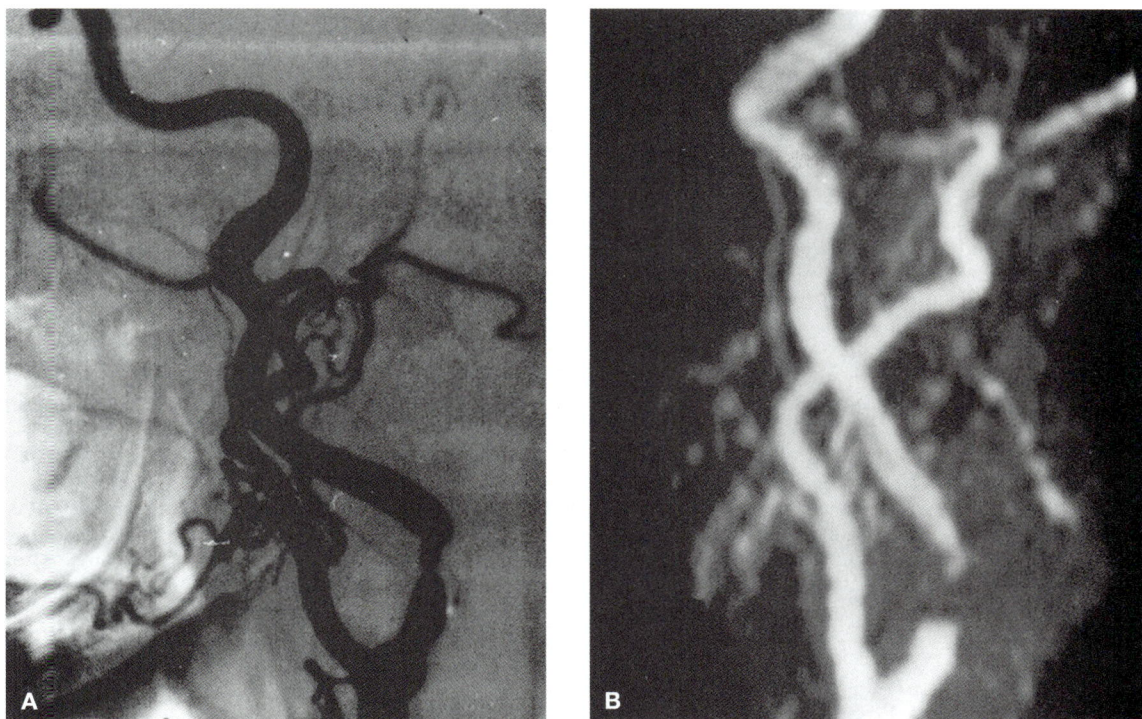

Figure 24-23. A. A conventional cerebral angiogram. B. A magnetic resonance angiogram in the same patient.

who underwent endarterectomy had fewer strokes but more MIs. More recent studies have shown that there is a significant learning curve associated with carotid artery stenting, and only experienced interventionalists should be performing these procedures, particularly in those patients who are not candidates for surgical revascularization. The most recent intervention developed to treat carotid stenosis is transcarotid artery revascularization (TCAR). In this procedure, a metallic stent is placed across the stenotic carotic lesion via a puncture in a surgically exposed common carotid artery. During this procedure, a sheath is placed in the common carotid artery and connected via a filter to the femoral vein, which allows "flow reversal" that decreases embolic complications associated with wire crossing of the carotid lesion.

All patients with carotid stenosis, whether asymptomatic or symptomatic, must be on antiplatelet (aspirin or clopidogrel) therapy, statins, and β-blocker therapy, unless one is contraindicated.

Vertebral Basilar Disease

The classic syndrome of vertebral basilar insufficiency is subclavian steal syndrome, which is associated with subclavian or innominate artery occlusive disease. Symptoms occur when an occlusive lesion that is located proximal to the origin of the vertebral vessel decreases perfusion pressure in the subclavian artery. The vertebral artery then functions as a collateral pathway to the arm circulation. During arm exercise, vascular resistance in the arm decreases, and flow is reversed in the vertebral artery. As a result, basilar arterial blood flow and perfusion pressure are decreased (Figure 24-24). Symptoms of posterior

cerebral and cerebellar ischemia are common and include light-headedness and syncope correlated with arm exercise. Supraclavicular bruits are often detected, and blood pressure in the ipsilateral brachial artery is usually reduced by at least 15 mm Hg. Because of the increased length of

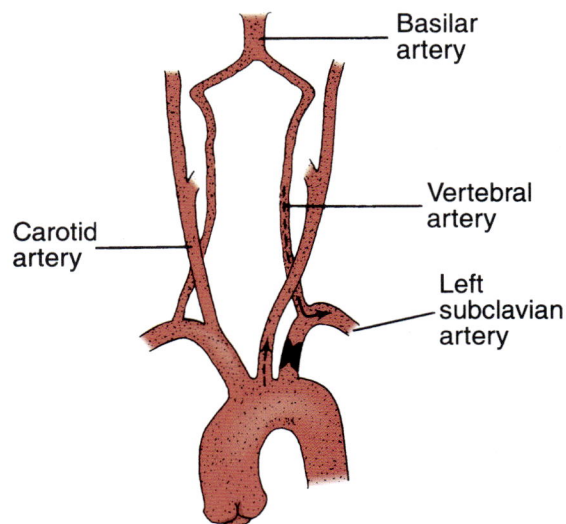

Figure 24-24. Subclavian steal syndrome. Proximal occlusion of the left subclavian artery causes retrograde flow of blood through the left vertebral artery, "stealing" blood from the basilar circulation and causing transient dizziness and syncope with arm exercise.

the left subclavian artery relative to the right, there is a 3 to 4 times increased incidence of left subclavian stenosis and subclavian steal syndrome.

In patients with associated carotid artery stenosis, CEA alone may relieve the symptoms of vertebral basilar insufficiency by increasing collateral flow to the posterior cerebral artery and cerebellum. However, in most symptomatic patients with subclavian steal syndrome, the most effective procedures are either carotid-subclavian bypass, reimplantation of the subclavian artery into the proximal common carotid artery, or subclavian angioplasty and stenting. These procedures restore normal blood flow to the subclavian artery and allow antegrade perfusion of the vertebral artery.

VENOUS DISEASE

Venous disease is one of the most common medical conditions affecting adults. Approximately 40% of adults have some form of venous diseases including varicose veins, postthrombotic syndrome, venous ulcers, and telangiectasias (spider veins). An adult has a 6% probability of having a venous ulcer within their lifetime. The incidence of venous diseases increases with age, so that 70% of adults over the age of 70 have some form of chronic venous disease.

Acute venous disease, primarily deep vein thrombophlebitis (DVT), is responsible for many unexpected deaths in hospitalized patients, particularly postsurgery. In 2008, the Surgeon General issued a "call to action" for physicians to reduce preventable deaths from DVT by using more aggressive prevention measures. Currently, all surgical patients must have consideration given to some form of prophylaxis when they undergo a procedure that has a significant risk of DVT.

Anatomy

The venous system is divided into central and peripheral systems. The central venous system includes the inferior and superior vena cava, iliac veins, and subclavian veins. The peripheral venous system includes the upper- and lower-extremity venous systems as well as the venous drainage of the head and neck region. The extremity veins are further classified as either superficial or deep (Figure 24-25). The superficial system of the lower extremity is composed of the great and small saphenous veins and their tributaries.

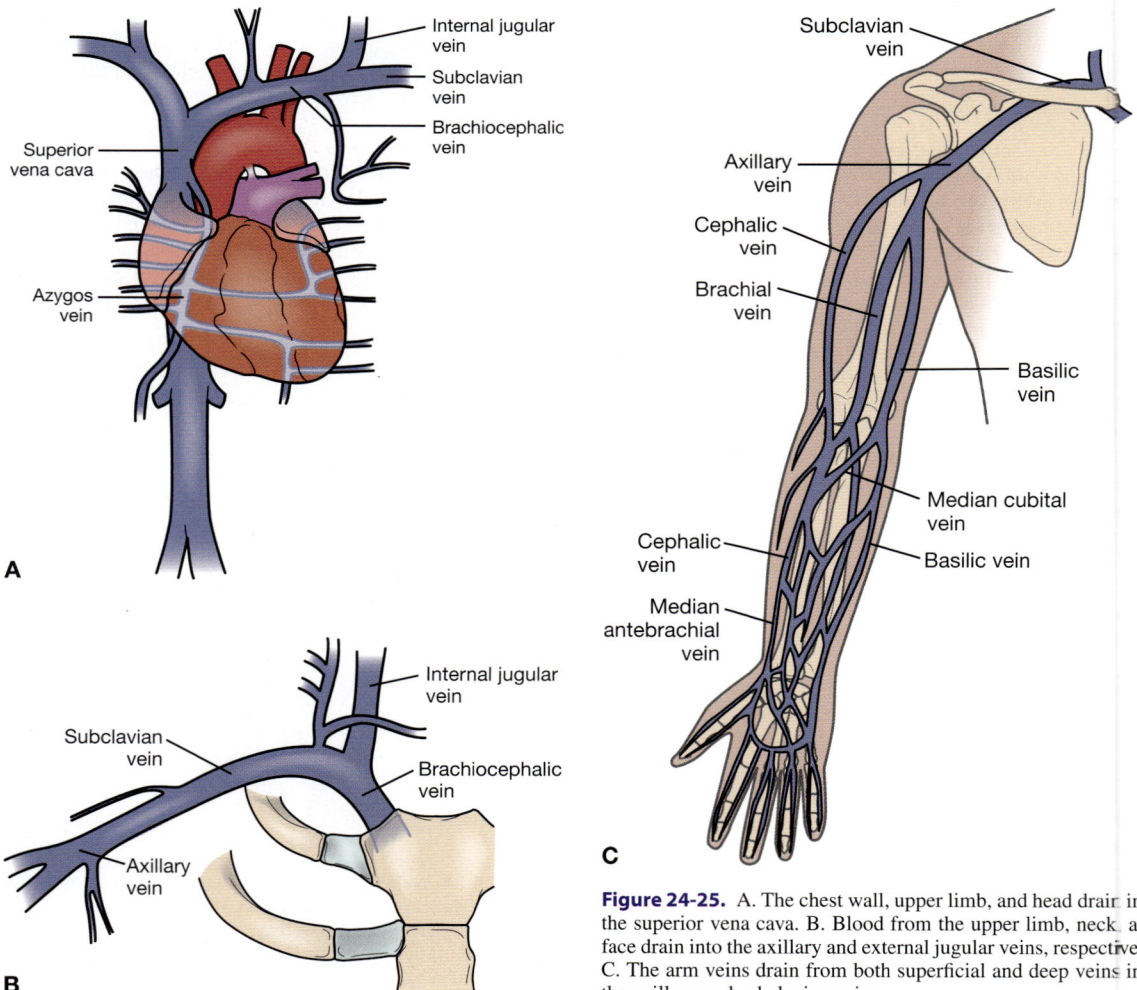

Figure 24-25. A. The chest wall, upper limb, and head drain into the superior vena cava. B. Blood from the upper limb, neck, and face drain into the axillary and external jugular veins, respectively. C. The arm veins drain from both superficial and deep veins into the axillary and subclavian veins.

The deep venous system is composed of large veins that travel with the major arteries of the extremity. The common femoral, femoral, and profunda femoral veins parallel the arteries of the same names. Recently, the "superficial femoral" vein was renamed the "femoral" to avoid confusion and assure appropriate concern for the risk of pulmonary embolism if this deep vein develops thrombosis. The anterior tibial, posterior tibial, and peroneal veins are almost always paired; therefore, the calf has six primary deep veins, in contrast to three primary arteries.

Unidirectional flow back to the heart is maintained by a series of bicuspid vein valves. These vein valves prevent the reflux of blood back toward the lower extremity during standing. The superficial and deep venous systems are connected by perforating veins that direct blood from the superficial system to the deep system. Incompetence of the valves in the deep or perforating veins, as a result of congenital defects, scarring, or distention, allows retrograde flow from the deep system into the superficial system. If severe and long-standing enough, such reflux will cause varicosities, chronic venous insufficiency, and eventually venous ulcerations. Venous ulcers are an important health care problem, resulting in disability, lost workdays, huge costs, and serious lifestyle changes.

Physiology

The muscular compartments of the calf are critically important in the venous circulation. Muscular contraction increases pressure within the compartments, forcing blood back to the heart. Unlike the deep veins, the superficial veins are not surrounded by muscular compartments and therefore are not emptied by muscular contraction. The venous pressures in the standing and supine positions reflect the critical role of the valves, muscular contraction, and the position of the patient (Figure 24-26).

Pathology

In 1856, Virchow identified a triad of risk factors for DVT. It included stasis, venous endothelial injury, and hypercoagulable states. Although many other risk factors,

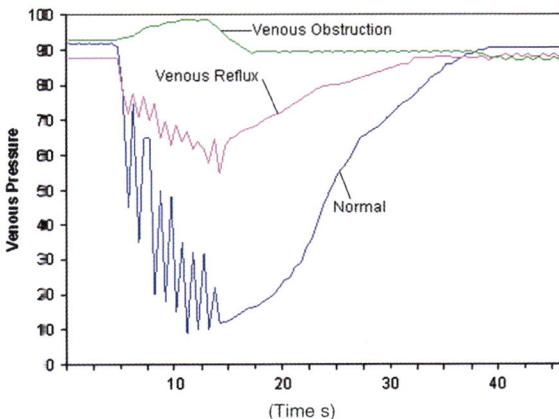

Figure 24-26. Graph showing venous pressure. The lower-extremity venous pressure starts high, but with walking, the pressure is significantly reduced. When walking is completed, the pressure rises gradually. When there is venous insufficiency, the pressure does not fall as rapidly and then returns to a higher pressure.

including pregnancy, the use of oral contraceptives, a history of DVT, surgical procedures, sepsis, and obesity, appear independent, they can all be placed into one of these categories. Bony and soft-tissue trauma to the legs is one of the most common causes of endothelial injury and DVT.

Once the valves are damaged from DVT, the ambulatory venous pressure becomes much higher and results in stasis and venous distention, which may injure the venous endothelium and allow the protein to leak into the subcutaneous tissue, causing inflammation in the interstitium. The end result of this process, which occurs over the years, is *lipodermatosclerosis* or scarring of the subcutaneous tissue in the limb. It invariably occurs in the region of the leg where the pressure is the highest in the standing position, which is called the "gaiter zone" of the leg (Figure 24-27). The pathophysiology of venous disease is generally caused by obstruction of the venous system, venous valvular insufficiency, or elements of both.

Superficial Vein Thrombosis

Superficial vein thrombosis (SVT) causes swelling, erythema, and tenderness along its course. Patients with varicose veins are at risk for thrombosis of the superficial veins and SVT. In addition, there are many iatrogenic causes of SVT, including insertion of IV catheters and sclerotherapy. When a superficial vein thromboses, there is often pain associated with swelling and inflammation around the vein. Patients who have superficial thromboses are managed with nonsteroidal anti-inflammatory agents and warm compresses. Low-molecular-weight heparins have also been used for 4 to 6 weeks to improve symptoms. Occasionally, the vein is so tender that the best treatment is excision of the involved vein. After the thrombosed vein is transected, the thrombus can be extracted and there is immediate pain relief. In addition, thrombectomy of superficial thrombosed veins improves the cosmetic appearance of the skin overlying the vein and reduces pigmentation of the skin.

Deep Vein Thrombosis

Approximately 900,000 patients per year have DVT, which is a risk factor for the development of pulmonary embolism. If pulmonary thromboembolism occurs, in-hospital mortality rates are as high as 10%.

Clinical Presentation

Up to 50% of hospital-acquired DVTs are asymptomatic. The remaining patients have local pain secondary to inflammation and edema. DVT of the left iliac venous system is more common than that of the right iliac venous system because of the potential for compression of the left iliac vein by the aortic bifurcation and crossing of the right iliac artery (May-Thurner syndrome; Figure 24-28). Unfortunately, in a small percentage of patients, the first symptom of DVT is pulmonary embolism.

Diagnosis

Physical examination of a patient with a lower-extremity DVT may show unilateral extremity swelling or pain. Calf pain precipitated by dorsal flexion of the foot (Homan sign) is present in fewer than 50% of cases. Because the accuracy of diagnosis based on clinical and physical examination alone is only 50%, more objective diagnostic studies are needed to confirm the presence of DVT before

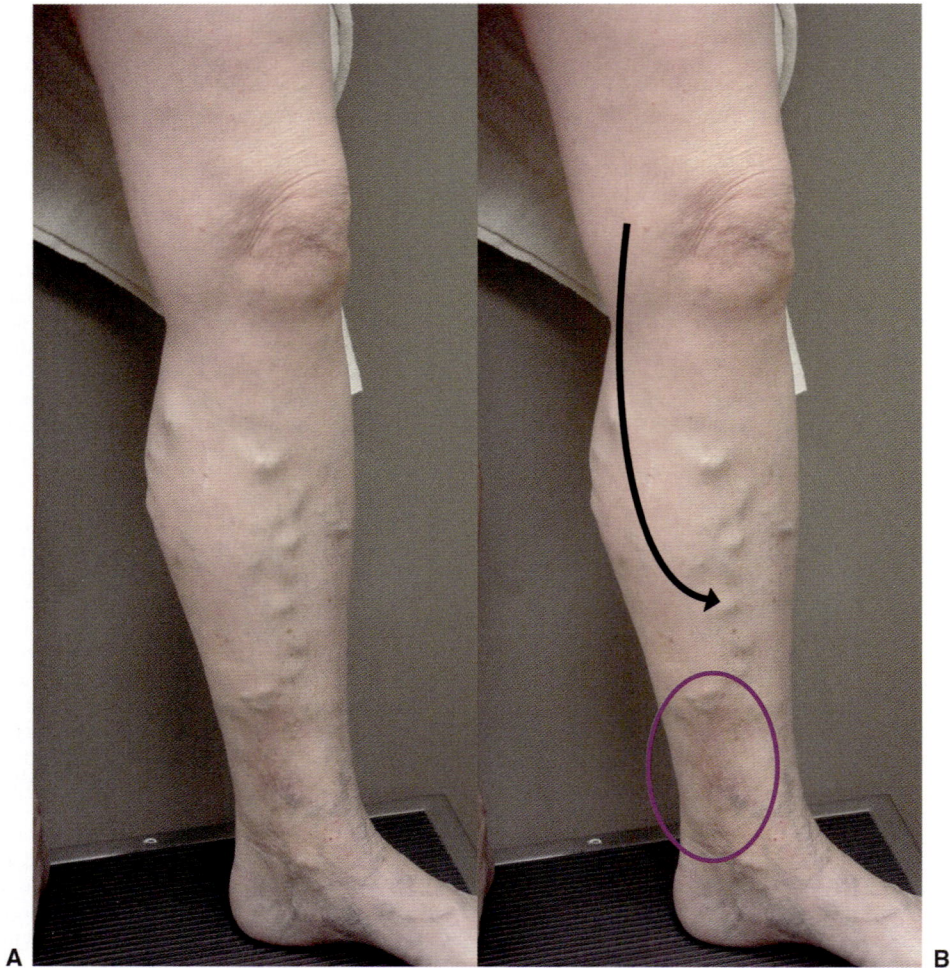

Figure 24-27. A. Varicose veins often occur when the proximal saphenous vein becomes incompetent, and there is reflux down the saphenous vein and into the tributaries. B. This reflux causes visible varicosities and even pigmentation in the "gaiter" zone at the level of the ankle, which is circled in purple.

treatment. In addition to DVT, the differential diagnosis of acute edema and leg pain includes trauma, ruptured plantaris tendon, infection, lymphangitis, muscle hematoma, and ruptured Baker cyst.

The accuracy of duplex ultrasound (duplex scan) is more than 95% in diagnosing DVT because it can characterize venous blood flow and visualize the venous thrombus (Figure 24-29). A Doppler ultrasound can document the loss of the normal augmentation of venous flow with distal compression and the variation of venous flow with respiration. Normally, lower-extremity venous flow decreases with inspiration as a result of increased intra-abdominal pressure. The accuracy of duplex scanning is reduced in the tibial veins because of the difficulty in visualizing these small veins within the muscular compartments. In unusual cases, CT scans of the abdomen and pelvis, with IV contrast material, may aid in the diagnosis of pelvic and vena caval thrombosis. The use of blood tests that measure the degradation of thrombus (D-dimer) can also be used as a screening test for DVT, particularly in the outpatient and emergency department setting where it is costly to bring in

a technician to test each patient with duplex ultrasound who has leg pain. D-dimer is a sensitive but not specific screening test for DVT and should be followed by duplex ultrasound if it is positive. Venography is rarely performed for a diagnosis of DVT but is frequently used prior to thrombolysis of DVT.

Evaluation for hypercoagulability with measures of protein C, protein S, antithrombin III, factor V Leiden, prothrombin mutation, and anticardiolipin antibodies should be performed in patients with spontaneous (unprovoked) DVT.

Prophylaxis

DVT and pulmonary embolus are significant risks for patients undergoing major surgery. Preoperative prophylaxis has an impact on reducing DVT and should be used routinely for patients who undergo major surgical procedures. Prophylactic measures include mechanical therapy (intermittent segmental compression device), early ambulation, and pharmacologic therapy (anticoagulants or antiplatelet agents). Patients can be stratified for risk of DVT; advanced age, long procedures, patients with cancer, and patients with prior DVT are particularly vulnerable.

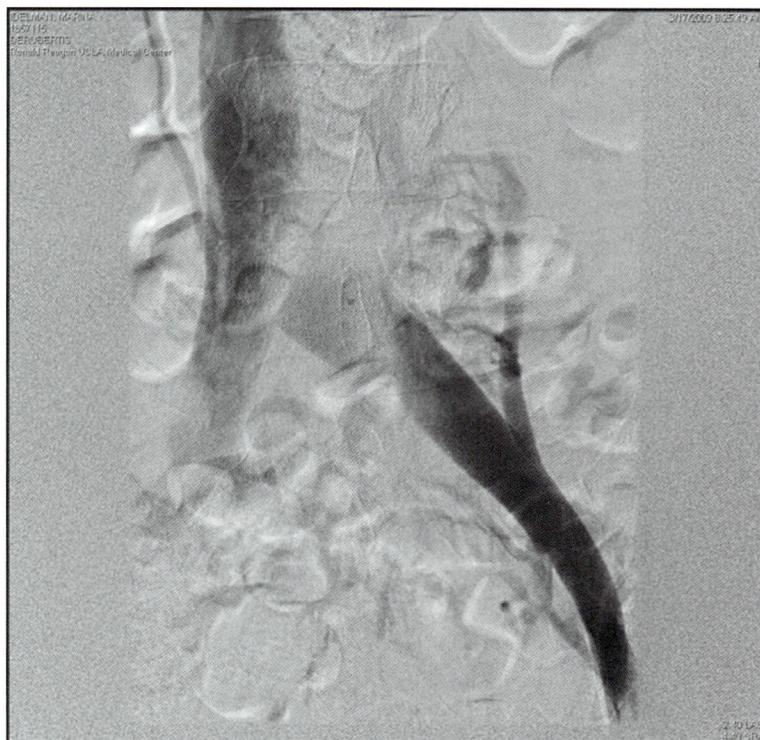

Figure 24-28. **This venogram of the iliac veins and vena cava shows compression of the left iliac vein by the right iliac artery.** The area of compression, when severe, leads to May-Thurner syndrome, in which a patient develops left leg swelling with exercise and venous thrombosis distal to the site of compression.

Treatment

The goals of treatment of DVT include reducing the risk of pulmonary embolus, preventing further propagation of the venous thrombus, and reducing the damage to the deep venous valves, so that long-term chronic venous insufficiency does not occur. The classic primary therapy includes anticoagulation with heparin; this can be administered in both inpatients and outpatients. After the patient is adequately anticoagulated with heparin, long-term anticoagulation is begun with warfarin (Coumadin). Warfarin therapy is monitored to maintain a therapeutic international normalized ratio of 2 to 3. Sodium warfarin inhibits the vitamin K–dependent factors for both the procoagulant factors (II, VII, IX, X) and the anticoagulant factors (protein C and protein S). Because the half-lives of protein C and protein S are less than those of the procoagulant factors, for a short time after the initiation of warfarin therapy, even appropriately treated patients may become hypercoagulable. Warfarin skin necrosis is a rare but catastrophic complication of this rare hypercoagulable state that can cause significant loss of skin. For this reason, heparin anticoagulation is maintained during the beginning of warfarin therapy. Contraindications to anticoagulation therapy include bleeding diathesis, GI ulceration, recent stroke, cerebral AVMs, recent surgery, hematologic disorders (eg, hemophilia), and bone marrow suppression as a result of chemotherapy.

In the last few years, several novel oral anticoagulant drugs have come to market that allow immediate anticoagulation. As such, they do not require heparinization prior to initiating the oral anticoagulant. These drugs also have the benefit over warfarin in that they do not require monitoring because they have stable bioavailability when taken as directed. They have similar risks of bleeding to warfarin, but it is important to be aware that currently all but one of these

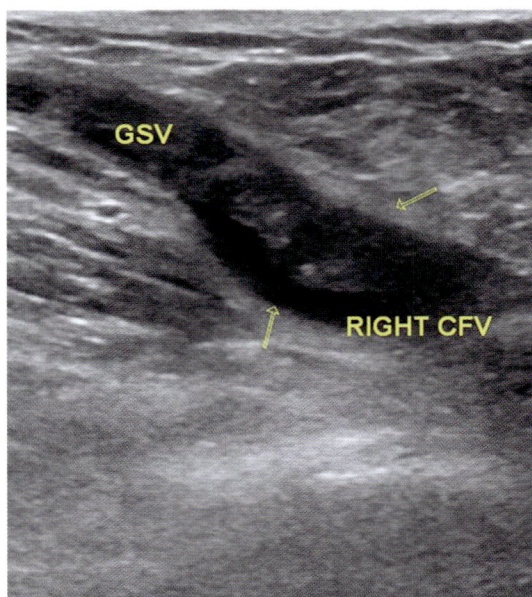

Figure 24-29. **Duplex scan.** CFV, central femoral vein; GSV, great saphenous vein.

drugs has no antidote. If there is a need for rapid reversal of the anticoagulant (as in trauma or emergent need for surgery), significant transfusions with fresh frozen plasma may be required, or prothrombin complex concentrates, which contain pooled human coagulation factors, may be useful.

Anticoagulation therapy prevents further propagation of the thrombus but does not actually dissolve or lyse the existing thrombus. Fibrinolysis occurs gradually through the endogenous plasminogen system or may be stimulated by the administration of an exogenous thrombolytic agent such as tPA. Definite indications for thrombolytic therapy include subclavian vein thrombosis, acute renal vein thrombosis, and acute superior vena cava occlusion by the thrombus. The American College of Chest Physicians recommends thrombolysis in patients with iliofemoral DVT, symptoms for less than 14 days, good functional status, life expectancy of more than 1 year, and a low risk of bleeding. In addition, mechanical thrombectomy devices are increasingly being used because they allow concentration of the agent in the vein that is occluded and limit the dissemination of the agent into the systemic circulation. Mechanical devices also reduce the time needed to recanalize the occluded deep vein and therefore reduce complications from thrombolysis. It is still uncertain whether venous valvular function can be preserved with successful thrombolytic therapy, but evidence supports a more aggressive approach for most patients with DVT who are otherwise healthy. Contraindications to thrombolysis include recent surgery or trauma, recent stroke, and recent bleeding. Mechanical thrombectomy has fewer contraindications because of the isolation of the thrombolytic agent in the thrombosed vein. Surgical venous thrombectomy is rarely indicated and is usually reserved for cases of limb-threatening ischemia. Even in complete iliofemoral thrombosis with massive edema (phlegmasia cerulea dolens or phlegmasia alba dolens), mechanical thrombectomy devices and thrombolysis are the primary treatment modalities.

Pulmonary Embolism

Pulmonary embolism results from the migration of venous clots to the pulmonary arteries. Clots may originate in any large vein, especially those that arise from the iliac, femoral, and large pelvic veins. Patients with hypercoagulable conditions are predisposed to DVT and pulmonary embolism.

Clinical Presentation

Patients with pulmonary embolism may have no specific clinical findings or may have massive cardiovascular collapse. The classic clinical presentation (Table 24-4) includes pleuritic chest pain, dyspnea, tachypnea, tachycardia, cough, and hemoptysis. Right-sided heart strain is seen on electrocardiogram (ECG).

Prevention

The use of support hose and prophylactic anticoagulation is indicated in patients who have a high risk of pulmonary embolism, with the indications being similar to those who have a high risk of DVT and were mentioned earlier.

Diagnosis

The definitive diagnosis of pulmonary embolism is made by a CT scan of the chest, ventilation-perfusion lung scan, or pulmonary angiogram. A wedge-shaped or lobar defect

TABLE 24-4. Clinical Presentations of Pulmonary Embolus
Pleuritic chest pain (70%)
Dyspnea and tachypnea (80%)
Tachycardia (45%)
Hemoptysis (25%-30%)

Associated findings
  Cough and rales
  Right heart failure

seen on a perfusion scan without a ventilation deficit indicates a high probability of pulmonary embolism. Chest CT scan often shows both the thrombus in the pulmonary artery and the infarcted lung parenchyma. Pulmonary angiogram has specificity and a sensitivity of greater than 98%, but it is an invasive procedure.

Chest radiography is rarely diagnostic for pulmonary embolus. A pleural effusion is present in as many as one-third of patients with pulmonary embolus. The classic wedge-shaped region of atelectasis from a pulmonary embolus is rarely noted. Chest radiography is most useful for ruling out other potential pulmonary pathology.

Treatment

The primary therapy for pulmonary embolism is anticoagulation to prevent further emboli and clot propagation. If the patient is hemodynamically unstable, inotropic support may be required. If the patient remains stable but is compromised as a result of the pulmonary embolus, thrombolytic therapy is considered. There is no direct correlation between clot size, cardiopulmonary dynamics, and other risk factors and survival in patients with acute embolism. Multiple small emboli cause cardiovascular collapse as often as massive emboli.

If a patient with lower-extremity or pelvic venous thrombus has a contraindication to anticoagulation or has had a pulmonary embolism while anticoagulated (failure of anticoagulation), a mechanical filter device can be placed in the inferior vena cava. This device traps emboli before they reach the pulmonary artery. Vena caval filters are designed to be removable and can be placed by a percutaneous technique from either the internal jugular vein or the femoral vein. These filters should be removed as soon as they are no longer needed, to prevent long-term complications such as filter migration, vena caval perforation, or occlusion.

Varicose Veins

Varicose veins are dilated branches of incompetent superficial veins, most commonly found in the legs.

Incidence

Venous disease, including varicose veins, spider veins, and postthrombotic limbs with edema and ulcers, is among the most common diseases in the United States. It is estimated that more than 40% of the adult population has varicose veins and that 6% of adults will develop a venous ulcer during their lifetime. In addition, the recurrence of the end-stage manifestation, venous ulcers, is high, and most patients live for long periods with open ulcers, punctuated with periods of healing. Consequently, venous problems are not only extremely common but also important to the entire health care system.

Anatomy

Knowledge of venous anatomy is critical to understanding venous disease. The superficial, perforating, and deep systems interconnect (Figure 24-30), with blood flowing from the superficial to the deep system, and with valves preventing reflux from proximal to distal and from the deep to the superficial systems. Because 85% to 90% of the venous return is in the deep system, establishing its presence and patency is a key to treatment, and removal of the superficial veins has little consequence on blood flow physiology as long as the deep system is patent.

Primary Varicose Veins

Superficial varicose veins are often not associated with other perforating or deep venous involvement and are therefore considered "primary." The most common cause of primary varicose veins is the development of incompetence of the venous valve at the junction of the saphenous vein with the femoral vein in the inguinal region. Incompetence of this valve results in proximal vein dilation and progressive incompetence of distal valves and veins. Eventually, the dilated vein results in incompetence of the entire saphenous vein as well as tributary (branch) veins. The visible portion of the incompetent veins is usually in the calf, where they are closer to the skin. In spite of proximal incompetence, many patients request treatment only when the calf veins become visible.

Symptoms

Superficial varicose veins cause symptoms of heaviness and fatigue after prolonged standing, night cramps, and occasionally ankle edema, superficial thrombophlebitis, or hemorrhage from superficial veins.

Diagnosis

Although physical examination is helpful in establishing the presence of varicose veins, the critical determinant of the approach to treatment is the competence of the saphenofemoral junction valve, which cannot be determined by physical examination. Duplex ultrasound is the best diagnostic test for valve incompetence and should be used in all patients with symptoms. If the saphenous vein is not assessed for competency, then an incompetent saphenous vein may be left in place, leading to recurrence. Venography is now rarely used and may cause phlebitis. Plethysmography assesses reflux in the superficial and deep system but has little role in primary varicose vein evaluation.

Treatment

The treatment of primary varicose veins has changed dramatically in the past 10 years and, like many areas of surgery, has become less invasive. The predominant mode of treatment is currently endovenous ablation, but there are multiple procedures that can be performed for this pathology.

1. "Stripping" of the saphenous vein. The saphenous vein may be removed by a technique of stripping, where the vein is exposed at each end and then removed by passing a disposable or metal catheter up the vein from the ankle or knee. A suture is tied around the vein at the saphenofemoral junction, and the vein is then removed or "stripped." This technique is being used less frequently because it is associated with a slightly longer patient recovery with more postoperative pain than minimally invasive approaches.

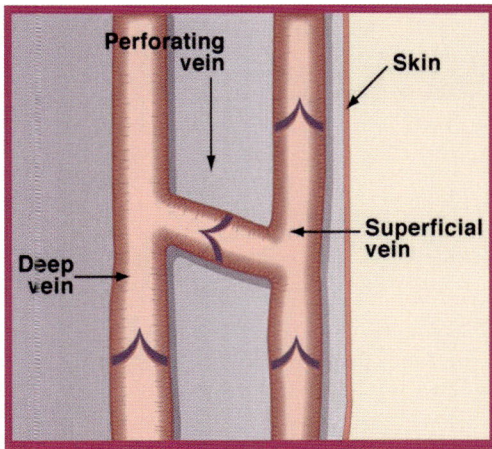

A

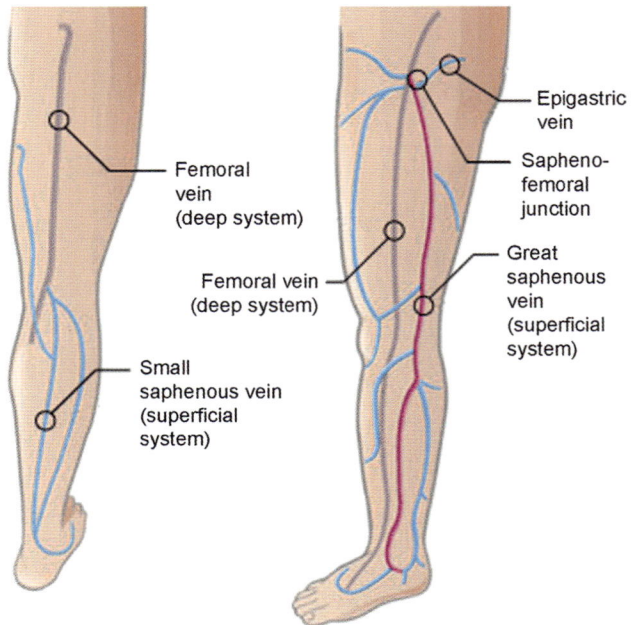

B

Figure 24-30. Venous anatomy. A. The superficial and deep venous systems are parallel, with multiple perforating veins connecting them. B. The superficial and deep venous systems are illustrated in two drawings of the leg.

2. Saphenous ligation. Ligating the saphenous vein flush with the femoral vein in the fossa ovalis can eliminate the saphenous reflux. Although this technique eliminates reflux, there is a higher recurrence with ligation than with stripping. Ligation is particularly indicated in patients with very large proximal saphenous veins that measure greater than 1.5 cm.

3. Endovenous closure with radiofrequency ablation (RFA) (Figure 24-31), endovenous laser therapy, ultrasound-guided foam sclerotherapy, or mechanico-chemical closure of the saphenous vein. These techniques are the least invasive and are performed by accessing the saphenous vein below the knee with a needle, using ultrasound guidance. In RFA or laser therapy, a wire is then passed into the vein, followed by a sheath and then a radiofrequency or laser catheter. After the catheter has been passed up to the saphenofemoral junction, the catheter is used to heat the vein. The heat contracts collagen and thromboses the vein, leading to closure.

4. Branch vein excision by micro incision (stab phlebectomy) (Figure 24-32). The tributary branches of the saphenous vein can be removed with small incisions that allow the vein to be visualized and removed with small crochet hooks, instruments, or clamps. The resulting scars are very small and nearly invisible.

Chronic Venous Insufficiency

Chronic venous insufficiency is a direct result of local venous HTN. Causes of venous HTN include deep venous valvular incompetence, venous obstruction as a result of intrinsic or extrinsic compression, and reflux from perforating veins.

The clinical manifestations of chronic venous insufficiency are chronically swollen legs, hyperpigmentation, and venous ulceration. The leg is typically swollen and pigmented in the "gaiter" zone of the ankle. The pigmentation is a reflection of inflammation and chronic venous HTN, which is worsened in the standing position. The term *lipodermatosclerosis* refers to the end stage of venous HTN when chronic venous HTN leads to pigmentation and fibrosis of the tissue around the ankle.

Diagnosis

Physical examination shows purple-brown skin discoloration at the level of the ankle (Figure 24-33) with

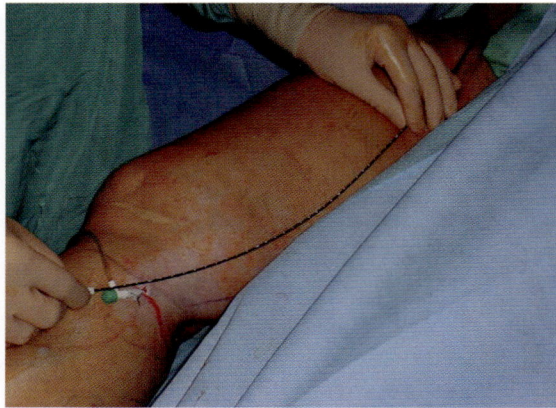

A

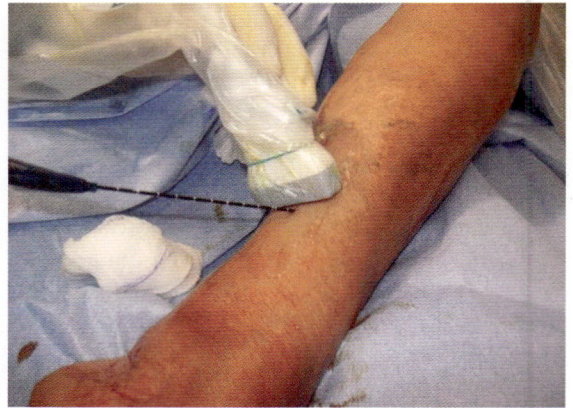

B

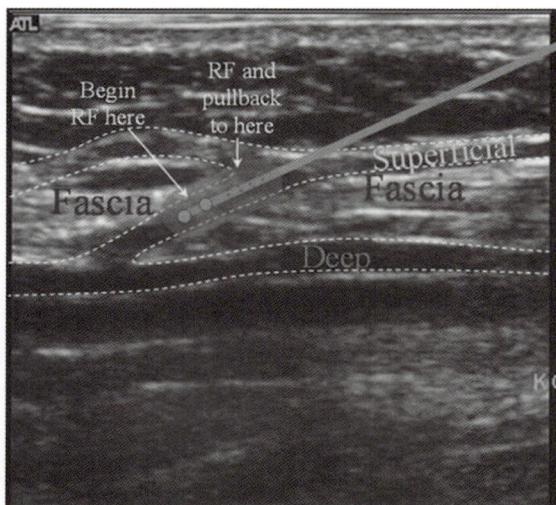

C

Figure 24-31. Endovenous closure with radiofrequency (RF) ablation. Endovenous ablation of the great saphenous and perforator veins is performed by placing a catheter into the vein (A) and then heating the tip of the catheter until the vein contracts, closing the incompetent perforator vein (B, C).

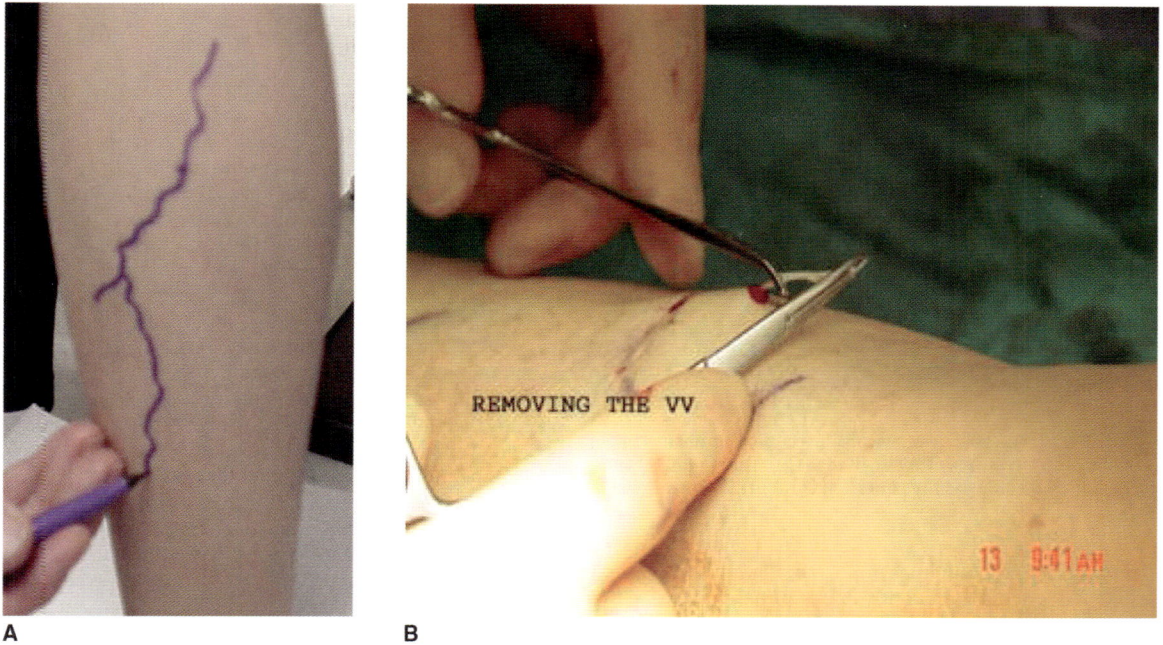

Figure 24-32. Microphlebectomy or "stab" phlebectomy is a technique for removing tributary or branch veins by making a small incision adjacent to the vein, which is marked in the standing position (A), and then removing it with a crochet-hook-like instrument (B). The ends of the avulsed veins are not tied, and bleeding is controlled with compression.

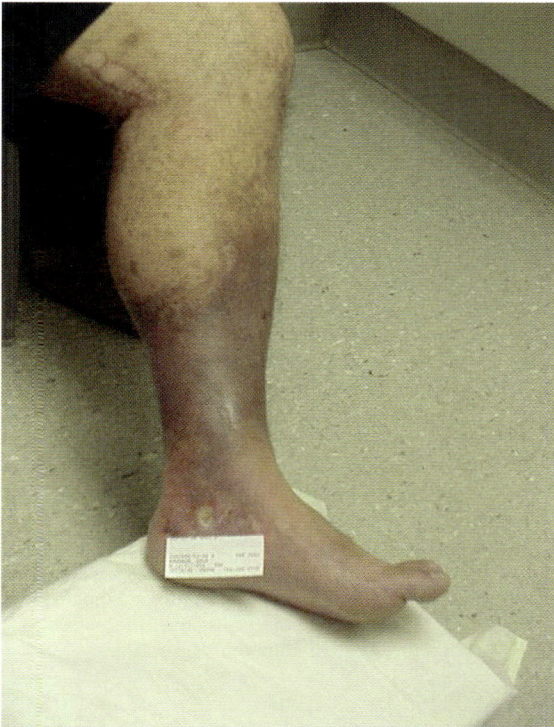

Figure 24-33. Lipodermatosclerosis occurs in the "gaiter zone" of the calf and ankle and is a combination of pigmentation and subcutaneous fibrosis.

hemosiderin deposition, lower-extremity edema, superficial varicosities, and/or ulceration. Venous stasis ulceration usually occurs at the medial and lateral malleoli of the ankle. These chronic changes in the lower extremity occur as a result of venous HTN and are usually postthrombotic, but may also be caused by congenital deep valvular incompetence and severe obesity.

Noninvasive vascular laboratory evaluation includes venous duplex ultrasonography, which allows visualization of venous flow as well as reflux through incompetent deep and perforator venous valves. Likewise, a duplex scan can directly visualize a deep vein chronic occlusion or note the inability of the vein to be compressed secondary to venous thrombus. If the noninvasive duplex scan is not diagnostic, an MRI/magnetic resonance venography (MRV) or CT venogram may be necessary.

Treatment

The initial management of chronic venous insufficiency with lower-extremity lipodermatosclerosis is the use of gradient compression stockings. Unfortunately, compliance is poor in many patients because they do not see the immediate benefit of the support hose and dislike the cost of the hose and the discomfort associated with wearing them. In patients with venous ulceration, wound care is required to promote healing. Proper wound care and a tightly applied dressing of three or four layers (Figure 24-34) should be used for compression. Stripping/removal or closure with RFA or laser of the refluxing superficial veins, as well as interruption of perforating veins, may be necessary to heal venous

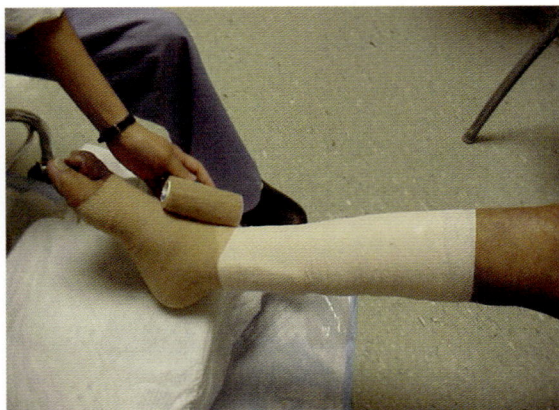

Figure 24-34. To heal, venous ulcers require uniform compression with pressures of 30 to 40 mm Hg, which reduces the leg edema and collapses the superficial and perforating veins.

ulcers. If the wound does not heal, but the refluxing veins and edema are controlled, split-thickness skin grafting may accomplish wound healing.

VASCULAR TRAUMA

Blood vessels are injured directly by penetrating trauma (eg, stab and gunshot wounds), blunt trauma (especially fractures of the long bones), and during surgical exposure to other structures adjacent to blood vessels. In high-speed collisions and falls, vessels may be torn by the shear stress of sudden acceleration or deceleration. Although patients with arterial injuries may have obvious signs such as hemorrhage and absence of distal pulses, the signs of vascular injury are often subtle. Hemorrhage may be occult and confined to soft tissue or body cavities. Other findings associated with the vascular injury include arteriovenous fistulae (associated with "to-and-fro" murmurs or palpable thrills), neurologic deficits and paresthesia (as a result of nerve compression by adjacent hematomas), or organ-specific deficits that reflect obstruction of the main arterial supply (eg, cerebral infarction with carotid artery injuries). A common misconception is that a patient who has an arterial injury must have a reduced or absent distal pulse; however, diminished pulses occur only if the injury restricts blood flow. Further, the presentation is commonly delayed; intimal flaps from deformation or stretching of the endothelial layer may not cause thrombosis for hours or days.

Immediate diagnosis and treatment of arterial injuries are indicated to avoid excessive blood loss and to restore extremity or organ blood flow. If the diagnosis is missed on initial evaluation, late complications may be much more difficult to treat. These late complications include pseudoaneurysms, high-volume arteriovenous fistulae with high-output cardiac failure, and delayed thrombosis from untreated intimal dissections.

The poor reliability of physical diagnosis in accurately assessing the location and extent of vascular injury mandates diagnostic studies whenever an arterial injury is suspected. If the patient has a viable extremity with an ABI

of 1.0, then limb-threatening arterial injury is unlikely and the vessels that are near the region of trauma can be further evaluated by duplex ultrasound studies. If the extremity is ischemic, angiography is indicated unless the delay puts the limb or organ at risk. Because of the tremendous concussive energy of high-velocity missiles, extensive damage can result even if the vessels are not in the direct line of the penetrating bullet. Certain types of blunt trauma (especially dislocation of the knees and elbows) are so often associated with arterial injury that duplex ultrasonography or arteriography is prudent even if no symptoms are present.

Although the consequences of venous injury are not as severe as those of arterial trauma, venous laceration must be considered in any patient who has evidence of excessive blood loss and no arterial lesion on angiography. MRV may be able to confirm and localize the injury although operative exploration to control bleeding may be more expedient. Venous injury also predisposes the patient to the development of deep venous thrombosis.

Repair of vascular injuries may be as simple as ligation of noncritical vessels or lateral suture (suture repair of the side of the vessel). In some cases, bypass grafts are needed, with resection of the vessel. In these cases, it is preferable to use an autologous vein from an uninjured extremity, because this type of conduit has higher patency and low infection rate, even in the face of contamination. When both arteries and veins of an extremity are injured, repair of both results in a higher limb salvage rate.

ANGIOACCESS FOR HEMODIALYSIS

Planning

Angioaccess for dialysis requires advanced planning by a multidisciplinary team to establish need, timing, type, and location. Early involvement of the vascular surgeon can reduce reliance on catheters and grafts with their attendant increase in infection, procedural complications, central venous stenosis, thrombosis, bleeding, and even mortality. Decisions should include judgments about social support, functional status, frailty, life expectancy, prospect for renal recovery or transplantation, and goals of care. On occasion, these lifestyle considerations may favor catheter or peritoneal dialysis. Since the time from creation to use is generally 2 to 3 months for surgically created arteriovenous fistulae, placement should be done in advance of anticipated need when creatinine clearance has decreased to less than 25 mL/min and even sooner for rapid rather than gradual functional deterioration. Options for dialysis access include tunneled hemodialysis catheters, autogenous arteriovenous fistulae, prosthetic arteriovenous grafts, and peritoneal dialysis. In general, catheters are placed in urgent settings and have a higher risk of infection, but can be used permanently in selective patients. Peritoneal dialysis is usually done in the home and requires the patient or family's involvement in the daily sessions. In this section, we'll focus on the surgical hemodialysis options.

History and Exam

Particular focus should be, in addition to the above factors, on the comorbidities of diabetes, HTN, and cardiac and peripheral vascular disease. Older patients and patients with diabetes with renal failure will often have multifocal calcific stenosis and distal small vessel arterial pathology, sometimes asymptomatic. Depressed cardiac output will impact flows and prospects for fistula-induced high-output cardiac failure.

On exam, bilateral brachial blood pressures, arm and leg pulse, Doppler assessments, and signs of proximal or distal venous occlusive disease—edema, large chest wall venous collaterals, stasis hyperpigmentation and lipodermatosclerosis—should be noted. Palmer arch and digital perfusion dependence on radial or ulnar artery integrity should be assessed by Allen test. Notation should be made of pacemaker, AICD, or central line placements. Use of extremities with current or prior indwelling catheters should trigger an imaging study for possible central venous stenosis. Ultrasound venous mapping for integrity and size of arm basilic, cephalic and, if lower-extremity use is anticipated, of greater saphenous and superficial femoral veins will assist in pre-op planning. If history or exam findings suggest upper- or lower-extremity arterial insufficiency, baseline noninvasive arterial studies should be used for localization and severity assessments. Arm venous diameters of at least 2 mm at wrist level, 2.5 mm at brachial level, and 3 mm at the saphenous are generally requisite to avoid problems of inadequate maturation.

Procedure

Following assessments of the relevant anatomic and physiologic variables, the selection of access should be individualized with initial placements as distal as possible to preserve proximal sites. Placement sequence should follow the algorithm of the first nondominant arm, first distal to proximal, with the inflow for vein beginning at the snuffbox for suitable arm vein, and then graft first forearm, then upper arm. Compulsion to use vein even if the size is inadequate needs to be avoided to prevent early thrombosis or maturation failure (Figure 24-35). If an adequate vein is not available, an arteriovenous graft with prosthetic material can be created, following a similar placement sequence. Other clinical scenarios are helpful in determining whether a patient will benefit from an arteriovenous fistula or graft (Figure 24-36).

The cephalic vein is preferred to avoid the need for superficialization of the basilic or brachial veins. Both the basilic and brachial veins are too deep to easily access and require a superficialization or transposition procedure where the vein is brought closer to the skin. This can be performed at the initial creation of the fistula anastomosis or often in a second-stage procedure. These veins also

Access Sequence

- Autogenous radial-cephalic
- Other forearm autogenous
- Autogenous brachial-cephalic
- Autogenous brachial-basilic
- Other upper arm autogenous
- Forearm prosthetic
- Upper arm prosthetic

Figure 24-35. Hemodialysis access placement algorithm.

require particular attention to avoid injury to the median or medial antebrachial cutaneous nerves. If arm access sites have been exhausted, femoral artery and saphenous or superficial femoral vein or chest wall axillary artery and vein options can be explored, with the understanding that these are more prone to wound, infectious, and thrombotic complications.

Postoperative Care

Access operations are generally performed as outpatient procedures with an initial postop visit, barring unanticipated complications, at 2 weeks. At this time, arteriovenous grafts with prosthetics may be ready for cannulation. If there are no wounds, perfusion, or patency problems on exam, surveillance of autogenous vein fistulas can be deferred to the time of anticipated maturation at 2 to 3 months. Ultrasound assessments for initiation of access are guided by the rule of 6's: flows in excess of 600 mL/min (to avoid recirculation with dialysis unit operating at about 400 mL/min), vein diameter greater than 6 mm, and depth from skin less than 6 mm to preclude cannulation problems.

Failing Access and Complications

Failing access may manifest as edema, collateral vein enlargement, bleeding, or inadequate flow at dialysis. Etiologies include failure of vein maturation, thrombosis, infection, neointimal hyperplasia, depressed cardiac output, inflow or outflow stenoses, formation of pseudo or true aneurysm, ulcerations at cannulation sites, or steal syndrome.

Vein maturation is a process of dilation and vein wall thickening induced by the rapid blood flow of the newly formed fistula. Vein grafts that fail to enlarge and mature can sometimes be rescued by balloon angioplasty. If vein diameters remain suboptimal, repetitive balloon dilations (balloon-assisted maturation [BAM]) may facilitate enlargement. Flows can be augmented by ligation of residual vein branches, and vein depth can be managed by superficialization or transposition techniques.

Infection is one of the more concerning complications of hemodialysis access and is more common in prosthetic grafts. If localized to a nonanastomotic segment, local excision and interposition or bypass grafting can be utilized. If the infection is at or includes an anastomosis, complete excision and native vessel repair or ligation are necessary to avoid blowout and hemorrhage. Open surgical rescue interventions for these complications include patch angioplasty, excision and interposition grafting, or bypass grafting around the thrombosed, infected, or nonfunctional segment.

In some cases, urgent or emergent intervention will be necessary to preclude either limb threat or serious life-threatening hemorrhage. Ulceration that extends from the skin level to the hemodialysis conduit needs urgent attention. Emergent revision or ligation should be performed in those cases where a sentinel bleed has been observed even if temporarily controlled by pressure. A rare complication that also requires emergent surgery is ischemic monomelic neuropathy (IMN). Manifestations are severe neuropathic pain and paresis with intact distal arm and digital perfusion. Immediate ligation is necessary to preclude permanent neuropathic symptoms and disability.

Selection Variables

Clinical scenarios favoring autogenous success	Young patient age
	Favorable vascular anatomy (artery >2.0 mm; vein >3.0 mm)
	Chronic skin diseases
	History of multiple previous access infections
	Immunosuppression/human immunodeficiency virus
	Hypercoagulability
	Multiple prior prosthetic access failures
Clinical scenarios favoring prosthetic access	Imminent need for or currently undergoing hemodialysis
	Short life expectancy
	Morbid obesity
	Unfavorable vascular anatomy
Factors that adversely influence autogenous access maturation	Diabetes mellitus (radial and ulnar-based accesses)
	Arterial diameter <2.0 mm
	Calcified radial artery
	Vein diameter <3.0 mm
	Congestive heart failure
	Advance patient age
	Female gender

Figure 24-36. Selection variables for fistula versus graft for hemodialysis access.

The more common immediate short- or longer-term problem that may occur and is also potentially limb threatening is arterial steal. Arterial steal syndrome is caused by a combination of flow diversion into the low-resistance venous limb and retrograde flow from the distal arterial bed, usually radial, ulnar, or both, into the vein away from hand and fingers. Ischemic manifestations that may occur with a frequency of up to 10% may be transient, present only during dialysis, or mild enough not to require treatment. Severe steal syndrome with intolerable painful paresthesias occurs with an incidence of only several percent. The most direct management is ligation of the fistula outflow or banding to constrict the arterial anastomosis and decrease the flow. However, banding is generally successful in only about 50% of cases. Therefore, other surgical options have been developed with higher success rates. Depending on experience and available conduits, options are moving the arterial inflow to a point more distally to the forearm brachial or radial artery (revision using distal inflow [RUDI]), more proximally on the brachial or to the axillary (proximalization of the arterial inflow [PAI]), or ligation of the brachial artery distal to the anastomosis and bypass from above the anastomosis to below the ligation (distal revascularization interval ligation [DRIL]). When applicable,

these procedures have reported success rates of 80% to 85% in eliminating or ameliorating ischemic symptoms or tissue loss while preserving the conduit for continued use (Figure 24-37).

OTHER VASCULAR DISORDERS

Arteriovenous Malformations and Arteriovenous Fistulae

AVMs result from abnormal embryologic development of the maturing vascular spaces, producing pathologic arteriovenous connections that involve small and medium-sized vessels. There is an equal male-to-female ratio, and the lower extremities are involved 2 to 3 times as often as the upper extremities. Although lesions are present at birth, most become clinically significant only in the second and third decade as they gradually enlarge. On palpation, a vibration or "thrill" is often noted over the level of the arteriovenous connection and an accompanying bruit can usually be auscultated. A mass may also be present, and cutaneous extension may result in a discolored or pigmented area marking the lesion. Intra-abdominal

Banding   **DRIL**   **RUDI**   **PAI**

Cephalic V.

Brachial
artery

Band

Bypass
graft

Artery
ligation

Fistula
ligation

Bypass
graft

Proximal
graft

Fistula
ligation

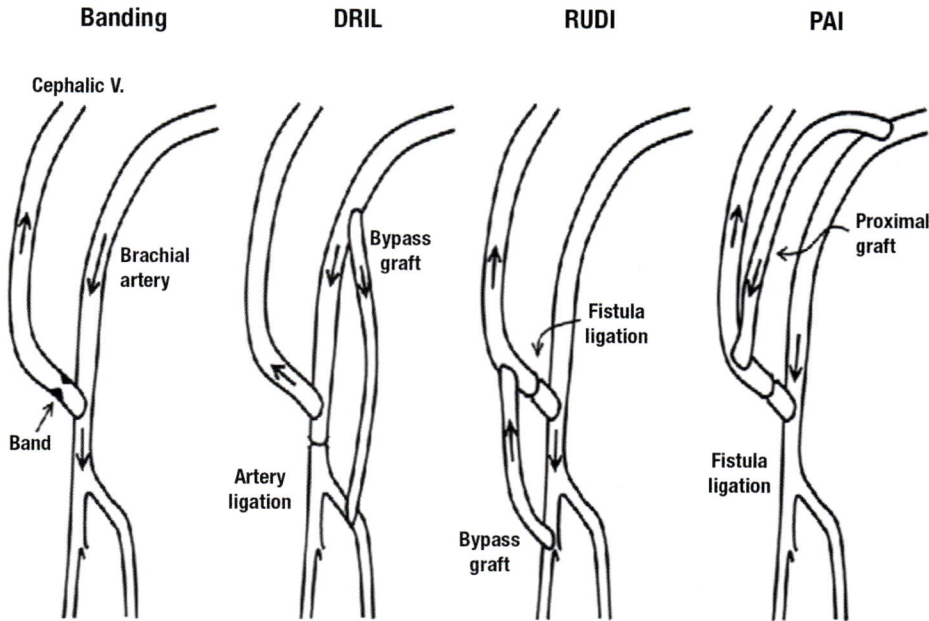

Figure 24-37. Options for surgical treatment of arterial steal syndrome.

and retroperitoneal AVMs are less common but can pose more complex diagnostic and management challenges. Symptoms usually consist of pain and swelling associated with the lesion. Significant musculoskeletal disability may result depending on the size and location of the AVM. In larger AVMs, skin ulceration and bleeding are troublesome complications. Rarely, congenital arteriovenous fistulae produce cardiac enlargement and heart failure as a result of increased blood flow. Diagnosis generally starts with a physical examination but is confirmed with duplex ultrasound and MRI/MRA. CTA/venography may also be useful for delineation of feeding vasculature, and conventional angiography/venography may be required for definitive diagnostic purposes as well as therapeutic intervention.

The management of symptomatic, localized congenital AVMs is surgical excision. The location and potentially disfiguring appearance of some AVMs may warrant treatment even in the absence of symptoms.

The treatment of large or diffuse lesions can be extremely difficult and is associated with a high recurrence rate. An alternative or adjunct to surgery is percutaneous intra-arterial embolization of the main feeding artery and/or IV sclerosis of the outflow veins to reduce the amount of blood that is shunted from the arterioles to the venules.

Treatment approaches can sometimes be directed by flow findings on duplex. High-flow lesions generally have a significant arterial component and require embolization prior to either surgery or sclerotherapy. Low-flow, primarily venous lesions can either be managed conservatively or be sclerosed primarily. In either case, significant soft-tissue necrosis and even marked skin ulceration and complex wounds can result. Therefore, these are best treated in a multidisciplinary fashion with a team including vascular, radiologic, plastic, and pediatric surgeons, along with other wound care specialists.

Acquired arteriovenous fistulae are abnormal communications between the arteries and veins, but they usually result from iatrogenic injuries (arterial catheterizations) or penetrating trauma (gunshot or knife wounds). These fistulae are often associated with a false aneurysm and involve large vessels (common femoral artery–common femoral vein fistula). A palpable thrill or audible bruit may be present. Diagnosis is confirmed by duplex ultrasound examination. Venous HTN, extremity swelling, and venous stasis changes may occur with long-standing arteriovenous fistulae.

All large acquired traumatic arteriovenous fistulae should be repaired to prevent the development of complications (eg, cardiac failure, local pain, aneurysmal formation, limb length discrepancy in children, chronic venous HTN). Direct ultrasound-guided compression of postcatheterization arteriovenous fistulae can be effective, especially if the patient is not anticoagulated. Operative intervention requires complete dissection and separation of the involved vessels and appropriate vascular repair. Depending on their location, some arteriovenous communications can be excluded via an interventional approach using covered stent grafts.

Vasospastic Disorders

Episodic digital vasospasm involving the hands and feet was first described by Maurice Raynaud in 1862. Raynaud syndrome is cold or emotionally induced episodic digital ischemia. As many as 90% of patients are female, and 50% have an associated autoimmune disease (eg, scleroderma, lupus erythematosus, rheumatoid arthritis, Sjögren syndrome). Some develop Raynaud syndrome from work-related overuse of vibratory machinery. Unilateral Raynaud syndrome is more common in men and is often associated with proximal arterial disease of the large vessels, such as subclavian stenoses or occlusions.

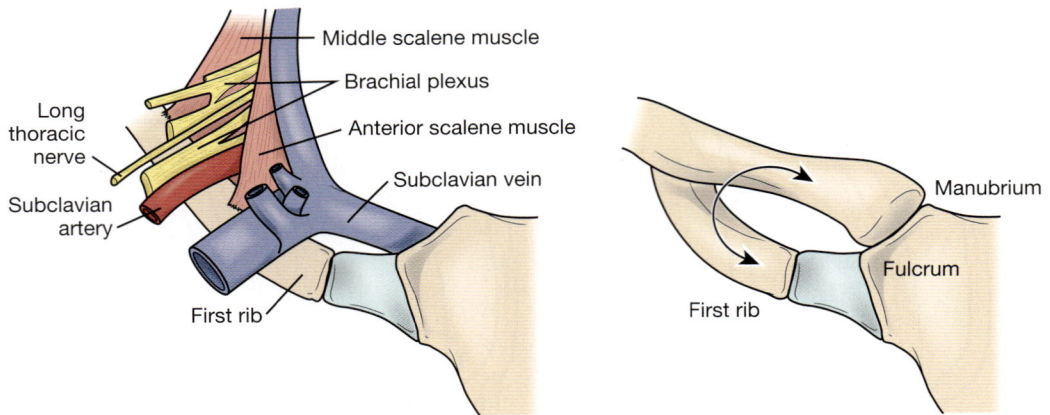

Figure 24-38. Anatomic causes of thoracic outlet syndrome.

The classic Raynaud attack has three distinct phases, which occur in sequence (white, blue, red). Exposure to cold initially causes profound vasospasm and blanching of the digits (white). After approximately 15 minutes, cyanosis is evident, caused by venous filling with delayed venous emptying (blue). Later, the digits and hands become hyperemic as vasospasm lessens and flow to the digits is restored (red).

The diagnosis of Raynaud syndrome is made from the history and physical examination. Coexistent symptoms of connective tissue disorders are often elicited. Laboratory tests (sedimentation rate, complement assay, antinuclear antibody assay) often confirm the immunologic disorders associated with the syndrome. It is important to document all pulses palpated. Doppler evaluation may be helpful if pulses are difficult to feel.

Treatment consists of discontinuing any medications that cause reduced cardiac output or promote vasospasm and that are associated with Raynaud syndrome (ergotamines and β-blockers). Other pharmacologic agents, especially α- and calcium channel–blocking agents, may be used to reduce the tendency toward vasospasm. Sympathetic blocks with xylocaine are occasionally used for temporary relief, although surgical sympathectomy is not a particularly effective treatment because sympathetic fibers regenerate over time. Revascularization of an ischemic extremity may markedly improve the symptoms in patients with concomitant arterial occlusive disease.

Thoracic Outlet Syndrome

Thoracic outlet syndrome (TOS) is a constellation of clinical problems related to compression of the brachial plexus (neurogenic), arteries (aneurysm and emboli), and veins (Paget-Schroetter syndrome). The neurogenic syndrome is often seen in young and middle-aged women. Symptoms are caused by compression or irritation of the brachial plexus as nerves pass through the thoracic outlet and the costoclavicular space.

Anatomic causes of the syndrome include an elongated transverse process of the seventh cervical vertebra; a fully developed cervical rib; congenital bands in the outlet related to the cervical rib, middle scalene muscle, or anterior scalene muscle; and a narrowed costoclavicular space, often because of a previously fractured rib or clavicle, with callus formation (Figure 24-38).

Paresthesia of the arm and hand reflects neurologic compression and is much more common than arterial symptoms. When arterial symptoms occur, they include coldness of the hand and arm, pallor, and muscle fatigue. In rare cases, stenosis of the subclavian artery causes an aneurysm (Figure 24-39) and/or emboli to the hand. Subclavian vein thrombosis (Paget-Schroetter syndrome) may also occur (Figure 24-40).

Evaluation of these patients involves a detailed history and a thorough physical examination to document localized scalene muscle tenderness and radicular phenomena. Adson test (disappearance of the radial pulse on arm abduction and external rotation of the shoulder), said in the early literature to be indicative of TOS, is now considered relatively nonspecific. Cervical spine radiographs are obtained to identify cervical ribs. Nerve conduction velocity across the outlet and local anesthetic injection of the anterior scalene muscle are used to determine the etiology of symptoms. Angiography is recommended only if arterial occlusion or embolization is suspected. Venography is used in patients with duplex scan confirmation of thrombosis of the subclavian vein.

After the diagnosis is confirmed, nonsurgical treatments, including physical therapy and Botox injection of the anterior scalene muscle, are attempted in patients with neurogenic TOS. If symptoms persist, surgical decompression of the

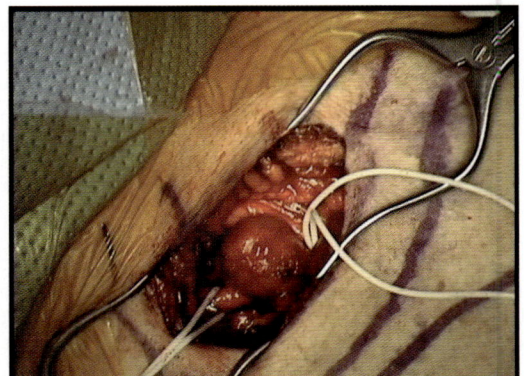

Figure 24-39. Aneurysm of subclavian artery. This photograph shows a subclavian artery aneurysm, which formed distal to compression from thoracic outlet syndrome.

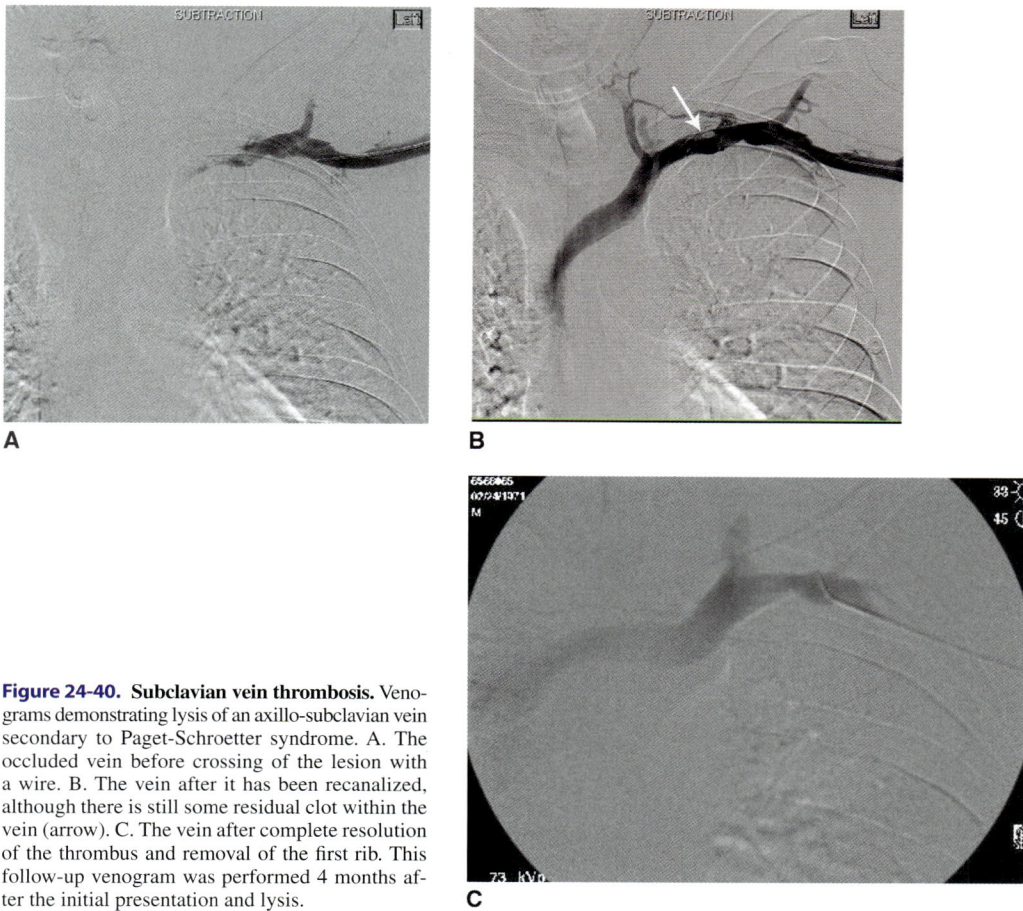

Figure 24-40. Subclavian vein thrombosis. Venograms demonstrating lysis of an axillo-subclavian vein secondary to Paget-Schroetter syndrome. A. The occluded vein before crossing of the lesion with a wire. B. The vein after it has been recanalized, although there is still some residual clot within the vein (arrow). C. The vein after complete resolution of the thrombus and removal of the first rib. This follow-up venogram was performed 4 months after the initial presentation and lysis.

outlet may be warranted. The most commonly used procedure is resection of the first thoracic rib, removal of any cervical ribs, and division of the anterior scalene muscle. Patients with TOS without a cervical rib can have either a transaxillary approach with first rib resection or supraclavicular anterior scalenectomy for decompression of the thoracic outlet. Patients with vasculogenic TOS (artery or vein) require a thrombolysis of the clot, followed by decompression of the thoracic inlet and occasionally surgical repair of the affected artery or vein.

Lymphatic Disorders

The lymphatic system serves a number of functions, including the return of proteins and extracellular fluid that are lost from the capillary circulation, and the removal of bacteria and foreign materials from the extracellular space. Lymphedema occurs when transcapillary fluid flux into the extracellular space exceeds the capacity of lymph transport to return that fluid to the circulation. In these situations, protein-rich fluid accumulates in the limb and relative stasis of the fluid ensues.

Primary lymphedema is classified as congenital lymphedema (present at birth), lymphedema praecox (usually starting at 10-15 years of age), or lymphedema tarda (starting after 35 years of age). The lymphangiographic appearance further divides primary lymphedema into hyperplasia, in which numerous dilated lymphatic vessels are present,

and hypoplasia, in which lymphatics are few in number and small in caliber. Secondary or acquired lymphedema occurs after recurrent infection, radiation, surgical excision, or neoplastic invasion of regional lymph nodes.

Patients with lymphedema usually have diffuse painless enlargement of the extremities. Elevation of the extremity is often of little help, as elevated venous pressures are not usually a major factor in the accumulation of fluid. Similarly, diuretics are often of little benefit. With time, the soft "pitting" edema becomes "woody" as progressive fibrosis of the connective tissue occurs. Superimposed infection (cellulitis) of the extremity will accelerate the fibrotic process and exacerbate lymphedema.

Treatment includes both medical and surgical management, neither of which can cure the process. The use of high-pressure support hosiery, avoidance of prolonged standing, lymphatic massage, sequential compression devices, and meticulous foot care to minimize infection are the primary medical therapies. If infection develops, erythema and lymphangitis may ensue. This should be treated aggressively with antibiotics, elevation, and bed rest. Patients with long-standing acquired lymphedema are at an increased risk of lymphangiosarcoma and should be followed closely with biopsy of any suspicious changes.

Surgical intervention is considered only if medical management fails to adequately control symptoms. Surgical approaches fall into two categories: reconstruction of the lymphatic drainage (lymphangioplasty) and excision of varying amounts of subcutaneous tissue and skin. Unfortunately, the results of surgery are often disappointing and should be reserved for patients with extensive edema who have failed medical therapy and are in such distress from the lymphedema that amputation is a viable consideration.

SUGGESTED READINGS

Cronenwett JL, Johnston KW. *Rutherford's Vascular Surgery*. 8th ed. Elsevier-Saunders; 2014.

Stanley JC, Veith FJ, Wakefield TW. *Current Therapy in Vascular and Endovascular Surgery*. 5th ed. Elsevier-Saunders; 2014.

SAMPLE QUESTIONS

QUESTIONS

Choose the best answer for each question.

1. A 68-year-old man comes to the office because he noted a pulsatile bulge in his abdomen for the past 2 years, and it is becoming more prominent. He has a remote history of MI, and his only risk factors are one pack per day of smoking and HTN, controlled with a diuretic. His physical exam is normal except for a pulsatile, nontender mass above his umbilicus, which measures 7 cm. What is the best initial test for this patient?

   A. CT scan with contrast of the abdomen and pelvis
   B. MRI/MRA of the abdomen and pelvis
   C. Duplex ultrasound of the abdomen
   D. Arteriogram
   E. Plain film of the abdomen

2. A 70-year-old woman responds to an advertisement for cardiovascular screening, which includes an ABI, an ECG, an ultrasound for AAA, and a carotid duplex ultrasound. She is told that she has a stenosis in her left carotid artery of 50% to 70%, and no significant stenosis in the right carotid bulb. What should your recommendation to her be?

   A. CEA
   B. Carotid angiogram
   C. Carotid stent
   D. High-dose aspirin
   E. Repeat carotid duplex ultrasound

3. A 50-year-old woman with type 1 diabetes has developed an ulcer that penetrates into the fat on the plantar aspect of the left foot, under the ball of her big toe. She has foot swelling, so pulses are not palpable, but she has good capillary refill in the toes. The ulcer is not painful and is not clinically infected. What is the next best step for this problem?

   A. Big toe amputation
   B. IV antibiotics
   C. Measure ABI and toe pressures
   D. Angiography
   E. Non-weight-bearing and continued observation

4. A 35-year-old woman comes to the office because of an ulcer on the skin of her left ankle. She developed pigmentation in her left medial ankle several years ago and then developed a superficial, painless ulcer in the center of the pigmented area 2 months ago. She had been in excellent health prior to that. She works as a schoolteacher and is on her feet most of the day. She has been unable to heal it with local wound care and comes to see you for treatment. Which of the following diagnostic tests would be most useful?

   A. ABI
   B. Wound culture
   C. Lab tests for autoimmune disease
   D. Venous duplex ultrasound
   E. Ulcer biopsy

5. An 80-year-old, frail woman with chronic renal insufficiency due to diabetes, HTN, and congestive heart failure (CHF) with an ejection fraction (EF) of 30% presents to your clinic for discussion of angioaccess planning for impending need for hemodialysis. Her renal function has worsened quickly, and her nephrologist thinks she'll need dialysis within a few weeks. On ultrasound, she has arm veins ranging from 1.5 mm in her lower arms to 2.0 mm in diameter in her upper arms. What is likely the most appropriate long-term angioaccess for this patient?

   A. Arteriovenous fistula with the 2-mm vein in her dominant upper arm
   B. Arteriovenous fistula with the 2-mm vein in her nondominant upper arm
   C. Percutaneously placed hemodialysis catheter
   D. Arteriovenous graft in her dominant arm
   E. Arteriovenous graft in her nondominant arm

ANSWERS AND EXPLANATIONS

1. **Answer: A**

   All of the tests offered will diagnose an aneurysm; an astute clinician needs to determine the most cost effective of available tests. The diagnosis of aneurysm, based on a large AAA by physical exam, is not in doubt, so the key to management is selecting the one test that can measure the aneurysm, determine the anatomy, determine whether he is a candidate for an endovascular graft, and allow for pre-op planning. Only a CTA provides all of this information. An ultrasound is the best and most cost-effective test for screening, which is not necessary in this situation because his aneurysm has already been diagnosed. MRI/MRA can show most aspects for planning, except for assessing the aortic wall for calcium, which can help determine whether he is a candidate for an endograft. Arteriography has been replaced by CTA because an arteriogram does not show the aortic wall or thrombus in the aneurysm sac, which is important for procedural planning. A plain film can assess for the presence and size of an aneurysm but does not allow for procedural planning. For more information on this topic, please see section "Clinical Presentation of Aneurysms."

2. **Answer: E**

Carotid stenosis is often found by screening studies but must be confirmed by another diagnostic test before treatment. Of the options available, only repeat duplex ultrasound is a low-risk diagnostic test. When a screening study is abnormal, confirmation of the findings with a repeat full-length study is often the best approach to confirm the findings. An angiogram carries a risk of stroke and has little additional information that cannot be obtained with an MR angiogram or CTA. The decision for treatment in an asymptomatic patient should be preceded by risk factor modification with low-dose antiplatelet therapy, statins, and β-blockers. Carotid stent is not approved in asymptomatic patients, and CEA should not be performed in asymptomatic women until their stenosis becomes greater than 80%. For more information on this topic, please see section "Cerebrovascular Insufficiency."

3. **Answer: C**

This patient has a mal perforans ulcer, which is a neuropathic ulcer on the ball of the foot caused by changes in the motor, sensory, and autonomic nerves in the extremity. The absence of ulcer pain, in itself, tells you that she has severe peripheral neuropathy. She is at risk for a major amputation unless she has adequate blood supply to heal, good local wound care with offloading of the ulcer, and then good footwear once the ulcer is healed. The presence of blood supply is critical to preventing amputation, and physical exam is not accurate

for assessing perfusion, so she needs noninvasive testing, including an ABI, toe pressures, and assessment of tissue perfusion around the ulcer. If she has a significant pressure deficit in the foot, then an angioplasty or bypass is needed to provide enough blood supply to heal the ulcer. Amputation and IV antibiotics will not be effective if there is inadequate blood supply. For more information on this topic, please see section "Evaluation" under the "Peripheral Arterial Occlusive Disease" heading.

4. **Answer: D**

On the basis of the location and description, as well as the age and absence of significant other medical problems, this patient has chronic venous insufficiency. The pigmentation represents lipodermatosclerosis, and the venous ulcer may be caused by reflux in the superficial, perforator, and deep venous systems. An ABI is unlikely to be helpful in a woman at her age, with the ulcer in its current location. Wound cultures are helpful occasionally in the management of venous ulcers, but not in diagnosing them, and the location and age make both serum autoimmune disease tests and biopsies unlikely to make the diagnosis. For more information on this topic, please see the section "Diagnosis" under the heading "Chronic Venous Insufficiency."

5. **Answer: E**

In this frail older adult woman with small veins, the best course of action would be an arterio-venous graft in her nondominant arm. Though the risks of infection are higher with prosthetics, her veins are very small and unlikely to mature enough for use. Furthermore, with early access grafts, she could be ready for dialysis 2 weeks postoperatively. For more information on this topic, please see section "Procedure" and Figures 24-35 and 24-36 under the heading "Angioaccess for Hemodialysis."

25

Otolaryngology: Diseases of the Head and Neck

Andrew M. Vahabzadeh-Hagh

Otolaryngology is the study of organ systems connected by the upper aerodigestive tract: the ear, vestibular system, cranial nerves, nose, paranasal sinuses, oral cavity, pharynx, larynx, esophagus, neck, and salivary and thyroid glands. These regions are critical for human interaction and communication, as well as for functions rudimentary to sustaining life (ie, breathing and eating).

The disorders discussed in this chapter have a great impact on the cost of health care and quality of life. More than 60% of all primary care visits for childhood illness and more than 50% of all adult primary care visits are for disorders of the ear, nose, and throat. Rhinosinusitis has the greatest financial impact on the economy of the United States through loss of job productivity and health care costs. Among the most common operations performed in the United States are tonsillectomy and/or adenoidectomy as well as myringotomy with tympanostomy tube placement.

THE EAR, THE VESTIBULAR SYSTEM, AND THE FACIAL NERVE

Anatomy

The ear is divided into the external, middle, and inner ears (Figure 25-1). The external ear includes the auricle, which has a cartilaginous framework, and the external auditory canal, which is cartilaginous in one-third of its lateral aspect and bony in two-thirds of its medial aspect. The skin of the cartilaginous external canal contains hair follicles and cerumen glands.

The middle ear is an air-containing space consisting of the eustachian tube, the tympanic membrane (ear drum), the ossicular chain (malleus, incus, and stapes bones), and the stapedius and tensor tympani muscles. The middle ear communicates with the mastoid cavity of the temporal bone (collections of air-containing sinusoids).

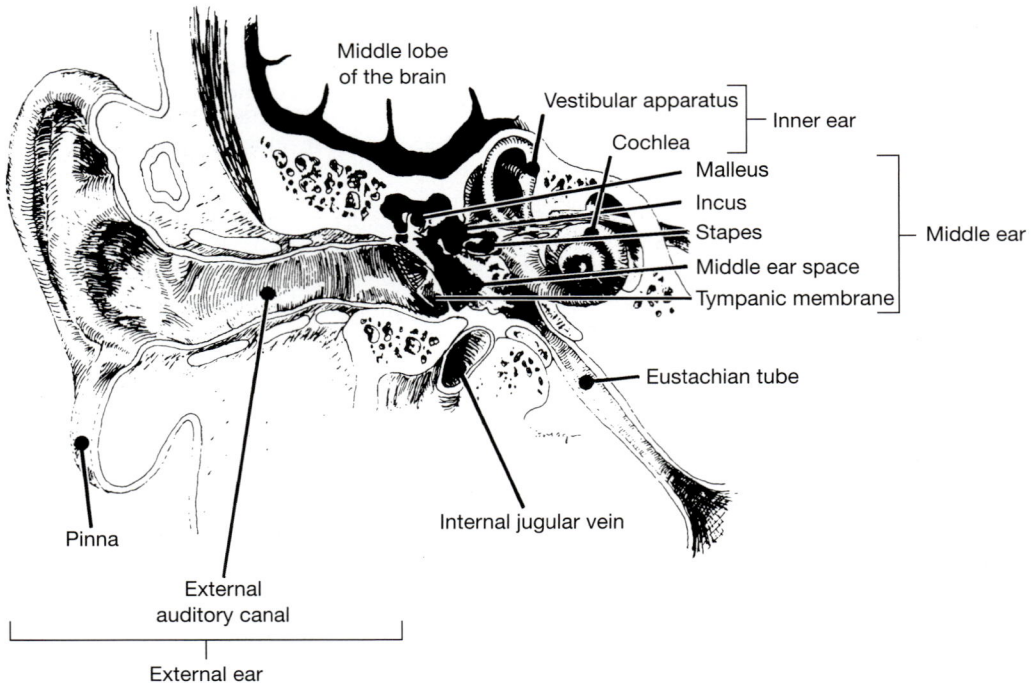

Figure 25-1. Cross-section of the ear. (From Lawrence PF. *Essentials of Surgical Specialties.* 3rd ed. Lippincott Williams & Wilkins; 2007.)

The inner ear consists of the cochlea, the semicircular canals, and the internal auditory canal. The inner ear is divided into the auditory and vestibular systems. Three types of sensory organ transducers are found in the inner ear: the organ of Corti (Figure 25-2), located in the cochlea; the macula, located in the utricle and saccule; and the crista, located in the semicircular canals.

The internal auditory canal, located on the posteromedial aspect of the temporal bone, houses cranial nerves VII (innervates the muscles of facial expression) and VIII (innervates the vestibular and cochlear portions of the inner ear). It also houses the nervus intermedius, which carries taste fibers from the tongue and parasympathetic secretomotor fibers from the brainstem to the sublingual, submandibular, and mucosal glands of the nose and palate and to the lacrimal glands. The facial nerve lies anterosuperior to the vestibular and auditory portion of the eighth cranial nerve in the internal auditory canal. It runs from the pons in the brainstem through the middle ear cavity and the mastoid, arising from the stylomastoid foramen. It innervates the stapedius, postauricular, and posterior belly of the digastric muscles. Its extratemporal component travels through the parotid gland to innervate the muscles of facial expression (Figure 25-3).

Physiology

The adnexal and ceruminous structures of the outer portion of the external auditory canal produce a waxy material that serves as a lubricant for the skin, a trap for foreign particles, and a protective acidic barrier against microorganisms.

The eardrum and the ossicular chain are responsible for conducting and amplifying sound waves from the external auditory canal to the inner ear through the oval window via the stapes footplate.

Under normal conditions, the air-containing space of the middle ear is periodically inflated when swallowing or chewing; this momentarily opens the eustachian tube, which is normally closed, and allows pressure equalization. The eustachian tube opens by the synergistic action of the tensor veli palatini (innervated by the third division of the trigeminal nerve) and levator veli palatini (innervated by vagus) muscles. Failure of the middle ear space to remain properly inflated with air may result in the accumulation of secretory fluids (effusion), affecting compliance of the tympanic membrane and the ossicles; this change in compliance may result in conductive hearing loss.

The inner ear houses three sensory organs (organ of Corti, macula, and crista) that contain hair cell transducers responsible for converting mechanical energy (vibratory, rotational, and gravitational) into electrical energy.

Vibratory energy (sound pressure), producing movement of the stapes footplate, causes the propagation of complex waves traveling through the inner ear fluid in the cochlea, which in turn causes the basilar membrane to move up and down. The movement of the basilar membrane with respect to the overlying gelatinous tectorial

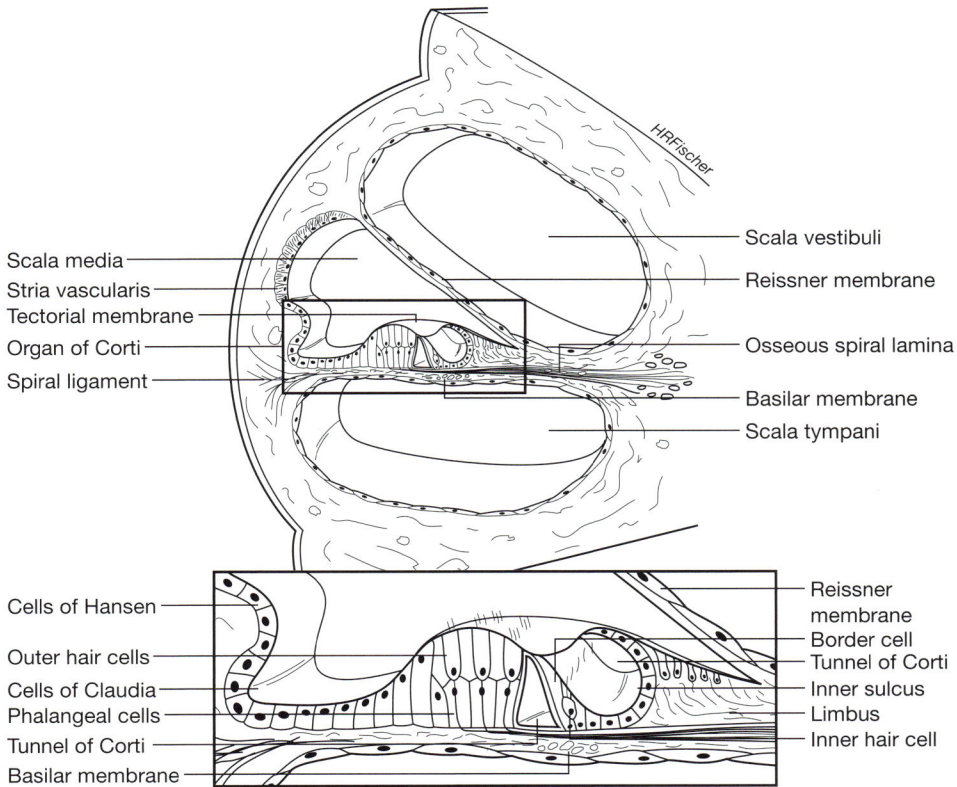

Figure 25-2. Cross-section of the cochlea showing the organ of Corti. (From Lawrence PF. *Essentials of Surgical Specialties.* 3rd ed. Lippincott Williams & Wilkins; 2007.)

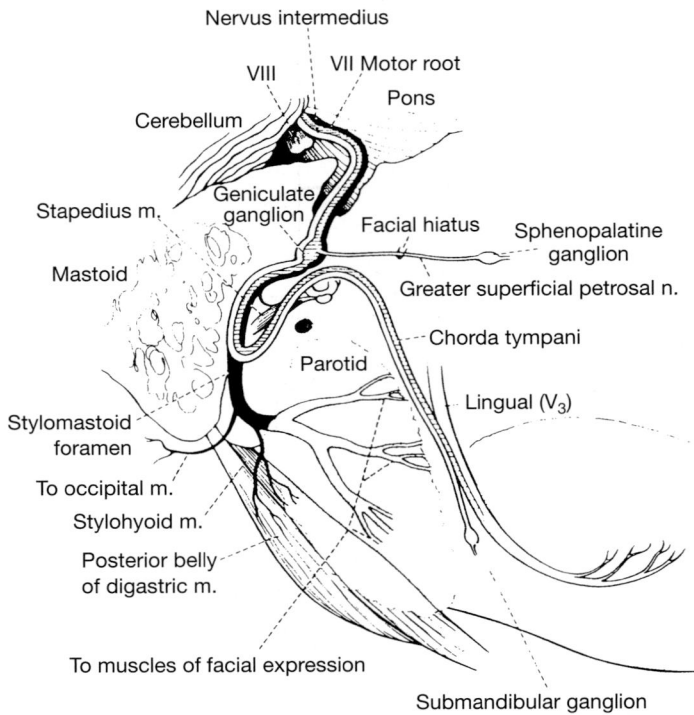

Figure 25-3. Anatomy of the facial nerve. (From Lawrence PF. *Essentials of Surgical Specialties.* 3rd ed. Lippincott Williams & Wilkins; 2007.)

membrane causes a shearing action, bending the stereocilia at the apical ends of the hair cells. This mechanical deformation triggers electrical energy in the form of nerve impulses emanating from the hair cells. This energy is transmitted to the central nervous system (CNS) through the auditory nerve, ultimately permitting the perception of sound. Hair cells maintain a tonotopic organization along the basilar membrane so that displacement by waves near the stapes (base of the cochlea) results in high-frequency perception while waves at the apex result in low-frequency perception (Figure 25-4).

Rotational acceleration of the head is detected by the semicircular canals, whereas linear acceleration is detected by the macula of the utricle and saccule. Hair cells are the basic element that transduces the mechanical forces to nerve action potentials in both systems, but their complex organization is different. Energy caused by the rotation of the head produces shifts in the fluid of the semicircular canal; these fluid shifts shake the gelatinous-like cupulae (within which hair cell cilia are embedded). This motion causes a temporary deformation of the cilia, resulting in stimulation of the hair cells. Energy from gravity or changes in linear acceleration produces movement of the utricular stone-like otoconia, resulting in temporary deformation of the cilia-like projections of the hair cells. These mechanical deformations trigger electrical energy in the form of nerve impulses emanating from the hair cells. This energy is transmitted through the superior and inferior vestibular nerves, permitting the sensation of either rotation or acceleration.

Vestibular input is one of three systems (ie, vestibular, ocular, proprioceptive) on which the body depends to maintain orientation in space. Under many circumstances one may be able to maintain relatively normal orientation without simultaneous input from all three systems; however, denying visual input (eyes closed) or proprioceptive input (weightlessness) to patients with vestibulopathy may significantly reduce a person's ability to orient.

Vertigo is a sensory phenomenon associated with the important relation between the input of the left and right vestibular systems into the CNS. If vestibular input is not symmetrical, it will result in discordant output, manifesting as vertigo, which is akin to a sensation of rotating in space. Vertigo is a hallucination of motion when objective motion does not exist. Because of the vestibular-ocular tracts, this fictitious motion produces a number of saccadic ocular tracking motions irrespective of visual input, referred to as "nystagmus." This type of asymmetrical input may occur whenever an insult occurs to one ear rather than both inner ears such as in vestibular neuritis. However, with time, the vestibular system, unlike the auditory system, may compensate for asymmetrical input.

The facial nerve is the motor nerve for muscles of facial expression. When nerve dysfunction exists, paralysis of these muscles occurs. Depending on the site of the paralyzing lesion, other dysfunction may also be present including loss of lacrimal secretions, absent stapedial reflex, loss of submandibular or nasal secretions or both, loss of sensation in the floor of the mouth, and loss of taste in the anterior tongue (Figure 25-5).

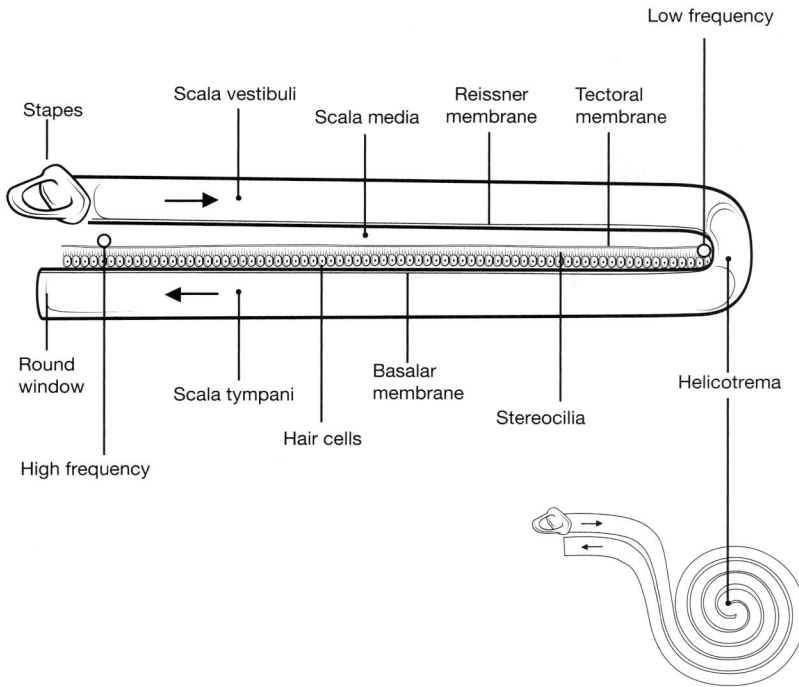

Figure 25-4. Schematic representation of the cochlea unwound. The arrows represent the initial fluid shifts as the stapes vibrates. Notice the tonotopic organization of hair cells. High-frequency sounds stimulate the hair cells near the stapes. Low-frequency sounds stimulate hair cells near the apex or helicotrema. (From Lawrence PF. *Essentials of Surgical Specialties.* 3rd ed. Lippincott Williams & Wilkins; 2007.)

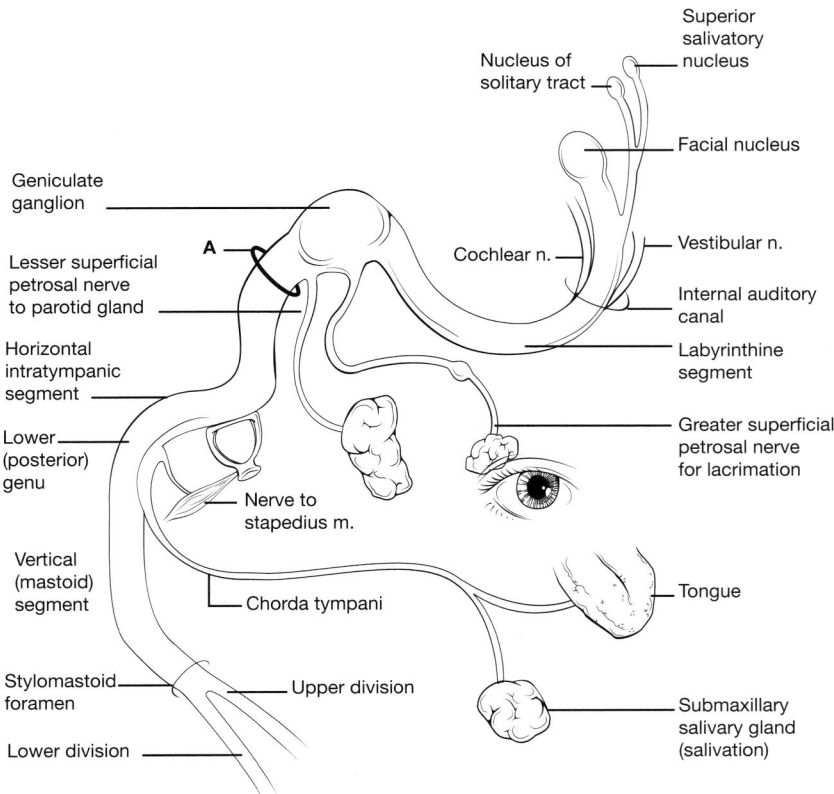

Figure 25-5. Schematic diagram of the facial nerve. Notice how damage to the nerve at site *A* would result in loss of function distal to the lesion, but lacrimation and parotid salivation would be preserved. (From Lawrence PF. *Essentials of Surgical Specialties.* 3rd ed. Lippincott Williams & Wilkins; 2007.)

If a facial nerve injury is severe, requiring significant regeneration, it is unlikely that normal anatomy will be reduplicated because not all nerve connections will reestablish. Aberrant reinnervation may result in very noticeable unintentional simultaneous contraction of multiple facial muscles (synkinesis).

Physical Examination

Examination of the ear begins with observation of the auricle. The examiner looks at its shape and the condition of the skin and surrounding area.

The external auditory canal is examined by using an otoscope fitted with a speculum. Pulling the pinna up and slightly away from the scalp straightens the external canal for easier examination and speculum insertion. The external auditory canal is observed for evidence of obstruction, otorrhea, or integumentary abnormality.

The eardrum, or tympanic membrane, should be evaluated for deviation from its normal translucent appearance (Figure 25-6). Often, one can see portions of the ossicular chain (malleus, incus, and stapes bones) through the tympanic membrane. The eardrum should be evaluated for thickness, opacification, inflammation, and abnormal deposits (eg, calcium). The presence of any unusually thin spots (monomer) should be determined. Perforations larger than 1 mm are quite easily seen but are often mistaken for the retraction pocket commonly seen in the ears of patients with chronic eustachian tube dysfunction. The eardrum should also be observed for any evidence of middle ear fluid, which may cause a loss of translucency and a speckled light reflex on the eardrum or may appear as air-fluid levels with bubbles in the middle air space. A pneumatic otoscope with a speculum large enough to occlude the ear canal is used to apply negative and positive pressure to the tympanic membrane to determine its freedom of movement, thus evaluating middle ear compliance.

During the course of the history and physical examination, the patient's hearing can be grossly assessed by determining whether the patient is able to understand normal conversational speech, which is at 55 dB and involves frequencies from 500 to 3,000 Hz.

In addition to a standard cranial nerve examination, patients with vestibular complaints should undergo further neurologic examination. The patient is observed for spontaneous or induced nystagmus with position changes. Because disorientation complaints may result from dysfunction of vestibular, ocular, or proprioceptive systems, Romberg testing attempts to "sort out" the cause by removing ocular influence. The Romberg test involves measuring a patient's ability to remain oriented in a standing position with eyes closed. Cerebellar testing (finger to nose, alternating hand test) is also helpful.

Evaluation

Hearing Loss

Although mixed hearing losses exist, pure losses are more common (ie, either conductive or sensorineural). Making this distinction and determining whether both ears are symmetrically affected are very important in simplifying the differential diagnosis. Table 25-1 categorizes some of the causes of hearing loss as they relate to the inner, middle, or outer ear.

TABLE 25-1. Etiologies of Conductive and Sensorineural Hearing Loss

Conductive Hearing Loss	Sensorineural Hearing Loss
External auditory canal obstruction	Cochlear pathology
Cerumen impaction	Presbycusis
Swelling from severe external otitis	Ototoxicity
Congenital stenosis or atresia	Temporal bone trauma
Noise-induced hearing loss	Meningitis
Ménière disease	Viral labyrinthitis
Acquired stenosis	Viral labyrinthitis
Neoplasm	Retrocochlear pathology
Middle ear pathology	Acoustic neuroma and other inner ear or skull-base neoplasms
Otitis media	Sudden sensorineural hearing loss
Tympanic perforation	
Unclear etiology	
Otosclerosis	
Ossicular trauma	

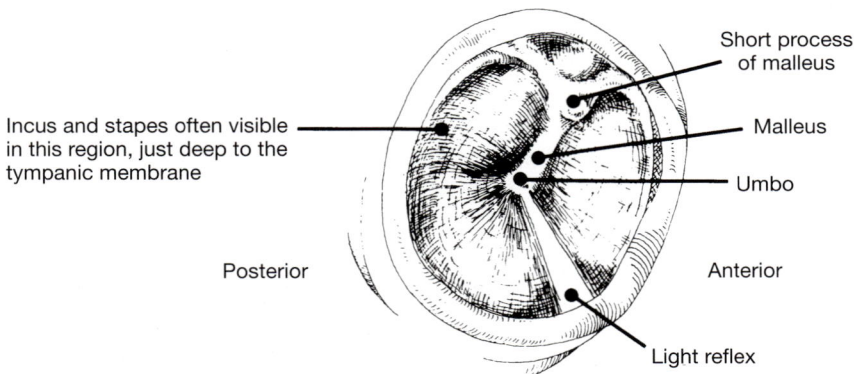

Figure 25-6. The tympanic membrane landmarks (right ear). (From Lawrence PF. *Essentials of Surgical Specialties.* 3rd ed. Lippincott Williams & Wilkins; 2007.)

As the term *conductive hearing loss* suggests, patients with this loss have inadequate means of properly conducting sound to the inner ear. This could be produced by any disorder related to the external auditory canal, tympanic membrane, middle ear space, or ossicles. This defect produces a loss of amplification, which is often described as "muffled hearing."

The most common complaint of patients with bilateral sensorineural hearing loss is difficulty hearing and understanding in large gatherings. Patients with sensorineural hearing loss generally have a distaste for loud music and loud conversation, which add further distortion and discomfort. Unilateral hearing loss commonly implies a local rather than systemic cause. This should prompt the clinician to rule out a neoplastic process.

Tuning fork tests help the clinician differentiate between conductive and sensorineural hearing loss. These tests are most helpful when the hearing loss is purely conductive or sensorineural, and unilateral. The Weber test is performed with a vibrating 512-Hz tuning fork, placed centrally on the forehead, bony nasal dorsum, or maxillary dentition. The patient is asked whether the sound is heard better in one ear or in the center of the head. If the patient hears the sound better in one ear, either a greater sensorineural hearing loss exists in the contralateral ear or a conductive loss is present in the ipsilateral ear. Conductive loss masks background sounds, resulting in enhanced body and skull sounds. In the Rinne test, the patient is asked to determine whether the tuning fork is heard louder when it is placed on the mastoid bone or when it is held approximately 2 cm from the external canal. A patient with normal hearing or with sensorineural hearing loss will hear the tuning fork better when it is placed adjacent to the ear canal, indicating air conduction. A patient with a significant conductive loss will hear the tuning fork better when it is placed on the mastoid bone because air-conducted sounds are masked and skull sounds are enhanced.

Pure-tone audiometry qualifies hearing loss according to frequencies, allocating and measuring the amount of loss according to sensorineural and conductive mechanisms. It does not assess speech recognition or discrimination. Pure-tone audiometry is performed by presenting a series of variable-intensity tone pips ("beeps") via earphones at six or more frequencies (250, 500, 1,000, 2,000, 4,000, and 8,000 Hz) to which the patient volunteers a response. The threshold is the lowest intensity of stimulus that the patient is able to hear. The zero-dB line on the audiogram is considered normal, and the patient's hearing levels are recorded as dB above or below the zero-dB point along each of the six frequencies.

A hearing threshold of 0 to 20 dB represents normal hearing; 25 to 40 dB, a mild loss; 40 to 70 dB, a moderate loss; 70 to 90 dB, a severe loss; and greater than 90 dB, a profound loss. Sensorineural hearing loss is determined by obtaining bone conduction thresholds. The tone pips ("beeps") are delivered to the cochlea by placing a sound-generating device on the mastoid bone bypassing the external and middle ear. Conductive hearing loss thresholds are measured by first delivering the "beeps" through the air via earphones. Sound stimuli delivered in this way must traverse the outer, middle, and inner ears to be heard, thus giving a set of air-conducted scores for each ear. These air-conducted scores are then compared with bone-conducted scores. If the scores match, no conductive hearing loss exists; if the air scores are worse than the bone scores (resulting in an "air-bone gap"), a conductive hearing loss equaling the size of the air-bone gap is present (Figure 25-7). The size of the air-bone gap can help predict the site of disruption.

The speech reception threshold (SRT) probably correlates best with one of the most important communication skills: understanding spoken words. The patient is presented with a series of two-syllable words. The SRT is the measure of the lowest dB hearing level at which the patient can successfully repeat these words 50% of the time. The speech discrimination or word recognition score is the percentage of phonetically balanced monosyllabic words the patient can successfully repeat when they are presented at 20 to 40 dB above the SRT. Pathology of the cochlea, auditory nerve, or CNS causes perceptual distortion impairing speech discrimination.

With electrophysiologic audiometry, the audiologist must interpret an involuntary or reflexive physiologic response. One of the most useful electrophysiologic tests is the **auditory brainstem response test,** which measures the electroencephalographic responses to sound stimuli. Another useful electrophysiologic test is the **evoked otoacoustic emissions (EOAEs) test.** EOAEs are sounds emitted by the cochlea in response to acoustic stimulation. The hearing of neonates, young children, and patients who are comatose, have intellectual disability, or are otherwise unreliable is assessed with these techniques because no volitional response is required.

Tympanometry measures the function of the eardrum with a multichannel probe (containing a speaker, a microphone, and a transducer) that fits into the ear canal. The transducer produces pressure changes from 400 mm H_2O of negative pressure to 200 mm H_2O of positive pressure, whereas the speaker delivers low-frequency sound. The microphone senses the amount of sound energy reflected and records it on a tracing. On the basis of the configuration of the tympanogram, inferences can be made about the function of the middle ear, the presence or absence of fluid, and the presence of a perforation (Figure 25-8).

Otalgia

Most causes of earache are easy to identify; however, because of the complex sensory innervation of the ear and the temporal bone, pain from many other sources may be referred to the ear and mistaken for an ear pathology. In addition to the obvious examination of the ear, the upper aerodigestive tract should be examined because pain at this site is frequently referred to the ear. Queries about exacerbating factors may be helpful. Increased otalgia on chewing, a history of temporomandibular joint (TMJ) trauma, or recent dental work point to the myofascial structures of the TMJ. Tenderness in these areas may be confirmatory in the absence of other physical findings (Table 25-2).

Tinnitus

Tinnitus is "ringing" or some other perceived noise in the ears. It usually occurs in the absence of an objective acoustic stimulus. The very nature of the sound is key to making a diagnosis. Pulsatile tinnitus is usually vascular in origin. Cochlear injury produces a continuous noise that may vary in intensity with background noise or the time

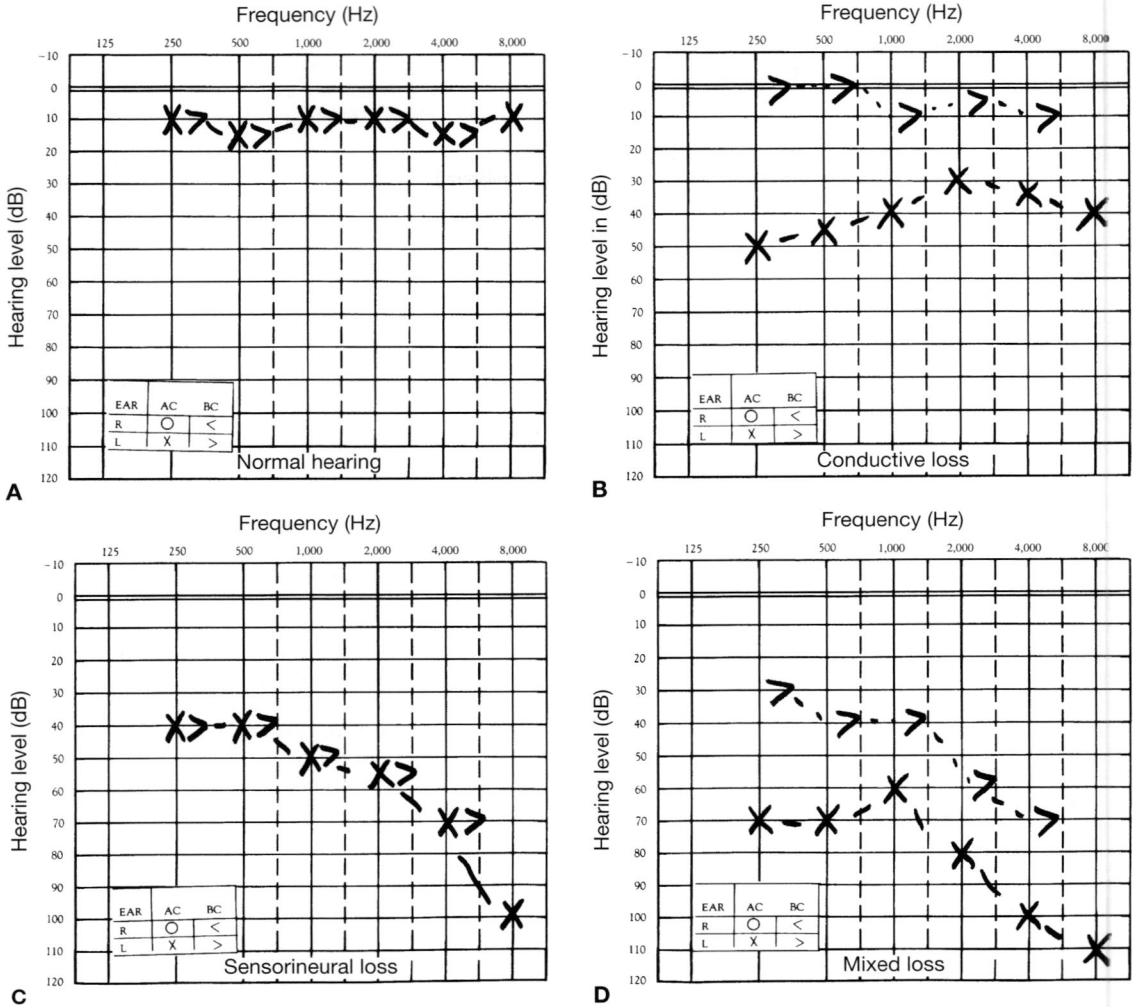

Figure 25-7. Examples of pure-tone audiograms of the left ear only. A. Normal hearing (normal air scores = normal bone scores). B. Conductive hearing loss (abnormal air scores and normal bone scores, indicating an air-bone gap). C. Sensorineural hearing loss (abnormal air scores = abnormal bone scores). D. Mixed or combined sensorineural and conductive hearing loss (abnormal air scores are worse than abnormal bone scores, indicating a conductive hearing loss [note air-bone gap] superimposed on a sensorineural hearing loss). The lower limit of normal hearing is about 20 dB. AC, air conduction; BC, bone conduction; L, left; R, right. (From Lawrence PF. *Essentials of Surgical Specialties.* 3rd ed. Lippincott Williams & Wilkins; 2007.)

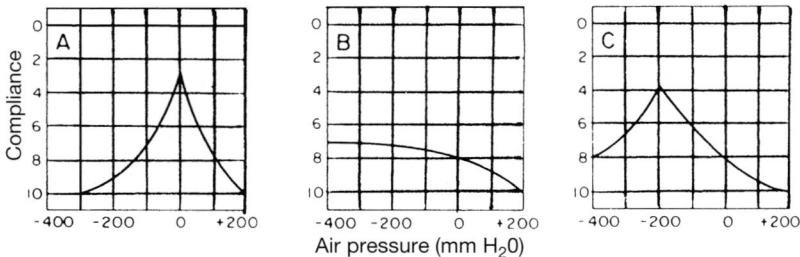

Figure 25-8. Typical patterns obtained with tympanometry. A. Peak efficiency occurs with no pressure manipulation. B. Often referred to as a flat tympanogram; peak efficiency is not realized at any tympanic position, suggesting fluid in the middle ear (effusion), perforation of the tympanic membrane, or occlusion of the external ear canal. C. Peak efficiency occurs only when the position of the tympanic membrane is manipulated outward, suggesting that its resting position is retracted, as would be seen with negative pressure in the middle ear space caused by poor aeration. (From Lawrence PF. *Essentials of Surgical Specialties.* 3rd ed. Lippincott Williams & Wilkins; 2007.)

TABLE 25-2. Causes of Otalgia	
Otogenic	**Nonotogenic**
External ear	Orofacial pain
Otitis externa	Temporomandibular joint disorders
Herpes zoster oticus	Dental pathology
Neoplasm	Parotitis
Middle ear and mastoid	Elongated styloid process (Eagle syndrome)
Otitis media	Visceral
Mastoiditis	Pharyngotonsillitis
Neoplasm	Tumors of the hypopharynx, larynx, esophagus

TABLE 25-3. Disorders Associated With Tinnitus	
Continuous	**Pulsatile**
Sensorineural hearing loss	Glomus tympanicum
Ménière disease (usually unilateral)	Glomus jugulare
Acute noise exposure (eg, rock concert, explosion)	Dural venous sinus fistula
Systemic disease (eg, diabetes, hypertension, thyroid disease)	Intracerebral aneurysms
Ototoxicity (eg, aminoglycosides, cisplatin, salicylates)	Arteriovenous malformations
Acoustic neuroma (unilateral)	Atherosclerotic disease
Viral labyrinthitis	Hydrocephalus
Bacterial labyrinthitis	

of day. Unilateral tinnitus infers pathology of the cochlear end organ or its nerve, whereas bilateral tinnitus may be from a systemic toxicity or binaural injury. When the onset is acute, other signs of labyrinthine injury (eg, vertigo, hearing loss, or facial weakness) should be sought. Patients with tinnitus need immediate attention because they may have a pathology that is reversible with early treatment (Table 25-3). Unfortunately, no medications have proven effective in treating tinnitus. The mainstay of treatment for persistent, bothersome tinnitus includes sound therapy and cognitive-behavioral therapy in addition to hearing aids for those with concomitant hearing loss.

Otorrhea

Drainage from the ear can be of many different consistencies. Thin, watery, and yellow-to-clear fluid may be nothing more than bath water mixing with cerumen if the examination reveals normal ear structures. However, when trauma has occurred, a cerebrospinal fluid (CSF) fistula must be considered. A mucoid and purulent discharge from the ear implies infection. Carefully cleaning the ear may reveal a long-standing perforation, an acutely inflamed tympanic membrane and middle ear, or evidence of squamous debris and retraction consistent with otitis media. Bloody discharge may be part of an infectious process, but trauma and neoplasm must also be considered. High-resolution computed tomography (CT) scans of the temporal bone will provide evidence of bony destruction; however, the usefulness of these scans is limited because the discharge will appear with the same density as soft tissue defects (eg, polyp, cholesteatoma, tumor).

Vertigo

Dizziness is a common symptom but is usually not otologic in origin. Spinning or whirling vertigo, on the contrary, such as is felt immediately after being spun around or with the nausea of motion sickness, should be distinguished from "lightheadedness." Cardiac history, symptoms or findings of orthostatic hypotension, changes in blood pressure medications, or a past history of cerebrovascular accident may point to decreased blood flow in the vertebrobasilar system. Complete neurologic examination may point to other CNS findings, especially those of cerebellar

pathology. The presentations of these conditions may be identical to those of labyrinthine pathologies (Table 25-4).

Electronystagmography takes advantage of the predictable saccadic eye movements (nystagmus) that accompany various types of stimulation of the semicircular canal. Periorbital electrodes are used to precisely sense and record nystagmus; cooling, warming, and head rotation techniques are used to stimulate the semicircular canals. The quantitated nystagmic response can thus be used to measure the integrity of the vestibular system.

Platform posturography alters a patient's visual and proprioceptive feedback to isolate the vestibular system's singular impact on the patient's orientation abilities. In this test, the patient is harnessed inside a chamber that systematically eliminates visual feedback, thus altering the patient's visual surroundings and proprioceptive feedback by eliminating platform stability.

Clinical Presentation, Diagnosis, and Treatment

Congenital Anomalies

During embryologic development, six small hillocks of cartilage (which arise from the first and second branchial arch) eventually fuse to form the pinna. Failure to complete

TABLE 25-4. Basic Differential Diagnosis of Vertigo	
Common	**Unusual**
Disequilibrium of aging	Viral or bacterial labyrinthitis
Vestibular neuronitis	Acoustic neuroma
Benign positional vertigo	Ototoxic or vestibulotoxic drugs
Benign brainstem ischemia (vasospastic, embolic, and atherosclerotic)	Degenerative neurologic disease (eg, multiple sclerosis)
Ménière disease	Systemic disease (eg, diabetes, hypertension, autoimmune disease, thyroid disease)

proper embryologic development results in the formation of cysts or sinus tracts in the pinna and the preauricular area. If these tracts become recurrently infected, they can be easily resected. More significant anomalies of the first branchial cleft and pouch may lead to marked deformities or the absence of the auricle, the external auditory canal, and the middle or inner ear structures. The most important interventions are early audiometric assessment and early placement of hearing aids, preferably within the first year of life. Later, the series of surgical reconstructions of the pinna, the external ear canal, and perhaps the middle ear can begin.

Ear Trauma

Auricular hematoma is caused by a blunt shearing injury that separates the auricular cartilage from the perichondrium, creating a space in which blood and fluid can collect. This collection of fluid eventually forms scar tissue and results in a "cauliflower ear" deformity. This fluid must be evacuated and the skin must be compressed to the cartilage for several days to prevent it from reaccumulating.

Frostbite and burns of the ear produce injuries that are not fully manifested until days later. It is important to debride eschar conservatively, to keep all exposed cartilage moisturized, to avoid pressure on affected areas, and to control infection topically.

Perforations may develop from previous otitis media. Approximately 90% of traumatic tympanic perforations heal uneventfully. Those that do not heal spontaneously are usually large or have edges curled in such a way that regrowth will not occur. If healing is not evident within several months, tympanoplasty using a temporalis fascia graft is indicated to close the perforation. This procedure is more successful in the absence of recurring otitis media.

Fractures of the base of the skull may traverse the temporal bone and damage the vestibular or auditory mechanisms or both. Classically, two types of fractures are described depending on the location of the fracture in relation to the petrous portion of the temporal bone (Table 25-5): longitudinal and transverse. Longitudinal fractures are far more common, resulting in about 85% of all temporal bone fractures (Figure 25-9). Physical findings may include hemotympanum, otorrhea containing CSF and blood, hearing loss, and nystagmus. Rarely, a fracture may affect the cochlea or the facial nerve. Balance disturbances and varying degrees of hearing loss may be observed. Ossicular disruptions may need surgical repair. Significant sensorineural hearing loss rarely recovers, but the vestibular system can compensate over a period of months.

Otitis Externa

The skin of the auricle and the external auditory canal is subject to most of the common dermatologic diseases and to some that are unique to the external ear. The most common infectious disease is otitis externa, which can be localized or diffuse. Localized otitis externa (folliculitis of the external auditory canal) may be caused by trauma (commonly from a fingernail or a hairpin). It produces pain out of proportion to findings on physical examination, which may range from a small red spot to a fluctuant swelling. The patient will complain of extreme pain when the ear is moved or the area is touched. Treatment involves antistaphylococcal antibiotics, drainage, or both.

The term *otitis externa* usually refers to a diffuse process that involves the entire external auditory canal. It is also known as "swimmer's ear" because moisture remaining in the external canal after swimming or showering may lead to this infection. Trauma to the delicate skin of the canal or exposure to purulent middle ear discharge through a perforation may initiate otitis externa. The most common causative agent is *Pseudomonas*, but *Klebsiella*, *Streptococcus*, and *Staphylococcus* are also frequently implicated. Fungus may appear but usually as a secondary growth on desquamated epithelium. Findings range from minimal inflammation and tenderness to complete closure of the ear canal, with surrounding cellulitis and adenopathy.

Management involves removing debris from the external auditory canal, so that topical ear solutions effective

TABLE 25-5. Classification of Temporal Bone Fractures

Fracture	Force of Injury	Location of Fracture	Examination	Hearing Loss	Facial Nerve Paralysis
Longitudinal	Blow to side of head	Parallels the long axis of the petrous bone	Disrupted ear canal skin and tympanic membrane	Usually conductive	Infrequent (~15%)
			Bloody otorrhea		
			Bruising behind ear (Battle sign)		
Horizontal	Blow to front or back of head	Transects the long axis of the petrous bone	Vertigo common	Usually sensorineural	Common (~50%)
			Intact tympanic membrane	May be mixed if hemotympanum present	
			Hemotympanum		

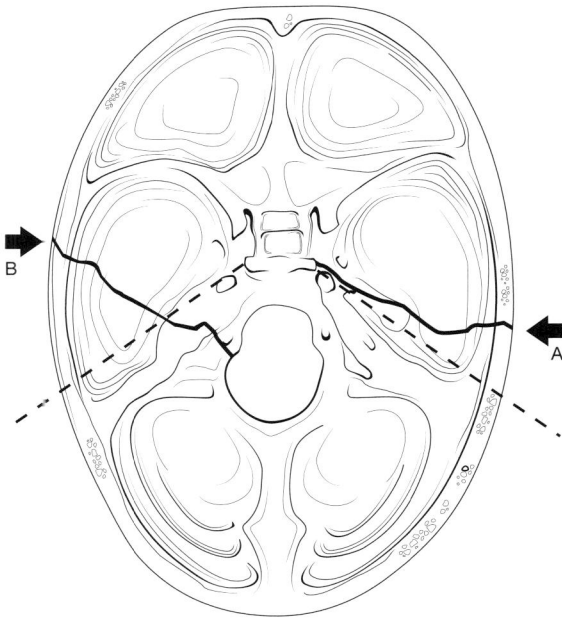

Figure 25-9. Classification of temporal bone fractures. *Dotted lines* represent the axis of the petrous portion of the temporal bone. Fracture *A* depicts a longitudinal fracture, whereas fracture *B* represents a transverse fracture. (From Lawrence PF. *Essentials of Surgical Specialties.* 3rd ed. Lippincott Williams & Wilkins; 2007.)

against *Pseudomonas*, *Staphylococcus*, *Candida*, and *Aspergillus* may reach the site of the infection. If the ear canal is so swollen that ear drops cannot be instilled, a small wick is placed into the external auditory canal. With the wick in place, the patient is instructed to use ear drops 2 to 4 times daily for several days. During the course of management, debris should be frequently removed from the patient's ear canal. If there is a marked cellulitis or inflammation involving the auricle and the tissues around the ear, systemic antibiotics and steroids are generally effective. Some patients may require hospitalization for treatment with intravenous antibiotics. Pain is a very significant part of the complex of symptoms, and narcotic analgesia is often required.

Necrotizing otitis externa, once called "malignant otitis externa," is an osteomyelitis of the temporal bone and skull base. The most common offending organism is *Pseudomonas aeruginosa*, but *Proteus* and *Klebsiella* may also be involved. Mortality is high. Patients at risk are those with simple otitis externa who have diabetes or those whose immune system is compromised. The patient develops persistent inflammation of the external auditory canal, persistent pain, and granulation tissue in the ear canal, often with exposed bone and cranial nerve involvement. This infection does not respond to topical therapy. Aggressive treatment with topical and systemic antibiotics over several months is mandatory. Surgical debridement may be helpful in very early cases. To prevent this condition, patients not responding to routine treatment of otitis externa must be referred early to the otolaryngologist.

Foreign bodies in the external ear canal are unfortunately all too common among preschool children. Fortunately, foreign bodies in the ear do not usually represent an emergency unless the object is caustic. However, all such foreign bodies, whether a soon-to-swell popcorn kernel, a bean, a toy bead, or a trinket, are somewhat difficult to remove. Children will usually allow physicians only one good try; if the attempt is unsuccessful, general anesthesia will almost certainly be required. In the meantime, the use of ear drops containing corticosteroids is prudent.

Otitis Media

Most of the infectious or inflammatory disease processes involving the middle ear space result from dysfunction of the eustachian tube. When the eustachian tube does not open frequently enough to allow equalization between the pressure in the middle ear and that of the atmosphere, a vacuum is created, and oxygen and nitrogen are absorbed into the mucous membranes of the middle ear and the mastoid air cell systems. The consequence is either increased capillary permeability and glandular activity with resultant middle ear effusion or retraction of the tympanic membrane with possible adherence to the ossicles and the medial wall of the middle ear space. If infectious agents are present, the transudate forms an ideal culture medium, leading to otitis media.

Acute otitis media (AOM) is the most common infection for which antibacterial agents are prescribed for children in the United States. It is defined by a history of acute onset, the presence of middle ear effusion, and signs and symptoms of middle ear inflammation. By their second birthday, 75% of all children will have had at least three episodes of AOM. The organisms that most commonly cause AOM are *Streptococcus pneumoniae*, *Moraxella catarrhalis*, and *Haemophilus influenzae*. A typical history is the onset of pain in one or both ears associated with behavioral changes, including crying, and often occurring in conjunction with an upper respiratory tract infection. Rarely, signs of meningeal irritation are present. Examination shows the eardrum to be red or opaque and possibly bulging, with a loss of normal landmarks secondary to an inflamed and often fluid-filled middle ear. Occasionally, infection results in a rupture of the tympanic membrane before a physician examines the child.

In 2004, the American Academy of Pediatrics (AAP) published updated guidelines for the management of AOM in an attempt to prevent unnecessary use of antibiotics, which can lead to bacterial resistance. If symptoms are not severe or diagnosis is unclear, only initial observation should be performed. The patients should be reevaluated in 48 to 72 hours. If antibiotics are used, then high-dose amoxicillin (90 mg/kg/d) should be used first. Azithromycin, clarithromycin, or erythromycin can be used if a penicillin allergy is present. After therapy is initiated, the pain usually resolves within 3 days and normal eustachian tube function usually returns in 2 weeks. If infection persists after 3 days of antibiotic therapy, then the antibacterial agent should be changed (high-dose amoxicillin-clavulanate). If this fails, a 3-day course of parenteral ceftriaxone should be used. Patients should be followed until the middle ear space is clear because approximately 10% of children will have persistent effusions for more than 10 and up to 12 weeks. Some patients might develop recurrent AOM, which is characterized by recurrent episodes of infection despite multiple rounds of antibiotics. Patients who experience six episodes of AOM in a 6-month period are considered candidates for tympanostomy tube placement. This allows direct access to the middle ear space so that topical antibacterial drops may be administered.

Untreated AOM can progress to acute mastoiditis, meningitis, brain abscess, facial nerve paralysis, and labyrinthitis. Drainage was standard therapy in the preantibiotic era; however, tympanocentesis is now infrequently indicated (Table 25-6). The procedure allows the infection to drain as well as material to be obtained for culture.

Otitis media with effusion (OME) is the second most common middle ear disease, with an estimated 2.2 million diagnoses annually in the United States. OME refers to fluid in the middle ear without signs or symptoms of an infection. Tympanometry is useful in its diagnosis. OME may occur spontaneously because of poor eustachian tube function or as an inflammatory response following AOM. The eustachian tubes of children are smaller and more horizontal in orientation than those of adults, thus restricting their ability to open and prevent nasopharyngeal reflux. The function of the eustachian tube may be impaired by edema of nasopharyngeal or eustachian tube mucosa caused by infection, allergy, adenotonsillar hypertrophy, nasopharyngeal neoplasm, or cleft palate. Risk factors for OME are listed in Table 25-7.

The American Academy of Otolaryngology-Head and Neck Surgery Foundation, the AAP, and the American Academy of Family Physicians published updated guidelines for the management of OME in 2016. It is a self-limiting disease, and watchful waiting is recommended for 3 months unless the child is at risk for speech deficit. Antibiotics, antihistamines, decongestants, and steroids have been shown to have no benefit. Seventy-five to ninety percent of cases resolve on their own by 3 months. A persistent effusion may create a significant hearing loss that can result in language development delay and learning disability. If fluid persists for more than 3 months despite treatment, myringotomy with placement of middle ear ventilation tubes should be considered. Ventilation tubes allow the middle ear to aerate, reducing the accumulation of fluid and restoring normal conductive hearing.

Some patients with chronic dysfunction of the eustachian tube will experience chronic otitis media associated with a nonhealing, chronically inflamed, draining perforation of the tympanic membrane. The middle ear and mastoid mucosa are involved and may be associated with destructive complications seen in AOM. Treatment is surgical, usually consisting of a combination of tympanoplasty (repair of the ear drum) and mastoidectomy (reestablishing an aerated mastoid cavity in communication with the middle ear space).

Cholesteatoma

Cholesteatoma is a skin-lined, keratin-producing middle ear cyst that may originate from a diseased tympanic membrane. Cholesteatoma tends to develop in a setting of chronic dysfunction of the eustachian tube and chronic negative pressure in the middle ear, resulting in persistent retraction of the tympanic membrane. This retraction yields a keratin-producing "pocket" of tympanic membrane that migrates into the middle ear and mastoid bone with time and growth. Osteolytic enzymes in the basement membrane of the cholesteatoma produce osteonecrosis. The ossicular chain, facial nerve, cochlea, semicircular canals, and skull base may be infected and eroded by this process. A patient with cholesteatoma commonly has chronic and recurrent infections with hearing loss. Facial nerve paralysis, vertigo, or intracranial abscesses may be seen. Otoscopic examination may reveal a white cheesy substance along the tympanic membrane with associated granulation tissue and tympanic membrane perforation. Surgical excision is necessary.

Otosclerosis

Otosclerosis is a spontaneous abnormality of the middle ear and occasionally the inner ear in far-advanced cases. It is most common in young adults causing an acquired conductive hearing loss. A small focus of spongy vascular bone involves a part or all of the stapes footplate. The result is fixation of the stapes footplate, with a conductive hearing loss. If the cochlea becomes involved, additional sensorineural hearing loss is produced. Otosclerosis occurs among both men and women, has a genetic predisposition, and may accelerate during pregnancy. A hearing aid may be used to amplify sound for affected patients. Most patients, however, prefer surgical replacement of the fixed stapes footplate by a prosthesis (stapedectomy).

Sensorineural Hearing Loss

Hearing loss affects 1 in 2,000 infants and may be either genetic (usually with a recessive mode of inheritance), developmental (anomalies affecting the temporal bone and the cochleovestibular apparatus), infectious in utero (cytomegalovirus, rubella, syphilis, herpes, and toxoplasmosis), or associated with other perinatal factors (meningitis, severe jaundice, prematurity, hypoxia, and ototoxic drugs). Early identification is imperative and rehabilitation

TABLE 25-6. Otitis Media: Indications for Urgent Myringotomy

Drainage and Culture	Culture
Otitis media with Significant sepsis Severe unresponsive otalgia Severe unresponsive headache Severe unresponsive fever or picket fence fever Facial paralysis Labyrinthitis Meningitis	Patient who are immunocompromised
Acute mastoiditis	Neonate

TABLE 25-7. Risk Factors for Otitis Media With Effusion

1. Day care
2. Male gender
3. Recent upper respiratory tract infection
4. Bottle feeding
5. Cigarette smoke in the house
6. Increased number of siblings in the home

through language interventions, hearing aids, cochlear implants, or other assistive listening devices may maximize the child's communication skills.

Acquired hearing losses may result from aging, noise exposure, ototoxic medications such as platinum based chemotherapy, and disease processes of the ear and the CNS. Presbycusis, or the hearing loss of aging, results from the degeneration of the cochlea. By age 80 years, 75% of people are affected. Exposure to noise in excess of 90 dB, especially if prolonged, may injure the cochlear hair cells, causing a localized loss in the mid to high-frequency range. Patients should be counseled on the use of noise protection. Damage to cochlear and vestibular hair cells by toxic levels of aminoglycosides has been well described. Other medications that can cause cochlear dysfunction are cisplatin, vancomycin, loop diuretics, opiates, and antimalarial agents. Erythromycin and aspirin can cause reversible sensorineural hearing loss. Patients will frequently complain of tinnitus and trouble hearing in the presence of background noise. Using hearing aids or assistive listening devices and optimizing the listening environment are usually helpful.

Vestibular Pathology

When the vestibular system is disrupted, problems ranging from imbalance to disabling vertigo are produced. As with sensorineural hearing loss, the causes vary. Vestibular neuritis involves inflammation of the vestibular nerve or the vestibular neuroepithelium believed to result from a viral cause. The condition is characterized by the acute onset of severe vertigo, which may last for a few days and gradually resolve over several weeks. It may be preceded by a viral upper respiratory tract condition or viral prodrome. Treatment is supportive and symptomatic, consisting of bed rest, short-term (1-2 days) use of vestibular suppressants (eg, antihistamines, benzodiazepines, and/or antiemetics), and vestibular rehabilitation.

Benign positional vertigo is an acute and rather severe vertigo lasting only a few minutes. The vertigo is reproduced by specific positioning of the head, such as looking up at a shelf, and is best diagnosed with the Dix-Hallpike maneuver. The condition is caused by canalithiasis or loose otoconia (eg, calcium debris) in the endolymph of one of the semicircular canals. Untreated episodes may resolve spontaneously over days to weeks while canalith repositioning maneuvers (ie, Epley maneuver) can be very effective with vestibular destructive procedures reserved for severe refractory cases.

Ménière disease, or endolymphatic hydrops, causes episodic hearing loss, incapacitating vertigo lasting for several hours, tinnitus, and a sensation of aural fullness. This disease is usually unilateral and is associated with bulging or rupture of the Reissner membrane (see Figure 25-2) and mixing of endolymphatic fluid with perilymphatic fluid; this mixture is toxic to vestibular and cochlear hair cells. Medical treatment consists of a low-salt diet and diuretics Surgical decompression of the endolymphatic sac or destruction of the nerves of the inner ear or vestibule is reserved for incapacitating vertiginous symptoms that do not respond to medical treatment.

Diseases of the Facial Nerve

Because of its long circuitous course (see Figure 25-5), the facial nerve may be affected at various intracranial or extracranial sites. In general, the prognosis for the recovery of facial nerve function is good if the paralysis is incomplete or caused by a reversible infection or inflammation. The prognosis is frequently poor if the paralysis is long standing, complete, or caused by cancer or trauma to the temporal bone. See Table 25-8 for a listing of diagnoses.

The most common process producing paralysis is idiopathic or Bell palsy. Viral infection of the nerve with herpes simplex is confirmed by polymerase chain reaction analysis. Facial paresis develops in a matter of hours and may progress to complete paralysis, often with associated mastoid pain, within a period of less than 72 hours. Most cases resolve spontaneously. Persistent or recurrent facial paralysis warrants imaging studies to rule out the presence of a tumor.

Other infectious or inflammatory diseases known to be associated with facial paralysis include AOM, chronic otitis media, herpes zoster oticus, Lyme disease, human immunodeficiency virus (HIV) infection, sarcoidosis, and Wegener granulomatosis. Treatment is generally medical and should be directed at the underlying cause. Facial paralysis caused by otitis media should be treated with wide myringotomy and with topical and systemic antibiotics.

Supranuclear lesions of the facial nerve, such as are seen in cerebrovascular ischemia, will frequently spare dysfunction of the forehead because these branches are connected to both crossed and uncrossed corticobulbar fibers.

Penetrating and blunt injuries involving the side of the face, the ear, or the temporal bone may affect the facial nerve. When the main trunk or one of the branches of the nerve is involved, paralysis of the muscles supplied by that portion of the nerve may be seen. Transection of the nerve proximal to the lateral canthus should be treated by primary reanastomosis or nerve grafting.

Facial paralysis significantly affects appearance; however, the most serious side effect is an ipsilateral exposure keratitis caused by the inability to close the upper eyelid. If ignored, this keratitis may lead to corneal scarring and even blindness. To protect the eye, application of artificial tears, ointment, and tape (to keep the eye closed while

TABLE 25-8. Differential Diagnosis of Facial Paralysis	
Inflammatory	**Other**
Infection	Tumors
Bell palsy	Parotid cancer
Acute otitis media	Skull-base cancer
Chronic otitis media	Trauma
Herpes zoster oticus	Temporal bone fracture
Lyme disease	Facial or parotid laceration
Human immune deficiency infection	Cerebral ischemia
Inflammation	
Wegener granulomatosis	
Sarcoidosis	

sleeping) is recommended. A tarsorrhaphy or the upper eyelid gold weight to allow better coverage of the cornea may be required.

Otologic Neoplasms

Because the skin of the external ear receives as much exposure to ultraviolet (UV) light as skin on any other area of the body, it is subject to the usual UV-light-induced skin neoplasms. Actinic keratosis is the most commonly seen. Benign neoplasms unique to the external auditory canal are osteomas and exostoses. Exostoses present as smooth, hard nodules, usually occurring multiply and bilaterally. Osteomas are single and unilateral. If either of these produces a marked obstruction, surgical excision is indicated. Of the malignant lesions, squamous cell and basal cell carcinomas, as well as malignant melanomas, are the most common. Surgical excision is usually the best treatment, although radiation therapy may also be useful for organ preservation.

Neoplasms of the middle ear and the mastoid are extremely rare. Glomus tympanicum is a vascular paraganglioma of the middle ear. It is histologically similar to glomus tumors of the carotid body, the vagus, and the jugular bulb. Patients classically complain of unilateral pulsatile tinnitus (see Table 25-3) and hearing loss. A reddish mass may be visible beneath an otherwise normal, translucent eardrum. Surgical excision is the best treatment.

Neoplasms of the inner ear are an unusual but important cause of unilateral sensorineural hearing loss. The most common tumor, vestibular schwannoma, is a benign intracranial tumor of the eighth cranial nerve. The hallmark symptom is unilateral sensorineural hearing loss with poor word discrimination, usually accompanied by tinnitus. Late symptoms are severe vertigo, facial nerve paralysis, and ataxia. Magnetic resonance imaging (MRI) is diagnostic, and treatment includes surgical excision or stereotactic radiosurgery.

NOSE AND PARANASAL SINUSES

Anatomy

The external nose is formed by a bony and cartilaginous framework covered by skin and facial muscles. The upper one-third, or bony vault, of the nose consists of the paired nasal bones supported by the frontal process of the maxilla and the nasal process of the frontal bone. The cartilaginous framework consists of the upper lateral cartilages that are fused to the septal cartilage medially and the lower lateral (alar) cartilages (Figure 25-10).

The nasal cavity extends from the anterior nares to the posterior choanae and is divided by the nasal septum. The internal nasal valve, located in the anterior nasal cavity, is composed of the inferior turbinate erectile tissue, the septum, and the upper lateral cartilage. This is the narrowest area of the adult upper airway. Common causes of nasal obstruction occur here, such as a deviated septum or enlarged turbinates. The roof of the nose is formed by the cribriform plate of the ethmoid bone. The lateral wall of the nasal cavity is configured by three overhanging scroll-like bones, namely, the turbinates. The turbinates subdivide the lateral nasal wall into a corresponding meatus or opening. Drainage from the nasolacrimal duct passes into the nose through the inferior meatus. The anterior ethmoid, maxillary, and frontal sinuses open into the middle meatus (Figure 25-11). The region containing the anterior ethmoid sinus and the middle meatus is known as the **osteomeatal complex**. Obstruction here is a common cause for sinus congestion because the maxillary, anterior ethmoid, and frontal sinuses can all be affected. The posterior ethmoid cells and sphenoid drain into the superior meatus.

Blood supply to the nose arises from both the external and the internal carotid artery systems (Figure 25-12). The sphenopalatine artery, a branch of the internal maxillary artery from the external carotid, is the primary vessel to the internal nose. It supplies the posteroinferior septum and turbinates. The anterior and posterior ethmoid arteries, branches of the ophthalmic artery from the internal carotid, supply the ethmoid and frontal sinuses, the nasal roof, and the anterosuperior septum and turbinates. Kiesselbach plexus, a highly vascular area on the anterior septum, receives its blood supply from both the internal and the external carotid artery systems and is the source for a vast majority of nosebleeds. Not unlike the skin, the turbinates contain erectile tissue composed of numerous arteriovenous shunts, referred to as "capacitance vessels." Regulation of blood volume in these capacitance vessels, in turn, regulates nasal lumen and airflow resistance.

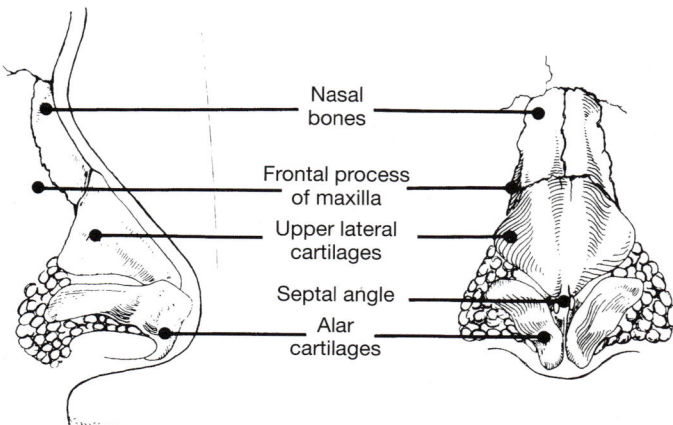

Figure 25-10. **Anatomy of the nasal vault.** (From Lawrence PF. *Essentials of Surgical Specialties.* 3rd ed. Lippincott Williams & Wilkins; 2007.)

Nasal bones

Frontal process of maxilla

Upper lateral cartilages

Septal angle

Alar cartilages

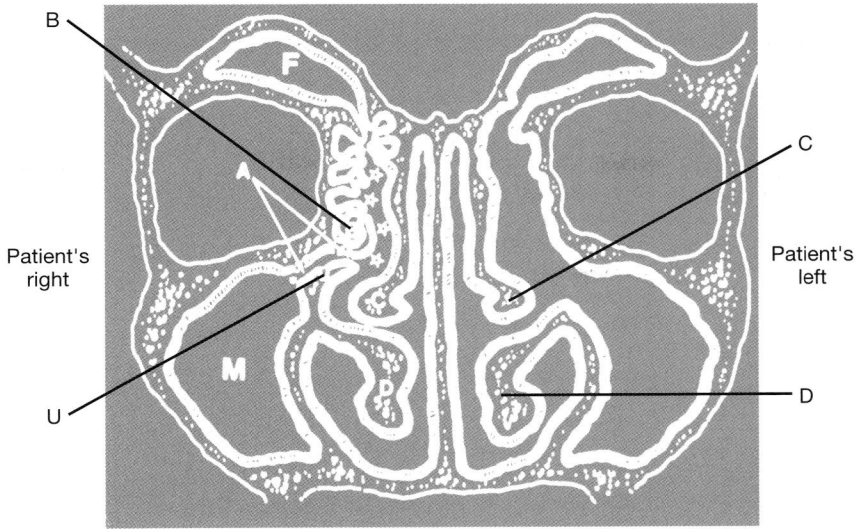

Figure 25-11. The anterior ethmoid sinus-middle meatus region (osteomeatal complex) in the coronal projection. On the patient's right, the middle meatus (*four stars*) receives drainage from the ethmoid bulla (*B*) and other anterior cells. Secretions from the frontal sinus (*F*) must pass through the ethmoidal regions, and maxillary sinus (*M*) secretions must pass through the ostium and the infundibulum (*A*) before reaching the middle meatus. The situation after functional endoscopic ethmoidectomy is shown on the patient's left. The uncinate process (*U*) has been removed, the anterior ethmoid cells opened, and the natural ostium of the maxillary sinus widened. The middle turbinate (*C*) is left intact. Also shown is the inferior turbinate (*D*).

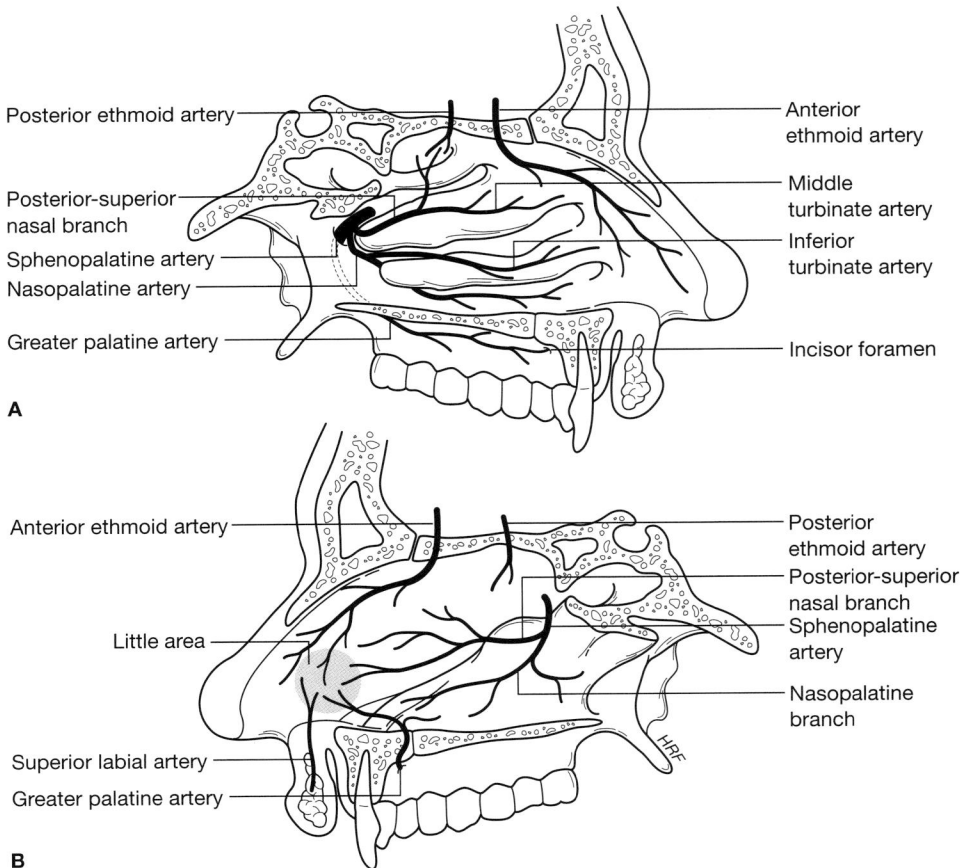

Figure 25-12. Blood supply to the nose. A. The arterial supply of the lateral wall of the internal nose. B. The arterial supply to the medial wall (septum) of the nose. (From Lawrence PF. *Essentials of Surgical Specialties*. 3rd ed. Lippincott Williams & Wilkins; 2007.)

Venous drainage from the nose passes through the sphenopalatine, facial, and ethmoid veins. The nose and the sinuses communicate with the orbit and the cavernous sinus through the pterygoid venous plexus of valveless emissary veins and with the anterior cranial fossa via the valveless diploic veins of the posterior frontal sinus wall. The absence of valves in this area is important to remember because simple infections of the face, nose, and sinuses can result in direct hematologic spread to the orbit and CNS. The nose is innervated by the first, fifth, and seventh cranial nerves and by fibers from the sympathetic and parasympathetic systems.

Physiology

Besides serving as the organ of olfaction, the nose is an integral part of the respiratory system. The nose filters, warms, and humidifies the air before it reaches the lungs. The optimal condition of inspired air is a temperature of 94 °F, a humidity level of 80%, and relative freedom from particulate matter. Achieving this condition requires the expenditure of an enormous amount of energy in the physical interaction of the air and the mucosal surfaces of the nose. This interaction disrupts laminar flow and ensures increased mixing and contact with respiratory mucosa, facilitating cleansing, humidification, and heating. Any inspired particulate matter is trapped on the mucous blanket overlying the nasal epithelium. The coordinated movement of the ciliated epithelial cells of the nasal mucosa transports secretions from the nose and the paranasal sinuses to the nasopharynx, where they are swallowed. Chronic contact between mucous membranes, as would occur with intranasal and sinus deformity and edema, disrupts mucociliary clearance, resulting in stasis of secretions with localized inflammation, facial pain and headache, and bacterial colonization.

Physical Examination

Physical examination of the nose begins with both inspection and palpation of the external dorsum. Any asymmetry or collapse (ie, from trauma) can cause narrowing of the nasal valve with resultant nasal obstruction. Complete inspection of the nasal cavities is difficult without the use of a topical decongestant, a nasal speculum, and a good light. The mucosa of the nasal cavity (septum and inferior and middle turbinates) should be inspected for signs of inflammation, telangiectasias, drainage, and lesions, including masses or polyps. Obstruction to airflow along the floor of the nose and to sinus mucociliary clearance more superiorly should be noted. Physical examination of the sinuses is also limited to inspection of the sinus ostia and to inspection and palpation of the overlying facial skin. The application of both flexible and rigid endoscopic instruments allows inspection of these concealed spaces and results in a more precise diagnosis of sinus disease.

Evaluation

Rhinorrhea

Liquid-like drainage from the nose can be unilateral, hemorrhagic, mucoid, or purulent. Patients may have obvious anterior discharge; however, postnasal drip is quite common, producing a variety of symptoms, including dysphagia, asthma exacerbations, sore throat, and hoarseness. Thin, clear-to-white secretions often imply allergic, vasomotor, or viral-induced rhinitis. Unilateral clear drainage

may come from a CSF leak, warranting collection and analysis of the discharge. Purulent and foul-smelling discharge indicates bacterial infection. Nasal examination may demonstrate the discharge, especially in the region of the middle meatus; however, the absence of discharge does not rule out sinusitis. Radiographic imaging, especially coronal noncontrast CT scans of the sinuses, visualizes areas hidden from endoscopic examination and displays anatomic variation that may predispose the patient to disease. This CT scan optimally evaluates the osteomeatal complex and can be a crucial reference during sinus surgery to safely treat the sinonasal disease.

Epistaxis

Bleeding from the nose most commonly occurs anteriorly from Kiesselbach plexus on the nasal septum. Anterior bleeding can be controlled by using a nasal decongestant spray on the affected side followed by firmly compressing the alar cartilages on both sides of the septum. Posterior epistaxis may be more often associated with arteriosclerotic cardiovascular disease, hypertension, and other systemic disorders; it requires more significant intervention, as explained later in the section on management.

The most common cause of epistaxis is trauma. Bleeding may develop after digital or penetrating injury to the nasal mucosa or as a result of blunt trauma to the nose that produces secondary mucosal laceration. Septal deviations and perforations cause excessive air turbulence, drying, and focal inflammation of nasal mucosa, increasing the potential for epistaxis. Acute or allergic rhinitis, especially among children, is another common cause of nasal bleeding. Intranasal foreign bodies, usually seen in pediatric patients or patients with mental health issues, should be suspected if there is unilateral purulent discharge or bleeding. Hereditary hemorrhagic telangiectasia, an autosomal dominant disorder exhibiting arteriovenous malformations of aerodigestive tract mucosa, is characterized by fragility of the vascularity of the nasal mucosa, with recurrent nasal hemorrhage. Epistaxis can be an early symptom of paranasal sinus neoplasm. **Juvenile nasopharyngeal angiofibroma** is a highly vascular, benign tumor of adolescent males, with the classic symptoms of unilateral epistaxis and nasal obstruction. This tumor should always be considered in pubescent males with recurrent unilateral epistaxis.

Epistaxis may also be a sign of systemic disease. Defects in coagulation caused by anticoagulation therapy, blood dyscrasias, lymphoproliferative disorders, and immunodeficiency may cause nasal bleeding. Chronic systemic diseases predisposing patients to epistaxis include nutritional deficiencies, alcoholism, and hereditary hemorrhagic telangiectasia. Recurring or atypical epistaxis warrants a coagulopathy workup.

The initial management of epistaxis focuses on the control of acute blood loss and airway relief if necessary. If the site of bleeding can be identified, it is cauterized electrically or chemically with silver nitrate. If the site cannot be identified, an anterior nasal pack (expanding sponge) is placed. If a well-placed anterior pack fails to control bleeding (often demonstrated by continued bleeding into the pharynx), a posterior pack may be required. Posterior bleeding is often more profuse than anterior. A posterior pack seals the choanae and provides a bolster against which anterior packing can be placed to tamponade posterior nasal vessels. Foley catheters or gauze packing is seated in the nasopharynx, against the choanae with anterior traction, while a formal anterior pack is placed. Several readymade posterior nasal pack balloons, which are easier to place and very effective, are available. Patients requiring posterior nasal packing need to be hospitalized so that they may be monitored for further bleeding, hypoxia, or bradycardia caused by the nasocardiac reflex, aspiration of blood, and for sedation if necessary. Further, these patients may require humidified oxygen, prophylactic antibiotics, narcotic analgesia, and bed rest.

If anterior and posterior packs fail to control bleeding, the arterial supply to the bleeding portion of the nose must be addressed. The profound collateral blood supply of the nasal cavity demands ligation or embolization close to the bleeding site. Ligation of the anterior and posterior ethmoid arteries may be performed for anterosuperior epistaxis, whereas ligation or embolization of the internal maxillary artery is performed for posterior bleeding.

Nasal Congestion and Obstruction

Nasal pathologies associated with congestion, obstruction, stuffiness, or the inability to clear, blow, or breathe through the nose are usually associated with obstruction along the floor of the nasal cavity. Shelf-like spurs along the base of the septum, deviation of the entire septum, and enlarged inferior turbinates or nasal masses are usually responsible. Turbinate swelling may be due to inflammatory pathology such as viral, bacterial, allergic, or vasomotor rhinitis. All intranasal masses deserve close attention to rule out neoplasm. Other entities in the differential diagnosis include nasal polyps, pyogenic granuloma, and hypertrophic or polypoid turbinates. Polyps are rarely unilateral; thus, unilateral polyps, especially in the presence of bleeding, increase the suspicion that the polyps may represent neoplasm. Polypoid sinusitis is rare among children and should prompt a workup to rule out cystic fibrosis and immunodeficiency.

Clinical Presentation, Diagnosis, and Treatment

Acute Viral Rhinitis

Acute viral rhinitis, or the common cold, is the most common infectious disease of human beings and is most prevalent among children younger than 5 years. The viral infection produces desquamation of ciliated epithelial cells. Symptoms, which vary significantly in severity, include nasal stuffiness, rhinorrhea, sneezing, and airway obstruction. There may be associated cough, headache, temperature elevation, sore throat, and generalized malaise. Mucopurulent drainage replaces the initial mucoid secretions, and resident flora may cause secondary bacterial infection. The disorder is self-limited; regeneration of epithelium occurs by approximately day 14, but the return of ciliary function and relief of rhinitis symptoms may lag for several weeks.

Bacterial Rhinitis

Acute bacterial rhinitis is most commonly seen among children, but adults may also develop the condition after nasal trauma, viral upper respiratory tract infection, or surgery. The clinical presentation of acute bacterial rhinitis may be identical to that of the common cold. Causative organisms include *S. pneumoniae, H. influenzae,* and *Staphylococcus aureus.* Clinical signs that distinguish bacterial rhinitis from acute sinusitis may be subtle, and both conditions may occur in a patient whose defenses have been compromised by a concurrent viral inflammatory process. Treatment with oral antibiotics may shorten the course of the disease.

Chronic bacterial inflammation of the nasal cavity is relatively uncommon, and the initial clinical manifestations of congestion, obstruction, and drainage are nonspecific. If these symptoms persist despite standard medical treatment, culture and biopsy should be considered to rule out infectious causes, such as tuberculosis, syphilis, rhinoscleroma (*Klebsiella rhinoscleromatis*), and leprosy. The clinician should also consider autoimmune diseases (eg, Wegener granulomatosis, lupus) and lymphoproliferative disorders. Children with an indolent history of unilateral purulent nasal discharge with or without blood may be harboring a nasal foreign body.

Allergic Rhinitis

Allergic rhinitis is the most common allergic disease, affecting 20% of the population. It is a disease of the immune system, mediated by immunoglobulin E (IgE). Allergic rhinitis is caused by hypersensitivity to inhaled particulates (eg, grass, ragweed, and tree pollens; animal dander; dust; mold spores). The disease most commonly affects children and young adults and is often associated with reactive lower respiratory tract disease. A positive family history is found in 50% of patients. Symptoms, which may be seasonal or perennial, include rhinorrhea, nasal obstruction, sneezing, and pruritus. Although pale-bluish, edematous mucosa is suggestive of the disease, no rhinoscopic findings are unique to allergic rhinitis. The results of skin tests, accomplished by injecting small amounts of extracts prepared from the culprit allergens, are usually positive, and elevated allergen-specific serum IgE levels are usually found.

Medical management begins with the identification and avoidance of offending allergens. If this measure fails to control symptoms adequately, pharmacotherapy with antihistamines, decongestants, and topical corticosteroid nasal sprays should be tried. Topical cromolyn sodium provides symptomatic relief by preventing the degranulation of mast cells.

Allergen immunotherapy should be considered to desensitize patients who are allergic and with symptoms that are not controlled adequately with medication and avoidance measures. Immunotherapy is usually accomplished by injecting into the patient progressively larger amounts of allergenic extract, which stimulates T-suppressor cell regulation of IgE synthesis. This treatment is effective only for diseases caused by IgE mechanisms and must usually be continued for several years.

Hormonal Rhinitis

Hormonal rhinitis (rhinitis of pregnancy) most commonly occurs in association with increasing endogenous estrogen levels during pregnancy. Estrogens, which cause vascular engorgement of the nose, cause nasal congestion and obstruction occurring in association with the immediate premenstrual period and with the use of oral contraceptives. Hormonal rhinitis may also be seen in hypothyroidism resulting from extracellular edema (myxedema).

Rhinitis Medicamentosa

Rhinitis medicamentosa is a drug-induced nasal inflammation, most commonly caused by the abuse of decongestant nasal sprays. Chronic use of these medications causes rebound congestion after use, resulting in more frequent medication use and reliance. Management requires gradual withdrawal of topical decongestants, which can be eased with systemic decongestants and/or steroids.

Mucociliary Dysfunction and Nasal Polyposis

The obstruction, congestion, and rhinorrhea so familiar to patients with chronic rhinosinusitis may be the result of mucociliary dysfunction, nasal polyposis, or both. Mucociliary dysfunction involves dysfunctional sinonasal mucociliary transport. Kartagener syndrome (immotile cilia syndrome) is a member of this group. Chronic smoke inhalation, viral rhinitis, chronic inflammatory disease, and trauma are some causes of acquired mucociliary dysfunction.

Nasal polyps are characteristically bilateral, multiple, and translucent masses that arise from the osteomeatal complex and extend into the nasal cavity. Although the cause of polyps is not well understood, multiple factors are probably implicated, including chronic mucosal inflammation, injury, and obstruction. Nasal polyps are seen in the presence of reactive airway disease and asthma, aspirin hypersensitivity, and cystic fibrosis. Initial management of nasal polyps can include both topical steroids and a short course of oral steroids. Surgical excision of the polyps is reserved for those patients for whom steroids are contraindicated or ineffective in restoring an adequate nasal airway. Recurrence is frequent; ethmoidectomy and the use of intranasal topical steroid sprays may help prolong the time to recurrence of polyps. For severe cases that have not improved despite medical and surgical standards of care, the biologic dupilumab can be considered to reduce polyp size and improve nasal congestion.

Nasal and Septal Deformity

The nasal bones are the most frequently fractured bones in the body. Clinical findings of a nasal fracture include edema, ecchymosis, epistaxis, crepitus, or a palpable bony deformity. The most frequent deformity is depression of one nasal bone and outward displacement of the contralateral bone, and it usually occurs after a lateral blow. Direct frontal blows may result in flattening and widening of the nasal dorsum. If the injury is severe, forces can be transmitted posteriorly to involve the ethmoid sinus, the medial orbital walls, and the cribriform plate, with resultant CSF rhinorrhea, hypertelorism (secondary to disruption of medial canthal tendons), and anosmia (eg, naso-orbitoethmoidal fracture).

Evaluation of a patient with suspected nasal fracture must include inspection of the septum for hematoma. Septal hematoma is caused by the accumulation of blood between the cartilage and the overlying mucoperichondrium, effectively separating this cartilage from its blood supply. Prompt drainage is required to prevent the formation of an abscess and resorption of cartilage, which can produce a saddle nose deformity. Nondisplaced fractures of the nasal bones do not require reduction. Minimal deviations of the bony dorsum, with no appreciable septal displacement, are managed with closed reduction. More complex injuries and those associated with septal displacement require open reduction with repositioning of the septum to achieve satisfactory functional and cosmetic results.

Septal deviations can be traumatic or congenital. Septal deviation may cause high velocity, excessively turbulent airflow or chronic contact with the lateral nasal wall or turbinate producing nasal obstruction, snoring, sleep apnea, epistaxis, facial pain, headache, or sinusitis. These are treated most often with endonasal septoplasty.

Choanal Atresia

Persistence of the nasobuccal membrane during gestation results in incomplete opening of the posterior nasal cavity or choanae. Resultant choanal atresia may be unilateral or bilateral. Because newborns are obligate nasal breathers, bilateral **choanal atresia** is a medical emergency. Diagnosis is suspected when a newborn's initial feedings result in progressive obstruction, cyanosis, choking, and aspiration. The airway obstruction is temporarily relieved by crying because that is the only time the neonate inhales through the mouth. An inability to pass a small catheter through the nose and into the nasopharynx is suggestive. Immediate treatment includes stenting with an oral airway or endotracheal intubation. The infant should also be evaluated for other craniofacial and upper aerodigestive anomalies (eg, cleft palate, subglottic stenosis, craniofacial synostosis, and tracheoesophageal fistula) because these anomalies often cluster together. Surgical opening of the choanae with prolonged stenting is required for correction.

Acute Sinusitis

Acute sinusitis most frequently develops as a complication of a viral upper respiratory tract infection (ie, the common cold). Symptoms such as periorbital tenderness, facial pain, headache, fever, hyposmia, and purulent nasal discharge are indicative of sinusitis. Acute sinusitis is caused by ostial closure as a result of inflammatory edema from a viral upper respiratory tract infection or allergies. The resultant stasis of secretions may lead to infection with bacteria. Common causative organisms in acute sinusitis are *S. pneumoniae, H. influenzae,* and *M. catarrhalis.* The diagnosis is usually established on the basis of clinical findings of mucopurulent nasal drainage, inflamed turbinates, pain over the anterior face, and fever. Medical therapy is begun empirically in the uncomplicated case. A 7- to 14-day course of amoxicillin-clavulanate, cefprozil, cefuroxime, clarithromycin, or loracarbef and a short course of topical decongestants and intranasal steroids are recommended. Other supportive measures include systemic decongestants, saline nasal sprays, expectorants, humidification, warm compresses, and analgesics.

Surgical treatment is indicated for acute sinusitis if the response to adequate medical therapy is poor or in the presence of a high risk for extranasal complications of sinusitis, such as orbital infection, meningitis, intracranial sinus thrombosis, and facial cellulitis. The maxillary sinus is aspirated and irrigated through a trocar that is punctured into the sinus. Aspiration and drainage of the frontal sinus are performed through an incision in the medial supraorbital region. Ethmoidal drainage can usually be accomplished through an intranasal approach.

Chronic Sinusitis

Chronic sinusitis is one of the most common health care complaints in the United States. It results when mucosal contact disrupts mucociliary clearance or forces closure of the sinus ostium. The resulting accumulation of secretions may cause chronic inflammation, ciliary injury, hyperplasia of seromucinous glands, and increasingly viscous mucus. Sinus hypoventilation interferes with local defense mechanisms and may lead to anaerobic infection and the development of biofilms. The region of the anterior ethmoid sinus and middle meatus (osteomeatal complex) is the site of inflammatory sinus disease in 90% of patients.

Although the symptoms of chronic sinus disease vary, most patients note a sensation of obstruction, facial pressure, pain, and/or hyposmia. The pain is often referred to areas supplied by the ophthalmic or maxillary division of the trigeminal nerve and is characterized as dull, deep, and nonpulsatile. Causes include ciliary dysfunction, immune deficiency, and nasal allergy. Structural variations that interfere with ventilation or mucociliary clearance in the osteomeatal complex will also produce chronic sinus disease.

The goals of medical therapy are to treat infection, to improve mucociliary clearance, and to maintain patency of sinus ostia. Antimicrobial treatment of chronic sinusitis is indicated in the presence of coexistent acute inflammation and for patients who have not received a prolonged course of a β-lactamase-resistant antibiotic. Topical intranasal steroid sprays are an important adjunct to antibiotic therapy because of their anti-inflammatory effect, which helps restore ostial patency. Saline nasal sprays, expectorants, smoking cessation, and increased fluid intake enhance mucociliary clearance by reducing the viscosity of mucus. Surgical treatment of chronic sinus disease focuses on the pivotal role of the osteomeatal complex and reestablishing normal ventilation, mucociliary clearance, and sinus outflow tracts (see Figure 25-11).

Nasal and Sinus Mycotic Infections

Fungal infections in the nose and paranasal sinuses are usually caused by the opportunistic organisms *Phycomycetes* (*Mucor, Rhizopus*) and *Aspergillus.* These normally innocuous organisms produce fulminant, invasive, frequently lethal diseases among patients who are immunocompromised. One should maintain a high clinical suspicion in this subset of patients because this disease can invade rapidly to involve the orbit or CNS. Characteristic clinical signs are nasal pain, facial hypesthesia, bloody nasal discharge, and black, necrotic turbinates. Diagnosis depends on the histologic identification of invasive fungus in biopsy specimens. Treatment requires radical surgical debridement of involved tissues, high-dose antifungal therapy, and a restoration of immune competence.

Nasal and Sinus Neoplasms

Benign neoplasms of the sinonasal tract are treated with simple excision, in most cases for cure. Squamous papilloma is a wart-like benign neoplasm occurring at the mucocutaneous junction of the nasal vestibule. Osteoma is the most common tumor involving the paranasal sinuses. It arises in the frontoethmoid region and is often an incidental finding of sinus radiographs. If the osteoma is asymptomatic, it can be monitored over time. Progressively growing osteomas are removed surgically. Although histologically benign, inverting papillomas are locally invasive, and 10% to 15% may develop into squamous cell carcinoma. For this reason, wide local excision is preferred. Juvenile nasopharyngeal angiofibroma arises in the pterygomaxillary fossa and presents as a unilateral nasal mass among adolescent boys, causing epistaxis and nasal obstruction. Diagnosis is clinical and radiographic because hemorrhage from biopsy may be hazardous. Hemorrhage after surgical excision is reduced by preoperative embolization.

Malignant neoplasms of the nose and sinus represent less than 1% of cancers. Bony destruction shown by CT scan is highly suggestive of malignancy; MRI scan distinguishes secondary inflammatory sinus disease from primary malignancy. Diagnosis depends on biopsy. Epithelial neoplasms, such as squamous cell carcinoma, adenocarcinoma, and salivary malignancies, are predominant in this rare group of tumors and are optimally treated with wide local excision combined with irradiation. The orbit, maxilla, and anterior fossa will be affected structurally to some extent by the treatment of these lesions. Local recurrence is the most common cause of treatment failure. Olfactory neuroblastoma (esthesioneuroblastoma), a rare malignant tumor of neuroectodermal origin, is often treated with a combination of surgery and radiation therapy. Rhabdomyosarcoma, a tumor of striated muscle, is the most common intranasal cancer among children. Advances in chemotherapy and radiation therapy techniques have reduced the role of surgery to a diagnostic procedure in most cases.

THE ORAL CAVITY AND PHARYNX

Anatomy

The oral cavity consists of the space posterior to the lips and anterior to the tonsils and soft palate (Figure 25-13). The vestibule is a space bounded by the lips anteriorly and by the cheeks, the gingiva, and the teeth posteriorly. The oral cavity is bounded anteriorly and laterally by the alveolar arches, superiorly by the hard and soft palates, and inferiorly by the tongue. The tongue is the predominant organ of the mouth and plays an integral role in chewing, swallowing food, and articulating speech. Its movements are controlled by paired extrinsic and intrinsic muscles, all of which are innervated by the hypoglossal nerve. Sensory innervation is supplied by both special visceral and general somatic nerves. The sensation of taste is transmitted from the anterior two-thirds of the tongue by the lingual nerve to the chorda tympani branch of the facial nerve. The lingual branch of the glossopharyngeal nerve carries special visceral afferent fibers from the posterior one-third of the tongue. General sensation is through branches of the fifth, ninth, and tenth cranial nerves.

Saliva is produced by a set of six paired major salivary glands and by hundreds of minor salivary glands. Most saliva is produced in the parotid, submandibular, and sublingual major salivary glands and flows through ducts into the oral cavity. The minor salivary glands empty directly into the oral cavity and are located in the palate, the lips, the tongue, the tonsils, and the buccal mucosa. The oral cavity ends at the fauces, the archway composed of the posterior soft palate and the palatoglossal folds.

The pharynx lies posterior to the nasal cavity, the mouth, and the larynx (see Figure 25-13). The three major muscles of the pharynx are the superior, middle, and inferior constrictor muscles, which play important roles in the process of swallowing. The nasopharynx lies above the level of the soft palate and communicates with the nasal cavity through the choanae. Opening into the lateral

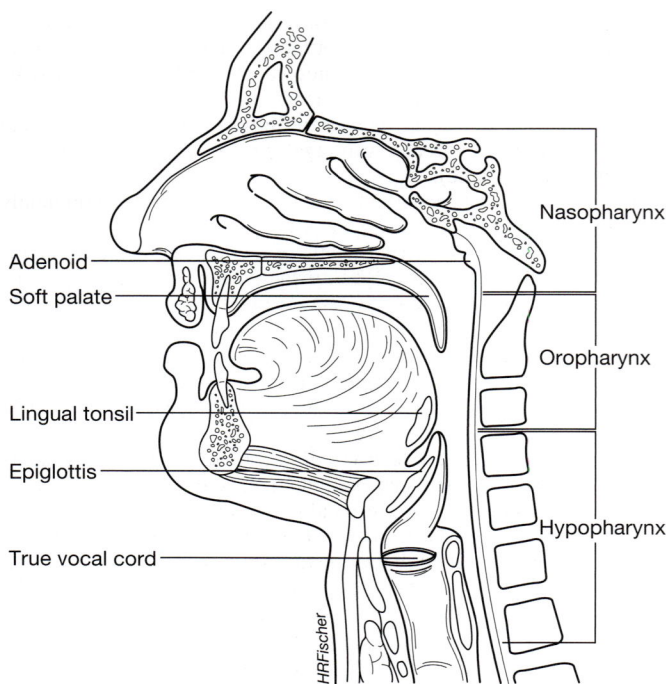

Figure 25-13. Sagittal view of the pharynx. (From Lawrence PF. *Essentials of Surgical Specialties*. 3rd ed. Lippincott Williams & Wilkins; 2007.)

walls of the nasopharynx are the eustachian tubes. On the posterior wall lies the adenoidal tissue.

The oropharynx extends from the level of the hyoid bone to the soft palate. It opens anteriorly into the oral cavity and contains the palatine tonsils laterally. The hypopharynx reaches from the hyoid bone to the lower border of the cricoid cartilage, where it narrows to become continuous with the esophagus. It communicates anteriorly with the larynx. Immediately lateral to the larynx are mucosal recesses called the "pyriform sinuses" that drain into the esophageal inlet through the upper esophageal sphincter or cricopharyngeus muscle.

Physiology

The oral cavity and pharynx play important roles in breathing, masticating, swallowing, and articulation. Each of these functions requires motor and sensory information for optimal performance.

Swallowing is divided into four phases. The first is the preparatory phase, in which a food bolus is crushed, macerated, and mixed with saliva. This preparation ensures an optimal consistency for passage to the stomach. In the second phase, voluntary control of the tongue sweeps the bolus posteriorly against the soft palate into the oropharynx. When the bolus traverses the fauces, the third phase, which is controlled involuntarily, begins. The larynx elevates, opening the pyriform sinuses and the upper esophageal sphincter. The epiglottis moves over the larynx, acting as a keel to direct food into the pyriform sinuses. The pharyngeal constrictors function as the soft palate elevates to seal the nose from the oral cavity. These movements drive the bolus to the esophageal introitus, which opens by relaxing the cricopharyngeus muscle. In the fourth phase, the esophagus drives the bolus to the stomach with primary peristaltic waves. Discoordination, lack of sensory feedback, or other anatomic derangements will lead to dysphagia, aspiration, or both.

The tongue, palate, and lips are key structures in shaping the sounds produced by the larynx into intelligible speech. Anatomic or neurologic dysfunction of these organs produces dysarthria.

Physical Examination

Physical examination of the oral cavity and pharynx is facilitated by ample lighting and the use of tongue blades for retraction of the cheeks and tongue. Congenital, inflammatory, or neoplastic abnormalities should be sought. Complete inspection includes a full examination of the buccal mucosal recesses, the palate, the floor of mouth, and the dental alveolar structures. Movement of the tongue and palate should be observed for symmetry. Most areas of the pharynx can be inspected with direct vision, mirrors, or fiberoptic endoscopes. Digital palpation of the oral cavity and oropharynx may be necessary as many lesions may be difficult or impossible to visualize but have palpable irregularity.

Evaluation

Sore Throat

Chronicity, concurrent systemic symptoms, patient age, and physical examination will help narrow the wide differential diagnosis. Sore throat for less than a week implies infection, whereas neoplasms usually cause symptoms for much longer periods and often refer pain to the ear. The presence of fever and malaise suggests infection, and weight loss over the months before treatment is sought raises the possibility of malignancy.

Snoring and Sleep Disturbance

Patients with disordered sleep may present with chronic fatigue, daytime somnolence, or right-sided heart failure. Snoring occurs more commonly as a person ages and is not necessarily pathologic in adults. More importantly, the physician must elicit any history of apnea (ie, cessation of breathing). Complete examination of the upper airway is mandatory. Any significant obstruction is exacerbated during sleep when the resting tone of the upper airway is decreased.

Dysphagia

Patients with trouble swallowing describe many different sensations. It is crucial to determine whether the dysphagia represents a mechanical obstruction or a neurologic coordination problem. Dysphagia for solids only, or a progressive dysphagia that began with solids and progresses to include liquids, implies mechanical blockage. Chronic odynophagia (painful swallowing) associated with this type of dysphagia may indicate a possible malignancy. Patients with this condition require laryngoscopy and esophagoscopy for evaluation and possible biopsy. Transnasal esophagoscopy is a visualization technique that allows evaluation of the esophagus and stomach in clinic without the need for general anesthesia or sedation. Barium swallow study also provides useful anatomic and functional information about the oropharyngeal to esophageal phases of swallowing. Patients may describe choking, especially with liquids, representing a loss of bolus control present in neurologic problems (central as well as peripheral). Some patients may have little difficulty swallowing yet complain of globus. Physical examination of these patients often reveals no significant findings; other causes of pharyngeal irritation, such as gastroesophageal reflux, postnasal drip, and inhaled irritants, must be considered.

Clinical Presentation, Diagnosis, and Treatment

Acute and Chronic Pharyngitis or Stomatitis

Inflammatory diseases of the oral cavity and the pharynx are common and frequently viral in origin. Viral upper respiratory tract infections may produce lesions of the pharynx, the oral cavity, or both. These lesions range from diffuse inflammation to vesicular eruptions. Various viruses, including parainfluenza, adenovirus, influenza, and Epstein-Barr, have been identified in pharyngotonsillitis. Viral pharyngitis or stomatitis is self-limiting and requires only symptomatic treatment. Herpes simplex virus type 1 or even type 2 may cause a painful, recurring, blistering infection that responds to early antiviral therapy. Aphthous ulceration is common in the oral cavity. Aphthous ulcers are single or multiple, shallow, painful ulcers presenting without other disease. When these lesions are recurrent or severe, topical steroids may shorten the course of the disease. If these lesions persist beyond a few weeks, biopsy should be considered.

Inflammation of the oral cavity and pharynx can also occur with the ingestion of caustic materials. Alkali ingestion causes liquefaction necrosis, which usually results in more severe damage to the esophagus, whereas acid ingestion causes a coagulation necrosis. It is important to remember that the severity of external and oropharyngeal damage may not correlate with the extent of esophageal or gastric injury. A seemingly benign oral examination may mask a more severe distal injury. If severe, the resulting mucosal necrosis can result in pharyngeal or esophageal perforation and airway obstruction caused by mucosal edema. Long-term strictures can require years of dilation or significant reconstructive surgery.

The most common fungal infection of the oral cavity is thrush, caused by *Candida albicans*. This infection is common in the neonate or in the adult during or following a course of systemic antibiotics or steroids as well as in patients who are immunocompromised. Thrush responds to topical therapy with agents such as miconazole or nystatin although more severe or recalcitrant infections may require systemic antifungal agents (eg, ketoconazole or fluconazole).

Streptococcal pharyngitis occurs more commonly in patients older than 2 years. The infection is caused by α-hemolytic streptococcus, which can be cultured from the exudate of the tonsils and the pharynx. It is characterized by fever, malaise, cervical adenopathy, exudative tonsillitis, and the notable absence of cough (eg, Centor criteria). Penicillin, administered intramuscularly or orally, provides adequate treatment against the organism. However, if the infection recurs frequently, removal of the tonsils may be necessary.

Bacterial infections of the tonsils can be caused by various organisms, including anaerobes. Patients whose infections do not respond to penicillin may have resistant bacteria and may require a different antibiotic. Chronic or repeated acute bacterial tonsillitis may require tonsillectomy. Occasionally, tonsillitis spreads to the peritonsillar region, resulting in peritonsillar abscess, parapharyngeal, or deep neck space infection. In most cases, these infections respond to systemic antibiotics, but peritonsillar abscess usually requires aspiration or surgical drainage. Peritonsillar abscess is characterized by an asymmetry of the tonsils and swelling of the soft palate, resulting in uvular deviation and a muffled or "hot potato" voice.

Adenoidal tissue can also be infected, producing recurrent purulent nasal discharge and obstruction of the nose. If the obstruction does not respond to antibiotic therapy or is recurrent, adenoidectomy is indicated. Young patients with recurrent tonsillitis have infection of the adenoidal tissue as well. For this reason, children usually undergo simultaneous tonsillectomy and adenoidectomy. Because the adenoid may contribute to recurrent otitis media, adenoidectomy will reduce recurring otitis in some cases. Table 25-9 summarizes current indications for tonsillectomy.

TABLE 25-9. Indications for Tonsillectomy

Infectious	Other
Tonsillitis	Upper airway obstruction
Recurrent acute tonsillitis	Symptomatic
7 episodes in 1 y	Obstructive sleep apnea
5 episodes/y in 2 y	Suspected malignancy
3 episodes/y in 3 y	
Chronic tonsillitis	
Peritonsillar abscess	
Recurrent peritonsillar abscess	
Peritonsillar abscess when general anesthesia is required for incision and drainage of first abscess	

Congenital Anomalies

The more common congenital disorders of the oral cavity include ankyloglossia, in which the tongue is bound to the mandible because of a shortened frenulum; cleft lip, cleft palate, or both; supernumerary teeth; micrognathia; cysts of the alveolar ridge or palate; lingual thyroid; and hemangioma. If the lesions neither obstruct the airway nor interfere with swallowing, most congenital defects can be corrected surgically when the child is older.

In addition to the esthetic consequences, cleft lip also impairs the child's ability to form an oral seal for suckling. Surgical correction begins during the first months of life. The rule of 10s is loosely applied to timing a cleft lip repair (when the child is >10 weeks old, weighs >10 lb, and has Hgb >10). Children with cleft palates due to the inability to constrict the velopharynx have no means of separating oral from nasal airflow or of controlling oral contents (ie, velopharyngeal incompetence). They are incapable of normal speech articulation, and they often experience reflux into the nasal cavity when eating. In addition, they have reduced swallowing pressures, hindering their ability to open the upper esophageal sphincter for bolus transit. Further, patients with clefts involving the soft palate routinely have chronic middle ear effusions because the palatal musculature is reoriented, causing the impaired opening of the eustachian tube. Cleft palate closure is performed before the age of 2 years to allow for more normal speech development. Ventilation tubes are usually inserted into the tympanic membranes to treat recurrent OME. (Cleft lip and cleft palate are further discussed in Chapter 22.)

Children with Pierre Robin sequence (characterized by mandibular hypoplasia, glossoptosis or ptotic tongue, and cleft palate) are at risk for airway obstruction caused by posterior displacement of the tongue. Infants with this problem have no mandibular support for the tongue and experience choking and aspiration during feeding. Special bottles, surgical fixation of the tongue, and tracheostomy may be necessary to treat more severe cases.

Obstructive Sleep Apnea and Snoring

Obstructive sleep apnea, characterized by recurring periods of apnea during sleep and associated with respiratory efforts, may be caused by a central loss of muscle tone, causing the upper airway to collapse during the negative pressure of inspiratory flow. Apnea is detected by a drop in the oronasal thermal sensor used in a sleep study by at least 90% of its baseline value for at least 10 seconds.

Obstructive sleep apnea is more common in obese adults, especially those with nasal airway obstruction and a large neck circumference. In children, body habitus is usually normal, and hypertrophied adenoids and tonsils are present. Neuromuscular diseases and craniofacial anomalies may also lead to the condition. Snoring at night and mouth breathing are common characteristics of patients with this condition. Long-term systemic problems include cor pulmonale (right-sided heart failure secondary to chronic upper airway obstruction and pulmonary hypertension) and growth retardation. Polysomnography (sleep study) monitors electroencephalography, respiratory efforts, heart rate, and oxygen saturation during sleep. A polysomnogram helps confirm the diagnosis and determine its severity and origins. The treatment of adult sleep apnea is continuous positive airway pressure (CPAP). For patients who are obese, weight loss to ideal body weight may be curative. For patients who cannot lose weight or tolerate CPAP, modification of the upper airway with septoplasty, turbinate reduction, tonsillectomy, or soft palate reduction (uvulopalatopharyngoplasty) is helpful. Other surgical procedures, such as tongue reduction, hyoid advancement, and mandibular advancement, may be helpful in selected cases. Select patients who are intolerant of CPAP may also qualify for a hypoglossal nerve stimulator, which is designed to activate the tongue protrusors during inspiration to open the oropharyngeal airway. In severe cases, tracheostomy may be necessary to bypass the obstructed airway.

Neoplasms

Benign neoplasms of the oral cavity and pharynx are frequently diagnosed by biopsy. Of malignant neoplasms in this region, 90% are squamous cell carcinomas. Like all head and neck carcinomas, they are strongly related to tobacco and alcohol use. These carcinomas may bleed or cause pain. New lesions are staged according to the tumor node metastasis (TNM) system proposed by the American Joint Committee on Cancer, taking into consideration tumor size and location, cervical nodal involvement, and distant metastasis. Patients whose tumors are small, with neither nodal involvement nor evidence of metastasis, have a much greater survival rate than those with evidence of tumor spread.

Squamous cell carcinoma of the lip is associated with sun exposure and tobacco use. Lip cancers have a better prognosis than oral cavity tumors but are more aggressive than similar cutaneous squamous cell carcinomas. Carcinomas of the oral cavity usually occur on the floor of the mouth and on the mobile tongue. They may present as enlarging masses or infiltrating ulcers. Neoplasms of the tonsillar area, the retromolar trigone, or the base of the tongue may cause hemoptysis, dysphagia, dysarthria, trismus (inability to open the mouth due to pterygoid muscle involvement), odynophagia, or referred otalgia. Patients with nasopharyngeal cancer may be seen with middle ear effusion caused by mechanical obstruction of the eustachian tube. Any adult with unilateral serous otitis should be evaluated for a nasopharyngeal tumor. These cancers, which are frequently asymptomatic, are often discovered during the workup of metastatic cervical lymph nodes.

Malignant neoplasms of the oral cavity and pharynx are treated by radiation therapy, surgery, or some combination of these treatments including adjuvant chemotherapy. Small, superficial lesions without nodal metastasis can be treated with either surgery or radiation therapy alone. Unfortunately, most cases of squamous cell carcinoma of the oral cavity and pharynx are associated with high rates of occult nodal metastasis, requiring cervical lymphadenectomy or radiation treatment. Larger primary tumors and those associated with cervical adenopathy usually require a combination of surgery and radiation therapy. Adjuvant chemotherapy can improve locoregional control and disease-free survival. Many patients show equivalent overall survival rates to those treated with surgery and postoperative radiation therapy. Therefore, specific treatment schemes are tailored to the individual patient's medical and psychosocial needs.

The oral cavity and the pharynx are functionally impaired after surgery or radiation therapy. Patients with this type of impairment require a large team of physicians and therapists for rehabilitation and functional preservation. The techniques of surgical reconstruction and irradiation continue to advance with the goal of minimizing morbidity associated with treatment.

THE LARYNX

Anatomy

The larynx occupies the central compartment of the neck and has muscular attachments to the tongue, mandible, skull base, sternum, and clavicles. The laryngeal framework consists of nine cartilage structures. There are three unpaired cartilage structures (epiglottis, thyroid, and cricoid) and three paired cartilage structures (arytenoids, corniculate, and cuneiform) (Figure 25-14). The epiglottis is an anterior leaf-like structure overlying the laryngeal inlet. The shield-shaped thyroid cartilage (ie, Adam apple) contains the anterior origin of the vocal ligaments and is readily palpated in the adult neck. The cricoid cartilage, the only complete cartilaginous ring in the larynx, is shaped like a signet ring. It lies below the thyroid cartilage and is attached posteriorly to the cricothyroid joint, laterally to the cricothyroid muscle, and anteriorly to the cricothyroid membrane. The paired arytenoid cartilages have a three-sided pyramidal shape and articulate with the cricoid inferiorly. They lie immediately below two small cartilages: the cuneiform and corniculate cartilages (Figure 25-15). Laterally, several intrinsic laryngeal muscles insert at the muscular process of the arytenoid. The vocal process arises medially and attaches to the vocal ligament and the vocalis muscle. Medial movement of the vocal processes adducts the vocal folds, closing the airway at the glottic opening.

The muscles of the larynx are classified as extrinsic or intrinsic. The extrinsic muscles elevate and depress the larynx as a unit, whereas the intrinsic muscles move the vocal folds. The posterior cricoarytenoid muscle rotates the arytenoid laterally, abducting (opening) the vocal folds for respiration. The remainder of the intrinsic muscles adduct (close) the vocal folds for phonation, coughing, and swallowing. The vocal folds have a unique and complex structure that facilitates their vibration during phonation. The vocalis muscle is lined by three connective tissue layers and a layer of squamous epithelium.

The nerve supply to the larynx derives from two branches of the vagus nerve: the superior laryngeal nerve, which provides sensory function and innervates the cricothyroid muscle, and the recurrent laryngeal nerve, which supplies motor functions to all remaining intrinsic muscles. The superior laryngeal nerve enters the larynx through the lateral thyrohyoid membrane. The recurrent laryngeal nerve leaves the vagus and courses around the aortic arch on the left and the subclavian artery on the right. It then ascends near the tracheoesophageal groove, branching to innervate the larynx. The left recurrent laryngeal nerve has a longer course in the chest and thus is more susceptible to injury.

Laryngeal lymphatic drainage is site dependent. The larynx is formed embryologically at the fusion of the respiratory diverticulum and the gut tube. The supraglottic larynx has a rich bilateral lymphatic drainage to the deep jugular lymph nodes. The glottic and subglottic larynx has sparse lymphatics, which drain to the pretracheal and paratracheal lymph nodes.

Physiology

The primary functions of the larynx are respiration, airway protection, and phonation. During normal respiration, the glottis opens widely, before the descent of the diaphragm. During deglutition, the larynx acts as a valve by carrying

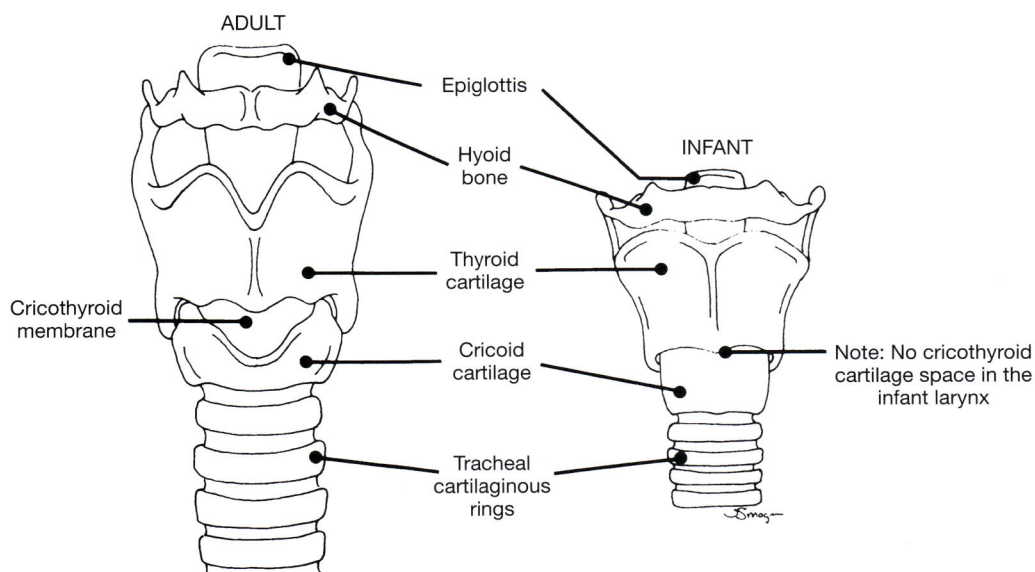

Figure 25-14. Laryngeal framework of the adult and infant. (From Lawrence PF. *Essentials of Surgical Specialties.* 3rd ed. Lippincott Williams & Wilkins; 2007.)

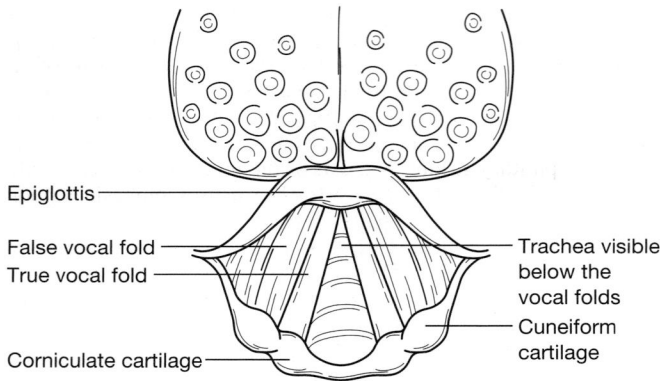

Figure 25-15. **Superior view of the larynx.** (From Lawrence PF. *Essentials of Surgical Specialties.* 3rd ed. Lippincott Williams & Wilkins; 2007.)

out a complex, intricately timed series of events to close the airway, preventing aspiration. Before the food bolus reaches the larynx, the extrinsic muscles of the larynx elevate and anteriorly displace it. This movement opens the pyriform sinuses widely, and the epiglottis covers the larynx to divert the bolus laterally into the pyriform sinuses. The false and true vocal folds also adduct to close off the airway.

Voice is produced by the movement of air through an adducted glottis. This air movement through the narrow, tense glottis produces a repeating wave of the vocal folds. Fine adjustments of the vocal fold tension and intrathoracic air pressure will then define both the frequency of this motion and the volume of the sound generated. This mechanism produces the rudiments of voice; however, the complex sounds of speech require the resonance of the pharyngeal, oral, and nasal cavities. Articulation of speech occurs when the voice is modified continuously by the musculature that shapes these three cavities.

Physical Examination

Special equipment is required for physical examination of the larynx and the hypopharynx. Most commonly a flexible fiberoptic laryngoscope is used; after the nasal cavity has been decongested, anesthetized, and/or lubricated, the scope is passed through the nose and over the soft palate. The base of the tongue, the epiglottis, and the larynx and pyriform sinuses should be visualized. The patient is asked to repeat the sound "eee" and then to take a deep breath, which allows visualization of the vocal folds in both adduction and abduction. For patients with a sensitive gag reflex, a topical spray anesthetic can be applied to the posterior pharynx.

Evaluation

In all complaints related to the larynx and the hypopharyngeal area, certain elements of the history are critical. Basic features, such as the duration of the complaint and exacerbating and relieving characteristics, are helpful in narrowing the differential diagnosis. Systemic signs of infection help confirm the presence of an inflammatory process, such as laryngitis or epiglottitis. Weight loss raises the suspicion of malignancy. Further, in a patient with odynophagia or dysphagia, weight loss will better define the degree of morbidity caused by the symptom. In the adult

population, neoplastic disease must be considered; thus, knowledge of risk factors such as tobacco use, alcohol use, and toxic exposure (eg, to carcinogenic chemicals) is key.

Hoarseness

Hoarseness is related to the disruption of the normal mechanisms of voice production. The characteristics of the vocal change help distinguish motor disturbances from a dysfunction of the vocal fold vibratory characteristics. Breathiness of the voice indicates incomplete adduction of the folds, which can be caused by denervation of the larynx, functional disorders, or senile atrophy of the vocalis muscle known as "presbylaryngis." Strained or strangled vocal characteristics imply spasticity of movement or laryngeal dystonia. A muffled quality ("hot potato voice") is present in patients with mass lesions or inflammatory conditions above the true vocal folds, typical of the oropharynx.

The patient with a rough vocal quality has pathology of the vocal fold. Inflammatory conditions are more likely to improve and deteriorate repeatedly over time. Neoplastic voice disturbance is usually progressive; however, patients with neoplasms may have elements of a concurrent inflammatory process. Hoarseness lasting longer than 6 weeks should prompt an otolaryngology evaluation with laryngeal visualization.

Chronic Cough

The patient with chronic cough can be very challenging to treat because the diagnosis is frequently difficult to confirm. Pulmonary causes, including bronchospastic disease without wheezing, must be carefully eliminated. Cough that occurs immediately after eating is usually the result of aspiration. The larynx is frequently irritated by a number of factors, such as postnasal drip, allergic rhinitis, and vasomotor rhinitis producing a chronic cough. Gastroesophageal reflux disease may cause inflammatory changes in the vocal folds, inducing cough. Children or adults with gastroesophageal reflux may develop pneumonitis when gastric secretions are aspirated, although this condition is uncommon. Drugs such as angiotensin-converting enzyme inhibitors may cause a mild edematous process of the vocal fold, inducing cough. Unfortunately, the continuous trauma of chronic cough usually induces mild edema or erythema of the larynx, leaving the physician to determine "Which came first?"

Hemoptysis

Although the classic teaching is that hemoptysis is caused by lung pathology, the condition may also indicate a bleeding lesion elsewhere in the upper aerodigestive tract. The physician must also rule out the possibility of aspiration of blood from an upper aerodigestive source, such as a posterior nasal bleed.

Stridor

Stridor is a high-pitched noise audible without a stethoscope that is a result of turbulent airflow through a narrowed portion of the upper airway. It represents significant obstruction of the airway. It can be characterized as inspiratory, expiratory, or biphasic (occurring during both inspiration and expiration). One can often determine the location of stenosis just by the nature of the stridor (Figure 25-16). In general, narrowing of the airway above the level of the vocal cords results in inspiratory stridor. Stenosis at the level of the vocal cords or in the extrathoracic trachea causes biphasic stridor and narrowing or partial obstruction of the intrathoracic trachea results in expiratory stridor. The latter is often mistaken for asthma, and patients may be improperly diagnosed and treated for some time. Patients who are not

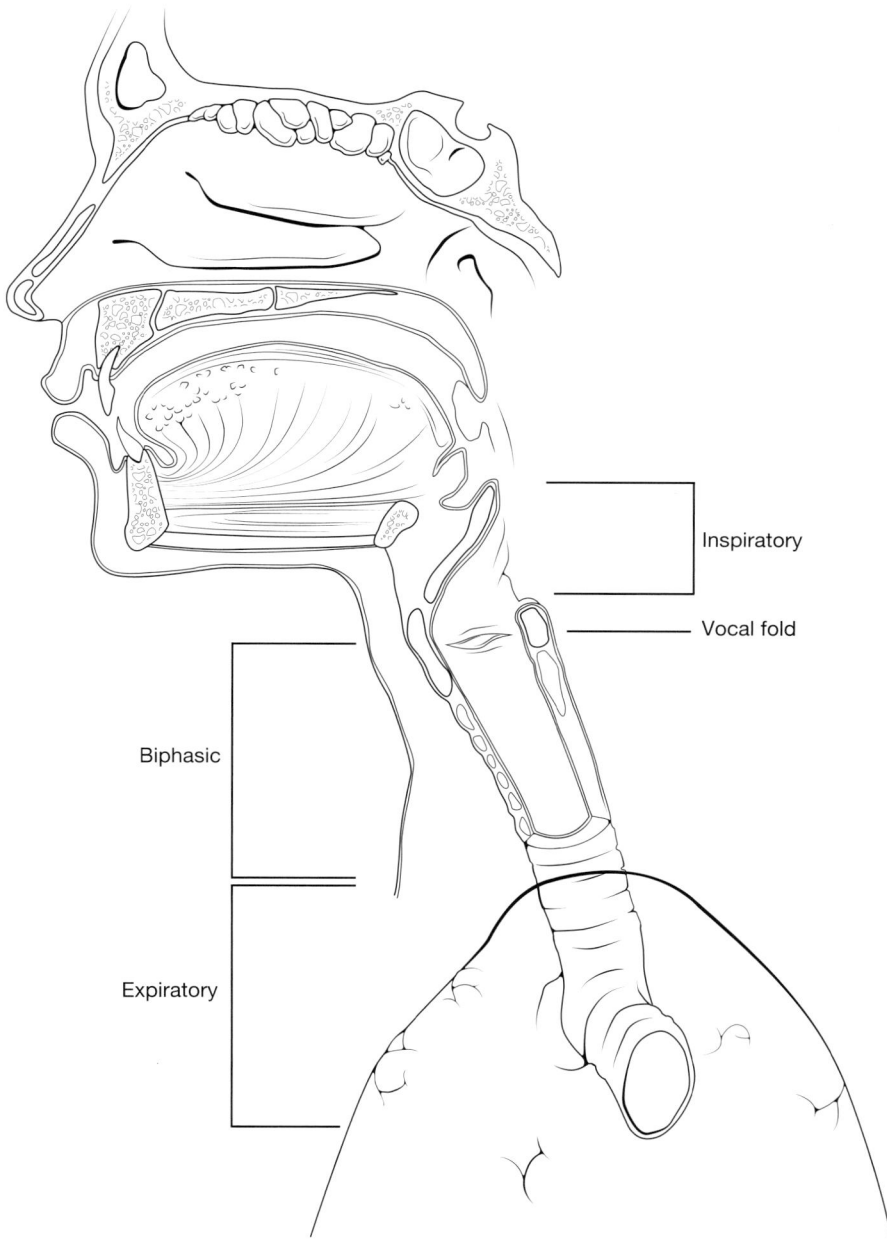

Figure 25-16. Location of airway obstruction with respect to the type of stridor. (From Lawrence PF. *Essentials of Surgical Specialties.* 3rd ed. Lippincott Williams & Wilkins; 2007.)

responding to asthma medications should be evaluated for possible other causes of airway narrowing.

In the infant, laryngomalacia, subglottic stenosis, laryngeal webs, and benign neoplasms are the most likely diagnoses; laryngoscopy or bronchoscopy is required for evaluation. Associated systemic illness in a child implies laryngotracheobronchitis or tracheitis and epiglottitis. In adults, these illnesses are less commonly associated with stridor and airway compromise because of the increased size of the adult glottis and its ability to tolerate the associated edema. In stridorous adults, neoplasm is more frequently diagnosed. Table 25-10 lists the common causes of stridor in adults and children.

Odynophagia and Dysphagia

Patients with difficulty swallowing describe an inability to pass food, pain with swallowing, or the feeling of something caught in the throat (known as "globus sensation"). The physician must first identify the consistency of the food that causes symptoms. Neuromuscular disorders will first affect the ability to swallow liquids and will eventually affect swallowing of foods of all consistencies. Difficulty in passing solid foods implies a mechanical obstruction, such as stricture, neoplasm, or diverticulum. An adult with chronic pain from swallowing requires careful evaluation to rule out malignancy. Unfortunately, superficial lesions can be quite painful and may escape radiologic assessment. Patients with risk factors for malignancies who have chronic unexplained odynophagia must undergo a complete assessment of the upper aerodigestive tract. Globus is quite common and can be associated with inflammation although frequently, no demonstrable pathology is found on further exam. A history of swallowing a sharp food

bolus that may have scratched the pharynx may be helpful. Symptoms that persist for longer than 1 month should be further evaluated.

Clinical Presentation, Diagnosis, and Treatment

Pediatric Structural Pathology

Laryngomalacia is the most common cause of stridor among infants, accounting for 60% of all cases. The supraglottic structures prolapse into the airway, producing inspiratory stridor. The condition is present at birth and is frequently noted in premature infants; most children will be seen during the first 2 months of life. The stridor worsens when the child is in the supine position or feeding but rarely results in severe distress. Diagnosis is permitted by flexible laryngoscopy, which demonstrates the airway collapse during spontaneous ventilation. Rigid laryngoscopy under general anesthesia will also demonstrate severe cases of malacia. The symptoms are usually self-limiting, with spontaneous recovery by the second year of life. Parents should be reassured but should also be advised to avoid keeping the baby in a supine position, especially during sleep. In the rare severe case, resecting redundant supraglottic tissue can be beneficial. This procedure, termed "supraglottoplasty," is generally reserved for patients with worrisome apnea spells or failure to thrive.

Tracheomalacia is seen as expiratory or biphasic stridor caused by collapse of the trachea in the anterior-posterior direction. The cartilage is often abnormally shaped and soft. Spontaneous resolution can usually be expected by the time the child reaches age 18 months. Occasionally, surgical treatment is required.

In the infant, the subglottic airway is the narrowest region of the upper airway. Stenosis of this region can occur congenitally but more commonly results from local trauma, such as prolonged intubation. If severe, this condition causes biphasic stridor. In most cases, children with mild stenosis are seen with stridor during upper respiratory tract infections or after intubation. Even the slightest circumferential narrowing of the airway results in significant reduction of the total area. The narrowed subglottis becomes critical with additional airway edema, and the child develops stridor or recurrent **croup**. These exacerbations usually respond to conservative measures, such as nebulized racemic epinephrine and systemic corticosteroids. The problem often resolves as the infant grows because the stenotic segment enlarges along with the rest of the larynx.

Vocal fold webs are membranous and usually involve the anterior true folds. Congenital webs are formed when normal embryonic laryngeal recanalization fails to occur. More commonly, they result from trauma and subsequent scarring of the anterior commissure. They may cause hoarseness or stridor, depending on their extent. The recommended treatment is endoscopic laser excision; however, an open surgical repair is rarely required.

Blunt and Penetrating Trauma of the Larynx

Laryngeal injuries can be immediately life threatening because they may cause airway obstruction. The upper airway must be carefully assessed for fractures or endolaryngeal trauma; if it is compromised, it should be secured by tracheotomy. A fractured larynx can lead to false passage or laryngotracheal separation on attempted oral intubation. Diagnosis of these injuries is facilitated by

TABLE 25-10. Common Causes of Stridor

Inspiratory	Pediatric	Adult
Inspiratory	Laryngomalacia	Neoplasm
	Epiglottitis	Angioedema
	Foreign body	Trauma to larynx
Biphasic	Croup	Vocal cord neoplasm
	Vocal cord web	Vocal cord paralysis
	Vocal cord paralysis	Laryngeal trauma
	Tracheomalacia	Subglottic stenosis
	Subglottic hemangioma	
	Vascular rings or slings	
Expiratory	Foreign body (tracheal or bronchus)	Tracheal neoplasm
	Asthma	Bronchial neoplasm
	Bronchomalacia	Foreign body

laryngeal examination. Findings such as neck tenderness, palpable laryngeal step-offs, voice change, the presence of subcutaneous emphysema, glottic mucosal disruption, or hematoma indicate possible laryngeal fracture. Blunt injuries causing fracture may escape detection if the patient is intubated for other reasons; the fracture may be discovered when attempts to extubate are unsuccessful. Penetrating injuries are readily apparent and usually require surgical repair.

Tracheal and Subglottic Stenosis

Trauma to the trachea can also occur from internal injury, the most common of which is prolonged endotracheal intubation. The pressure of the endotracheal tube can cause local ischemia and subsequent mucosal damage. If perichondritis and chondritis follow, significant scarring may occur. Occasionally, the cartilage is damaged, leaving a malacic segment that dynamically collapses on inspiration. A tracheostomy may also cause tracheal narrowing. These conditions may occur days to months after extubation as the scar matures. Treatment with segmental tracheal resection may be necessary. Occasionally, endoscopic laser excision with dilation can be curative. Subsequent serial steroid injections to the region of stenosis can decrease the likelihood of recurrence.

Inflammatory Conditions

Patients of all age groups can suffer inflammatory processes of the larynx, usually causing hoarseness. Infectious conditions may cause odynophagia and systemic symptoms. The larynx of a child is substantially smaller than that of an adult, and the swelling caused by laryngeal infections can produce life-threatening airway compromise.

Epiglottitis

Epiglottitis is a potentially lethal inflammation of the supraglottis, usually caused by the bacteria *H. influenzae*. The incidence of epiglottitis has reduced substantially with the introduction of the *H. influenzae* vaccine. The condition occurs most commonly among children 3 to 6 years old but may also occur well into adulthood. The child is seen with a sudden onset of fever and stridor. Physical examination reveals a child in moderate to severe distress sitting upright with the head hyperextended to straighten the upper airway in an effort to facilitate air exchange. The child may be drooling and may also have severe odynophagia. A tongue blade must not be used to examine the child's throat because this may produce severe laryngospasm and loss of the airway. The child should be kept calm; if the child's condition permits, a portable lateral neck radiograph should be made to look for loss or blunting of the usual sharp borders and thin contour of the epiglottis.

If epiglottitis is considered, the child is taken to the operating room for anesthesia, direct laryngoscopy, and oral intubation. A nasotracheal tube is often inserted later because it is more stable and less likely to become displaced. In addition to an experienced anesthesiologist, an otolaryngologist or pediatric surgeon should be in attendance in the event that intubation cannot be carried out and bronchoscopy, tracheostomy, or both become necessary. Once the airway is established, cultures are taken, and treatment with intravenous antibiotics effective against *H. influenzae* is instituted. From the operating

room, the child is taken to the intensive care unit, where the nasotracheal (preferable) or orotracheal tube is kept secure. The edema usually resolves rapidly, and the child can be extubated within 72 hours.

Croup

Laryngotracheobronchitis, frequently referred to as croup, most commonly affects children of age 2 years or younger. It is viral in origin and generally affects the subglottic larynx although it may extend the length of the trachea. The child is seen with symptoms of an upper respiratory tract infection of a few days' duration. Over a period of several hours, the child develops a barking cough as the primary symptom. Fever is usually low grade or absent. Physical examination reveals an irritable infant with mild stridor and barking cough. A lateral neck film reveals a normal epiglottis but a narrowed subglottic air column (known as a "steeple sign"). Treatment is based on the severity of symptoms. In mild cases, cool humidified air alone suffices. In moderate cases, racemic epinephrine treatments may be required in the emergency department (ED). In severe cases, the child may require hospitalization, with frequent racemic epinephrine treatments and intravenous or aerosol administration of steroids to reduce inflammation. Rarely, the airway distress is so severe that endotracheal intubation is required to secure the airway. The edema from croup resolves more slowly than that from epiglottitis, often requiring 5 to 7 days for full resolution. Because several viruses cause croup, recurrence is common. Rarely, bacterial tracheitis is seen and is associated with a more virulent course, requiring intubation and therapeutic bronchoscopy.

Laryngitis

The most common inflammatory condition of the larynx among adults is acute laryngitis. It is usually viral in origin, causing hoarseness and symptoms of upper respiratory tract infection. Examination of the vocal cords reveals edema and erythema. The disease usually resolves spontaneously, but improvement can be expedited with humidification and voice rest. Fungal laryngitis in patients on inhaled steroid therapy may require systemic treatment because this area is difficult to treat with topical antifungals. It should be emphasized that an adult with hoarseness that persists for longer than 1 month should undergo an examination of the vocal cords and possible biopsy.

Chronic laryngitis is precipitated by chronic irritation of the larynx, usually resulting in painless dysphonia. The vocal cords are erythematous, with some degree of edema. In some patients, the edema becomes quite pronounced and is described as "polypoid degeneration"; occasionally, classic polyps form and should be excised. The treatment is removal of the irritating condition, which is usually an inhaled irritant (eg, tobacco smoke, an allergen, or some noxious compound). Gastroesophageal reflux and postnasal drainage of inflammatory mucus may also lead to chronic laryngitis.

Vocal Fold Paralysis

Unilateral vocal fold paralysis usually causes a weak, breathy voice and sometimes aspiration. The patient will commonly relate coughing when swallowing thin liquids. The recurrent laryngeal nerve is susceptible to injury during carotid, thyroid, or thoracic surgical procedures. Central lesions, such as brainstem stroke, amyotrophic lateral sclerosis, and multiple sclerosis, will usually have other neurologic manifestations. Tumor at the base of the skull or within the lung, thyroid, esophagus, hypopharynx, or larynx may disrupt the innervation of a vocal fold if it extends to involve the nerve. Unilateral vocal fold paralysis can be a congenital defect, usually caused by trauma resulting from stretching the recurrent laryngeal nerve during pregnancy or delivery. Often, the workup will reveal no cause (ie, idiopathic vocal fold paralysis). Idiopathic vocal fold paralysis is probably viral related and behaves similarly to other cranial nerve neuropathies in that it may reverse itself without treatment. If after 6 to 12 months no function returns and the patient has an uncompensated paralysis, the paralyzed vocal fold can be medialized. This procedure allows the mobile contralateral vocal fold to approximate the paralyzed fold, producing voice and protecting the airway (Figure 25-17).

Bilateral vocal fold paralysis is quite uncommon and may be caused by central and systemic pathologies. Adults with this condition will have a near-normal voice and a marked biphasic stridor. Both vocal folds can be paralyzed at birth because of a brainstem lesion, such as Arnold-Chiari malformation. Initial treatment for airway distress is intubation. Tracheotomy is usually performed in patients with airway distress. Tracheotomy can preserve voice while providing an adequate airway. Frequently, patients find the secretions and management associated with a long-term tracheostomy unsatisfactory. In such patients, vocal fold lateralization procedures, unilateral arytenoidectomy, or unilateral vocal cordotomy can be performed. These procedures will compromise the voice, as they enlarge the glottic airway.

Chronic Lesions of the Vocal Folds

Vocal fold nodules are a common cause of chronic hoarseness and occur in children and adults. They are usually the result of localized chronic inflammation from improper vocal use and vocal abuse. Also known as "singer's nodules," they may occur among vocalists, especially those without

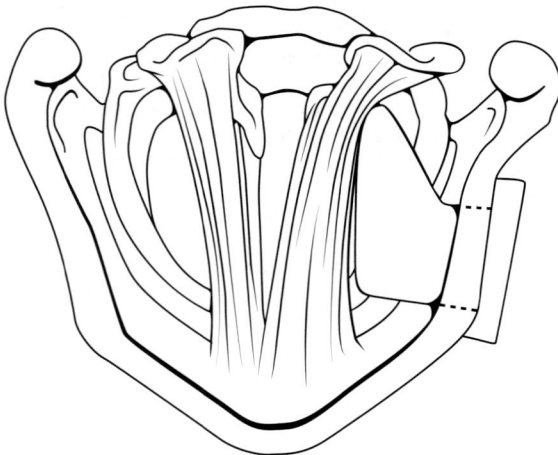

Figure 25-17. Coronal section of the larynx at the level of the vocal cords. An implant has been surgically placed on the left inside of the thyroid cartilage to medialize the left vocal cord. (From Lawrence PF. *Essentials of Surgical Specialties*. 3rd ed. Lippincott Williams & Wilkins; 2007.)

voice training. Examination reveals symmetrical white nodules at the junction of the anterior and middle third of the true vocal cords, the site of the highest amount of mucosal trauma during phonation. Correcting the patterns of voice use and abuse through diligent voice training will in many cases enable spontaneous clearing of nodules. Without speech or voice therapy, the nodules are likely to recur.

Granuloma formation can occur at the posterior true vocal cord near the vocal process of the arytenoid cartilage as a result of local trauma, usually in the presence of gastroesophageal reflux. Granuloma formation is frequently associated with endotracheal intubation or repeated vocal trauma, such as throat clearing and chronic cough. The condition will frequently respond to aggressive treatment of gastroesophageal reflux, antibiotics, and a short course of corticosteroids. Lesions that do not respond to the abovementioned measures can be treated by injection of botulinum toxin (Botox) into the laryngeal adductors (thyroarytenoid and lateral cricothyroid muscles). Botox provides neuromuscular paralysis by preventing the release of presynaptic acetylcholine. This results in a less forceful adduction of the vocal cords, which allows the granuloma to resolve and the area to heal. In rare instances, granulomas are removed surgically because they cause airway obstruction, or to rule out malignancy.

Benign Neoplasms of the Larynx

The most common benign tumor in children is squamous papilloma, which can also involve the trachea and the bronchi. The papilloma is an epithelial lesion of connective tissue covered by squamous epithelium that may be keratinized. Papillomas are believed to be caused by viruses and to be influenced by hormonal changes, as evidenced by their tendency to remit spontaneously around the time of puberty. Papillomas usually involve the anterior portions of the vocal cords but can also involve the false cords superiorly and the immediate subglottic area. In children, onset usually occurs before the age of 5 potentially via vertical transmission from the mother, and the condition can persist until late adolescence. Papillomas arising in adults are not as aggressive. Papillomas spread by manipulation and can seed up and down the respiratory tract. For this reason, tracheostomy should be avoided unless absolutely necessary for severe disease burden.

Treatment is endoscopic laser ablation of the papilloma. Radiation therapy is not helpful. Systemic therapies, such as α-interferon, ribavirin, acyclovir, and indole 3, are currently under investigation for more severe cases. It is difficult to determine the best treatment because the natural history of this disease involves waxing and waning of severity.

Subglottic and tracheal **hemangiomas** are vascular lesions seen during the first year of life in association with stridor and cutaneous hemangiomas. Like hemangiomas of the skin, they usually regress by 4 years of age; thus, a conservative approach is warranted. If these lesions cannot be managed with a β-blocker, surgical treatment in the form of endoscopic laser excision or tracheotomy may be necessary. Steroids have also been used with varying degrees of success.

Malignant Neoplasms of the Larynx

The most common laryngeal malignancy is squamous cell carcinoma; all other malignancies combined make up less than 5% of laryngeal malignancy. In most populations, the incidence of laryngeal malignancy is 10% of that seen for lung cancer. Tobacco smoking and alcohol are strong risk factors. The peak incidence is in the sixth and seventh decades of life; men are affected more commonly than women.

A diagnosis of carcinoma of the larynx requires a biopsy of the lesion or an obvious lymph node metastasis. In addition to indirect mirror and fiberoptic examination of the dynamic larynx in the awake patient, direct operative laryngoscopy under general anesthesia best delineates the extent of mucosal involvement. CT or MRI scans can demonstrate the depth of invasion and lymph adenopathy. New lesions found in the larynx are then staged according to the system proposed by the American Joint Committee on Cancer considering the tumor size and location, cervical nodal involvement, and metastasis. Patients whose tumors are small, with no nodal involvement and no evidence of metastasis, have a much greater survival rate than those with an evidence of tumor spread.

Primary treatment methods are surgery and radiation therapy. Chemotherapy given in conjunction with radiation therapy improves the survival rates for advanced stages of larynx cancer and obviates the need for surgery in select cases. For end-stage malignancies, chemotherapy has been used palliatively with limited success. To determine the therapeutic modality, the size and location of the tumor, the presence or absence of cervical lymph node involvement, and the patient's own desires and physical status are considered.

The surgery for laryngeal carcinoma is dictated by the primary tumor and the patient's premorbid conditions. Endoscopic excision or partial laryngectomy is used with good success for small tumors. Total laryngectomy is reserved for larger lesions and for smaller lesions in patients with marginal pulmonary lung function who could not tolerate aspiration. This completely disconnects the airway from the alimentary tract. The trachea is matured as a stoma to the skin at the base of the neck above the sternal notch. Once laryngectomy has been performed, it is important to note that the patient cannot be intubated orally. Postoperatively, verbal communication is accomplished by using an electrolarynx or by using the esophagus and the neopharynx to produce a vibratory noise. A one-way prosthetic valve may be placed into a surgically created fistula between the esophagus and tracheostoma, thus allowing the patient to produce this esophageal speech.

Radiation therapy can be delivered to the larynx alone with little morbidity. Small tumors are usually treated with radiation therapy, particularly when they involve the true vocal cords without paraglottic spread. For small superficial cancers of the larynx with no cervical node involvement, either surgery or radiation therapy will produce a 3-year survival rate greater than 90%. Tumors of the supraglottic larynx are associated with a high rate of lymph node metastasis, and even small lesions without palpable adenopathy will necessitate treatment of the neck. Patients treated with radiation for supraglottic cancers must have a much larger proportion of the neck treated than those with glottic cancers. Therefore, the morbidity rates associated with irradiation increase. Surgical treatment is used for patients whose disease recurs or does not respond to therapy.

The presence of cervical adenopathy in laryngeal carcinoma is an indicator of a much poorer prognosis, reducing the predicted 5-year survival rate by as much as 70%.

These advanced-stage lesions are frequently treated with a combination of irradiation and surgery. Chemotherapy may also be used to increase the radiosensitivity of the tumor in certain cases.

THE NECK AND SALIVARY GLANDS

Anatomy

A significant part of any gross anatomy course is spent covering the complex structures of the neck. The neck serves two basic functions. It is a portal through which a vast array of visceral and neurovascular structures traverse, and it also serves as the fifth limb, allowing movement of the head. The musculature connects the cervical vertebrae to move the head and to elevate the ribs and the shoulder girdle. The sternocleidomastoid muscle divides the neck into two triangles—anterior and posterior. The anterior triangle of the neck is bounded medially by the midline of the neck, superiorly by the angle of the mandible, posteriorly by the sternocleidomastoid muscle, and inferiorly by the clavicle. The posterior triangle is bounded medially by the sternocleidomastoid muscle, superiorly by the mastoid tip and the superior nuchal line, posteriorly by the trapezius muscle, and inferiorly by the clavicle. Normal structures in the anterior triangle that can be seen or palpated include the sternocleidomastoid muscle, the hyoid bone, the larynx, the trachea, the thyroid gland, the parotid gland, and the submandibular gland. Deep to the sternocleidomastoid muscle in the anterior triangle lies the carotid sheath, which contains the common, external, and internal carotid arteries; the internal jugular vein; the vagus nerve; the sympathetic chain; and the deep jugular lymph nodes. The lymphatics drain the mucosal surfaces of the upper aerodigestive tract (Figure 25-18). This leads to a somewhat predictable spread of infection or tumor into the cervical lymphatics.

Four distinct layers of cervical fascia envelop the contents of the neck. Deep to the skin is the superficial cervical fascia encompassing the platysma muscle. Immediately below the platysma is the investing, or superficial, layer of the deep cervical fascia, which splits to envelop the sternocleidomastoid and strap muscles. The visceral, or middle, layer of deep fascia envelops the thyroid, pharynx, larynx, and trachea. Laterally, the middle layer forms the carotid sheath. The deepest layer is the prevertebral fascia, enveloping the paraspinous musculature of the neck.

The major salivary glands are the parotid, the submandibular, and the sublingual glands (Figure 25-19). These paired glands are located outside the mucosa of the oral cavity, to which they are connected by ducts. The minor salivary glands are scattered throughout the oral cavity and the oropharynx. They lie just deep into the mucosa and connect with the oral cavity and the pharynx by way of rudimentary ducts.

The parotid gland is the largest salivary gland. It lies anterior to the ear, overlying the masseter muscle, and has a tail part that extends inferiorly to the mandibular angle and posteriorly below the mastoid tip. Its duct (Stensen) arises anteriorly approximately 1 cm below the zygoma. It traverses the masseter muscle and terminates orally in an

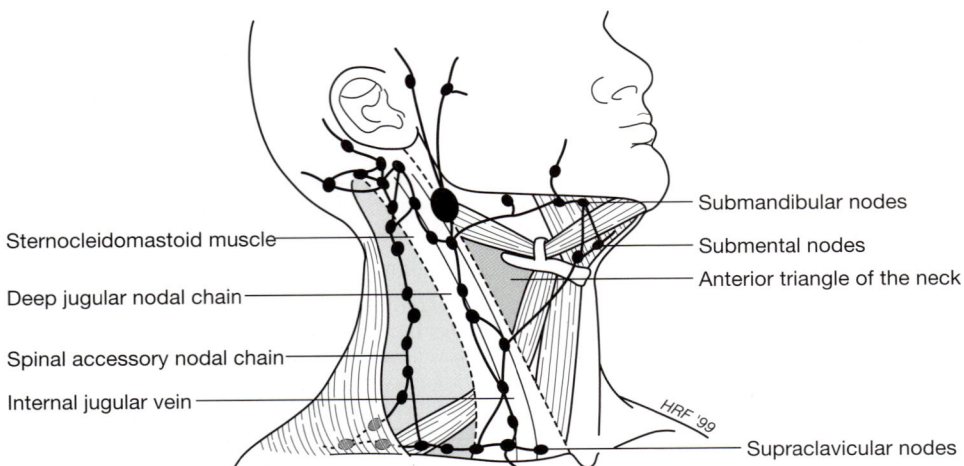

Figure 25-18. The cervical lymphatics. (From Lawrence PF. *Essentials of Surgical Specialties.* 3rd ed. Lippincott Williams & Wilkins; 2007.)

ampulla opposite the second maxillary molar tooth. The most important of the multiple nerves associated with the parotid gland is the facial nerve, which exits the mastoid bone through the stylomastoid foramen and passes through the center of the gland, where it branches into the cervical, marginal mandibular, buccal, zygomatic, and temporal motor nerves. The secretomotor supply to the gland is parasympathetic via the ninth cranial nerve from the inferior salivatory nucleus in the brainstem.

The submandibular gland lies in a concavity inferior to the mandible, between the anterior and posterior bellies of the digastric muscle. Its duct (Wharton) runs anteriorly from the gland between the mylohyoid and hyoglossus muscles. It ends in an ampulla immediately adjacent to the lingual frenulum in the anterior floor of mouth. The parasympathetic secretomotor nerve supply is derived from the superior salivatory nucleus by way of the chorda tympani and the lingual nerves.

The sublingual gland, the smallest of the major glands, lies directly under the oral mucosa, forming a ridge next to the tongue in the lateral floor of mouth. The gland empties directly into the oral cavity through several ducts on its superior surface. It lies close to the superior part of the submandibular gland, and minor sublingual ducts may enter the submandibular gland. The secretomotor nerve supply is the same as that of the submandibular gland.

Physiology

The salivary glands produce approximately 500 mL of saliva per day, of which 90% is secreted by the parotid and submandibular glands. Saliva acts both as a lubricant and as a protective agent throughout the upper aerodigestive tract. It promotes clearing of debris and bacteria, sweeping these contaminants into the lower gastrointestinal tract. It also helps maintain oral and dental hygiene and indirectly aids in maintaining hydration. The main digestive enzyme of saliva is β-amylase, which is important for the enzymatic breakdown of starch.

Physical Examination

The physical examination must be performed in a systematic way to avoid omitting a structure. Visual inspection for lesions and scars on the skin and for signs of muscular atrophy or deformity must always precede palpation.

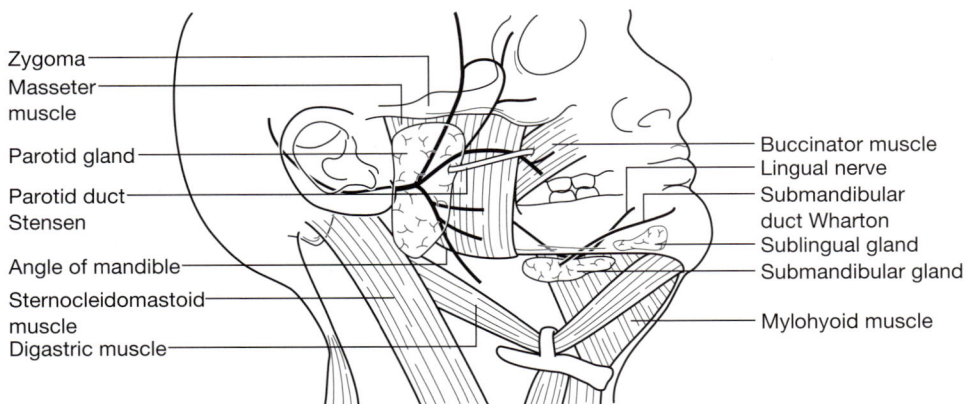

Figure 25-19. Anatomy of the parotid and submandibular glands. (From Lawrence PF. *Essentials of Surgical Specialties.* 3rd ed. Lippincott Williams & Wilkins; 2007.)

Then the parotid gland should be palpated. To allow complete assessment of the submandibular triangle, a gloved finger should first be inserted into the floor of the mouth, allowing bimanual palpation. Otherwise, the contents of the submandibular triangle will elevate on palpation. The anterior triangle should be palpated to assess the cervical lymphatics and anterior airway cartilages. Then the posterior triangle should be palpated for masses. The thyroid gland should be palpated anteriorly by insinuating the fingers between the trachea and the sternocleidomastoid muscle. Having the patient swallow will cause the gland to move under the palpating fingers, facilitating the detection of nodules.

Evaluation

Patients with a neck mass present a diagnostic challenge due to the lengthy differential diagnosis. In broad categories, these lesions are traumatic, congenital, inflammatory, or neoplastic. The temporal history of the lesion, associated pain, systemic manifestations of disease, and other symptoms of aerodigestive pathology are quite important. Past medical history and patient demographics complete the information required to shape the differential diagnosis. The location of the lesion is also important. The tail of the parotid and the submandibular gland are frequently confused with adenopathy. It is important to note that with age the submandibular gland may descend in the neck to become "low lying" or ptotic. Certain bony protuberances, such as the angle of the jaw and the transverse process of C-1, can be mistaken for neck masses. The physician should carefully feel for the characteristics of the lesion. If it is pulsatile, is there a symmetrical mass on the contralateral side (does it represent a prominent carotid bulb)? Is there a thrill or bruit, as in a vascular tumor? Is the mass discrete, fixed, or infiltrating surrounding structures? Are there other masses palpable nearby?

Nontender Neck Mass

In an adult older than 40 years, a nontender neck mass indicates a neoplasm until proven otherwise. Squamous cell carcinoma commonly metastasizes to the cervical lymph nodes from the upper aerodigestive tract. In the era of human papillomavirus (HPV)-related oropharyngeal cancer, cystic metastatic lymph nodes may be incorrectly identified as a branchial cleft cyst. Distant metastasis from infraclavicular sites, such as the lung or abdomen, may occur within the supraclavicular fossae. Thyroid carcinoma may also metastasize to the cervical lymph nodes without obvious palpable nodularity in the thyroid gland. A careful examination of the head and neck should be performed. If a primary site is identified, a biopsy of the primary tumor should be performed. If no primary site can be found, a fine needle biopsy performed properly and read by a skilled cytopathologist is quite accurate in providing a diagnosis. An open excisional biopsy of a neck mass is performed only as a "last resort" because it may compromise future treatment. Incisional biopsy is best avoided given the risk of tumor seeding. Therefore, it is to be performed only after repeated fine needle aspiration is nondiagnostic, and examination of the upper aerodigestive tract under anesthesia (including ipsilateral tonsillectomy and biopsies of the nasopharynx and base of tongue) fails to discover a primary site of malignancy. CT scans and MRI provide detailed information about nonpalpable pathology; these imaging methods also allow good visualization of the nasopharynx, which can be difficult to assess fully.

In adolescents and young adults, cancer for an isolated neck mass is a less common diagnosis. A compliant patient with a neck mass smaller than 3 cm in size may be followed. Reactive lymph nodes do not always return to normal size. Certain infectious conditions may produce nontender adenopathy. A history of exposure to tuberculosis, HIV, and animal bites and scratches may be helpful. Larger and solid lesions that enlarge over time raise the suspicion of lymphoma and demand fine needle aspiration. It is diagnostic and can provide tissue for flow cytometry to aid in defining the subtype of lymphoma. Occasionally, a lymphoma may depend on histologic architecture, making open biopsy necessary. Cystic congenital lesions are seen most commonly among patients in this age group. Because of the thick fascial layers of the neck, differentiating cysts from solid lesions can be difficult. Ultrasound and CT or fine needle aspiration will help make the diagnosis.

Tender Neck Mass

Inflammatory processes that lead to reactive lymphadenopathy are usually more recent in onset and shorter in duration; they may be accompanied by fever and symptoms related to an upper respiratory tract infection, such as sore throat or congestion. Tender adenopathy that is not responsive to antibiotics may imply granulomatous infections, which may be identified through fine needle cytopathology and culture. Useful laboratory tests include a complete blood cell count with differential, an erythrocyte sedimentation rate, and a serum test as appropriate for mononucleosis (Epstein-Barr virus), cat scratch disease (*Bartonella*), and HIV.

Clinical Presentation, Diagnosis, and Treatment

Acute and Chronic Sialadenitis

Inflammatory diseases of the salivary glands include mumps, acute suppurative **sialadenitis**, parotid abscess, chronic sialadenitis, and Sjögren syndrome. Acute sialadenitis is a bacterial infection most frequently involving the submandibular gland. Adults are more commonly affected. Debilitated and dehydrated patients are particularly susceptible. The gland becomes hard and tender, and purulent discharge can be seen from the duct, producing a foul taste in the patient's mouth. Causative organisms include *S. aureus*, *S. pneumoniae*, and hemolytic streptococcus. Treatment includes hydration and appropriate antibiotics targeting gram-positive organisms. Abscesses of the salivary glands are treated by incision and drainage.

Chronic sialadenitis is characterized by recurrent tender enlargements of the glands and is frequently associated with strictures or calculi involving the ductal system. These conditions can be treated with ductal dilation, removal of stones, or sialodochoplasty (reconstruction of the duct). Treatment of chronic sialadenitis is usually conservative, including sialagogues (saliva stimulants, such as sour candy), gland massage, and antibiotics. When conservative measures are unsuccessful, superficial parotidectomy or excision of the submandibular gland may be the most appropriate means of treatment.

Sjögren syndrome is an autoimmune disease of the salivary glands and includes xerostomia, keratoconjunctivitis sicca, and connective tissue disorders. The cause of the syndrome is unknown, but most patients exhibit hypergammaglobulinemia with elevated immunoglobulin G fraction and positive SS-A and SS-B antibodies. Rheumatoid arthritis is a common characteristic of the syndrome, and antinuclear antibodies are present in 50% of the cases, with or without clinical arthritis. The diagnosis may be confirmed with a minor salivary gland biopsy, and treatment generally includes local measures to counteract xerostomia and conjunctivitis. If the salivary glands are infected, antibiotic therapy is also recommended. Patients with this syndrome should be observed for increasing the size of the glands because they are at significantly higher risk for developing salivary lymphoma.

Benign Neoplasms of the Salivary Glands

Tumors of the salivary glands account for approximately 1% of all head and neck tumors, and 85% of them arise from the parotid gland. Of these, 75% are benign; in comparison, 50% of submandibular gland tumors and 30% of minor salivary gland tumors are benign. Diagnostic procedures for tumors of the salivary glands include fine needle aspiration, sialography, scintillation scanning, CT scanning, and MRI. The introduction of CT scanning and MRI over the past 15 years and the increased use of fine needle aspiration for obtaining tumor information have resulted in a dramatic reduction in the use of other diagnostic techniques.

Benign tumors usually display painless, slow growth and tumor mobility; they may occasionally cause secondary fibrosis or inflammation. Because of secondary infection or cystic degeneration, pain may be present but is not common. Minor salivary gland tumors usually occur on the palate but may occur anywhere in the upper aerodigestive tract. They are firm, nontender, mucosally covered masses.

Approximately 80% of benign tumors are mixed tumors or pleomorphic adenomas, which tend to occur in the third and fourth decades of life and do carry a small potential risk of malignant transformation. Warthin tumor occurs 8% of the time, primarily in the tail of the parotid gland and principally among male smokers. Treatment of these benign tumors consists of total removal of the submandibular gland or minor salivary gland, or removal of the appropriate portion of the parotid gland while preserving the facial nerve.

The most common benign parotid gland tumor among children is hemangioma, which usually resolves spontaneously. Surgery should be reserved for rapidly growing tumors or those that do not resolve by the time the patient has reached the age of 2 or 3 years.

Lymphoepithelial parotid cysts occur frequently among patients with acquired immunodeficiency syndrome (AIDS). These cysts may respond to laser treatment, sclerotherapy, or low doses of radiation. Surgical excision is reserved for symptomatic cysts for which other treatment methods have failed.

Malignant Neoplasms of the Salivary Glands

Malignant lesions of the salivary glands share many of the characteristics of their benign counterparts. However, certain signs and symptoms indicate malignancy: rapid growth, large size, fixation of the tumor to the overlying skin, facial pain, facial nerve dysfunction, and cervical node enlargement. Children tend to have a higher rate of malignancy than adults with salivary gland tumors.

Fine needle aspiration allows diagnosis of malignancy in 85% to 95% of cases. Open or partial biopsy is performed only when mucosal or skin involvement is noted. Minor salivary gland biopsy may be performed if the tumor is not accessible by fine needle aspiration. Biopsies of small tumors of the submandibular gland are best performed by removal of the gland. New lesions found in the salivary glands are staged according to the TNM system, described earlier, proposed by the American Joint Committee on Cancer.

The most common malignancy of the major salivary glands is mucoepidermoid carcinoma, followed by adenoid cystic carcinoma and acinic cell carcinoma. Each of these tumors shows a wide spectrum of biologic behavior. They are histopathologically classified into low- and high-grade tumors. Low-grade cancers usually have a favorable prognosis, grow locally, and metastasize to upper neck nodes infrequently and late in the course of the disease. High-grade cancers commonly metastasize to the neck nodes and lungs. Adenoid cystic carcinoma, the most common malignancy in all but the parotid gland, tends to have a high degree of perineural invasion. This tumor is also characterized by late distant metastasis; the 10- to 20-year survival rate is poor. Other malignant tumors of the salivary glands include adenocarcinoma and squamous cell carcinoma. The primary treatment of malignancies of the salivary glands is removal of the tumor and the involved lymph nodes, followed by radiotherapy. If possible, the facial nerve should be spared in this resection. If there is preoperative facial nerve paralysis, or obvious nerve involvement with tumor, the nerve should be sacrificed to provide adequate tumor resection. Numerous plastic surgery techniques are available to reanimate the paralyzed face, if needed.

Cervical Adenitis

Most inflammatory neck masses are inflamed lymph nodes, especially in children. Nearly every person has lymphadenitis at some point in life, most commonly during childhood; the inciting disease may be bacterial, viral, or granulomatous. In children, concurrent viral upper respiratory tract illness is associated with swollen tender adenopathy.

Frequently, staphylococcal and streptococcal bacteria species infect the cervical nodes, requiring treatment with appropriate antibiotics. The source of initial infection is often the adenotonsillar tissue of the Waldeyer ring; however, bacterial adenitis may appear without obvious initiating sources. Posterior cervical nodes may be enlarged as a result of scalp lesions, such as those associated with head lice or other cutaneous infections. The treatment is appropriate oral antibiotic therapy, with resolution expected in days to weeks.

Occasionally, lymphadenitis may become suppurative, particularly in infants and children. In children, a trial of intravenous antibiotics is often curative. If the suppuration becomes more superficial or fails to improve within 24 to 48 hours of antibiotic therapy, incision and drainage are appropriate. Rarely, suppurative adenitis involves one or more of the deep jugular lymph nodes; in these cases, patients are toxemic with fever and leukocytosis, and they exhibit diffuse erythema and swelling of the lateral neck with a brawny edema. Fluctuance is not present in most cases because of the deep location of the purulence. In adults, deep neck infections frequently result from dental pathology. CT scanning is of great benefit in diagnosing the extent of the deep neck abscess. In children, the CT scan can be misleading, indicating an abscess when there is only phlegmon. Because these nodes and resultant abscesses are within the carotid sheath, careful incision and drainage through a lateral neck incision are indicated. If these potentially dangerous, deep neck abscesses are not drained adequately, the infection may tract along tissue planes into the mediastinum, with a significant additional morbidity and risk of mortality.

Granulomatous Cervical Adenitis

Cat scratch fever is a bacterial granulomatous adenitis, often occurring after exposure to or a scratch from a cat or a dog. Usually, the lymph node on the ipsilateral side of the scratch becomes enlarged and tender. Initial systemic symptoms include low-grade fever, malaise, and myalgia. The adenopathy may resolve spontaneously over months, and management is usually supportive. Antibiotics for gram-negative infections may shorten the clinical course. If suppuration occurs, needle aspiration and, rarely, excision of the node or nodes are indicated.

Mycobacteria produce granulomatous adenitis, usually without systemic symptoms. The majority of mycobacterial cervical infections in adults are caused by *Mycobacterium tuberculosis*. Cases involving atypical organisms, most commonly *Mycobacterium avium-intracellulare*, occur more frequently in children and are more common than tuberculous cervical adenitis. Affected patients may have a weakly positive tuberculin skin test. They often present with a nontender fluctuant mass, usually around the parotid or submandibular glands. The overlying skin develops a violaceous hue, and, if left alone, the mass will often progress to rupture and drainage. These highly resistant organisms are best treated with surgical excision of the involved nodes. Antibiotic therapy is reserved for recurrent disease or for disease that can only be partially excised to prevent the development of a chronic draining fistula. Tuberculous cervical adenitis, historically known as "scrofula," is best treated with antibiotic therapy. Surgery is helpful in making the diagnosis if culture material is unobtainable through needle biopsy. Curiously, most patients exhibit no evidence of pulmonary tubercular infection.

Benign Cervical Cysts

Thyroglossal duct cysts occur as soft, painless, persistent midline neck masses (Figure 25-20). Physical examination shows that the cyst elevates on swallowing or on protruding the tongue; this occurs because the cyst or tract is tethered to the hyoid bone. The thyroid develops embryologically at the tuberculum impar at the base of the tongue and descends through the neck to its final location, creating a thyroglossal tract of tissue. Thyroglossal duct cysts are caused by failure of this cyst to obliterate. Excision is usually performed because these cysts may enlarge, become infected, or undergo malignant degeneration. Before the cyst is excised, the normal position and function of the thyroid gland should be carefully documented. On

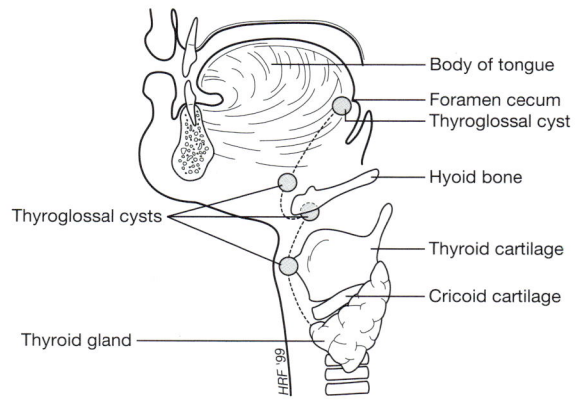

Figure 25-20. **Localization of thyroglossal duct cysts.** (From Lawrence PF. *Essentials of Surgical Specialties.* 3rd ed. Lippincott Williams & Wilkins; 2007.)

rare occasions, the cyst may contain the only functioning thyroid tissue.

Branchial cleft anomalies arise from a failure of the embryologic cervical sinus of His to obliterate during fetal development. Branchial anomalies can involve the first through fourth arches but most commonly involve the second branchial arch. They usually present as persistent, painless (unless infected) cysts just anterior to the middle third of the sternocleidomastoid muscle. They may also be seen as sinuses or fistulae. These cysts may occur in a patient of any age; however, fistulae and sinuses usually occur during infancy, and cysts commonly occur during the second and third decades of life. A second branchial arch anomaly classically courses superiorly between the internal and external carotid arteries, superior to the hypoglossal nerve. The tract of the second branchial cleft begins in the central cleft of the pharyngeal tonsil and courses above the hypoglossal nerve between the internal and external carotid arteries, and out to the skin of the lower third of the neck, anterior to the sternocleidomastoid muscle. These masses or tracts are subject to recurrent infection, usually in conjunction with an upper respiratory tract infection. Surgical excision of the cyst, the fistula tract, or both is recommended during a quiescent period. See Table 25-11 for a comparison of thyroglossal duct cysts and branchial cleft cysts.

Dermoid cysts, like thyroglossal duct cysts, are soft, painless, persistent midline neck masses occurring during the first or second decade of life. Unlike thyroglossal duct cysts, however, they do not elevate with swallowing because they are not attached to the hyoid bone, and they are often found superficial to the strap musculature. Pathophysiologically, they are developmental anomalies involving pluripotent embryonal cells that become isolated and subsequently undergo disorganized growth. They are composed of ectoderm and mesoderm and often contain hair follicles, sweat glands, and sebaceous glands. The treatment of choice is complete surgical excision.

Lymphangioma and Hemangioma

Lymphangioma and hemangioma are pathologically similar; **hemangiomas** contain blood-filled channels, and **lymphangiomas** contain lymph-filled channels. These lesions are classified as capillary, cavernous, or mixed.

TABLE 25-11. Thyroglossal Duct Anomalies Versus Branchial Cleft Anomalies

	Thyroglossal Duct Anomalies	Branchial Cleft Anomalies
Presentation	Cysts/sinuses/fistulae	Cysts/sinuses/fistulae/cartilaginous rests
Age	Most present in childhood or in early adult life	Commonly present in young adults
Histology	Usually lined by stratified squamous epithelium or pseudostratified columnar epithelium with mucus-secreting glands	Lined by squamous or columnar epithelium and often have lymphoid tissue
Anatomic location	Almost always in the midline, from the tongue base to the thyroid isthmus; when adjacent to the thyroid cartilage, may lie slightly to one side of the midline	Lateral along the anterior border of the sternocleidomastoid, anywhere from the angle of the mandible to the clavicle
Physical	Cyst moves upward not only on swallowing but also on protrusion of the tongue because it is attached by the tract remnant to the foramen cecum.	Not so
Clinical	Cyst does not have a sinus opening to the skin unless infection has resulted in spontaneous drainage or an incomplete excision or incision and drainage procedure has previously been performed.	Sinuses present as cutaneous openings marked by skin tags or subcutaneous cartilaginous remnants.
	Discharges mucus	Nonpurulent drainage (before infection) cysts contain a yellow fluid, which on microscopy is rich in cholesterol, hence they do not transilluminate.
Origin	Thyroglossal fistula is never congenital; it follows infection or inadequate removal of a thyroglossal cyst.	Congenital
	Characteristically, the cutaneous opening of a thyroglossal fistula is drawn upward on protrusion of the tongue.	Not so
Risk	Infection	Infection
	Malignant potential of the dysgenetic thyroid tissue	
Treatment	Sistrunk operation	McFee step-ladder technique
Differential diagnosis	Dermoid inclusion cyst	Pathologic lymph nodes
	Pathologic lymph nodes	
	Cervical thymic cysts	
	Bronchogenic cysts	
	Ectopic thyroid tissue	

Table courtesy of Mohammed I. Ahmed, MBBS, MS (Surgery).

Cystic hygromas are soft, painless, often very large multiloculated masses that are usually evident at birth or occur during the first year or two of life. These masses are cavernous lymphatic malformations that can occur anywhere in the body but are most common in the posterior triangle of the neck. They often enlarge during upper respiratory tract infections. When allowed to enlarge massively, they may compress the larynx, the trachea, or the esophagus. These masses are unencapsulated arcades of disorganized, thinly lined, fluid-filled spaces that often surround vital nerves and blood vessels, making excision difficult. Before the lesions are excised, MRI scanning should be performed to delineate their extent and to rule out thoracic involvement. Complete surgical excision, although desirable, should not sacrifice important neurovascular structures. With large hygromas, multiple excisions are likely to be necessary over the course of the first several years of life.

Congenital hemangiomas, usually easily diagnosed, are developmental abnormalities present at birth. They appear as bluish masses in the oral cavity, the pharynx, the parotid gland, or the neck, and they generally increase in size when the infant cries or strains. Because most hemangiomas regress spontaneously by the time the patient reaches the age of 5 years, a conservative approach is warranted. Laser surgery or excision may be beneficial when hemangiomas do not resolve. Steroids have also been used with varying degrees of success. Cutaneous hemangiomas of the head and neck are sometimes associated with hemangiomas of the airway, particularly of the subglottis. This diagnosis should always be considered in an infant with breathing difficulties and known facial hemangioma. Subglottic hemangioma can often be treated with a carbon dioxide laser or medical therapy in the form of β-blockers.

Other Benign Neoplasms

Typically, benign neoplasms are slow growing, nontender neck masses that are often present for a number of years. Lipomas are common asymptomatic mobile soft masses located in the subcutaneous tissues or the deeper spaces of the neck; they are usually quite characteristic on physical examination and may occasionally arise intramuscularly. Lesions that enlarge or that are troublesome to the patient are excised. Neurogenic tumors consist primarily of schwannomas and neurofibromas. They arise from the peripheral nerve sheath of cranial nerves (eg, the vagus or glossopharyngeal nerve) or from the cervical sympathetic chain. They usually occur as solitary lesions in the neck. Of the two neurogenic tumors, schwannomas are the more clinically benign. Because the individual nerve axons drape around the tumor, nerve-sparing excision should always be attempted. Neurofibromas are more difficult to treat because nerve fibers pass through the tumor rather than around it. Removing the tumor thus requires sacrificing the involved nerve. Patients with multiple neurofibromas should be suspected of having neurofibromatosis (von Recklinghausen disease).

Malignant Tumors

Malignant lymphomas are the most common neoplastic neck mass among children and young adults, accounting for more than 50% of cases. The masses may be bilateral, are usually nontender, and solid without significant central necrosis. Other signs and symptoms of lymphoma include hepatosplenomegaly, abnormal chest radiograph with hilar adenopathy, and weight loss. Lymphomas are classified as Hodgkin or non-Hodgkin. The nodular sclerosing histologic type of Hodgkin disease is the most common and is often localized to the cervical and upper mediastinal lymph nodes. Pathologic confirmation is mandatory, and this is usually the only role played by surgery in treating this condition. Treatment generally consists of chemotherapy, irradiation, or both.

Rhabdomyosarcoma, usually the embryonal form, is the most common solid primary tumor of the neck in children. This lesion was once considered universally fatal, but the combined treatment of surgery, radiation, and chemotherapy has significantly improved survival rates.

Squamous cell carcinoma is the type of cancer that most commonly metastasizes to the neck; the primary site is usually in the upper aerodigestive tract. The mucosa of the upper aerodigestive tract should be carefully examined during a search for the primary tumor site. A chest radiograph should be obtained to check for lung metastasis and rule out the lung as a primary tumor site, particularly for supraclavicular masses. A CT scan or MRI can help determine the extent of large masses and their relation to the base of the skull, the prevertebral fasciae, and the carotid artery. Recently, positron emission tomography (PET) scanning has become popular for evaluating tumor extent and metastasis and even for identifying unknown primary site locations. PET scanning utilizes a radiolabeled glucose molecule that is injected into the patient. The glucose is "taken up" by rapidly dividing cells (either due to inflammation or malignancy), therefore concentrating the radioisotope so that it can be identified on scanning. Fine needle aspiration can often be used as part of the early evaluation to confirm the cytologic features. Treatment for the primary tumor site generally consists of irradiation, surgery, or both, depending on the site and size; neck dissection is performed to remove the nodal contents of the anterior and posterior triangles of the ipsilateral neck. For 5% to 10% of patients with metastatic squamous cell cancer of the neck, no primary tumor can be identified by examination or endoscopy. Treatment for these patients consists of modified radical neck dissection with possible irradiation treatment of the most likely primary tumor site. For 30% of these patients, the primary tumor will manifest itself within 2 years, making regular surveillance imperative.

Cancer metastatic to the neck from more distant sites—such as the lungs, kidneys, or gut—is usually treated with radiotherapy or chemotherapy. Melanoma metastatic to the neck will usually require neck dissection. Adjuvant postoperative radiotherapy for cervical melanoma metastasis may also be beneficial although potentially less so than in other head and neck malignancies. Metastatic thyroid cancer may first be seen as a nodal metastasis. See Chapter 18 for a discussion of thyroid malignancy.

The Surgical Airway

The indications for a surgical airway are listed in Table 25-12. In most instances, a tracheotomy is performed in a controlled setting as a planned procedure.

Cricothyrotomy

In cases of acute airway obstruction, when attempted orotracheal intubation fails, the fastest, safest surgical airway is a **cricothyrotomy**. The technique involves making a vertical skin incision directly over the cricothyroid membrane. The cricothyroid membrane is incised horizontally, opening the airway to allow the insertion of an available endotracheal tube. In young children, this is not possible, and the airway is best entered between the cricoid and the first tracheal ring (see Figure 25-14). Because there is a higher incidence of subglottic stenosis associated with cricothyrotomy, prompt conversion to a tracheostomy is prudent if the airway is needed longer than a few days.

Tracheotomy

Tracheotomy is the act of cutting the trachea to create an airway that bypasses the upper aerodigestive tract and assists with ventilation and pulmonary hygiene. The hole, or stoma, connecting the trachea to the skin is known as a "tracheostomy." After the tracheostomy is created, an

TABLE 25-12. Indications for Tracheotomy
Bypass upper airway obstruction.
Expect prolonged ventilatory dependence (usually over 2 wk).
Allow direct access for irrigation and suctioning of the airway (pulmonary toilet).
Prevent chronic aspiration.
Reduce the dead space to overcome in patients with poor ventilatory effort or central nervous system depression.

appropriately sized tracheostomy tube is inserted. In the patient with a tracheostomy tube, the nasal functions of warming and humidifying air are bypassed. Humidified air and frequent suctioning are important, especially in the early postoperative period, to keep the secretions from drying and creating mucous plugs in the airway. Potential early complications of tracheostomy are bleeding, pneumothorax, accidental decannulation, false passage into the mediastinum, and cardiac arrest. Late complications include peristomal or tracheal granulation tissue formation with bleeding and airway obstruction, persistent tracheocutaneous fistula following decannulation, tracheal stenosis, tracheoinnominate fistula, and tracheoesophageal fistula.

SUGGESTED READINGS

Baugh RF, Basura GJ, Ishii LE, et al. Clinical practice guideline: Bell's palsy executive summary. *Otolaryngol Head Neck Surg.* 2013;149(5):656-663.

Rackley T, Palaniappan N, Owens D, Evans M. Adjuvant treatment decisions for oropharyngeal cancer—is it time for a change? *Clin Otolaryngol.* 2014;39(5):316-321.

Rosenfeld RM, Piccirillo JF, Chandrasekhar SS, et al. Clinical practice guideline (update): adult sinusitis executive summary. *Otolaryngol Head Neck Surg.* 2015;152(4):598-609.

Rosenfeld RM, Shin JJ, Schwartz SR, et al. Clinical practice guideline: otitis media with effusion (update). *Otolaryngol Head Neck Surg.* 2016;154(1 Suppl):S1-S41.

SAMPLE QUESTIONS

QUESTIONS

Choose the best answer for each question.

1. A 71-year-old man describes acute onset of the room spinning as he rolled over to awaken this morning. The symptoms lasted a few minutes and then dissipated with rest. He describes a similar episode when he looked up to grab something off of the shelf before coming into the ED. He denies any headaches, weakness, fevers, or recent viral illness. This happened once before 10 years ago and got better on its own. Aside from clinical history, what is the next best step to secure the diagnosis?

   A. MRI of the brain with contrast
   B. Romberg test
   C. Visual acuity test
   D. Dix-Hallpike maneuver
   E. CT of the head with contrast

2. A 55-year-old man presents with right complete facial paralysis that started 2 days ago. He describes right-sided ear pain that progressed to gradual and now complete immobility of his right face. He denies any headaches, visual changes, or peripheral weakness. This has never happened before. What is the best treatment for this patient and when should it be implemented?

   A. Oral steroids, within 2 weeks of symptom onset
   B. Oral steroids, within 72 hours of symptom onset
   C. Oral steroids with an antiviral, within 72 hours of symptom onset
   D. Oral steroids with an antiviral, within 2 weeks of symptom onset
   E. Antiviral alone, within 72 hours of symptoms onset

3. A 30-year-old man presents with several months of right ear malodorous drainage and some muffled hearing. He denies fevers, headaches, or facial weakness. He reports having a lot of ear infections as a child. Examination of his right ear demonstrates a white cheesy material on the tympanic membrane with some adjacent pink fleshy tissue. What is the next best step in the diagnosis of this patient's condition?

   A. CT of the temporal bone without contrast
   B. CT of the temporal bone with contrast
   C. MRI of the internal auditory canals with contrast
   D. MRI of the internal auditory canals without contrast
   E. Audiogram

4. A 5-year-old child presents with muffled hearing for 1 month. He is otherwise healthy and developing normally. Communication skills are not impaired. Examination shows bilateral middle ear effusions. What is the next best step in managing this patient?

   A. Myringotomy
   B. Myringotomy with tympanostomy tube placement
   C. Antibiotics
   D. Observation
   E. CT of the temporal bones

5. A 13-year-old boy has presented to the ED a few times over the last 3 months with nosebleeds. He denies any trauma but says they happen spontaneously and always come from the left side. He denies any fevers, headaches, or weight loss. He says his sense of smell is normal, but he does have some difficulty breathing through his left nostril sometimes. What is the next best step in the workup of this patient's problem?

   A. CT of the sinus with contrast
   B. CT of the sinus without contrast
   C. Angiogram
   D. Incisional biopsy
   E. Nasal endoscopy

ANSWERS AND EXPLANATIONS

1. **Answer: D**

   The Dix-Hallpike maneuver begins with the patient sitting upright. The head is turned 45° to one side and the patient is then placed supine rapidly with the head slightly extended and the ear toward which the patient is turned facing down. The patient is observed for nystagmus for 30 seconds, then brought back upright and observed for another 30 seconds. When paroxysmal vertigo and nystagmus are resulting from posterior canal dysfunction (most common), one would observe downbeating nystagmus that fatigues with time. A brain MRI or head CT would be indicated if the patient's symptoms are more intractable and suggest a central origin or if the patient has signs suggestive of a possible stroke or mass lesion. The Romberg test is a test of balance resulting from proprioception, vestibular function, and vision. It can be impaired in vitamin deficiencies and peripheral neuropathies. Visual acuity tests would not help narrow the diagnosis. For more information on this answer, please see section "Vestibular Pathology."

2. **Answer: B**

This patient has an apparent right-sided Bell palsy. Oral steroids should be initiated as soon as possible, preferably within 72 hours of symptom onset. Two weeks would be too long to wait. Clinical practice guidelines no longer recommend an antiviral. For more information on this answer, please see section "Diseases of the Facial Nerve."

3. **Answer: A**

This patient has a right ear cholesteatoma. Definitive diagnosis occurs with excision, but before that, one would need a CT of the temporal bone without contrast to best characterize the lesion and the extent to which it has involved the middle ear and temporal bone. CT of the temporal bone is performed with contrast if the patient demonstrates signs of complicated otomastoiditis, such as swelling over the mastoid, malaise and altered mental status,

or meningismus. MRI of the internal auditory canals is best for ruling out a lesion in the cerebellopontine angle such as a vestibular schwannoma. Audiogram will be necessary before any surgical intervention, but it is not the next best step. For more information on this answer, please see section "Cholesteatoma."

4. **Answer: D**

This is a child not at risk for communication or developmental delay who has had OME for at least 1 month. Nearly 90% of children will have resolution of their OME by 3 months. As such, it is prudent to continue observation in this child. Myringotomy with or without tympanostomy tube would be indicated if the child had hearing loss and was at risk for communication and developmental delay, such as a child with Down syndrome. Antibiotics are not indicated as OME is defined by a lack of infection. Imaging at this stage is not warranted. For more information on this answer, please see section "Otitis Media."

5. **Answer: E**

This patient is demonstrating a classic case of juvenile nasopharyngeal angiofibroma, which typically occurs in adolescent boys. Although imaging plays an important part in the diagnosis and treatment planning for these patients, there is no substitute for taking a look in the nose via nasal endoscopy and seeing the lesion directly. Additionally, nasal endoscopy does not require any radiation and can be performed easily at bedside. Angiogram would be performed preoperatively because these lesions are routinely embolized before surgery. Incisional biopsy would not be advised because this can lead to severe hemorrhage. For more information on this answer, please see section "Epistaxis."

26

Orthopedic Surgery: Diseases of the Musculoskeletal System

John J. Murnaghan

The musculoskeletal system is composed of connective tissue of mesodermal origin. Bones, joints, muscles, tendons, ligaments, and aponeurotic fascia constitute 70% of total body mass. Although disorders of the musculoskeletal system do not usually affect longevity, they frequently interfere with the quality of life and consume a significant portion of U.S. health care resources. Musculoskeletal problems are the second most frequent cause of visits to a physician and are second in the consumption of health care dollars. Forty percent of emergency department visits are related to musculoskeletal problems. It is estimated that **osteoporosis** affects more than 20 million postmenopausal women and that associated hip fractures occupy almost 20% of surgical hospital beds. Back pain is the most common cause of time lost from work and disability in patients younger than 45 years. The annual cost of treatment and compensation for back conditions is greater than $14 billion. These statistics make it clear that a working understanding of the musculoskeletal system is necessary for all physicians, especially those who practice primary care.

TRAUMA

FRACTURES (BONES), SUBLUXATIONS, AND DISLOCATIONS (JOINTS)

A fracture is a break or loss of structural continuity in a bone. In a subluxation of the acromioclavicular joint, the normally **apposing** joint surfaces are partially out of contact (Figure 26-1A). In a dislocation of the acromioclavicular joint, those surfaces are completely out of contact (see Figure 26-1B). Joint subluxation may be a transient phenomenon in which the joint surfaces approach dislocation but reduce spontaneously.

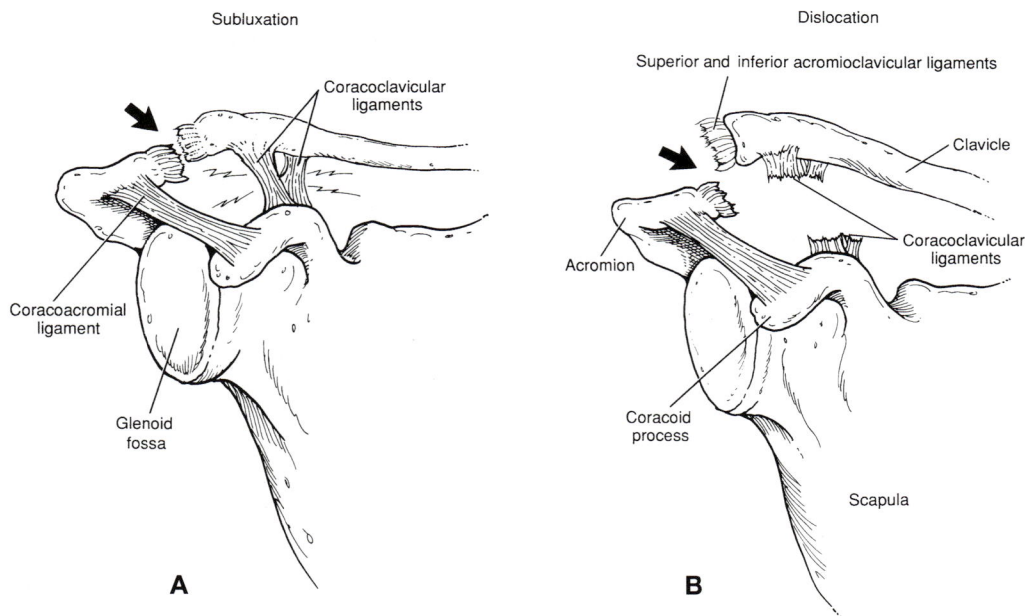

Figure 26-1. A. Subluxation is a partial displacement of opposing joint surfaces. This phenomenon may be transient and reduce itself. B. Dislocation is complete displacement of opposing joint surfaces. A reduction maneuver is often needed to restore joint alignment. (Modified with permission from Rockwood C, Green D. *Fractures in Adults*. 3rd ed. JB Lippincott; 1982:1193.)

Fractures

Description

Knowledge of the accepted fracture nomenclature allows for communication between medical colleagues and may affect decision-making. It is essential to describe fractures in a precise and detailed manner. Fractures are described according to the type, site, pattern, amount of displacement, and angulation. In children, injuries can affect the growth plate and are described according to the **Salter-Harris classification**.

Type

Fractures are either **open** or **closed**. A fracture is open when there is a break in the surrounding skin or mucosa that allows the fracture to communicate with the external environment. Although most open fractures are obvious to cursory inspection, others, such as pelvic fractures, may communicate with the rectum or vagina and are discovered only in the course of a thorough physical examination. All open fractures are, by definition, contaminated and require emergency treatment to prevent infection. A fracture is closed when the skin or overlying mucosa is intact.

Fractures are usually the result of a single forceful impact. However, repeated submaximal stress can produce microscopic fractures, which, if not allowed to heal, will coalesce into a **stress fracture**. Stress fractures are frequently seen in army recruits or in insufficiently conditioned patients who participate in vigorous athletic training routines. A fracture produced by minimal trauma through abnormal bone is termed a **pathologic fracture**. Pathologic fractures occur in bone that is weakened by metabolic bone diseases (eg, osteoporosis) or in bone weakened by primary or metastatic tumors.

Site

When describing the location of a fracture, the bone affected is identified, as well as the specific site involved, such as the proximal or distal **epiphysis, metaphysis,** or **diaphysis** (Figure 26-2). A fracture in the epiphyseal region suggests intra-articular fracture extension that would violate the joint surface and could result in traumatic arthritis. By convention, the diaphysis of a long bone is described in thirds: proximal, middle, or distal (Figure 26-2). Fracture location has implications for healing and treatment. Fractures of metaphyseal or cancellous (spongy) bone with a rich blood supply and high bone turnover rates usually heal quite rapidly. In contrast, the cortical, diaphyseal bone heals more slowly. Diaphyseal fractures, therefore, require lengthier periods of stress protection by immobilization or protection from weight bearing.

Pattern

The fracture pattern suggests the type and amount of kinetic energy imparted to the bone. A transverse fracture (Figure 26-3A) is a low-energy injury, usually the result of either a direct blow to a long bone or a ligament avulsion. A "nightstick" fracture is a transverse fracture of the ulna that occurs when the forearm receives a direct blow. Stress and pathologic fractures usually have a transverse pattern. Spiral or oblique fractures (see Figure 26-3B and C) result from a rotatory, twisting injury. These fractures have a tendency to displace and shorten after reduction and immobilization. A fracture with more than two fragments is

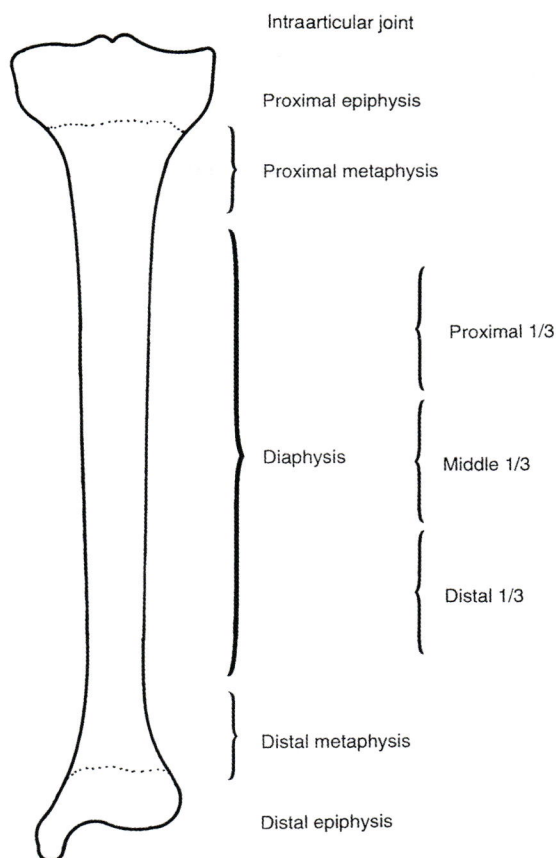

Figure 26-2. Anatomic regions of a long tubular bone. (From Lawrence PF. *Essentials of Surgical Specialties*. 3rd ed. Lippincott Williams & Wilkins; 2007.)

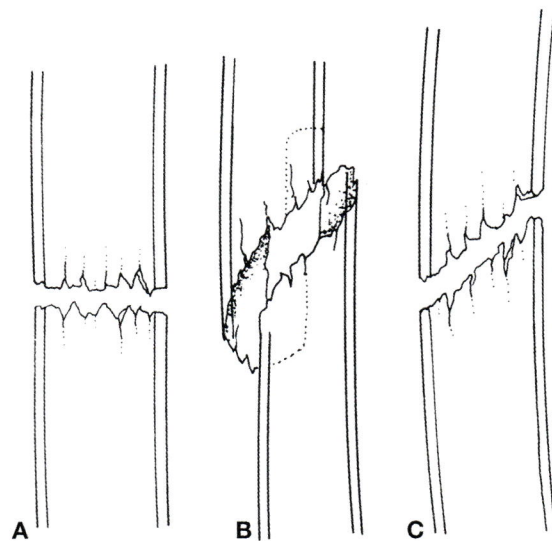

Figure 26-3. Common fracture patterns. A. Transverse fracture. B. Spiral fracture. C. Oblique fracture. (From Lawrence PF. *Essentials of Surgical Specialties*. 3rd ed. Lippincott Williams & Wilkins; 2007.)

termed *comminuted or multifragmented*. The middle fragment may be triangular and is called a butterfly fragment (Figure 26-4A); when cylindrical in configuration, it is described as segmental (Figure 26-4B). Comminuted fractures occur as a result of larger forces and imply greater degrees of damage to the intramedullary blood supply to the bone and surrounding soft tissues, which may compromise the healing of one or both fracture sites. An impacted fracture (Figure 26-5A; also see Figure 26-15) is commonly seen in the metaphyseal bone, such as with femoral neck, distal radius, or tibial plateau fractures. These are low-energy injuries in which two bone fragments are jammed together. A compression fracture signifies that the trabecular or cancellous bone is crushed; it often occurs in vertebral bodies (Figure 26-5B). Although most bone fractures are complete, an incomplete buckling of only one cortex is seen in children and is known as a greenstick fracture (Figure 26-6).

Displacement

Fractured bone fragments may be displaced by the force of an injury, gravity, or muscle pull. Displacement is described in terms of distance or bone diameters in the anterior-posterior (AP), mediolateral, and length (either shortening or distraction).

Displacement is measured in both the mediolateral (coronal) and AP (sagittal) planes. The position of the distal fragment is always named relative to the proximal fragment. This naming convention is helpful, because

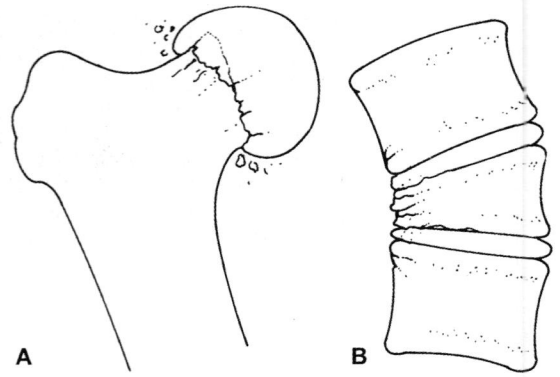

Figure 26-5. A. Impacted femoral neck fracture. B. Anterior compression fracture of the vertebral body. (From Lawrence PF. *Essentials of Surgical Specialties*. 3rd ed. Lippincott Williams & Wilkins; 2007.)

most fractures are aligned by reducing the displaced distal fragment to the proximal one. Fracture displacement is customarily quantified as a percentage (Figure 26-7). This description can be misleading because 50% posterior (Figure 26-7B) and 50% lateral displacement (Figure 26-7A) may, when viewed in three dimensions, represent only 25% bone apposition (Figure 26-7C). Angulation is the relationship between the long axis of the distal fragment to the long axis of the proximal fragment. It may be described by one of two conventions. In the first convention, the direction to which the distal fragment is inclined is identified (Figure 26-8). In the second convention, the location of the fracture angle apex is described. Reference to either the distal fragment or apical angulation should be mentioned in reports of fracture alignment. For example, in Figure 26-8, the distal fragment is inclined in the posterior and lateral directions, or the fracture apex is angled anteromedially.

The terms **varus** and **valgus** are also used in the descriptions of fractures and limb deformity. These terms refer to the direction of an angular deformity in relation to the midline of the body. If the deformity apex is pointed away from the midline (Figure 26-9A), the term varus is used. If the deformity apex is directed toward the midline (Figure 26-9B), it is called valgus. Thus, bowlegs in which the deformity apex at the knee (genu) is away from the midline are called **genu varum,** whereas knock-knees are called **genu valgum.**

Fracture apposition, angulation, and shortening are quantified in percentage, degrees, and centimeters, respectively, from radiographs. Rotation describes angular shifts around the long axis of the bone. It is best judged clinically. Rotational deformity is expressed by identifying the position of the distal fragment as it relates to the proximal one. For example, if the foot is twisted outward, the fracture is externally rotated.

The Salter-Harris Classification of Growth Plate Fractures

In children, the growth plate (physis) is the growing zone of cartilage situated between the epiphysis and the metaphysis of long bones. Cartilage is weaker than bone; thus, it is a common site of injury. The Salter-Harris classification of

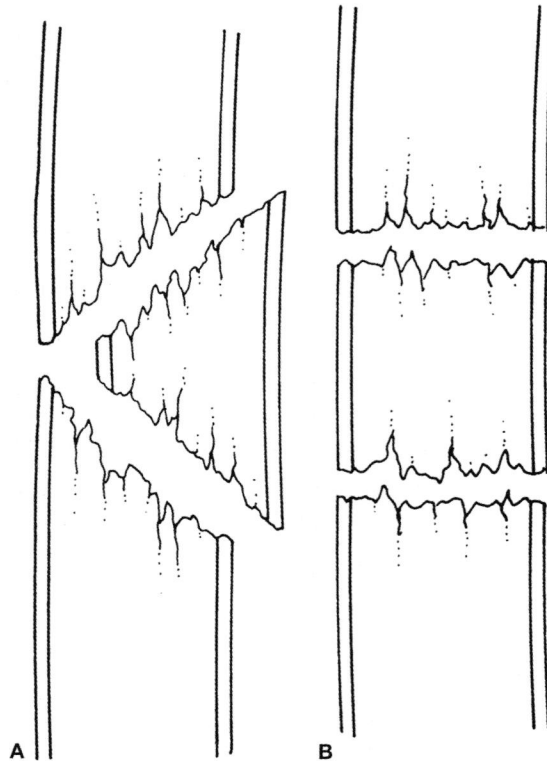

Figure 26-4. Comminuted fractures. A. Triangular butterfly fragment. B. Cylindrical segmental fracture. (From Lawrence PF. *Essentials of Surgical Specialties*. 3rd ed. Lippincott Williams & Wilkins; 2007.)

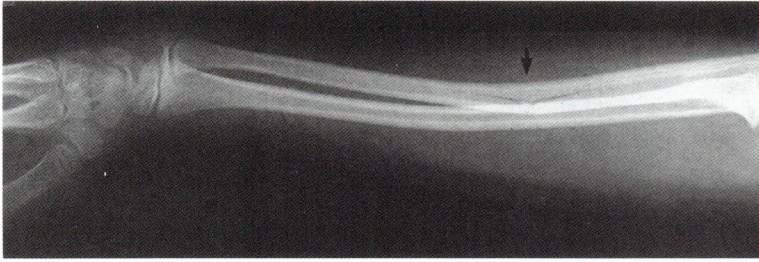

Figure 26-6. Greenstick fracture of the ulna in which only one cortex is broken (arrow) and the bone is bowed with its apex anterior. The fracture must be completed (the other cortex broken) to prevent angular deformity. Greenstick fractures typically occur in children whose bones are more plastic and less brittle than those of adults. (From Lawrence PF. *Essentials of Surgical Specialties*. 3rd ed. Lippincott Williams & Wilkins; 2007.)

growth plate injuries is descriptive, is generally recognized, and has important prognostic implications (Figure 26-10).

The Salter-Harris type I fracture is a separation of the epiphysis from the metaphysis (Figure 26-10). If the periosteum is not torn, the fracture remains undisplaced. In this injury, there is tenderness over the growth plate. The Salter-Harris type II fracture passes through the growth plate and exits through the metaphysis. This fracture is due to a bending movement that tears the periosteum on the side opposite the triangular metaphyseal fragment. In a Salter-Harris type III injury, the fracture extends from the growth plate through the epiphysis to enter the joint. This fracture is intra-articular and requires a perfect reduction to avoid arthritic sequelae. The Salter-Harris type IV fracture line extends from the metaphysis through the growth plate cartilage into the epiphysis. This fracture pattern is also intra-articular. These fractures must be operatively fixed to prevent nonunion and joint surface incongruity. The Salter-Harris types III and IV fractures have the highest incidence of growth disturbance if not properly managed. A Salter-Harris type V fracture involves a crushing of the epiphyseal growth plate. These injuries may not be apparent on radiographs and are, therefore, difficult to identify prospectively. The type V injury causes a bony bar to replace the injured section of the growth plate, which will result in asymmetrical, angular growth.

Growth plate injuries, no matter how trivial, have the potential to cause growth disturbance of the involved long bone. The larger Salter-Harris numbers represent greater degrees of injury to the growth plate. Consequently, the type IV fracture has a poorer prognosis and higher incidence of growth disturbance than the type I injury. The possibility of a growth disturbance requires that all growth plate fractures be followed radiographically for at least 1 year after injury.

Evaluation of Patients With Musculoskeletal Trauma

The patient usually has a history of injury, although, in pathologic fractures, the injury may be minimal. In children, either a limp or the refusal to use an extremity suggests a possible fracture. Symptoms of musculoskeletal injury include pain, swelling, and deformity. Bony tenderness, crepitus, or deformity strongly suggests a fracture. The examiner should inspect the extremity circumferentially for small puncture wounds. Vascular integrity (pulses, capillary return) and neurologic status (sensory, motor, and reflex functions) must be assessed and documented. Active motion of articulations distal to the fracture site implies an element of soft tissue integrity and neurologic function. The two most important clinical features of the fracture (whether it is open and whether the neurovascular status is compromised) are determined by clinical examination before x-ray films are obtained.

A complete radiologic evaluation includes the following:

1. Two views of the affected bone or joint at right angles to each other must be taken. Because fractures occur in three dimensions, a single radiographic view will not permit an accurate description (ie, displacement and angulation) of the injury (see Figure 26-7). Two views taken perpendicular to each other, usually an AP and a lateral view, meet these requirements.

2. The joint above and the joint below the injured area must be visualized. It is not uncommon for a knee injury or hip fracture to be associated with a fracture of the femoral shaft.

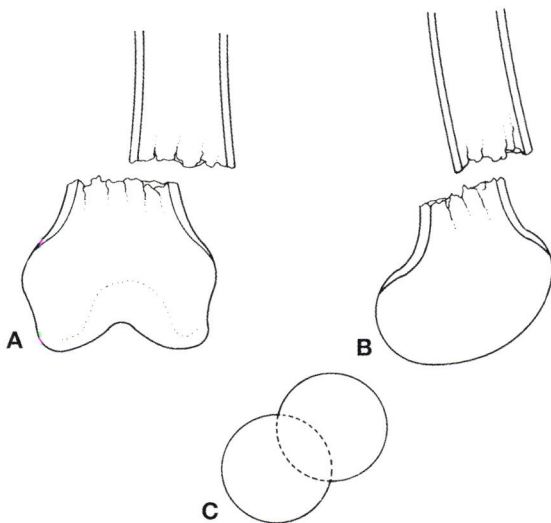

Figure 26-7. Fracture displacement. A. The anteroposterior view shows approximately 50% lateral displacement of the distal fragment. B. The lateral view shows 50% posterior displacement of the distal femur. C. Additively in three dimensions, the amount of bone apposition is approximately 25%, an amount that is underestimated by either view (A or B) in isolation. (From Lawrence PF. *Essentials of Surgical Specialties*. 3rd ed. Lippincott Williams & Wilkins; 2007.)

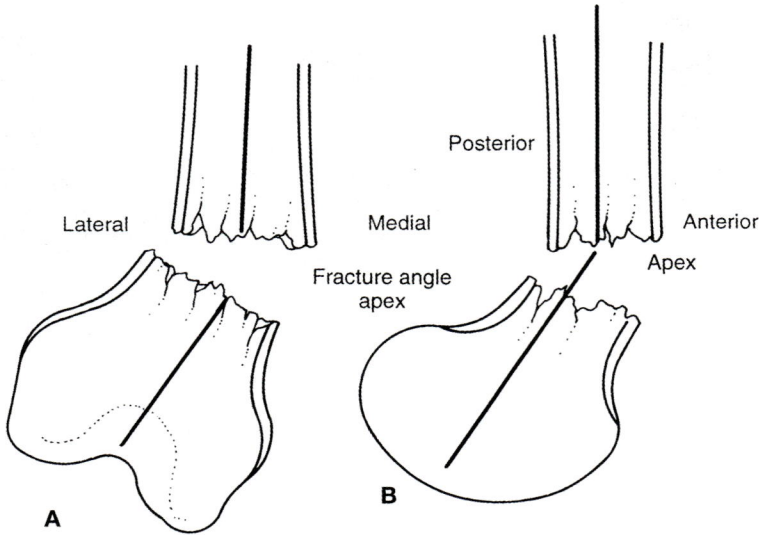

Figure 26-8. A. On the anteroposterior view (coronal plane), the distal fragment is angulated laterally, and the fracture angle apex is medial. B. On the lateral view (sagittal plane), the distal fragment is angulated posteriorly, and the angle apex is anterior. (From Lawrence PF. *Essentials of Surgical Specialties*. 3rd ed. Lippincott Williams & Wilkins; 2007.)

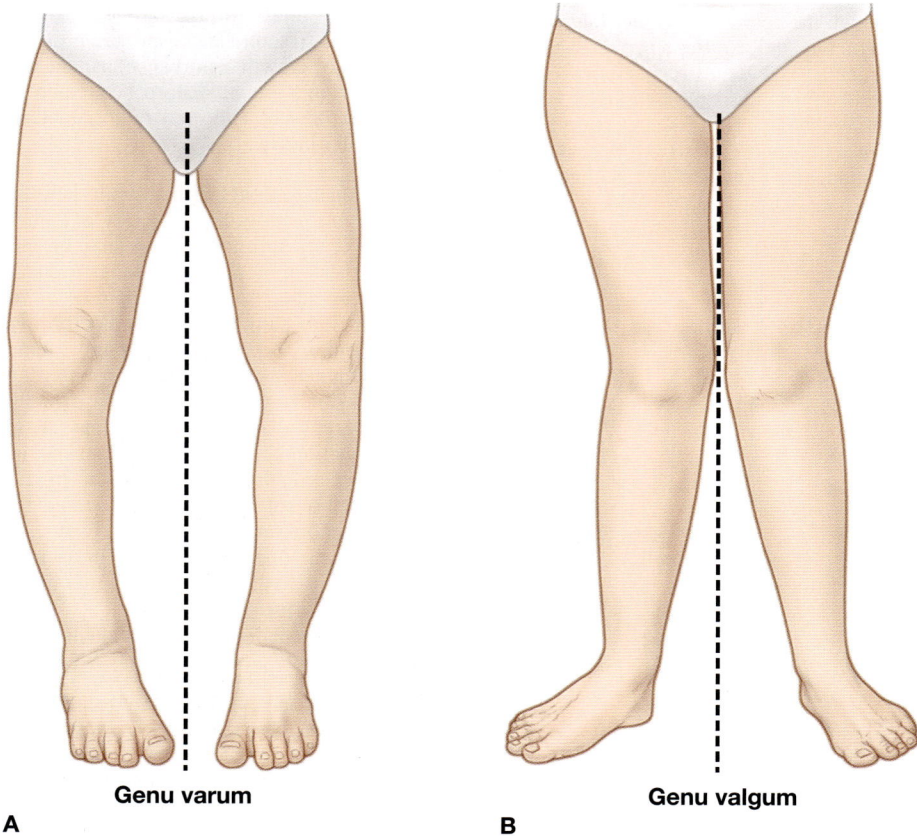

Figure 26-9. **The terms *varus* and *valgus* refer to the relation of a deformity to the midline of the body.** A. Genu varum, or bow-legs, occurs when the deformity apex is pointing away from the midline. B. Genu valgum, or knock-knees, occurs when the deformity apex is directed toward the midline; it is called valgus. In knock-knees, the knee resembles the letter L, which is a helpful mnemonic in distinguishing between these confusing terms.

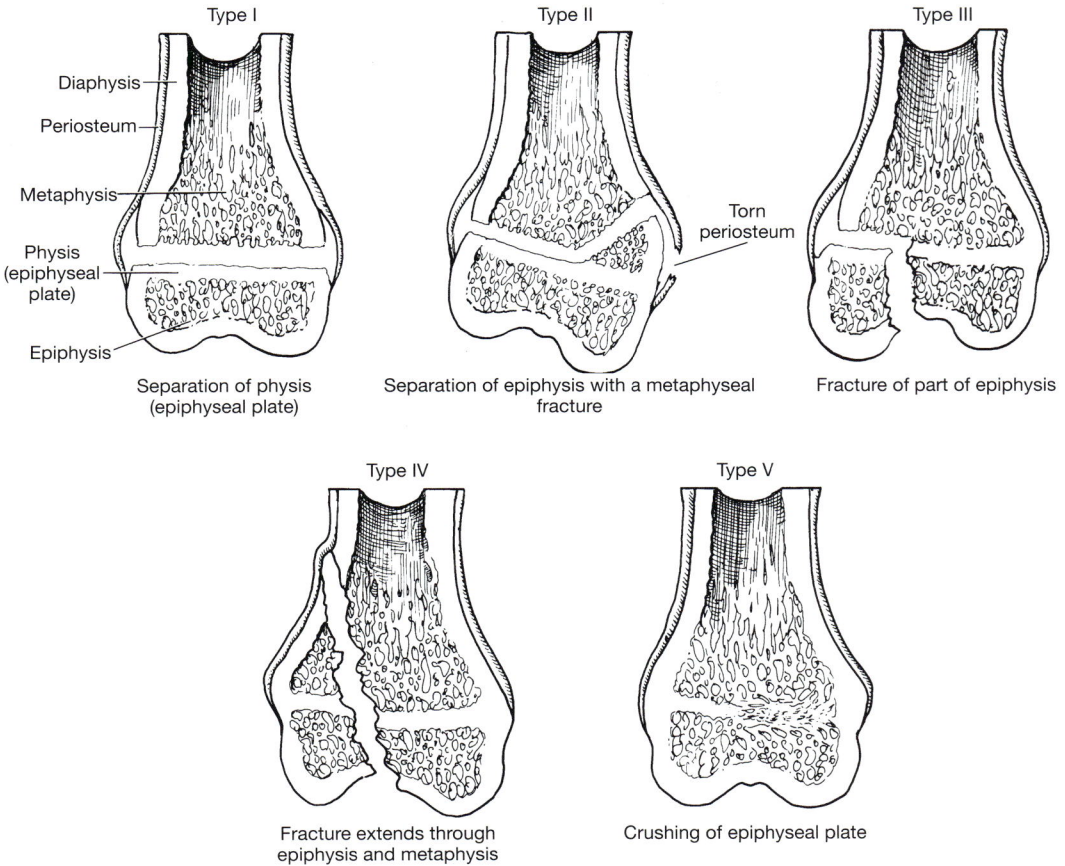

Figure 26-10. Salter-Harris classification of pediatric growth plate fractures. The greater the classification number, the more violent the injury to the epiphyseal plate and the greater the risk for long bone growth and healing problems. (Reprinted with permission from Rang MC. *Children's Fractures*. 2nd ed. JB Lippincott; 1983.)

3. Known injury associations warrant special radiographic examination. Cervical spine radiographs are mandatory in all patients with facial and head injuries; hip dislocations are associated with high-energy injuries to the knee. Fractures of the axial skeleton (spine and pelvis) occur with injuries to the thoracic, abdominal, or pelvic viscera, as well as neural structures.

4. If a fracture is not evident radiographically but is suspected clinically (eg, scaphoid fracture), the patient will not be harmed if the extremity is immobilized and reassessed. Repeated radiographs, stress views, or other imaging techniques—such as bone scan, computed tomography (CT), or magnetic resonance imaging (MRI)—may be needed to establish the diagnosis.

Although rare, patients with trauma with long bone fractures are prone to fat embolism. Clinical examination should watch for petechiae in conjunction with alteration of mental status. Patients are often dyspneic and have low oxygen saturation. Chest x-ray films reveal diffuse opacification without focal findings. Fat embolism syndrome is a clinical diagnosis because there is no specific laboratory finding. Treatment is supportive and, in severe cases, may require intubation and positive pressure ventilation with up to 100% O_2.

Principles of Fracture Management

A patient with a fracture should be initially managed as a patient with trauma (see Chapter 7) with life-threatening conditions treated first. All musculoskeletal injuries must be splinted in the field, and splints should remain in place whenever the patient is transported. Splinting prevents fracture motion, thus minimizing further damage to the surrounding soft tissues (nerves, blood vessels, and muscle; see Figure 26-16); limits blood loss; and decreases the pain of injury. Proper splinting requires that the joint above and the one below the fracture site be immobilized. Similarly, with a dislocation, the bone above and the bone below the joint should be splinted. It is essential to check the integrity of neural and vascular structures distal to any fracture site. Repeat evaluation of these clinical examination findings should be performed after any reduction or manipulation of the fractured extremity.

All open fractures are considered contaminated with bacteria, and treatment is aimed at preventing subsequent infection. The wound is examined once, covered with a sterile dressing, and the extremity is splinted. Tetanus prophylaxis is administered if necessary (see Chapter 6) and antibiotic treatment initiated. Intravenous first-generation cephalosporin is used for mildly contaminated wounds.

Extensive open wounds or those that occurred in barnyards should receive an aminoglycoside and metronidazole (Flagyl) in addition. If needed, surgical debridement and irrigation are usually performed in the operating room under general anesthesia. All tissue layers are examined, foreign material and devitalized tissue are removed, and the wound is copiously irrigated. The severity of the wound determines the closure technique: primary versus orthoplastics soft tissue reconstruction; however, not until a clean healthy wound is achieved can fracture treatment be performed.

Fracture management requires knowledge of the stages of fracture healing (Table 26-1). The two principles of fracture care are obtaining a reduction and maintaining this reduction until the bone heals while preserving the bone's blood supply.

Reduction

Fracture deformity is reduced to restore bone apposition and alignment and can be achieved by either closed or open methods. Closed reduction involves the manipulation of the fracture into a functional position with traction applied to the distal segment to separate the impacted fragments and force applied to provide realignment. When an open reduction is required, the fracture is surgically exposed, and bone fragments are manipulated directly. Open reduction is indicated when closed reduction methods fail, or with most displaced fractures in weight-bearing bones, or with intra-articular fractures in which the joint surface must be perfectly restored to prevent the development of posttraumatic arthritis.

Maintenance of Reduction

Once the fracture has been reduced, alignment must be maintained until the process of bone healing is completed. Maintaining alignment requires some form of fracture immobilization, which may include casting, traction, functional bracing, and internal or external fixation. The type of immobilization employed depends on fracture stability or its propensity for displacement, with the traditional method of immobilization most commonly being a circumferential plaster or fiberglass cast. A cast protects and maintains fracture alignment until healing occurs. Early clinical and radiographic follow-up is necessary to ensure that fracture reduction is not lost as swelling diminishes.

Continuous traction applied through the skin, the skeleton, or by gravity is a technique that can both affect

and maintain reduction. Skin traction is useful in small children or to temporarily splint an adult with a hip fracture before surgery. Skeletal traction requires that a pin be inserted through bone distal to the fracture site. Large **distraction** forces can then be applied directly to the bone and can overcome the contractile forces of large muscles in patients with pelvic, femoral, or tibial fractures (Figure 26-11). Gravity acting through a dependent extremity can also act as a traction force. In humeral fractures, the weight of the distal arm applies traction if the body is kept upright (Figure 26-12A). Application of a forearm cast can augment this type of traction (Figure 26-12B). This technique is rarely used and largely replaced by functional bracing.

Several complications are associated with casts and traction. Circumferential bandages may cause circulatory impairment in acutely traumatized limbs in which further swelling is expected. To prevent this complication, a splint is generally used in the acute treatment of fractures, which is then replaced by a circumferential cast after the initial swelling subsides. A cast or dressing that is too tight must be completely released to the level of skin. Excessive traction can cause nonunion and peripheral nerve injury. Ulcerative skin problems may occur with both skin and skeletal traction. Skeletal traction causes frictional shearing forces between the patient's sacrum and the bed, which can result in a sacral decubitus ulcer. A poorly applied cast can cause a pressure ulcer over an inadequately padded bony prominence or a displaced bone end. Joint stiffness and muscle atrophy are common problems after prolonged immobilization.

Functional braces that are used most often for humeral shaft fractures allow for early joint motion while maintaining fracture alignment through a compressive hydraulic effect on the soft tissues. Conversion from a cast or splint to a functional brace after early evidence of fracture healing hastens both healing and rehabilitation.

Internal fixation devices include pins, screws, plates (Figure 26-13), circumferential wires or bands, and intramedullary rods (see Figure 26-19). Indications for internal fixation are listed in Table 26-2. Metallic fracture fixation implants may appear sturdy on radiographs. However, like a cast, they simply position the fracture until healing is complete. Fracture fixation hardware should be considered an internal splint that must respect the biology of fracture healing. The mere presence of an internal fixation device does not guarantee fracture healing. If the fracture does not unite, repetitive (cyclic) loading of a fracture implant will ultimately lead to its loosening or to breakage. Whenever internal fixation is employed, there is a race between fracture healing and implant failure. Although internal fixation enhances early patient mobility, it has a number of potential complications. Internal fixation requires a surgical exposure that itself can devitalize tissue and adds to the risk of infection and nonunion. A second surgical procedure may be needed if the implant is to be removed. Finally, after hardware removal, the bone can refracture through screw holes, especially when they are in the cortical, diaphyseal bone.

External fixation is a minimally invasive method of maintaining fracture alignment. Threaded pins are placed into the bone above and below the fracture site and are attached to an external frame to immobilize the fracture

TABLE 26-1. Stages of Fracture Healing
Hematoma formation (immediate)
Inflammation and cellular proliferation (hours to weeks)
Soft callus formation (2 d-6 wk)   Chondrogenic and osteogenic cell proliferation; formation of woven or fibrous bone
Hard callus formation (10 d-4 mo)   Consolidation; transformation of woven bone to lamellar bone
Bone remodeling (2-24 mo)   Callus remodeling and resorption, with reconstitution of the medullary cavity

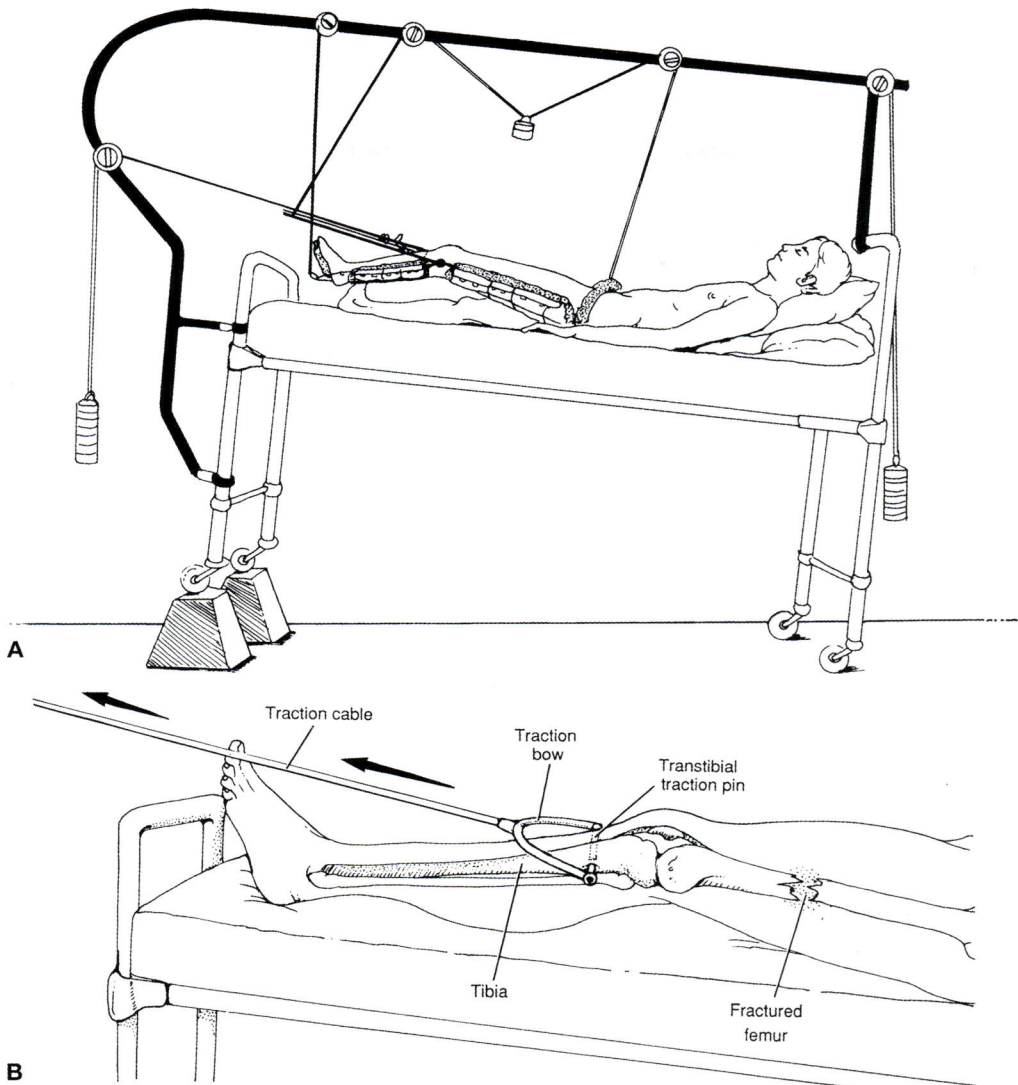

Figure 26-11. A. Skeletal traction applied through a pin placed in the tibia is useful for treating some femur or pelvic fractures. B. The leg is supported in a suspension apparatus, and the foot of the bed is raised to permit body weight and gravity to act as countertraction. (From Lawrence PF. *Essentials of Surgical Specialties.* 3rd ed. Lippincott Williams & Wilkins; 2007.)

(Figure 26-14). Indications for external fixation are listed in Table 26-3. Complications include pin-track infection and delayed union.

Rehabilitation of Function
Rehabilitation planning begins with the initial phases of fracture management. To avoid joint stiffness common to periarticular and intra-articular fractures, the limb is immobilized in a position of maximum function. Isometric exercises of immobilized muscles are started to avoid excessive atrophy. Range of motion exercises for adjacent joints that are not immobilized are encouraged from the onset of care. After a cast or brace is removed, active range of motion and resistive muscle-strengthening exercises are initiated.

The speed of rehabilitation depends on the rate and quality of fracture healing. Exuberant rehabilitative activities or exercises may result in delayed healing, implant failure, and loss of reduction. A rational rehabilitation plan incorporates those factors that influence the speed and success of fracture healing. These factors include the amount of energy imparted to the bone during injury (open, multi-fragmented, and displaced fractures heal slowly), the type of bone involved (cancellous or cortical), the integrity of the soft tissue envelope, and the patient's general health or nutritional status and age (children heal more rapidly than adults).

Bone healing is evaluated clinically and radiologically. Clinically, healing is evident when the fracture is no longer tender to palpation or mobile when stressed.

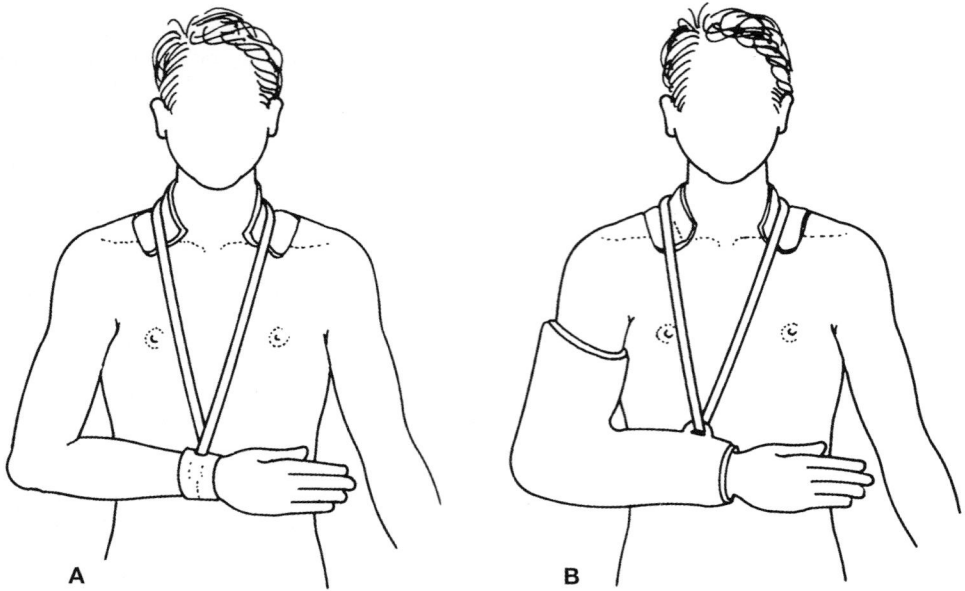

Figure 26-12. Gravity traction. A. With the weight of the arm supported by a collar and cuff. B. With a hanging cast that adds weight to the arm and increases the traction. (From Lawrence PF. *Essentials of Surgical Specialties*. 3rd ed. Lippincott Williams & Wilkins; 2007.)

Radiographically, healing is evident when distinct bony trabeculae are seen crossing the fracture site on radiographic images.

Complications of Fracture Healing
Local Complications

Local complications of fracture healing include infection, delayed union, nonunion, malunion, avascular necrosis, and, in children, growth disturbances. Fractures that are open, either from injury or from surgical intervention, have a higher incidence of infection than closed fractures. Delayed union is characterized by fracture healing that appears to be taking longer than usual. Nonunion is characterized by incomplete fracture healing. The nonunited fracture gap may be filled with fibrous tissue or, if subjected to significant motion, may form a synovial membrane with joint fluid called a pseudarthrosis (a "false joint"). Delayed unions and nonunions are caused by fracture separation, soft tissue interposition,

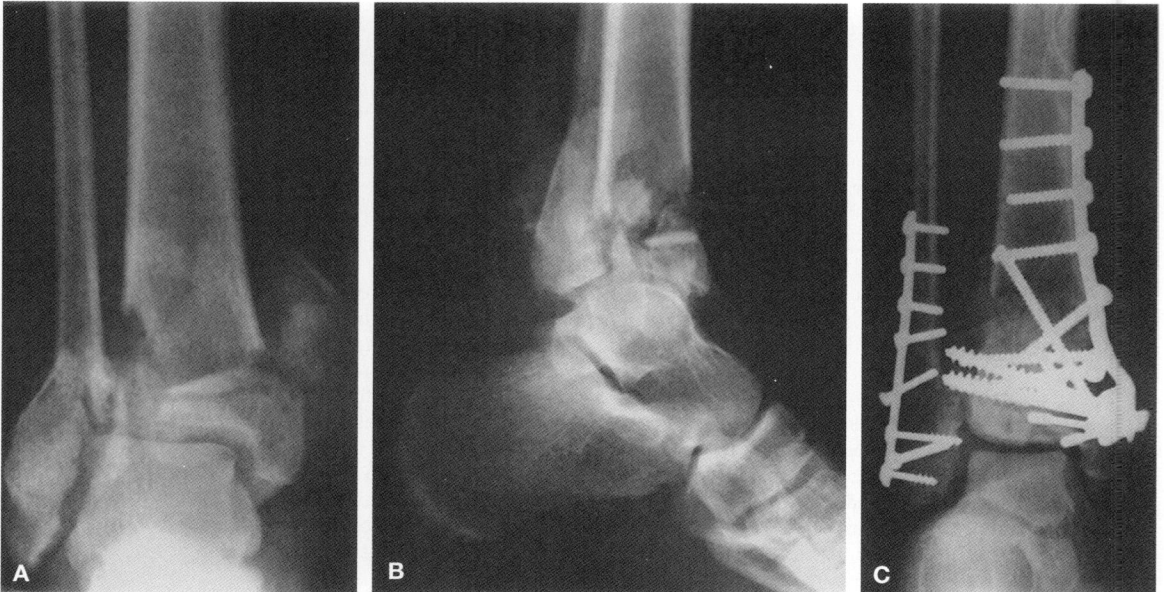

Figure 26-13. Radiographs of a comminuted ankle fracture. A. Anteroposterior radiograph. B. Lateral radiograph. C. Intra-articular fracture treated with a complex array of internal fixation plates and screws. (From Lawrence PF. *Essentials of Surgical Specialties*. 3rd ed. Lippincott Williams & Wilkins; 2007.)

TABLE 26-2. Indications for Internal Fixation of a Fracture

Failure of nonoperative reduction methods

Anatomic reduction of intra-articular fractures

Fractures not amenable to traction or cast immobilization (eg, femoral neck fractures, intertrochanteric fractures in older patients)

Pathologic fractures

Multiple fractures in the same extremity or same patient

Fractures in paraplegics (to assist nursing care)

excessive fracture motion, inadequate vascularization of the fracture segments, or infection. When a fracture heals with a deformity that causes cosmetic or functional impairment, it is called a malunion. Malunited fractures can be shortened, angulated, or rotated. A corrective osteotomy may be required to regain alignment and function.

Avascular necrosis occurs when the blood supply to a bone is injured by a traumatic event (see section "Bone Necrosis"). Bones that are extensively covered by articular cartilage and have a minimal muscular envelope are particularly vulnerable to osteonecrosis (eg, the femoral head, the scaphoid, or the talus).

Growth disturbance is a fracture complication specific to children. The epiphyseal plate is composed of cartilage and is the site of longitudinal growth in bones. Because cartilage is weaker than bone, the growth plate is often involved in pediatric fractures. Fractures in children may damage the growth plate, especially by compressive or shearing mechanisms. When the entire growth plate is damaged, growth will cease, and the affected limb will be shorter than the unaffected limb by the end of growth. If only part of the epiphyseal plate is damaged, the bone may grow asymmetrically and cause an angular deformity. A growth plate injury can be detected only by serial radiographs. Most growth plate problems can be identified by

radiographs taken at the 1-year anniversary of the injury, a date that parents should mark down so they are reminded to present for follow-up radiographs. Lower limb shortening of less than 1 cm is well tolerated; shortening between 1 and 2 cm can be managed by a shoe lift. A leg length discrepancy of more than 2 cm can be corrected by fusion of the opposite growth plate, a procedure known as epiphysiodesis. The timing of this procedure is calculated from growth tables. Angular deformity from a partial growth plate arrest is managed surgically and is best handled when diagnosed early.

Posttraumatic arthritis is a complication of displaced intra-articular fractures. Articular cartilage has no blood supply and depends on synovial fluid for nourishment. When injured, articular cartilage has minimal healing potential. If intra-articular fractures are not anatomically reduced, the irregular surface may cause rapid arthritic change.

Arthritis can also develop indirectly from a severe angular deformity. Weight-bearing forces can be concentrated in the part of the joint causing abnormal stress concentration and joint wear. Depending on the magnitude of injury, posttraumatic arthritis can occur rapidly or slowly over a decade or more. Patients who have had a traumatic hip dislocation, for example, usually have hip arthritis 10 to 20 years later.

Systemic Complications

Systemic complications are unusual following a fracture and usually result from trauma in general and not from the fracture itself. These complications include shock, sepsis, tetanus (in open injuries), gas gangrene, venous thrombosis, and fat embolism. The emergent stabilization of spine, pelvic, and long bone fractures is necessary to minimize blood loss and to allow a patient to sit upright and receive proper pulmonary physiotherapy. Accomplishing this can significantly decrease the incidence of respiratory insufficiency in patients with multisystem trauma.

Joint Subluxation and Dislocation

Diagnosis and Evaluation

Subluxation of a joint is usually a transient phenomenon, when articular surfaces of a joint become partially separated. When a joint is dislocated, the articular surfaces of a joint are no longer in contact with each other, and the patient is reluctant to move it. The limb may be held in a typical posture (eg, when a hip is posteriorly dislocated, the

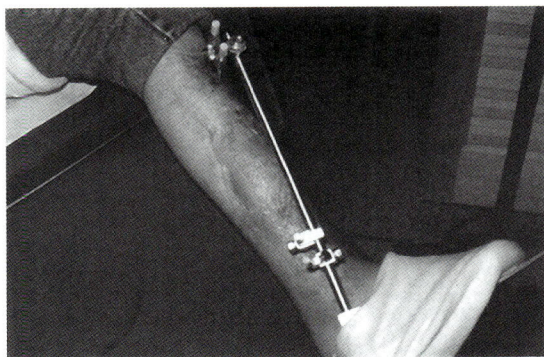

Figure 26-14. Severely comminuted open tibia fracture treated with an external fixator. This form of fixation immobilizes the fracture yet permits access to the wound for observation and care. (From Lawrence PF. *Essentials of Surgical Specialties.* 3rd ed. Lippincott Williams & Wilkins; 2007.)

TABLE 26-3. Indications for External Fixation of a Fracture

Open, unstable fractures (to allow access to and care of the wound and to avoid the use of internal fixation devices in contaminated wounds)

Infected fractures

Unstable pelvic fractures

Severely comminuted or unstable fractures not amenable to internal fixation

Fractures involving bone loss in which bone length must be maintained until a bone graft can be performed thigh is held in flexion, adduction, and internal rotation). Neurovascular structures, in close proximity to joints, can be injured with dislocations, especially in older patients whose arteries may be thickened by atherosclerotic plaque. Not all vascular injuries are acute occlusive phenomena. An intimal tear of the artery may slowly cause thrombus formation, delaying the presentation of vascular compromise. Therefore, serial neurovascular evaluations are essential after the reduction of a dislocated joint. Asymmetry in pulses, which is detected by palpation, Doppler ultrasonography, or ankle-brachial index (ABI) determination, warrants further vascular workup, especially in young patients who have had little stimulus to develop collateral circulation.

Radiographs of the involved joint are obtained in the dislocated posture. This radiograph demonstrates the pathology and allows the treating physician to infer which specific ligamentous structures are damaged. Like a fracture, a dislocation can be described as open or closed and according to the position of the distal fragment relative to the proximal fragment. If radiographic assessment will be delayed and if skin is compromised (eg, ankle fracture or dislocation) or if neurovascular integrity is in question (eg, knee dislocations), then reduction should be attempted immediately.

Treatment

Dislocations are usually realigned by traction along the normal axis of the extremity. Occasionally, bone or soft tissue may be interposed between joint surfaces and will require a surgical (open) reduction. Postreduction radiographs must be taken to ensure the adequacy of reduction and rule out an associated fracture.

Common Musculoskeletal Injuries

Upper Extremity
Distal Radius Fracture

A distal radius fracture is caused by falling on an outstretched hand. When this injury causes a transverse fracture of the distal radius just proximal to the wrist, it is referred to as a Colles fracture. It is a common fracture in older patients with osteoporosis. Radiographically, dorsal comminution can be noted, and the distal fragment is impacted and shortened with apex palmar angulation (Figure 26-15), and the ulnar styloid is often fractured as well.

Reduction is obtained by longitudinal traction applied to the hand, disimpacting the fracture. The wrist and distal fragment are manipulated into flexion and ulnar deviation to correct the dorsal and radial displacement. After reduction, a splint is applied from the elbow to the palm. A repeat radiograph should be taken following the reduction at approximately 10 days to assess whether the reduction has been maintained. If it has not, repeat manipulation or external fixation is required. The deformity tends to recur because of dorsal cortical comminution. Occasionally, Kirschner wires, or K-wires, are inserted percutaneously to prevent the loss of fracture alignment.

The median nerve is in proximity to the volar aspect of the wrist. Its function must be documented before and after fracture manipulation. Shoulder-hand syndrome is a common complication of a Colles fracture in the older

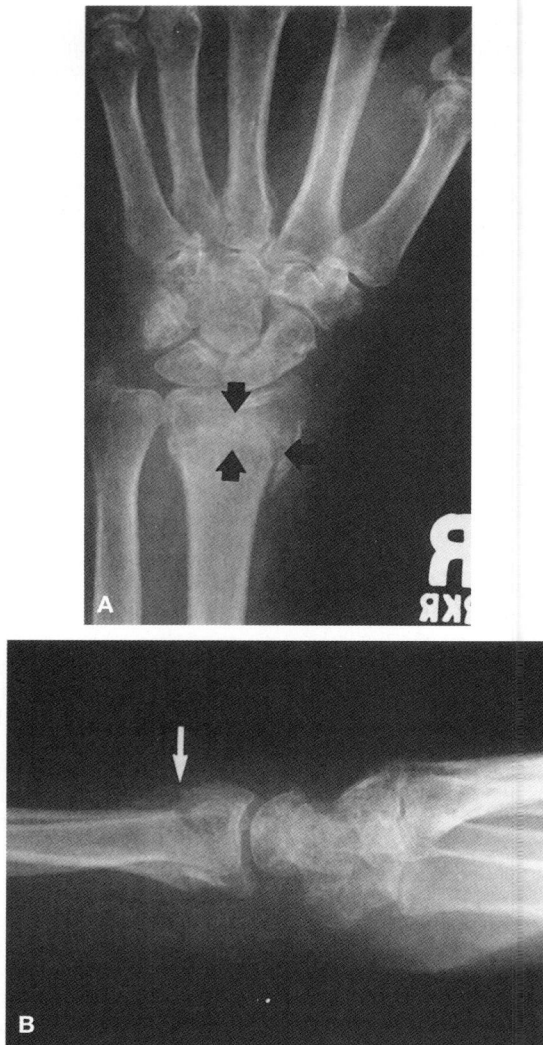

Figure 26-15. Colles fracture of the distal radius is common to patients with osteoporosis. The fracture occurs from a fall on an outstretched dorsiflexed hand. A. The anteroposterior view demonstrates the impaction and shortening of the distal fragment (arrows). B. The lateral radiograph shows the dorsal cortex of the radius to be comminuted and impacted, which results in apex palmar angulation. (From Lawrence PF. *Essentials of Surgical Specialties*. 3rd ed. Lippincott Williams & Wilkins; 2007.)

patients. In this syndrome, shoulder and finger stiffness results from disuse during the treatment period. Patients are encouraged to exercise their shoulders and fingers during the early phases of fracture healing.

Olecranon Fracture

An olecranon fracture is usually caused by a fall in which there is a direct blow to the point of the elbow. The fracture is displaced by contraction of the triceps muscle. Thus, there is a loss of active elbow extension. The fracture also involves the elbow joint surface, and any displacement of the fracture fragments requires an open reduction to restore the articular surface and triceps integrity.

Carpal Scaphoid Fracture

The scaphoid is the bone most frequently fractured of the carpal bones. A fracture through the waist of the scaphoid usually occurs after a fall on the outstretched hand, with the wrist positioned in dorsiflexion and radial deviation. If a fracture is suspected from the mechanism of injury and tenderness in the anatomic snuff box, the patient should be treated as if there were a fracture (even if radiographic views do not indicate a fracture). A bone scan, CT scan, or follow-up radiographs at 7 to 14 days will confirm or disprove the diagnosis. The scaphoid bone is extensively covered by hyaline cartilage and has limited soft tissue attachments and blood supply. Complications of avascular necrosis, delayed union, and nonunion are increased by failure to treat a scaphoid fracture initially. Undisplaced fractures are treated in a thumb spica cast (a forearm cast extended to incorporate the thumb in the pinch position). Displaced scaphoid fractures are treated by open reduction and internal fixation.

Pulled Elbow

This is a painful condition that affects young children aged 1 to 4 years. It occurs frequently when the child has been pulled forcibly by the hand. The child tends to hold the elbow slightly flexed and avoids moving it. The pain is believed to be due to impingement of the annular ligament of the radial neck. Treatment is to flex the elbow slightly and supinate the child's hand, which repositions the annular ligament around the radial neck and relieves the symptoms.

Supracondylar Humerus Fracture

A supracondylar humerus fracture is commonly seen in children aged 5 to 10 years. It occurs from a fall on an outstretched hand with the elbow extended. The distal fragment is usually displaced posteriorly. It can cause significant neurovascular complications by entrapping the brachial artery and the median and radial nerves, either at the time of injury or during reduction (Figure 26-16). This fracture is a frequent cause of forearm **compartment syndrome** because of ischemia (Volkmann ischemic contracture). It must be treated with great care and vigilance. Usual management of displaced fractures is with prompt reduction and percutaneous pin fixation in the operating room.

Forearm compartment syndrome can be caused by kinking of the brachial artery at the site of the supracondylar fracture. If the flow of blood with the delivery of oxygen and removal of metabolic waste from the muscles is not restored, severe and even permanent muscle injury can occur. If muscle is ischemic at normal body temperature for more than 2 hours, there is some permanent muscle damage. If the warm ischemia time exceeds 8 hours, then the muscle is likely dead, and revascularizing the limb can lead to systemic complications from hyperkalemia and release of myoglobin. The flexor compartment of the forearm is completely dependent on the blood supply from the brachial artery. If the muscles die, the fibers contract and leave a nonfunctional hand because the fingers and thumb become flexed into the palm. There is no effective tendon transfer to restore hand and wrist function when the entire flexor compartment has stiffened and scarred.

Shoulder Dislocation

The shoulder is the most frequently dislocated joint in the body. In more than 90% of traumatic dislocations, the humeral head is anterior to the scapular glenoid fossa

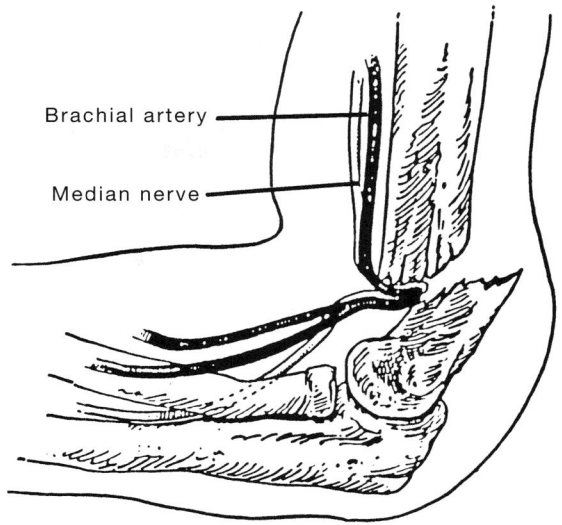

Figure 26-16. The dangerous supracondylar distal humerus fracture may entrap the brachial artery and the median and radial nerves. This fracture is associated with forearm compartment syndrome and warrants cautious and frequent neurovascular monitoring. (Reproduced with permission from American Academy of Orthopaedic Surgeons. *Athletic Training and Sports Medicine*. 2nd ed. American Academy of Orthopaedic Surgeons; 1991:277.)

(Figure 26-17A), which can endanger the axillary nerve and artery. The integrity of the axillary nerve should be documented by testing sensation over the deltoid patch and motor function of the deltoid muscle before and after reduction of the shoulder dislocation. An anterior shoulder dislocation occurs with forced external rotation of the abducted arm. This type of injury may be caused by an arm tackle in football or by blocking a basketball shot.

Reduction can be achieved by gradual shoulder abduction while longitudinal traction is placed on the arm and countertraction is placed through the axilla with a sheet (Figure 26-17B). Sedation and muscle relaxation facilitate the manipulation.

Posterior shoulder dislocations, although rare, are often missed because of improper interpretation of the AP radiograph, which appears to show the humeral head aligned with the glenoid. An axillary view shows the humeral head to lie posterior to the glenoid, which should reinforce the principle that two radiographs taken in perpendicular planes are needed for proper radiographic evaluation of any bony structure. Clinically, the arm is held internally rotated and cannot be externally rotated beyond the neutral position. A posterior dislocation should be considered in all patients with shoulder symptoms after an electrocution or a seizure caused by epilepsy, alcohol withdrawal, electroconvulsive therapy, or electrocution.

Lower Extremity
Hip Fractures

Low-energy hip fractures are common in older patients with osteoporosis. They account for about 33% of admissions to large orthopedic centers. The common types are femoral neck (see Figure 26-5A) and intertrochanteric hip fractures (Figure 26-18). In both fractures, the affected limb is externally rotated and shortened. The patient cannot bear weight, and slight amounts of hip motion cause pain.

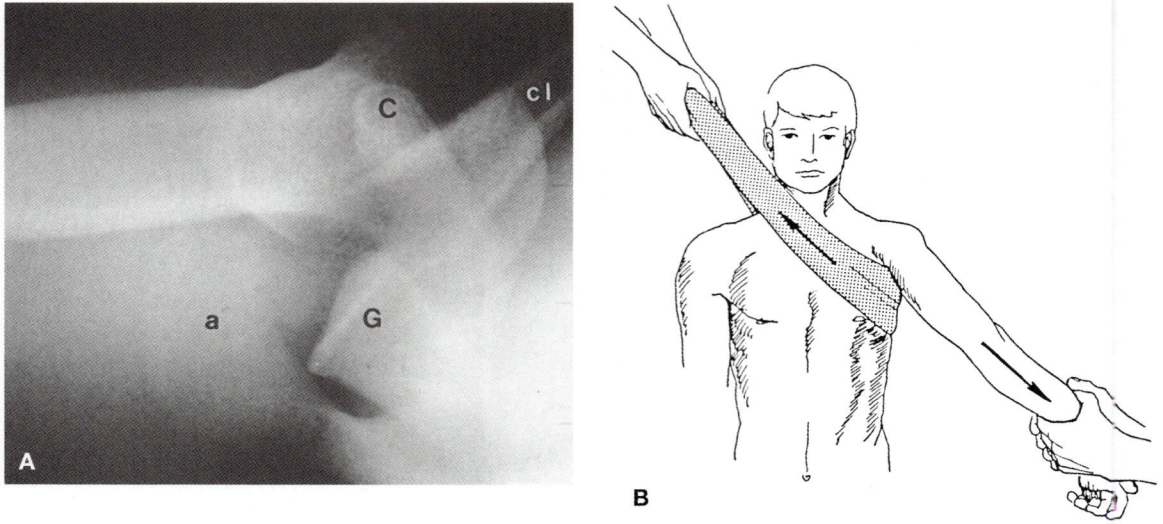

Figure 26-17. A. Axillary lateral radiograph of an anterior shoulder dislocation. The humeral head lies out of the glenoid fossa (*G*). The coracoid process (*C*) is an anterior scapular structure and orients the film. B. Closed reduction of an anterior shoulder dislocation via traction countertraction. a, acromion; cl, clavicle. (Reprinted with permission from Rockwood C, Green D. *Fractures in Adults*. 3rd ed. JB Lippincott; 1982:1092.)

The blood supply to the femoral head comes from vessels that run along the posterior femoral neck. These vessels can be damaged by a femoral neck fracture. If the femoral head is rendered avascular, the bone cells die. When dead bone is subjected to repetitive weight-bearing loads, it will collapse and fragment. Femoral neck fractures have a higher incidence of nonunion because the fracture is within the hip joint (intracapsular), with a thin periosteum and no muscle envelope. Femoral neck fractures are either reduced and surgically fixed or, because

of attendant complications, replaced with a metal hemiarthroplasty. An intertrochanteric hip fracture occurs outside the hip joint (extracapsular). There is a good blood supply, and the fracture usually heals (Figure 26-18A). Intertrochanteric fractures are reduced under radiographic guidance and fixed with a sliding screw and sideplate device (Figure 26-18B). Surgical treatment allows for early patient mobilization and decreases problems related to prolonged bed confinement (eg, pneumonia, thrombophlebitis, decubitus ulcers).

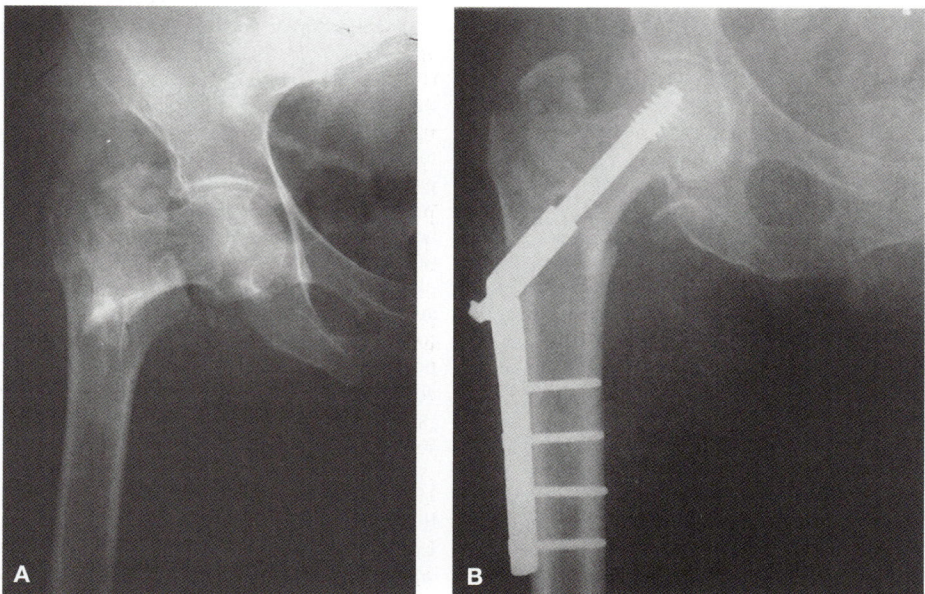

Figure 26-18. A. Intertrochanteric hip fracture. The bone is osteopenic and rarefied. B. This fracture has been reduced and internally fixed with a screw and sideplate device. This type of fixation will permit early patient mobilization. (From Lawrence PF. *Essentials of Surgical Specialties*. 3rd ed. Lippincott Williams & Wilkins; 2007.)

Femoral Shaft Fractures

The femoral shaft is the largest and strongest bone in the body. In young patients, femur fractures require high-energy trauma and are incurred by motor vehicle accidents and falls from heights. Blood loss may be considerable. In a closed fracture, 1 to 3 units of blood may be lost into the thigh, and the patient may present in hypovolemic shock. Other sources of hypovolemia (such as intra-abdominal and intrathoracic injuries or pelvic fractures) must be excluded. In all patients with a fractured femur, the pelvis and hip must be assessed radiologically to rule out associated fractures or dislocations. Knee stability should be evaluated.

Closed, interlocked intramedullary nailing is the preferred treatment (Figure 26-19). Because the nail can be locked proximally and distally, the fracture can be rendered quite stable and allow early ambulation. This approach prevents the lengthy periods of bed rest required with skeletal traction (see Figure 26-11) and minimizes the risks of venous thrombosis, knee stiffness, quadriceps contracture, muscle atrophy, and disuse osteoporosis.

Hip Dislocation

Hip dislocation often occurs in motor vehicle accidents when the knee strikes the dashboard. Seated posture places the hip in adduction and 90° of flexion. The longitudinal load of unrestrained dashboard impact drives the hip posteriorly out of the acetabular socket and may stretch the sciatic nerve. All patients with posterior hip dislocations should be assessed for a foot drop. The hip should be reduced urgently and associated fractures repaired to restore stability of the hip joint. Delays in treatment beyond 8 to 12 hours from injury can increase the risks for avascular necrosis of the femoral head and posttraumatic arthritis of the hip.

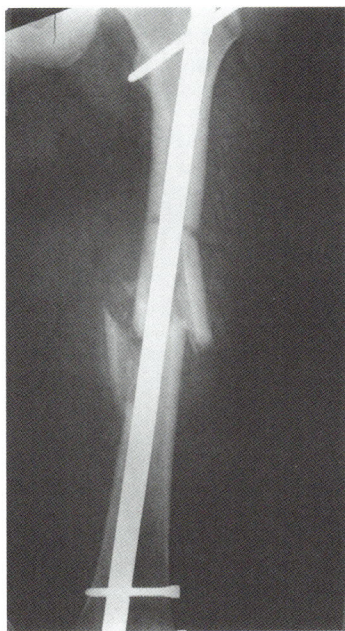

Figure 26-19. Comminuted femoral shaft fracture after internal fixation with an interlocked intramedullary nail. (From Lawrence PF. *Essentials of Surgical Specialties*. 3rd ed. Lippincott Williams & Wilkins; 2007.)

Tibia and Fibular Shaft Fracture

Shaft fractures of the tibia and fibula occur 9 times more often than femoral shaft fractures. Almost 33% of the tibial surface is subcutaneous. For this reason, tibia fractures are often open and contaminated. The limited blood supply to the tibia causes fractures of this bone to have delayed union and nonunion. Tibia fractures are at risk for compartment syndrome (discussed later), which requires attentive observation and early diagnosis. The key clinical sign in a conscious patient is pain that is out of proportion to the injury. Complications associated with tibia fracture management are the most frequent cause of trauma-related orthopedic malpractice suits.

Closed reduction and above-the-knee cast immobilization are the standard treatment for uncomplicated closed fractures of the tibia and fibula. Open reduction and internal fixation are considered only when an acceptable reduction cannot be achieved by closed means or the reduction cannot be maintained by a plaster cast. External fixation (see Figure 26-14) is frequently used in managing open fractures of the tibia: Stability and alignment of the fracture fragments are maintained while allowing access to treat the soft tissue wound. Current trends are toward adequate surgical debridement at the time of injury followed by internal fixation. The implant of choice is a reamed intramedullary nail.

Ankle Injuries

Ankle injuries are common in young, athletic individuals and may involve both ligamentous and bony structures. The ankle is a mortise and tenon joint. The three-sided mortise is composed of the tibial malleolus, the tibial plafond (ceiling), and the fibular malleolus. The talus represents the tenon. The mechanism of injury can be inferred from the plane of the fracture line (Figure 26-20). A transverse fracture line occurs from a tensile or "pulling off" force. Thus, when the medial malleolus fracture is transverse, it suggests an abduction (eversion or pronation) force of the foot on the leg (Figure 26-20B and C). If the lateral malleolus fracture is transverse, the force applied to the foot is adduction (inversion or supination; Figure 26-20A). A spiral fracture configuration implies a rotatory force. A coronal plane spiral fracture is a common lateral malleolar fracture pattern and is seen when the foot is externally rotated on the leg and body (Figure 26-20C). Bimalleolar ankle fractures are common. When a posterior tibial fragment is seen on the lateral radiograph, it is called a trimalleolar fracture, and it results from vertical loading of the plantar flexed ankle (Figure 26-20D).

Because ankle fractures are intra-articular, anatomic restoration of the joint congruity is an essential treatment principle. One millimeter of ankle displacement can reduce joint surface contact by 40%. Anatomic open reduction with internal fixation is the ideal treatment for displaced ankle fractures.

Spinal and Pelvic Fractures

Spinal and pelvic fractures in young people result from high-velocity trauma and are associated with intrathoracic, intra-abdominal, and extremity injuries. In the older patients, spine fractures may occur after minimal trauma in bone that is weakened by osteoporosis or tumor.

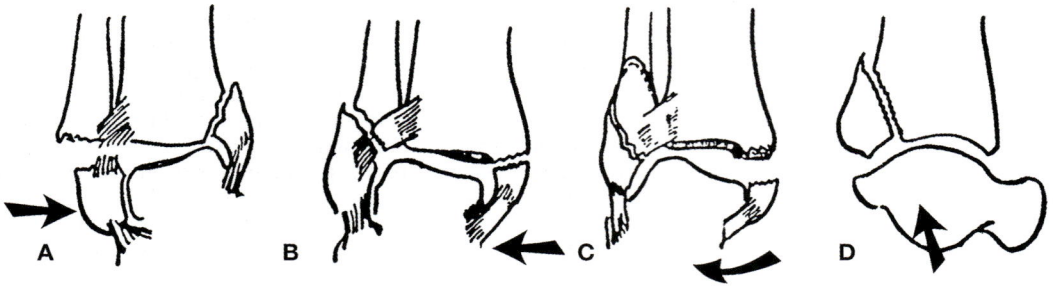

Figure 26-20. Ankle fractures. The basic mechanism of injury can be identified by the characteristic fracture patterns. A transverse fracture line implies that tensile, avulsive force was applied to the bone and is usually the first fracture to occur in the injury pattern. A. Adduction (inversion), in which the lateral malleolus is pulled off transversely and the medial malleolus is pushed off obliquely by the talus. B. Pure abduction (eversion), in which the medial malleolus is pulled off transversely and the fibula pushed off obliquely by the talus. The lateral malleolus is fractured in the sagittal plane. In some cases, the fibula is fractured above the joint line, indicating a tear in the interosseous membrane. C. Abduction (eversion) and external rotation (common), in which the medial malleolus is pulled off transversely, whereas the lateral malleolus is obliquely fractured by the talus as it externally rotates and abuts the fibula. The fibular fracture is in the coronal plane. D. Vertical load, in which the posterior malleolus, seen best on a lateral x-ray film, can be fractured by a vertical compression load as the talus impacts the posterior tibia. The addition of this fracture fragment to any of the above constitutes a trimalleolar fracture. (Reprinted with permission from Rockwood C, Green D. *Fractures in Adults*. 3rd ed. JB Lippincott; 1982.)

Spinal Fractures

Spinal stability is the critical concept in the treatment of spinal fractures. The spine is unstable if unprotected movement causes fracture displacement that can compromise the integrity of neural structures. In all cases of suspected spinal injury, a complete and detailed baseline neurologic assessment should be performed and documented as soon as the patient's condition permits. In unconscious patients or in those with any injuries above the level of the clavicle (facial), the cervical spine is presumed to be injured until proven otherwise (see Chapter 7). Patients with minor wedge compression fractures (see Figure 26-5B) of the lower thoracic or lumbar spine often develop an ileus from retroperitoneal bleeding and should not be fed enterally until the ileus has resolved. If paraplegia results from a catastrophic spinal column injury, the signs of other injuries are masked by the lack of sensation. A systematic and thorough examination of all vital structures must, therefore, be carried out in patients with paraplegia. The patient with suspected spine trauma is properly splinted at the site of injury in a cervical collar with the head secured by taped sandbags. The thorax, abdomen, and extremities are strapped to a spine board. Consultation with a neurosurgeon or an orthopedic surgeon is indicated if the physician has any doubt about the stability of the spine injury.

Pelvic Fractures

The pelvis transfers body weight through the sacroiliac joints and acetabula in stance and through the ischial tuberosities in seated postures. The pelvis also protects the lower abdominal and genitourinary tracts. The pelvis houses the extensive vascular arborizations of the iliac vessels and the lumbosacral plexus of nerves. Pelvic fractures usually occur after high-velocity blunt trauma and can be associated with massive blood loss and multiorgan system injuries (Figure 26-21). Therefore, in a hemodynamically

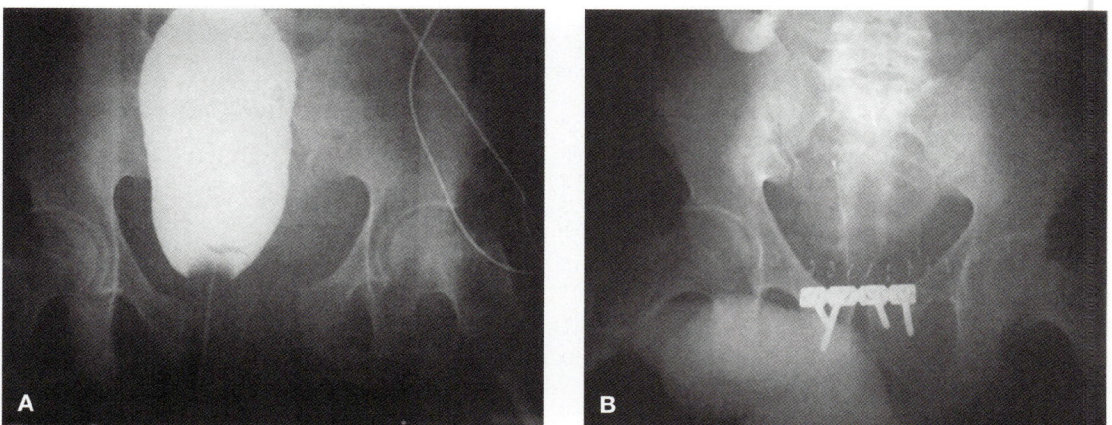

Figure 26-21. A. Anteroposterior (AP) pelvis radiograph depicting diastasis of the symphysis pubis. The retrograde cystogram demonstrates bladder compression from a large pelvic hematoma. This type of pelvic injury can cause massive amounts of internal hemorrhage. B. AP pelvis radiograph after internal fixation with a plate and screws. Fracture reduction decreases pelvic volume, which both stabilizes and facilitates tamponade of bleeding fracture surfaces. (From Lawrence PF. *Essentials of Surgical Specialties*. 3rd ed. Lippincott Williams & Wilkins; 2007.)

unstable patient, emergency pelvic stabilization with external fixation is considered essential to the trauma resuscitation. The two goals of acute pelvic fracture surgery are to stop bleeding and permit sitting stability to facilitate pulmonary physiotherapy.

Almost one in five pelvic fractures has a concomitant bladder or urethral injury in males. When blood is seen at the external urethral meatus or when the patient cannot pass urine, a retrograde urethrogram is obtained to evaluate the integrity of the urethra before an indwelling catheter is placed. With hematuria, an intravenous pyelogram is performed to show renal function. If blood is detected in the rectum or vagina, the pelvic fracture may be open. Open pelvic fractures are treated with a diverting colostomy after debridement and external fixation to prevent ongoing fecal contamination of the fracture.

TRAUMATIC AMPUTATIONS AND REPLANTATION

With the advent of microsurgical techniques, completely severed digits and limbs can be surgically reattached. Limb replantation is most successful if the part is amputated cleanly with a minimum of crushed tissue. Children enjoy better nerve regeneration than adults and are ideal candidates for replantation. A general rule applies to replantation: Because muscle tissue is sensitive to ischemic injury, the greater the amount of muscle attached to the amputated part, the poorer the prognosis for its function after replantation.

The best amputation levels for replantation in adults are the thumb, multiple digits, and the wrist or metacarpal level of the hand. In children, amputations at any level have a good chance of successful replantation. Contraindications to replantation include amputations with large crush or avulsive components; body parts that have been amputated at multiple levels; individual digit amputations (other than the thumb), especially proximal to the middle phalanx; and amputation in older patients who have concurrent disease or mental instability.

An amputated part may remain viable for approximately 6 hours of warm (36 °C) ischemia. Cooling decreases tissue metabolism and increases the duration of viability. Amputated tissues can tolerate up to 16 hours of cold (10 °C) ischemia. Thus, preparation of a severed part for transportation should include cleansing of superficial contamination, wrapping in moist gauze, and placement in an air-tight plastic bag that is then immersed in ice water. Dry ice is never used because it causes frostbite and further tissue damage.

Of digital replants, 85% remain viable. Joint motion is usually about 50% of normal, and two-point sensory discrimination is protective (>10 mm) in half of adults yet almost normal (>5 mm) in children. All digits are cold intolerant for a period of at least 2 years, and 80% of epiphyses will continue to grow after replantation.

COMPARTMENT SYNDROME

Muscles are surrounded by a relatively stiff fascial membrane composed of fibrous collagen. These fibrous envelopes separate various muscles into anatomically distinct compartments (Figure 26-22). Bleeding and tissue swelling inside these membranes cause increased pressure within the fascial compartment. Under these circumstances, capillary blood flow to muscle and nerve is thus reduced, causing local acidosis, cell injury, and further edema. Compartment pressures can become so elevated

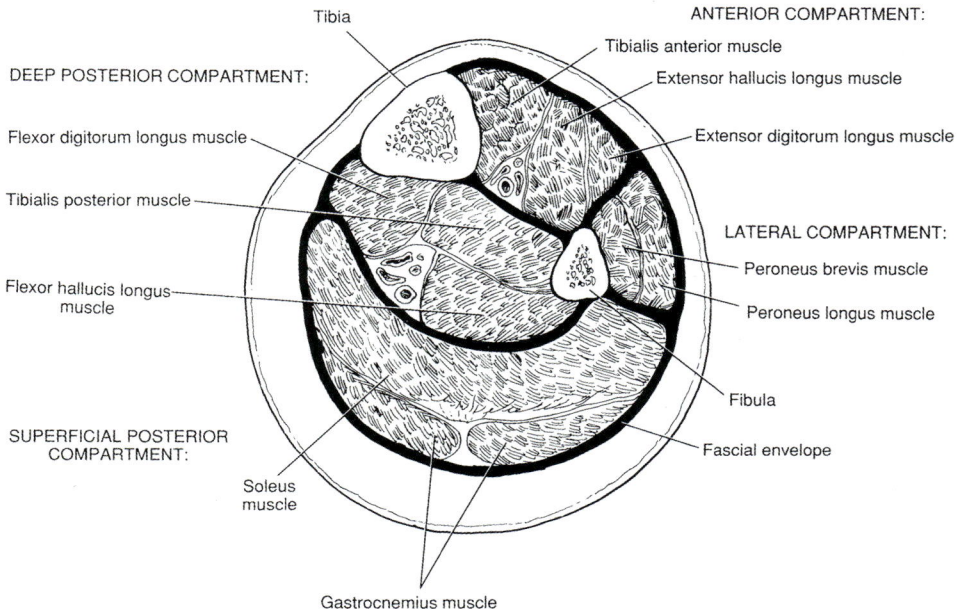

Figure 26-22. Four distinct leg compartments are separated by thick, unyielding fascial planes. (From Lawrence PF. *Essentials of Surgical Specialties.* 3rd ed. Lippincott Williams & Wilkins; 2007.)

that muscle and nerve necrosis result. Dead fibrotic muscle will cause joint contractures, and the limb function will be severely impaired.

Compartment syndrome can be caused by fractures, severe muscle contusions, crush injuries, and acute vascular occlusion followed by revascularization. They may be aggravated by casts. Fractures that cause the most compartment syndromes are supracondylar distal humerus (see Figure 26-16), both bones (radius and ulna) of the forearm, and proximal third tibia fractures.

The classic signs of compartment syndrome caused by tissue ischemia are described by the four Ps: pain, paresthesia, paralysis, and pallor. Pain is the most useful clinical sign. It is intense and usually disproportionate to the injury. In addition, the pain is intensified on passive stretching of the muscles within the suspected compartment. If these symptoms and signs occur in the presence of one of the high-risk injuries, an urgent orthopedic consultation should be obtained regarding possible fasciotomy. It is important to remember that compartment syndrome can occur in the presence of normal pulses and sensation. Systolic arterial pulse pressures are usually much higher than the 30 mm Hg interstitial compartment pressure at which myonecrosis begins.

A high index of suspicion and pain out of proportion to the injury should lead to the removal of all circular bandages or casts. The clinician should not wait for paresthesia, paralysis, or pallor. Decompression by open fasciotomy is indicated if compartment pressure is greater than 30 to 40 mm Hg in an unconscious or paralyzed patient. (Compartment syndrome is also discussed in Chapters 8 and 24.)

SPORTS-RELATED INJURIES

The recent emphasis on physical fitness has led to an increase in sports-related injuries. These injuries can be classified as those caused by acute trauma or repetitive stress. All musculoskeletal tissues are composed of living cells that are stimulated by physical stress to become stronger. When these tissues are not stressed, bones, ligaments, muscles, and tendons will atrophy. The goal of exercise is to produce beneficial increases in physical strength and endurance through the controlled application of stress. Tissues gain strength following stress-induced microscopic breakdown by a process of hypertrophic repair. When the stresses of exercise overwhelm the normal reparative process, tissues become chronically injured and inflamed and ultimately fail. There is much to be learned about the proper duration, frequency, and intensity of physical training. For example, the "no pain, no gain" attitude toward exercise often exacerbates many injuries. Although pain may be an annoyance, it is also appropriate biofeedback signifying injury and the need for rest.

It has been calculated that, while running, the foot strikes the ground between 800 and 2,000 times per mile at a force of 2 (bid) to 4 times body weight. An average 140-lb man generates between 110 and 560 tons of ground reaction force per mile. This tremendous amount of force is dissipated by the shoe, the small joints of the foot, and the bones and muscles of the leg. Any of these tissues can and do fail with injudicious exercise.

This section describes the more common injuries related to acute trauma and chronic, repetitive overuse. Many of these syndromes can occur as occupational injuries in which a given task is repeated with great frequency and without adequate periods of restorative rest.

Stress Fractures

Stress fractures are the classic overuse injury. They occur when individuals are subjected to increased activity levels or changes in habits and training methods. Historically, stress fractures were first identified in the metatarsals of military recruits who were expected to endure arduous marches (march fracture syndrome). Stress fractures have been identified in most bones of the body, including femur, tibia, calcaneus, and metatarsals in runners; humerus in throwers; ribs in oarsmen; and wrists and L5 vertebrae in gymnasts.

Stress fractures are postulated to occur as a consequence of muscle fatigue. Not only do muscles cause locomotion, but they also absorb shock. Eccentric muscle contraction, or controlled muscle lengthening, decelerates the body, absorbs shock, and diffuses stress away from bone. When muscles tire, this stress-shielding effect is negated and stress is transferred directly to bone. Repeated submaximal stress will cause bone as a material to fatigue. Microfractures result and may cause achy discomfort. The traditional treatment of rest and stress protection permits these microscopic fractures to heal. Normal cellular bone healing mechanisms permit the bone to strengthen in response to increasing demands. If the bone's ability to heal itself is overwhelmed by repeated, unremitting stress, these microfractures will coalesce, resulting in a gross, macroscopic fracture. Because stress fractures are initiated on a microscopic level, radiographs lack diagnostic sensitivity and have high false-negative rates, missing as many as 70% of these injuries. Radioisotope-labeled technetium pyrophosphate bone scans, which detect cellular bone formation, can identify a stress fracture at an earlier stage of its pathogenesis (Figure 26-23).

Lateral Epicondylitis (Tennis Elbow)

Lateral epicondylitis, or tennis elbow, is an overuse injury of the wrist extensor muscle origin. This condition affects players of racket sports, as well as laborers who use their hand in repetitive forceful gripping. Wrist extension is necessary for power grip (try to grip with your wrist flexed!).

The wrist extensor muscles also dissipate force when a handheld object is used in striking. In tennis elbow, the common wrist extensors are damaged and inflamed at their lateral humeral epicondyle origin. The majority of these injuries respond to nonoperative methods that include rest, heat, anti-inflammatory agents, wrist extensor muscle stretching, and antagonist (wrist flexor) strengthening exercises. In the few cases that are managed operatively, chronic granulation tissue is found in the origin of the extensor carpi radialis brevis and is resected.

Rotator Cuff Tendonitis (Shoulder Bursitis)

The glenohumeral joint of the shoulder is the most mobile joint in the body. The four rotator cuff muscles—subscapularis, supraspinatus, infraspinatus, and teres minor—all take broad origin from the scapular body and insert just lateral to the and tearing (Figure 26-24). Painful inflammatory changes may also affect the subacromial bursa. It is difficult to distinguish which structure is painful, the bursa or the tendon proper. A rotator cuff tear may show weakness of shoulder external rotation strength. Pain can mask the reliability of strength testing. A shoulder arthrogram, ultrasound, or MRI scan can diagnose a rotator cuff tear with good dependability.

Factors that contribute to rotator cuff pain include overuse, weakness, muscle imbalance, improper throwing technique, strenuous training techniques, and an unstable glenohumeral joint. Treatment consists of rest, eccentric rotator cuff strengthening exercises, and anti-inflammatory medication. Surgical decompression of the coracoacromial arch is indicated if the condition becomes chronic or if it is necessary to repair a torn rotator cuff tendon.

Plantar Fasciitis (Calcaneal Bursitis)

Plantar fasciitis is a problem common to runners. The plantar fascia is a thick, fibrous structure attached to the calcaneus that fans distally along the sole of the foot to envelop the metatarsal heads. It increases and stiffens the longitudinal arch of the foot during the propulsive toe-off phase of gait. When the inflexible plantar fascia is repeatedly impacted and stretched by running, it is injured at its calcaneal origin, becoming inflamed and painful. The inflammatory reaction can produce a traction spike of new bone, which, on radiograph, is called a heel spur. It is not clear how much of the heel pain can be attributed to the spur. Many patients who have had foot x-rays for other reasons have evidence of heel spurs but no symptoms of heel pain.

Classically, plantar heel pain is worse when gait is initiated in the morning, after sitting, or at the start of jogging. Contributory factors include both flat (planus) and high-arched (cavus) feet, toe or sand running, obesity, and improper shoe wear (eg, slippers). Nonoperative treatment includes rest, medication, weight loss if applicable, proper shoe wear, heel padding, or cushioned shoe orthoses. If the condition has been of long duration, recovery may be slow. Surgical release of the plantar fascia from its calcaneal origin is reserved for the most recalcitrant cases.

Patellar Overload Syndrome

Anterior knee pain is common to sports participants. The patella is embedded in the quadriceps muscle and glides through the femoral groove. The patella functions much like a pulley to increase the mechanical efficiency of the quadriceps in extending the knee joint. When the patella is abnormally loaded or malaligned, abnormal patellar wear and irritation can produce chondromalacia, or cartilage (*chondro-*) softening (*malacia*).

Patellofemoral knee pain is located anteriorly and is aggravated by climbing or descending stairs and hills, squatting, kneeling, arising from a chair, or after prolonged sitting. These activities all stress the knee extensor (quadriceps) mechanism. As the quadriceps muscle is inhibited by discomfort, it may atrophy. Nonoperative treatment is often effective. Avoidance of aggravating activities and anti-inflammatory medications and the use of patellar orthotics known as "knee sleeves" are effective treatment adjuncts. Straight-leg raising and quadriceps-strengthening exercises are important to successful rehabilitation. Quadriceps exercises over a full arc of motion are to be avoided

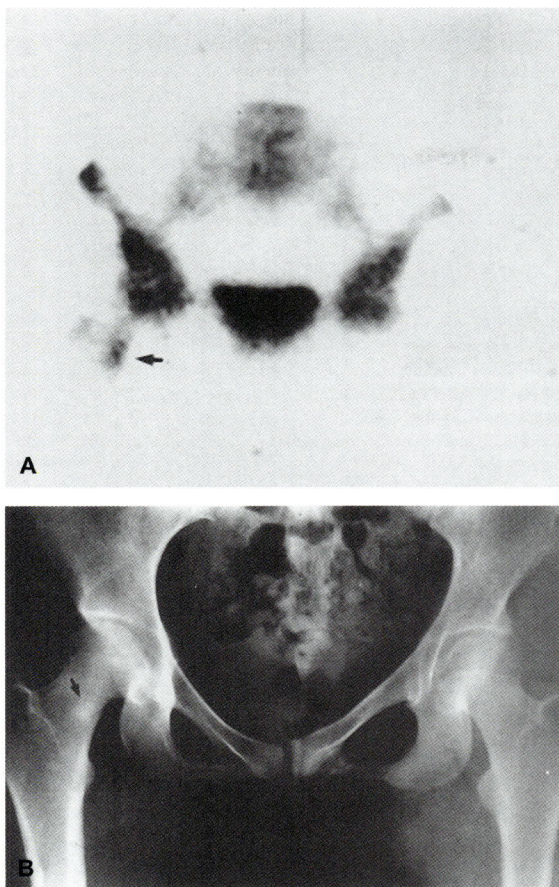

Figure 26-23. A. Femoral neck stress fracture detected by increased radioisotopic uptake on bone scan (arrow) 2 weeks before (B) radiographic evidence of the fracture (arrow). (From Lawrence PF. *Essentials of Surgical Specialties*. 3rd ed. Lippincott Williams & Wilkins; 2007.)

articular surface of the humeral head. These muscles act to stabilize the joint by pulling the humeral head into the shallow scapular glenoid fossa. The combined cross-sectional area of the rotator cuff musculature is equal to that of the deltoid muscle. Because cross-sectional area is directly related to muscle strength, it is interesting that the amount of shoulder muscle strength expended on joint stability through the rotator cuff is equal to that of the deltoid, which is responsible for joint mobility.

Rotator cuff tendonitis, or subacromial bursitis, is common to people involved in sports (eg, swimmers, throwers) or who have jobs in which the arm is used overhead (eg, mechanics). As the shoulder abducts away from the body, the rotator cuff muscles (especially the supraspinatus) contract under the coracoacromial arch. As the arm is raised, this arch becomes narrower, impinging on and mechanically irritating the tendons of the rotator cuff muscles. The subacromial bursa, which is a fluid-filled synovial sac, may become inflamed under these conditions of friction and can contribute to the pain. However, pathologic changes can also affect the tendon and run the gamut from edematous inflammation to calcific degeneration to tendon thinning

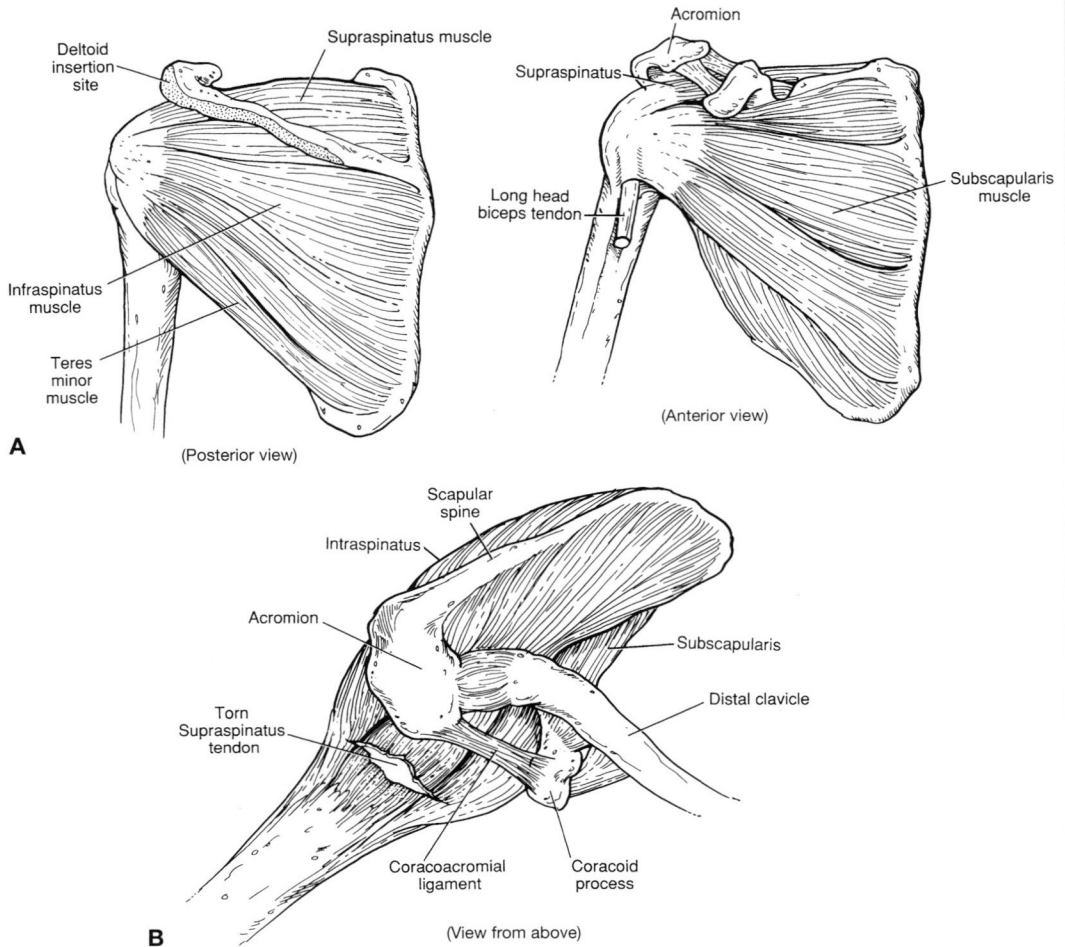

Figure 26-24. A. Viewed from the posterior and anterior perspectives, the cowl of rotator cuff muscles takes broad origin from the scapula and inserts close to the articular margin of the humeral head. The rotator cuff acts to pull the humeral head into the glenoid fossa as the arm is abducted away from the body. B. Viewed from its superior surface, the supraspinatus tendon is torn near its humeral insertion. The tear results from acromion and coracoacromial ligament attrition, when the shoulder is abducted and forward flexed. (Reproduced with permission as modified from American Academy of Orthopaedic Surgeons. *Athletic Training and Sports Medicine*. 2nd ed. American Academy of Orthopaedic Surgeons; 1991:235.; B. Modified from Rowe CR. *The Shoulder*. Churchill Livingstone; 1988:142.)

because they place excessive load on the patella and exacerbate the condition. The diagnosis of chondromalacia should be reserved for injury to the articular cartilage observed either by MRI or by arthroscopy.

Exercise Compartment Syndrome (Shin Splints)

Shin splints are leg pain that is intensified during exercise. In recreational runners, the pain is usually localized to the anterior leg compartment (see Figure 26-22) containing the tibialis anterior, extensor digitorum, and extensor hallucis longus muscles. In competitive runners, the pain often emanates from the distal medial leg in the deep posterior compartment musculature (posterior tibialis, flexor digitorum, and flexor hallucis longus). Intramuscular pressures increase during contraction, which decreases blood flow. Muscle perfusion, therefore, occurs primarily during muscle relaxation. Sustained increases in compartment pressure decrease muscle perfusion, producing pain and the cessation of exercise. This phenomenon is known as exercise compartment syndrome. When measured, compartment pressures can increase to well over 100 mm Hg with exercise. In the asymptomatic individual, pressures return to normal levels very rapidly during periods of rest. In patients with exercise compartment syndromes, interstitial tissue pressures fall off slowly and have a delayed return to normal values. Tibia stress fractures, periostitis, nerve entrapment, and fascial muscle hernias have a similar clinical presentation. The diagnosis of exercise-related compartment syndrome is based on objective pressure measurements. When conservative treatments (eg, rest, cushioned shoe orthotics, and changes in training patterns and running surfaces) fail, the condition can be successfully treated with a surgical fasciotomy of the involved leg compartment.

Sprains

A sprain is a ligament injury. Ligaments are collagenous structures that originate from and insert on bone. Ligaments stabilize joints, and they are injured under tensile or stretching loads. Sprains are classified according to

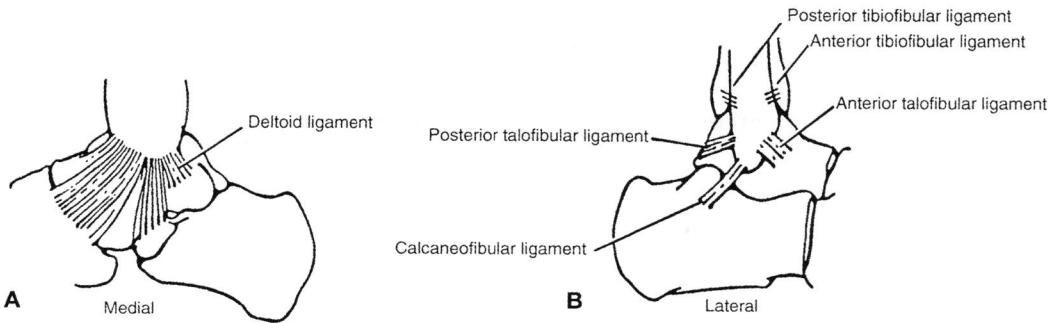

Figure 26-25. A. Extensive medial deltoid ligament of the ankle. B. The lateral ankle is supported by three discrete ankle ligaments. The most commonly sprained anterior talofibular ligament, the calcaneofibular, and the posterior talofibular ligaments. The anterior talofibular ligament resists anterior translation of the ankle (anterior drawer test); the calcaneofibular resists inversion stress (talar tilt). (Modified with permission from Wilson FC, ed. *The Musculoskeletal System: Basic Processes and Disorders.* 2nd ed. JB Lippincott; 1983.)

the three grades of damage. Grade I sprains exhibit microscopic ligament damage, which produces ligament tenderness but no change in joint stability when the joint is subjected to stress. Grade II sprains show a greater degree of damage, with rupture of entire fascicles of ligament collagen. The ligament is in macroscopic continuity but is stretched or partially torn and, therefore, demonstrates joint laxity when stressed. There is a firm end point to clinical testing. When grossly disrupted with total loss of joint stability, the ligament injury is classified as a grade III sprain.

Ankle Sprains

The lateral ankle ligaments are the most commonly sprained ligaments in the body. The lateral ankle is supported by three discrete ligaments: the anterior talofibular, calcaneofibular, and posterior talofibular ligaments (Figure 26-25). Because the longer fibular malleolus buttresses the ankle from abduction or eversion stress, the broad deltoid ligament that connects the medial tibial malleolus to the talus is not commonly injured.

When the ankle is subjected to an inversion stress, the anterior talofibular ligament is the first lateral ligament to be torn. With more severe injury, the calcaneal-fibular ligament will also be disrupted. These two ligaments resist anterior talar displacement on the tibia (anterior drawer test, Figure 26-26) and abnormal inversion talar tilt, respectively.

The diagnosis of a lateral ankle ligament sprain and its severity is determined by the extent of ligament tenderness and by manual and radiographic stress tests. Treatment consists of ice, elevation, compressive wraps, and early weight bearing. Primary surgical ankle ligament repair is rarely indicated because most ankle sprains have no residual joint instability and the outcomes of early versus late ankle reconstruction are similar. Ligaments contain proprioceptive nerve endings that are also injured by a sprain. Recurrent ankle sprains may be the result of inadequate proprioceptive feedback, and thus, balance board proprioceptor retraining is an effective component of ankle rehabilitation.

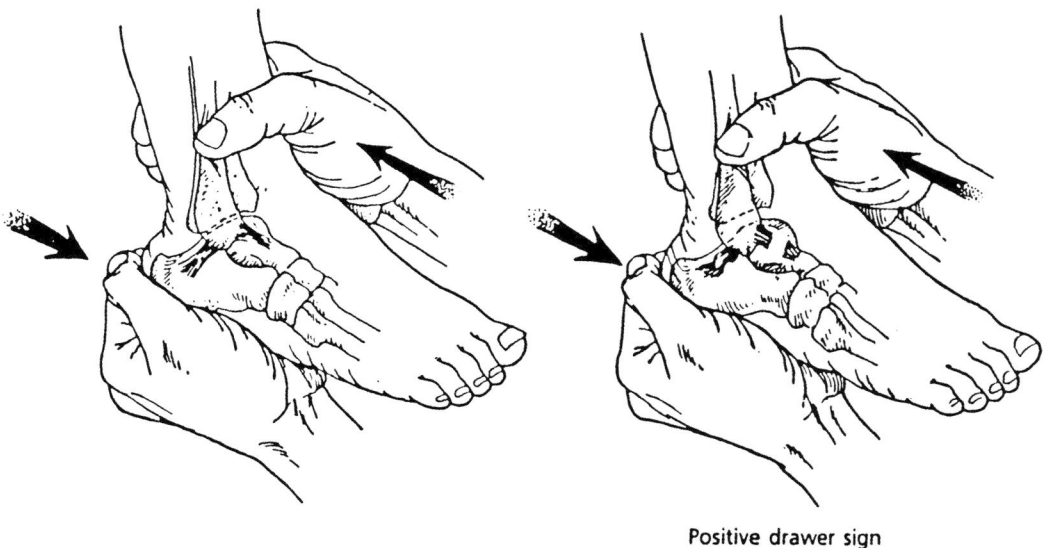

Positive drawer sign

Figure 26-26. Anterior drawer test. The anterior talofibular ligament resists anterior ankle stress. The anterior drawer test is positive when this ligament is disrupted and will detect excessive anterior translation of the foot on the leg. (Reproduced with permission from American Academy of Orthopaedic Surgeons. *Athletic Training and Sports Medicine.* 2nd ed. American Academy of Orthopaedic Surgeons; 1991:414.)

Knee Ligament Sprains

The knee is situated between the two largest bones, the femur and the tibia, and is spanned by the body's strongest muscles, the quadriceps and hamstrings. In general terms, the knee is stabilized by four ligaments: the two collateral ligaments that resist varus and valgus stress and the two cruciate ligaments that primarily resist AP motion (Figure 26-27).

The collateral ligaments are usually damaged by trauma. The anterior cruciate ligament (ACL) can be injured in isolation in twisting with hyperflexion or hyperextension noncontact modes. The ACL is the only one of the four ligaments that is intrasynovial. In patients with bloody effusions (hemarthrosis) following knee injury, 70% have an ACL injury. In those with an acute ACL tear, 50% have a concomitant meniscus tear. The medial collateral ligament and ACL are frequently injured in combination from a valgus stress (eg, as occurs from a blow to the lateral thigh). When a collateral ligament is severely injured, the knee joint capsule and synovial lining are disrupted. The knee may not contain an effusion because hemorrhage leaks through the torn capsule.

Collateral ligament damage can be detected by local tenderness, pain, and laxity when the knee is manually stressed in a mediolateral (varus/valgus) plane. Laxity tests of an injured knee are always judged in comparison to the normal side. Valgus force on the knee will stress the medial collateral ligament, whereas varus force will test the integrity of the lateral collateral ligament. Full knee extension places the joint in a position of maximal geometric stability. Joint laxity in knee extension, therefore, implies a greater degree of collateral ligament damage. Subtle differences between the laxity on the normal side and that on the injured side can best be detected with the knee at 20° of flexion.

The **anterior drawer test** is used to evaluate cruciate ligament integrity. With the knee flexed 45°, the tibia is pulled forward like a drawer (Figure 26-28). If there is abnormal anterior tibial translation, the anterior drawer test suggests that the anteromedial fibers of the ACL are torn. Conversely, abnormal posterior tibial translation to a posteriorly directed tibial force indicates a posterior cruciate ligament (PCL) injury. Anterior knee laxity may be better appreciated in the 20° knee-flexed position, which is called the Lachman test. This suggests injury to the posterolateral fibers of the ACL.

Isolated medial collateral ligament injuries heal well with immobilization in a hinged cast-brace, which protects the knee from valgus stress. An ACL injury is disabling to most athletes. With cutting and twisting movements, the knee will transiently sublux and give way. PCL-deficient knees are associated with patellar overload and arthritis, because the quadriceps muscle attempts to compensate for increased posterior tibial displacement. The less stout lateral collateral ligament (LCL) is often injured in conjunction with one of the two cruciate ligaments. Acute repairs of combination knee ligament injuries should be strong enough to tolerate early motion to prevent the common postoperative complication of joint stiffness.

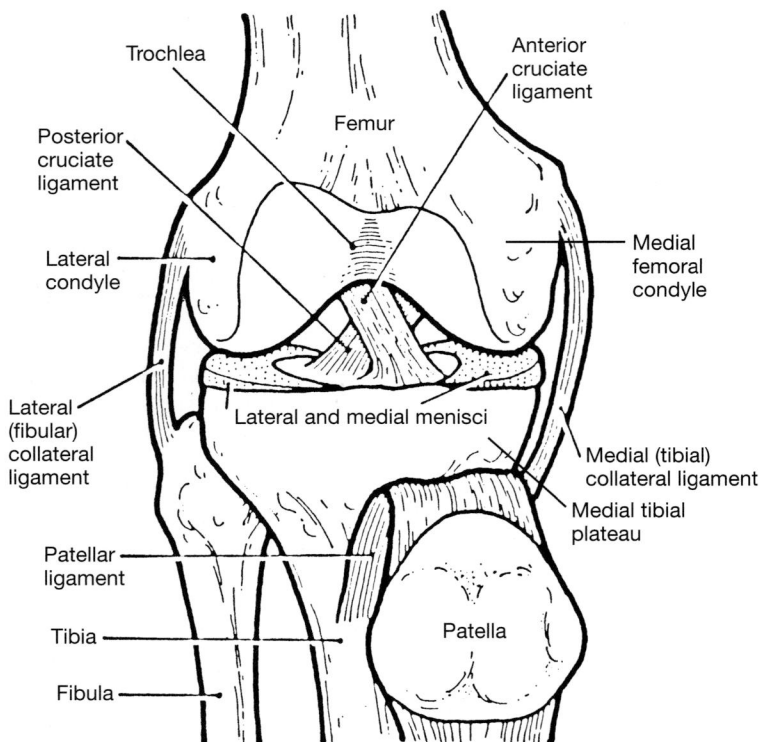

Figure 26-27. Knee joint stability depends on the two collateral and cruciate ligaments. The medial collateral ligament is broad and large and resists varus or abduction stress. The anterior cruciate ligament resists anterior tibial translation, whereas the posterior cruciate prevents posterior tibial shear. (From Lawrence PF. *Essentials of Surgical Specialties.* 3rd ed. Lippincott Williams & Wilkins; 2007.)

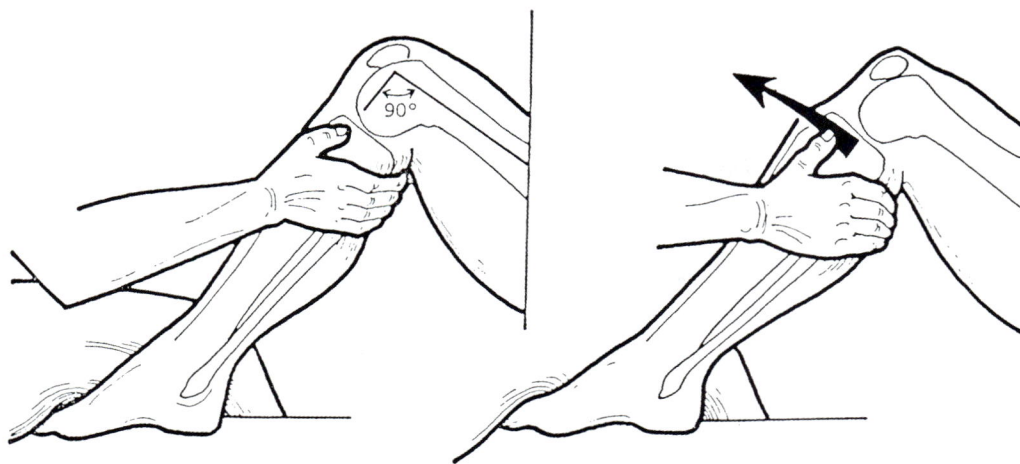

Figure 26-28. **The anterior drawer test is performed with the foot stabilized and the knee flexed 90°.** With the examiner's thumb placed on the joint line, the tibia is pulled anteriorly. Excessive anterior tibial shift suggests that the anterior cruciate ligament is incompetent. The contralateral side can be used as a comparative reference. A similar test performed in 20° of knee flexion is called the Lachman test and is more sensitive in the evaluation of acute injuries. (From Lawrence PF. *Essentials of Surgical Specialties*. 3rd ed. Lippincott Williams & Wilkins; 2007.)

The indications for surgical ligament repair and reconstruction are controversial. In general, younger patients whose activities cause symptoms of instability are candidates for surgery. The ACLs heal poorly and are generally reconstructed with soft tissue autografts from the patellar tendon, hamstrings tendon, or fascia lata.

Meniscal Injury

The knee joint is minimally constrained by virtue of its bony geometry. The medial and lateral meniscal fibrocartilages increase joint surface contact and aid in joint stability. In stance, the menisci transmit 40% to 60% of the weight-bearing load placed across the joint. The menisci also assist with joint lubrication and hyaline cartilage nutrition. The menisci move anterior to posterior as the knee is flexed. In flexion, the menisci are trapped between the femoral condyle and the tibial plateau. If a twisting, rotatory motion occurs when the knee is flexed, the menisci may split longitudinally (Figure 26-29C and D). Meniscal tissue loses hydration and becomes more brittle with age. Shearing, horizontal cleavage tears not seen on the meniscal surface are frequently found in older patients (Figure 26-29A).

Patients with meniscal pathology may have pain and tenderness localized to the joint line (ie, the palpable gap between the femur and the tibia). There may be recurrent effusion. A history of painful giving way suggests a tear located in the posterior portion of the meniscus. Symptoms of intermittent joint locking occur with displaceable and bucket handle tears (Figure 26-29C), in which the torn component of the meniscus becomes trapped between the condyle and acts as a mechanical block to joint motion.

Clinical examination should check for loss of terminal extension (locking), localized joint line tenderness, and provocative test for displaceable meniscus (McMurray test). McMurray test involves flexion of the knee to 90°, followed by internal rotatory movements of the tibia, and then followed by extension into valgus. The test is repeated with tibial rotation in the opposite direction, followed by extension into varus. The test tries to trap a displaceable fragment of the meniscus between the articular surfaces of the tibia and femur. The test is positive if the patient experiences joint line pain and the examiner feels a snap or rub at the joint line.

Longitudinal tears (Figure 26-29D) in the peripheral third of the meniscus will heal when repaired, because this zone is well vascularized. Total meniscectomy leads to the slow

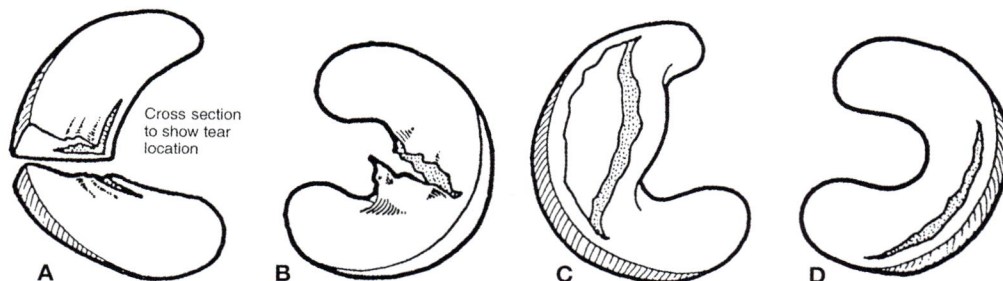

Figure 26-29. **Meniscal tears.** A. Degenerative horizontal tear. B. Radial tear. C. Displaced bucket handle tear. D. Longitudinal tear. (Reproduced with permission from American Academy of Orthopaedic Surgeons. *Athletic Training and Sports Medicine*. 2nd ed. American Academy of Orthopaedic Surgeons; 1991:365.)

development of tibiofemoral arthritis. Irreparable and displaceable meniscal tears causing mechanical symptoms are best treated by arthroscopy and partial excision of the meniscus, leaving the stable, untorn meniscus in situ. Meniscal surgery is performed arthroscopically because it is less traumatic, more precise, and can be performed on an outpatient basis.

Acromioclavicular (Shoulder) Separation

In addition to the glenohumeral articulation, the shoulder is composed of three other joints: the acromioclavicular, sternoclavicular, and scapulothoracic articulations. The acromioclavicular joint rotates approximately 20° with flexion and extension of the shoulder. It is stabilized in this AP (horizontal) plane by the acromioclavicular ligaments (see Figure 26-1). In the craniocaudal direction (coronal plane), the joint is constrained by the stronger coracoclavicular ligaments.

The acromioclavicular joint is injured after a blow or fall onto the point (acromion) of the shoulder. The scapular acromion is driven caudally, whereas the clavicle remains fixed to the chest. If the acromioclavicular ligaments alone are torn and the coracoclavicular ligaments stretched, the injury is classified as grade II; the clavicle is partially displaced (subluxed) from the acromion (see Figure 26-1C). This may not be obvious but can be determined by stress radiographs taken with weights strapped to the patient's wrists. The distance between the clavicle and the coracoid process will be widened on the affected side. When both acromioclavicular and coracoclavicular ligaments are disrupted (grade III), the joint will be dislocated. The distal clavicle will be elevated above the acromion, which is obvious to inspection (see Figure 26-1B). Treatment of a grade III shoulder separation is controversial. Both surgical and nonsurgical methods yield functional results.

Gamekeeper Thumb

The ulnar collateral ligament of the thumb metacarpophalangeal (MCP) joint is a critical structure because it stabilizes the thumb during grip and index finger pinch. As the thumb is out of the plane of the hand, this ligament is vulnerable to abduction stress. It is injured in skiers who fall while still gripping their pole or in ball handling sports (Figure 26-30). Loss of the stabilizing effect of the thumb

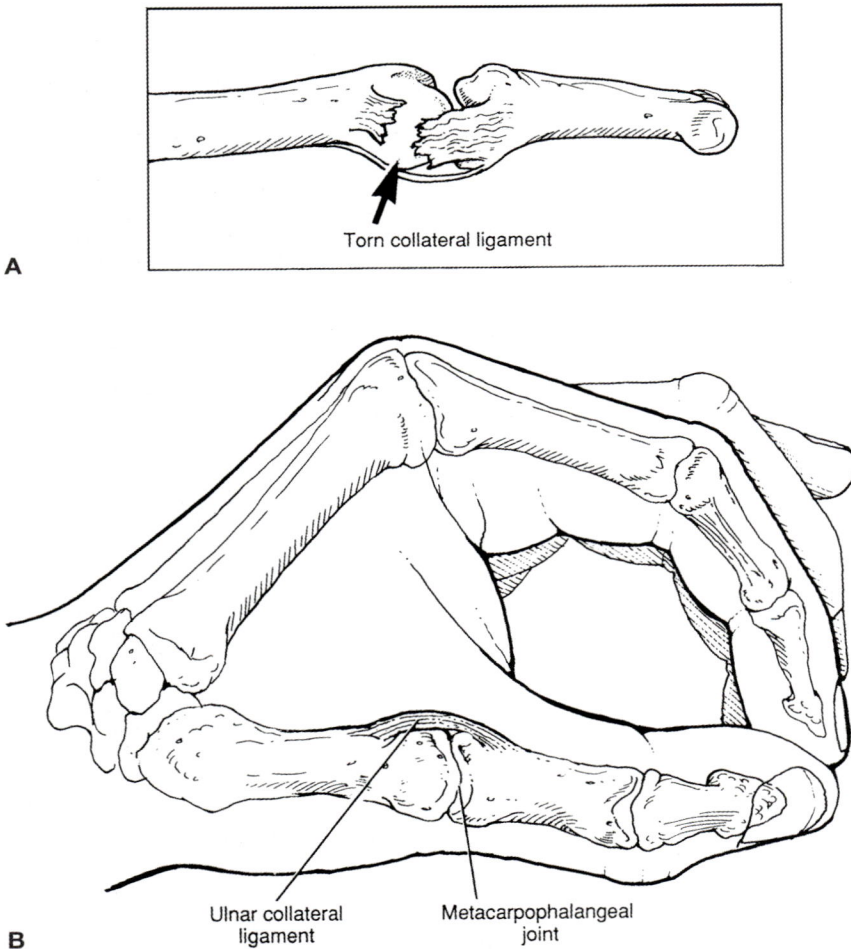

Figure 26-30. A. Lateral depiction of a torn collateral ligament metacarpophalangeal joint. B. The ulnar collateral ligament of the thumb metacarpophalangeal joint is critical to opposable thumb function. Injury to this ligament (gamekeeper thumb) renders the thumb unstable and weakens its contribution to pinch and grip strength. (From Lawrence PF. *Essentials of Surgical Specialties.* 3rd ed. Lippincott Williams & Wilkins; 2007.)

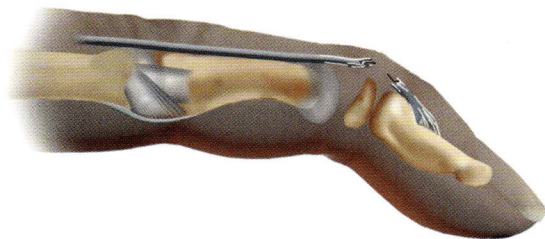

Figure 26-31. Mallet or baseball finger, which results from rupture of the extensor tendon. (Reprinted with permission from Brinker MR. *Review of Orthopaedic Trauma.* 2nd ed. Lippincott Williams & Wilkins; 2013.)

MCP ulnar collateral ligament renders pinch weak and painful. To stress test the ligament, the thumb MCP joint is positioned in 35° of flexion to relax the volar plate and the short thumb flexor. Adductor pollicis aponeurosis may be interposed between the ligament and the proximal phalanx, and this can prevent ligament healing. Ligament exploration with repair or reattachment is performed. Good clinical results are also reported with use of a hand-based adduction splint for 6 weeks.

Mallet (Baseball) Finger

A sudden blow causing flexion to the tip of an extended finger can cause rupture of the digital extensor tendon. The finger distal interphalangeal (DIP) joint is in a flexed position, and the patient cannot actively extend this joint (Figure 26-31). This injury heals well if splinted in full DIP extension for 6 weeks.

Boxer Fracture

The index and long finger metacarpals have limited mobility and act as rigid posts for the fine precision work of the hand. In contrast, the ring and little finger metacarpals are more mobile and are important to power grip because motion is needed for these fingers to surround an object. For a fist to impart maximal kinetic energy, the more rigid radial side of the fist should strike the object. When the ulnar fist strikes an object, the little finger metacarpal neck often fractures (**boxer fracture**). With marked amounts of fracture angulation (>45°), closed reduction and plaster immobilization is the preferred and usually successful treatment. Occasionally, percutaneous pins may be required to stabilize a very unstable fracture.

Achilles Tendon Rupture

Achilles tendon ruptures occur in the middle-aged athlete who stresses the tendon beyond its tolerance. Systemic and local steroid injections weaken tendinous tissue and predispose it to rupture. With an Achilles tendon rupture, the athlete feels a severe pain in the calf. There may be swelling, ecchymosis, and, sometimes, a palpable gap between the tendon ends. Active plantar flexion of the ankle is weak but present because the tibialis posterior and long toe flexors are still functional.

The **Thompson test** (Figure 26-32) verifies whether the gastrocnemius-soleus complex is intact. With the patient lying prone and the foot hanging free over this end of the stretcher, the examiner squeezes the calf muscle belly. Normally, the foot plantar flexes. Lack of plantar flexion indicates that the Achilles tendon is torn. The diagnosis can be easily confirmed by ultrasound.

Nonoperative treatment in a long leg cast with the foot in plantar flexion permits excellent tendon healing. This method is cumbersome. Surgical treatment may be more expeditious for athletes. Both types of treatment are effective.

Turf Toe

Turf toe is a hyperextension injury to the great toe metatarsophalangeal (MTP) joint (Figure 26-33). The flexor hallucis brevis tendon is ruptured either at its proximal phalangeal insertion or by a fracture of its sesamoid

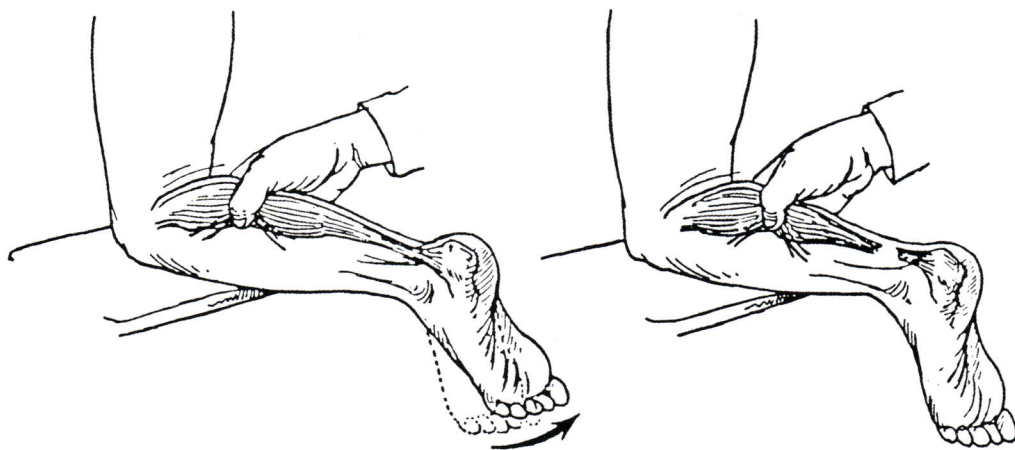

Figure 26-32. The Thompson test will provoke ankle plantar flexion when the gastrocnemius-soleus Achilles tendon complex is intact. Absence of this response indicates a tear of the Achilles tendon. (From Lawrence PF. *Essentials of Surgical Specialties.* 3rd ed. Lippincott Williams & Wilkins; 2007.)

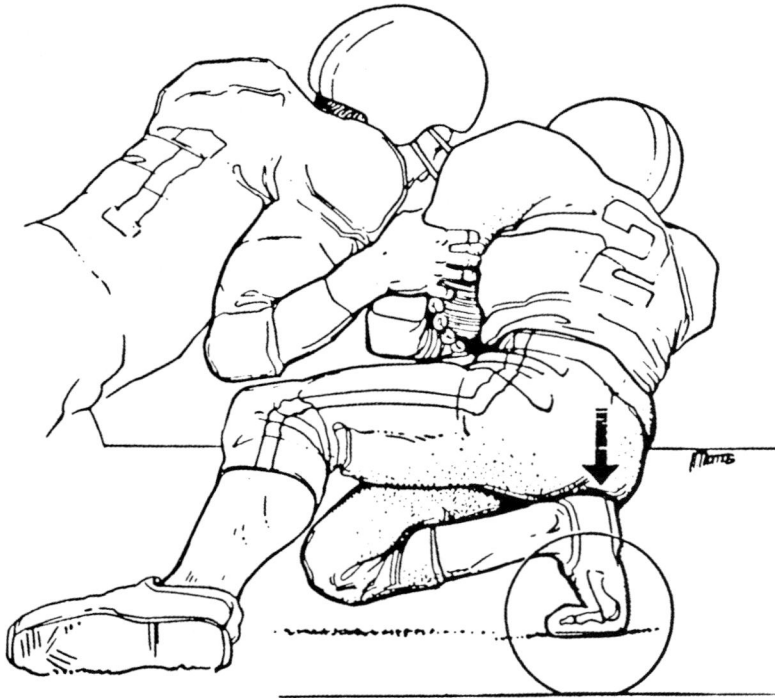

Figure 26-33. A turf toe injury occurs from hyperdorsiflexion of the great toe metatarsophalangeal joint and ruptures the flexor hallucis brevis mechanism through the tendon or its sesamoid bone. (Reprinted with permission from Rodeo SA, O'Brien S, Warren RF, Barnes R, Wickiewicz TL, Dillingham MF. Turf toe: an analysis of metatarsophalangeal joint sprains in professional football players. *Am J Sports Med.* 1990;18:280-285.)

bones. The plantar plate may also be torn. The injury occurs during football pileups, in which a player falls on the posterior aspect of a prone player's foot, hyperextending the great toe. The injured player experiences exquisite plantar great toe pain exacerbated by passive extension of the MTP joint. The toe-off, propulsive phase of gait is painful. Treatment consists of rest, taping of the toe in plantar flexion, and the use of a stiff forefoot, in-shoe orthosis. Untreated turf toe has been implicated as the cause of great toe MTP arthritis and loss of extension known as hallux rigidus.

Myositis Ossificans

Bone deposited in a muscle after a blunt injury is known as traumatic myositis ossificans (Figure 26-34). When a deep muscle (often the quadriceps) is contused, the muscle closest to bone has the greatest amount of direct damage. Either a metaplasia of muscle cells or a release of osteogenic material from the underlying bone causes bone to form within the injured muscle. Early symptoms are deep muscle tenderness and loss of joint motion. The condition is self-limited and may be decreased by nonsteroidal anti-inflammatory agents. If the lesion is large or causes mechanical problems, surgical excision is indicated. When a lesion is resected early (ie, before 18 months), there is a high rate of recurrence. A systemic form of myositis ossificans occurs in patients with traumatic paralysis or extensive burns.

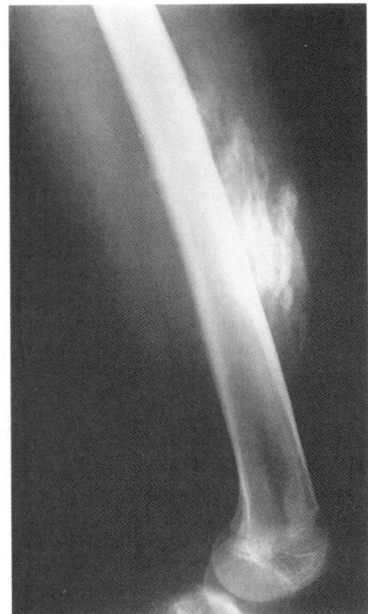

Figure 26-34. Myositis ossificans. Bone deposition in the quadriceps muscle after an anterior thigh contusion. (From Lawrence PF. *Essentials of Surgical Specialties.* 3rd ed. Lippincott Williams & Wilkins; 2007.)

PEDIATRIC MUSCULOSKELETAL PROBLEMS

The term **orthopedic** is derived from the Greek word for straight, *orthos,* and the word for child, *pais.* The diagnosis and treatment of pediatric deformities thus represent the origin of the specialty of orthopedics. This section deals with common pediatric musculoskeletal disorders.

LOWER LIMB TORSION: IN-TOEING AND OUT-TOEING

The most common childhood "deformities" are actually normal variations of musculoskeletal development. Flat feet, bowlegs, knock-knees, in-toeing, and out-toeing are commonly seen in young children but are unusual in adolescence. Because these conditions seem to resolve spontaneously, they must be considered part of the natural process of skeletal growth and development. The first 2 years of life are a remarkable period of physical growth. The average child attains almost half of its adult size and stature during these first 2 years. Body structure also changes radically as the skeletal frame is subjected to the demands of locomotion and bipedal gait.

The common rotational deformities of in-toeing and out-toeing can be ascribed to one of three lower limb sites: the femur (anteversion or retroversion), the tibia (internal or external torsion), or the forefoot (metatarsus adductus). Although rotational variations may run in families, the most common cause is the intrauterine positioning (Figure 26-35). Certain sleeping or sitting postures may accentuate these conditions and delay their resolution. The femoral version describes the anatomic relationship of the femoral head and neck with the femoral shaft. The femoral neck is offset from the shaft in the coronal plane. This relation, called femoral anteversion, is seen if one looks down the shaft of the femur as one would a gun barrel: The femoral neck is canted an average of 10° to 15° anterior (Figure 26-36). At birth, femoral anteversion averages about 40°. It decreases to 10° by adulthood, with most of the change occurring in the first 3 years of life (Figure 26-37).

All rotational deformities are best evaluated with the child placed prone. Femoral anteversion is present when medial or inward rotation of the femur is in excess of 30° more than external femoral rotation (Figure 26-38). When external (outward) femoral rotation is excessive, femoral retroversion is present.

When the prone child is viewed from above with their knee flexed, the angle that the sole of the foot makes with the thigh (ie, the thigh-foot angle) allows for assessment of internal versus external tibial torsion (Figure 26-39A). The normal lateral border of the foot is straight. If it is curved inward or its lateral border is convex, metatarsus adductus is present (Figure 26-39B). If the foot is flexible and can be passively corrected to neutral alignment, treatment is probably unnecessary. When the deformity is rigid, corrective serial casting is beneficial. Metatarsus adductus is often associated with internal tibial torsion. Both result from fetal positioning, the latter being the most common cause of rotational lower extremity problems (see Figure 26-35).

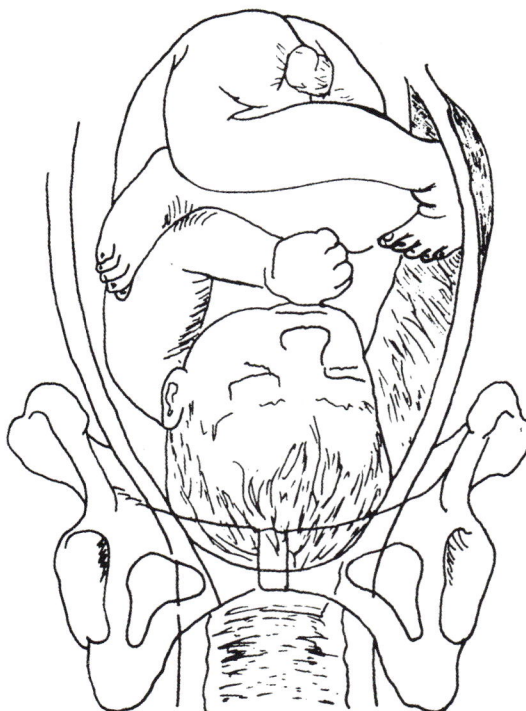

Figure 26-35. Cramped intrauterine confines often mold the child's plastic bone structure. Note that in utero fetal posture forces the tibias to be internally rotated and the forefeet adducted. (From Lawrence PF. *Essentials of Surgical Specialties.* 3rd ed. Lippincott Williams & Wilkins; 2007.)

As the skeleton adapts to growth and bipedal posture, these torsional "deformities" resolve. A slight amount of in-toeing has been noted in the better athletes. In-toeing is advantageous during cutting maneuvers because a limb that is internally rotated will be aligned with the intended change of direction and is more effective in push-off acceleration.

ANGULAR LIMB DEFORMITIES: BOWLEGS AND KNOCK-KNEES

Angular lower limb alignment, bowlegs and knock-knees (genu varum and valgum; see Figure 26-9), are another common cause for an orthopedic consultation. For most children, these conditions represent the spectrum of normal development. It is rare for limb malalignment to persist and cause functional or cosmetic impairment sufficient to require surgical intervention. Normal, nonambulatory infants have physiologic bowlegs with tibiofemoral angles of 20° or more of varus (bow). At approximately 18 months of age, the angle corrects as the femur and tibia become collinear. After 3 years of age, the limbs assume the normal adult alignment of 7° of skeletal valgus (Figure 26-40).

Pathologic conditions can cause knee bowing, including growth arrest of the medial tibial metaphysis, chondrodysplastic dwarfism, and vitamin D–resistant (hypophosphatemic or renal) rickets. These systemic conditions also cause deformities of other bones and joints. If bowlegs persist beyond 2 years of age, radiographic evaluation may be warranted.

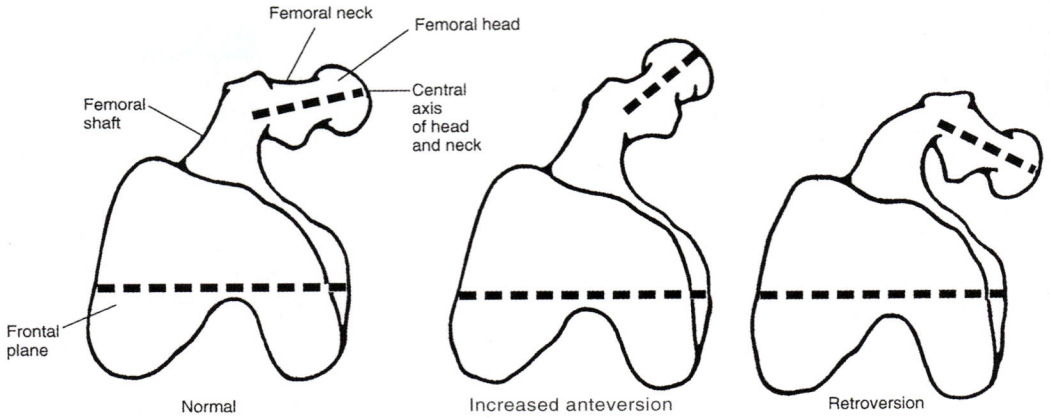

Figure 26-36. **Femoral neck version or torsion as seen from the distal femoral condyles.** (Reprinted with permission from Wilson FC, ed. *The Musculoskeletal System: Basic Processes and Disorders.* 2nd ed. JB Lippincott; 1983.)

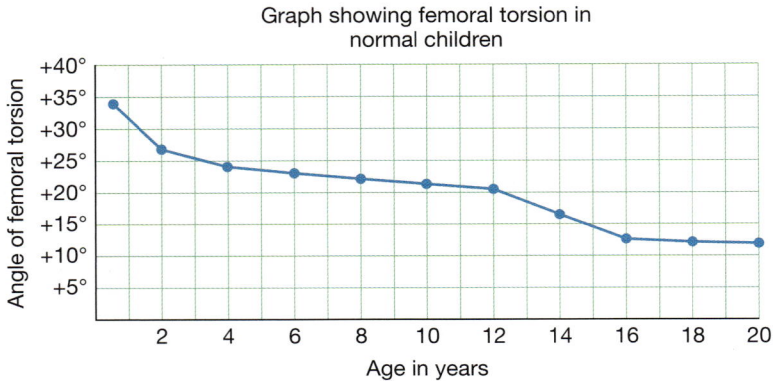

Figure 26-37. **The average amount of femoral anteversion decreases from about 40° at birth to the normal 10° in adulthood.** The most dramatic change occurs within the first 2 years of life. (Reprinted with permission from Dunlap K, Shands AR, Hollister LC, et al. A new method for determination of torsion of the femur. *J Bone Joint Surg.* 1953;35(2):289-311.)

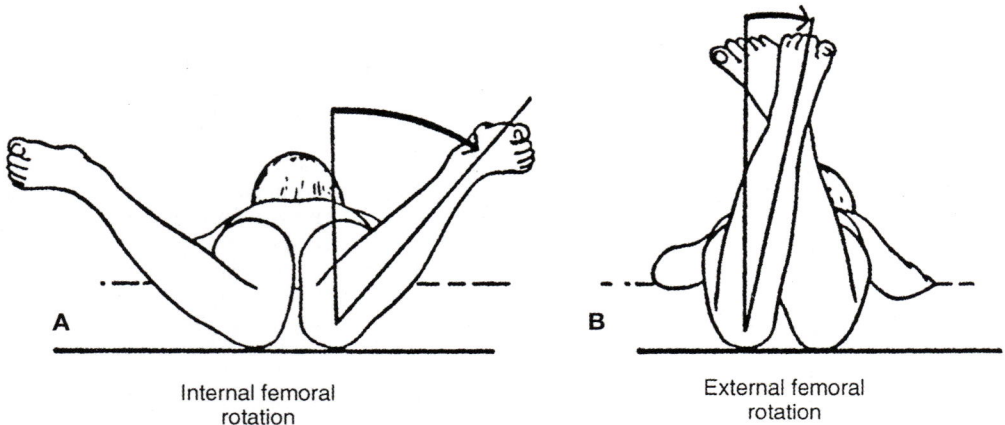

Figure 26-38. **Clinical evaluation of a patient with in-toeing caused by femoral anteversion.** A. Internal femoral rotation is in greater excess than in part B. B. External femoral rotation. (Reprinted from Staheli L. Rotational problems of the lower extremities. *Orthop Clin North Am.* 1987;18:503-512. Copyright © 1987 Elsevier.)

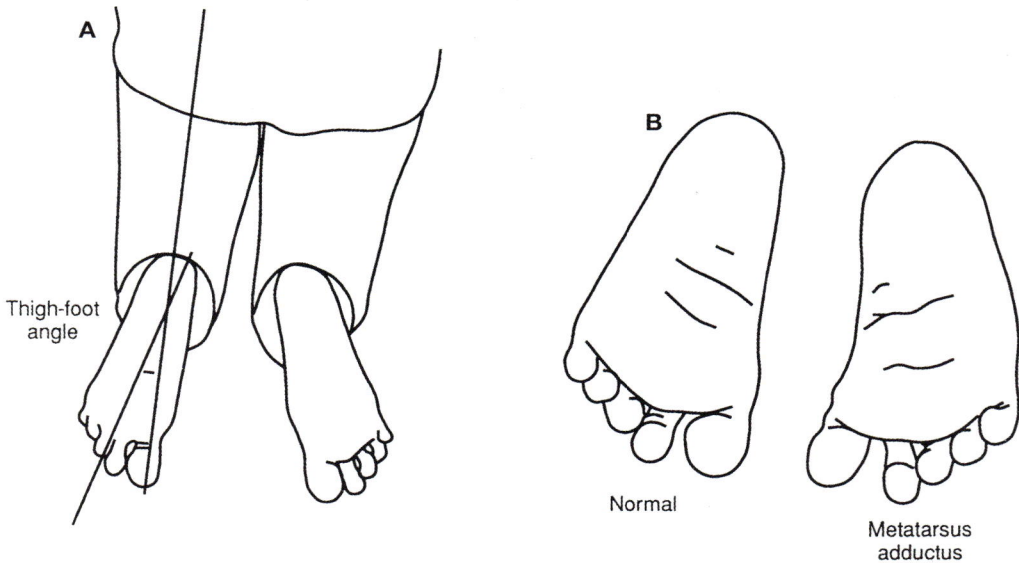

Figure 26-39. A. External tibial torsion is detected by a thigh-foot angle pointed away from the midline. B. Metatarsus adductus as a cause of in-toeing is noted by a convex lateral foot border. If the foot cannot be passively corrected to neutral, the deformity is rigid and may require serial casts for correction. (Reprinted from Staheli L. Rotational problems of the lower extremities. *Orthop Clin North Am.* 1987:18:503-512. Copyright © 1987 Elsevier.)

FLAT FEET

Flat feet are another common skeletal variation. The most common type is the flexible flat foot. The longitudinal arch of the foot is absent or flat in stance but reconstitutes when the foot is non–weight bearing. Most flexible flat feet are asymptomatic and result from ligamentous laxity affecting the many small joints of the midfoot. A flat foot that is rigid and has little passive motion may be caused by a congenital coalition of the tarsal bones. A flat foot associated with a tight heel cord may be caused by muscular dystrophy or cerebral palsy. High-arched feet (pes cavus) with clawed toes are the sequelae of peripheral neuropathies, such as hereditary motor and sensory neuropathy (formerly known as Charcot-Marie-Tooth disease).

DEVELOPMENTAL DYSPLASIA OF THE HIP

The incidence of developmental dysplasia of the hip, previously referred to as congenital dislocation of the hip, is 1.5 per 1,000 newborns. One-third of cases are bilateral. The condition shows a familial predisposition and is associated with intrauterine breech presentations. Girls are affected much more often than boys, possibly because their ligaments are more sensitive to the relaxing effects of maternal estrogen released in preparation for birth.

The early diagnosis of developmental dysplasia of the hip allows early treatment. All newborns and infants must be examined for hip instability. The diagnosis is never obvious but must be sought by careful examination. Limited or asymmetrical thigh abduction suggests a hip abnormality

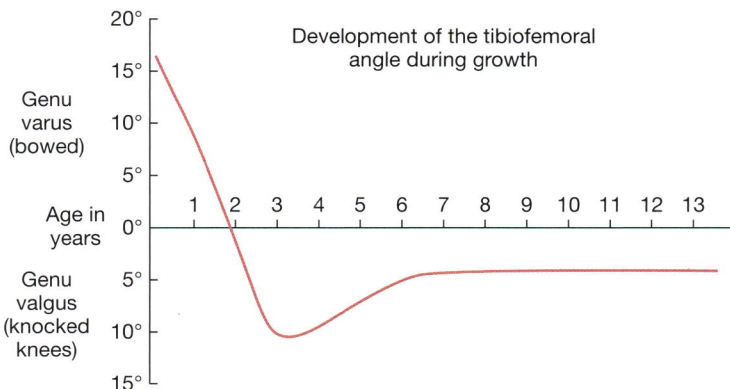

Figure 26-40. Changes in tibiofemoral alignment with growth show that there is a natural progression from bowlegs at birth to physiologic knock-knees by the age of 3. (Modified from Kling T. Angular deformities of the lower limb in children. *Orthop Clin North Am.* 1987;18:513-527. Copyright © 1987 Elsevier.)

(Figure 26-41). The infant's thigh is gently grasped by the long finger and thumb. With the hip and knee flexed 90°, the thigh is abducted, whereas the greater trochanter is gently pressed forward in an anterior direction. A palpable jump or click during this maneuver—Ortolani sign—signifies that the femoral head has been reduced into the acetabulum and that the hip was dislocated. An opposite, provocation maneuver, in which adduction and posterior pressure is applied by the thumbs over the femoral head, will lever the hip out of the acetabulum (Barlow sign) if the hip is unstable. These two tests are useful in the first 2 weeks of life when the child's ligaments are under the relaxing influence of maternal hormones. Treatment is most successful early in life and is accomplished by manipulative reduction (Ortolani maneuver) and immobilization with the hips in a stable position of flexion and abduction using a Pavlik harness. If the hip remains dislocated, the acetabular socket does not develop normally and remains shallow.

After 1 month of age, limited hip abduction is the most reliable sign of developmental dysplasia of the hip (Figure 26-41). Asymmetry of thigh and buttock folds or telescoping of the flexed femur are other signs of late hip dislocation. When the condition is bilateral, all physical signs that depend on noting asymmetry will be absent, making diagnosis more difficult. When the child begins walking, a short leg limp is evident when the hip dislocation is unilateral. A waddling, hyperlordotic gait is apparent if the condition is bilateral. Treatment after walking age is more difficult. Contracted hip muscles are gradually stretched with traction or an adductor muscle release. Operative hip reduction is likely needed, and the reduced hip must be maintained in a cast.

The head of the femur is cartilaginous until almost 9 months of age and is not visible on radiograph. (Radiographs are, therefore, of limited early diagnostic value.) Ultrasonography shows cartilage well and is useful in the first 9 months. Hip joint ultrasound can dynamically evaluate the hip under positional stress. After the femoral head ossifies, radiograph shows a dislocated hip to be displaced lateral and superior to a shallow acetabulum.

The management of developmental dysplasia of the hip requires prompt attention by an orthopedic specialist.

When treatment is initiated early and followed closely, the prognosis for normal hip development and function is good.

LEGG-CALVÉ-PERTHES DISEASE

Legg-Calvé-Perthes is a condition of uncertain etiology that results in osteonecrosis of the femoral head in children aged 4 to 8 years. Boys are affected 8 times more commonly than girls. Hip discomfort may be referred to the medial knee in the distribution of the obturator nerve. Therefore, pediatric patients complaining of knee pain should have their hips examined. The hip will display a subtle decrease in range of motion, especially in abduction and internal rotation. Hip abduction strength is also decreased and may cause a Trendelenburg limp, in which the child leans the torso over the affected hip.

Legg-Calvé-Perthes disease is self-limited and runs a 2- to 4-year course. Initial radiographs show minimal findings and may show disuse osteoporosis and hip joint space widening. Later, when the dead bone is being resorbed and revascularized, new bone is laid down on dead bone, causing the femoral head to appear dense (sclerotic). During this revascularization stage, radiographic changes are most dramatic. Pathologic fractures of dead trabeculae may occur with weight-bearing loads, causing a flattening of the femoral head. The femoral head may appear fragmented and laterally displaced. The metaphysis may be rarefied and broadened. A child with Legg-Calvé-Perthes disease should be referred to an orthopedic surgeon. Treatment consists of traction to regain motion followed by bracing or surgical osteotomy to keep the articular portion of the femoral head within the weight-bearing portion of the acetabulum. This may involve femoral or pelvic osteotomies.

SLIPPED CAPITAL FEMORAL EPIPHYSIS

A cause of limping in adolescence is a fracture of the proximal femoral growth plate or slipped capital femoral epiphysis. A slipped capital femoral epiphysis is more common in

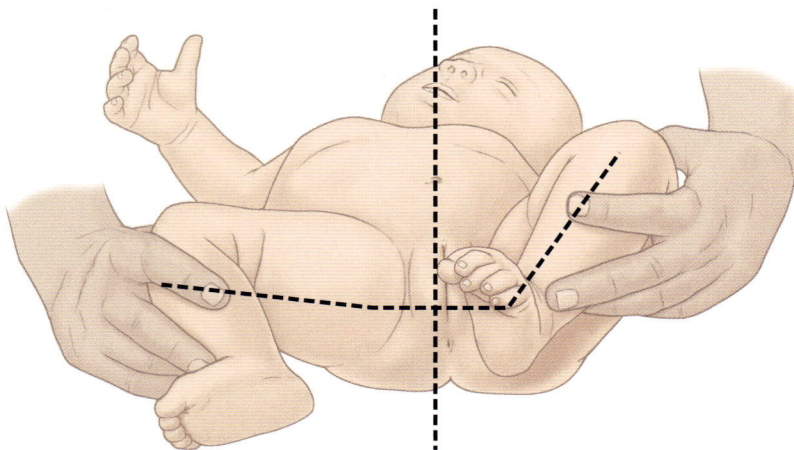

Figure 26-41. Limited hip abduction in congenital hip dislocation. The perineum should be perpendicular to the table. The limit of true hip joint motion is evidenced by concomitant movement of the perineum.

boys than girls, is bilateral in approximately 33% of cases, and usually occurs during the prepubescent growth spurt (ie, 10-14 years of age). Two distinctly different body types are susceptible to the condition. One group consists of children who are obese with delayed gonadal development; the other includes very tall children who have grown rapidly.

In addition to a limp, patients may have pain localized to the knee or, less frequently, to the groin. The affected leg is held externally rotated. Internal hip rotation is limited and painful. An AP and Frog lateral pelvis radiograph is ordered to compare the painful hip to the other side. It is common for this condition to affect both hips. On AP radiographs, a line drawn tangential to the superior femoral neck does not intersect the femoral head epiphysis as it does in a normal hip (Figure 26-42A). Displacement is more apparent on the lateral radiograph, in which the femoral head appears posteriorly on the femoral neck (Figure 26-42B). Untreated, this femoral head/neck slippage can continue until growth ceases. To prevent further displacement, the femoral head is fixed with multiple pins.

OSGOOD-SCHLATTER DISEASE

Osgood-Schlatter disease affects the insertion of the patellar tendon onto the tibial tubercle. It is believed to represent partial avulsion of the tibial tubercle in active children with avascular necrosis of the avulsed portion. The patient complains of pain over the tibial tubercle aggravated by kneeling, direct pressure, and running. The area is prominent and tender. Radiographs show irregular areas of bone deposition and resorption in the tibial tubercle. The condition is usually self-limiting and resolves as the growth plates close. Occasionally, a painful ununited nodule persists and is treated by excision.

CONGENITAL CLUB FOOT

The etiology of congenital club foot (**talipes equinovarus**) is unknown. It occurs in approximately 1 per 1,000 births and is twice as common in males as in females. Club feet are bilateral in 33% of cases. The condition is characterized by three deformities: the ankle or talus is plantar flexed (equinus), the hindfoot or calcaneus is inverted into varus, and the navicular bone and forefoot are shifted medially and supinated (metatarsus adductus; see Figure 26-39B). Untreated, this deformity causes the patient to walk on the lateral border of the foot, not upon the sole. The posterior muscles of the leg are atrophic and contracted. Neuromuscular abnormalities must be excluded in children with a club foot. Corrective casts are applied immediately with the gradual application of force directed to correct each of the three deformities. When a club foot is refractory to serial cast correction, surgical release of the tight soft tissue structures of the posteromedial foot and ankle is indicated.

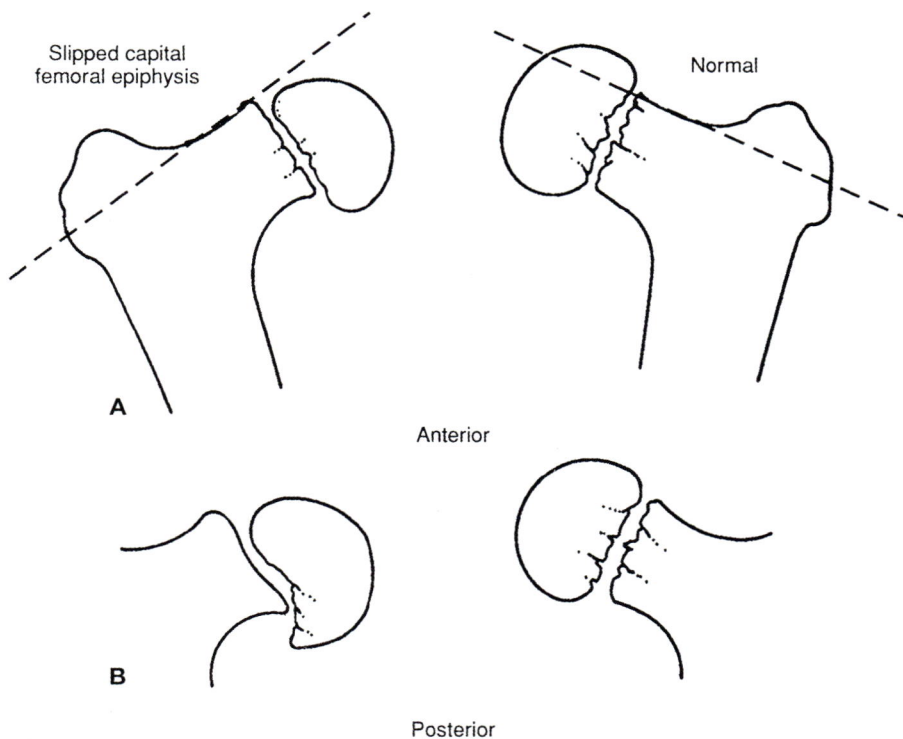

Figure 26-42. Slipped capital femoral epiphysis. The slipped capital femoral epiphysis on the left is compared to the normal hip on the right. A. On anteroposterior radiograph, a line drawn tangential to the top of the femoral neck should pass through the normal femoral head (right). In a slipped femoral epiphysis, the line does not intersect the head but passes above it (left). B. On a lateral radiograph, the head of the femur has slipped posterior to the femoral neck (left). (From Lawrence PF. *Essentials of Surgical Specialties.* 3rd ed. Lippincott Williams & Wilkins; 2007.)

SCOLIOSIS

Scoliosis is a curvature of the spine that is either flexible (correctable) or fixed (structural). A mobile form of scoliosis may be due to poor posture, the muscle spasm secondary to a prolapsed disk, or as compensation for a shortened leg. A fixed, structural scoliosis is accompanied by a rotational vertebral deformity that is not correctable by a change in posture. Scoliosis causes an asymmetry of the rib cage that is most noticeable when the patient bends forward. In stance, if the trunk is laterally shifted and not centered over the pelvis, the scoliotic curve is said to be decompensated. Decompensated scoliosis may be associated with a higher incidence of back pain.

Structural scoliosis can be caused by congenital vertebral deformities, neuromuscular diseases (eg, myelomeningocele, cerebral palsy), or neurofibromatosis. Congenital scoliosis is due to abnormalities of vertebral formation. It is manifested at a young age and is rapidly progressive. These children frequently have associated neural tube, genitourinary, and cardiovascular malformations that occur at the same stage of embryologic development. A comprehensive assessment of these organ systems is mandated in the child in whom congenital scoliosis is identified. Neuromuscular scoliotic curves usually involve the full length of the spine. These curves result from paraspinal muscle imbalance produced by diseases such as polio, spinal muscle atrophy, cerebral palsy, and muscular dystrophies. The scoliosis of neurofibromatosis is characterized by a short but severe curve.

The most common cause of scoliosis is idiopathic. It causes a painless progressive deformity of the thoracolumbar spine during adolescence. Girls are affected 9 times more frequently than boys. The spinal deformity begins before puberty but increases most rapidly during the adolescent growth spurt. As the scoliotic curvature increases, the shape of the vertebrae and the attached ribs change. The vertebral bodies become wedge shaped, and the ribs prominent on the convex side of the curve. These changes of vertebral structure explain why the curves become inflexible over time. Aside from cosmetic concerns, severe thoracic spinal curves can compromise cardiopulmonary function. Some patients with large curves also develop degenerative spinal joint pain. Curve progression is more likely in young patients with larger curves. The goal of treatment is to prevent the scoliotic curve from increasing in magnitude. Spinal braces work well in smaller curves but must be worn until the cessation of growth. Larger curves or scoliosis that occur with congenital or neuromuscular conditions that progress rapidly in severity despite bracing are managed with surgical correction and spinal fusion.

INFECTIOUS DISEASES OF THE MUSCULOSKELETAL SYSTEM

Musculoskeletal infection involves either bone (osteomyelitis), joints (septic arthritis), or soft tissues. Gram-positive organisms, primarily staphylococci, are usually the causative microbes. Gram-negative organisms have been increasing as a cause, especially in compromised hosts and in the nosocomial environment.

OSTEOMYELITIS

Bacteria may infect bone by one of the following four mechanisms:

1. Hematogenous spread from a distant site
2. Contamination from an open fracture
3. After an operative procedure on bone
4. Extension from a contiguous infected foci

Acute Hematogenous Osteomyelitis

Acute osteomyelitis occurs most commonly in children and is due to hematogenous spread from a distant site of infection. In the 0- to 3-month age group, the common causative organisms are coliforms from the maternal birth canal to which the infant is exposed during delivery. *Haemophilus influenzae* from otitis media and pharyngeal sources is common until age 3. *Staphylococcus aureus,* which predominates in skin infections, is common in all age groups.

Pathology

In children, metaphyseal capillaries turn back toward the diaphysis at the level of the growth plate, forming a turbulent area where organisms may be deposited. Because of this peculiarity of intraosseous vascular anatomy the metaphyses of long bones are the most common foci of acute hematogenous osteomyelitis. Metaphyseal vessels cross the epiphyseal plate during a brief period of neonatal development, which permits epiphyseal infection to occur in infancy.

As trapped bacteria multiply and pus forms in metaphyseal tissue, the pressure within the unyielding bone causes intense pain, forcing the infection through the thin metaphyseal cortex to elevate and spread beneath the periosteum as a subperiosteal abscess (Figure 26-43). Periosteal stripping stimulates new bone formation that is seen on radiographs. The infection may envelop the bone or burst through the periosteum into the soft tissues.

Clinical Presentation

The onset is acute, and progression can be rapid, even life-threatening. The child experiences severe pain near the end of a long bone and guards the limb, unwilling to move it. With septicemia, there may be fever, increased irritability, or malaise. Soft tissue swelling occurs late and indicates that the infection has spread beyond the bone. The white blood cell (WBC) count and erythrocyte sedimentation rate (ESR) are usually elevated. Radiographic changes occur late and may not provide evidence of infection for 1 week or more. A three-phase technetium pyrophosphate bone scan can distinguish among soft tissue cellulitis, rheumatic fever, and acute hematogenous osteomyelitis earlier in its clinical course.

Evaluation and Treatment

Blood cultures should be obtained along with a bone marrow aspirate for cultures and Gram stain. Parenteral antibiotic treatment should be initiated to cover organisms common to the child's age group, and final antibiotic selection will depend on the results of bacteriologic cultures and sensitivities. If local and systemic manifestations of the infection have not improved within 24 hours, open surgical drainage of subperiosteal pus is indicated, as is

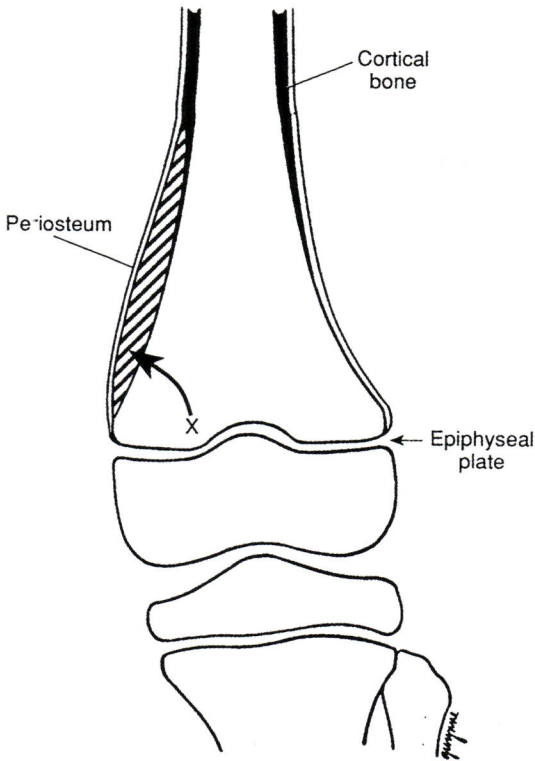

Figure 26-43. Osteomyelitis begins in the bony metaphysis, where hematogenous spread leaves bacteria entrapped in the end arteriolar system of interosseous blood vessels. With exponential bacterial reproduction, pressure within the unyielding bone causes pain and forces the infection through the thin metaphyseal cortex to form a subperiosteal abscess. The epiphyseal plate and periosteum provide a temporary barrier to the infection. X, infected foci; arrow, path of infection; shaded area, periosteum stripped from bone. (Modified with permission from Salter RB. *Textbook of Disorders and Injuries of the Musculoskeletal System.* 3rd ed. Lippincott Williams & Wilkins; 1999.)

bone drilling. Antibiotic therapy should be continued for at least 3 weeks to fully eradicate the organism. Serial sedimentation rates are useful in monitoring the therapeutic response: Elevated rates should return to normal values as the infection resolves. Late complications of hematogenous osteomyelitis include the development of persistent or recurrent chronic osteomyelitis, pathologic fractures, and growth disturbances from epiphyseal plate injury.

Adult osteomyelitis typically occurs after an open fracture or as a complication of surgery. Proper management of open fractures with aggressive and repeated debridement of devitalized tissue, wound irrigation, appropriate antibiotic coverage, fracture stabilization, and delayed wound closure serve to decrease the incidence of posttraumatic infection. A clean operative environment (eg, room, air, personnel), nontraumatic tissue handling, adequate hemostasis, and prophylactic antibiotic administration—especially in implant surgery—are surgical methods that prevent postoperative infections. Effective treatment of an infected implant requires surgical removal of the implant, debridement, and parenteral antibiotics. *S. aureus* remains

the leading cause of bone infection in adults. Some infections can result from less virulent organisms, such as *Staphylococcus epidermidis*. Diabetic foot infections tend to be due to mixed aerobic and anaerobic bacteria.

Chronic Osteomyelitis

The incomplete eradication of a previous bone infection results in chronic osteomyelitis. Bacteria that have been protected from leukocytes and antibiotics by a surrounding wall of avascular dead bone (sequestrum) remain dormant in the dead bone. Many years after the initial infection, the bacteria can suddenly multiply, form a sinus, and drain, or they can cause an acute recurrence of osteomyelitis. Infected, sequestered bone needs to be surgically debrided (saucerized). Soft tissue coverage may be required to enhance local blood supply and antibiotic delivery. A bone graft or bone transport (distraction osteogenesis) may be necessary if radical amounts of infected bone have been resected.

SEPTIC ARTHRITIS

Pathology

When bacteria invade a synovial joint, the inflammatory process can cause rapid, severe destruction of the articular cartilage. In children, septic arthritis occurs as an extension of hematogenous osteomyelitis. The joints commonly involved are those in which the metaphysis resides within the joint capsule: the hip, elbow, and shoulder. Because the metaphysis is enclosed in the joint capsule, what begins as osteomyelitis can erupt through the cortex to involve the joint in the septic process (Figure 26-44). Thus, in children, the causative organisms of septic arthritis are the same as those involved with osteomyelitis. *Staphylococcus* predominates in all age groups. Gram-negative organisms affect children younger than 3 years. In adults, joint infections occur via hematogenous spread, after penetrating wounds, and rarely as a manifestation of disseminated gonorrhea.

Evaluation

If a newborn is profoundly ill and unresponsive, the diagnosis of septic arthritis may be difficult to establish. The major finding on physical examination is restricted, painful joint motion. The joint is also tender to palpation. Early radiographs and peripheral WBC counts are usually nonspecific. Because treatment delay has dire consequences, the clinical suspicion of septic arthritis is enough to warrant emergency joint fluid aspiration for cell count, culture, and Gram stain. To document that the joint has been entered, an arthrogram should be performed after aspiration. Joint aspiration through an area of cellulitis is contraindicated, because it may introduce organisms into the joint.

In patients with active inflammatory arthritides on suppressive medications, acute septic arthritis can be mistaken for an acute flare of inflammatory arthritis. Joint aspiration for cell count, crystal evaluation, and Gram stain and culture should be performed to rule out infection. A WBC count less than 50,000 is typically noninfectious, whereas greater than 100,000 is infectious. However, a WBC count in the 50,000 to 100,000 range can be either inflammatory or infectious. Once an aspirate of the joint is performed, the patient should be treated with antibiotics pending results of the cell count and Gram stain.

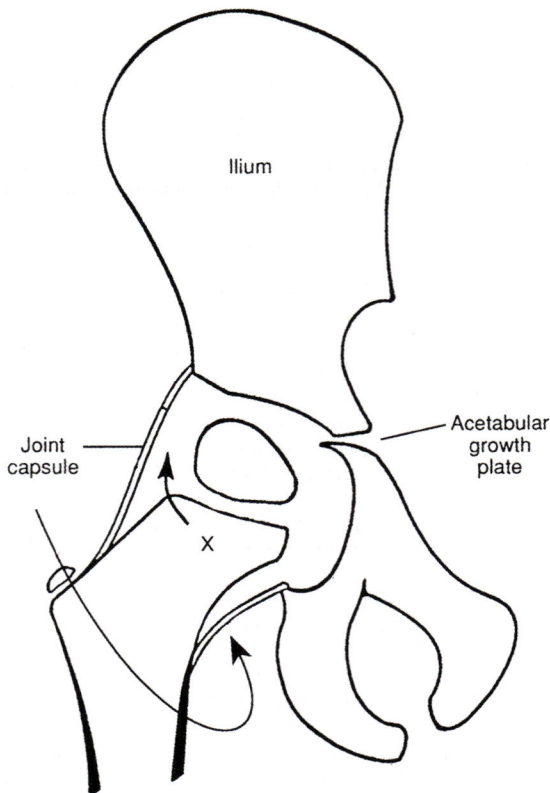

Figure 26-44. In children, septic arthritis occurs as a consequence of hematogenous osteomyelitis. The joints involved are those in which the bony metaphysis resides within a joint capsule, such as the hip. When osteomyelitis erupts through the metaphyseal cortex, it will infect the joint space. X, infected foci; arrow, path of infection. (Modified with permission from Salter RB. *Textbook of Disorders and Injuries of the Musculoskeletal System.* 3rd ed. Lippincott Williams & Wilkins; 1999.)

Treatment

To prevent the rapid degradation of articular cartilage by pyogenic toxins, treatment of a septic joint is an emergency. The most effective treatment is surgical incision of the joint capsule (arthrotomy), drainage, debridement of infected tissue, and joint irrigation. Intravenous antibiotic therapy is started, and the wound is loosely closed over a drain. In the knee, arthroscopic drainage, irrigation, and synovectomy have proven equally effective in the treatment of joint sepsis. The potential complications from septic arthritis include arthritis, epiphyseal necrosis, pathologic joint dislocation, growth disturbances, leg length discrepancies, and limb deformity.

INFECTED HAND FLEXOR TENOSYNOVITIS

Improperly treated hand infections can cause severe disability. A flexor tendon sheath infection is especially serious because it can rapidly destroy the tendon's gliding mechanisms, create adhesions, and cause severe loss of joint motion. Tendon sheath infection can even cause tendon necrosis.

The prevailing infecting organism is *S. aureus*. Pyogenic flexor tenosynovitis is commonly caused by a penetrating palmar injury but can also occur by means of hematogenous seeding.

Kanavel described the four classic physical signs of infected flexor tendon sheaths as follows:

1. The entire digit is enlarged and swollen (looks like a sausage).
2. The finger is held in a flexed posture.
3. There is tenderness over and limited to the course of the tendon sheath (tender with AP pressure, but not with mediolateral pressure).
4. There is exquisite pain with passive digital extension.

Pyogenic hand infections are limb-threatening and require emergency care. If treated early with parenteral high-dose antibiotic therapy, the infectious process may be halted. Failure of symptoms and signs to improve over 24 to 48 hours warrants surgical drainage with irrigation. Early active range of motion exercise is needed to rehabilitate hand function.

NECROTIZING FASCIITIS

Necrotizing fasciitis ("flesh-eating bacteria") is a rare but potentially deadly soft tissue infection of the fascia that occurs most commonly in an immunocompromised host (eg, those with diabetes). Its diagnosis may be complicated by the fact that it can mimic cellulitis or compartment syndrome, and it is rapidly progressive and usually requires emergent diagnosis and treatment. Typically, necrotizing fasciitis develops after a wound has occurred, most commonly the foot, but it can begin without a break in the skin.

There are three types of necrotizing fasciitis. Type 1 is polymicrobial, which is most common in immunocompromised people. Type 2 is the classic group A β-hemolytic *Streptococcus* with or without *S. aureus* and usually seen in previously healthy patients. Type 3 is caused by marine bacteria.

The early clinical presentation involves swelling, erythema, and pain out of proportion to the appearance of the limb. These may rapidly progress to bullae, necrosis of skin and underlying soft tissues, and subcutaneous crepitus. As the infection spreads, signs and symptoms of systemic septic shock may develop. The Laboratory Risk Indicator for Necrotizing Fasciitis (LRINEC) score emphasizes the following abnormal laboratory values as a diagnostic aid: elevated WBC count, glucose, C-reactive protein, and creatinine and low sodium and hemoglobin.

Treatment consists of a combination of emergent wide surgical debridement and intravenous antibiotics. Necrosis of fascia and superficial soft tissues can result in gray, watery, foul-smelling "dishwater" pus, as seen at the time of debridement. Time-to-surgical debridement is the most important factor for limb salvage and survival.

The diagnosis of necrotizing fasciitis should be considered for any individual who has unexplained limb pain and the above abnormal laboratory values. Because of its fulminant course, loss of limb and life are not uncommon, and even today, mortality rates can approach 25%.

INFLAMMATORY DISEASES OF THE MUSCULOSKELETAL SYSTEM

Arthritis means joint inflammation. The two common forms are **osteoarthrosis** and **rheumatoid arthritis**. The management of arthritis as it affects specific joints is well described in orthopedic and rheumatology texts. In this section, treatment is discussed in general terms.

OSTEOARTHROSIS

Osteoarthrosis, also called degenerative joint disease, is the most prevalent form of arthritis affecting adults and is characterized by the progressive narrowing of articular cartilage, sclerosis in the subchondral regions, and a hypertrophic response of bone and cartilage (osteophyte formation). In the adult population older than 65 years, there will be radiographic evidence of joint degeneration affecting one or more joints. Its incidence increases with age and has no sex predilection. The etiology of osteoarthrosis is not clearly understood; however, mechanical joint stresses are related to its development, and arthrosis results from joint surface incongruity, malalignment, and joint instability.

Pathology

Articular cartilage has physical properties that tolerate a limited amount of stress per unit surface area. When these forces are exceeded, the cartilage will show signs of wear. Pathologically, articular cartilage becomes softened, frayed, and eventually fibrillated. Focal cartilage erosions become widespread and expose the underlying subchondral bone. This bone becomes sclerotic and stiff as the trabeculae thicken and cysts form. At the periphery of the joint, spur-like bony outgrowths covered by hyaline cartilage (osteophytes) develop. Osteophytes are a biologic attempt to decrease joint stress by increasing joint surface area and decreasing motion.

The radiologic hallmarks of **osteoarthrosis** are as follows (Figure 26-45):

Localized joint space narrowing
Subchondral bone sclerosis
Osteophytes
Subchondral cysts

Symptoms of degenerative joint disease begin gradually with joint pain brought on by activity and relieved by rest. The patient may report a history of joint swelling, stiffness, and slow, progressive loss of joint motion. Because the articular cartilage has no nerve supply, the pain of osteoarthritis is believed to originate in the periarticular structures. Pain and crepitus (a grinding sensation) occur with joint motion, and signs and symptoms often correlate with the degree and extent of radiographic abnormalities. It must be emphasized that osteoarthrosis is generally a local disease. Multiple joint involvement suggests a systemic process (inflammatory arthritis).

While weight-bearing joints (eg, hip and knee) are most frequently involved, degenerative joint disease may also occur in the hand or in the great toe at the MTP joint. If present in the hand, it commonly affects the trapeziometacarpal joint in the thumb, and pain occurs at the base of the thumb with pinching.

Treatment

Nonsurgical Treatment

The goal of nonsurgical treatment of osteoarthrosis is to relieve pain and maintain strength and function. Reduction of joint load by means of activity modifications, weight loss, or walking aids (eg, a cane) may provide some relief from symptoms. Physical therapy alleviates pain with the use of heat while attempting to maintain joint motion and muscle strength through exercise. Medications for osteoarthritis may include simple analgesics, nonsteroidal anti-inflammatory drugs, dietary supplements, or intra-articular injection of steroids of lubricating agents. Simple analgesics (eg, acetaminophen) have been shown to be efficacious in the management of musculoskeletal pain and are recommended. Nonsteroidal anti-inflammatory drugs that interfere with the pain-producing products of inflammation (eg, prostaglandins, lymphokines, kinins) can reduce pain and swelling. These drugs can have adverse effects, including rashes, peptic ulceration, elevation of blood pressure, and tinnitus. Intra-articular steroid injections provide dramatic relief of acute arthritic symptoms. However, the repeated use of steroids may accelerate joint deterioration by deleterious effects on the metabolism of the cartilage. The injection of intra-articular lubricating agents (hyaluronic acid) may provide short-term symptomatic relief of arthritis. There are numerous dietary supplements (eg, glucosamine and chondroitin sulfate) whose benefits in the management of degenerative joint disease have been claimed but have not been substantiated in scientific studies. The role of platelet-enriched plasma on the course of arthritis is not clear at this time.

Surgical Treatment

The selection of surgical procedures depends on the stage, site, and debility caused by the arthrosis. There are four categories of bony procedures: osteotomy for joint realignment, partial joint replacement, total joint replacement, and joint fusion (or arthrodesis). An osteotomy realigns the extremity, corrects deformity, and shifts weight-bearing forces from worn joint surfaces to healthier cartilage. This procedure should be considered in younger patients with degenerative arthrosis of the knee. An example would be a valgus-producing tibial osteotomy for a varus knee with symptomatic medial compartment arthrosis.

Partial joint replacement uses prosthetic components to resurface either the medial, lateral, or patellofemoral compartments of the knee. These devices are used in the presence of single compartment disease with intact cruciate ligaments and functional range of motion. Total joint arthroplasty (Figure 26-45C) involves the replacement of articulating surfaces with low-friction metal and high-molecular-weight polyethylene surfaces. Total joint arthroplasty is an extremely successful procedure that profoundly relieves pain in more than 90% of cases. Joint replacement is not without complications: Prosthetic components wear out, loosen, become infected, and cause local osteoporosis and periprosthetic fractures. Therefore, joint replacement is reserved for patients with advanced **arthrosis** and a relatively sedentary lifestyle.

Joint arthrodesis is an effective procedure that converts painful arthritic joint motion into a painless, stable, stiff joint. Arthrodesis is a durable procedure that is indicated in young, very active patients with isolated joint involvement

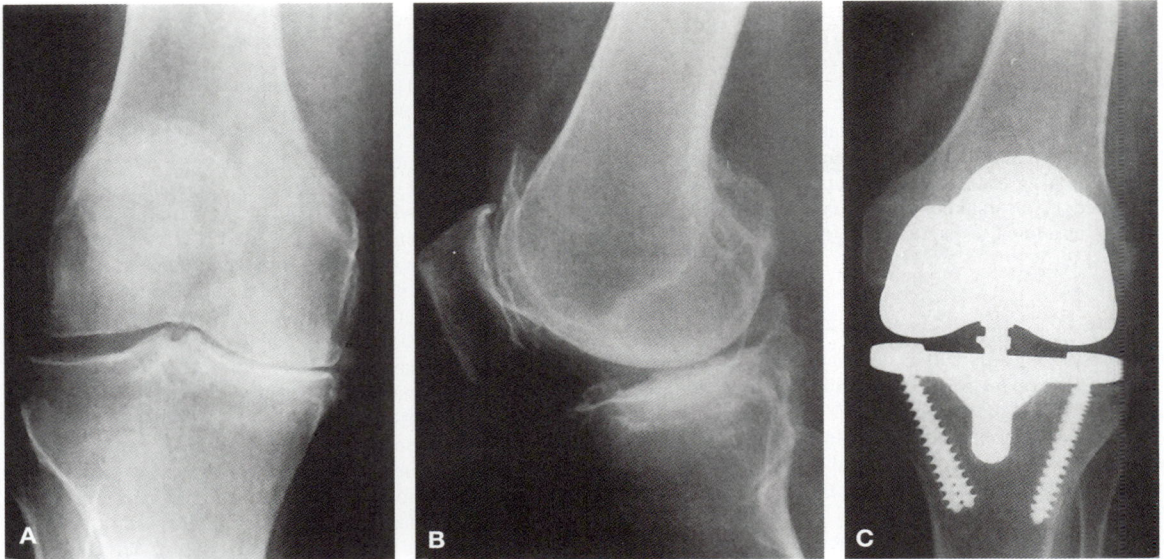

Figure 26-45. Osteoarthritis affecting the knee joint. A. The anteroposterior radiograph shows joint space narrowing, subchondral sclerosis, and a hypertrophic osteophytic response of the bone at the joint margins. B. Osteophytes (seen better on this lateral radiograph) decrease joint motion and increase joint surface area, in a biologic attempt to decrease excessive joint surface stresses. C. The knee ultimately required total joint replacement. (From Lawrence PF. *Essentials of Surgical Specialties.* 3rd ed. Lippincott Williams & Wilkins; 2007.)

(eg, great toe, spine, or ankle). Large joint arthrodesis is contraindicated in patients with systemic multiple joint inflammatory arthritis.

RHEUMATOID ARTHRITIS

Rheumatoid arthritis is an inflammatory disorder of unknown etiology. It is a chronic symmetrical polyarthritis with a relapsing course that frequently leads to progressive joint destruction, deformity, and incapacitation. The disease occurs in women more commonly than men (3:1 predominance) and has a genetic basis with individuals with the HLA-DR4 haplotype having a risk of developing the disease. Regardless of the inciting factor, the immune system is involved in the disease process; 80% of patients have autoantibodies to the Fc region of immunoglobulin G (IgG), and the immunoglobulin M (IgM) autoantibody is termed the rheumatoid factor. Although the presence of the rheumatoid factor is not diagnostic of the disorder (1%-5% of normal subjects have it), high titers are associated with severe joint disease, multisystem involvement, and a poor prognosis.

Pathology

The pathology of rheumatoid arthritis results from synovial inflammation of joints and tendon sheaths. As the synovial membrane becomes infiltrated by macrophages and lymphocytes, it undergoes hypertrophy and causes joint swelling and effusions. The byproducts of the inflammatory process injure adjacent bone and cartilage. Hypertrophic synovial cells proliferate, forming a "pannus," and damage the articular cartilage. Recurrent joint swelling stretches the capsule and supportive ligaments, which causes joint instability, deformity, and further mechanical injury. Adjacent inflammatory processes weaken tendons and cause muscle imbalance in the complex joint

systems of the hand. Joint and tendon subluxation is common in rheumatoid hands that become weak and deformed (Figure 26-46). The systemic nature of the disease is made evident by its extra-articular manifestations, which include vasculitis, neuropathy, iritis, lymphadenopathy, splenomegaly, and polyserositis.

Just as the pathophysiology of rheumatoid arthritis differs from that of osteoarthrosis, so do the radiologic features. Soft tissue swelling and periarticular osteoporosis are the early signs of rheumatoid arthritis. Diffuse cartilage destruction leads to generalized joint space narrowing and bone erosions at the site of synovial attachments (Figure 26-46). Joint deformity, cystic bone destruction, and joint ankylosis mark end-stage disease. Hypertrophic osteophytes are rare in rheumatoid arthritis.

Treatment

The treatment of rheumatoid arthritis is directed toward pain relief, suppression of the inflammatory synovitis, prevention of joint deformities, and early joint reconstruction. In its early stages, synovitis is inhibited by drug therapy or managed by surgical removal of the diseased synovium (synovectomy). Splinting the involved joints in functional positions during acute flare-ups rests the joint, prevents contractures, and minimizes deformity. Exercises to maintain range of motion and muscle strength—although painful and frustrating to the patient—are encouraged. With advanced joint destruction, tendon ruptures are repaired, and excisional or replacement arthroplasty helps to restore mobility and function.

To optimize the patient's function, it is often necessary to use mechanical aids and adaptive apparatus and to modify the physical layout of both the home and the workplace. The proper management of rheumatoid arthritis requires the multidisciplinary teamwork of a rheumatologist, surgeon, physiotherapist, occupational therapist, and social worker.

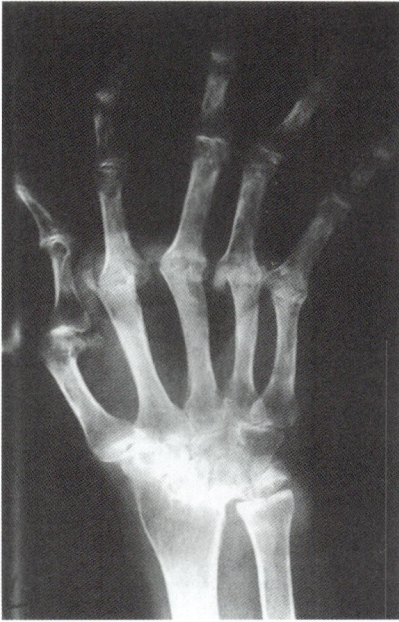

Figure 26-46. Radiographic evidence of rheumatoid arthritic joint involvement, with soft tissue swelling and multiple meta-carpophalangeal joint palmar dislocations. Disuse osteoporosis is evident. Actual cartilage destruction causes joint space narrowing, as exemplified at the proximal interphalangeal and wrist joints. Bone erosions occur at the site of synovial attachments. Osteophytic changes of bone hypertrophy typical of osteoarthrosis are unusual with rheumatic diseases. (From Lawrence PF. *Essentials of Surgical Specialties*. 3rd ed. Lippincott Williams & Wilkins; 2007.)

Anti-tumor necrosis factor (anti-TNF) preparations have been added to the treatment of patients with systemic inflammatory arthritis. There are reports of dramatic reduction in pain for some patients. The effects of long-term use of drugs of this class are not known.

OTHER ARTHRITIDES

Although osteoarthrosis and rheumatoid arthritis are the most common arthritic conditions, there are a myriad of other arthritic diseases, including infections, gout, chronic juvenile arthritis, spondyloarthropathies of ankylosing spondylitis, Reiter disease, and psoriatic arthritis. In addition, neuropathies, hemophilia, and many other diseases may have arthritic manifestations. Complete medical histories and review of the system are thus crucial in determining the underlying etiology of a patient's joint pain.

Some arthritides, such as gonococcal arthritis and Lyme disease, are caused by infectious agents. Systemic gonococcal infection may be associated with petechial and pustular rashes on the palms and soles of the feet, and joint aspiration and culture reveal typical gram-negative diplococci. Infection usually involves small joints, especially of the hands and feet. Treatment with cefuroxime 1 g intravenously daily for 7 days or penicillin 10 to 20 million units daily for 7 days, if sensitive, usually leads to full recovery, because the organism does not produce collagenase.

Lyme disease is caused by the spirochete *Borrelia burgdorferi*. The infective agent is carried by ticks that live on deer. The clinical course tends to be migratory polyarthralgia with or without a rash. The symptoms usually subside after antibiotic treatment with doxycycline 100 mg PO bid or amoxicillin 500 mg PO q6h for 10 days.

With gouty arthritis, microscopic analysis of joint fluid under polarized light reveals splinter-like, monoclinic, negatively birefringent uric acid crystals. In pseudogout, positively birefringent, rhomboid-shaped, calcium pyrophosphate dihydrate crystals are apparent. Radiographs of the latter may show typical articular cartilage or meniscal calcification. Acute flares of crystal-induced arthritis are treated with high doses of nonsteroidal anti-inflammatory drugs or colchicine. Long-term preventive treatment of gout involves the use of allopurinol to decrease systemic uric acid levels.

BONE NECROSIS

Interruption of the blood supply to bone results in bone cell death (osteonecrosis or avascular necrosis). Traumatic causes of osteonecrosis have been discussed and involve vascular injury or interruption of the blood supply to bones. The femoral head, talus, carpal lunate, and scaphoid are prone to avascular necrosis. These bones are all extensively covered by articular cartilage and have limited soft tissue attachments. Legg-Calvé-Perthes disease of the femoral head represents a form of avascular necrosis in developing skeleton. Nontraumatic causes of osteonecrosis involve intraosseous microvascular disturbances that result from either arterial emboli or impairment of venous outflow. There is MRI evidence that some forms of osteonecrosis of the knee in adults may arise from fractures in subchondral bone. All of these mechanisms can compromise bone perfusion.

Patients on glucocorticoid therapy (especially those with systemic lupus erythematosus and/or those who have had a renal transplant) are at higher risk for developing osteonecrosis. The thrombi of hemoglobinopathies (eg, sickle cell disease), the nitrogen bubbles of decompression sickness (dysbarism), the glucocerebroside deposits of Gaucher disease, hyperuricemic crystals, fat emboli of alcoholism, and pancreatitis may cause an occlusive form of bone infarction. Affected bones have a paucity of arterial anastomoses. The femoral head of the hip is the most frequently affected by avascular necrosis.

PATHOLOGY

Bone is a living tissue that is in a dynamic state of homeostasis involving bone resorption, replacement, and remodeling. Unlike other tissues, normal bone turnover occurs slowly. Following a loss of blood supply, bone cell and marrow necrosis occur within 24 hours. Although these changes can be detected microscopically by the absence of osteocytes from their lacunae, there is often a delay of as much as 5 years between the onset of symptoms and the appearance of radiologic abnormalities. MRI is the most sensitive method of detecting early osteonecrosis.

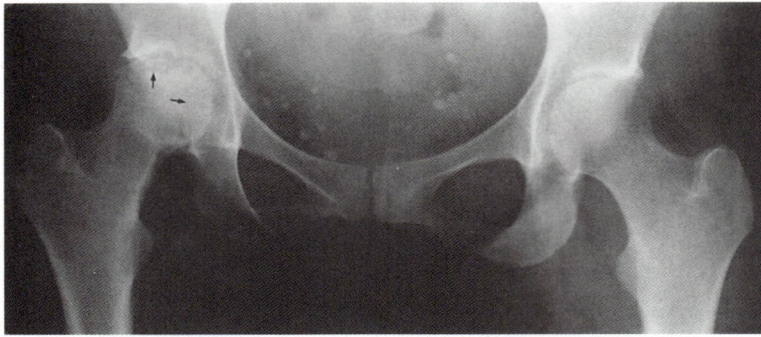

Figure 26-47. **Advanced avascular necrosis of the femoral head in a patient with sarcoidosis who had been treated with systemic steroids.** The femoral head is dense (sclerotic). There is evidence of a subchondral lucency (arrows) with joint surface flattening, collapse, and marginal osteophyte formation. (From Lawrence PF. *Essentials of Surgical Specialties*. 3rd ed. Lippincott Williams & Wilkins; 2007.)

The revascularization process is slow. The living bone surrounding the infarction becomes hypervascular. The hyperemia of the surrounding bone causes local bone mineral resorption appearing as osteopenia on x-ray. Dead tissue retains its density and appears white (sclerotic) on x-ray. As vessels invade and try to repair the necrotic zone, new bone is laid down on the old trabeculae, and dead bone is removed by osteoclasts. This reparative process weakens the femoral head at the margins of the infarct. With persistent weight-bearing stress, the necrotic subchondral bone may fracture, leading to severe pain and rapid joint degeneration (Figure 26-47). Initially, the articular cartilage remains intact because it is nourished by synovial fluid. When a subchondral fracture occurs, the bone support is lost. The articular cartilage becomes separated from the subchondral bone, and a process similar to osteoarthrosis causes joint destruction.

EVALUATION AND TREATMENT

The symptoms of osteonecrosis may not become manifest until a subchondral fracture occurs. Symptoms begin with painful limited active motion. Two-thirds of patients complain of pain at rest, which can occur at night. In the older patients, spontaneous osteonecrosis of the femoral condyle occurs with the sudden onset of severe knee pain not associated with trauma. Many cases show increased bone scan activity over the femoral condyle adjacent to the necrotic zone. MRI scans show bone edema and subchondral fracture.

The prevention of joint loading until natural healing processes are completed on the basis of conservative treatment. Core decompression, in which a hole is drilled through the dead cancellous bone, may be of benefit. Intraosseous pressure is decreased as the biopsy tract creates an avenue for revascularization.

Although the inciting agent is vascular, the joint deterioration results from the loss of mechanical support for the articular surface. The management principles for advanced disease are similar to those employed in the treatment of osteoarthrosis. If the volume of dead bone is large, total joint replacement is a reasonable treatment option. Unfortunately, avascular necrosis occurs in younger patients, whose high activity levels place stresses that can exceed the design tolerance of implants.

DEGENERATIVE DISEASES OF THE SPINE

LUMBAR SPINE

Low back pain is the most common musculoskeletal complaint for the 30- to 65-year age group. Eighty percent of adults experience an episode of low back pain severe enough to interfere with normal daily activities. In the United States, the annual cost of back-related medical payments is estimated at $16 billion. An additional $50 billion is attributed each year to lost worker productivity.

Anatomy and Physiology

Degenerative joint disease is far more common to the joints of the spine than to the joints of the limbs. The spine is an articulated column of vertebrae that protects the spinal cord and nerve roots. The neural elements also can be affected by degenerative spinal pathology. The motion segment of the spine is composed of two bony vertebrae covered with cartilage end plates and the intervertebral disk. Vertebral motion takes place through a three-joint complex: the intervertebral **disk** and two posterior synovial facet joints (Figure 26-48A). The disk is composed of a central gelatinous nucleus pulposus and an elastic **annulus fibrosus** (Figure 26-48B). In flexion-extension and lateral bending, the vertebrae moving through the spatial orientation of the paired facet joints direct spinal motion. The lumbar vertebral facets are in the sagittal plane and permit flexion and extension. The thoracic facets are oriented in more of a horizontal plane, allowing lateral bending and rotatory motion. Degenerative spine disease anatomically affects the two sites of spinal motion—the disk and/or the facet joints. The ligaments that tether the vertebrae together include the AP longitudinal ligaments attached to the vertebral bodies. The ligamentum flavum connects the laminae with the interspinous and supraspinous ligaments between the spinous processes (Figure 26-49). The paraspinal muscles are complex and span two to five vertebral segments. These muscles power spinal motion and help absorb the stresses of erect bipedal posture.

Etiology of Low Back Pain

Contrary to popular opinion, the vast majority of low back pain is not due to a "slipped disk." In 80% to 90% of patients with low back pain, the pain is of unknown etiology

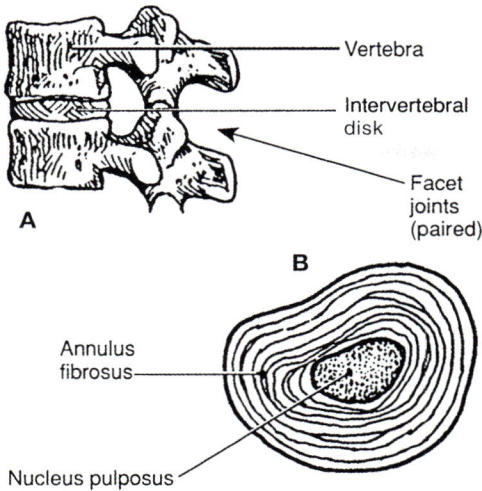

Figure 26-48. A. The spinal motion segment consists of two vertebral bodies and the intervening disk. Motion occurs through two paired facet joints and the disk. The vertebrae rock or pivot over the disk in flexion and lateral bending. B. The disk comprises a central gelatinous nucleus pulposus and its peripheral fibrous encasement, the annulus fibrosus. (Reprinted with permission from American Academy of Orthopaedic Surgeons. *Athletic Training and Sports Medicine*. 2nd ed. American Academy of Orthopaedic Surgeons; 1991:515.)

and the pathology remains obscure. Fewer than 10% of patients experience pain in the sciatic nerve (L5-S3) distribution ("sciatica"). Only 1% to 2% of patients require surgical treatment for disk herniation. With symptomatic care, 50% improve in 2 weeks and 90% in 3 months.

Pathophysiology

Lumbar Strain (Mechanical Back Pain)

Most cases of back pain result from minor events, not from significant trauma. Many injuries involve myofascial strains, minor ligament injury, or overuse. Lack of exercise, poor muscle tone, and obesity contribute to minor postural injuries of the spine. This type of mechanical back pain is common in women during or after pregnancy. The pain of mechanical strain rarely radiates beyond the knee and remains localized to the spine and buttocks. More than 80% of these back problems resolve within 6 weeks of onset.

Spondylolysis and Spondylolisthesis

The facet joints of the lumbar spine are oriented in the sagittal plane, which permits flexion and extension while resisting rotational and lateral bending motion. When the spine is hyperextended, the facet joints are engaged. If a rotational twisting force is added, the lamina may fracture, either after an acute injury or from the stress of repetitive microtrauma. The fracture occurs immediately caudal to the superior facet in a region called the pars interarticularis (Figure 26-50A). This injury, **spondylolysis,** occurs 10 times more often in gymnasts than in age-matched controls and may result from back extension during dismount landings.

If the fracture is bilateral, the superior vertebral body, lacking facet support, may slide forward on the inferior vertebra. This anterior shift of one vertebra on another is called spondylolisthesis (Figure 26-50B). In young patients, the condition may be painful and the slippage can progress. Spinal fusion is the standard treatment for progressive, painful spondylolisthesis.

Disk Herniation

Disk herniation is the result of extrusion of the nucleus pulposus through the annulus fibrosus. It occurs in adults aged 30 to 50 years (ie, during the prime working years). The most frequently involved disks are at L4-L5 and L5-S1, the most mobile lumbar spinal segments. A ruptured L4-L5 disk will affect the L5 nerve root, and a ruptured L5-S1 disk affects the S1 root. In adults, the nucleus pulposus loses proteoglycans and water content, making it less resilient. In the aging process, the annulus fibrosus loses its elasticity, especially posteriorly, where it is thinnest. The combination of age-related changes and repeated minor trauma can cause tears in the annulus. If an annular tear is large, it will permit the extrusion of the nucleus pulposus. In some cases, the herniated disk material causes minimal symptoms. In others, the herniated disk material exerts direct pressure on the nerve root (Figure 26-51).

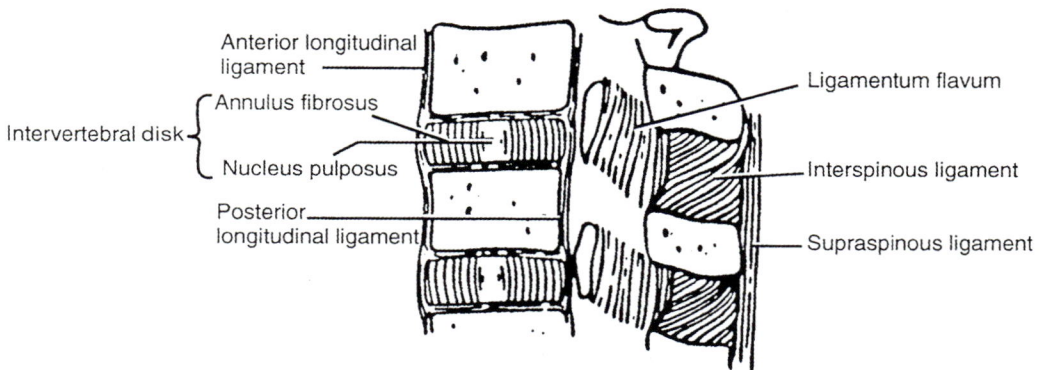

Figure 26-49. The ligaments of the spinal column. (Reprinted with permission from Wilson FC, ed. *The Musculoskeletal System: Basic Processes and Disorders*. 3rd ed. JB Lippincott; 1983.)

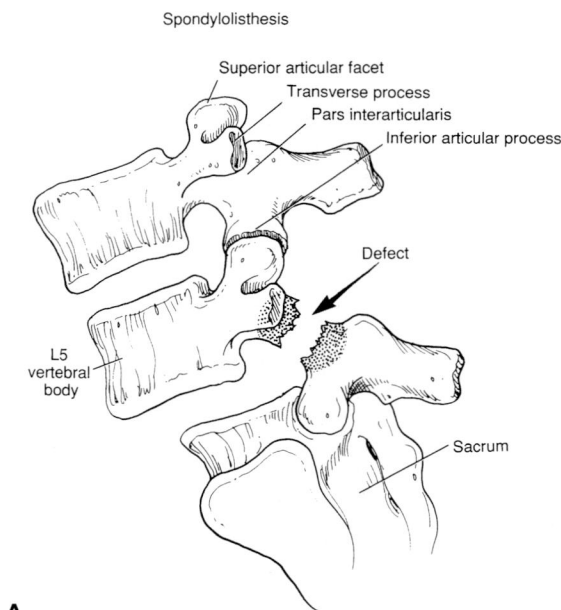

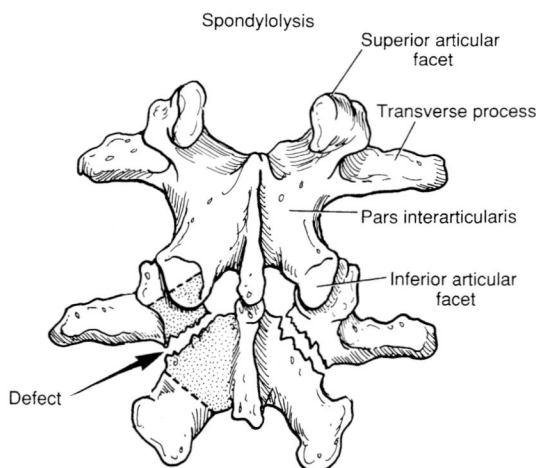

Figure 26-50. The lumbar facet joints are oriented in the sagittal plane and allow flexion and extension. With lumbar extension, the facet joints engage; when a significant rotatory force is added, the lamina just inferior to the facet may fracture. A. If spondylolytic fractures occur bilaterally, the unsupported superior vertebrae may translate anteriorly, producing spondylolisthesis. B. This fracture is called spondylolysis, which literally means spine lysis. (Modified from McNab I, McCullough J. *Backache*. 2nd ed. Lippincott Williams & Wilkins; 1990.)

Clinically, patients complain of severe pain, often after bending to lift or while twisting with a heavy object. The pain emanates from the back or buttock and radiates into the leg and foot in a radicular (nerve root), dermatomal distribution. The pain is accentuated by bending, sitting, and coughing. The supine straight-leg raising test places traction on the S1 nerve root and, to a lesser degree, the L5 root. This test reproduces the pain, which should radiate below the knee to be considered positive. Ankle dorsiflexion

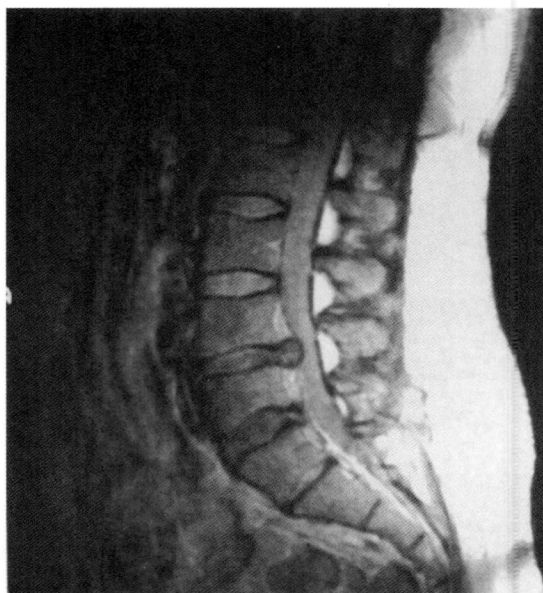

Figure 26-51. Magnetic resonance scan of a large L4-L5 herniated disk. The epidural fat plane is obliterated as the disk exerts extradural pressure on the thecal space. (From Lawrence PF. *Essentials of Surgical Specialties*. 3rd ed. Lippincott Williams & Wilkins; 2007.)

accentuates the pain (Lasègue maneuver), whereas ankle plantar flexion should not affect it. The latter test is helpful to exclude malingerers. Radicular motor weakness, numbness, and reflex diminution provide objective evidence of nerve root compression (Table 26-4). When a large amount of disk is extruded into the spinal canal, it may compress more than one nerve root. When multiple nerve roots are involved, the clinical picture may be confusing because of overlapping patterns of pain and functional losses. Loss of bowel and bladder continence is a result of a central disk herniation compressing multiple S1-S4 roots. Called the **cauda equina syndrome**, this condition is a surgical emergency demanding decompression to prevent permanent incontinence.

MRI of the lumbosacral spine is the diagnostic test of choice to define the anatomic location of disk material for patients considered for surgery with unremitting leg pain or progressive neurologic deficit. CT is less sensitive and specific but may localize pathology. Myelography, the injection of water-soluble dye into the epidural space, is rarely used unless MRI is not available.

Spinal Stenosis

The spinal facets are synovial joints and are subject to degenerative arthritic changes. As the disks narrow, there are increased forces on the facet joints. The facet joints narrow and develop marginal osteophytes. The development of hypertrophic facet joint osteophytes narrows the space available for existing nerve roots and may irritate or compress them. The narrowing of the disk may allow the ligamentum flavum to buckle into the spinal canal. This combination of folds of ligamentum flavum posteriorly and hypertrophic osteophytes anteriorly can cause encroachment of spinal canal or foraminal contents, causing symptoms of **spinal stenosis**.

TABLE 26-4. Lumbar Lesions and Associated Radicular Abnormalities

Location	Abnormality
L4 Nerve Root	
Pain/numbness	Medial leg and ankle
Sensory	Hypesthesia, medial leg, and ankle
Motor	Weak ankle dorsiflexion or weak quadriceps (knee extension)
Reflex	Decreased knee jerk
L5 Nerve Root	
Pain/numbness	Lateral calf and dorsal foot
Sensory	Hypesthesia, dorsal foot, great toe
Motor	Weak extensor hallux longus
Reflex	Usually none; decreased posterior tibial tendon reflex possible (but that reflex is present in only 20% of normal patients)
S1 Nerve Root	
Pain/numbness	Posterior calf, lateral and plantar foot
Sensory	Hypesthesia, lateral foot
Motor	Weak toe and ankle flexors, foot evertor
Reflex	Decreased ankle jerk

Spinal stenosis is a pattern of back and leg pain attributed to narrowing of the spinal canal. The pain tends to begin after being upright or walking for a period of time. It does not tend to diminish unless the patient sits down or lies down. This feature usually distinguishes it from vascular claudication, where the pain usually dissipates by standing still for a short period. This pattern of pain is referred to as neurogenic claudication. It tends to affect people with extensive degenerative disk disease who are usually over 65 years of age.

Surgery for spinal stenosis involves decompression of the spinal cord and roots. Careful preoperative evaluation is necessary to properly identify the location and extent of pathology. CT and MRI scans of several spinal levels are needed to define the pathology and extent of neural canal and foraminal compromise. Each disk space is evaluated for herniation and each facet joint for stenosis of the lateral recess of the spinal canal.

Other Conditions

There are many other causes of back pain. Medical history is extremely helpful in identifying the etiology of low back disorders. The differential diagnosis includes the following:

1. Disk herniation with nerve root irritation or neurologic deficit
2. Spinal stenosis
3. Vertebral infection
4. Primary or metastatic neoplasms; especially thyroid, lung, breast, renal, and prostate

5. Trauma (see Chapter 7)
6. Rheumatologic conditions (eg, ankylosing spondylitis, rheumatoid arthritis, Reiter disease)
7. Vascular disorders (eg, aortic aneurysm, aortic dissection)
8. Psychogenic or malingering pain (vague history and bizarre gait with inconsistent physical findings suggest psychogenic causes)

Treatment

Nonsurgical Treatment

Most cases of back pain are mechanical. Nonsurgical measures that include analgesics, anti-inflammatories, and stretching and strengthening exercises are often effective. Patient education about the causes and nature of back pain is important. Instruction in proper postural mechanics and lifting techniques will prevent reinjury. Patients should be encouraged to take an active interest in and responsibility for their own back care.

Patients with back and referred leg pain may benefit from a short period of rest, analgesic and anti-inflammatory medications, and heat followed by an active back exercise program. A brace may provide symptomatic relief. The brace acts as a proprioceptive device, reminding the patient to lift and bend properly. The excessive use of bed rest and back braces is to be avoided because both can cause paraspinal muscle atrophy.

Nonsteroidal anti-inflammatory medications are useful for their analgesic and anti-inflammatory effects. Narcotic analgesics and antispasmodic agents are used with caution, especially with chronic back pain. Both of these classes of drugs mask symptoms and may cause chemical dependency.

The two absolute indications for surgical decompression are as follows:

1. When disk herniation causes a progressive neurologic deficit
2. When cauda equina syndrome is suspected with loss of bowel or bladder continence

The majority (>80%) of patients with a symptomatic lumbar disk herniation will improve with conservative treatment and not require surgery.

Surgical Treatment

Approximately 10% of patients with leg pain do not respond to conservative treatment. If leg pain persists for more than 2 months of conservative care, surgery may be considered. The results are better if surgery is performed within 6 months of the onset of symptoms. After 6 months, the patient becomes physically deconditioned and psychologically dependent. The candidate for surgery should have consistent physical and radiographic findings. Spinal surgery treats symptoms and does not reverse the degenerative processes of spinal aging and arthritis. Operations for disk herniations should be precisely defined. In patients with spinal stenosis, decompression is more extensive. All structures causing nerve root pressure, herniated disks, osteophytic spurs, and calcified ligaments are surgically removed from each involved spinal level. The indications for spinal fusion in this setting are controversial. In patients with spinal instability from progressive spondylolisthesis or after anatomically extensive decompression, spinal fusion can be an effective stabilizing and palliative procedure.

CERVICAL SPINE

Degenerative disk disease and disk protrusion also occur in the cervical spine. The erosive synovitis of rheumatoid arthritis has an affinity for the mobile cervical spine.

Cervical Disk Protrusion

The combined effects of age-related disk degeneration and abnormal stresses can cause cervical disk herniations. When disk material presses on the posterior longitudinal ligament, symptoms of stiffness and neck pain may be referred to the scapular region. When the herniated disk material protrudes posterior and lateral to the posterior longitudinal ligament, it may impinge on a cervical nerve root. Consequently, it may cause radicular pain, numbness, focal motor weakness, and diminution or loss of upper extremity deep tendon reflexes (Table 26-5). The most commonly ruptured disks are at the C5-C6 and C6-C7 interspaces, where cervical flexion-extension motion is the greatest. Likewise, the respective C6 and C7 nerve roots are most often affected by cervical disk pathology.

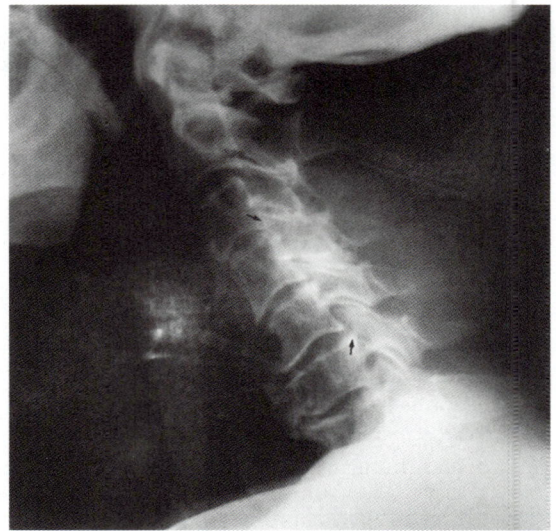

Figure 26-52. Osteoarthrotic cervical spondylosis with anterior vertebral body osteophyte formation and disk space narrowing. Posterior vertebral body osteophytes, also called Luschka (or uncovertebral) joints (arrows), can cause encroachment on the spinal cord. This is known as a hard disk. (From Lawrence PF. *Essentials of Surgical Specialties*. 3rd ed. Lippincott Williams & Wilkins; 2007.)

Nonoperative treatment involves rest, immobilization with a soft cervical collar, heat, and anti-inflammatory medication. Traction may help to alleviate nerve root pressure. Indications for surgical intervention are similar to those in the lumbar spine. Emergency decompressive surgery is indicated if there is spinal cord involvement (myelopathy) with hyperreflexia, ipsilateral weakness, contralateral numbness, or the presence of pathologic long tract reflexes (eg, **Babinski** or **Hoffmann sign**).

Cervical Spondylosis

Degenerative disk changes cause disk space narrowing and increase the forces on the facet joints and joints of Luschka. Osteophytes form at the posterior disk margin, creating a "hard disk." These bone spurs, called **Luschka joints,** can encroach on the spinal cord or peripherally on an individual nerve root (Figure 26-52). The clinical picture is similar to the herniation of the nucleus pulposus (soft disk), except that the onset of symptoms is more gradual. Treatment for degenerative cervical spondyloarthrosis is similar to that for cervical disk protrusion. When refractory to conservative treatment modalities, both conditions respond to anterior cervical discectomy with a fusion.

Rheumatoid Arthritis of the Cervical Spine

Rheumatoid arthritis often involves the synovial joints of the cervical spine. Progressive inflammatory destruction of bone, ligaments, and articular cartilage may cause cervical spine instability or neural compression.

Rheumatic cervical spine involvement usually assumes one of the following three patterns:

1. Rheumatoid inflammation and swelling of the small synovial joint between the atlas and the odontoid process can stretch the stabilizing transverse ligament and cause

TABLE 26-5. Cervical Lesions and Associated Radicular Abnormalities	
Location	**Abnormality**
C5 Nerve Root	
Sensory	Hypesthesia of the lateral arm
Motor	Weak deltoid, biceps
Reflex	Decreased biceps reflex
C6 Nerve Root	
Sensory	Hypesthesia of the lateral forearm and palmar thumb
Motor	Weak wrist extension
Reflex	Decreased brachioradialis reflex
C7 Nerve Root	
Sensory	Hypesthesia of the long finger
Motor	Weak finger extension, triceps
Reflex	Decreased triceps reflex
C8 Nerve Root	
Sensory	Hypesthesia of the medial forearm and little finger
Motor	Weak finger flexion
Reflex	None
Myelopathy	**Diffuse Hypesthesias**
Sensory	Diffuse weakness, increased muscle tone, rigidity
Motor	Hyperreflexia with clonus
Reflex	Positive Hoffmann or Babinski sign

the atlantoaxial joint (C1-C2) to subluxate with flexion. The two vertebrae no longer move in synchrony, and this causes spinal canal narrowing and potential cord compromise by the posteriorly displaced dens.

2. Erosive synovitis between the atlas (C1 vertebra) and the occipital condyles causes cranial settling, and this may result in the protrusion of the odontoid process of the axis (C2) into the foramen magnum. This phenomenon is termed *occipitoatlantoaxial impaction,* and it can compress the spinal cord, causing long tract signs.

3. Finally, facet joint synovitis affecting any cervical vertebrae below the axis can cause segmental instability known as subaxial subluxation. This instability is demonstrated on lateral radiographs by abnormal vertebral body tilt or displacement in the AP direction.

The prevalence of cervical instability in patients with polyarticular rheumatoid arthritis is such that flexion-extension lateral cervical spine radiographs must be obtained for any rheumatoid patient undergoing intubation for a general anesthetic. Neurologic involvement does not necessarily correlate with the degree of cervical vertebral subluxation. However, when neurologic impairment is caused by cervical instability, the treatment of choice is stabilization through surgical spine fusion. Most cases of rheumatoid neck pain, however, are successfully managed by nonoperative treatment modalities.

TABLE 26-6. Causes of Osteoporosis

Type	Examples
Involutional	Postmenopausal age
Nutritional deficiencies	Scurvy
Endocrine disorders	Hypogonadism
	Hyperparathyroidism
	Cushing disease
	Hyperthyroidism
Drug use	Corticosteroids
	Methotrexate
Disuse	Prolonged bed rest
	Weightlessness
Inflammatory arthritis	Rheumatoid arthritis
	Ankylosing spondylitis
	Chronic infection (tuberculosis)
Malignant disease	Multiple myeloma
	Leukemia
Idiopathic	

METABOLIC ENDOCRINE DISORDERS

Bone is a biphasic material consisting of an inert mineral and an organic matrix. The mineral is composed of calcium and phosphorus in a hydroxyapatite crystal $Ca_{10}(PO_4)_6(OH)_2$. The organic matrix (osteoid) is composed primarily of type I collagen, which has high tensile strength. The mineral phase of bone resists compressive forces, whereas the organic collagen fiber phase provides reinforcement and resistance to bending and twisting stress (like the meshed wire in cement). Normal bone is 70% mineral and 30% organic matrix.

OSTEOPOROSIS

Bone strength depends on the amount of bone mineral per unit volume. In osteoporosis, the chemical composition of the bone is normal, but total bone mineral is more than 2 standard deviations below an age-matched control. The ratio of bone mineral to organic matrix is normal, but the absolute value of each is decreased. The bone is, therefore, weak, less dense, and predisposed to fractures with minimal trauma. The most common type of osteoporosis is the involutional senile type and is seen in postmenopausal White females. The cause is unknown. Other conditions also result in osteoporosis (Table 26-6).

Osteoporosis is second to arthritis in causes of musculoskeletal morbidity in the older patients. The symptoms occur when bone mass is so compromised that the skeleton fractures as a result of the mechanical stresses of everyday life. Compression fractures of vertebral bodies or fractures of the proximal femur (hip; see Figure 26-18),

humerus, and distal radius (Colles; see Figure 26-15) are often the first manifestations of osteoporosis. These patients should be screened for the medically treatable causes of osteoporosis, and a bone mineral density scan should be obtained to help quantify the severity of their disease. Exercise, dietary calcium, and vitamin D supplements (and estrogen in early postmenopausal women) can be effective prophylaxis against the bone loss of osteoporosis. Diphosphonates and calcitonin can be used to treat this condition and have been shown to increase bone mineral density and decrease fracture rates. Adequate calcium intake during the growing years as well as a healthy level of physical activity are the current long-term prevention strategies.

OSTEOMALACIA

Osteomalacia is the result of a deficiency in the mineral content of bone. In contrast to osteoporosis, the amount of bone matrix per unit volume is normal. However, the matrix that is present is incompletely calcified. Clinically and radiographically, osteoporosis and osteomalacia are similar. Often, the distinction is made by bone biopsy and histomorphometry, an analytic technique that requires ultrathin, nondecalcified, tetracycline-labeled bone biopsy specimens. In osteomalacia, wide osteoid seams of unmineralized bone are detected. The ratio of bone mineral to organic bone matrix is decreased because there is a mineral deficiency. In osteoporosis, the ratio of bone mineral to matrix is normal because the quantity of both is deficient.

TABLE 26-7. Causes of Osteomalacia

Type	Examples
Dietary	Vitamin D deficiency (rickets)
Hereditary	Hypophosphatemic rickets
Gastrointestinal	Biliary disease
	Pancreatitis
	Celiac sprue
	Milk alkali syndrome
	Cirrhosis
Drug use	Phenytoin
	Barbiturates
Chronic renal disease	

Inadequate bone mineralization can result from inadequate dietary vitamin D or calcium intake, gastrointestinal malabsorption of calcium, problems with the enzymatic conversion of vitamin D, or defective renal calcium and phosphorus handling (Table 26-7). Correctable defects in the calcium pathway can be screened by obtaining levels of serum calcium and phosphorus, blood urea nitrogen, and creatinine, which may detect gastrointestinal, endocrine, or renal causes. In addition to the generalized decrease in bone density seen radiologically, a band of bone rarefaction, called a Looser zone, is typical of osteomalacia (Figure 26-53). The Looser zone represents a healing stress fracture and is most often noted in the femoral neck or pubic rami.

The pediatric form of osteomalacia is called rickets and is caused by dietary vitamin D deficiency and lack

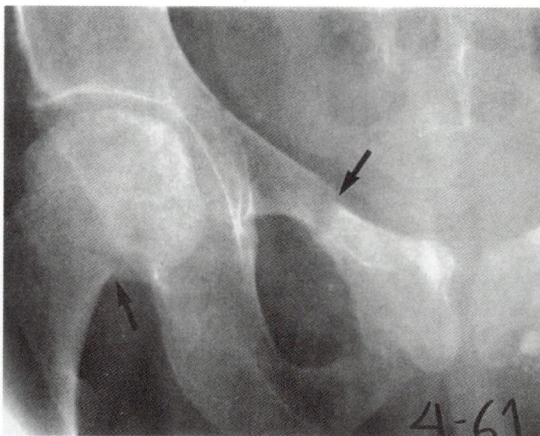

Figure 26-54. Rickets, the pediatric form of osteomalacia, is noted by diffuse osteopenia and abnormally wide growth plates. The soft bones may be bowed. (From Lawrence PF. *Essentials of Surgical Specialties.* 3rd ed. Lippincott Williams & Wilkins; 2007.)

of exposure to sunlight. This disease was common during the industrial revolution before the advent of child labor laws. Today, rickets is seen primarily in a genetic disease called vitamin D–resistant (hypophosphatemic) rickets, which is transmitted in an autosomal dominant pattern. In growing children, radiographs of osteomalacia (rickets) demonstrate widened growth plates and cupped metaphyses (Figure 26-54). Soft, undermineralized long bones may be abnormally bowed.

HYPERPARATHYROIDISM

Hyperparathyroidism causes diffuse bony osteopenia. Parathyroid hormone is involved with the homeostasis of ionized calcium levels in the blood. In response to low serum calcium or high serum phosphorus concentrations, parathyroid hormone increases calcium release from bone, calcium absorption by the intestines, and calcium reabsorption by the kidney (while decreasing renal absorption of phosphate). These changes cause a net increase in plasma calcium and a decrease in plasma phosphate levels. Primary hyperparathyroidism is due to an adenoma or hyperplasia of the parathyroid gland. Secondary hyperparathyroidism is due to chronic renal insufficiency with decreased phosphate excretion. Radiographs of hyperparathyroidism show not only diffuse bony rarefaction but also include disseminated focal osteolytic lesions of cortical bone called osteitis fibrosis cystica (Figure 26-55).

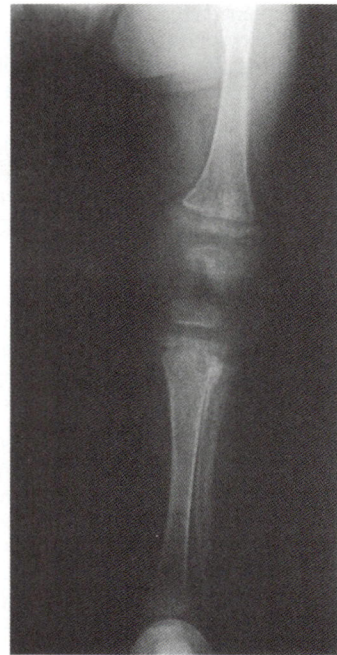

Figure 26-53. Looser line seen with osteomalacia. The band of rarefaction in the superior pubic ramus and in the femoral neck (arrows) represents a stress fracture and is due to inadequate bone mineralization. (From Lawrence PF. *Essentials of Surgical Specialties.* 3rd ed. Lippincott Williams & Wilkins; 2007.)

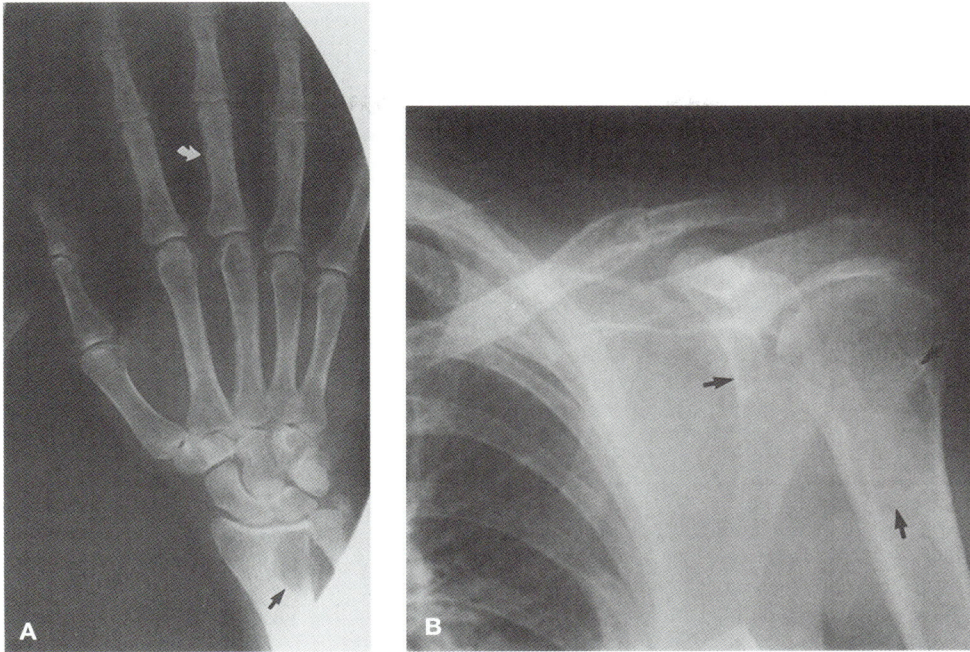

Figure 26-55. Primary hyperparathyroidism causes increased bone resorption to increase serum calcium levels. Radiographs of primary hyperparathyroidism show diffuse bone rarefaction. Note the phalangeal cortices (curved arrow in A) and multiple focal osteolytic lesions of cortical bone (straight arrows in A and B). This explains why the radiographic picture is described as osteitis fibrosis cystica. (From Lawrence PF. *Essentials of Surgical Specialties*. 3rd ed. Lippincott Williams & Wilkins; 2007.)

PAGET DISEASE

Paget disease (osteitis deformans) is a disorder of unknown etiology characterized by excessive bone resorption and unregulated abundant bone formation. The involved areas of bone are highly vascular and can cause massive arteriovenous shunting with high-output cardiac failure. In the early (osteolytic) phase of the disease, bone resorption exceeds deposition. The bone is weak and may fracture and bend. Later, bone formation predominates (osteosclerotic phase) but is poorly organized. The bones become enlarged and thickened.

Patients with Paget disease complain of bone pain, progressive lower limb bowing, or skull enlargement. Fractures through pagetic bone are prone to nonunion. Serum alkaline phosphatase levels secreted by bone-forming osteoblasts can be markedly elevated with Paget disease. Microscopically, the bone is irregular, with a mosaic pattern of mature and immature bone. Radiographs show dense and irregular sclerotic bony trabeculae (Figure 26-56). Long bone fractures are characteristically transverse and begin as a crack on the convex or tension side of the deformed bone. In less than 1% of all cases of Paget disease, these bone-forming cells undergo malignant degeneration into osteosarcomas. The majority of cases are asymptomatic and are discovered incidentally on pelvic radiographs, the pelvis being a frequent site of Paget disease.

The medical treatment of Paget disease with calcitonin or diphosphonates is reserved for intractable bone pain, malignant hypercalcemia, cardiac failure, or neural involvement from bony foraminal hypertrophy in the spine.

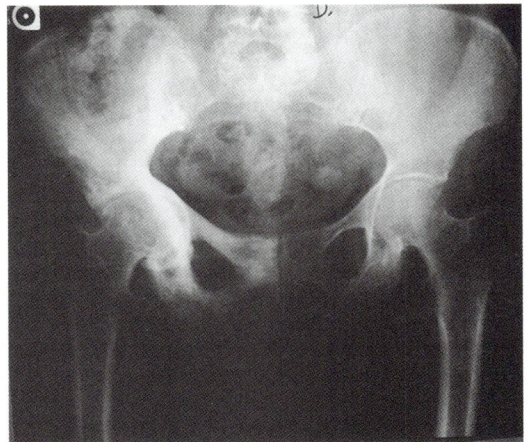

Figure 26-56. Paget disease. The dense irregular sclerotic bony trabeculae signify the excessive, unregulated formation of bone. The bone is brittle and may fracture pathologically. (From Lawrence PF. *Essentials of Surgical Specialties*. 3rd ed. Lippincott Williams & Wilkins; 2007.)

NEOPLASMS OF BONE

Tumors arising from musculoskeletal tissues are rare. However, bone involvement with metastatic tumor is common in patients older than 50 years. Primary tumors of breast, prostate, lung, kidney, and thyroid often metastasize to bone. The sites of tumor metastasis are typically those bones involved with hematopoiesis and those with a rich blood supply, such as the spine, ribs, skull, pelvis, and long bone metaphyses. Metastases from breast and prostate may be either osteoblastic (inducing bone formation) or osteolytic (inducing bone resorption). Metastases from lung, kidney, thyroid, or gastrointestinal tract are usually osteolytic.

The most frequent primary bone tumors and their tissue of origin are listed in Table 26-8. Table 26-9 describes their salient features. The evaluation of primary or secondary bone tumors should be systematic and multidisciplinary. Before treatment is initiated, the physician must define the tumor according to its histology, its anatomic relationships to neuromuscular compartments and perivascular spaces, and the likelihood and mode of its metastatic spread.

The most common primary tumor of bone is multiple myeloma. It occurs in late adulthood. Patients may present with fatigue, bone pain, or, rarely, with a pathologic fracture. Clinical assessment involves general physical examination, routine blood work (including ESR), and urine for Bence Jones proteins. Protein electrophoresis should also be carried out. A medical oncologist should be consulted as soon as the diagnosis of multiple myeloma is suspected.

TABLE 26-8. Primary Bone Tumors and Their Tissue of Origin

Tissue of Origin	Bone Tumor	
	Benign	**Malignant**
Bone	Osteoid osteoma	Osteosarcoma
Cartilage	Osteochondroma	Chondrosarcoma
	Enchondroma	
Fibrous tissue	Fibroma	Fibrosarcoma
Marrow elements	Eosinophilic granuloma	Myeloma
		Ewing sarcoma
Uncertain	Giant cell tumor	Aggressive giant cell tumor

TABLE 26-9. Salient Features of Common Bone Tumors

Tumor	Main Symptoms	Age	Common Sites	Radiographic Appearance	Other
Benign					
Osteoid osteoma	Pain, often relieved by aspirin	<30 y	Femur and tibia	Small, radiolucent area <1 cm surrounded by zone of dense sclerosis	–
Osteochondroma	Palpable lump; may interfere with tendon function	Adolescence	Long bone metaphysis	Sessile or pedunculated bone excrescence; cartilage not seen unless calcified	Pain or increase in size suggests malignant change.
Enchondroma (chondroma)	Swelling or pain with a pathologic fracture	Any age	Metaphysis of tubular bones of hands and feet; may be single or multiple (Ollier disease)	Well-demarcated area of radiolucency that may contain specks of calcification	Malignant transformation is more common with multiple cartilage lesions (osteochondromas or enchondromas).
Nonossifying fibroma (fibrous cortical defect)	Asymptomatic unless pathologic fracture occurs through it	<30 y	Cortical metaphysis of the distal femur or tibia	Well-demarcated, radiolucent, multilocular area adjacent to cortex	Ossifies with skeletal maturation
Giant cell tumor (osteoclastoma)	Pain and swelling near joint	20-40 y	Epiphyseal, especially distal femoral, radius, or proximal tibial epiphysis; after growth plate has closed	Epiphyseal, eccentric expanding; expands to involve metaphysis	Often aggressive; should be treated as a malignant lesion

TABLE 26-9. Salient Features of Common Bone Tumors (*continued*)

Tumor	Main Symptoms	Age	Common Sites	Radiographic Appearance	Other
Malignant					
Osteosarcoma	Tender mass; pain worse at night	Bimodal; before 30 y and after 50 y because of malignant change in Paget disease	Metaphyseal; half affect distal femur and proximal tibia	Irregular, destructive lesion with radiodense osteoblastic or radiolucent osteolytic areas; periosteal new bone formation juxtaposed to a cortex that is permeated and destroyed; neoplastic bone spicules perpendicular to bone radiating in a sunburst pattern	Slightly more common in men than women
Chondrosarcoma	Increasing mass; dull, aching pain	40-60 y	Central sites; pelvic and shoulder girdle	Permeative radiolucent lesion with calcific densities	Malignant transformation of preexisting enchondroma or osteochondroma, especially if multiple
Fibrosarcoma	Painful, destructive lesion	Adolescence and young adulthood	Metaphyseal regions of long bones	Poorly defined, destructive, radiolucent lesion	–
Myeloma	–	45-65 y	Red marrow areas of the skeleton	Osteopenia, spinal compression fractures with minimal trauma	Most common primary malignant bone tumor of plasma cell origin; Bence Jones proteinuria, serum and urine protein electrophoresis
Ewing sarcoma	Enlarging, painful, soft tissue mass	10-15 y	Diaphysis of femur; ilium, tibia, humerus, fibula, ribs	Destructive bony lesion; onion skin layers of periosteal new bone formation	May be mistaken for osteomyelitis clinically and histologically

EVALUATION

History is of great importance. It should include the patient's age, medical conditions associated with bone tumors (eg, Paget disease, dermatomyositis, prior radiation exposure), systemic symptoms (eg, weight loss, bleeding diathesis, fever), and occupation (which may explain an unusual environmental exposure). Lifestyle and personal expectations are also important in selecting therapy. The physical examination should note the color and temperature of overlying tissues and the size, degree of tenderness, and mobility of the tumor if it is palpable. A tumor that is confined to bone may have no abnormal physical findings.

A complete blood count and differential help to exclude infection and hematologic malignancies. Usually, laboratory studies can detect other organ system involvement and determine the patient's overall medical condition. Liver function studies and measurements of uric acid (DNA turnover), alkaline phosphatase, calcium, and phosphorus are helpful in the evaluation of processes that form or destroy bone. With carcinoma of the prostate, a prostate-specific antigen level is measured before a rectal examination is undertaken. If myeloma is suspected, serum protein electrophoresis is obtained.

The plain-film radiograph provides many clues about the behavior of the tumor. It may show a well-demarcated lesion with a reactive zone of bone formation or undemarcated lesion with bone destruction and little surrounding bone formation (Figure 26-57). Defining the specific bone and region of involvement (epiphysis, metaphysis, or diaphysis) aids in diagnosis (see Table 26-9) and staging. Subsequent radiographic investigation with

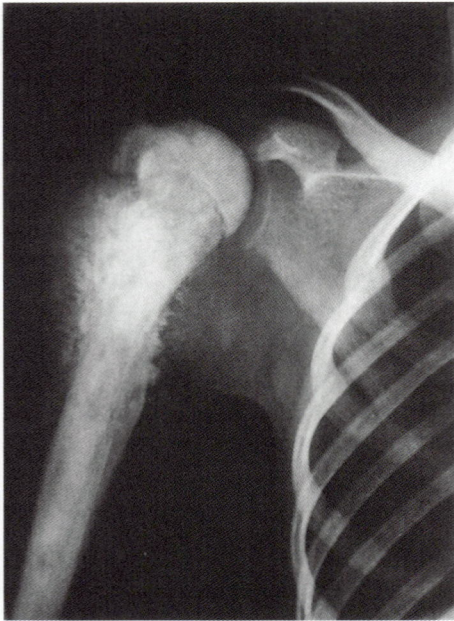

Figure 26-57. Osteogenic sarcoma of the proximal humerus metaphysis showing an aggressive, expanding, poorly demarcated, bone-forming lesion. (From Lawrence PF. *Essentials of Surgical Specialties*. 3rd ed. Lippincott Williams & Wilkins; 2007.)

bone scan, CT, MRI, or other specialized techniques is directed by suspicions generated from the plain-film radiograph. A bone scan is often an excellent screening test for metastatic disease. Radioactive, isotopically labeled technetium-99m pyrophosphate is incorporated into regions of active bone formation or increased vascularity. In multiple myeloma, however, the bone scan is characteristically negative and shows no increased uptake. CT provides the best definition of cortical bone. It can detect cortical penetration and intraosseous detail. The CT scan is the preferred method of evaluating the lung for small pulmonary lesions. With contrast enhancement, a CT scan can define the relation between a tumor and the surrounding neurovascular structures. MRI is used to evaluate the intramedullary (marrow) extent of a tumor. The MRI also yields the best definition of soft tissue and neurovascular tumor relationships. Angiography is used to identify vascular lesions, which can then be embolized to shrink tumor mass and decrease blood loss before a surgical resection. These special imaging techniques are obtained before biopsy.

A surgical biopsy is performed to obtain tissue for histologic diagnosis. A biopsy may be obtained with open or closed (needle) techniques and should be performed by the surgical team responsible for definitive tumor treatment. The biopsy incision is placed so that it can be resected in total and not compromise the definitive procedure. An open biopsy incision is generally directed in the longitudinal bone axis over the tumor. To prevent contamination and tumor spread, extensive muscular dissection and neurovascular structures are avoided, although meticulous hemostasis is maintained. When possible, an intraoperative

frozen section is obtained to ensure that an adequate tissue specimen has been sampled. In closed biopsies, either a fine-needle aspiration is used to remove cells for cytology or a tissue core is obtained for routine histologic preparation.

TREATMENT

The treatment of bone tumors depends on the tissue diagnosis, the degree of cell anaplasia, the extent of spread, the patient's medical condition, and the sensitivity of the tumor to treatment modalities. These modalities include surgery, chemotherapy, and radiotherapy.

Benign tumors are cured by local excision. If tumor resection compromises the structural integrity of the bone (ie, femoral neck), bone grafting or implant reinforcement will be necessary. Metastatic lesions may be palliated with local radiation. When a lesion occupies greater than 50% of a bone's cortical diameter, a pathologic fracture is imminent. Prophylactic fixation is preferable with impending pathologic fractures because patient morbidity and mortality are higher after fracture.

Generally, malignant bone tumors are resected with wide or radical surgical margins. Adjuvant chemotherapy and radiation therapy are used to eradicate tumor micrometastases that are assumed to be present. In some centers, reconstructive techniques using bone and joint allografts either alone or in combination with customized prosthetic joint replacement are used to salvage limbs (limb sparing) and maximize patient function. Limb salvage techniques should never compromise the eradication of the neoplasm.

GAIT

Normal ambulation is efficient and conserves energy. Abnormal ambulation is inefficient, requires increased energy expenditure, and usually is a manifestation of neuromuscular pathology. Gait observation and analysis is thus an essential part of the musculoskeletal examination.

A normal gait cycle (Figure 26-58) extends from the heel strike of one foot to the next heel strike of the same foot. The normal cycle is divided into the stance phase (60% of the cycle), when the foot is in contact with the ground, and the swing phase (40% of the cycle), when the foot is off the ground. The stance phase begins at heel strike, is followed by foot flat, and ends with toe-off. The swing phase is marked by advancement of the limb to the next heel strike. The stride length is the distance covered during one gait cycle (heel strike to ipsilateral heel strike). The step length is the distance between the heel strike of one foot and the heel strike of the contralateral foot. Because the pelvis and trunk as well as the muscles and joints of the lower limb are involved in gait, abnormalities in these regions may indicate gait abnormalities.

An abnormal gait is often called a limp. Most gait abnormalities are detectable during the stance phase, when body weight is supported by one lower extremity. During stance, pain, muscle weakness, and joint abnormalities produce their maximal effect. The typical reaction to pain is to quickly unload the affected leg. Thus, an antalgic

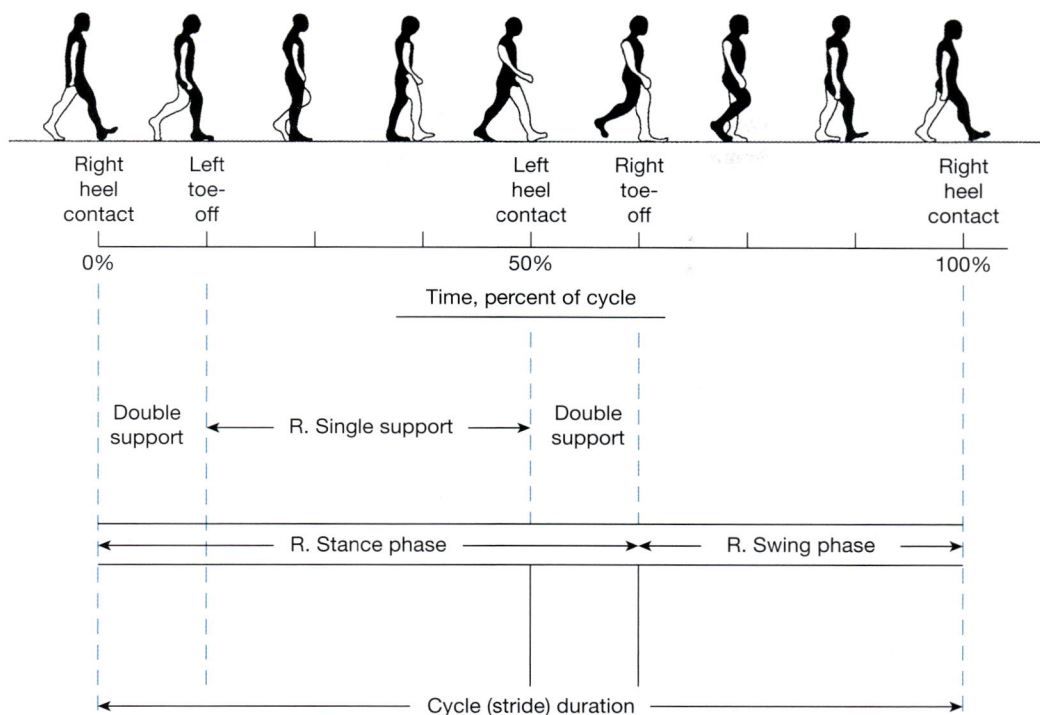

Figure 26-58. The gait cycle. (Modified from Phillips WA. The child with a limp. *Orthop Clin North Am*. 1987;18:489-501. Copyright © 1987 Elsevier.)

(pain-relieving) gait is manifested by a decreased stance phase of the affected limb. The swing phase of the limb opposite is also decreased, resulting in a shortened step length.

Muscle weakness has significant effects on gait. Quadriceps weakness interferes with the ability to lock the knee in full extension before heel strike. To compensate, the patient will push the thigh backward with the hand. Weakness of the foot and ankle dorsiflexors will not allow the controlled placement of the foot after heel strike to the foot flat position. This results in a foot slap gait as the foot slaps to the ground after heel strike. Likewise, paralysis of the foot and ankle dorsiflexors caused by peroneal nerve palsy will cause the patient to bring the knee up higher than normal during the swing phase so the toes clear the ground. This motion may result in a steppage gate. Other compensatory mechanisms for clearing a dropped foot include elevating the ipsilateral pelvis (hip-hike gait) or swinging the leg out to the side (circumduction gait). A weak gluteus maximus, which serves as a hip extensor, causes the trunk to collapse forward during midstance. The patient will compensate by thrusting the trunk posteriorly in what is called an extensor lurch or gluteus maximus gait. Weakness of the hip abductor muscles (gluteus medius and minimus) allows the contralateral pelvis to sink downward during stance. To compensate, the patient's torso lurches laterally over the weak hip in what is known as Trendelenburg or gluteus medius gait. Weakness of the calf muscles (gastrocnemius and soleus) prevents the normal propulsive toe-off push and is manifest as a flat-footed or calcaneal gait.

Joint abnormalities that interfere with the normal range of toe, metatarsophalangeal, ankle, knee, or hip joint motion also adversely affect gait. For example, an equinus (plantar flexion) ankle contracture causes knee hyperextension during the stance phase of ambulation.

Armed with knowledge of gait mechanics and a critical eye, the clinician can distinguish many of these gait patterns when observing a group of people. An abnormal gait pattern may provide the first clue in the diagnosis of a neuromuscular disease process.

SUGGESTED READINGS

American Academy of Orthopaedic Surgeons. Primary total hip arthroplasty: everything you need to know. AAOS Instructional Course Lectures; March 2016; Orlando, FL.

American Academy of Orthopaedic Surgeons. Principles of open fracture management. AAOS Instructional Course Lectures; March 17, 2017; San Diego, CA.

Bronstein RD, Schaffer JC. Physical examination of the knee: meniscus, cartilage, and patellofemoral conditions. *J Am Acad Orthop Surg*. 2017;25(5):365-374.

Lieberman JR, Heckmann N. Venous thromboembolism prophylaxis in total hip arthroplasty and total knee arthroplasty patients: from guidelines to practice. *J Am Acad Orthop Surg*. 2017;25(12):789-798.

Morris BJ, Mir HR. The opioid epidemic: impact on orthopaedic surgery. *J Am Acad Orthop Surg*. 2015;23(5):267-271.

Ochi J, Nozaki T, Nimura A, Yamaguchi T, Kitamura N. Subchondral insufficiency fracture of the knee: review of current concepts and radiological differential diagnoses. *Jpn J Radiol*. 2022;40(5):443-457.

SAMPLE QUESTIONS

QUESTIONS

Choose the best answer for each question.

1. Which of the following joints are most prone to septic arthritis during childhood?

   A. Ankle
   B. Knee
   C. Hip
   D. Wrist
   E. Base of thumb

2. Radiographic features of degenerative joint disease include all of the following except one. Which of the following is the exception?

   A. Localized joint space narrowing
   B. Marginal erosions
   C. Subchondral sclerosis
   D. Osteophytes
   E. Subchondral cysts

3. Radiographic features of inflammatory joint disease include all of the following except one. Which of the following is the exception?

   A. Generalized joint space loss
   B. Periarticular osteopenia
   C. Marginal erosions
   D. Osteophytes
   E. Soft tissue swelling

4. Which of the following bone or portion of bone is LEAST likely to be affected by osteonecrosis?

   A. Femoral head
   B. Talus
   C. Olecranon
   D. Lunate
   E. Scaphoid

5. The majority of episodes of low back pain resolve over time. What percentage of low back pain episodes resolve by 3 months following onset?

   A. 51%
   B. 60%
   C. 70%
   D. 80%
   E. 90%

ANSWERS AND EXPLANATIONS

1. **Answer: C**

   In children, septic arthritis occurs as an extension of hematogenous osteomyelitis. The joints commonly involved are those in which the metaphysis resides within the joint capsule: the hip, elbow, and shoulder. Because the metaphysis is enclosed in the joint capsule, what begins as osteomyelitis can erupt through the cortex to involve the joint in the septic process. For more information on this topic, see section "Septic Arthritis."

2. **Answer: B**

   Marginal erosions are not a feature of degenerative joint disease. Erosions are typical of inflammatory joint disease. The radiologic hallmarks of osteoarthrosis are localized joint space narrowing, subchondral bone sclerosis, osteophytes, and subchondral cysts. For more information on this topic, see section "Osteoarthrosis."

3. **Answer: D**

   Osteophytes are typical of degenerative joint disease. All the other features are typical of inflammatory joint disease. Soft tissue swelling and periarticular osteoporosis are the early signs of rheumatoid arthritis. Diffuse cartilage destruction leads to generalized joint space narrowing and bone erosions at the site of synovial attachments. Joint deformity, cystic bone destruction, and joint ankylosis mark end-stage disease. Hypertrophic osteophytes are rare in rheumatoid arthritis. For more information on this topic, see section "Rheumatoid Arthritis."

4. **Answer: C**

   The olecranon is not prone to osteonecrosis, whereas the other bones are prone to it. Interruption of the blood supply to bone results in bone cell death (osteonecrosis or avascular necrosis). Traumatic causes of osteonecrosis have been discussed and involve vascular injury or interruption of the blood supply to bones. The femoral head, talus, carpal lunate, and scaphoid are prone to avascular necrosis. These bones are all extensively covered by articular cartilage and have limited soft tissue attachments. For more information on this topic, see section "Complications of Fracture Healing."

5. **Answer: E**

   The vast majority of episodes of low back pain resolve within 3 months. Contrary to popular opinion, the vast majority of low back pain is not due to a "slipped disk." In 80% to 90% of patients with low back pain, the pain is of unknown etiology, and the pathology remains obscure. Fewer than 10% of patients experience pain in the sciatic nerve (L5-S3) distribution ("sciatica"). Only 1% to 2% of patients require surgical treatment for disk herniation. With symptomatic care, 50% improve in 2 weeks and 90% in 3 months. For more information on this topic, see section "Etiology of Low Back Pain."

27 Urology: Diseases of the Genitourinary System

Joseph Shirk and Patrick Lec

Urology is the field of medicine focusing on the surgical and medical treatment of diseases of the male and female genitourinary systems as well as the reproductive systems of men. This chapter reviews the anatomy, diseases, and treatments of common urologic conditions.

PROSTATE

Anatomy and Physiology

The normal prostate gland is located just distal to the bladder neck and surrounds the urethra for a distance of 2 to 3 cm. The membranous urethra, which is surrounded by the external urinary sphincter, is located just distal to the prostatic urethra. The ejaculatory ducts empty into the prostatic urethra at the level of the verumontanum (pronounced *VEE-roo-mon-TAN-um*), a small midline portion of the prostate that protrudes into the prostatic urethra seen readily during cystoscopy (Figure 27-1). The prostate gland is divided anatomically into discrete segments—the central, transition, and peripheral zones. From the bladder neck to the striated sphincter runs the anterior fibromuscular stroma. The transition zone enlarges substantially in men with benign prostatic hyperplasia. The peripheral zone is the origin of nearly 90% of prostatic cancers.

The blood supply to the prostate originates primarily from branches of the hypogastric artery that enter the prostate posterolaterally (Figure 27-2). A large dorsal vein complex draining the penis is located on the anterior surface of the prostate. The puboprostatic ligaments anchor the prostate gland anteriorly to the pubic bone. Microscopically, the prostate gland is composed of glandular epithelium contained within a fibromuscular stroma.

Secretions from the prostate gland constitute approximately 20% of the volume of a normal ejaculate. The prostatic fluid provides nutrients that are necessary for normal sperm motility and function. The prostate remains relatively dormant from birth until puberty and then begins to function as an exocrine gland. Enlargement begins in the fourth decade of life and may lead to benign prostatic hyperplasia.

Prostatitis

Prostatitis is an inflammatory condition of the prostate that may be bacterial or noninfectious in origin but often has no defined etiologic agent. Symptoms include prostatodynia, a symptom complex consisting of an aching perineal discomfort, urinary frequency, urgency, and dysuria, as well as more classic obstructive symptoms (eg, urinary

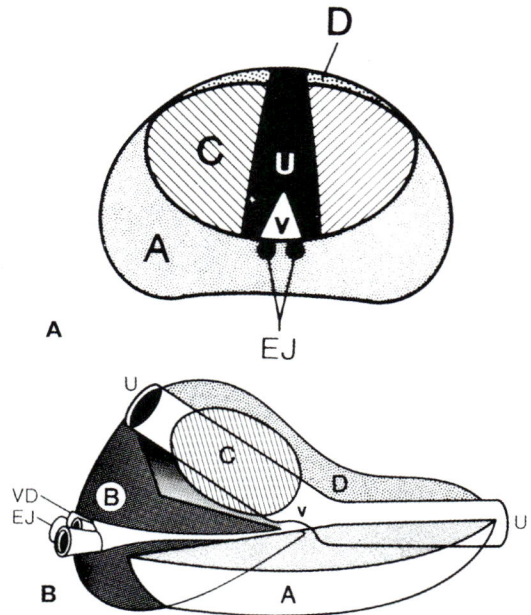

Figure 27-1. A. Schematic transverse image of the midportion of the prostate. B. Schematic longitudinal representation of the prostate. A, peripheral zone; B, central zone; C, transition zone; D, anterior fibromuscular stroma; U, urethra; V, verumontanum; EJ, ejaculatory ducts; VD, vas deferens. (From Lawrence PF. *Essentials of Surgical Specialties*. 3rd ed. Lippincott Williams & Wilkins; 2007.)

hesitancy, dribbling, and difficulty emptying the bladder). A distinction between bacterial and nonbacterial prostatitis cannot reliably be made on the basis of symptoms alone.

Acute Prostatitis

Acute prostatitis is a relatively unusual bacterial infection of the prostate that may have protean manifestations. The disease typically occurs after the second decade of life and is characterized by rapidly developing symptoms of fever, back and perineal pain, chills, and dysuria. On physical examination, the prostate gland is swollen and often described as boggy, sometimes warm to the touch because of inflammation, and often exquisitely tender. The urine sediment shows white blood cells and the serum white blood cell count may be increased. Patients may present with acute urinary retention because of severe prostatic edema.

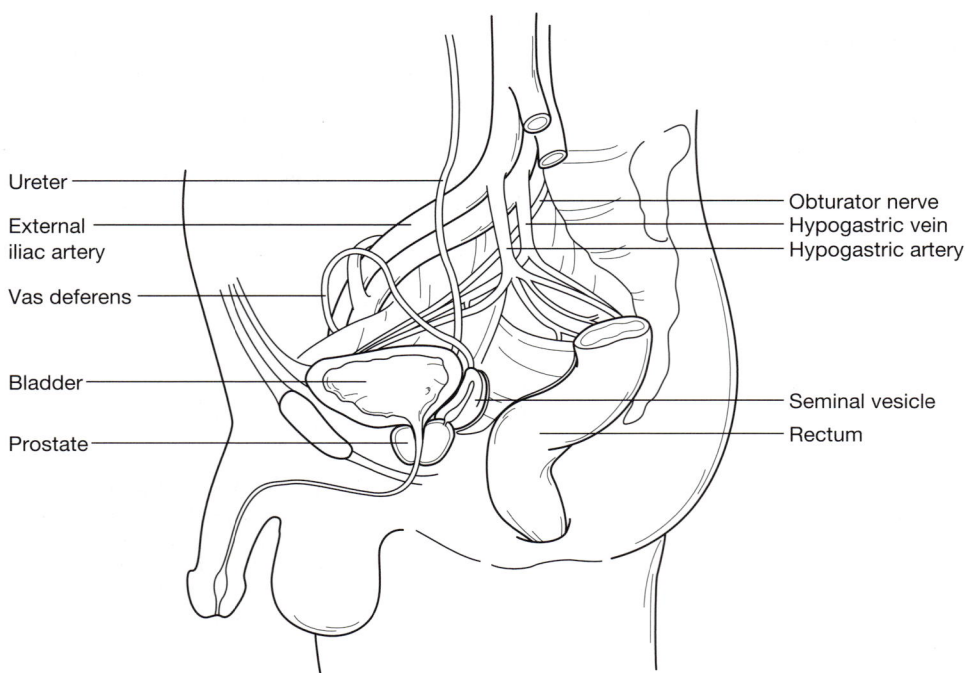

Figure 27-2. Sagittal view of the male pelvic anatomy showing the relation of the prostate gland to adjacent pelvic structures. (From Lawrence PF. *Essentials of Surgical Specialties*. 3rd ed. Lippincott Williams & Wilkins; 2007.)

Gram-negative bacteria (eg, *Escherichia coli*) are the most common organisms found in bacterial prostatitis. Treatment consists of broad-spectrum antibiotics dosed for several weeks due to poor tissue penetration into the prostate. Bladder decompression is recommended in cases associated with urinary retention. Suprapubic cystostomy is preferred in this setting given the risk of septicemia with passing a transurethral catheter across the prostate. Acute and chronic prostatitis can be complicated by the formation of a prostate abscess. Prostate abscess can be evaluated with cross-sectional imaging (ie, computed tomography [CT] scan) when clinically indicated, including patients who do not improve with antibiotics or show fluctuance on digital rectal examination. Prostate abscesses can be treated with transurethral unroofing with a resectoscope and transrectal or transgluteal aspiration with or without drain placement.

Chronic Prostatitis

Chronic prostatitis has a more indolent clinical course than acute prostatitis. It is uncertain whether chronic bacterial prostatitis is a consequence of recurring independent infections or of failure to adequately eliminate an initial infection. Most often, there is no antecedent history of acute prostatitis. Patients typically present with discomfort in the perineum, back, or pelvis that is associated with urinary frequency, hesitancy, and dysuria. A voided urinalysis may show white blood cells. Expressed prostatic secretions can be obtained for analysis by "milking" the urethra after a digital prostatic massage. This fluid characteristically has more than 12 white blood cells per high-power field in patients with prostatitis, even after previous treatment with antibiotics. Cultures of prostatic fluid should be positive

for bacteria before a diagnosis of chronic bacterial prostatitis can be made. Treatment consists of oral broad-spectrum antibiotics (eg, trimethoprim-sulfamethoxazole and quinolone), often for a 6-week course. Voiding symptoms usually improve on antibiotics but may recur after antibiotics are discontinued. Caution should be exercised when prescribing prolonged courses of quinolones given the risk of tendon rupture.

Nonbacterial Prostatitis

Nonbacterial prostatitis is a common and often frustrating problem for patients and physicians. The subjective manifestations may be indistinguishable from those associated with chronic prostatitis. However, no bacterial or other etiologic agent has been consistently identified, although *Chlamydia trachomatis* has been isolated in some patients. Frequently, there are no objective findings and the prostatic fluid is normal on microscopic examination. Treatment options may include antibiotics (despite the absence of a documented bacterial etiology), prostatic massage, α-blockers, and pelvic floor physical therapy for patients in whom concomitant pelvic floor dysfunction is suspected. Symptomatic treatment consists of sitz-baths and nonsteroidal anti-inflammatory drugs.

Benign Prostatic Hyperplasia

Epidemiology

Benign prostate hyperplasia (BPH) is a degenerative process of hyperplasia (proliferation in the number of cells) and hypertrophy (enlargement of the cells) of the prostate associated with voiding symptoms. The pathologic process primarily occurs in the transition zone and can be demonstrated histologically as early as the third decade of life. Symptomatic manifestations of BPH are uncommon before 50 years of age. There is no apparent causal association between BPH and other pathologic conditions of the prostate (eg, prostatitis, cancer). The natural history of BPH is poorly understood and variable. Significant spontaneous symptomatic improvement is relatively uncommon, but not all patients have progressive symptoms if left untreated. Histologic evidence of BPH is almost universal in aging men, but there is no direct correlation between prostate size and symptoms.

Clinical Presentation and Evaluation

Because of its anatomic position surrounding the urethra, enlargement of the prostate typically results in a relative obstruction of bladder outflow. Classic obstructive symptoms are hesitancy in initiating voiding, a decrease in the force of the urinary stream, terminal dribbling, intermittency, or a feeling of incomplete bladder emptying. Because of compensatory bladder changes that may result from obstruction, typical irritating voiding symptoms (eg, frequency, urgency, and nocturia) are also common. The symptoms are usually of gradual onset and may progress to the point of acute urinary retention.

Digital rectal examination of the prostate often shows palpable enlargement. There may be some asymmetry of the prostate, but BPH characteristically has a smooth contour and a soft consistency. It is important to remember that a marked enlargement of the prostate can occur without associated symptoms, and urologic consultation and evaluation are not indicated simply because of prostate enlargement on physical examination alone. Moreover, symptoms may occur without marked enlargement. In the absence of infection, a voided urinalysis is normal. A urine flow rate test shows diminished force of the urinary stream (usually <15 mL/s in symptomatic patients). An abnormal amount of urine in the bladder after voiding, termed postvoid residual (PVR), may be demonstrable by direct catheterization or ultrasonography. Intravenous pyelography (IVP), when obtained for other symptoms or signs, may suggest thickening of the bladder detrusor muscle (trabeculation); it may also show J-hooking of the distal ureters, which is caused by cephalad displacement by the enlarged prostate. However, IVP is not routinely obtained or indicated in the evaluation of uncomplicated BPH. A decompensated bladder with poor emptying and/or impaired compliance is a relatively unusual manifestation of long-standing BPH; it could result in hydronephrosis and renal failure because of the chronically increased intravesical pressure. An endoscopic examination of the lower urinary tract called cystoscopy usually reveals trilobar hyperplasia or not infrequently a median lobe that causes obstruction of urinary outflow via a "ball valve" mechanism.

Invasive urodynamic studies utilize intracavitary pressure catheters to measure intravesical pressure changes during the storing and emptying phases of micturition. This study can help diagnose bladder outlet obstruction secondary to BPH. However, its use should be restricted to patients in whom the results are likely to change management, particularly in those for whom invasive intervention (ie, surgery) is being considered. This includes patients with lower urinary tract symptoms (LUTS) refractory to treatment, mixed LUTS, and upper tract compromise.

Treatment

Occasionally, patients may have objective indications for treatment (eg, renal failure and poor bladder emptying resulting in recurrent infection or bladder stones). More commonly, treatment of BPH aims to alleviate the symptoms and improve the quality of life. Patients should be counseled that symptomatic improvement can be achieved with treatment, but that a lack of treatment does not necessarily imply progressive symptoms or detrimental consequences. Symptoms are usually quantified by administering the American Urological Association (AUA) Symptom Score test. Improvement in symptom score is often used as an objective measure of treatment response. As some patients tolerate marked symptoms with little bother, the degree of patient annoyance or bother with symptoms is most often the initiating factor for treatment.

Medical Therapy

With the advent of modern medical therapy that provides symptomatic benefit in most patients with BPH, surgical treatment is much less frequently performed and is usually reserved for patients who do not tolerate or are unresponsive to medical management. α_1-Adrenergic blockers are usually the first-line agent in medical management of BPH. The exact mechanism of action is uncertain, although α-adrenergic receptors are present in the bladder neck and prostatic urethra. Currently, five α blockers are used to treat lower urinary tract voiding symptoms: terazosin (Hytrin), alfuzosin (Uroxatral), doxazosin (Cardura), tamsulosin (Flomax), and silodosin (Rapaflo). Each agent is administered as a single daily dose. A favorable response can occur rapidly, sometimes within 24 hours of dose administration. Each of the available drugs is usually well tolerated, although drug-related weakness may occur and postural hypotension is occasionally observed. Patients planning to undergo cataract surgery should be cautioned about the risks of floppy iris syndrome if taking an α-blocker.

Finasteride (Proscar) and dutasteride (Avodart) are 5α-reductase inhibitors used for the treatment of symptomatic BPH. 5α-Reductase converts testosterone to the active intracellular metabolite dihydrotestosterone. Consequently, these agents act by blocking androgenic activity on the prostate cells. A modest decrease in prostatic size (20%-30%) occurs, and some patients have mild symptomatic improvement or a small increase in urinary flow rates. The drugs are well tolerated, with very few side effects, although a small percentage of patients notice sexual dysfunction (eg, decreased libido, impotence). Finasteride and dutasteride usually lower serum prostate-specific antigen (PSA), a marker for prostate cancer. When a patient is taking one of these drugs, serum PSA should be doubled to calculate a useful relative value. Further, any increase in PSA while taking 5α-reductase inhibitors should raise an alarm for an underlying prostatic malignancy. In comparative studies, finasteride was less effective than α-adrenergic blocking drugs in relieving LUTS when the overall prostate size is less than 50 g. Thus, 5α-reductase inhibitors should only be offered to patients with prostate glands larger than 30 g on imaging, a PSA value greater than or equal to 1.5 ng/dL, or a palpably enlarged prostate on digital rectal examination. These patients may also be offered a combination of α_1-adrenergic blockers and 5α-reductase inhibitors, especially in the setting of single-drug failure.

Surgical Therapy

The surgical removal of obstructing prostatic tissue may be performed through an open/robotic or a transurethral route. An open/robotic surgical approach is usually chosen for patients with a very large (>100 g) prostate size. The enlarged prostatic adenomatous tissue is enucleated by sharp and blunt dissection through either the bladder (suprapubic prostatectomy) or the prostatic capsule (simple retropubic prostatectomy). During surgery for BPH, the capsule of the prostate is not removed and there is no disruption of urethral continuity.

More often, the transurethral route is chosen for the performance of transurethral prostatectomy (TURP). An electrocautery loop is used to successively remove prostatic tissue under direct visualization. The resection is usually carried to the level of the prostatic capsule, and all obstructing tissue is removed. Alternatively, a transurethral incision of the prostate may be performed in patients with small glands or an elevated bladder neck. With either technique, hemostasis is obtained with electrocautery. The risk of incontinence is low (1%-2%) and treatment-related impotence occurs in less than 5% of patients.

Photoselective vaporization of the prostate can be offered as an alternative to TURP, whereby a green light laser is utilized to ablate prostate tissue. This procedure carries a hemostatic advantage and can be performed in patients on therapeutic anticoagulation, in contrast to all other forms of surgical BPH treatments.

Enucleation of the prostate utilizing a holium (HoLEP) or thulium (ThuLEP) laser is a transurethral surgery in which the prostatic adenoma is surgically dissected from the capsule and removed via intravesical morcellation. This surgical option can be offered to patients irrespective of prostate size by surgeons with adequate experience performing this procedure.

More recently, waterjet ablation offers an alternative to traditional TURP. Using this technique, a transrectal ultrasound (TRUS) probe is used to map the prostate, and then the gland is ablated using a hypersonic transurethral waterjet. This technique has been shown to be as efficacious as TURP in reducing urinary symptoms while decreasing the risk of retrograde ejaculation, another common side effect for patients undergoing transurethral prostate surgery.

Office-Based Procedures

Less invasive procedures for the treatment of LUTS have proliferated. These procedures may carry fewer side effects than those of surgery and can be conducted on an outpatient basis.

Transurethral microwave thermotherapy and transurethral needle ablation have been advocated as office-based procedures. However, these techniques are no longer used widely because of a relatively modest improvement in symptoms. However, data suggest the efficacy of transurethral water vapor thermal therapy in patients with prostate glands measuring 30 to 80 g.

Prostatic urethral lift procedures utilize surgical clips deployed cystoscopically to pin the prostate adenoma laterally, thereby augmenting the diameter of the prostatic urethra. This procedure should be offered to patients with a prostate gland measuring 30 to 80 g in the absence of a large median lobe. This procedure offers the advantage of preserved ejaculatory and erectile functions, albeit with relatively decreased efficacy relative to surgical treatments.

Malignant Diseases

Epidemiology

Carcinoma of the prostate is among the most common cancers in men in the United States. More than 95% of prostatic cancers are adenocarcinomas arising from the prostatic acinar structures. The incidence of prostate cancer increases with age and a familial pattern has been identified, with the disease more common in African Americans than in European Americans. A high-fat diet has been implicated as a contributing factor in some studies and a pattern of autosomal dominant inheritance has been identified in some patients, especially those with an early age of onset.

Histologically, an adenocarcinoma can be identified at autopsy in over 30% and 70% of men over the age of 50 and 80 years, respectively. Thus, there is a large discrepancy between histologic and clinically significant diseases.

Clinical Presentation and Evaluation

Most men with early-stage prostate cancer have no disease-related symptoms. Prostate cancer and BPH may occur simultaneously, but there is no apparent causal relation. Obstructive voiding symptoms may be from BPH or, as the cancer enlarges, from malignant tissue. Patients with advanced disease may have weight loss, pelvic pain, ureteral obstruction, gross hematuria, or bone pain from local invasion and distant metastasis.

Digital Rectal Examination

Digital rectal examination is an important method for screening and early detection of prostate cancer. A normal prostate is smooth, symmetrical, and has a consistency similar to that of the muscles of the thenar eminence of the hand. About 80% of prostate cancers arise in the peripheral zone and, once they attain sufficient size, are palpable as an area of induration or nodularity within the substance of the prostate (Figure 27-3).

For digital rectal examinations, patients are directed to lie in the knee-chest position or to stand while bending forward at the waist. A gloved and lubricated index finger is inserted into the rectum. The prostate gland is palpable beneath the anterior rectal wall (normal seminal vesicles are usually not palpable). The margins of the prostate should be distinct, and any areas of induration, nodularity, or asymmetry should be noted.

Prostate-Specific Antigen Testing

PSA is a serine protease enzyme whose function is to cleave the proteins and liquefy postejaculatory semen. Serum PSA is specific for the prostate but not prostate cancer because PSA is expressed by both benign and malignant prostatic epithelial cells. In normal conditions, PSA is secreted into the prostatic lumen. With any conditions that destroy the normal prostatic architecture, the cellular polarity is lost and PSA is secreted both into the prostatic lumen and the blood vessels. Thus, the PSA level may be elevated in men with prostatitis, BPH, prostate cancer, or any conditions that result in a dysregulation of cellular polarity.

PSA has remained the cornerstone of prostate cancer screening since its widespread implementation in the early 1990s, during which time deaths due to prostate cancer decreased by approximately 40%. For those at high risk—African Americans and those with a family

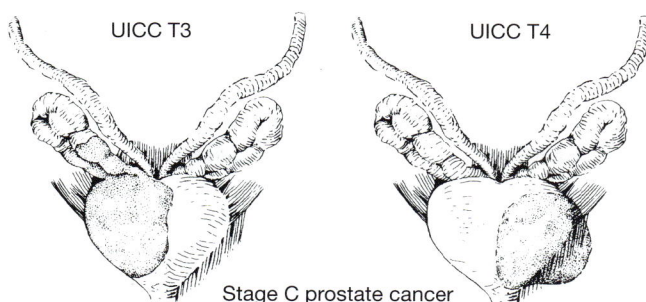

Figure 27-3. Schematic representation of a palpable prostate cancer with extension into the seminal vesicle (left) and the levator ani muscle (right). Most prostate cancers arise in the peripheral zone and, once they attain sufficient size are palpable by digital rectal examination as an area of induration or nodularity. UICC, Union for International Cancer Control. (From Lawrence PF. *Essentials of Surgical Specialties*. 3rd ed. Lippincott Williams & Wilkins; 2007.)

history of prostate cancer or known germline mutations—screening should be considered at 40 to 45 years of age. In older patients and those with a life expectancy of less than 10 years, there may not be a significant benefit to prostate cancer screening. In fact, two large-scale clinical trials have demonstrated that an annual population-wide screening for prostate cancer (rather than just those at high risk) may not be beneficial. Nevertheless, many feel that screening should begin at age 55 years in all patients. Ultimately, the decision to screen for prostate cancer with PSA should be a shared decision between the patient and doctor.

PSA values differ somewhat depending on the assay used. In general, a level less than 4.0 ng/mL is considered normal. However, prostate cancer is present in 20% to 25% of patients with "normal" PSA levels. A number of factors can be used to adjust PSA levels to increase specificity. The PSA level increases gradually with age, probably because of overall prostate enlargement. By age-adjusted PSA standards, a PSA level of 3.9 ng/mL is considered high for a man in the sixth decade of life, whereas a level greater than 4.0 ng/mL is within the normal range for older men.

Serum PSA occurs in two dominant forms: one conjugated to α_1-antichymotrypsin and the other unconjugated, or free. The relative proportion of the two forms can be used to improve the specificity of PSA testing. A greater proportion of free PSA is seen in men with a modest increase in PSA from BPH compared with those with prostate cancer. In general, a percent-free fraction of less than 20% to 25% is more commonly associated with prostate cancer than higher levels. PSA density (serum PSA [ng/dL]/prostate volume [cc]) can help distinguish between elevated PSA due to benign enlargement and prostatic adenocarcinoma. The PSA density cutoff measures have been proposed ranging from greater than or equal to 0.07 to greater than or equal to 0.15 that are associated with an increased risk of clinically significant prostate cancer diagnosis.

Transrectal Ultrasonography

TRUS can distinguish the zonal anatomy of the prostate and accurately measure the prostate size. Prostatic cancers are typically located in the peripheral zone and classically have a hypoechoic pattern. However, because of its lack of sensitivity and specificity, TRUS is not used as a screening test. Rather, it is used to direct prostate biopsy in men with a palpable abnormality of the prostate or an abnormal PSA reading.

Magnetic Resonance Imaging

With recent advances in technology, magnetic resonance imaging (MRI) has been advocated by some investigators as a diagnostic tool for patients with an elevated PSA or abnormal digital rectal examination. To establish standards for MRI interpretation, the PI-RAD (Prostate Imaging—Reporting and Data System) scoring system has been adopted by most centers. Prostate cancers may be seen as dark areas in the peripheral zone on T2 imaging (Figure 27-4).

Prostate Biopsy

Obtaining a biopsy for the detection of prostate cancer can be via the transrectal or transperineal route under TRUS guidance. A spring-loaded automatic gun is used to obtain cores of tissue in a systematic fashion. Usually, 10 to 14 cores are obtained. Patients are usually given an enema on the morning of the examination. In addition, premedication with a broad-spectrum antibiotic such as fluoroquinolones or cephalosporin with an aminoglycoside for a single dose is recommended. Increasingly, biopsies are performed by fusing the lesions identified on MRI to the live ultrasound images, resulting in better biopsy yield.

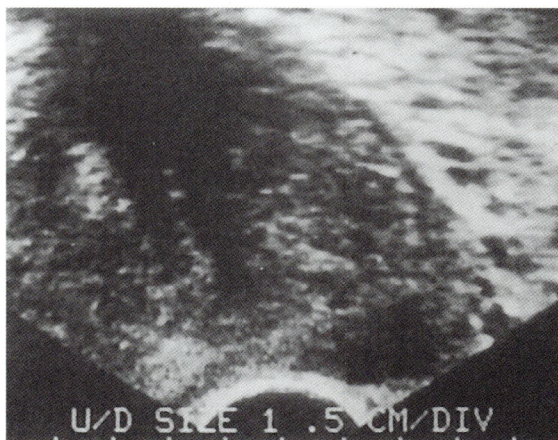

Figure 27-4. T2 magnetic resonance imaging (MRI) scan of the prostate showing an area in the peripheral zone suspicious for cancer. MRI can help direct biopsies to specific areas of the prostate that may be suspicious for cancer.

Tumor Grade

The degree of differentiation of the tumor provides important prognostic information. Most often, the Gleason grading system is used. This system assigns a number (1-5) to the dominant grade and a secondary number to arrive at a Gleason sum or score. By convention, pathologists omit assigning scores of 2 to 5, with a Gleason score of 6 representing the lowest grade malignancy. Combined with other clinical information, such as PSA, the Gleason score allows the stratification of prostate cancer into low, intermediate (favorable and unfavorable), and high risks. Most cancers found through early detection or screening programs are low risk. More recently, a new classification system (Gleason Grade Group) that divides prostate cancer into five risk strata is being advocated.

Staging of Prostate Cancer

Staging of prostate cancer defines the local, regional, and distant extent of disease. The tumor, node, metastasis (TNM) system is the current standard that allows categorization of nonpalpable tumors detected because of PSA or ultrasound abnormalities. (For detailed information on the staging of prostate cancer, see the American Joint Committee on Cancer's *Cancer Staging Manual*. 8th edition.)

The primary staging modality for local disease is digital rectal examination. TRUS is used primarily to direct biopsy and is of limited value for staging. Serum PSA levels correlate only roughly with disease extent. However, bone metastasis is quite uncommon in patients with a PSA value less than 20 ng/mL. Radionuclide bone scanning is the most sensitive method for the detection of bone metastases (Figure 27-5). Prostate cancer, when metastatic, typically affects the axial skeleton and forms osteoblastic metastases visible on plain radiography (Figure 27-6). Soft

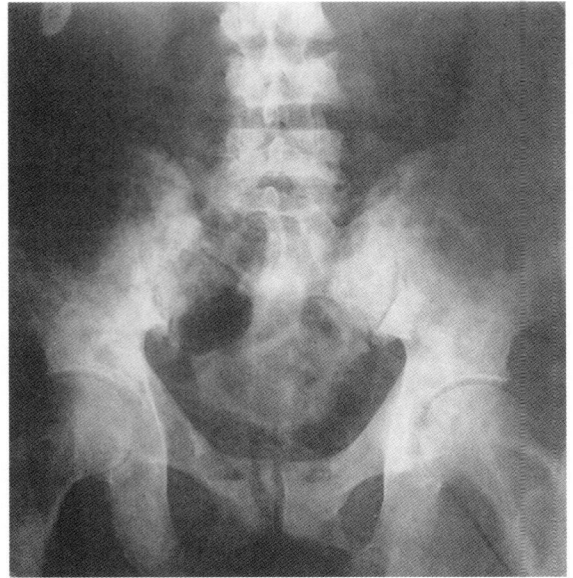

Figure 27-6. Radiograph of the pelvis showing characteristic osteoblastic metastases from prostate cancer. (From Lawrence PF. *Essentials of Surgical Specialties*. 3rd ed. Lippincott Williams & Wilkins; 2007.)

tissue metastasis may also occur but is unusual without concomitant bone metastasis. Prostate-specific membrane antigen positron emission tomography (PET) imaging has emerged as a sensitive and specific diagnostic tool, with applications established in the setting of biochemical recurrence (discussed later) and being investigated in the initial staging of prostate cancer.

CT scanning may show enlarged lymph nodes in patients with high-volume or high-grade primary tumors. Lymph node dissection is performed simultaneously with radical prostatectomy. The anatomic limits of a staging lymph node dissection for prostate cancer are the bifurcation of the common iliac artery proximally, the circumflex iliac vein distally, the midportion of the external iliac artery laterally, and the bladder wall medially. The dissection is carried posteriorly to below the obturator nerve (Figure 27-7).

Treatment

Localized Disease

The optimal therapy for localized prostate cancer is uncertain and a point of continual controversy. For men with a life expectancy of less than 10 years, observation alone (ie, "watchful waiting") may be appropriate. In patients with a longer life expectancy, active surveillance, involving periodic PSA testing, digital rectal examinations, and biopsy, is the preferred treatment for low-risk prostate cancer (Gleason score 6 or less). Active surveillance refers to the active surveillance of a diagnosed cancer with the intent of cure at a later date if it becomes more aggressive (stage or Gleason score progression). In contrast, watchful waiting involves the observation of prostate cancer with the intent of treating symptoms of disease progression without the intent of cure, if and when they arise.

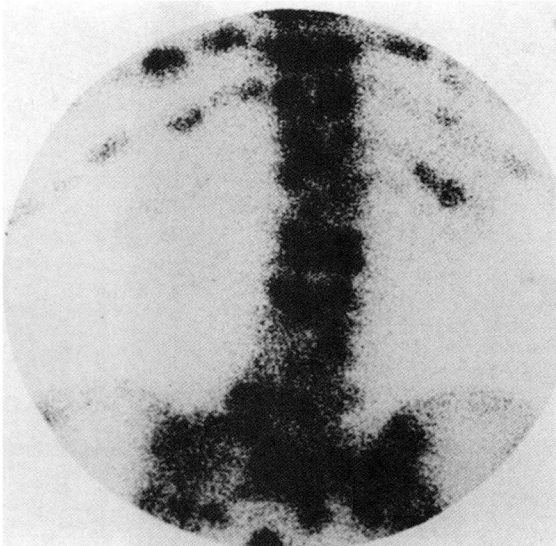

Figure 27-5. Radionuclide bone scan showing multiple areas of abnormal uptake in the pelvis and spine, typical of metastatic prostate cancer. (From Lawrence PF. *Essentials of Surgical Specialties*. 3rd ed. Lippincott Williams & Wilkins; 2007.)

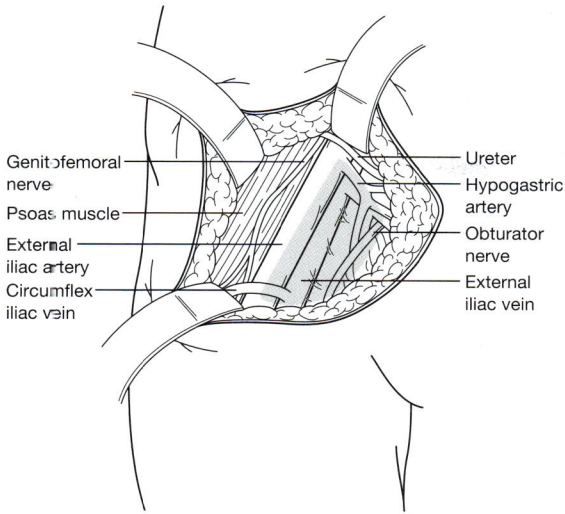

Figure 27-7. Anatomic boundaries of a staging pelvic lymph node dissection for prostate cancer. (From Lawrence PF. *Essentials of Surgical Specialties*. 3rd ed. Lippincott Williams & Wilkins; 2007.)

Surgical removal of the prostate (ie, radical prostatectomy) and radiation therapy are the most commonly used treatments with curative intent in patients with longer life expectancies or more aggressive tumors. Ten-year survival rates are similar after external beam radiation or surgery, but valid comparisons are difficult and follow-up beyond 10 years is important. Brachytherapy using interstitial implantation of either iodine-125 or palladium-103 is also used for low- and intermediate-risk disease. Cryotherapy (ie, freezing of the prostate) is being utilized in some centers, but results published to date indicate that this method is inferior to established treatments for intracapsular tumors.

Historically, radical prostatectomy is accomplished by a retropubic route. An incision is made from the umbilicus to the pubis. Usually, pelvic lymphadenectomy is performed. During radical retropubic prostatectomy, the entire prostate—including the prostatic capsule, the seminal vesicles, and the ampullary portion of the vas deferens—is removed. After the prostate is removed, a direct anastomosis is performed between the reconstructed bladder neck and the urethra (Figure 27-8). In patients who are sexually active before therapy, potency can be retained in nearly two-thirds by the preservation of the neurovascular bundle that lies immediately posterolateral to the prostate and urethra. In patients with negative surgical margins, a 15-year, disease-free survival rate of nearly 50% can be anticipated. In patients who have positive surgical margins or histologically positive lymph nodes, adjuvant radiation treatment or hormonal therapy may be used.

Robotic prostatectomy, the most common surgical technique today, involves the removal of the prostate using multiple small incisions. Available data suggest that robotic radical prostatectomies have the following advantages over open surgery: (a) better cosmesis, (b) reduced risk of transfusion, (c) shorter time to recovery, and (d) earlier return to continence. Short-term results indicate that this technique is equivalent to the open approach in controlling the cancer.

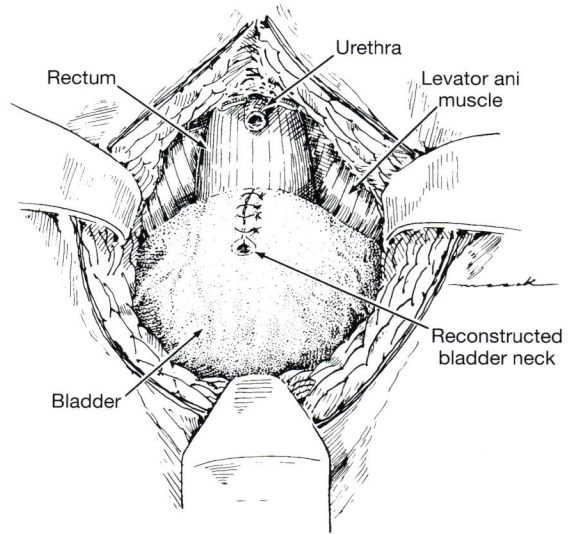

Figure 27-8. Radical retropubic prostatectomy. The surgical specimen has been removed and the bladder neck reconstructed. A direct anastomosis is performed with the stump of the urethra. (From Lawrence PF. *Essentials of Surgical Specialties*. 3rd ed. Lippincott Williams & Wilkins; 2007.)

Serum PSA levels should decrease to an undetectable range after radical prostatectomy because all PSA-producing cells, both benign and malignant, are ideally removed. After radiation therapy, superior results are achieved in patients in whom the PSA level decreases to less than 1.0 ng/mL or, perhaps, less than 0.2 ng/mL. An increasing serum PSA is evidence of tumor recurrence, although other studies may not identify metastatic disease initially. There is controversy and uncertainty about when to initiate hormonal therapy in men with an increasing PSA level after treatment.

Metastatic Disease

Prostate cancer is initially an androgen-dependent disease. Therefore, the primary treatment for metastatic carcinoma of the prostate is deprivation of androgens from the cancer cells. Suppression of serum testosterone can be achieved by bilateral surgical orchiectomy or medical castration. Oral administration of estrogens effectively lowers serum testosterone but is associated with cardiovascular side effects in up to 20% of patients. Estrogen therapy, common in the past, has been replaced by luteinizing hormone-releasing hormone (LHRH) analogues, which effectively suppress testosterone to the castrate range within 1 month of administration. LHRH analogues are associated with few serious side effects; however, they cause vasomotor hot flashes in approximately two-thirds of patients. Loss of libido and impotence are consequences of orchiectomy or LHRH administration.

Less than 10% of circulating androgens in men are of adrenal origin. The contribution of these androgens to the growth of prostate cancer is uncertain. Some studies have shown that antiandrogen can prolong the duration of response when used in conjunction with LHRH analogues or orchiectomy. However, other studies have shown conflicting results. The drug is administered orally and can cause some degree of gynecomastia and gastrointestinal side effects (usually diarrhea). Hepatotoxicity is seen occasionally.

If disease progression occurs, second-line antiandrogen therapies (ie, abiraterone, enzalutamide, apalutamide, and darolutamide) and taxol-based chemotherapy have been shown to be moderately effective in castration-resistant prostate cancer. Radiation can be effective for isolated sites of bone metastasis. In the PSA era, the median survival of patients with hormone-refractory prostate cancer is 53 months.

KIDNEYS

Anatomy

The kidneys are paired retroperitoneal organs that lie on either side of the vertebral column, opposite T12 and L1 through L3. They are bordered by the diaphragm posteriorly and superiorly, and by the psoas and quadratus lumborum muscles posteriorly. The right kidney is bordered by the right lobe of the liver anteriorly and superiorly and by the right colon inferiorly (Figure 27-9). The duodenum lies over the anteromedial portion of the right kidney. The left kidney lies adjacent to the spleen, with the left colon over its anterior lateral surface. The stomach borders the anterior surface of the upper pole, the jejunum overlies the anterior lower pole, and the tail of the pancreas overlies the hilum. Normally, the left kidney lies more cranially than the right one. The dimensions of the average kidney are approximately 11 cm in length, 6 cm in breadth, and 3 cm in anteroposterior thickness. Each kidney typically weighs 150 g in men and approximately 135 g in women.

Each kidney is enveloped by a renal capsule composed of fibrous tissue that is closely applied to the renal cortical surface. At the hilum, this layer becomes continuous with the fibrous sheaths of the renal and great vessels. The capsule is easily stripped from the parenchyma. The layer of adipose connective tissue surrounding the kidney and its vessels, the perirenal fat, is thickest at the borders of the kidney. Surrounding the perirenal fat is a layer of fibroareolar connective tissue, the renal fascia (Gerota). Superiorly, the fascial layers envelop the adrenal glands. Inferiorly, the layers remain separate and surround the ureters. Medially, the layers fuse and adhere to the renal vessels and kidney pelvices, limiting extravasation of urine, blood, or purulence.

Physiology

A clear understanding of renal and acid-base physiology is the basis for the management of many urologic disorders. Examples include hyponatremia as a complication of fluid absorption during TURP (TUR syndrome), renal tubular acidosis, hyperchloremic metabolic acidosis after urinary diversion using intestinal segments, acute tubular necrosis after renal ischemia, and renal artery stenosis. A complete discussion of renal physiology should be reviewed in a physiology text.

Blood Supply

About 20% of cardiac output is directed to the kidneys. The renal vascular pedicle is anterior to the renal pelvis, entering at the hilum (Figure 27-10). Usually, a single renal artery supplies each kidney. Later, this artery divides into branches that supply the various kidney segments. Variation in number and configuration of the renal arteries is extremely common. In one study, 65% of kidneys examined had at least one aberrant vessel. Interruption of these end arteries may result in ischemia and infarction of that part of the kidney. The potential long-term sequela of this type of injury is hypertension. Additionally, aberrant lower pole arteries may be associated with congenital ureteropelvic junction obstruction.

Trauma

Blunt trauma accounts for 70% to 80% of all renal injuries. It usually results from motor vehicle accidents or, less commonly, from accidental falls or contact sports. The mechanism of injury arises from the forces of rapid deceleration or actual impact on the upper abdomen, flank, or back. Hematuria occurs in many patients. Associated

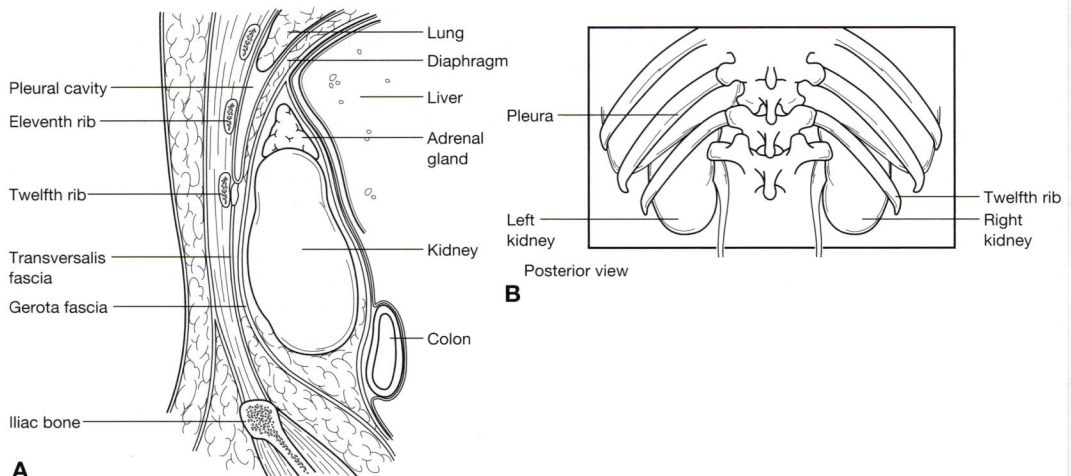

Figure 27-9. Anatomic relation of the pleural cavity and some intra-abdominal structures to the kidneys (A and B). (From Lawrence PF. *Essentials of Surgical Specialties.* 3rd ed. Lippincott Williams & Wilkins; 2007.)

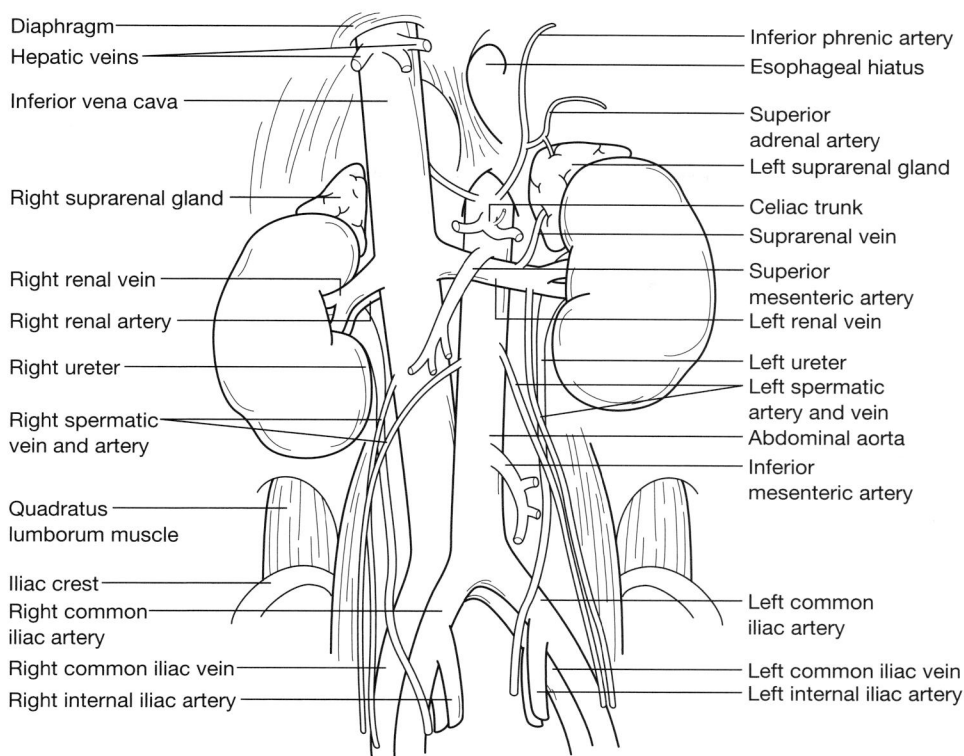

Figure 27-10. Blood supply to the kidneys. (From Lawrence PF. *Essentials of Surgical Specialties*. 3rd ed. Lippincott Williams & Wilkins; 2007.)

injuries can include rib fractures, vertebral body and transverse process fractures, and flank contusions and abrasions. Retroperitoneal hematoma secondary to renal injury must be considered in patients who present in shock.

Evaluation

In the past, imaging was routinely performed when a renal injury was suspected on the basis of the mechanism of injury, microhematuria, or gross hematuria. It has subsequently been shown that adults with microhematuria after blunt renal trauma but with no history of a major deceleration injury or hypotension do not necessarily need renal imaging. Children and patients with gross hematuria, hypotension, or a major deceleration injury require evaluation. A concern in children with rapid deceleration injury is an avulsion of the ureteropelvic junction; urinalysis can be negative in this situation.

A patient in trauma with a suspected renal injury should be promptly evaluated for hemodynamic instability. The evaluation of a stable patient with a suspected renal parenchymal injury includes a CT scan. Any renal injury noted is classified as shown in Figure 27-11. Minor contusions are the most common, and lacerations may be minor or major. In minor lacerations, the injury extends no further than the renal cortex, there is no urinary extravasation or large hematoma, and the capsule may remain intact. In major lacerations, there is a transcapsular rupture through the corticomedullary junction of the kidney and, often, associated with urinary extravasation or a large perirenal hematoma.

A patient who is unstable should be taken to the operating room for an emergency laparotomy regardless of whether a renal injury is suspected. In this situation, renal imaging may be accomplished with a "one-shot" IVP. One protocol for this test involves administering an intravenous bolus of 2 mL/kg contrast, with a film taken 10 minutes later.

Treatment

In the stable patient who sustains blunt trauma, renal exploration is required only if the CT scan shows a major renal injury. There is no general agreement as to exactly what CT findings justify exploration; however, the trend is toward observation if the patient is hemodynamically stable. Hemodynamic instability is an indication for immediate intervention, either in the form of angioembolization or exploratory surgery. In a patient who is unstable and undergoes surgery, indications for renal exploration include an expanding or pulsatile retroperitoneal hematoma or a major abnormality on the IVP. The technical approach during renal exploration includes incision of the posterior peritoneum medial to the inferior mesenteric vein, anterior to the aorta, with isolation of the renal vessels before reflection of the colon and exploration of the kidney. This avoids exsanguinating hemorrhage.

The patient with penetrating injury is managed similarly to the patient with blunt trauma. However, patients who have penetrating injuries more often require exploration, and the threshold to explore the kidneys tends to be lower.

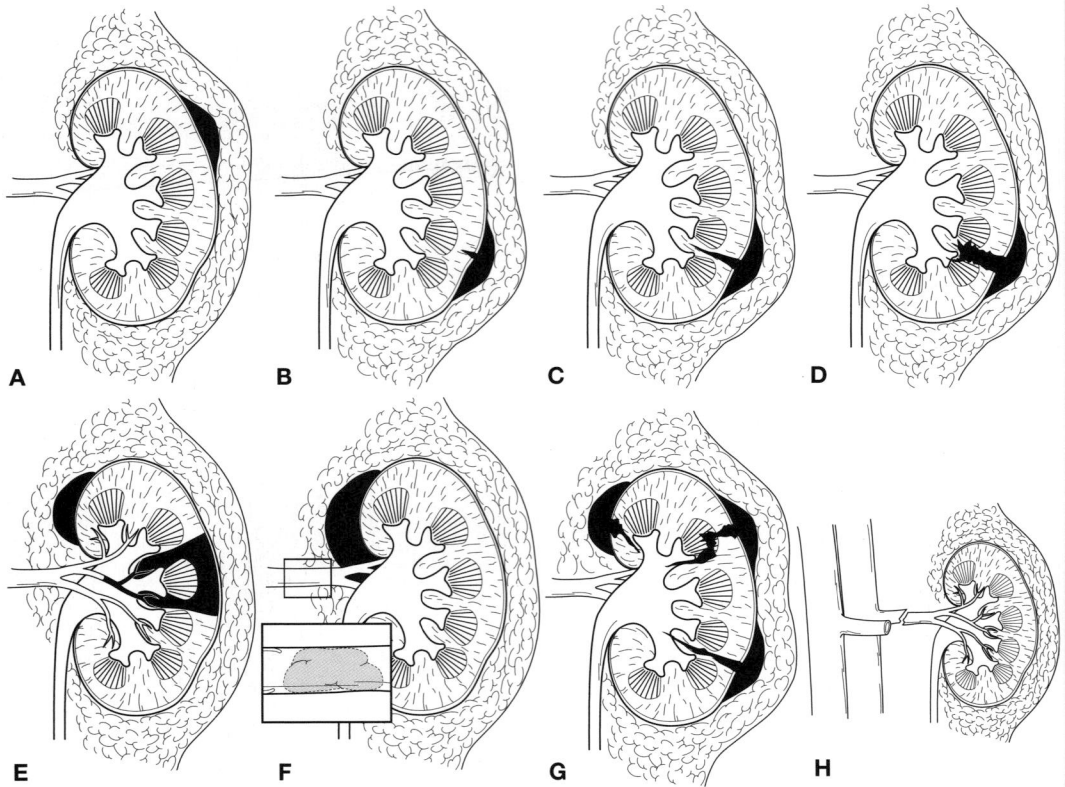

Figure 27-11. Grades of renal trauma. Grades I and II are considered minor. Grades III, IV, and V are considered major. A. Grade I trauma showing microscopic or gross hematuria. A contusion or a contained subcapsular hematoma is present. There is no parenchymal laceration. B. Grade II trauma showing a nonexpanding, confined perirenal hematoma or cortical laceration that is less than 1 cm deep. No urinary extravasation is present. C. Grade III trauma showing laceration of the parenchyma that extends less than 1 cm into the cortex. No urinary extravasation is present. D. Grade IV trauma showing laceration of the parenchyma that extends through the corticomedullary junction and into the collecting system. Laceration of a segmental vessel may also occur. E. Grade IV trauma showing thrombosis of a segmental renal artery. There is no laceration of the parenchyma, but there is ischemia of the corresponding parenchyma. F. Grade V trauma showing thrombosis of the main artery of the kidney. An intimal tear and a distal thrombosis are seen in the inset. G. Grade V trauma showing a kidney that is shattered because of multiple lacerations. H. Grade V trauma showing avulsion of the main artery or vein of the kidney. (Modified from Tanagho EA, McAninch JW, eds. *Smith's General Urology*. 13th ed. Appleton & Lange; 1992.)

Congenital Disorders

Scores of congenital anomalies are found in the urinary tract. These range from early symptomatic disorders which are diagnosed in children, asymptomatic and discovered incidentally, and delayed symptomatic not diagnosed until adulthood. Two common disorders that may require intervention are horseshoe kidneys and congenital obstruction of the urinary tract.

Horseshoe kidneys occur in 1:400 to 1:1,800 live births. A horseshoe kidney is the most common type of renal fusion anomaly and usually occurs at the lower pole, resulting in halted ascent of the renal unit at the level of the inferior mesenteric artery. Symptoms are usually associated with obstruction or infection and include hematuria and vague abdominal discomfort. Diagnosis is usually made by CT or ultrasonography. When intervention is necessary, the renal isthmus connecting the kidneys is divided surgically (symphysiotomy). Revision of the ureteropelvic junction may need to accompany symphysiotomy.

Congenital obstruction of the urinary tract occurs most often at the junction between the ureter and the renal pelvis—the ureteropelvic junction. The etiologic factors in this obstruction are myriad and complex and result in varying degrees of hydronephrosis. Bilateral involvement occurs in 10% to 40% of cases. An intrinsic obstruction caused by maldevelopment of the ureteropelvic junction is the likely cause of obstruction in children. In patients presenting in adulthood or late childhood, an aberrant vessel that crosses the ureteropelvic junction may also cause obstruction. The resulting stenosis or functional obstruction leads to hydronephrosis. The presenting signs and symptoms include palpable abdominal mass, intermittent pain, hematuria, urinary infection, fever, hypertension, and renal stones. Today, many cases of ureteropelvic junction obstruction are diagnosed by antenatal ultrasonography. Diagnosis of functional obstruction is made by nuclear scan (Lasix renography). Surgical repair of the obstruction is performed to prevent loss of renal function and recurrent urinary tract infections (UTIs).

Inflammatory Diseases

Pyelonephritis

Pyelonephritis is a clinical diagnosis. Patients commonly present with fever, flank pain, and costovertebral angle tenderness on the side of the involved kidney in the setting of ascending bacterial cystitis. In 80% of cases, *E. coli* is the causative organism. Chronic pyelonephritis often leads to renal failure and is a common reason for renal transplantation. Findings on IVP, usually nonspecific, include diffuse renal enlargement with calyceal distortion. If the infection is uncomplicated, treatment is outpatient oral antibiotic therapy. When the patient has evidence of sepsis or significant compromise requiring hospitalization, intravenous antibiotics are administered. It is not uncommon for fever and flank pain to persist for several days. If symptoms persist for a longer period, it is reasonable to image the kidneys with a CT or ultrasound to exclude an abscess. If upper tract obstruction is suspected, renal imaging must be immediately obtained and any obstruction emergently relieved (eg, obstructive pyelonephritis associated with an obstructing ureteral stone) with a ureteral stent or a percutaneous nephrostomy. Obstructive pyelonephritis is a urologic emergency due to pyelovenous back flow from elevated intrarenal pressure causing bacterial translocation and sepsis. These patients can rapidly decompensate, and antibiotics alone do not provide adequate therapy. Removal of the stone is contraindicated during active infection because stone manipulation can lead to worsening sepsis. When emergently treating obstructive pyelonephritis, the goal is to relieve the obstruction. Renal abscess usually requires percutaneous drainage in addition to antibiotics.

Emphysematous Pyelonephritis

Emphysematous pyelonephritis is a life-threatening infection in which bacteria, often *E. coli,* form gas in the renal parenchyma. Mortality rates for this condition have been reported as high as 40%. The condition is associated with poorly controlled diabetes. Patients are frequently septic and can deteriorate rapidly. A CT scan is diagnostic. Patients are managed with intravenous antibiotics, supportive measures, and appropriate percutaneous drainage. However, in patients who are unstable or when conservative measures fail, nephrectomy remains the standard treatment option. In contrast to emphysematous pyelonephritis, emphysematous pyelitis refers to a gas-forming infection limited to the collecting system of the kidneys. Although pyelitis is also a high-risk infection that should be treated aggressively, these patients have favorable outcomes relative to patients with emphysematous pyelonephritis.

Xanthogranulomatous Pyelonephritis

Xanthogranulomatous pyelonephritis (XGP) is another inflammatory disease of the kidneys. Women are affected more often (75% of cases). Patients with XGP, a disease generally involving patients in the fifth to seventh decades of life, often have a history of failure to thrive and chronic UTI. The diagnosis can be difficult because the symptoms are usually nonspecific. There is often a delay in the diagnosis of XGP, and it is important for primary care physicians to consider this disease with the described presentation. When urine culture shows UTI, *E. coli* and Proteus species are the most common causes. Currently, a

CT scan is the imaging test of choice to diagnose XGP. The lesions in the kidney, which may be quite large, are characterized by diffuse enlargement, central nephrolithiasis, and spherical areas surrounding the kidney in a hydronephrotic pattern. The affected kidney is usually nonfunctional. The treatment is usually a nephrectomy. The kidney can be adherent to adjacent structures, and the nephrectomy is frequently technically challenging.

Genitourinary Tuberculosis

Painless frequency, especially at night, is a common complaint in patients with genitourinary tuberculosis (TB). In a patient with sterile pyuria, TB should be suspected. A purified protein derivative (PPD) skin test can help establish the diagnosis. A positive test does not necessarily indicate active disease. A definitive diagnosis is made by urine culture with isolation of *Mycobacterium tuberculosis.* Further tests include chest films and spine imaging. When genitourinary TB is diagnosed, an upper tract imaging with CT or IVP is mandatory. Findings may include calcifications at any point along the genitourinary tract, and extensive renal calcifications can be seen. Ureteral obstruction can occur secondary to a stricture of the ureter. The management of genitourinary TB begins with antituberculosis drugs. Subsequent nephrectomy may be indicated in some cases where extensive renal destruction results in a nonfunctioning kidney. Ureteral stricture management options may include temporary internal stenting, corticosteroids, or ureteral reimplantation in distal ureteral strictures. Treatment depends on the location and length of the stricture and the response to medical management.

Neoplasms

Renal masses are classified as benign or malignant; malignant tumors are primary or metastatic. The most commonly encountered renal lesion is a simple cyst (70% of cases). Renal cell carcinoma (RCC) is the most common primary neoplasm of the kidney and accounts for more than 85% of all primary renal cancers in adults. This chapter discusses only the most frequently encountered tumors.

Clinical Presentation and Evaluation

Patients with renal cancer often have painless hematuria, but the cancer is most frequently discovered with CT and ultrasounds as an incidental finding. Many texts refer to the classic triad (a complex of flank pain, abdominal mass, and hematuria) as characteristic of renal cancer. However, patients seldom have all three findings.

CT plays a prominent role in the workup of solid renal masses and may be valuable in characterizing some atypical cystic masses. Arteriography, once a standard preoperative study, is recommended only in selected patients in whom the diagnosis is in doubt or aberrant vasculature is expected. If tumor invasion of the inferior vena cava is suspected, an MRI or CT/MR venogram is indicated to define the extent of involvement.

Benign Neoplasms

Most simple cystic lesions are asymptomatic and benign and require no intervention. However, some are complex (eg, septations, wall thickening and/or enhancement, or calcifications) and require further investigation to rule out malignancy. Benign simple renal cysts are usually asymptomatic. Simple cysts are found in as many as 33% of adults. A simple cyst noted on imaging (eg, CT, ultrasound) is managed by observation. A complex cyst is usually considered cancerous until proven otherwise, and partial or radical nephrectomy may be indicated. A needle biopsy or cyst aspiration is usually of little value in most cases because a negative result may be a false negative and does not rule out malignancy. Benign solid tumors of kidneys are encountered occasionally. An angiomyolipoma is usually diagnosed by the characteristic appearance of fat within the lesion on CT scan. Fat is black on CT, and when fat is seen within a renal mass, angiomyolipoma is almost always the diagnosis.

Malignant Neoplasms
Renal Cell Carcinoma
RCC, a tumor that usually arises from the proximal convoluted tubules, is by far the most common primary solid malignancy affecting the kidneys. Although etiologic factors are not well delineated, nitrosamines and cigarette smoke carcinogens have been implicated. RCC has a 2:1 male-to-female preponderance. Typically unilateral, this lesion is spherical with a pseudocapsule of parenchyma and fibrosis. About 5% of RCC may be bilateral.

Although RCC is most commonly found incidentally, hematuria is the single most common sign, occurring in 29% to 60% of reported cases. Flank pain and palpable flank mass occur next most often, but the classic triad of hematuria, flank pain, and a palpable abdominal mass is reported in only 4% to 17% of cases. Other common signs and symptoms are fever, anemia, and elevated sedimentation rate. Although serum lactate dehydrogenase and alkaline phosphatase may be elevated, there are no reliable tumor markers for RCC. Renal cell cancers may present only with nonspecific symptoms such as weight loss, fever, or weakness.

In later stages, this tumor invades the renal vein and vena cava and may even extend into the right atrium. A staging system such as the TNM system is used to determine the extent of the primary lesion, the involvement of contiguous structures, the extent of vascular involvement, and whether the tumor has metastasized. (For detailed information on the staging of kidney cancer, see the American Joint Committee on Cancer's *Cancer Staging Manual*, 8th edition. A summary of the stages can be found at https://www.cancer.org/cancer/kidney-cancer/detection-diagnosis-staging/staging.html.)

RCC metastasizes most often to lungs, bone, and brain, in that order. Metastatic lesions may appear in the ipsilateral or contralateral kidney or both, and late metastasis may occur to the liver. Five-year survival rates for stages I and II are 80% to 90%, and for stages III and IV are 40% to 60%.

Treatment for localized RCC is radical or partial nephrectomy (Figure 27-12). Partial nephrectomy is the preferred option for small tumors, even in the presence of a normal contralateral kidney. As with radical prostatectomy, robotic surgery has significantly reduced the perioperative and postoperative morbidity associated with the traditional open approach. Preoperative evaluation should include a chest radiograph and liver function tests. A bone scan is required in the presence of bone pain or elevated alkaline phosphatase. The kidney, perinephric fat, Gerota fascia, ipsilateral adrenal gland, and ipsilateral regional lymph nodes are removed during a radical nephrectomy. The renal vessels should be controlled before manipulation and dissection. In the case of vena cava involvement, the incision may need to be extended or a median sternotomy performed for adequate exposure. The vena cava, which is controlled superiorly and inferiorly, may need to be incised to remove a tumor thrombus. The lumbar and contralateral renal veins must be controlled as well. Postoperative complications include bleeding, retroperitoneal abscess, ileus, and wound infection, as well as recognized complications of abdominal surgery (eg, pulmonary embolism).

Urothelial Cell Carcinoma
Urothelial cell carcinoma of the renal collecting system may present as a renal mass or a filling defect on CT. Urine cytology may be negative but usually shows abnormal cells. Ureteroscopy is usually necessary to visualize or biopsy suspicious lesions for definitive diagnosis. Many upper urinary tract lesions seed the lower urinary tract, making upper tract evaluation paramount when urothelial cell carcinoma is found in the lower tract.

Upper tract urothelial carcinoma is stratified into low and high risk based on several factors including tumor size, multifocality, grade and histologic subtype, and imaging characteristics. Recent data support attempts at kidney-sparing interventions for low-risk disease, such as laser ablation or upper tract instillation of chemotherapeutic agents. The mainstay of therapy for high-risk disease is radical nephroureterectomy with the removal of a cuff of bladder at the ureteral orifice.

Urinary Stone Disease
Urinary tract calculi represent a significant cause for morbidity in the United States. More than 500,000 people are affected yearly, with men affected more often than women, and the 30- to 50-year age group having the highest incidence. The majority of urinary stones are composed of calcium oxalate.

Risk factors are associated with specific types of stone formation. Factors that lead to the formation of calcium stones include underlying metabolic disorders (eg, renal tubular acidosis and hyperparathyroidism). Other risk factors include poor hydration, immobilization, and a family history of renal stones. Risk factors for uric acid stones include a high dietary intake of purines, a history of gout, poor hydration, and hyperuricosuria. Cystine stones are usually seen in families with a history of cystinuria, an inherited disorder affecting the renal reabsorption of four amino acids, including cysteine. Cysteine, ornithine lysine, and arginine are the four involved amino acids. Cystine stones represent a true inherited disorder, in which the renal tubules do not transport the four amino acids. These patients develop stones early in life and require aggressive stone prevention with urine alkalinization or thiol therapy. Struvite (magnesium ammonium phosphate) stones (infection stones) develop in patients with chronic UTIs. Patients with chronically indwelling catheters are at a particular risk for the development of these stones. When these stones grow to occupy the entire collecting system, they are termed staghorn stones.

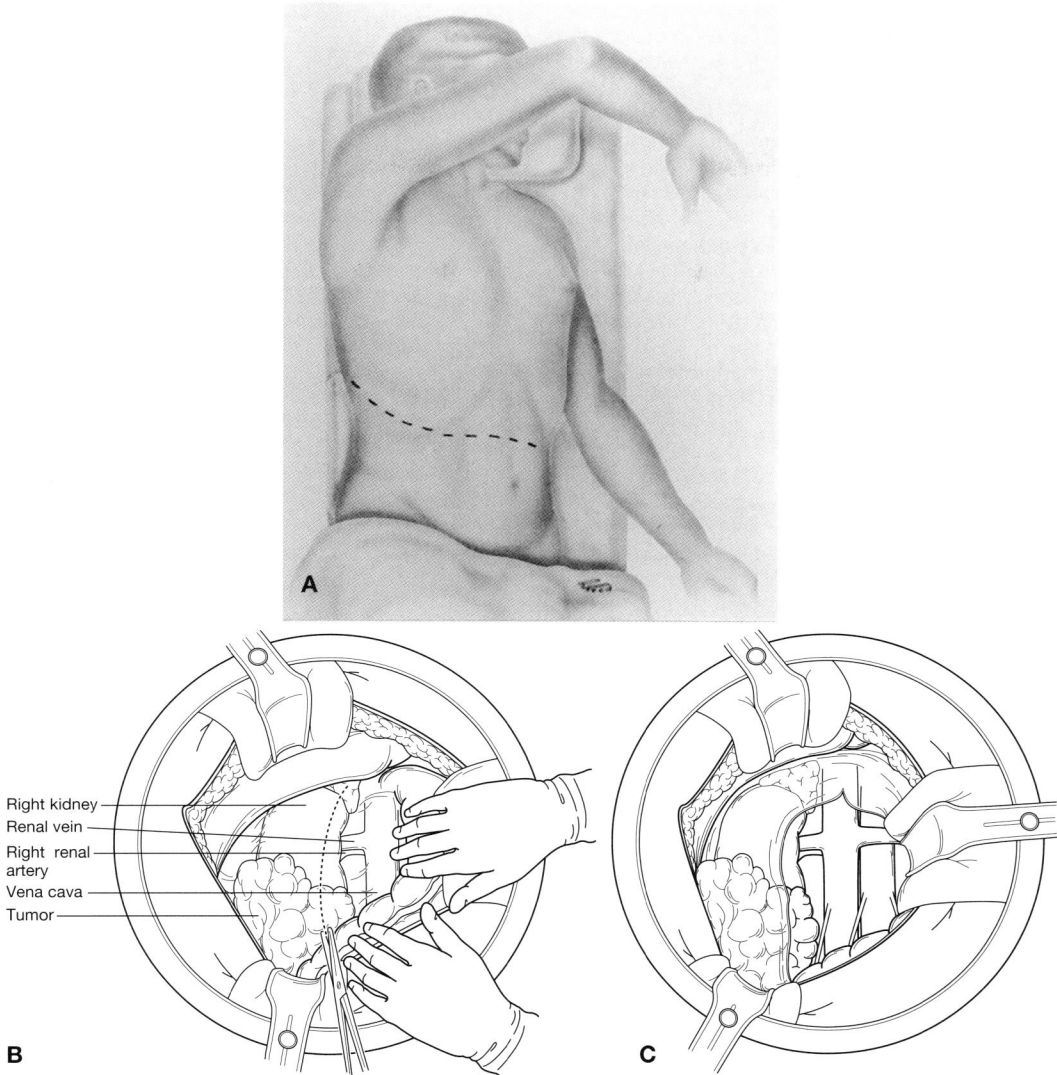

Figure 27-12. A. Eleventh rib surgical approach for radical nephrectomy. B. Right kidney, renal artery, and tumor identified. C. Line of incision in the retroperitoneum to expose the right kidney. (From Lawrence PF. *Essentials of Surgical Specialties.* 3rd ed. Lippincott Williams & Wilkins; 2007.)

Several theories have been proposed to describe the mechanism of calcium stone formation. A widely accepted theory proposes that urine becomes supersaturated with calcium oxalate. Normal urine contains substances that inhibit crystallization. If an individual has an inadequate amount of one or more inhibitors, or an inhibitor does not function properly, spontaneous crystallization follows. Moreover, if there is a high calcium concentration in the urine through increased calcium absorption from the intestine, or increased excretion (renal leak), crystallization is promoted. These crystals are either passed harmlessly through the kidneys into the ureter or become lodged in the collecting system. Once they lodge, the crystals develop rapidly, forming a stone. If the stone obstructs the ureteropelvic junction or ureter, hydronephrosis can result.

Clinical Presentation and Evaluation

Urinary tract stones are usually diagnosed in the emergency room. Renal colic is the presenting symptom in most patients with symptomatic stones. It is described as an intermittent pain in the flank often radiating to the groin, accompanied by nausea and vomiting. The pain can be acute and so severe that even large doses of narcotics cannot completely control it. The cause of the pain is usually not the stone itself, but the obstruction caused as the stone passes along the ureter.

Emergency room evaluation always includes urinalysis. Microhematuria is commonly associated with stone disease. The diagnosis of stone disease requires an imaging study. The optimal study used to image the upper urinary tract for stones is noncontrast CT. A uric acid stone is lucent on a plain film but is bright white on a noncontrast CT. A renal ultrasound is noninvasive but lacks the anatomic accuracy of a CT, especially for evaluation of the ureters.

The elective metabolic workup for renal stones is usually obtained in children with stones and patients with recurrent stones but may be obtained in any patient with urolithiasis. This evaluation is obtained after passage of the stone, when the patient is on a regular diet. There is no standard metabolic evaluation. Some urologists obtain a more comprehensive evaluation initially, whereas others obtain screening laboratory data and obtain further testing if the initial studies are abnormal. Laboratory testing includes determining values for serum calcium, parathyroid hormone, electrolytes, urine pH, and 24-hour urine collections to measure calcium and other electrolyte concentrations.

Treatment

Treatment of urinary calculi depends on the size, location, and composition of the stones. Obstructive pyelonephritis is one situation that deserves particular attention, as discussed in the section "Pyelonephritis." This condition occurs when a patient has an obstructing stone associated with infection of the affected upper urinary tract, causing "pus under pressure"; it is a true urologic emergency. Patients come to the emergency room with flank pain, fever, and infected urine. This is similar to the presentation of a patient with pyelonephritis not associated with stone disease. In this setting, it is important to rule out obstructive pyelonephritis by imaging the kidneys. When a patient has obstructing pyelonephritis, antibiotics alone do not effectively treat the problem. The treatment must include relief of the obstruction, with emergency placement of an internal stent (placed cystoscopically) or a percutaneous nephrostomy. No attempt is made to manipulate or remove the stone because manipulation can lead to septic complications. The goal of emergency intervention is a prompt drainage.

Ureteral stones smaller than 5 mm usually pass spontaneously. Larger ureteral stones usually do not pass without urologic intervention. When intervention is indicated for ureteral stones, treatment may involve stent placement alone because a stent in the ureter can lead to passive dilation of the ureter and subsequent stone passage. Another option is flexible or rigid ureteroscopy with stone fragmentation and extraction. When ureteral stones are approached endoscopically and require fragmentation before removal, a HoLeP or ThuLeP laser is the most commonly used technology.

Selected ureteral stones can be managed with extracorporeal shock wave lithotripsy to fragment the stones into pieces small enough to pass spontaneously. The technology involves transmission of a focused shock wave from outside the body to the calculus. A high-voltage underwater spark gap initiates the shock wave. The gap or discharge, occurring in approximately 1 μs, results in vaporization of the fluid surrounding the arc, developing a plasma-like state. This explosive vaporization of fluid propagates a high-energy shock wave, which is focused by surrounding the spark gap with a semi-ellipsoid, allowing concentration of the energy at a second focal point, F2 (Figure 27-13). By placing the calculus at this second focal point, the destructive energy is transmitted to the stone, causing it to fragment.

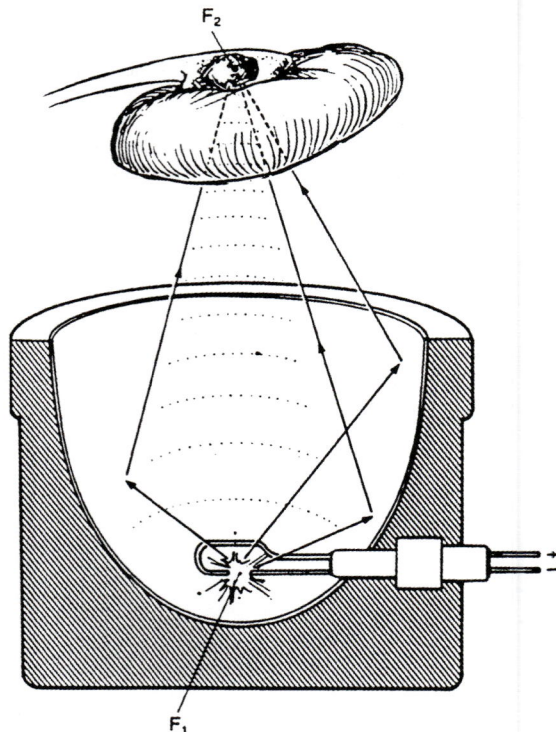

Figure 27-13. Spark gap electrode and semiellipsoid for focusing shock waves. The electrode is placed at the first focus inside the ellipsoid with the stone placed at the second focus. (From Lawrence PF. *Essentials of Surgical Specialties*. 3rd ed. Lippincott Williams & Wilkins; 2007.)

Management of stones in the collecting system is usually accomplished with extracorporeal shock wave lithotripsy. Alternatively, percutaneous removal is an option, especially when there is a large stone burden. Unlike calcium stones, uric acid stones can be treated medically because they dissolve when pH is increased. The treatment of uric acid stones, therefore, consists of urinary alkalization and increased fluid intake. Open surgery, commonly performed in the past, is rarely indicated today.

THE URETERS

Anatomy

The ureters are the conduits for urine between the kidneys and the bladder. Each ureter enters the bladder posterolaterally on its inferior portion and courses obliquely for 1.5 cm through the bladder wall. For half that distance, the ureter traverses the muscularis; for the other half, it is submucosal. The lower portion of the ureter is anchored and supported by special fibromuscular tissue called the Waldeyer sheath. The normal anatomy of the ureter allows free efflux of urine into the bladder but prevents reflux. This one-way flow depends on the complex relation between the ureteral muscle, the bladder base, and the ureteral route through the bladder wall. In its upper part, the ureteral muscle has an irregular helical pattern. Near the bladder and in its intramural part, the muscle fibers run parallel to the lumen. Vermiculation of the ureteral wall propels urine toward the bladder. As the contraction approaches the bladder, the longitudinal fiber arrangement causes the intramural ureteral lumen to open and shorten, allowing urine to enter. When a ureteral contraction is not present, increasing bladder pressure compresses the submucosal ureteral lumen against the underlying bladder muscle and prevents reflux (Figure 27-14).

Ureteral Obstruction

Ureteral obstruction can be caused primarily by diseases directly involving the ureters, including stones, extrinsic masses, gynecologic malignancy, vascular aneurysm, inflammatory disease of the colon, and retroperitoneal fibrosis. Both CT and IVP are excellent tests to diagnose

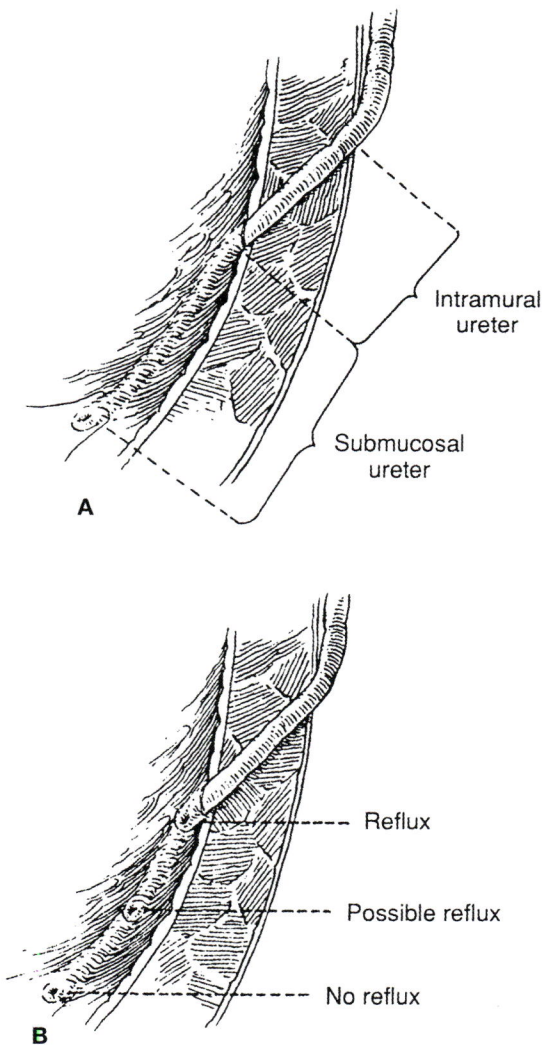

Figure 27-14. A. Normal ureterovesical junction. B. Refluxing ureterovesical junction and ureterovesical junction showing inadequate submucosal tunnels. (From Lawrence PF. *Essentials of Surgical Specialties*. 3rd ed. Lippincott Williams & Wilkins; 2007.)

ureteral obstruction because they provide both anatomic and functional information. Treatment depends on the underlying etiology. In patients with nonurologic malignancy causing ureteral obstruction, treatment is influenced by the overall prognosis. Initial management usually includes stenting of the ureter.

Ureteral obstruction can also be secondary to other diseases. In obstruction of bladder outlet secondary to BPH, prostate cancer, urethral stricture, impaired bladder compliance, or other lower tract pathology, the effects are transmitted to the upper tracts. Ultrasound findings often include bilateral hydronephrosis with bilateral hydroureter along the entire length of both ureters. The patient should initially be managed with bladder catheterization.

Iatrogenic Injuries to the Ureters

Iatrogenic injury to the ureters can occur during general, vascular, and gynecologic surgery. Diverticulitis, aortic or iliac artery aneurysms, and ovarian or uterine tumors often exist in close proximity to the distal third of the ureter. The ureters are occasionally injured inadvertently during surgery for a large pelvic mass. Ureteral stents may be temporarily placed through the bladder before surgery to help with intraoperative identification of the ureters when the risk of injury is high. A ureteral injury can often be repaired with a primary end-to-end anastomosis and then stented. When the injury occurs to the distal ureter, a ureteral reimplantation is the preferred repair. If a ureter is injured in a contaminated surgical field, however, proximal urinary diversion with percutaneous nephrostomy or open nephrostomy becomes necessary. If the ureter is injured during repair of an intra-abdominal aortic aneurysm, the ureter is often repaired primarily and then wrapped with omentum.

THE BLADDER

Anatomy

The bladder is a hollow muscular organ that functions to store urine and then evacuate it. When empty, the bladder lies just behind the pubic symphysis. As it fills, its superior part protrudes into the peritoneal cavity and can often be palpated suprapubically. It is lined with transitional epithelium that lies on a loose, elastic connective tissue bed—the lamina propria. The muscle of the body of the bladder, the detrusor, is composed of interlacing smooth muscle bundles with no distinct layers. An exception is the trigone, a triangular area that lies between the ureteral orifices and the urethral opening. In this area, the muscle wall has two layers, a superficial one fusing with the ureteral musculature and a deeper one indistinguishable from the detrusor. Although only the superior most portion of the bladder is covered with peritoneum, the entire bladder is covered with the loose fascia of the pelvic cavity. The bladder is firmly attached to the posterior aspect of the pubic bone by condensations of this fascia, called the "puboprostatic ligaments" in men and "pubovesical ligaments" in women. The median umbilical ligament, the fibrotic remnant of the urachus, attaches the bladder to the anterior abdominal wall. Condensation of the pelvic fascia in the dorsolateral aspect of the bladder also serves as an anchor and neurovascular conduit. Blood is supplied by the superior, middle, and inferior vesical arteries and branches of the hypogastric artery. In women, blood is also supplied by the vaginal and uterine arteries. The bladder is surrounded by a rich plexus of veins that drains into the hypogastric veins. Bladder lymphatics drain to the external iliac, hypogastric, common iliac, and sacral lymph nodes.

Evaluation

Endoscopic Evaluation

The bladder and urethra are evaluated endoscopically by flexible and rigid cystoscopes. These contain an optical fiber-lens system for visualization—fibers to carry illumination and ports for instruments, catheters, and irrigation fluid. The rigid cystoscope consists of a telescope, a bridge, and a sheath available in various sizes, with input and output ports for irrigation. The bridge, forming a watertight connection between the sheath and telescope, may have one or two ports for the introduction of tools, catheters, or electrodes. The cystoscopic lenses range in viewing angles from 0° (straight ahead) to 120° (retro view). Flexible cystoscopes have a maneuverable tip for examining the bladder.

A systematic survey is used during cystoscopy to ensure the entire urothelium is adequately visualized. The entire bladder mucosa is examined for mucosal irregularities, tumors, lesions, or unusual vascularity. Trabeculation (ie, the formation of hypertrophic bands of muscle tissue) of the bladder wall, cellule formation (ie, the formation of small diverticula that have not yet protruded beyond the bladder wall), and diverticula are noted. Ureteral orifices are checked for position and configuration. Ureteral urine, as it effluxes into the bladder, can be observed for evidence of hematuria from the upper tract. In addition, the bladder neck is evaluated for contracture, the prostatic fossa is checked for mucosal lesions and anatomic occlusion from prostatic tissue, and the urethra is examined for stricture formation, mucosal lesions, and tumors. Retrograde pyelography can be performed through the cystoscope by inserting a catheter into the ureteral orifice and injecting radiographic contrast to evaluate the anatomy of the ureteral and renal collecting systems. Although cystoscopy provides information about the anatomy of the lower urinary tract, its ability to assess lower urinary tract function is extremely limited.

Urodynamic Evaluation

Urodynamics is a collection of studies used to evaluate the reservoir and micturition function of the lower urinary tract. Urodynamic tests include PVR urine volume, cystometrogram (CMG), urinary flow rate (uroflow test), urethral pressure profile, sphincter electromyography (EMG), and fluoroscopic cystography. The PVR is the volume of urine that remains in the bladder after voiding. One way to measure the PVR is to catheterize the bladder immediately after voiding and record the output. Ultrasound is a less invasive but less precise test that also can be used to measure the PVR. Normal individuals void to completion; significant residual urine occurs with bladder outlet obstruction and/or detrusor underactivity. The CMG evaluates intravesical pressures during filling and voiding. The CMG measures bladder sensation, capacity, compliance, and voiding pressures; it can also detect premature detrusor

contractions. The normal bladder should fill to a capacity of 350 to 500 mL without a significant increase in pressure or detrusor contraction. The first sensation of needing to void occurs around 150 to 250 mL of filling, and definite fullness is sensed at 350 to 450 mL.

Urinary flow rate measures the rate of urine flow from the urethra. Normally, flow rates occur around a tight, bell-shaped curve. Men have a peak flow rate of 20 to 25 mL/s and women 20 to 30 mL/s. Low-flow rates indicate either bladder outlet obstruction or poor detrusor function. Urethral pressure recordings measure intraluminal pressures of the urethra. EMG is used to evaluate sphincter activity. Normally, sphincter EMG activity increases during the guarding reflex and decreases with initiation of the voiding reflex. Fluoroscopic cystoscopy visualizes the bladder neck and sphincter and can be used to detect cystocele, descensus (bladder prolapse), reflux, and other conditions, such as primary bladder neck obstruction.

Congenital Anomalies

Vesicoureteral Reflux

Primary vesicoureteral reflux (VUR) is the result of an abnormally short intramural ureteral tunnel. Developmentally, this is thought to be due to a laterally placed origin of the ureteral bud from the fetal bladder. This anomaly results in a very short tunnel through the bladder wall and compromises the natural result of bladder distension that compresses the intramural ureter to prevent reflux. Such anatomy allows potentially infected urine to reflux up the ureter, resulting in kidney damage. The ensuing inflammatory reaction causes permanent tubular damage and loss of renal function.

VUR is graded as a function of the level of refluxing urine and degree of upper tract dilatation (Figure 27-15). Lower grades of reflux (grades I and II) usually resolve as a child grows and the ureterovesical junction matures. Because higher grades of reflux are less likely to resolve spontaneously and present an increased risk of renal damage, surgical correction is often necessary. Secondary reflux can occur after resection of the ureteral orifice during the removal of an overlying tumor, after ureteral meatotomy to aid in stone removal, after kidney transplantation, or after dilation of the intramural ureter for ureteroscopy. Occasionally, secondary reflux may require operative intervention. During episodes of cystitis, marginally competent ureteral orifices may reflux, but this transient reflux usually subsides after resolution of the bladder inflammation.

Clinical Evaluation

VUR is often discovered on routine prenatal ultrasound, or during the workup of pediatric UTI. In children, the prevalence of VUR is inversely proportional to age; it is associated with 29% to 50% of children evaluated for UTI. The voiding cystourethrogram (VCUG) is the primary diagnostic test for reflux. The bladder is filled with contrast and visualized fluoroscopically to detect reflux as the bladder fills and voids. The VCUG may be performed as soon as the urine has been sterilized after an acute infection. This study can also be performed with a radioisotope (radionuclide cystogram), which allows a smaller total dose of radiation and can detect smaller degrees of reflux. However, the anatomic detail is inferior to that obtained with a fluoroscopic VCUG. Renal ultrasound and IVP detect

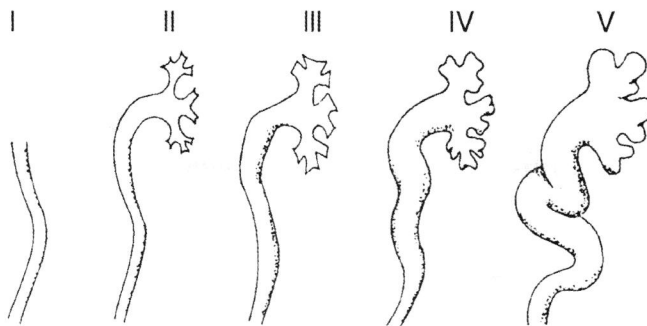

Figure 27-15. Grading of reflux based on findings on voiding cystourethrogram. (From Lawrence PF. *Essentials of Surgical Specialties*. 3rd ed. Lippincott Williams & Wilkins; 2007.)

upper tract dilatation but cannot alone diagnose reflux. Cystoscopy is not indicated routinely in children with reflux. However, it may be useful if there is suspicion of an associated anatomic abnormality (eg, an ectopic ureter).

Treatment

The therapeutic goal in VUR is prevention of UTIs and renal damage. In children with reflux but without dilated ureters (ie, grade I or II reflux), reflux spontaneously resolves in 20% to 30% of children every 2 years, with 80% ultimately resolving. Continual low-dose antibacterial agents can be used prophylactically to prevent UTI. However, the benefit of prophylactic antibiotic therapy in preserving renal function has been questioned. Nevertheless, the child should have a careful follow-up with each febrile illness, and with urinary symptoms. Routine renal ultrasonography should be performed to monitor for progression of hydronephrosis and/or renal scarring, and repeat VCUG performed as indicated. If there is suspected new renal scarring, a radionucleotide renal scan is more sensitive than ultrasound. Serum creatinine, blood urea nitrogen, height, weight, and blood pressure should also be checked yearly.

Surgical repair is undertaken in patients who have severe reflux or in those who fail medical management, either by poor compliance, repeated UTIs despite prophylaxis, or by loss of renal function. An endoscopic therapy for reflux is the transurethral injection of dextranomer/hyaluronic acid copolymer (Deflux) into the bladder wall just within the ureteral orifice. This is an outpatient procedure performed under general anesthesia and generally takes less than 30 minutes. Early results for grade II to IV reflux show that between 70% and 91% of patients are cured after a single injection. Although this therapy may be emerging as a "middle ground" between antibiotic prophylaxis and open surgery, long-term data are lacking. Another mode of therapy for reflux is the transurethral injection of collagen or Teflon into the bladder wall just below the ureteral orifice. This method is effective in milder forms of reflux or after failed reimplantations. With these endoscopic interventions, concern exists regarding migration of particles to distant sites, such as the brain, lungs, and lymph nodes.

The goals of ureteral reimplantation (or ureteroneocystostomy) include lengthening the intramural portion of the ureter 4 to 5 times its diameter, immobilizing the ureteral meatus by anchoring it to the underlying detrusor, and supporting the intramural ureter with the firm underlying bladder wall. In cases with severe reflux and marked ureteral dilation, the ureter may require plication or tapering before reimplantation.

Several techniques are used to perform a ureteroneocystostomy, allowing the operation to be tailored to fit the patient's needs and anatomy. Ureteral advancement procedures (eg, the Glenn-Anderson technique) can be applied when the ureteral meatus is high and lateral enough to allow the creation of a tunnel of adequate length without placing the new meatus too close to the bladder neck. The ureteral orifice is approached transvesically and the surrounding mucosa circumscribed. A stent is placed up the ureter and sutured to the mucosa next to the orifice (Figure 27-16). The Cohen procedure is a cross-trigonal tunneling of the ureter that can be used when there is insufficient space between the ureteral hiatus and the bladder neck (Figure 27-17). The Politano-Leadbetter technique is often used when reoperation is required. Although originally a transvesical procedure, it is now most often approached as a combined transvesical and extravesical procedure, in which the ureter is completely mobilized from the bladder. The submucosal tunnel is lengthened by creating a new hiatus superolaterally. The old hiatus is closed, and the new orifice is created nearer the bladder neck. The ureter is then brought through the new hiatus and passed submucosally to the new orifice and secured there (Figure 27-18). Ureteral reimplantations can also be performed laparoscopically or robotically, with results similar to those with open surgery.

Other Anomalies

Exstrophy of the bladder is the result of improper development of the anterior abdominal wall, pelvic girdle, and anterior wall of the bladder. It results in exposure of the posterior wall of the bladder through the abdominal wall and a separation of the symphysis pubis. It is an uncommon anomaly, occurring in 1:30,000 births, and has a 3:1 male predominance. Besides disfigurement and total incontinence, bacterial colonization and UTIs are common. Often, total urinary tract reconstruction including bladder augmentation and bladder neck reconstruction is necessary to preserve renal function and provide urinary continence. There is an increased risk of adenocarcinoma of the bladder in patients with exstrophy, and they need lifelong follow-up by a urologist.

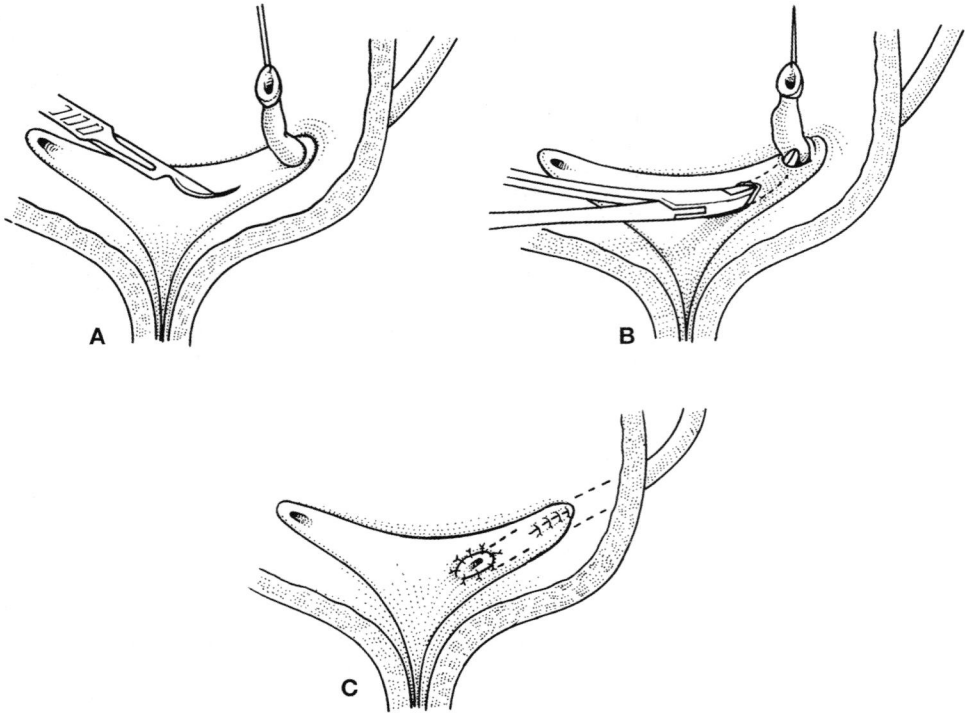

Figure 27-16. Glenn-Anderson technique. A. Ureter has been mobilized and the new site for the meatus is incised. B. Ureter is brought through a new, longer submucosal tunnel to the new meatus site. C. Completed procedure showing the longer submucosal tunnel. (From Lawrence PF. *Essentials of Surgical Specialties*. 3rd ed. Lippincott Williams & Wilkins; 2007.)

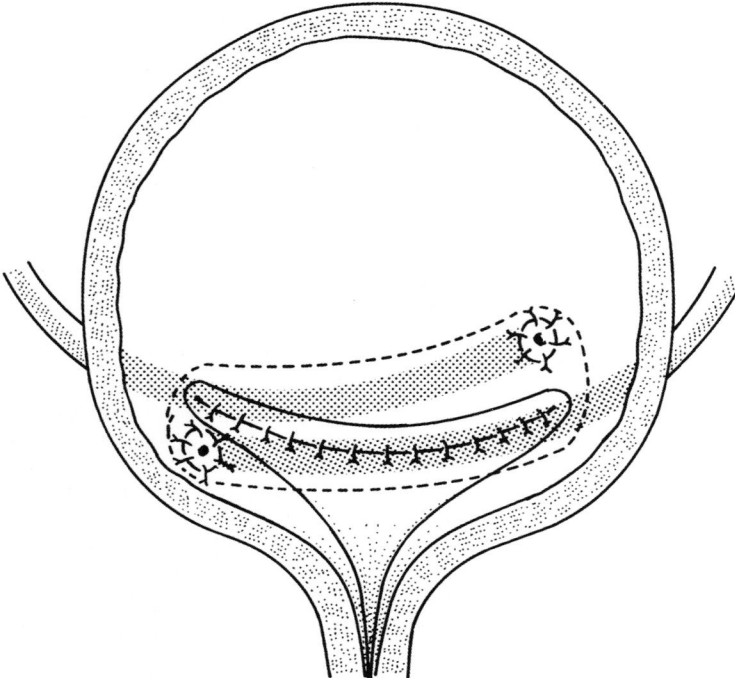

Figure 27-17. Cohen procedure. Cross-trigonal ureteral advancement (bilateral reimplantations using this technique are shown). (From Lawrence PF. *Essentials of Surgical Specialties*. 3rd ed. Lippincott Williams & Wilkins; 2007.)

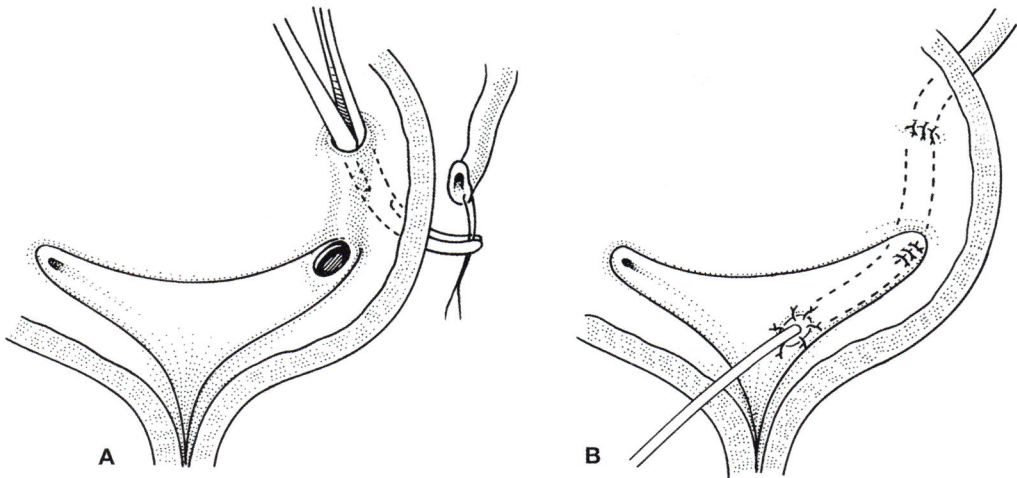

Figure 27-18. Politano-Leadbetter procedure. A. The ureter has been dissected completely and a new hiatus made superolaterally. B. The finished procedure with stent in place. (From Lawrence PF. *Essentials of Surgical Specialties*. 3rd ed. Lippincott Williams & Wilkins; 2007.)

Urachal persistence can occur as umbilical sinus, abdominal wall cyst, diverticulum at the bladder dome, or fistula from bladder to umbilicus. These are best treated with simple excision. Persistent urachal remnants are also associated with adenocarcinomatous changes. Congenital diverticula are difficult to differentiate from acquired ones. Previously, the presence of muscle in the wall of the diverticulum was considered to indicate a congenital origin, but this is no longer believed to be true. Excision of the symptomatic diverticulum is the treatment of choice in most situations.

Trauma

Bladder injury can occur as a result of penetrating or blunt trauma. Common causes of penetrating bladder injuries are gunshot wounds, stab wounds, and instrumentation. Pelvic fractures can cause puncture of the bladder wall by either sharp fracture edges or bone fragments. Blunt trauma, as occurs in motor vehicle accidents, causes a sudden increase in intravesical pressure, resulting in a bladder wall contusion or rupture. Bladder contusions often result in hematuria, whereas bladder tears may result in intraperitoneal or extraperitoneal extravasation. Traumatic bladder ruptures are often associated with damage to other pelvic and intra-abdominal organs.

Evaluation

Conscious patients with a bladder rupture usually complain of severe suprapubic or pelvic pain with an inability to void. In unconscious patients, however, a high degree of suspicion is essential to make the diagnosis. Bladder ruptures almost invariably cause hematuria, and, if associated with pelvic fractures, a urethral disruption must be suspected. The most dependable diagnostic study for a bladder rupture is a cystogram. However, if accompanying urethral damage is suspected (eg, because of blood at the meatus), a retrograde urethrogram must be performed to exclude a urethral tear before catheterization (Figure 27-19). To perform a cystogram, a scout

film is taken: Approximately 350 mL of sterile contrast is instilled into the bladder (adults), the catheter is clamped, and films are taken (Figure 27-20). Views may include oblique and lateral films in addition to a posterior-anterior image. A post-drainage film must be obtained because approximately 15% of bladder ruptures are diagnosed with this image.

Treatment

Small, extraperitoneal ruptures can be managed with 1 to 2 weeks of Foley catheter drainage, with complete healing anticipated. Intraperitoneal bladder ruptures and large or complicated extraperitoneal bladder ruptures require surgical repair.

Repair consists of exploration through a midline intraperitoneal incision, with care exercised to avoid the pelvic hematoma, careful inspection of the bladder, closure of the bladder with absorbable suture, and placement of a catheter to provide adequate urinary drainage. Because bladder ruptures are often associated with damage to other intra-abdominal organs, repair is often part of an exploratory laparotomy.

Inflammatory Diseases

Bacterial Cystitis

Patients who have bacterial cystitis classically experience irritative voiding symptoms, including dysuria, worsened urgency and frequency of urination from baseline symptoms, and, if the inflammation is severe enough, gross hematuria. Fever is not common with uncomplicated cystitis, and, if present, may indicate an upper tract infection. These symptoms in conjunction with a urine culture growing more than or equal to 100,000 CFU of a uropathogen are required to formally diagnose bacterial cystitis. Bacterial cystitis is much more common in women, with bacteria ascending to the bladder by way of their shorter urethra. Women who are prone to recurrent UTIs may be predisposed to infections because of increased vaginal and bladder mucosal bacterial adherence. In men, bacterial cystitis

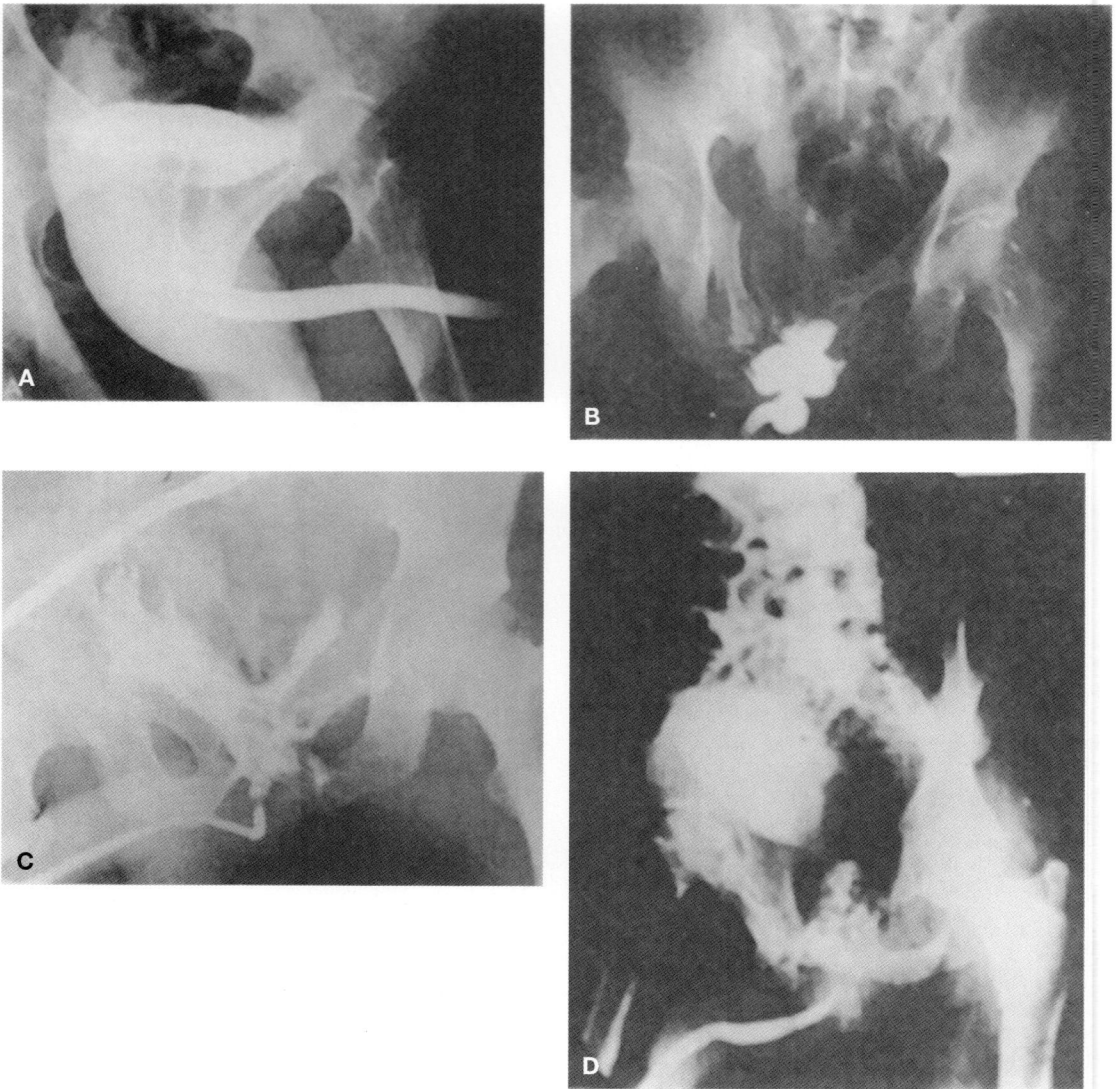

Figure 27-19. A. Normal retrograde urethrogram. The contrast material has been injected during the exposure to ensure delineation of deep bulbar, membranous, and prostatic urethra. B-D. Disruption of the posterior urethra in the man. (From Lawrence PF. *Essentials of Surgical Specialties*. 3rd ed. Lippincott Williams & Wilkins; 2007.)

is usually the result of incomplete emptying of the bladder. The most common offending bacteria are the gram-negative rods of the family Enterobacteriaceae. *E. coli* causes more than 80% of all UTIs.

Evaluation includes a urinalysis to determine the presence of bacteria, leukocytes, and red blood cells. A properly collected urine specimen (ie, a "clean catch") for culture and sensitivity is necessary for accurate diagnosis. The initial antibiotic is chosen empirically, usually a drug effective against a broad range of gram-negative organisms. Antibiotic therapy is then adjusted depending on the culture and sensitivity results. With appropriate therapy, symptoms should resolve in 3 to 5 days.

Further evaluation of the urinary tract, including cystoscopy and radiologic studies, is indicated in children, in men, and in women who do not respond to antibiotic therapy or have multiple recurrent infections despite appropriate prophylactic measures. The purpose of evaluation is to detect correctable causes of recurrent infections (Table 27-1). Carcinoma should be considered in patients in whom irritative voiding symptoms persist even after sterilization of the urine. To prevent bacteremia, manipulation of the urinary tract should be delayed until after the acute infection has resolved. Evaluation in adults includes a CT urogram (a study that combines CT with a postcontrast abdominal film to outline the ureters) or renal ultrasound, urinary cytology, cystoscopy, and possibly a VCUG when reflux is suspected. Children are usually evaluated with a renal ultrasound and a VCUG. Although cystoscopy is of little value in diagnosing bacterial cystitis, it can detect the presence of a neoplasm or stone and may suggest anatomic bladder outlet obstruction.

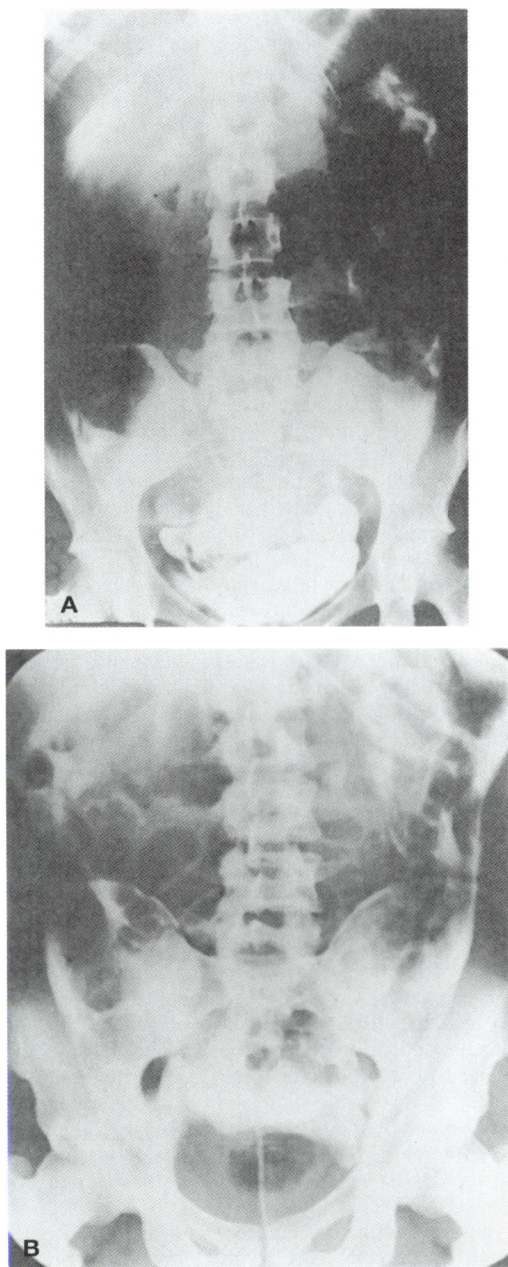

Figure 27-20. Intraperitoneal urinary bladder rupture. A. Pooling of contrast media in the right upper quadrant of the peritoneum. B. The contrast material outlines the peritoneal surface that the bowel interfaces. (From Lawrence PF. *Essentials of Surgical Specialties*. 3rd ed. Lippincott Williams & Wilkins; 2007.)

Bladder Pain Syndrome

Bladder pain syndrome is a diagnosis of exclusion that is characterized by a spectrum of often waxing and waning symptoms, including lower abdominal pain and irritative voiding symptoms. It predominantly affects women and can be difficult to manage given the varied potential etiologies and inconsistent response to therapy. Urinalysis occasionally shows microhematuria. Typically, urine cultures for bacteria, fungi, and viruses are negative. Cystoscopically, submucosal petechiae (glomerulations) may be seen. Rarely, a mucosal ulceration (Hunner ulcer) is seen; however, when present responds well to fulguration. In some patients, the pain and urinary frequency become debilitating. Histologically, the bladder may be chronically inflamed, and in severe cases, the bladder becomes fibrotic and contracted. Carcinoma in situ, which can also cause irritative symptoms in patients with sterile urine, is excluded by urinary cytology and bladder biopsy. Cystoscopy may show a Hunner ulcer or glomerulations after hydrodistension of the bladder. Biopsies often show evidence of chronic inflammation, mast cell infiltration, and fibrosis. Therapeutic options may include bladder hydrodistension under general anesthesia with or without instillation of various substances (including dimethyl sulfoxide, heparin, and amitriptyline), neuroleptic medications, urinary analgesics, and pelvic floor physical therapy. These therapies often bring temporary relief of symptoms. A subtotal cystectomy and augmentation with bowel or a cystectomy with diversion may be necessary in patients with a severely contracted bladder whose symptoms are incapacitating.

Degenerative Diseases

Bladder Fistulae

A fistula between the bowel and the bladder is most commonly caused by sigmoid diverticulitis, neoplasm, Crohn disease, or penetrating abdominal injury. Patients often present with symptoms of UTI, hematuria, pneumaturia, or fecaluria. Tests that can detect a fistula include water-based contrast enemas, cystogram, cystoscopy, and CT without bladder catheterization (air in the bladder confirms the diagnosis). Treatment usually involves resection of the

TABLE 27-1. Correctable Urologic Causes for Recurrent Urinary Tract Infections
Causes
Prostatic hypertrophy
Urethral stricture
Calculus
Chronic bacterial prostatitis
Ureteral reflux
Foreign body
Infected dysplastic or atrophic kidneys
Urethral diverticulum
Papillary necrosis
Vesicovaginal or vesicointestinal fistula
Urachal cyst
Ureteral duplication or ectopy
Perivesical abscess

Adapted from Dairiki L, Stamey T. Infections of the urinary tract. In: Walsh PC, Retik AB, Stamey TA, eds. *Campbell's Urology*. 7th ed. WB Saunders; 1998.

involved part of the bowel, with either primary anastomosis or colostomy, depending on the etiology. The edges of the bladder fistula are debrided and closed. Vesicovaginal fistulae can occur from pressure necrosis during prolonged labor or from surgical injury. Incontinence, the usual presenting symptom, is typically continuous. Diagnosis can be made by physical examination, a cystogram, and cystoscopy. IVP or bilateral retrograde pyelography is sometimes necessary to evaluate the upper tracts for obstruction or a ureterovaginal fistula. Small fistulae may be particularly difficult to delineate and may require additional maneuvers, including instillation of methylene blue into the bladder followed by the insertion of a vaginal tampon to detect leakage. Repair of a simple vesicovaginal fistula can often be performed by a vaginal approach.

Urinary Incontinence

Urinary incontinence is the involuntary loss of urine. It is classified as stress, urge, overflow, or total incontinence, according to the symptoms associated with the leakage of urine.

Stress urinary incontinence (SUI) occurs when an increase in the intra-abdominal pressure from coughing, sneezing, laughing, or straining causes urine leakage. The etiology of female SUI stems from diminished resistance between the bladder neck and the urethra, either due to urethral hypermobility or intrinsic sphincter deficiency. In men, SUI most commonly is a sequela of prostate surgery, notably radical prostatectomy. Urge incontinence is an irritative symptom in which leakage is preceded by an involuntary detrusor contraction with the urge to urinate. This manifests with the patient's inability to "make it to the restroom in time." Overflow incontinence occurs when the bladder overfills, usually from urinary retention, and uncontrollably empties. Urinary retention can be caused by an obstruction to outflow or detrusor underactivity. Total incontinence occurs when there is continuous leakage of urine. This type of incontinence is characteristic of a fistula (eg, a vesicovaginal fistula).

Evaluation

Taking an accurate history is essential in the evaluation of incontinence. The amount of leakage, associated activities, and voiding symptoms must be characterized. A voiding and incontinence diary that records the frequency, timing, and severity of episodes is helpful. In particular, when a patient wears pads, it is helpful to document the number of pads used daily and the degree of saturation that occurs. The medical history should be reviewed for medications, trauma, pelvic or urinary tract surgery, difficult deliveries, malignancy, neuromuscular disorders, diabetes, UTIs, and abnormal bowel habits. In men, a review of erectile and ejaculatory function may reflect underlying neurologic dysfunction.

The physical examination should include special attention to the abdomen, back, pelvis, and rectum. Perianal sensation, anal sphincter tone, as well as lower-extremity motor and sensory function and reflexes should be evaluated. Women with suspected stress incontinence should undergo a pelvic exam with a cough stress test with a full bladder. Laboratory evaluation should include urinalysis. Other studies that can be performed include a PVR measurement, cystoscopy, and urodynamic evaluation. Most patients with SUI do not benefit from formal invasive urodynamic studies, and this test should be reserved for patients in whom management is likely to be impacted by its results. Upper tract evaluation should be carried out when indicated but is not a routine part of an incontinence workup.

Treatment

The cause of incontinence dictates the mode of therapy. Overactive bladder (OAB) with urgency incontinence but without associated obstruction, bladder malignancy, infection, or neurogenic pathology can be treated with a number of modalities. First-line treatments include behavioral modification and pelvic floor physical therapy with bladder training exercises. Second-line therapy includes pharmacotherapy, with anticholinergics, β-3 agonists, or combination therapy. Patients who fail or cannot tolerate pharmacotherapy may progress to third-line treatments including intravesical injection of onabotulinum toxin A, posterior tibial nerve stimulation, or sacral neuromodulation. Rarely, patients will progress to invasive surgical management of OAB, with augmentation cystoplasty or urinary diversion.

SUI is treated by increasing the bladder outlet resistance and/or restoring support to the urethra. For women, noninvasive treatment options include pelvic floor physical therapy and vaginal inserts (ie, incontinence pessaries). Office-based procedures include urethral bulking, whereby one of several agents (eg, coaptite and polyacrylamide gel) is injected cystoscopically into the submucosal layer of the urethra. These procedures offer office-based convenience at the expense of some efficacy and durability (relative to surgical techniques). The gold standard treatment for stress incontinence is a mesh mid-urethral sling, which comes in retropubic and trans-obturator varieties. This procedure can be thought of as a modification of a bladder neck suspension procedure in which the fascia or anterior vaginal wall is fashioned as a sling around the urethra. The upward traction of sutures attached to the sling bilaterally reestablishes coaptation and increases urethral resistance.

The Marshall-Marchetti-Krantz procedure uses an anterior abdominal approach. The bladder and urethra are dissected off the posterior aspect of the pubic symphysis. Heavy, absorbable sutures are placed into the vaginal fascia on either side of the bladder neck and the urethra. These sutures are then placed in the posterior aspect of the symphysis to reposition and anchor the bladder and urethra superiorly and anteriorly (Figure 27-21).

Elevation of the bladder neck into the proper position can also be accomplished with a suspension procedure using a combined vaginal and suprapubic approach. The Stamey, Raz, and other similar procedures place nonabsorbable sutures through a vaginal incision into the tissue on each side of the bladder neck. In the Stamey procedure, a small piece of Dacron vascular graft placed on the suture near the bladder neck serves as a bolster to prevent the suture from tearing out. In the Raz procedure, the suture is passed several times helically through tissue lateral to the bladder neck, including the urethropelvic ligament. In both of these procedures, suprapubic incisions are used and a needle ligature carrier is passed from the suprapubic incision immediately behind the pubic symphysis through the vaginal incision. Both ends of the bladder neck sutures are passed by this needle into the suprapubic incision.

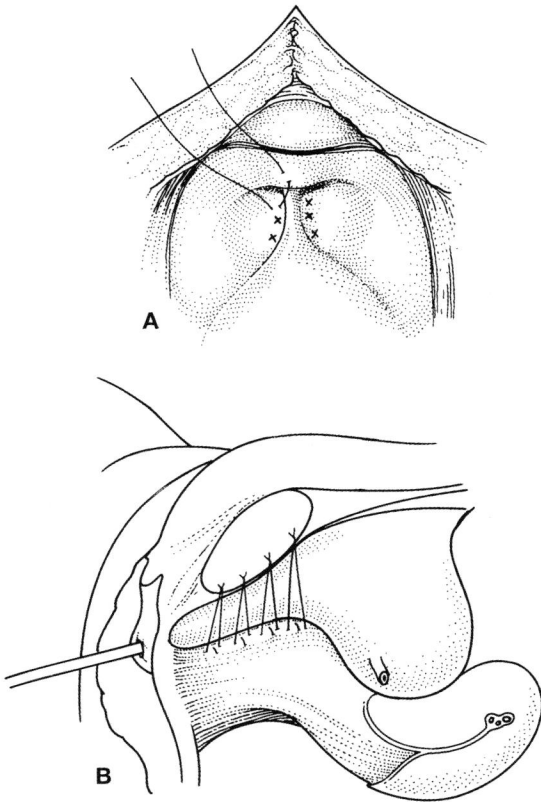

Figure 27-21. Marshall-Marchetti-Krantz procedure. A. Placement of absorbable sutures lateral to urethra and bladder neck as seen intraoperatively. B. Lateral view of completed repair with bladder neck and urethra in proper position. (From Lawrence PF. *Essentials of Surgical Specialties*. 3rd ed. Lippincott Williams & Wilkins; 2007.)

The suspension sutures are then tied over the anterior rectus fascia with enough tension to correct the anatomy but not kink or obstruct the urethra. A suprapubic tube, placed at the time of surgery by some surgeons, serves postoperatively as the primary bladder drainage. Later, as the patient begins to void, it serves to empty any PVRs until normal voiding returns (Figure 27-22).

A myriad of management options exist for men with post-prostatectomy SUI. Pelvic floor physical therapy with pelvic floor strengthening can be sufficient in cases of low-volume incontinence. While controversial, off-label pharmacotherapy with duloxetine has been utilized in this cohort of patients as well. All patients considering surgical management should undergo cystourethroscopy to rule out underlying bladder neck contracture and measurement of PVR bladder volume to ensure adequate incomplete bladder emptying. In men with low-volume SUI and no previous history of pelvic radiation, male slings can be considered. For those with high-volume SUI and/or prior radiation or those men who desire the most definitive form of surgical therapy, an artificial urinary sphincter is preferred. An artificial urinary sphincter is a prosthetic device comprising a cuff that encircles the bulbar urethra,

a reservoir that contains fluid, and a pump in the scrotum. The cuff is inflated at rest, causing the urethra to coapt and increase outflow resistance. When the patient wishes to void, he uses the pump to transfer fluid from the cuff to the reservoir.

Neurogenic Bladder Dysfunction

Micturition is a complex event requiring coordination between different levels of the central nervous system, the somatic and autonomic systems, and the detrusor and sphincter muscles of the bladder. During the filling phase, the bladder "relaxes" to accommodate an increasing urine volume. This ability to store appropriate urine volumes without a significant increase in pressure is called "compliance." Also, during bladder filling, sphincter muscle tone is increased. Normal micturition, a voluntary event involving complex coordination of the detrusor and sphincter muscles, begins with relaxation of the external sphincter followed by relaxation and opening of the bladder neck, sympathetic inhibition, and parasympathetic activation with detrusor contraction. The normal detrusor contraction lasts long enough to empty the bladder. In the central nervous system, there are highly integrated interrelations between the cerebral motor cortex, basal ganglia, cerebellum, pontine nuclei, and sacral cord nuclei that control voiding. Peripheral detrusor innervation is parasympathetic, mostly from S3 and some from S4. The trigone and bladder neck receive sympathetic output from T11 to L2. The external sphincter (somatic) receives most of its input from S2 via the pudendal nerve. Disruption of any one of these pathways can result in a neurogenic bladder dysfunction (Table 27-2).

Classification

Several classification systems have been devised to help categorize the etiology and phenotypes of neurogenic bladder dysfunction. It can be helpful to categorize types of neurogenic bladder dysfunction by the level of neurologic defect, with its resultant symptomatology and urodynamic findings.

Classically, patients with suprapontine lesions present with detrusor overactivity, due to a lack of inhibition of the pontine micturition center (Barrington nucleus). These lesions include brain tumors, cerebrovascular accidents, Alzheimer and Parkinson dementia, cerebral palsy, and multiple sclerosis. Of note, multiple sclerosis can present with lesions across the central nervous system. Also, Parkinson dementia has been associated with a cog-wheeling pattern of sphincteric relaxation, which manifests with obstructive LUTS.

Suprasacral neurologic defects below the pons may result in detrusor-sphincter dyssynergia, or dyscoordination between detrusor contraction and sphincter complex relaxation during micturition. This can be appreciated on urodynamic studies with an increase in the perineal EMG activity during attempted voiding and leads to obstructive voiding symptoms. This can also be associated with detrusor overactivity. Common lesions in this region include spinal cord injuries, transverse myelitis, spina bifida, and again multiple sclerosis. Notably, lesions above the T6 spinal cord level may result in autonomic dysreflexia due to excessive sympathetic outflow from the thoracolumbar trunk.

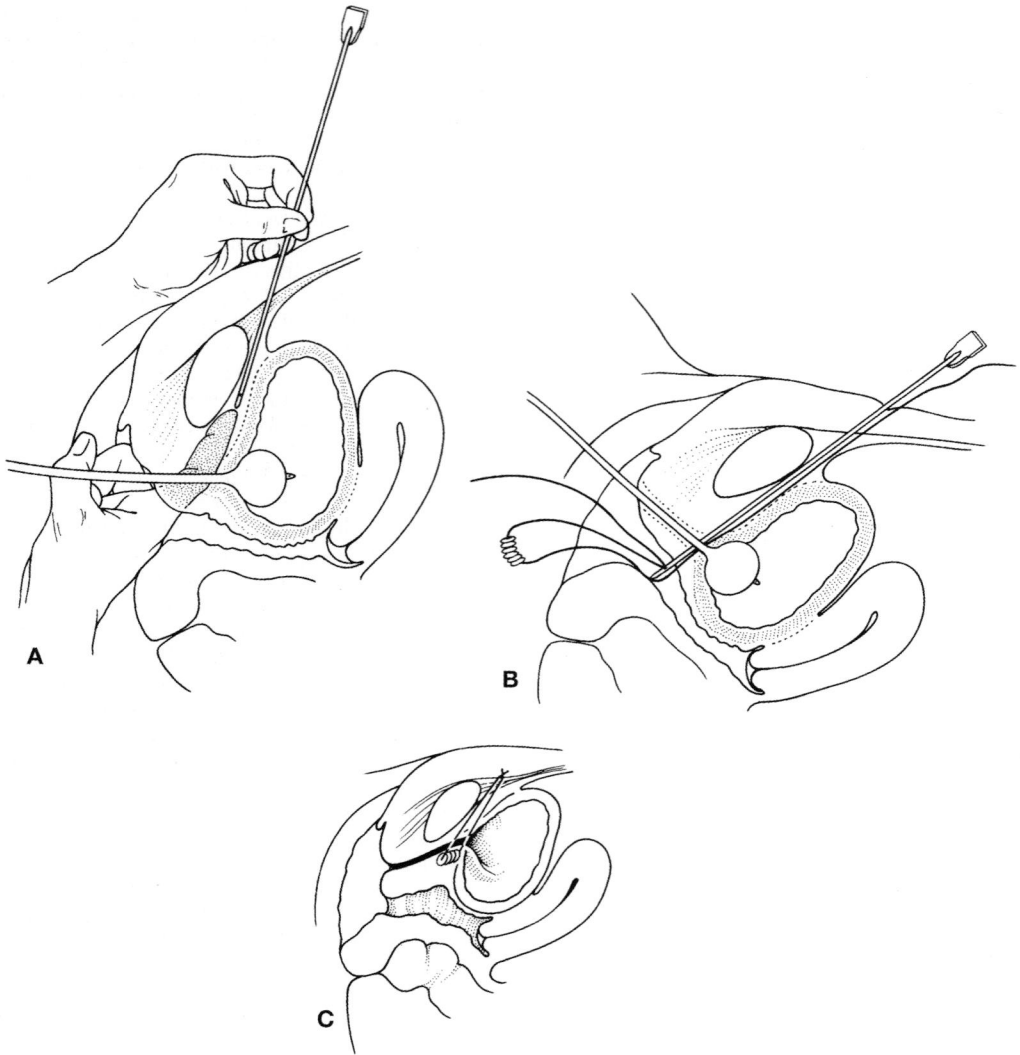

Figure 27-22. Stamey cystourethropexy. A. Lateral view showing passage of ligature carrier from the suprapubic incision, behind the pubic symphysis, and down to the vaginal incision (surgeon's finger is in the vaginal incision). B. Lateral view of ligature carrier with ready-to-pass second end of a suspension suture (note Dacron bolster). C. Lateral view of completed Stamey procedure with corrected position of bladder neck. (From Lawrence PF. *Essentials of Surgical Specialties*. 3rd ed. Lippincott Williams & Wilkins; 2007.)

Defects in the sacral spinal cord, namely resulting from conditions such as spina bifida, may result in a flaccid bladder (ie, detrusor underactivity). This may or may not be associated with an underactive sphincter complex. It is important to note that decreased bladder compliance can occur over time in this setting.

Evaluation

Invasive urodynamic studies are utilized to evaluate a patient with suspected, or a history of, neurogenic bladder. Again, this study should be reserved for cases where results will impact patient management. An invasive urodynamic study involves intracavitary measurement of bladder and abdominal pressures during the storage and emptying phases of micturition. Perineal EMG monitoring and urethral pressure catheters can also evaluate sphincter activity.

Video urodynamic studies involve concomitant utilization of fluoroscopy to better delineate bladder and bladder outlet anatomy, and rule out VUR.

Bladder compliance is defined as Δ bladder volume/Δ bladder pressure during filling. As such, an increase in the bladder pressure readings during filling reflects a decrease in compliance, reflecting compromise of the bladder's viscoelastic properties. Impaired bladder compliance with elevated bladder pressure is important to identify, as this pressure can be translated to the upper tracts and result in renal compromise. The detrusor leak point pressure refers to the detrusor pressure at which leakage occurs in the absence of a bladder contraction or an increase in the abdominal pressure. A detrusor leak point pressure of more than 40 cm H_2O is associated with an increased risk of upper tract deterioration.

TABLE 27-2. Effects of Neurologic Lesions on Bladder Functions

Neurologic Lesion	Urodynamic Findings
Lesions above the brainstem	Involuntary bladder contractions
Complete lesions of the spinal cord above S2	Involuntary bladder contractions with smooth sphincter synergia and striated sphincter dyssynergia
Brain tumors	Detrusor hyperreflexia, urinary incontinence
Parkinson disease	Detrusor hyperreflexia, urgency, frequency, urge incontinence
Shy-Drager syndrome	Detrusor hyperreflexia
Lesions above T6	Autonomic dysreflexia
Multiple sclerosis	Detrusor hyperreflexia, urgency, frequency
Diabetes mellitus	Impaired bladder sensation, decreased bladder contractility, impaired urinary flow, residual urine
Tabes dorsalis	Loss of bladder sensation, decreased bladder contractility
Herpes zoster	Urgency, frequency, urinary retention
Disc disease	Detrusor areflexia
Radical pelvic surgery	Urinary retention
Myelodysplasia	Urinary retention, bladder dysfunction

Detrusor overactivity can also be identified during a urodynamic study, visualized as unintentional detrusor contractions during filling. Detrusor underactivity can also be diagnosed during the voiding phase if diminished detrusor pressures are observed. Detrusor-sphincter dyssynergia can be diagnosed as described earlier, as also other forms of bladder outlet obstruction.

In addition to urodynamics, renal ultrasound should be performed to monitor for hydronephrosis and/or stone disease, particularly in patients with spinal cord injuries who are at risk for stones. Serum creatinine should be obtained to evaluate renal function.

Treatment

The therapeutic goals in the management of neurogenic bladder dysfunction are to preserve renal function and to normalize urinary tract function as much as possible, especially with respect to continence, bladder emptying, and infection prevention. Anticholinergics (eg, tolterodine tartrate and oxybutynin chloride) act on muscarinic (M3) receptors to inhibit involuntary detrusor contractions to improve OAB symptoms. More recently, β-3 agonists (eg mirabegron and vibegron) have emerged as alternatives to anticholinergics, with a favorable side effect profile. In patients who fail to improve with pharmacotherapy, intravesical botox is an option to treat symptoms of detrusor overactivity. The use of sacral neuromodulation in the management of patients with neurogenic bladder is still under investigation.

Patients with incomplete bladder emptying often require some form of urinary drainage. Clean intermittent catheterization is generally the preferred method of drainage in these patients although suprapubic cystostomy or an indwelling Foley catheter can also be utilized.

It is important to identify patients who have poorly compliant bladders that fill and store at a high pressure, causing ureteral reflux. Intervention is mandatory to prevent the patient from developing irreversible renal damage. When conservative management options fail, the patient may progress to bladder augmentation (with small intestine or sigmoid colon) or urinary diversion (eg, ileal conduit and continent catheterizable pouch). Alternatively, high-pressure filling and storage can be treated in certain cases with a sphincterotomy, an endoscopic procedure that cuts the sphincter. This usually promotes incontinence, which is managed with a condom catheter external drainage device; this device connects through tubing to a drainage bag. In the past, sphincterotomy or chronic indwelling catheterization were common treatments for neurogenic bladder dysfunction from spinal cord injury. The current trend is toward bladder augmentation and intermittent catheterization.

Regardless of the regimen used, patient compliance and close follow-up are essential. These patients need an annual evaluation of renal function and upper tract anatomy and possibly cystoscopy. Urodynamic evaluations are repeated as necessary to detect deleterious changes in bladder function that require a change in management.

Malignant Diseases

Bladder carcinoma is the fourth most common malignancy in men—the lifetime risk of bladder carcinoma in men is approximately 1.1%, in contrast to 0.27% in women. This disease is primarily diagnosed in persons 70 to 84 years of age, and is about 5 times more prevalent among cigarette smokers. Pure urothelial cell carcinoma represents approximately 75% of tumors, while the remaining 25% of tumors are composed of variant histologic subtypes. These subtypes include but are not limited to adenocarcinoma, which may occur with a patent urachus and tumors of the bladder dome, and squamous cell carcinoma, which can be associated with inflammation from chronic indwelling Foley catheters or schistosomiasis infection. That said, it is important to appreciate that variant histologies can be present in the absence of these less common risk factors.

Evaluation

Gross, painless hematuria is a common presenting sign of bladder cancer. However, approximately 20% of patients may present with only microscopic hematuria ($\geq$3 RBC/HPF [red blood cells per high-power field] on well-collected microscopic urinalysis in the absence of an inciting cause). Irritative voiding symptoms may also suggest a bladder tumor. The evaluation of gross hematuria usually includes imaging of the upper tracts (eg, IVP or a CT urogram), cystoscopy, and urine cytologic study. Microscopic hematuria evaluation varies by AUA risk stratification and ranges from repeat urinalysis to cystoscopy with upper tract imaging (renal ultrasound vs cross-sectional imaging).

Bladder cancer is staged primarily according to the depth of tumor invasion, as follows:
Tis = Carcinoma in situ
Ta = Noninvasive papillary tumor
T1 = Extension to lamina propria
T2 = Invasion of the detrusor muscle
T3 = Perivesical fat invasion
T4 = Adjacent organ involvement

Treatment

Management of bladder carcinoma depends on the extent of tumor invasion, with significant differences in treatment strategies between nonmuscle-invasive (≤T1) and muscle-invasive (≥T2) disease. Nonmuscle-invasive bladder cancer (NMIBC) is further stratified into low-, intermediate-, and high-risk categories based on a number of tumor characteristics, including but not limited to tumor grade (low vs high), tumor size and focality, presence of variant histology or carcinoma in situ, presence of lymphovascular invasion, history of recurrence, or prior treatment failure.

The initial treatment of any bladder tumor is surgical resection (transurethral resection of bladder tumor [TURBT]). This is accomplished transurethrally using a surgical instrument called a resectoscope. This procedure is both diagnostic and therapeutic, although adjunctive treatments are often required. For patients with low-risk NMIBC, TURBT alone and with or without a single dose of intravesical chemotherapy (mitomycin C or gemcitabine) is the recommended first-line treatment. Patients subsequently are enrolled into a strict surveillance program. Those with intermediate-risk NMIBC are recommended to undergo repeat resection if pathology reveals T1 disease. Subsequently, patients are recommended to undergo intravesical chemotherapy or immunotherapy, followed by surveillance. Finally, the gold standard treatment of patients in the high-risk category is radical cystectomy. Alternatively, patients can undergo repeat TURBT followed by a regimen of intravesical immunotherapy with bacillus Calmette-Guérin (BCG). Patients with disease persistence or recurrence with this therapy should be counseled on salvage radical cystectomy.

BCG is the mainstay intravesical therapy for patients with NMIBC; however, alternative regimens to this have emerged in recent years. Patients typically undergo initiative treatment with a 6-week induction course, followed by a maintenance regimen for 1 to 3 years. Systemic infection occurs in a small percentage of patients, and fever, dysuria, and hematuria are common during treatment. The risk of progression to muscle-invasive disease is relatively low (<10%) for Ta tumors, but increases as tumor stage advances (T1) or with high-grade lesions. As stated above, alternative intravesical therapies have demonstrated efficacy in clinical trials. These include sequential gemcitabine-docetaxel, nadofaragene firadenovec, and ALT-803. Further, the systemic checkpoint inhibitor pembrolizumab was granted U.S. Food and Drug Administration's (FDA) approval for treatment of BCG-unresponsive NMIBC.

In patients who can tolerate major surgery, radical cystectomy is the recommended treatment for muscle-invasive bladder cancer (MIBC). In men, this entails removing the bladder, prostate, perivesical fat, and pelvic lymph nodes; in women, it involves removing the bladder, anterior vaginal wall, uterus, and lymph nodes (however, vaginal and uterine-sparing approaches may have a role in select cases). Neoadjuvant systemic therapy with either chemotherapy or immunotherapy before radical cystectomy has been demonstrated in clinical trials to improve survival in patients with MIBC. For those who refuse or cannot tolerate surgery, bladder-sparing approaches can be considered. Trimodal therapy is principal among these and takes the form of maximal TURBT in concert with chemotherapy and radiation.

For patients who undergo radical cystectomy, the urine must be diverted in some manner. The most common form of urinary diversion is the ileal conduit, whereby the ureters are anastomosed to a segment of ileum which is brought up to the skin as a urinary stoma. Continent cutaneous diversions are urinary reservoirs constructed most often from the right colon with a tapered and catheterizable efferent limb of ileum. An orthotopic neobladder allows the creation of a reservoir using detubularized bowel with direct anastomosis to the urethra. This procedure avoids any cutaneous diversion, and patients can void per urethra or via clean intermittent catheterization.

THE PENIS

Anatomy

The penis is composed of two corpora cavernosa and one corpus spongiosum, which are bound by fibrous tissue called Buck fascia and covered by skin (Figure 27-23). Each corpus cavernosum has a thick fibrous capsule—the tunica albuginea—which forms around the cavernous sinuses. Distal to the symphysis pubis, the corpora cavernosa run side by side, divided by a septum. More proximally, the corpora cavernosa separate and fuse to the ischial rami. The corpus spongiosum is positioned ventrally, with its distal portion expanding to form the glans penis. The urethra is enclosed by the corpus spongiosum, traverses the glans penis, and opens as the external urethral meatus. The corpora cavernosa and corpus spongiosum are enveloped by Buck fascia and covered with skin that is virtually hairless and devoid of fat. The penile skin extends over the glans to form the prepuce or foreskin.

The major blood supply of the penis is from branches of the internal pudendal artery, which in turn is a branch of the internal iliac artery. Venous drainage from the penis is into the iliac veins by way of the deep and superficial dorsal veins. The lymphatics of the glans penis, corpus spongiosum, and distal corpus cavernosum drain into the external iliac, superficial, and deep inguinal lymph nodes. The proximal corpus cavernosum and posterior urethra drain into the internal iliac lymph nodes.

Trauma

Penile injury may result from blunt or penetrating trauma, avulsion, strangulation, burns, fracture, and, occasionally, biting. When the mechanism of injury indicates that there

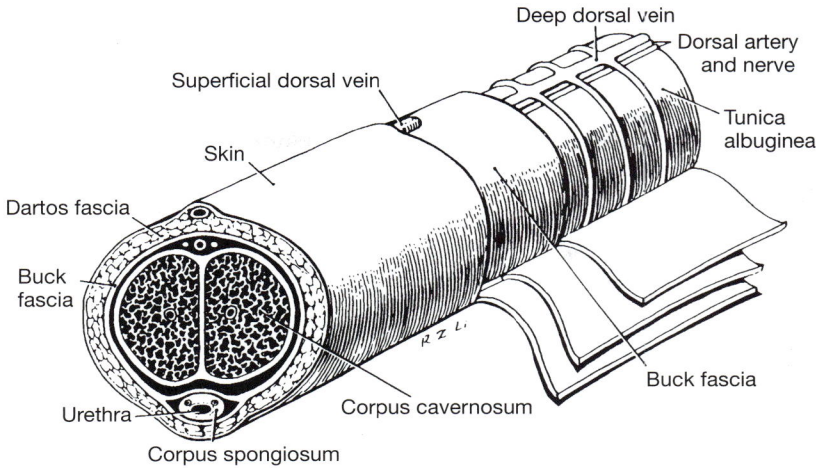

Figure 27-23. Anatomy of the penis. (From Lawrence PF. *Essentials of Surgical Specialties*. 3rd ed. Lippincott Williams & Wilkins; 2007.)

is a possibility of urethral injury, assessment of urethral integrity with a retrograde urethrogram is mandatory. A careful physical examination is of prime importance. Retrograde urethrography is indicated in all cases of suspected urethral injury, and scrotal ultrasound is helpful when testicular injury is suspected.

The management of penetrating penile injuries is variable depending on the presence, extent, and location of urethral or corporal injury. Knife injuries resulting in superficial lacerations may be closed if the wound is clean. Urethral injuries along the anterior urethra can occasionally be immediately repaired or can be managed with suprapubic catheter placement and delayed urethral repair. Repair of complete penile amputations using microsurgical techniques can be attempted if the penis has been properly preserved in cold saline. If repair of the amputated penis is not feasible, then partial penectomy is performed. Injuries that involve the testes require surgical exploration.

Avulsion injury to the skin of the penis may be caused by the patient's clothing and penis becoming entrapped in industrial machinery. Usually, the skin and loose areolar tissue superficial to Buck fascia are avulsed and deeper tissues are left intact. When sufficient skin remains, the injury can be treated with primary closure. With circumferential penile avulsions, complete interruption of the lymphatic drainage results in chronic lymphedema of the skin distal to the injury. Superior cosmetic results are obtained if the skin distal to the injury is removed up to the coronal sulcus and replaced with a split-thickness skin graft.

Penile burns may be caused by thermal, chemical, or electric injury and are managed similarly to burns in other areas of the body. As penile preservation is the prime objective, extensive debridement should be approached cautiously. One consideration is to avoid prolonged urethral catheterization because this can result in urethral sloughing. When bladder drainage is indicated, especially for longer than 72 hours, a suprapubic tube should be placed.

Fracture of the penis involving rupture of the tunica albuginea of the corpus cavernosum can occur during intercourse. The patient typically reports experiencing a cracking sensation or noise in association with a misguided thrust followed by pain, detumescence, and rapid penile shaft swelling. The immediate management of penile fracture consists of surgical exploration with evacuation of the hematoma and repair of the tunica albuginea. Patients who suffer penile fractures should be counseled regarding the risks of subsequent erectile dysfunction.

Malignant Diseases

Premalignant Lesions

Four penile lesions have been identified as premalignant: leukoplakia, Bowen disease, erythroplasia of Queyrat, and giant condyloma acuminatum (Table 27-3). Leukoplakia appears grossly as a white plaque and is characterized microscopically by acanthosis, hyperkeratosis, and parakeratosis. The treatment is local excision. Bowen disease typically appears as a solitary, erythematous plaque on the penile shaft. Approximately 25% of patients with Bowen disease will have a concomitant visceral malignancy. Erythroplasia of Queyrat consists of raised, red, velvety, and well-marginated areas of the glans penis or coronal sulcus. Both Bowen disease and erythroplasia of Queyrat histologically appear as carcinoma in situ and may be treated with Nd:YAG (neodymium-doped yttrium aluminum garnet) laser fulguration, local excision, or topical application of 5-fluorouracil. Giant condyloma acuminatum (Buschke–Löwenstein tumor and verrucous carcinoma) is a large, exophytic lesion often grossly indistinguishable from squamous cell carcinoma. Histologically, these lesions are similar to condyloma acuminatum except that the tumor extends into the underlying tissue. Local excision is required, often necessitating partial or total penectomy. Balanitis xerotica obliterans (BXO), also referred to as lichen sclerosus et atrophicus, has been classified as a "premalignant" condition but is generally benign. BXO presents as white, atrophic, and edematous lesions involving the glans penis or prepuce. Histologically, the dermis is composed of abundant amorphous collagen and a lymphocytic infiltrate in the underlying reticular dermis. BXO is often associated with urethral stricture disease that can become progressive to involve the

TABLE 27-3. Premalignant Penile Lesions

Penile Lesion	Gross Characteristics	Microscopic Characteristics	Treatment
Leukoplakia	White plaque	Acanthosis, hyperkeratosis, and parakeratosis	Excision
Balanitis xerotica obliterans	White, atrophic red lesion of glans or prepuce	Abundant, amorphous collagen and lymphocyte infiltrate of reticular dermis	Excision, topical steroids
Bowen disease	Solitary, red plaque on penile shaft	Carcinoma in situ	Laser fulguration, excision, topical 5-fluorouracil
Erythroplasia of Queyrat	Raised, red velvety lesion of glans or coronal sulcus	Carcinoma in situ	Laser fulguration, excision, topical 5-fluorouracil
Giant condyloma acuminatum	Large, exophytic lesion	Similar to condyloma acuminatum with invasion into underlying tissue	Excision

entire anterior urethra. Treatment of BXO consists of topical steroids, and, if there is associated urethral stricture disease, extended meatotomy or open-staged urethral reconstruction is the standard of care.

Squamous Cell Carcinoma

Although rare in the United States, penile cancer is more common in men living in hot, humid regions. Poor personal hygiene and retained phimotic foreskin have been implicated in the etiology of penile carcinoma. Penile cancer is extremely rare in men circumcised at birth. Squamous cell carcinoma of the penis occurs most commonly in the sixth decade of life. The symptoms are ulceration, necrosis, suppuration, and hemorrhage of the penile lesion. The clinical evaluation of patients with penile cancer includes physical examination with palpation of the inguinal region, liver function tests, chest radiographs, CT of the abdomen and pelvis, and bone scans. The most widely used staging system is the TNM staging system. (For detailed information on the staging of penile cancer, see the American Joint Committee on Cancer's *Cancer Staging Manual*, 8th edition. A summary of the stages can be found at https://www.cancer.net/cancer-types/penile-cancer/stages-and-grades.)

Small penile cancers limited to the prepuce can be treated by circumcision alone. Partial penectomy with at least a 2-cm margin of normal tissue is used to treat smaller (2-5 cm) distal penile tumors (Figure 27-24). The remaining penis should be long enough to permit voiding in the standing position. The 5-year cure rate for patients treated with partial penectomy is 70% to 80%. Larger distal penile lesions or proximal tumors require total penectomy and perineal urethrostomy. If the scrotum, pubis, or abdominal wall is involved, radical en bloc excision may be necessary.

Many patients have inguinal lymphadenopathy at presentation. The superficial and deep inguinal nodes are often the first involved nodes. Removal of involved nodes

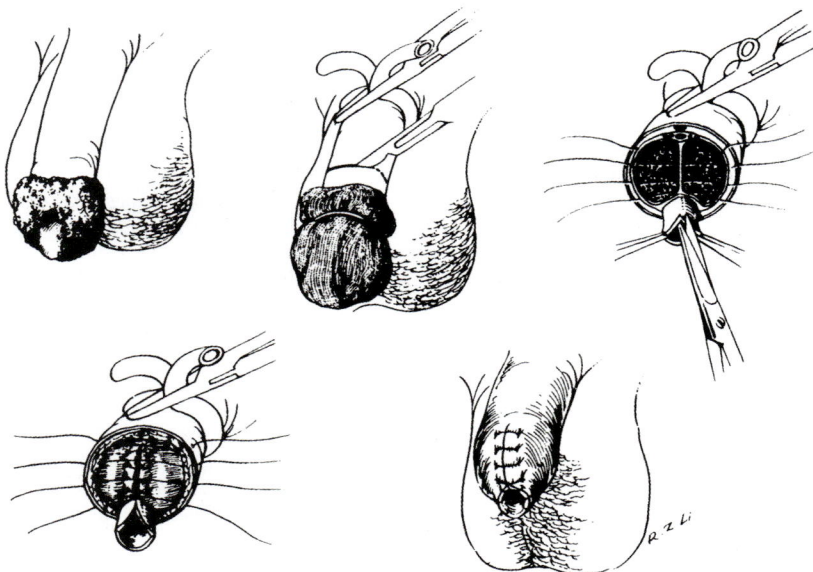

Figure 27-24. **Technique of partial penectomy.** (From Lawrence PF. *Essentials of Surgical Specialties*. 3rd ed. Lippincott Williams & Wilkins; 2007.)

can be curative in penile cancer. The next location of spread is often to the pelvic nodes, including the iliac and obturator. However, inguinal lymph node enlargement before excision of the primary tumor may be the result of infection and not metastatic disease. Thus, clinical assessment of the inguinal region should be delayed 4 to 6 weeks, during which time the patient is treated with antibiotics. If inguinal lymphadenopathy persists or subsequently develops, there is a high likelihood of metastatic lymph nodal disease, and ilioinguinal lymphadenectomy should be performed. Furthermore, if nodes are found in the inguinal region, pelvic lymph node dissection may be indicated.

Radiation of the primary tumor and regional lymph nodes is an alternative to surgery in patients with small (<2 cm), low-stage tumors. The advantage of radiotherapy over surgery is preservation of the penis. However, control rates are slightly lower than those of surgical excision. Similarly, radiation therapy can cure some patients with inguinal nodal metastases, but at a rate lower than those with ilioinguinal lymphadenectomy. Chemotherapy is also used in some cases.

Acquired Disorders

Priapism

Priapism is the pathologic prolongation of penile erection. Unlike normal tumescence, in priapism only the corpora cavernosa are turgid, whereas the corpus spongiosum (including the glans penis) remains flaccid. Priapism is characterized as either low flow or high flow. In low-flow priapism, the penile venous outflow is obstructed, which produces sludging and thrombosis of cavernosal blood. Left untreated, prolonged ischemic injury may result in corporal fibrosis and/or erectile dysfunction. Etiologies include sickle cell anemia, leukemia, metastatic disease, pharmacologic secondary effect, and intracorporeal injection of vasoactive substances for the treatment of impotency. In high-flow priapism, there is increased blood flow to the penis. It can be caused by injury to the pelvic vasculature, as in pelvic trauma, with increased blood flow to the penis secondary to a vascular fistula.

The treatment of patients with sickle cell anemia should be directed at the underlying cause. Such patients should be treated with hydration, alkalinization, analgesics, and exchange transfusions.

Patients with priapism may respond to intracorporeal injection of phenylephrine, especially when the duration of priapism is shorter than 6 hours. Otherwise, treatment requires aspiration of the corporal blood with a large needle and corporal irrigation with saline. If this treatment fails, another option is the Winter procedure, as illustrated in Figure 27-25. This procedure involves placing a biopsy needle into the corpora through the glans bilaterally and removing a core of tissue. In this way, a communication between the corpora cavernosa and the corpus spongiosum is created, allowing the blood trapped in the corpora

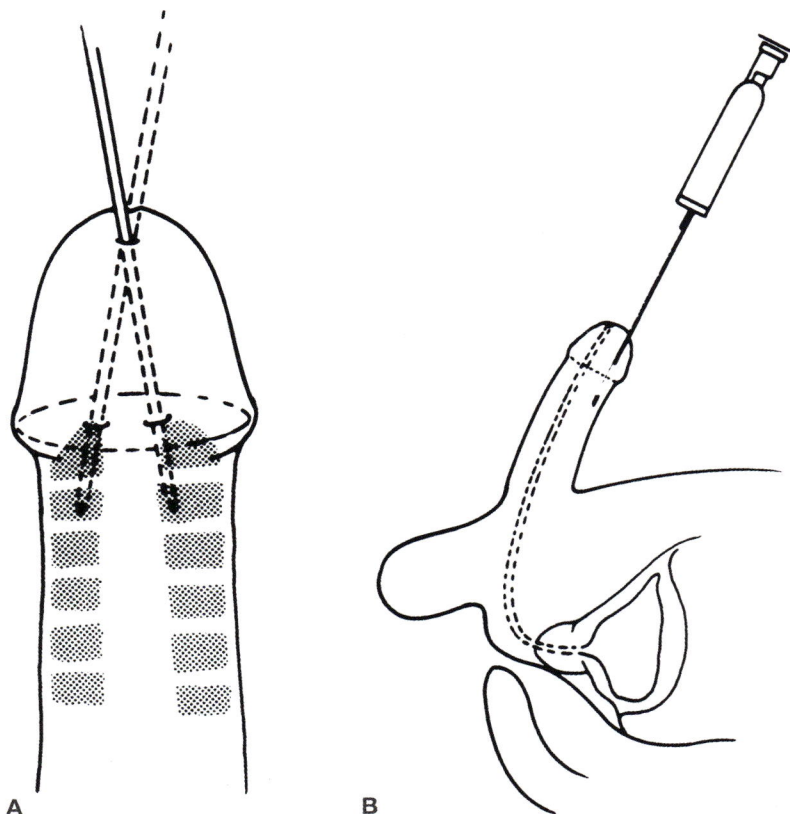

Figure 27-25. **Winter shunt for the treatment of priapism.** A Travenol biopsy needle is used to create fistulae between the glans penis (corpus spongiosum) and the corpora cavernosa. A. Dorsal view. B. Sagittal view. (From Lawrence PF. *Essentials of Surgical Specialties.* 3rd ed. Lippincott Williams & Wilkins; 2007.)

cavernosa to drain through the unobstructed outflow of the corpus spongiosum. In the rare patient for whom the abovementioned maneuvers fail, open surgery is an option: A formal communication is made between the corpora cavernosa and the corpus spongiosum.

When high-flow priapism is suspected, a corporal blood gas determination should be obtained. In low-flow ischemic priapism, the Po_2 is low. In high-flow priapism, the Po_2 is high and management is pudendal arteriography with selective embolization of the fistula.

Phimosis

Phimosis is the fibrotic contracture of the penile foreskin, prohibiting retraction of the prepuce over the glans penis. The cause is poor hygiene or infection beneath redundant foreskin, resulting in chronic irritation. Diabetes mellitus is a predisposing factor. Phimosis is often effectively managed with improved hygiene and steroid cream to allow the skin to stretch. Elective circumcision is often indicated.

Paraphimosis

When mild preputial contracture is present, the retracted foreskin forms a constricting band proximal to the coronal sulcus that over a prolonged period of time results in edema. The inability to place the foreskin back over the glans is termed "paraphimosis." Initially, venous occlusion results in edema, which leads to arterial occlusion, and eventually, glandular ischemia. Paraphimosis is a urologic emergency. Manual compression of the glans usually reduces the edema, allowing the foreskin to be reduced (Figure 27-26). If manual compression fails, the constricting preputial band of tissue requires incision. Circumcision should follow the resolution of edema and inflammation.

Peyronie Disease

Peyronie disease is a process involving scarring of the tunica albuginea of the corpora cavernosa, resulting in plaques. Peyronie plaques are typically located on the dorsal penile surface. During tumescence, these plaques restrict corporal expansion leading to variable degrees of penile curvature that may be sexually incapacitating. The acute or "immature" form of this disease is variable in duration but often lasts longer than 6 months. It is characterized by painful erections, progressive curvature, and

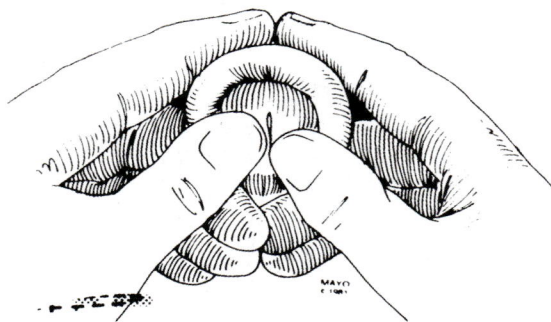

Figure 27-26. Manual reduction of paraphimosis. (From Lawrence PF. *Essentials of Surgical Specialties.* 3rd ed. Lippincott Williams & Wilkins; 2007.)

induration of the plaque on physical examination. During this immature phase, surgery is contraindicated and management is conservative. Conservative approaches include collagenase, vitamin E, and perhaps potassium *p*-aminobenzoate (Potaba) or colchicine. Peyronie disease can often resolve spontaneously. If conservative management fails and a patient has mature disease (generally defined as unchanged curvature for a 6-month duration with resolution of pain) and curvature that prevents satisfactory intercourse, the erectile function is assessed. If the patient has good erectile function, surgical options to correct the curvature include plication opposite the plaque or incision/excision of the plaque with grafting (eg, dermis or saphenous vein, or other biomaterials). Erectile dysfunction is often associated with Peyronie disease; when this occurs, therapy is directed at treating the erectile dysfunction. As a last resort in a patient with erectile dysfunction, a penile prosthesis is sometimes placed to correct impotency and ensure penile straightening.

Circumcision and Dorsal Slit

Circumcision is the most common operation performed on men in the United States (Figure 27-27). Indications include parental decision, phimosis, cosmetic effect, and malignancy. Contraindications to circumcision include myelodysplasia and hypospadias (because the foreskin may be needed for use during hypospadias repair). In newborns, a Gomco clamp or Plastibell is usually used without anesthesia. Adults often obtain excellent anesthesia from a local penile block; circumcision is performed as an outpatient procedure.

After appropriate preparation and draping, a straight hemostat is placed on the middle of the dorsal surface of the prepuce. The hemostat is removed, and a dorsal slit is performed by cutting the crushed foreskin proximally to within 1 cm of the coronal sulcus. The prepuce should now easily retract to expose the glans penis. If only a dorsal slit is to be performed, the cut edges are hemostatically approximated by absorbable interrupted sutures. If a circumcision is to be performed, the cut edges of the dorsal slit are not sutured. A similar incision is made in the ventral surface of the prepuce to the frenulum. Occasionally, bleeding from a frenula artery will require ligature. With the foreskin divided in two, redundant prepuce is excised. Hemostasis is secured with electrocautery or absorbable sutures. It should be stressed that cautery should not be used in conjunction with Gomco or similar metal clamps because it can result in severe cautery injuries to the glans penis. The mucosal and cutaneous surfaces of the foreskin are then approximated using interrupted absorbable sutures.

THE URETHRA

Anatomy

The male urethra is divided into posterior and anterior portions (Figure 27-28). The posterior portion includes the prostatic urethra and the membranous urethra (which is the location of the external striated sphincter). The anterior portion consists of the urethral meatus, the fossa navicularis, the penile urethra, and the bulbar urethra. The prostatic urethra is lined by transitional epithelium; the membranous, bulbous, and penile sections of the urethra

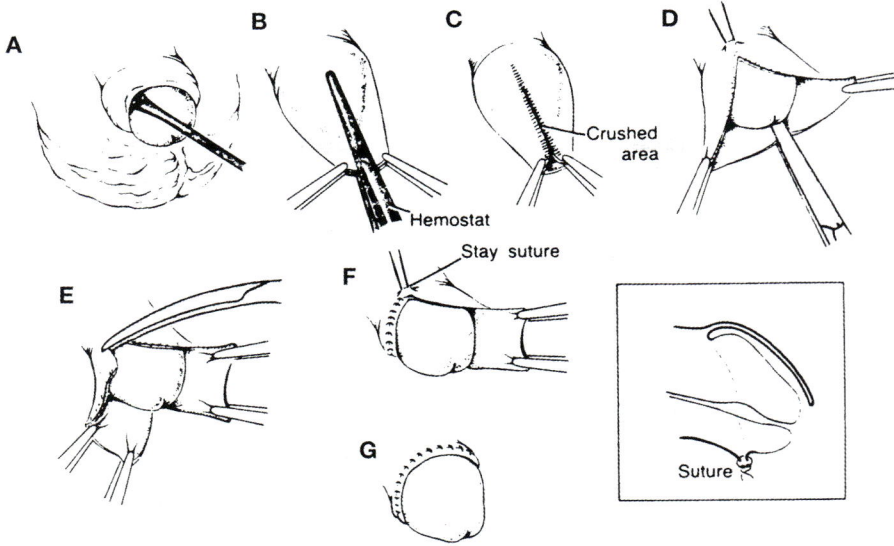

Figure 27-27. **Freehand circumcision (A–G).** (From Lawrence PF. *Essentials of Surgical Specialties*. 3rd ed. Lippincott Williams & Wilkins; 2007.)

are lined by pseudostratified or stratified columnar epithelium; and the external urethral meatus is lined by squamous epithelium. Paired bulbourethral (Cowper) glands, located in the membranous urethra, produce a clear viscous fluid (sometimes called the "pre-ejaculatory fluid") and secrete into the bulbous urethra. Multiple glands of Littre, which also produce a pre-ejaculatory fluid, line the penile urethra. The lymphatic drainage of the posterior urethra is directly into the obturator and iliac nodes, whereas that of the anterior urethra is through the deep inguinal nodes into the iliac nodes.

The female urethra, about 4 cm long (Figure 27-29), lies immediately anterior to the vagina; its external urethral meatus opens 2 cm posterior to the clitoris. Transitional epithelium lines the proximal third of the female urethra and stratified squamous epithelium lines the distal two-thirds. The periurethral glands of Skene are homologues of the male urethral glands and empty into the distal urethra. The proximal female urethra drains into the iliac lymph nodes and the distal portion into the inguinal lymph nodes.

Trauma

Anterior urethral injuries usually result from blunt trauma, such as straddle injuries, in which the bulbous urethra is injured. Prostatomembranous urethral injuries occur in approximately 10% of patients who sustain pelvic fractures in motor vehicle accidents or occupational injuries. Urethral injury should be suspected in patients with blood at

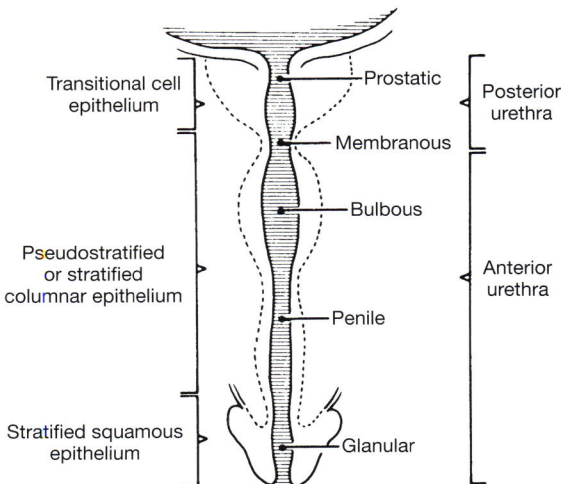

Figure 27-28. **Anatomy and cell types lining the male urethra.** (From Lawrence PF. *Essentials of Surgical Specialties*. 3rd ed. Lippincott Williams & Wilkins; 2007.)

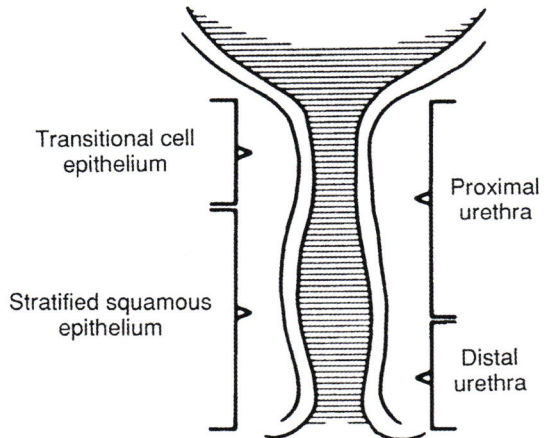

Figure 27-29. **Anatomy and cell types lining the female urethra.** (From Lawrence PF. *Essentials of Surgical Specialties*. 3rd ed. Lippincott Williams & Wilkins; 2007.)

the urethral meatus, inability to void, or penile or perineal edema and ecchymosis. If Buck fascia remains intact, extravasation of blood and urine are confined to the penile shaft (Figure 27-30).

Evaluation

On retrograde urethrography, a partial urethral rupture is suggested when there is both urethral extravasation and passage of contrast into the bladder. Extravasation without passage of contrast into the bladder suggests a complete urethral rupture (Figure 27-31).

Treatment

Small, incomplete anterior urethral ruptures with extravasation limited by Buck fascia are initially treated by draining with a urethral catheter or by performing a suprapubic cystostomy. Patients who sustain a posterior urethral injury associated with a pelvic fracture require a suprapubic tube. In addition, an aligning urethral catheter can be placed, if possible, but this procedure is controversial. In general, posterior urethral disruptions are managed by a minimum of 3 months of suprapubic diversion and delayed urethral reconstruction via a perineal approach with excision of the stricture and a primary anastomosis.

Malignant Diseases

Male Urethral Carcinoma

Urethral carcinoma is rare and usually occurs after 60 years of age. Approximately 80% are squamous cell cancers. In the absence of metastatic disease, partial or total penectomy is the treatment of choice when the distal urethra is involved. Proximal urethral cancers are managed with urethrectomy.

Female Urethral Carcinoma

Urethral cancer is the only genitourinary malignancy that occurs in women more often than in men. The usual presenting symptom is a papillary or fungating urethral mass or urethral or vaginal bleeding. Local tumor extension into the vagina and bladder neck is common. Lymphatic spread of distal urethral lesions is by way of the inguinal nodes, whereas that of proximal urethral tumors is by way of the iliac nodes. When present, inguinal lymphadenopathy usually indicates metastatic disease. Noninvasive distal urethral lesions are often squamous cell cancers and can be managed with distal urethrectomy. Proximal and panurethral cancers are managed by chemotherapy or radiation therapy followed by radical excision. The aforementioned represents general guidelines for the management of localized disease. The treatment of an individual patient may vary depending on a number of factors, including general health status, nodal status, and the extent of involvement of the primary tumor.

Urethral Strictures

Urethral strictures were once considered to be most often caused by gonococcal urethritis. The most common causes of anterior urethral strictures today are straddle injury (eg, a bicycle accident long ago) and instrumentation of the urethra. Obstructive voiding symptoms (eg, those encountered with prostatism) are common complaints. Occasionally, UTI or inability to pass a urethral catheter may lead to the initial diagnosis.

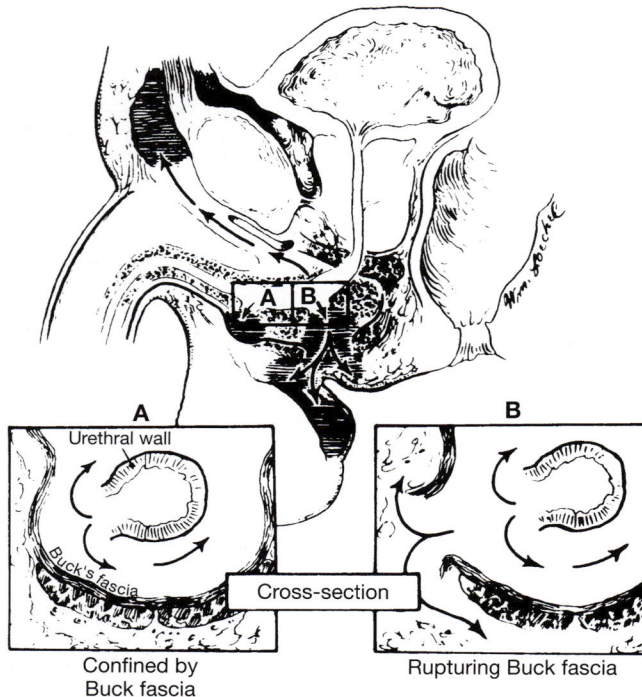

A
Urethral wall
Buck's fascia
Cross-section
Confined by
Buck fascia

B
Rupturing Buck fascia

Figure 27-30. **Straddle injury to the bulbous urethra demonstrating pathways of blood and urine extravasation (A and B).** (From Lawrence PF. *Essentials of Surgical Specialties.* 3rd ed. Lippincott Williams & Wilkins; 2007.)

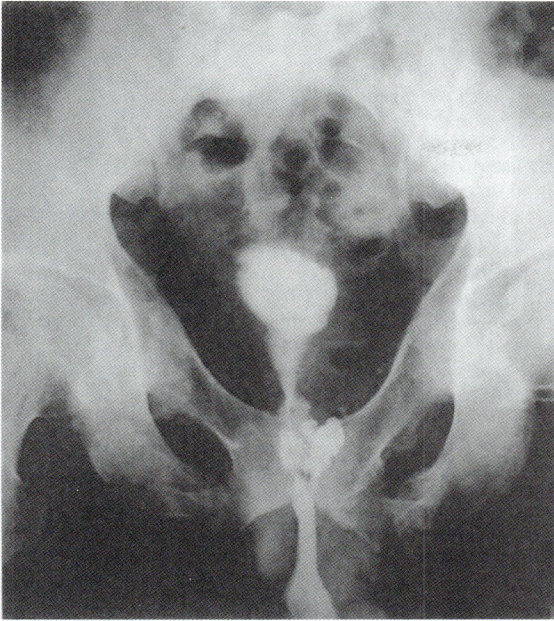

Figure 27-31. Retrograde urethrogram showing retroperitoneal extravasation of contrast caused by a traumatic posterior urethral rupture. (From Lawrence PF. *Essentials of Surgical Specialties*. 3rd ed. Lippincott Williams & Wilkins; 2007.)

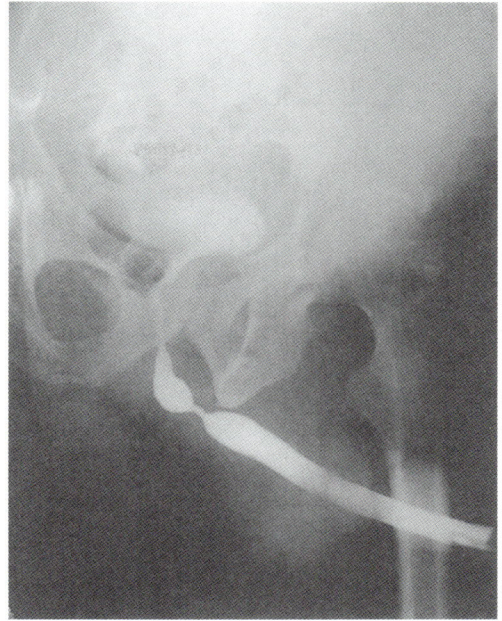

Figure 27-32. Retrograde urethrogram showing bulbar urethral stricture. (From Lawrence PF. *Essentials of Surgical Specialties*. 3rd ed. Lippincott Williams & Wilkins; 2007.)

Evaluation

When a urethral stricture is suspected, cystoscopy will diagnose a stricture. However, the urethra is usually seen only up to the point of narrowing, and the scope cannot be passed proximally. A retrograde urethrogram along with a VCUG will outline the exact location, caliber, and length of a urethral stricture.

Treatment

In the past, most strictures, regardless of the length, were initially managed with one or more dilations or endoscopic incisions (direct visual internal urethrotomy) of the strictures. These treatments were often performed without preoperative imaging studies. The modern management of urethral stricture disease requires complete diagnostic evaluation with retrograde and antegrade imaging and urethroscopy before a discussion of treatment options. The treatment that is best for a patient depends on the length and location of the stricture. If the stricture is truly discrete (<1 cm) and mucosal in character, dilation or urethrotomy may be curative. Longer strictures and recurrent strictures can also be managed with the abovementioned modalities. However, the recurrence rate is high, approaching 100% when multiple previous endoscopic treatments have failed. The advantage of dilation and urethrotomy is that they are less invasive than open surgery. These procedures are an excellent option when the patient wants to "manage" the stricture.

When the goal is to permanently cure the disease, open urethral reconstruction offers the highest success when properly performed using dedicated equipment and instruments. For example, a short bulbar urethral stricture (Figure 27-32) can be treated with open excision and primary anastomotic repair, with a permanent cure rate of

more than 98%. When strictures are long or more distally located, open repair requires tissue transfer. Tissues that can be used to enlarge the narrowed urethra include preputial skin as a flap or graft, or a graft of buccal mucosa.

Congenital Disorders

Posterior Urethral Valves

The most common type of posterior urethral valve anomaly (type I) consists of paired folds of mucous membranes that extend from the distal portion of the prostatic verumontanum and meet anteriorly in the membranous urethra (Figure 27-33). Posterior urethral valves cause a variable degree of urethral obstruction, with resultant bladder distension, VUR, hydroureteronephrosis, and renal damage. Today, it is commonly diagnosed on antenatal ultrasound, with bladder distension, echogenic hydronephrotic kidneys, and oligohydramnios. In severe cases, placing a vesicoamniotic shunt may reverse the oligohydramnios, allowing the lungs to develop and the pregnancy to be carried to term. The diagnosis is suggested in newborns with poor urinary streams or inability to void, and suprapubic or flank masses. VCUG may show the valves, but a more consistent finding is a dilated posterior urethra, with secondary findings of bladder and upper urinary tract obstruction.

Initial treatment consists of placing either an 8F infant feeding tube as a urethral catheter or a percutaneous suprapubic tube. Fluid, electrolyte, and acid-base status must be optimized. After the patient is stable, endoscopic valve ablation may be performed; alternatively, the bladder dome may be opened onto the lower abdomen (cutaneous vesicostomy) and endoscopic valve ablation performed another time.

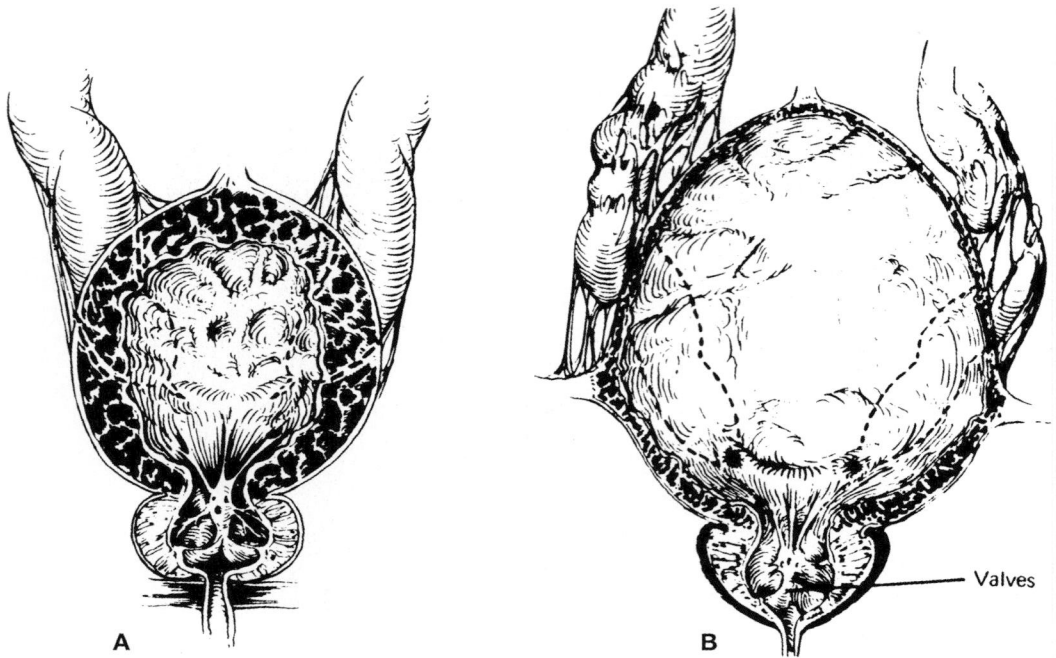

Figure 27-33. Posterior urethral valves. A. Dilation of the prostatic urethra, hypertrophy of vesical wall, and trigone in stage of compensation; bilateral hydroureters caused by trigonal hypertrophy. B. Attenuation of bladder musculature in stage of decompensation; advanced ureteral dilation and tortuosity, usually secondary to vesicoureteral reflux. (From Lawrence PF. *Essentials of Surgical Specialties*. 3rd ed. Lippincott Williams & Wilkins; 2007.)

Hypospadias

Hypospadias is one of the most common congenital anomalies, occurring in 1:300 live male births. In hypospadias, the urethral meatus is located on the ventral penile surface proximal to its normal position at the tip of the glans penis (Figure 27-34). Classification is based on the location of the meatus, which may be perineal, penoscrotal, shaft, coronal, or glanular. Usually, the prepuce is incompletely developed and is present as a dorsal hood. Additionally, remnants of the corpus spongiosum distal to the urethral meatus form fibrous bands termed "chordee," producing ventral penile curvature. When the chordee is released during hypospadias repair, the meatus often retracts more proximally, resulting in a greater distance between the hypospadiac and normal meatal positions. In boys with perineal hypospadias, the scrotum is bifid (resembling labia majora), the testes are often undescended, and the penis is small (resembling a hypertrophied clitoris); gender assignment may be difficult.

The goals of hypospadias repair are 2-fold. First is the correction of penile curvature, which is usually accomplished by releasing the chordee, either by simply degloving the phallus or by placing dorsal plication sutures in the dorsal corpora cavernosa. Second is the creation of a new urethra to bridge the gap between the hypospadiac meatus and the tip of the penis. Numerous techniques of hypospadias repair exist, including dorsal urethral incision with ventral urethral tubularization (Snodgrass repair), penile skin flap repairs, and in complex and revision cases, reconstruction with the use of buccal or split-thickness skin

grafts. To minimize the psychological effects of genital surgery, it is best that hypospadias repair be performed before the child is 1 year old.

Infectious Diseases

Gonococcal Urethritis

Gonorrhea is caused by the pathogen *Neisseria gonorrhoeae*, an anaerobic gram-negative diplococcus, which is transmitted during sexual intercourse. After an incubation period of 2 to 14 days, most men present with a yellowish urethral discharge caused by anterior urethritis. Other symptoms may include dysuria, urethral itching, and urinary frequency. About 25% of infected men remain asymptomatic and serve as a reservoir. Diagnosis is made by obtaining a urethral specimen (swab) for culture using Thayer-Martin medium. If rectal or oral intercourse is suggested by the history, rectal and pharyngeal cultures are recommended. If a presumptive diagnosis of gonococcal urethritis is made, patients and their sexual contacts are treated without waiting for the culture reports. Ceftriaxone 500 mg given once intramuscularly is considered the treatment of choice.

Nongonococcal Urethritis

Nongonococcal urethritis is characterized by dysuria, urinary frequency, periurethral itching, and a clear or white mucoid discharge. *C. trachomatis* is the most common causative agent. The incubation period is 1 to 3 weeks. The diagnosis of nongonococcal urethritis is made by cultures of the urethral swab, not the exudate. *C. trachomatis*

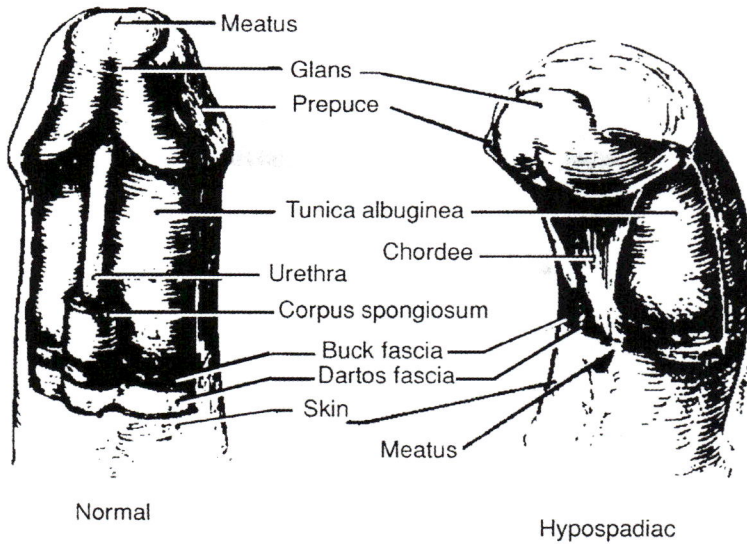

Figure 27-34. **Comparison of normal and hypospadiac penis showing chordee.** (From Lawrence PF. *Essentials of Surgical Specialties.* 3rd ed. Lippincott Williams & Wilkins; 2007.)

and *Ureaplasma urealyticum* are sensitive to doxycycline; 100 mg is given orally twice daily for 7 days. It has recently been shown that a single dose of azithromycin (1 g orally) is equivalent in efficacy to a 7-day course of doxycycline and is currently the treatment of choice. In clinical practice, patients suspected of having a sexually transmitted disease from gonorrhea or chlamydia are usually managed for both agents with swabs for both pathogens and then treated with both ceftriaxone and azithromycin.

THE TESTES, MALE INFERTILITY, AND IMPOTENCY

The Testes

Embryology and Anatomy

The testes develop embryologically from a long band of mesoderm on the posterior abdominal wall (retroperitoneum), that is, the genital ridge. Because of differential growth, by the seventh month of gestation, the testicle lies just inside the internal inguinal ring. The gubernaculum is a thick, inelastic structure connecting the lower pole of the testicle to the genital eminence, which leads the testicle through the inguinal canal into the scrotum during the eighth month of gestation. During its descent, the testicle becomes invested with a number of coverings (Figure 27-35). The peritoneum surrounds the anterior four-fifths of the testicle and becomes the tunica vaginalis. The superior part remains as the tubular processus vaginalis, which shortly collapses and obliterates. The internal oblique fascia becomes the cremasteric (suspender) fibers, which act as a thermoregulator, elevating the testicle during periods of cold.

The main arterial supply to the testicle, the internal spermatic artery, arises from the aorta below the renal artery. Additional arterial inflow arises from the deferential

artery, a branch of the inferior vesical artery, and from the external spermatic (cremasteric) artery, a branch of the inferior epigastric artery. The venous drainage parallels the arterial supply. A deferential vein drains into the hypogastric vein, an external spermatic vein drains into the epigastric vein, and an internal spermatic vein drains into the vena cava on the right and the renal vein on the left. Because of the juxtaposition of the mesonephric and genital ridges, the lymphatic drainage of the testicles is to the preaortic and precaval region. This knowledge is essential in considering the spread of testicular malignancy.

Congenital Disorders
Testicular Abnormalities
One of the more common abnormalities seen in newborn boys is cryptorchidism, which is a nonpalpable testicle. The incidence of this abnormality decreases with age, from 3.4% seen in term infants to 0.7% seen in infants at 9 months of age. The incidence is high with prematurity. If an empty scrotum is found, anorchia, nondescent, or retractile testis is possible. (See Chapter 10.)

Anorchia occurs in 3% to 5% of all cases explored for nonpalpable testes. Most are caused by prenatal torsion or vascular accidents, rarely by agenesis. At exploration, a vas deferens is found adjacent to the spermatic vessel, with a bud of scar representing the infarcted testicle (blind-ending vas). Unilateral anorchia is of minimal concern; the contralateral testicle is usually larger, and spermatogenesis and hormonal function do not appear to be affected. Bilateral anorchia leads to sterility and the need for hormone replacement at puberty.

Retractile testes are caused by overactivity of the cremasteric musculature. They are easily pulled into the scrotum but retract promptly into the groin. Most descend properly at puberty. This phenomenon underlines the need to examine the infant in a warm environment with gentle manipulation of the inguinal region.

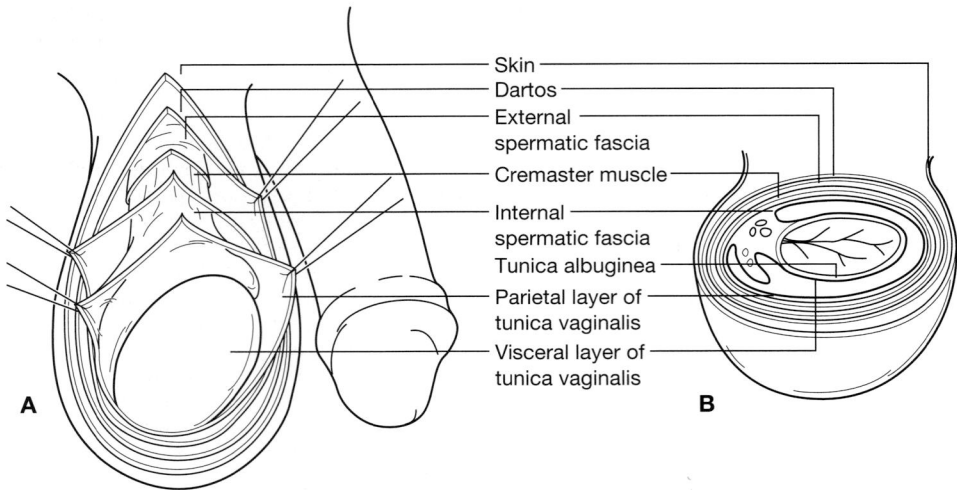

Figure 27-35. **Coverings of the testicle** (A and B). (From Lawrence PF. *Essentials of Surgical Specialties*. 3rd ed. Lippincott Williams & Wilkins; 2007.)

Undescended testicles usually lie along the usual course of descent, from the retroperitoneum to the external inguinal ring. Rarely, the testicular descent is aberrant and the testicle may be found in the perineum in front of the anus. Most commonly, if the undescended testicle is not palpable within the inguinal canal, it is found just inside the internal inguinal ring. If neither testicle is palpable but present, a stimulatory test with human chorionic gonadotropin (hCG) will cause an increase in serum testosterone. If no surge is noted, the diagnosis of an intersex condition should be considered. If a surge is noted with bilateral, and sometimes unilateral, cryptorchidism, treatment with exogenous hCG may occasionally lead to descent. In general, studies such as CT and ultrasound are not useful for locating nonpalpable testicles. Laparoscopy is often useful to locate intra-abdominal testes or to confirm the diagnosis of an absent testis. An intra-abdominal testicle must be brought down because the undescended testicle has 48 times greater incidence of testis malignancy. The contralateral descended testicle also has an increased risk of malignant degeneration. Unfortunately, surgical orchidopexy (movement of the testicle into its normal position) does not reduce these risks but does allow earlier diagnosis of future malignancies. Men with a history of testicular maldescent also have an increased risk of subfertility. A number of epididymal abnormalities are also seen with testicular nondescent, including an elongated epididymis, detachment from the testicle, and partial disruption.

Patent Processus Vaginalis

The processus vaginalis, the tube of peritoneum extending from the abdominal cavity to the tunica vaginalis, usually closes and involutes before birth. When it does not, the child presents with an inguinal hernia. A patent processus vaginalis is found in 4.4% of full-term and up to 13% of premature infants. If the processus is completely open, herniation of abdominal viscera may occur with possible strangulation, dictating emergency surgical correction. If the processus partially closes, a hydrocele forms, which increases in size if the infant is upright or cries. If a hydrocele is not apparent, gentle examination may show

a fuller cord on one side. During examination, rubbing the cord between the thumb and forefinger may give the sensation of silk rubbing on silk (ie, the "silk glove" sign) when the peritoneal sac is palpated. Spontaneous obliteration of the processus vaginalis may occur after birth. If the hydrocele persists after 1 year of age, varies in size (communicating hydrocele), or is symptomatic, repair is necessary. Repair consists of simple high ligation of the patent processus vaginalis at the internal inguinal ring.

Testicular Cord Torsion

Neonates who present with an acutely hard, enlarged scrotal mass that does not transilluminate may have incarcerated inguinal hernia, torsion of a testicular appendage, trauma-induced scrotal hematoma, or testicular torsion. In the newborn, torsion is extravaginal; that is, the epididymis, testicle, and tunica vaginalis all twist within the internal spermatic fascia with resultant organ infarction. Examination of the scrotum in the early phase of torsion will sometimes demonstrate a testicle lying in the transverse plane rather than in the normal longitudinal position. Occasionally, the epididymis may be palpable in the abnormal anterior position rather than in the normal posterior medial position. Loss of cremasteric reflex can be seen in 95% of patients with testicular torsion. An incarcerated hernia is sometimes diagnosed with ultrasound. On physical examination, auscultation of bowel sounds in the scrotum indicates trapped bowel contents.

Intravaginal torsion occurs more commonly in the adolescent period. In this entity, the tunica vaginalis surrounds the testicle instead of being fixed posterolaterally. The testicle is then free to twist inside the tunica, like the clapper within a bell. The patient presents with an acutely swollen, tender testicle that may preclude examination. The testicle may be retracted high in the scrotum, or the epididymis may be in an abnormal position. A thorough history may elicit previous episodes of transient testicular pain. Torsion may follow vigorous activity, but it is rarely caused by it. Differential diagnosis includes trauma, epididymo-orchitis, torsion of a testicular appendage, scrotal insect bites, viral orchitis (chickenpox, mumps, coxsackievirus, infectious mononucleosis), or testicular cord torsion. Torsion of a testicular appendage may have a blue dot sign, in which the infarcted appendage is seen through the scrotal skin as a blue infarcted area. Epididymo-orchitis is extremely rare in the adolescent age group and in the absence of pyuria should be low on the list of differential diagnoses.

If the diagnosis is in doubt, color Doppler ultrasonography should be performed to evaluate testicular blood flow and intrascrotal anatomy. If testicular cord torsion is a possible diagnosis, the patient should undergo surgical exploration. Temporizing maneuvers of icing the scrotum, blocking the cord with an anesthetic, or attempting manual detorsion may be used while awaiting operating room availability. Because prolonged torsion (>6 hours) may lead to irreversible testicular damage with resultant subfertility, correction should proceed quickly. If a bell clapper deformity is noted at surgery, it should be assumed to be present bilaterally, and simultaneous contralateral testicular fixation can prevent subsequent contralateral torsion.

Trauma

Although the testicles hang freely within the scrotum and are relatively resistant to trauma, a direct blow to the organ may lead to injury. It is important to determine if the tunica albuginea of the testicle is intact because this influences the management. If a patient has a scrotal hematoma and an intact testicle, conservative management is the standard of care. If the tunica albuginea is torn, the patient is managed with scrotal exploration, with the removal of the defunctionalized seminiferous elements and closure of the tear. An ultrasound examination is often helpful in assessing the integrity of the tunica albuginea.

Scrotal Infections

Infections involving the scrotal skin include cellulitis caused by gram-positive bacteria, which is treated with antibiotics such as cefazolin or cephalexin, and candidal fungal infection, which is treated with a topical antifungal medication.

A rare but dreaded infection involving the scrotum is necrotizing fasciitis (Fournier gangrene), a process associated with a mixed infection involving the subcutaneous tissue. Associated conditions may include diabetes, obesity, urethral stricture, and perirectal disease. The scrotum becomes erythematous, tense, and moist. The gangrene spreads rapidly and can progress along the anterior abdominal wall with associated crepitus. Wide debridement and drainage of the affected area, as well as the administration of broad-spectrum antibiotics, is essential. Delay of care and failure to adequately debride the necrotic tissue can worsen already considerable morbidity and mortality associated with this disease.

Scrotal Masses

Testicular cancer is the most common solid malignancy in men between the ages of 18 and 35. Finding a scrotal mass is a frightening experience for a young man, and fear of malignancy may lead to denial.

Evaluation

The patient presenting with a scrotal mass should be questioned as to how long the mass has been present and whether it is increasing in size or painful or has been preceded by infection, trauma, or surgery. After the scrotum is examined manually, a bright light is placed behind the mass in an attempt to transilluminate it. Transillumination implies

fluid with probable hydrocele or spermatocele as the etiology. If the testes are seen to float in the middle of the cystic mass, the mass is a hydrocele, caused by decreased absorption of fluids by the parietal layer of the tunica vaginalis, leading to a fluid collection between the two leaves of the tunica. If, however, the mass sits above or below the testes, it is probably a spermatocele. Both entities are benign, but the distinction is important if surgical correction is entertained. If the mass is adjacent to the spermatic cord and is tubular with a bag of worms sensation, it is probably a varicocele: a dilated segment of the internal spermatic vein. Varicoceles are seen in approximately 15% to 20% of all men and need correction only if there is ipsilateral pain, testicular atrophy, or subfertility. The etiology of this abnormality is unknown, but because of its predilection for left-sided occurrence, a valve abnormality is a common explanation. If the mass does not transilluminate but appears to be localized to the head or tail of the epididymis, it most likely is a sperm granuloma, an epididymal cyst, a benign epididymal adenomatoid tumor, or, rarely, a mesothelioma of the epididymis, which has malignant potential.

A mass that involves the testicle has a high probability of malignancy. Real-time ultrasonography of the mass can be performed to help differentiate the various causes of scrotal masses, but surgical exploration is usually necessary for both diagnosis and treatment. Because of the lymphatic drainage of the testicle, a scrotal incision is contraindicated. If a malignancy is present, lymphatic drainage patterns are altered and future treatment is compromised. Therefore, a groin incision should be made in the region of the midinguinal canal. The spermatic cord is atraumatically occluded and the testicle brought into the surgical field and exposed. If a tumor is present, the cord structures are ligated with a silk suture, and the testicle is removed.

Treatment

Testicular malignancies can be divided into germ cell (which arise from the germinal elements) and nongerm cell tumors (which arise from the mesodermal elements of the testicle). Germ cell tumors, the most common, are discussed in the following section.

Germ cell tumors of the testicle are divided into seminomas and nonseminomas. Seminomas do not undergo further neoplastic transformation, whereas nonseminomas differentiate along extraembryonic lines (eg, in choriocarcinoma or yolk-sac tumors) or intraembryonic lines (eg, in a teratoma). Before radical orchiectomy, certain tumor markers are obtained. α-Fetoprotein (AFP) has a half-life of 5 to 7 days and when elevated is diagnostic of nonseminomatous tumor components. β-hCG has a shorter half-life and may be elevated in either seminoma or nonseminomatous tumor. Because AFP is produced by endodermal cells lining the yolk sac, it will not be elevated in a pure seminoma. β-hCG, however, is produced by the syncytiotrophoblastic cell and may be found in 30% to 40% of seminomas.

Tumor markers are important in the management of testicular cancer. For example, if the AFP (made by a nonseminomatous tumor only) is elevated after orchiectomy and the testicle has pure seminoma, either the pathologist missed nonseminomatous cells in the specimen or there are nonseminomatous cells elsewhere. If the AFP or β-hCG is elevated before orchiectomy, extragonadal cancer is indicated.

After radical orchiectomy (removal through an inguinal incision), tumor staging is performed with abdominal CT, chest radiographs (with or without CT scan), and postoperative tumor markers. Clinical and pathologic staging is complicated but usually follows the outline in Table 27-4.

Seminomas usually cause diffuse enlargement of the testes. The cut tissue is glistening white. Microscopically, there is a monotonous overgrowth of large round cells with clear cytoplasm. Lymphocytic infiltration is found in 20% of cases. After the histologic diagnosis is made, staging is completed (according to Table 27-4).

Seminoma is an exquisitely radiosensitive tumor. Stages I and IIa seminoma were traditionally treated with moderate doses of retroperitoneal radiation therapy, but platinum-based chemotherapy is now the first-line treatment.

For stage I nonseminomatous disease, retroperitoneal lymph node dissection is a good option. In this procedure, lymph node packets adjacent to the aorta and vena cava medial to the ureters are removed. (Additional details regarding this technique, including templates of the dissection, can be found in the urologic atlas and textbooks listed at the end of this chapter.) Preservation of sympathetic nerve fibers within the dissection preserves ejaculatory function in most men. Careful surveillance without node dissection is an option for some men but is usually not recommended. These surgeries are now performed robotically at more advanced centers, resulting in quicker recovery times.

Platinum-based chemotherapy is the most commonly used systemic agent. A 5-year survival rate exceeding 70% is achieved, even in the presence of metastatic disease. Resection of any abdominal mass is required after chemotherapy to identify any residual cancer or to remove mature teratoma, which may gradually enlarge.

Male Infertility

Of all newly married couples, 15% experience difficulty conceiving a child. Statistically, 60% of fertile couples will conceive within 3 months of unprotected intercourse, and 90% within 1 year. Therefore, each partner merits evaluation if no pregnancy occurs within 1 year of unprotected intercourse. This section will limit itself to male infertility. A male factor is causative in 40% of cases, and partially responsible in an additional 20%.

Male infertility can be classified as primary (the person was never fertile, eg, congenital etiologies) or secondary (infertility was acquired following a period of prior fertility). The etiology of male factor infertility can be further stratified by the location of the anatomic abnormality as well as semen parameters.

Evaluation

A complete history should include obtaining information about the following:

Childhood illnesses (eg, mumps) and previous groin, scrotal, or bladder surgical procedures
Problems with delayed or premature puberty
Previous viral illnesses (because spermatogenesis takes approximately 90 days)
Medications that may cause fertility abnormalities (eg, cimetidine, Macrodantin, Azulfidine)
Toxin exposure and marijuana or cigarette smoking
Knowledge of fertility timing (the couple may be having intercourse too often, not often enough, or timing it incorrectly)
Use of lubricants (some are spermicidal)

Physical Examination

The physical examination includes the following: examining the genitalia; the body habitus for Klinefelter syndrome; the visual fields and olfactory sense to ascertain possible pituitary or hypothalamic lesions; the chest for gynecomastia; the penis for lesions; the urethral meatus for position and size; the vas deferens and epididymis (palpated for abnormalities); and the testicles (palpated and sized with an orchidometer, noting consistency and abnormalities). The presence of a varicocele should be documented.

Semen Analysis

The mainstay of male evaluation is semen analysis. Because the findings of this analysis may vary, three fresh ejaculates, obtained after 24 hours of sexual abstinence, are examined within 1 hour of collection. Semen analysis results should be discussed in terms of adequacy as determined by the World Health Organization (Table 27-5), rather than in terms of average or normal. Parameters of interest include sperm density, motility and morphology, and ejaculate volume. Problems with fertility can occur in the setting of low or normal/high volume. Causes of a low volume include decreased serum testosterone, retrograde ejaculation into the bladder, and ejaculatory duct obstruction.

Treatment

Patients with retrograde ejaculation can be diagnosed by an evaluation of a postejaculatory urine specimen for the presence of sperm. The treatment of retrograde ejaculation is sympathomimetic medication, such as pseudoephedrine. If this fails, sperm can be harvested from the bladder, washed, and used for intrauterine insemination. Tests for ejaculatory duct obstruction include fructose ejaculatory analysis because fructose is normally produced by the seminal vesicles. Its absence in the ejaculate indicates a

TABLE 27-4. Staging of Germ Cell Tumors

Stage I	Metastatic workup negative; preoperative markers, if positive, normalize; tumor isolated to the testicle
Stage IIA	Microscopic retroperitoneal disease
Stage IIB	Minimal retroperitoneal disease on radiographic studies (<5 cm)
Stage IIC	Bulky retroperitoneal disease (>5 cm)
Stage III	Disease beyond retroperitoneal lymph drainage, or positive markers after retroperitoneal lymph node dissection

TABLE 27-5. Standards for Adequate Semen Analysis

Ejaculate volume	1.5-5.0 mL
Sperm density	>20 million/mL
Motility	>60%
Grade of motility	>2 (scale 1-4)
Morphology	>60% normal

As determined by the World Health Organization.

lack of seminal vesicle fluid in the ejaculate. TRUS is now used more often to evaluate patients for ejaculatory duct obstruction, which can often be successfully treated with transurethral resection of an ejaculatory duct stenosis.

Patients with azoospermia without the abovementioned etiologies may have vasal agenesis, a condition that warrants an evaluation to rule out cystic fibrosis. These patients may be candidates for microsurgical epididymal sperm aspiration. Patients with azoospermia, atrophic testicles, and a high follicle-stimulating hormone level usually have intrinsic testicular failure. Testicular biopsy may show sperm that can be extracted. Unfortunately, these patients are usually infertile and adoption may be the best option. Normal testicular biopsy findings and azoospermia with a normal ejaculate volume suggest obstruction at the level of the vas deferens or epididymis. These patients may be candidates for scrotal exploration, vasography, and vasovasostomy or vasoepididymostomy.

If a varicocele is present in a patient with a low sperm count or abnormal functional parameters (oligoasthenospermia), varicocele repair is an option.

Impotency

In the past, most men with erectile dysfunction were thought to have an underlying psychological abnormality. However, recent advances in the knowledge of the mechanisms of erections have led to findings of organic impairment in over 85% of these men.

The ability to achieve and maintain an erection involves neurologic, endocrine, psychological, and vascular events. Physiologically, adequate arterial inflow, smooth muscle relaxation in the erectile corporal tissues, and storage of blood within the corpora cavernosa at high pressures are required. Sexual stimulation and arousal, associated with libido that is in part mediated by testosterone, lead to neurologic events with nitric oxide release from nonadrenergic, noncholinergic neurons. This leads to increased cyclic guanosine monophosphate (cGMP) production, leading to corporal smooth muscle relaxation. Dilation of arteries and arterioles and blood flow to the penis increases, and venous outflow decreases, trapping the blood in the corporal tissue. A disturbance of one or more of the abovementioned processes causes erectile dysfunction. Erectile impotence is classified according to four main categories: vasculogenic, endocrinologic, psychogenic, and neurogenic. However, several of these components are often present in a given patient.

Vasculogenic

Vasculogenic disorders probably are the most common cause of erectile dysfunction. Arterial insufficiency is worsened by hypertension, hyperlipidemia, diabetes mellitus, and cigarette smoking. Pelvic trauma can lead to a focal arterial injury. An inability to store venous blood in the corporal tissue may occur secondary to a venous leak, where inflow is adequate but the blood does not become trapped.

Endocrinologic

Endocrinologic syndromes associated with a low-serum testosterone, decreased libido, and erectile dysfunction include hypogonadotropic hypogonadism and pituitary adenoma. The first hormonal test in the evaluation of impotence is a serum testosterone level, keeping in mind the circadian nature of testosterone release. If the testosterone level is low, gonadotrophins and prolactin levels are drawn. Hyperprolactinemia (associated with a low testosterone)

may be caused by a pituitary lesion; when this condition is found, an MRI of the brain is indicated. Although rare, a pituitary adenoma can present as erectile dysfunction.

Psychogenic

Psychogenic factors may contribute to, or may be entirely responsible for, erectile dysfunction. Testing to determine if impotence is psychogenic is performed selectively. One test, nocturnal penile tumescence, uses rapid eye movement sleep erections, which occur in otherwise healthy men. The absence of erectile function during normal sleep suggests organic impairment, whereas normal erectile function at night indicates psychogenic impairment.

Neurogenic

The most common neuropathic lesions are caused by spinal cord injury, multiple sclerosis, alcoholism, and diabetes. Surgery (eg, radical prostatectomy) may lead to injury to the neurovascular bundles as they course posterolaterally between the prostate and the rectum.

Evaluation

A number of tests can be performed to evaluate erectile dysfunction. Nocturnal tumescence testing, duplex ultrasound of the penis before and after a pharmacologically induced erection, cavernosometry/cavernosography, and pudendal arteriography are used for evaluation. These tests are not routinely performed in most patients because the results may not affect treatment decisions. Exceptions include young patients with pelvic trauma who may benefit from revascularization if a discrete arterial injury is the etiology of impotence.

Treatment

Phosphodiesterase-5 (PDE-5) inhibitors such as sildenafil, vardenafil, and tadalafil are the first-line therapy for most erectile dysfunction. These agents work by inhibiting PDE, a compound that breaks down cGMP, which is necessary for smooth muscle relaxation in the penis. The result is that cGMP level is increased, promoting smooth muscle relaxation and erectile function. This medication is highly effective in most patients, and alternative treatments should be considered only if PDE-5 inhibitors fail.

Other treatment options include observation and a vacuum erection device (pump placed over the penis that can cause an erection as a vacuum is created), with or without the use of a constriction band at the base of the penis to maintain the erection induced by the vacuum pump. Another option is the administration of a urethral suppository of alprostadil or the intracavernous injection of vasoactive medications. These treatments involve the administrations of medications that cause smooth muscle relaxation in the penis. Penile prosthesis is an excellent surgical option for patients who fail conservative therapies.

SKILLS

Bladder Catheterization (Male)

1. Have all materials to be used opened and ready to use before beginning any aspect of the procedure. Once the procedure is initiated, one hand is always holding the penis or spreading the labia; therefore, it is essential that everything be ready for use and available within reach

of the other hand. Items needed are the catheter (usually 16F) and a drainage bag, lubrication (to coat the tip of the catheter or inject into the urethra), a cleansing agent (eg, povidone-iodine [Betadine]) and an applicator, a 10-mL syringe filled with water, drapes, and sterile gloves.

2. Drape the field with the patient in the supine position. With one hand, grasp the penis with upward traction, retracting the foreskin completely if the patient is uncircumcised. With the other hand, clean the meatus and glans with antiseptic solution. The hand that is not holding the penis is used to perform the remainder of the procedure.

3. Coat the catheter tip with a water-soluble lubricant. Excellent lubrication of the urethra facilitates catheter passage. Gently injecting 10 mL of lubricant into the urethra, as well, is recommended. Prefilled tapered-tip syringes that contain a lubricant and lidocaine are commercially available (Uro-jet). Alternatively, a 10-mL syringe can be filled with lubricant during the setup.

4. Slowly pass the catheter to the end until only the part of the catheter in the area of the balloon port remains visible (2-3 inches) (Figure 27-36). Do not stop when urine is first visible. The catheter must be inserted all the way to the bifurcation of the Foley balloon port.

5. Look for urine return, then inflate the balloon with 10 mL of water, or per instructions on the catheter.

6. Connect the catheter to the drainage bag, and tape the catheter to the thigh.

Bladder Catheterization (Female)

1. Place the patient in the frog-leg position. When practical, the lithotomy position is preferred.

2. Perform the procedure as stated earlier, except for the following: Use one hand to spread the labia (Figure 27-37). Alternatively, have an assistant perform this maneuver. When the catheter is placed, it needs to be advanced for only half its length before the balloon is inflated.

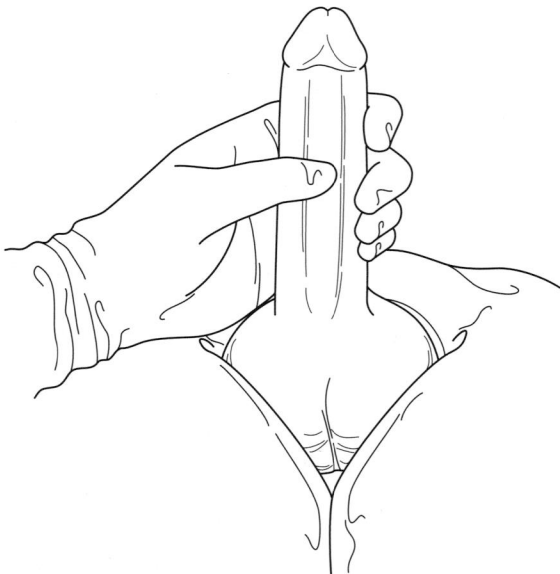

Figure 27-37. Catheterization of a female patient. (From Lawrence PF. *Essentials of Surgical Specialties*. 3rd ed. Lippincott Williams & Wilkins; 2007.)

Difficulties

The main problem encountered is resistance to passage of the catheter in the man. This commonly occurs at the level of the prostate where the urethra courses upward toward the bladder (Figure 27-38). If the catheter cannot negotiate this curve, it will poke into the median lobe of the prostate. Moreover, enlargement of the lateral lobes of the prostate inhibits efforts to pass the catheter. When resistance is encountered, do not use force because doing so will only cause urethral trauma and false passages. Instead, attempt to overcome the resistance by injecting additional lubricant into the urethra and placing a larger (18-20F) coudé catheter (Figure 27-39), which has an upwardly curved tip.

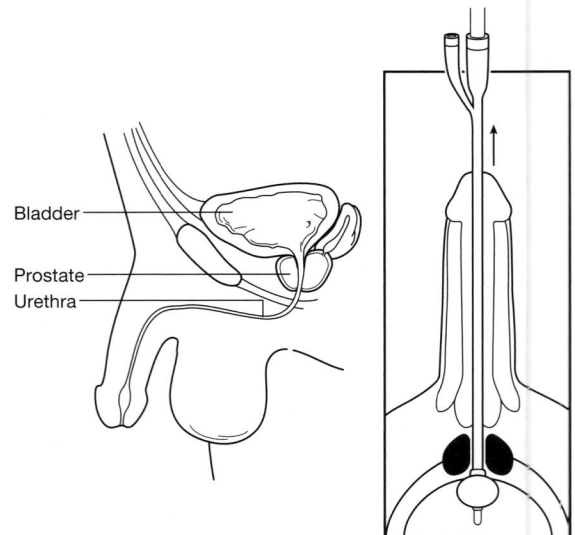

Figure 27-36. Catheterization of a male patient. (From Lawrence PF. *Essentials of Surgical Specialties*. 3rd ed. Lippincott Williams & Wilkins; 2007.)

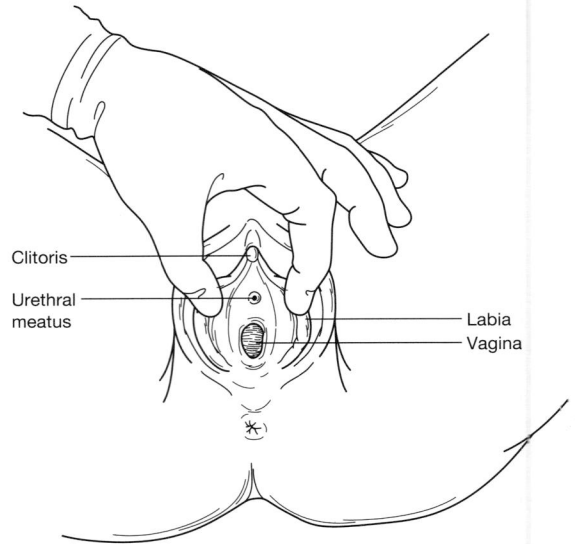

Figure 27-38. Difficulty in passage of the catheter because of the prostate. (From Lawrence PF. *Essentials of Surgical Specialties*. 3rd ed. Lippincott Williams & Wilkins; 2007.)

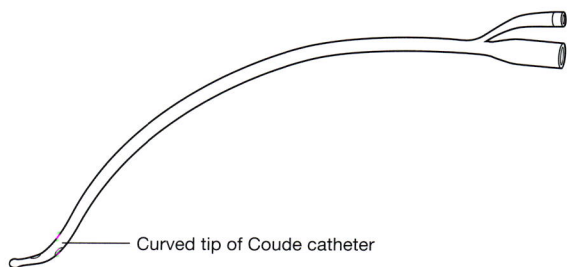
Curved tip of Coudé catheter

Figure 27-39. Coudé catheter. (From Lawrence PF. *Essentials of Surgical Specialties*. 3rd ed. Lippincott Williams & Wilkins; 2007.)

As the catheter is advanced, orientation is maintained by keeping the balloon port facing upward. The most important points are never force the catheter in and never inflate the balloon unless the catheter advances all the way in and urine output is seen.

If urine output is not seen, the catheter lumen may be temporarily blocked with lubricant. The lubricant usually dissolves within a minute. If urine output is still not seen, irrigate the catheter with 60 mL of saline using a catheter-tip syringe (Toomey) without inflating the balloon. Appropriate catheter position is confirmed when saline can be easily instilled and withdrawn without resistance.

A urethral stricture can also cause resistance to catheter passage. At times, a smaller catheter (12-14F) can be placed. However, the urethral lumen in the area of a stricture is often too narrow to permit the passage of a catheter. In such a case, urologic consultation is mandatory.

SUGGESTED READINGS

Coughlin GD, Yaxley JW, Chambers SK, et al. Robot-assisted laparoscopic prostatectomy versus open radical retropubic prostatectomy: 24-month outcomes from a randomised controlled study. *Lancet Oncol.* 2018;19(8):1051-1060.

James ND, Sydes MR, Clarke NW, et al. Systemic therapy for advancing or metastatic prostate cancer (STAMPEDE): a multi-arm, multistage randomized controlled trial. *BJU Int.* 2009;103(4):464-469.

Kaplan SA, Lee JY, Meehan AG, Kusek JW; MTOPS Research Group. Long-term treatment with finasteride improves clinical progression of benign prostatic hyperplasia in men with an enlarged versus a smaller prostate: data from the MTOPS trial. *J Urol.* 2011;185(4):1369-1373.

SAMPLE QUESTIONS

QUESTIONS

Choose the best answer for each question.

1. Which of the following is NOT correct concerning PSA?

   A. PSA is a serine protease that liquefies postejaculatory semen.
   B. A high serum-free fraction of PSA is associated with a reduced incidence of prostate cancer.
   C. An elevated serum PSA is associated with benign and malignant prostate diseases.
   D. A serum PSA of 0.5 after radical prostatectomy for prostate cancer is considered to be no evidence of disease.
   E. Serum PSA after successful radiation therapy for prostate cancer should be less than 1.0.

2. Which of the following patients does NOT require renal imaging for trauma?

   A. A 7-year-old child with microhematuria after a car accident
   B. A 40-year-old man with microhematuria and hypotension after a motorcycle accident
   C. A 50-year-old woman pedestrian hit by a car with gross hematuria
   D. A 30-year-old hemodynamically stable man with microhematuria after falling down two steps with no external signs of injury
   E. A 25-year-old man with microhematuria after a gunshot wound to the left flank area

3. A 35-year-old male develops flank pain and is found to be anemic. There is tenderness to palpation of the right flank area. A CT scan of the abdomen/pelvis is performed showing a 6-cm mass within the right kidney that is composed of macroscopic fat (verified by negative Hounsfield unit measurement). There is evidence of hemorrhage around the mass. No other masses or lymphadenopathy are noted. Which of the following is the diagnosis?

   A. RCC with hemorrhage
   B. Angiomyolipoma of the kidney with hemorrhage
   C. Complex renal cyst
   D. Simple renal cyst
   E. Metastatic disease to the kidney

4. Which of the following patients requires immediate treatment to prevent significant illness or death?

   A. A patient with a 3-mm distal ureteral stone and flank pain
   B. A patient with a 1-cm renal pelvis stone who is asymptomatic
   C. A patient with a 3-mm ureteral stone, fever, and urine Gram stain showing gram-negative rods
   D. An asymptomatic patient with a 1-cm ureteral stone
   E. A patient with nausea and vomiting due to a 5-mm distal ureteral stone

5. Squamous cell carcinoma of the penis typically metastasizes to which of the following lymph node chains first?

   A. Obturator
   B. Iliac
   C. Periaortic
   D. Pericaval
   E. Inguinal

ANSWERS AND EXPLANATIONS

1. **Answer: D**

   Serum PSA after radical prostatectomy for prostate cancer should be "undetectable," which in most labs means less than 0.04. Any value above 0.2 is considered to be a recurrence. This is referred to as biochemical recurrence if all imaging studies are negative. Serum PSA after radiation therapy should remain very low, such as less than 1.0, but will still be "detectable" because the prostate is still intact. A high serum percent–free PSA is associated with a lower incidence of prostate cancer in men with a PSA between 4.0 and 10.0. PSA is specific to prostate tissue, not only to cancerous tissue of the prostate. For more information on this topic, please see the section "Malignant Diseases" under the heading "Prostate."

2. **Answer: D**

   Adults with microhematuria after blunt renal trauma but no history of a major deceleration injury or hypotension do not necessarily need renal imaging. Children and patients with gross hematuria, hypotension, or a major deceleration injury require evaluation. Patients with penetrating trauma in the area of urologic organs also need evaluation. For more information on this topic, please see the section "Trauma" under the heading "Kidneys."

3. **Answer: B**

   An angiomyolipoma is usually diagnosed by the characteristic appearance of fat within the lesion on CT scan. Fat is black on CT, and when fat is seen within a renal mass, angiomyolipoma is almost always the diagnosis. RCC is typically heterogeneous, solid, fat poor, and enhances with contrast. Simple cysts contain only simple fluid. Complex cysts have septations or calcifications within the cyst. For more information on this topic, please see the section "Benign Neoplasms."

4. **Answer: C**

   Obstructive pyelonephritis is one situation that deserves particular attention. This condition occurs when a patient has an obstructing stone associated with infection of the affected upper urinary tract, causing "pus under pressure"; it is a true urologic emergency. Patients come to the emergency room with flank pain, fever, and infected urine. When a patient has obstructing pyelonephritis, antibiotics alone do not effectively treat the problem. The treatment must include relief of the obstruction, with emergency placement of an internal stent (placed cystoscopically) or a percutaneous nephrostomy. Ureteral stones smaller than 5 mm usually pass spontaneously. Large stones may not pass and require treatment but are not life threatening, unless there is obstruction and infection present. For more information on this topic, please see the section "Urinary Stone Disease."

5. **Answer: E**

   The superficial and deep inguinal nodes are often the first involved nodes. Removal of involved nodes can be curative in penile cancer. The next location of spread is often to the pelvic nodes including the iliac and obturator, which carries a very poor prognosis. For more information on this topic, please see the section "Squamous Cell Carcinoma."

28

Neurosurgery: Diseases of the Nervous System

Isaac Yang and Sanah Vohra

Neurologic surgery is a young specialty field that evolved as a separate discipline from general surgery during the early 1900s. Although often referred to as "brain surgery," modern practice management surveys reveal that general neurosurgical practice comprises spinal, cranial, cerebrovascular, and peripheral nerve surgery. This chapter presents an overview of neurosurgical diseases and interventions.

CRANIAL AND CEREBROVASCULAR DISEASE

Anatomy and Physiology

Unlike other organs such as the liver, lungs, kidneys, and muscles, in which cells are organized into repetitive identical units (eg, lobules, alveoli, glomeruli), the central nervous system (CNS) is heterogeneous and is hierarchically organized at many different levels. The involuntary motive force for activities such as consciousness, breathing, blood pressure, and heartbeat has intrinsic pacemakers within the brain stem, which is divided into the midbrain, pons, and medulla (see Figures 28-1 and 28-2; shown in Figure 28-12). Voluntary activities including thinking, communicating, motor movements, and behavior have their origin in the lobes of the cerebral hemispheres (frontal, parietal, temporal, and occipital), which send motor efferent and receive sensory afferent signals down through the brain stem and the spinal cord to reach the rest of the body via the cranial and peripheral nerves, as well as the autonomic nervous system. These afferent and efferent connections are modulated and modified by superimposed secondary circuitry from the cerebellum, striatum, subthalamus, and red nucleus. The thalamus serves as a relay station and connection module for afferent primary and all secondary circuitries. Through its control of the pituitary gland, the hypothalamus serves as the source of autonomic tone and impulses, the modulator of body homeostasis (temperature, serum osmolarity), and the master regulator of hormonal levels and temporal rhythms. Knowledge of CNS functional organization and regional specialization, along with a thorough neurologic examination, is key to determining the level and location of a CNS lesion.

The intracranial cavity is divided into two chambers by a fibrous curtain called the "tentorium." The tentorium has an opening (tentorial incisura) through which the brain stem travels to connect with the cerebral hemispheres. Both cerebral hemispheres occupy the **supratentorial** space. The supratentorial space is divided into two lateral compartments by an incomplete curtain of dura called the "falx cerebri," which extends the length of the interhemispheric fissure. The hemispheres are composed of an outer cortical layer (gray matter—containing neurons), a middle layer of white matter (containing axons), and an inner mass of gray matter (diencephalon, thalamus, and hypothalamus—containing neurons) (Figures 28-1 to 28-3). The outer cortex is folded into ridges (gyri) separated by fissures (sulci). The frontal lobe, which occupies the anterior cranial fossa, is separated from the parietal lobe by the Rolandic fissure (ie, central sulcus—see Figure 28-1) and from the temporal lobe, which sits in the temporal bone and the tentorium, by the Sylvian fissure (Figure 28-1). The occipital lobe occupies the posterior pole of each hemisphere.

The frontal lobe is the primary source of motor function. Lesions in the posterior portion cause contralateral weakness and hyperreflexia. The primary motor strip lies just in front of, and the primary sensory strip is just behind, the central sulcus. Lesions of the anterior parietal lobe cause contralateral sensory dysfunction. The visual pathways course from the optic nerves through optic chiasm and tracts to the lateral geniculate body of the thalamus. From there, the white matter connections course through the posterior temporal lobe (Meyer loop) and through the parietal lobe to finally end on the primary calcarine cortex in the interhemispheric surface of the occipital lobe. Lesions of the temporal lobe visual pathways lead to a contralateral superior visual field defect (superior quadrantanopsia), lesions of the parietal visual connections cause an inferior visual defect (inferior quadrantanopsia), and lesions of the primary visual cortex cause a contralateral complete visual field defect (hemianopsia).

Although primary motor and sensory functions are symmetrically organized bilaterally, some higher cortical functions are represented only in one hemisphere or the other. Speech dominance is an example. Ninety-five percent of naturally right-handed people have speech located in the left hemisphere, whereas around 25% of naturally left-handed people have speech located in the right hemisphere. For left brain–dominant humans, lesions of the inferior-lateral left frontal lobe, just above the root of the Sylvian fissure (Broca area), can cause an **expressive (nonfluent) aphasia**. Lesions in the left posterior-superior temporal lobe, just below the end of the Sylvian fissure (Wernicke area), can cause loss of speech comprehension and a fluent aphasia consisting of meaningless sounds or words. Lesions of the connection between the two areas lead to a conductive aphasia, in which speech is understood but the patient is unable to repeat the understood phrase. Other examples include calculations, which localize to the

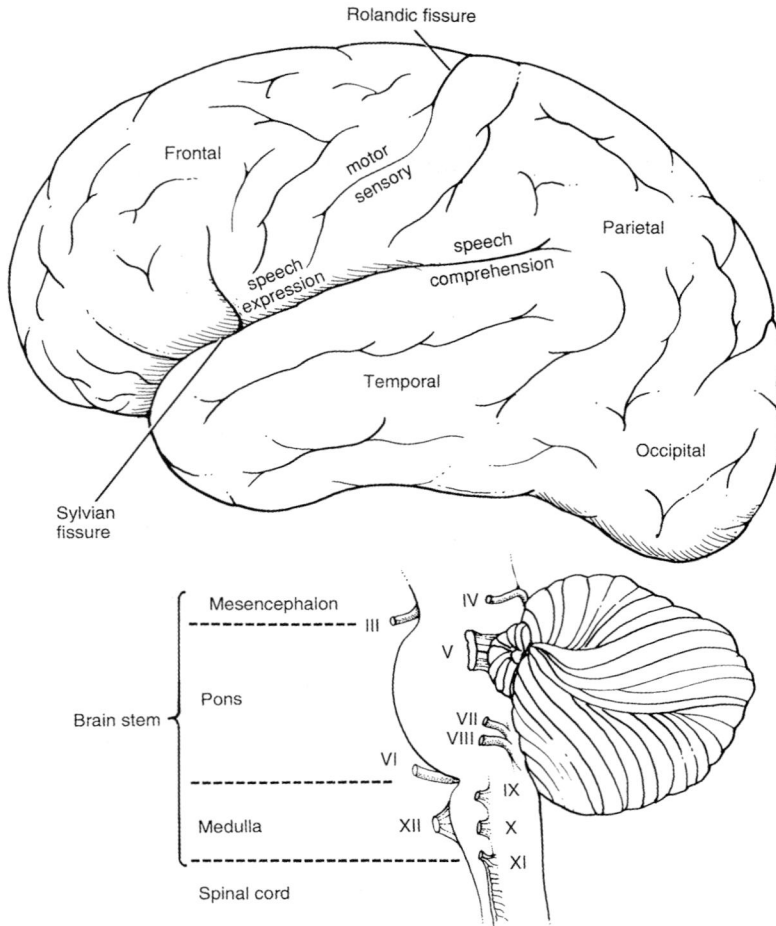

Figure 28-1. Medial aspect of the left side of the brain. The brain stem is displaced caudally for purposes of illustration. (From Lawrence PF. *Essentials of Surgical Specialties*. 3rd ed. Lippincott Williams & Wilkins; 2007.)

parietal lobe, and pattern recognition and spatial orientation, which also localize to the parietal lobe (Gerstman syndrome).

The cortical functions of the four lobes within one hemisphere connect with one another via subcortical white matter tracts oriented anteriorly-posteriorly, including the superior and inferior longitudinal fasciculi. They connect one hemisphere to the other by way of laterally oriented white matter tracts across the corpus callosum, as well as the anterior and posterior commissures. They connect with the brain stem and spinal cord by way of a condensation of white matter tracts called the "internal capsule" (Figure 28-3; shown in Figure 28-9E), which are oriented in a rostral-caudal direction. The internal capsule passes through the diencephalon between the basal ganglia. The caudate and putamen (striatum) lie laterally and the thalamus medially to the internal capsule (Figure 28-3; shown in Figures 28-9E and 28-10). Even very small vascular lesions in this tight condensation of white matter connections can lead to severe weakness (lacunar strokes).

The infratentorial compartment of the cranium (the **posterior fossa**) contains the brain stem and the cerebellum. The brain stem connects inferiorly with the spinal cord

by way of an opening in the skull called the "foramen magnum." The cerebellum lies on the back of the brain stem like a papoose and connects with the brain stem by way of three axially oriented white matter tracts on each side (the superior, middle, and inferior cerebellar peduncles, respectively—Figure 28-1; shown in Figure 28-12). The cerebellum is involved with the modulation and coordination of motor movements by means of inhibitory modulatory inputs. The paired lateral hemispheres control the limbs, and lesions here lead to dysmetria. The central vermis controls the axial musculature, and lesions here cause ataxia. The inferior tonsils, as well as the inferior-lateral flocculus and nodulus, control vestibular-ocular coordination, and lesions here cause nystagmus.

The brain stem is divided into a dorsal component (tectum) that contains the reticular formation, cranial nerve nuclei, and lemniscal sensory tracts. The level of lesions in the brain stem can be determined from the level of cranial nerve involvement. Cranial nerves III and IV arise from the midbrain. Cranial nerves V, VI, VII, and VIII come from the pons. Cranial nerves IX, X, XI, and XII arise from the medulla (see Figure 28-2). All cranial nerves exit the brain stem ventral-laterally except for the fourth cranial nerve,

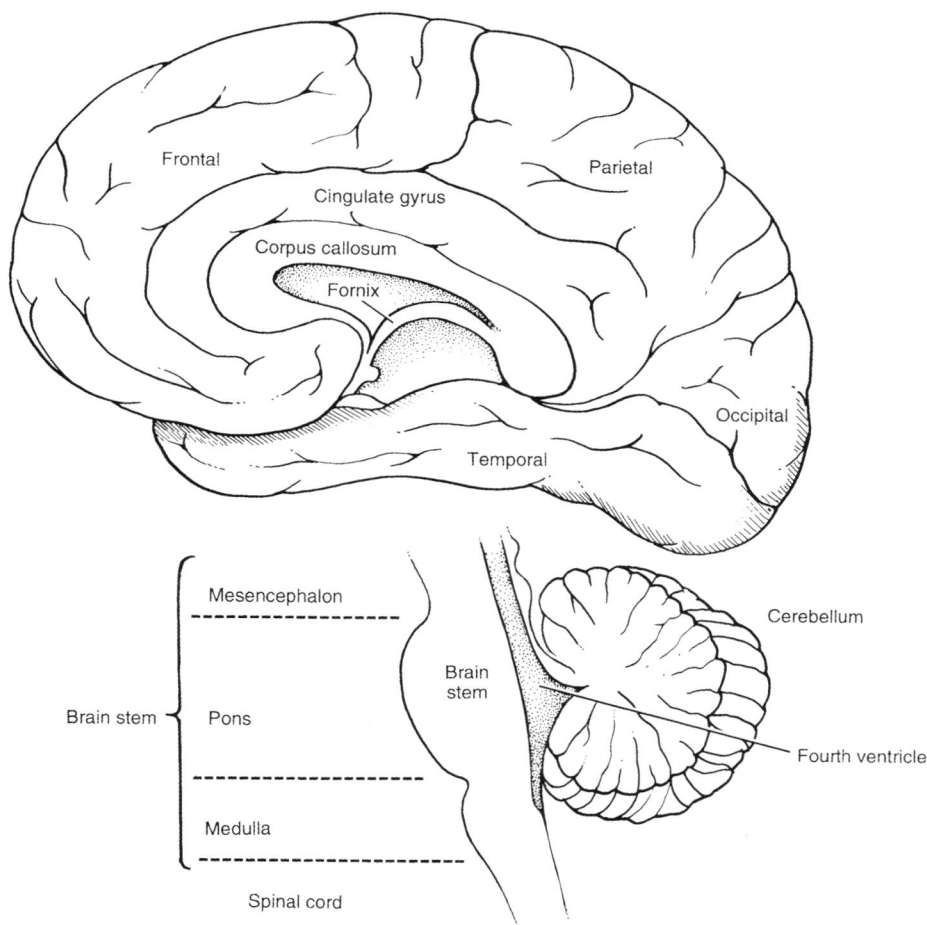

Figure 28-2. Lateral view of the left side of the brain. The brain stem is displaced caudally for purposes of illustration. (From Lawrence PF. *Essentials of Surgical Specialties.* 3rd ed. Lippincott Williams & Wilkins; 2007.)

which exits dorsally. The reticular formation of the brain stem controls respiration, heart rate, blood pressure, and consciousness.

Blood Supply

The brain receives 20% of the stroke volume of each heartbeat. Four major blood vessels course through the neck from the apical chest vessels to supply the brain. The two common carotid arteries divide at the carotid bifurcation into the internal carotid artery (ICA) and external carotid artery (ECA). The ECA supplies blood to the face, the scalp, and the meningeal covering of the brain by way of several terminal arteries, including the middle meningeal artery (MMA). The major ECA scalp terminal branches are the superficial temporal artery (STA) coursing just in front of the ear and the occipital artery coursing just behind the ear. The ICA courses through the petrous canal of the skull base to the cavernous sinus located on either side of the pituitary gland. It supplies the ophthalmic branch to the orbit and then penetrates the dura covering of the brain. The carotid system supplies 80% of the blood supply to the brain, with each ICA supplying approximately 40%. The two vertebral arteries (VAs) together supply 20% of

the brain's blood volume. The VAs enter the transverse foramen of the cervical vertebra at C6 and segmentally course through each transverse foramen all the way up through C2. They penetrate the dura between the arch of C1 and the posterior-lateral rim of the foramen magnum. The VA is susceptible to injury (dissection or occlusion, with subsequent ischemia or embolization) with sudden spinal movements or with spine fractures involving the transverse foramen.

The posterior fossa is the only location in the human body where vessels (in this case the VAs), instead of branching as they extend further from the heart, join to form a single distal posterior circulation artery, the basilar artery (BA). Before joining to form the BA, each VA gives off a posterior inferior cerebellar artery (PICA), which supplies the lateral medulla and the inferior-lateral cerebellum. At the mid-pons level, the BA gives off bilateral anterior-inferior cerebellar arteries, which supply the lateral pons and cerebellum. Near its terminus, the BA gives off bilateral superior cerebellar arteries, which supply the lateral brain stem and the superior and superior-lateral cerebellum. The BA ends in a bifurcation consisting of the initial segments of the posterior cerebral arteries (PCAs), which supply the

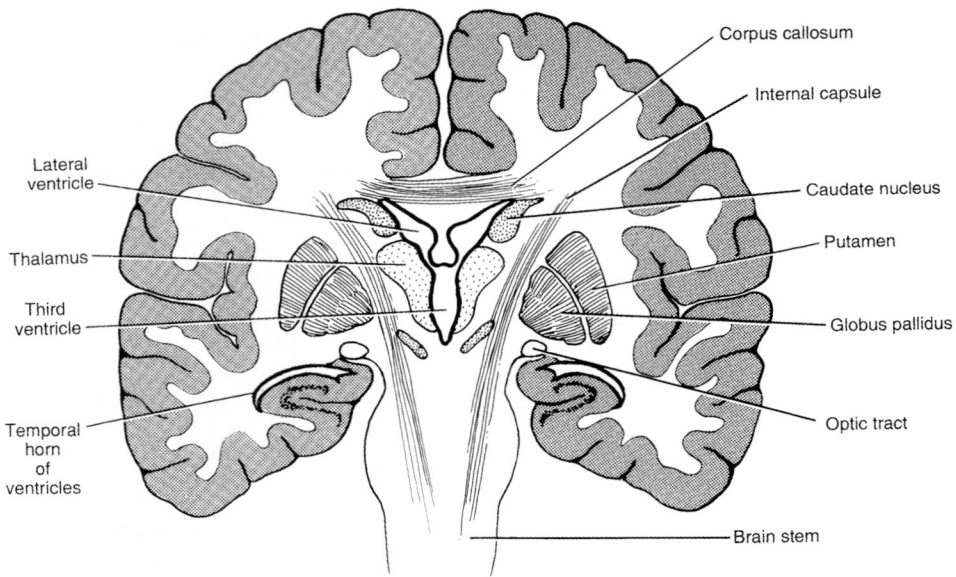

Figure 28-3. **Coronal section of the brain showing the gray matter (stippled).** (From Lawrence PF. *Essentials of Surgical Specialties* 3rd ed. Lippincott Williams & Wilkins; 2007.)

inferior temporal lobe, the occipital lobe, and the posterior-medial parietal lobe. The third nerve is found in between the PCA and the superior cerebellar artery.

The ICAs give off posteriorly coursing posterior communicating arteries (pCom A) on each side, which join with the PCAs at the level of the midbrain. They then continue, bifurcating into the middle cerebral artery (MCA) and the anterior cerebral arteries (ACAs). The ACAs course medially under the frontal lobes and connect with each other by way of an anterior communicating artery (aCom A), before continuing up the interhemispheric fissure to supply the frontal pole and the medial frontal and medial anterior parietal lobes. The MCA courses up the Sylvian fissure to supply the whole lateral portion of the frontal, temporal, and parietal lobes. Because it carries the largest volume of blood flow and supplies the largest volume of the brain, the MCA distribution is the most common to receive a vascular embolus (embolic stroke or metastatic brain tumor). Normal, average, mixed cortical cerebral blood flow (CBF) to the brain is 55 mL/100 g/min (SD $\pm$ 12); white matter values are approximately 22 mL/100 g/min.

The base of the brain in the arachnoid cisterns contains a unique collateral supply system called the "circle of Willis." It consists of the ICA, the first segments of both ACAs, the aCom A, both pCom As, and the first segments of both PCAs. These segments connect in a geometric pentagon, with the short aCom A segment constituting the blunted apex. Through the circle of Willis, any one ICA and one VA could theoretically supply blood to any area of the brain. In reality, the circle of Willis is quite variable in integrity and symmetry, and even angiographic demonstration of an intact ring does not guarantee adequate collateral potential. Only 75% to 80% of people will tolerate the sudden loss or occlusion of one ICA without stroke. Five percent will become symptomatic within 5 to 15 minutes of occlusion from flow-related ischemia, and 15% to 20% will initially be asymptomatic, but will have marginal

reserves that carry a high risk of delayed stroke with any subsequent episode of dehydration or hypotension.

Venous drainage of the brain has both deep and superficial components. Deep in the brain, the two paired thalamostriate and intracerebral veins drain the diencephalon and join the two basal veins of Rosenthal, which drain the upper brain stem to form the single, short, and deep vein of Galen. The inferior sagittal sinus, which runs along the inferior edge of the falx cerebri dural reflection separating the hemispheres, joins the vein of Galen. Here, the falx joins the tentorium to form the straight sinus. The straight sinus runs along the falx-tentorium insertion to join the torcula. Superficially, the Sylvian vein (the vein of Labbé), coursing in the Sylvian fissure, drains the brain. This vein runs from the top of the Sylvian fissure down along the posterior-lateral aspect of the temporal lobe to join the transverse sinus. The vein of Trolard runs upward from the top of the Sylvian fissure along the central sulcus to join the superior sagittal sinus.

Multiple smaller lateral cortical veins run upward to join the sagittal sinus by bridging across the subarachnoid space to the dura. These "bridging veins" are particularly prone to tearing with lateral shear forces. They are a major source of both acute traumatic and spontaneous chronic subdural hematomas. Ultimately, the sagittal sinus flows back to join the two transverse sinuses, along with the straight sinus at a junction called the "torcula," which is adjacent to the posterior occipital protuberance (the inion). The two transverse sinuses then flow laterally to join the sigmoid sinuses behind each ear, which then flow down to finally become the internal jugular veins bilaterally.

Cerebrospinal Fluid Circulation

Cerebrospinal fluid (CSF) performs a structural and cushioning role; it also forms a second circulation for the brain, helping maintain and regulate cerebral and systemic homeostasis. It is produced by choroid plexus in an energy-dependent, carbonic anhydrase–dependent, active process at the rate of 0.3 mL/min (totaling 432 mL/d). Because the total volume of CSF in the cranium and spinal canal is approximately 150 mL, this means that the total volume of CSF is completely replenished 3 times per day.

The cerebral hemispheres contain paired lateral ventricles that form the internal core of all four lobes. They form a large medial-leaning C with a posterior extension into the occipital lobe (occipital horn). The two lateral ventricles drain into a single midline third ventricle, which lies between the two diencephalons just above the midbrain by way of the paired foramen of Monroe (Figure 28-4). The third ventricle drains through the midbrain by way of the single narrow aqueduct of Sylvius to join the fourth ventricle, which lies in the posterior fossa between the brainstem in front and the cerebellum behind. Fluid then exits the ventricular system either by way of the single medial foramen of Magendie (located between the paired tonsils of the cerebellum and the obex), draining into the cisterna magna, or laterally via two foramina of Luschka, draining into the cerebellopontine angle on either side. The CSF flows down the spinal canal, under the brain through the basal arachnoid cisterns, and over the convexity of the brain in the subarachnoid space. It is absorbed into the venous system at the dural venous sinuses by way of the arachnoid villi.

Intracranial Pressure, Cerebral Perfusion Pressure, Cerebral Autoregulation, and Brain Herniation

The skull is a closed, rigid chamber with both fixed and variable content volumes. Under normal conditions, the cranial cavity contains only the brain, CSF, and blood.

Normal intracranial pressure (ICP) in an adult is less than 10 to 15 cm of H_2O (14-20 mm Hg). In children, before skull growth plate fusion, it is much lower. According to the Monroe-Kellie hypothesis, in a fixed, enclosed space, adding additional masses to the fixed volume (eg, blood clots, swollen contusions, tumors, large strokes, excess CSF) will lead to stable ICP only so long as the buffering capacity of increased CSF absorption can keep up. At some point, this buffering capacity is saturated, and at this point, even small extra-volume increases will lead to very large increases in ICP. Indeed, ICP will rise exponentially with additional volume increases from this point onward.

The brain volume is fixed in both the supratentorial and infratentorial compartments. It is also fixed in each lateral compartment of the supratentorial space (separated by the falx cerebri). The CSF volume is relatively fixed, with only small increases in CSF absorption possible by increasing the pressure gradient across the arachnoid villi–dural sinus interface. The blood volume is the most variable of the three because elevated ICP can prevent the inflow of blood into the cranial cavity. It is, therefore, the most susceptible to pathologic derangement resulting from conditions that raise ICP, with the potential for secondary ischemic injury to the brain. Cerebral perfusion pressure (CPP) is the difference between mean systemic arterial pressure (MAP) and ICP (CPP = MAP − ICP). Normal CPP is greater than 50 mm Hg (usually in the range of 55-65 mm Hg). In general, when CPP falls below 45 mm Hg, the brain is at risk for developing areas of reduced CBF.

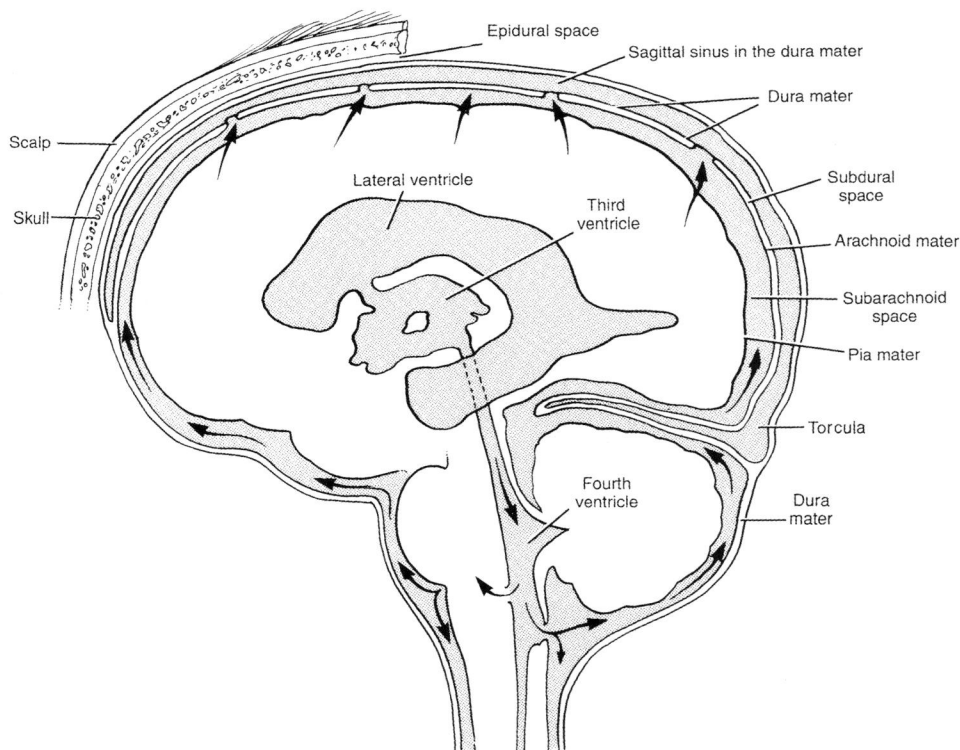

Figure 28-4. Circulation of the cerebrospinal fluid. (From Lawrence PF. *Essentials of Surgical Specialties.* 3rd ed. Lippincott Williams & Wilkins; 2007.)

Cerebral autoregulation is a vasoconstriction-dilatation compensation mechanism that normally keeps CBF constant over a wide range of blood pressures (MAP 40-140 mm Hg). In addition to the actual CBF, the arterial level of CO_2 is the second main arbiter of the degree of cerebral vascular tone (vasoconstriction with low levels of CO_2 and vasodilation with high levels). ICP can be lowered by hyperventilating the patient and lowering arterial CO_2, but only at the expense of lowering CBF to a brain that may be very susceptible to secondary injury with any further ischemia. With brain injury from trauma or ischemia, autoregulation can be disrupted in local regions of the brain, and with repeated or prolonged elevations of CPP, autoregulation can fail throughout the brain. When this occurs, CBF is dependent on CPP in a linear manner.

A hernia is the physical displacement of tissue from one compartment into another usually caused by a pressure gradient across the opening between the chambers in question. Because the cranium has several compartments, several types of herniation are possible, including the following: (a) transtentorial herniation (tissue moving downward from the supratentorial space through the tentorial incisura into the infratentorial space); (b) tonsillar or downward herniation (tissue moving from the posterior fossa through the foramen magnum); (c) subfalcine herniation (tissue moving from one side of the supratentorial space to the other under the falx cerebri); (d) upward central herniation (tissue moving upward from the infratentorial space through the tentorial incisura into the supratentorial space); and (e) herniation of tissue outside the skull through a craniotomy or traumatic skull defect. With herniation syndromes, it is the physical mass effect from the herniating tissue pressing on the tissue in the recipient compartment that causes dysfunction and damage. High ICP alone will not lead to herniation so long as the pressures are equal across compartments. Patients with pseudotumor cerebri routinely exhibit ICPs in the 20 to 30 cm H_2O range without herniation because the pressures are equal across all compartments.

Evaluation

The Neurologic Examination

An organized and systematic approach to the neurologic examination is the best way to ensure thoroughness. The examination should include an assessment of the following: (a) mental status, (b) cranial nerves, (c) cerebellar function, (d) motor and reflex function, and (e) sensory function. Initial elective evaluations require detail and depth in each portion.

The mental status examination includes an assessment of the level of consciousness; orientation to person, place, and time; speech comprehension and expression (often tested with repetition of phrases); immediate and short-term memory; mental arithmetic; writing; and drawing. Descriptions should include the specifics of both the stimulus attempted and the response obtained. For patients with head injury, the Glasgow Coma Scale (GCS) with scores extending from 3 to 15 is very useful and has been verified for reproducibility and interobserver variability (Table 28-1). A patient with a score of 8 or less is considered to be comatose. For nontrauma patients, a useful objective and quantifiable format is the Mini-Mental Status Examination (Table 28-2).

TABLE 28-1. Glasgow Coma Scale

Activity	Score
Eye opening	
Spontaneous	E4
To speech	3
To pain	2
Nil	1
Best motor response	
Obeys	M6
Localizes	5
Withdraws	4
Abnormal flexion	3
Extensor response	2
Nil	1
Verbal response	
Oriented	V5
Confused conversation	4
Inappropriate words	3
Incomprehensible sounds	2
Nil	1

Glasgow Coma Scale score (E + M + V) = 3 to 15.

Olfaction is tested in conscious and cooperative patients in each nostril separately with a nonvolatile, nonirritating odor (eg, coffee grounds, cinnamon, vanilla). Eyes are checked for pupil size, shape, and reactivity; fullness of visual fields; the presence of atrophy, papilledema, or hemorrhages on funduscopic examination; ptosis of the eyelids; fullness and absence of diplopia on extraocular movements (EOMs); and the presence or absence of nystagmus. Trigeminal nerve examination includes testing facial sensation in all three trigeminal divisions, symmetry of the muscles of mastication, and the presence and symmetry of corneal reflex. Facial nerve testing includes distinguishing between peripheral cranial nerve weakness (all branches) and central CNS upper motor neuron weakness (weakness limited to the mid and lower face). Hearing can be tested with a 712-Hz tuning fork for both bone conduction symmetry (midline—Weber test) and an air-bone conduction gap on either side (mastoid tip vs ear canal—Rinne test). In an unconscious patient, vestibular function can be assessed with the oculocephalic reflex ("doll's eyes") or caloric testing. In a normal state, rotating the head suddenly from side to side leads to the eyes maintaining a straight-ahead gaze. If they move with the rotation of the head, then they have an abnormal oculocephalic reflex. With caloric testing, cold water irrigated through a small tube in one ear canal, with the patient's head elevated 30°, depresses the vestibular function of that ear, permitting unopposed function of

TABLE 28-2. Mini-Mental Status Exam		
Maximum Score	**Score**	**Mini-Mental State**
		Orientation
5	()	What is the (year) (season) (date) (day) (month)?
5	()	Where are we: (state) (county) (town) (hospital) (floor)?
		Registration
3	()	Name three objects: allow 1 s to say each. Then ask the patient all three after you have said them. Give 1 point for each correct answer. Then repeat them until the patient has learned all three. Count trials and record.
		Attention and calculation
5	()	Count by serial 7s. Give 1 point for each correct answer. Stop after five answers. Alternatively, spell "world" backward.
		Recall
3	()	Ask for the three objects named earlier. Give 1 point for each correct answer.
		Language
9	()	Name a pencil and a watch (2 points).
		Repeat the following: "No ifs, ands, or buts" (1 point).
		Follow a three-stage command: "Take a paper in your right hand, fold it in half, and put it on the floor" (1 point).
		Read and obey the following: "Close your eyes" (1 point).
		Write a sentence (1 point).
		Copy a design (1 point).
30	___	Total score

Assess the level of consciousness along a continuum.

the opposite ear and conjugate deviation of the eyes toward the irrigated ear. The absence of response is pathologic. Glossopharyngeal function is tested by both symmetry of the uvula with palate elevation and gag reflex on either side. In patients who are intubated, vagal nerve function can be tested by the presence of cough reflex to deep tracheal suctioning. Shoulder shrug symmetry and tongue protrusion symmetry assess cranial nerve XI (spinal accessory) and XII (hypoglossal) functions, respectively.

Cerebellar function testing includes stance and gait assessment, stability of stance with eyes closed and arms extended (Romberg sign), as well as appendicular assessments for dysmetria (finger-to-nose with eyes closed) and dysdiadochokinesia (finger-nose-finger with eyes open and changing target positions). The cerebellum does not function in isolation. Thus, abnormal gait can also be seen with motor hemiparesis, and nystagmus or poor balance can also indicate vestibular dysfunction.

Motor assessment in conscious patients includes an analysis of the symmetry of muscle bulk and tone as well as muscle strength on a scale of 0 to 5. Zero means no palpable muscle contraction, whereas 5 is normal strength. Three means strong enough to resist gravity but no additional resistance. Two and four are any assessments between 0 and 3 or between 3 and 5. In patients with altered consciousness, motor response is assessed in response to stimuli (localization, purposeful coordination, symmetry of response). A pathologic flexor response (**decorticate**) must be distinguished from a pathologic extensor response (**decerebrate**). Reflexes are rated on a scale of 0 to 4. Zero is absent reflexes, 1 is a weak reflex, and 2 is a normal reflex. Three is an overly active reflex with up to 1 to 3 beats of clonus. Four is a reflex associated with more sustained clonus. Pathologic reflexes associated with upper motor neuron lesions include extensor plantar responses (**Babinski reflex**), finger flexion response with sudden flexion of the distal interphalangeal joint (**Hoffmann response**), and ankle clonus.

The sensory examination includes both the spinothalamic pathway (pain-pin response) and the lemniscal pathway (joint position sense and symmetry of vibration sensation). Testing for pronator drift (Barré sign—arms extended, palms up with fingers spread, with eyes closed) is a rapid way to test for both asymmetry of motor strength and integrity of joint position sense. A pathologic response includes both unilateral pronation and asymmetrically dropping one arm.

For supratentorial cerebral lesions, bilateral symmetry of examination takes on paramount importance, and "lateralizing signs" (either motor, reflex, or sensory) are key findings assisting in hemispheric localization. For brain stem lesions, the level of cranial nerve involvement and the presence of decorticate or decerebrate posturing in comatose patients are critical for localizing the level of the lesion. For cerebellar lesions, lateral asymmetry of findings for hemispheric lesions and defining truncal versus appendicular findings are critical for distinguishing midline vermis versus lateral hemispheric lesions. Coma (GCS score ≤ 8) occurs only with diencephalic or brain stem reticular activating system dysfunction, or with global, bilateral, and diffuse cortical dysfunction.

Brain Death

Brain death is a legal definition of death that recognizes an irreversible physiologic state in which the brain has no function, but heartbeat and blood pressure are maintained. The determination is best made by a neurologist or neurosurgeon. At the time of examination, there should be no evidence of significant hypothermia or potential pharmacologic cause of CNS suppression. Brain stem reflexes (pupillary, corneal, oculovestibular, caloric, gag, and respiratory) should be absent. There should be no response to trigeminal painful stimuli and no more than local motor responses (spinal) to body or limb stimulation. Disconnection of the respirator to test for the absence of spontaneous respiration is essential. This determination is carried out after a period of ventilation that allows the P_{CO_2} to normalize. When the respirator is disconnected, an adequate, steady flow of oxygen is delivered through a catheter that is introduced well down the endotracheal tube. The patient is observed for the absence of spontaneous respirations. The determination is carried out until the arterial P_{CO_2} is greater than 59 mm Hg.

Laboratory tests (electroencephalographic silence; cerebral radionuclide brain scans, cerebral angiography, or possibly, transcranial Doppler confirmation of absent CBF) are usually considered optional unless hypotension occurs and forces discontinuation of apnea testing. Usually, two complete examinations, which are separated in time and show no evidence of brain activity by the previously described criteria, are performed by licensed physicians before the patient is pronounced brain dead.

Lumbar Puncture

The CSF is a separate homeostatically regulated physiologic fluid that is unique to the CNS. Laboratory evaluation of CSF is just as important as systemic blood work in evaluating patients with CNS pathology. It is usually accessed by means of a lumbar puncture (LP) at either L4-L5 or L5-S1. At these levels, there is less risk of spinal cord injury because only the cauda equina lies in the thecal sac at these levels. An LP can give a diagnostic opening pressure, which will be elevated in cases of pseudotumor cerebri, CNS infection, or high ICP from mass lesion. Standard CSF examination includes measurement of glucose level (lowered in the setting of infection), protein level (elevated in many pathologic settings), Gram stain and culture (infection), and cell count (both white cell and red cell). In the emergency department, if community-acquired and potentially infectious meningitis is suspected, the CSF can be screened for antigens to the common community-acquired infectious meningitis agents. The CSF cell count assessment is particularly important. Although white cells will be elevated (>5) in the setting of many infections, a neutrophil predominance suggests a bacterial process, whereas a mononuclear predominance suggests a viral, fungal, or noninfectious inflammatory condition. An elevated CSF red blood cell (RBC) count may be the only indication that a patient has had a subarachnoid hemorrhage (SAH). Computed tomography (CT) scans are only 90% to 95% sensitive for SAH in the acute setting, but a CT scan, coupled with an LP, increases sensitivity to approximately 98%. It is important in this setting to send both the first and fourth tubes of a fluid sample for cell count because a high RBC count in the first tube that clears by the fourth tube suggests a traumatic LP rather than an SAH. The CSF should also be assessed for xanthochromia (straw color), which indicates a subacute SAH (minimum 2-3 days previously) with subsequent RBC lysis, a high protein content, or both.

Neuroimaging

In 1976, CT revolutionized the ability to directly see brain lesions and brain and skull anatomy. Magnetic resonance imaging (MRI) followed in the late 1980s, offering even better resolution of CNS tissue. Few medical disciplines are as critically dependent on imaging for achieving best clinical practice benchmarks as neurosurgery. Neurosurgeons are experienced at interpreting CT and MRI neuroimages and usually work closely with their affiliated neuroradiologist(s).

Cerebral Angiography, Embolization, Thrombolysis, and Embolectomy

Although MR angiography and CT angiography are less invasive and can usually be obtained more quickly, cerebral angiography is the gold standard for detailed resolution of CNS vascular anatomy and diagnosis of CNS vascular lesions. Such lesions include cerebral aneurysm, arteriovenous malformation (AVM), arteriovenous fistula, and arterial embolus. Originally performed by direct needle stick of the cervical common carotid artery (CCA) and VA, it is now routinely performed by catheters introduced into the femoral artery in the groin and navigated cephalad. Diagnostic cerebral angiography is a very powerful tool; however, it is an invasive test and carries an approximately 1% risk of stroke for anterior circulation assessment, increasing to a 1% to 3% stroke risk for posterior circulation assessment. Diagnostic cerebral angiography can be used to visualize CNS lesions and to assess collateral circulation by assessing the status of the circle of Willis. It can also be used to perform a temporary balloon test occlusion of an artery while the patient is assessed clinically, electrophysiologically, or with CBF imaging.

Cerebral angiography can even be used therapeutically. Endovascular embolization of CNS vascular lesions (eg, aneurysms and AVMs) is currently performed by both endovascular neurosurgeons and interventional radiologists. With endovascular access, selected cases of aneurysms can now be partially or completely occluded by either coil embolization or glue casting. Some AVMs and vascular tumors, such as meningiomas, can now be temporarily (in preparation for microsurgical excision) or permanently embolized with resorbable particles, permanent coils, or casting glue. Endovascular applications of treatment for cerebrovascular disease have now expanded to include angioplasty and stenting for cervical and intracranial carotid, VA disease, and arterial dissections. Intraluminal chemical and mechanical cerebral angioplasty for post-SAH vasospasm, catheter-directed chemical thrombolysis, and endovascular embolus retrieval for stroke are also frequently performed.

CT Scanning

CT scans are the study of choice for neurosurgical emergencies because they are readily available at most hospitals (even during late nonbusiness hours), can be obtained very quickly, and provide a wealth of important information for emergent decision making. They can show bone more clearly than MRI and therefore are excellent when used in evaluating cases of skull fracture. They are very sensitive for detecting acute blood (which appears white—hyperdense), and are, therefore, useful in assessing patients for SAH, intraparenchymal hemorrhage (IPH), hemorrhagic stroke, spontaneous or posttraumatic extra-axial blood clot (**epidural** or **subdural hematoma**), or traumatic contusion. They show the ventricular system very well (hypodense) and thus aid in detecting communicating or obstructive hydrocephalus. They can show differentiation between ventricular system displacement and a space-occupying mass lesion. They are useful in detecting abnormal calcium deposits in a blood vessel or brain mass. They are moderately sensitive for detecting swelling or vasogenic edema surrounding a pathologic lesion. CT scan disadvantages include poorer resolution of parenchymal brain structures than MR scarring, less sensitivity for identifying brain tumors (even with intravenous contrast agents), and an inability to show an acute ischemic stroke (hypodensity can take 12-36 hours to develop on CT scans). Administration of iodine-based intravenous contrast dye improves the sensitivity of the CT scan for detecting brain tumors and areas of focal infection. Administration of dye into the CSF (CT cisternography) improves its ability to show lesions in the CSF compartments and detect CSF leaks. The development of CT angiography has been a major step forward in assessing suspected SAH for the presence of an aneurysm without the time delay and risks of more invasive cerebral angiography. CT angiography at many centers has now become so good that in some cases neurosurgeons are able to take patients directly to the operating room to clip an aneurysm microsurgically without ever performing a preoperative diagnostic cerebral angiogram.

Magnetic Resonance Imaging

MRI scans do not show bone well and are thus inferior to CT scanning for assessing patients for fractures or osseous involvement of tumors or infection. Although MRI is very sensitive for detecting subacute or chronic bleeding, it is relatively insensitive compared with CT scanning for detecting acute blood and is, therefore, not the ideal study for evaluating acute hemorrhage or head trauma.

MR scanning provides the best resolution of intracranial soft tissue. Gray matter, white matter distinctions, deep gray matter structures, major cerebral vessels, the meninges, the ventricular lining, and even cranial nerves are very well shown. Flow-attenuated inversion-recover sequences and long time-to-response (TR), or "T2-weighted," sequences provide excellent sensitivity to even small amounts of vasogenic cerebral edema or demyelination. Gradient response sequences with long TRs provide very good sensitivity to ever small amounts of deposited extracellular blood products. Administration of contrast leads to significant improvements in sensitivity over contrast CT scanning for detecting meningeal, ventricular, or cranial nerve pathology, as well as brain tumors, areas of cerebritis, and abscesses. MRI diffusion studies can almost immediately detect the early cytotoxic edema associated with a stroke, well before the area becomes hypodense on a CT scan. As a result, MRI scanning has become the diagnostic procedure of choice for neuro-oncology, stroke neurology, and for assessing patients for inflammatory lesions or multiple sclerosis. MR angiography also serves as an excellent noninvasive screening tool without iodine dye load for screening patients for cerebral aneurysm, AVM, atherosclerotic cerebrovascular disease (both cervical and intracranial), and vascular dissection.

Further advances in MRI are rapidly being made with exciting potential applications for clinical neuroscience. High-field 3-tesla magnets have increased soft-tissue resolution further while allowing the high signal-to-noise ratios necessary to perform metabolic tissue sampling through single- and multivoxel MR spectroscopy (MRS). MRS is an excellent technique for distinguishing a mass lesion from tumor, radiation necrosis, infarction, or infection. It can also assess the likelihood of tumor invasion beyond imaging apparent tumor borders into the surrounding normally appearing brain. Functional MR can localize sensory and motor speech areas as well as the primary motor strip and determine their relationship and degree of direct involvement versus displacement with regard to adjacent

mass lesions. Diffusion tensor imaging is a way of mapping the major CNS white matter association tracts (corpus callosum, side to side, superior and inferior longitudinal fasciculus, anterior-to-posterior, and the primary motor and sensory long tracts, rostral-to-caudal). It does this by detecting the integrity of the selective movement of water within the parallel-oriented cleavage planes along these white matter tract connections. It has the potential to determine whether a mass lesion has invaded and disrupted these cleavage planes within the relevant tracts or merely compressed or displaced them (and if so, demonstrate where they are located relative to the lesion in question). All of this information is very important for clinical decision making and preoperative surgical planning.

Head Injury

In the United States, approximately 2 million people every year suffer a head injury and approximately 150,000 people per year become comatose from head injury. Annually, head injury accounts for approximately 1% to 2% of all deaths in the United States, 25% of all trauma-related deaths, and up to 60% of all motor vehicle–related deaths. Head injuries can be acute, subacute, or chronic. Acute head injuries include scalp lacerations, contusions, and abrasions, skull fractures (basal and cranial vault), CSF leakage, extraparenchymal hematomas (subdural and epidural hematomas), brain contusions and intraparenchymal hematomas, traumatic arterial dissection leading to SAH or stroke, and axonal connection shear injuries. Subacute and chronic problems include postconcussive syndrome, chronic subdural hematomas, persistent CSF leak, growing skull fracture, arteriovenous fistulae, infection from a retained foreign body, hydrocephalus, posttraumatic epilepsy, and permanent cognitive and neurologic deficits.

Evaluation of Acute Injuries

Evaluation of an acutely head-injured patient begins with a primary survey that focuses on the ABCs (airway, breathing, and circulation). Neurologic examination is not reliable or predictive until the patient has been stabilized from the standpoint of ventilation, hypoxemia, and circulatory shock. Careful note should be taken of the need to administer pharmacologic paralytic agents or sedatives during initial resuscitation because these will significantly affect neurologic assessment. The neurologic assessment begins with a rapid initial survey that determines the patient's GCS score (see Table 28-2), pupillary response, and the symmetry of motor and papillary findings on either side. The degree of impairment and the presence or absence of pending herniation syndrome determine the need to proceed immediately to a CT scan for head examination versus the ability to proceed with a secondary neurologic survey before the CT scan. Often, portions outlined in this paragraph are assessed simultaneously or in parallel to save time and expedite the logistics of transport and imaging acquisition. If the patient has a GCS score of 12 or less, the operating room and anesthesiologist should probably be notified to be standing by for possible emergent craniotomy or ICP monitoring procedures.

During the secondary neurologic survey, a careful history from the emergency medical technicians is desirable. The mechanism of injury provides valuable information regarding associated injuries and the severity of force transmission to the patient. Whether the patient had a safety belt on, whether the airbag deployed, the structural state of the car, the location the patient was found in the car, and whether the patient was ejected from the car (if the incident was a motor vehicle accident) are all very useful information. Knowing whether the patient had a predisposing medical event (eg, myocardial infarction, drug ingestion) and whether there was a period of hypotension, hypoxemia, or even cardiac arrest is helpful in the clinical assessment. The timing of intubation, if required (in the field vs on arrival), may give valuable clues as to potential secondary hypoxemic injury.

During this portion of the evaluation, a more detailed systematic neurologic examination is obtained if the patient is conscious and cooperative. If the patient is unconscious or sedated, cranial nerve reflexes (pupils, corneas, gag, and cough) are assessed. The scalp is assessed for signs of bleeding from laceration or abrasion, subgaleal hematoma, projectile wound, or palpable fractures. If an open wound is located, it is noted but is not probed or explored for fear of causing further bleeding and increasing the risk of infection. The patient's mastoid and periorbital areas are assessed for ecchymosis indicating basilar skull fracture (mastoid—Battle sign; periorbital—raccoon eyes). The nose is assessed for signs of CSF rhinorrhea, and, if noted, the trauma surgeon or emergency department physician is instructed (a) to be careful with any subsequent bag-mask pressure ventilation for fear of introducing intracranial air and raising ICP because of ball-valve cranial air entry and (b) not to insert a nasogastric tube if stomach decompression is required, but to decompress the stomach using an orogastric tube (danger of intracranial penetration by way of an anterior basal skull fracture). The ear canals are examined bilaterally for otorrhea, and the tympanic membranes are assessed for hemotympanum. Given the risk of cervical spine injury in a patient with an acute head injury, oculocephalic reflex testing is usually deferred until cervical spine injury is excluded.

An unconscious patient should be assessed for a history of loss of consciousness, as well as anterograde or retrograde amnesia, which correlates with the degree and risk of concussion. Any patient with a history of head injury with a loss of consciousness or a GCS score less than 13 should probably be assessed by CT scan if it is readily available. Patients with a GCS score of 13 to 15 can be assessed with a CT scan or observed for at least 23 hours (the time a patient can be held in the emergency department before that patient must be admitted to the hospital). Observation consists of repeated neurologic examinations every 2 hours, with a CT scan obtained rapidly if the patient worsens clinically. A patient with a history of a head injury, a GCS score of 15, and a normal neurologic examination with a normal CT scan of the head can probably be discharged home so long as the patient is returning to a stable social situation with an identified caretaker who has been instructed in how to monitor and assess the patient for the next 23 hours. The patient should return to the hospital if there is hemiparesis, pupillary inequality, increase in headache, sleepiness, reduction in consciousness, or persistent vomiting.

Intracranial Pressure Monitoring and Control

In general, monitoring of ICP is indicated for patients with a GCS score of 8 or less. ICP monitors usually take the form of either a ventriculostomy or an intraparenchymal fiberoptic pressure probe. A ventriculostomy consists of a percutaneous Silastic tube inserted through a burr hole in the skull that courses through the brain tissue to the lateral ventricle. The tube provides a continuous column of fluid from the ventricular CSF to an external drainage system and can be transduced like an arterial line. A ventriculostomy is the preferred means of ICP monitoring because it is therapeutic at the same time that it provides the necessary ICP data. Given the conditions of the Monroe-Kellie hypothesis, outlined previously, nothing reduces ICP faster or more effectively than actual CSF drainage. Unfortunately, some ventricular systems are too small to safely intubate, and ventricular chambers can collapse to the point where the ventriculostomy no longer effectively transduces pressure. There are also borderline situations in which the need for ICP monitoring is equivocal or uncertain. In these situations, an intraparenchymal fiberoptic ICP monitor is another option. It provides accurate readings of ICP. However, it cannot drain CSF and becomes increasingly less accurate over time because of zero baseline "drift," which can gradually lead to inaccuracies of approximately 5 mm Hg over the course of 5 to 10 days. With the ICP known and tracked, the actual CPP for the patient can be determined at any given time (CPP = MAP − ICP) and adjustments made to maintain it on a running basis.

Acute or persistent elevations of ICP are treated as described in Table 28-3. Once CT scanning has ruled out the presence of an acutely reversible surgical mass lesion, and other measures have had a chance to take effect, hyperventilation to even moderate degrees is avoided whenever possible, to prevent secondary ischemic CNS injury. The mainstay of ICP management in the acute head injury situation is CSF drainage through a ventriculostomy. In the presence of reduced brain compliance, even intermittent removal of volumes as small as 1 to 2 mL can have a dramatic and sustained ICP reduction effect. Mannitol is given in intermittent intravenous boluses of 0.125 to 0.25 g/kg (usually 12.5-25 g at a time) every 4 to 6 hours as needed, taking care to follow serum osmolality closely (not allowing it to rise above 315 mOsm/L). The ICP-reducing effects of mannitol can be accentuated by premedication with small intravenous doses of furosemide

TABLE 28-3. Medical Treatment of Increased Intracranial Pressure

Method	Treatment
Osmotic diuretics	Mannitol 20%, 1 g/kg IV single dose or 0.25 g/kg every 8 h as needed for repeated usage
Renal diuretics	Furosemide 1 mg/kg IV single dose or 0.25-0.5 mg/kg every 8 h or more as needed
Maintain normovolemia[a]	IV infusion of crystalloid
Hyperventilation	P_{CO_2} 30-35 mm Hg
Elevation of the head	30°: elevation

IV, intravenous.

[a]Some protocols favor normovolemia or even hypervolemia and hypertension rather than dehydration and normotension.

(10-20 mg/bolus) given 5 to 10 minutes before the mannitol dose. Intravenous infusion sedation with an agent that is short acting and that can be quickly stopped to allow for neurologic examination (eg, fentanyl or propofol) will reduce the incidence of struggling against the ventilator, endotracheal tube, or other Valsalva maneuvers, and thus help keep ICP down. Both intravenous sedation and pharmacologic paralysis will reduce muscular tone, thereby increasing venous return from the head and decreasing CO_2 production from muscle contractions, all of which will help with ICP control. Physiologic levels (up to 5 mm Hg) of positive end-expiratory pressure (PEEP) are not likely to have major negative effects on cerebral venous return and ICP, but higher levels of PEEP should be avoided when possible. Serum sodium needs to be carefully monitored because the syndrome of inappropriate antidiuretic hormone secretion (SIADH) or cerebral salt wasting, and the accompanying hyponatremia can accentuate cerebral edema and ICP problems. Maintenance fluids should consist of normal saline solution with consideration given to the judicious use of intravenous 3% NaCl solution if SIADH or cerebral salt wasting is confirmed with elevated ICP. Occasionally, 23% saline bullets can be given intermittently in severe and dire head injury. When all else fails, induction of barbiturate coma by bolus injection, followed by continuous infusion, is sometimes necessary. When utilized, the minimum infusion necessary to maintain electrical activity burst suppression should be confirmed by electroencephalogram (EEG). Induction of barbiturate coma must be considered carefully because it tends to lead to hypothermia, systemic hypotension due to cardiac suppression (which fights against CPP maintenance efforts), and impaired pulmonary ciliary function, which makes patients susceptible to pneumonia. It can also take significant time to wear off.

Cerebral Perfusion Pressure

In general, under normal autoregulatory conditions, CBF is not impaired with normal ICP down to MAP as low as 40 mm Hg (CPP ~30-32 mm Hg). Even within the globally high ICP situation of pseudotumor cerebri (in which ICP is routinely 27-34 mm Hg), the brain functions normally with a CPP of approximately 36 to 43 mm Hg. However, in head injury, cerebral autoregulation has been shown to be dysfunctional and impaired both globally and in the microenvironment at the site of injury, so that CBF can become directly dependent on CPP. Although normal CPP is 50 to 60 mm Hg, in the setting of head injury, a desirable target is a minimum CPP of 60 to 70 mm Hg. CPP is maintained by ensuring adequate cardiac preload (CVP 8-10 mm Hg or pulmonary artery wedge pressure 12-15 mm Hg) without volume overload (which could accentuate cerebral edema). Early use of systemic vasopressors is implemented once preload is optimized if a CPP of 60 to 70 mm Hg is not spontaneously achievable. Dopamine has the added advantage of dilating cerebral surface collateral vessels; however, epinephrine or norepinephrine can also be used and may need to be used if dopamine is insufficient.

Closed Head Injury

Closed head injury (CHI) describes conditions in which the intradural contents of the cranium are not exposed to the outside environment and are not herniating out through a traumatic cranial defect. CSF leak from a basilar skull fracture is one exception that is still considered a CHI. In the civilian sector, and certainly in times of peace, CHI is the most common form of head injury seen in the US health care system.

Concussion

A concussion is a clinical syndrome of temporary global brain dysfunction that can be inferred from a history of brief loss of consciousness or a period of anterograde or retrograde amnesia surrounding a CHI. A patient with a history suggestive of a concussion and a history of head injury with a GCS score of 13 to 15 is classified as having a minor CHI. Very few of these patients, if imaged, will be found to have a pathologic lesion on CT scan, and the vast majority of these will be nonsurgical in consequence. A concussion does, however, imply significant force transmission to, and absorption by, the brain. Given the delicacy of the CNS, it is not surprising that many of these patients will continue to have symptoms for weeks to months (occasionally for up to 6-12 months after injury) until they finally resolve. The condition is known as postconcussive syndrome. To prevent unwarranted anxiety in patients and assist them in coping with it, counseling should be offered regarding the likelihood of syndrome symptoms. These symptoms include persistent recurring headaches, difficulty concentrating, reduced attention span, short-term memory and learning dysfunction, disturbance in the normal wake-sleep rhythms, social disinhibition, emotional lability, depression, and social withdrawal. These symptoms tend to be self-limited and usually resolve given sufficient time.

Closed Skull Fractures

Skull fractures can occur in the skull base or the cranial vault. Skull-base fractures involving the anterior cranial fossa may manifest with unilateral or bilateral periorbital swelling and ecchymosis (raccoon eyes). If they involve the orbit roof, floor, and walls, vision acuity and EOMs should be carefully checked to rule out extraocular muscle entrapment by the bone fragments. Involvement of the posterior wall of the frontal sinus, cribriform plate, or planum sphenoidale could indicate a risk of early or delayed anterior CSF leak. Anterior cranial fossa skull-base fracture is a relative contraindication for positive pressure bag-mask ventilation and for nasogastric tube placement. The potential risks are intracranial air introduction, elevation in ICP if introduced air cannot subsequently escape (ball-valve mechanism), and intracranial passage of the gastric tube. Basal skull fractures involving the middle cranial fossa are at risk for damaging the ICA in its parasellar/cavernous sinus location. Fractures that extend through the petrous carotid canal exit into the cavernous sinus, or lateral sphenoid sinus wall fractures with sphenoid sinus air-fluid levels may warrant further investigation with CT angiography, MR angiography, or conventional cerebral angiogram. Fractures of the temporal bone can lead to CSF leak through the tympanic membrane (otorrhea) or down the back of the throat via the middle ear and eustachian tube. Visualization of fluid within the mastoid air cells on a CT scan should lead to a careful search for a temporal bone fracture. Horizontal temporal bone fractures run parallel to the course of the internal auditory canal. Although they can cause CSF leak, they rarely cause cranial nerve dysfunction.

Transverse temporal bone fractures run perpendicular to the course of the internal auditory canal. They imply a much larger transmission of force to the skull base and are much more likely than horizontal fractures to be associated with facial, vestibular, and cochlear nerve dysfunction. They are also occasionally associated with mechanical disruption of the middle ear ossicles. Every patient with a temporal bone fracture should be carefully evaluated for facial nerve function, nystagmus, and hearing loss, as well as CSF leak. Fractures that extend through the petrous carotid canal of the temporal bone may warrant further investigation to rule out ICA injury with CT angiography, MR angiography, or a conventional cerebral angiogram.

Cranial vault fractures can be linear or comminuted (several fragments). They can be diastatic (gap between the fracture edges) or even depressed. Closed cranial vault fractures require surgical exploration only if they are depressed and the depression is greater than the cross-sectional width of the skull (unlikely to heal cosmetically through remodeling alone), occur in a cosmetically obvious area (eg, forehead), are associated with an underlying mass lesion that needs to be excised, or are associated with an area of intracranial air suggesting dural penetration. Diastatic fractures in very young children can lead to a special situation called a "growing skull fracture." In this situation, the dura gets trapped between the edges of the skull fracture and begins to act as a new skull growth plate, preventing proper healing and promoting further diastasis. Growing skull fractures are detected with a 4- to 6-week follow-up skull x-ray and require surgical exploration.

Subdural Hematomas

Subdural hematomas can be acute, subacute, or chronic. Acute subdural hematomas can be spontaneous or traumatic. Subdural hematomas occur between the arachnoid of the brain and the dura of the meninges (Figure 28-5). They are hyperdense on CT scans (white) because of the presence of fresh blood. On CT scans, they appear to follow the curve of the hemispheric surface like the rind of a watermelon. Spontaneous subdurals usually occur because of the tearing of a parasagittal bridging vein caused by shearing forces associated with even minor CHIs or cerebral acceleration-deceleration. They are more common in older adult patients who have an accentuated distance between their brain and dura because of cerebral atrophy. They are also more common in patients taking anticoagulant medications (eg, non-vitamin K oral anticoagulant [NOACs], warfarin, aspirin, clopidogrel, dual antiplatelet therapy [DAP]). Posttraumatic subdural hematomas are usually associated with an underlying cortical brain injury (eg, cortical laceration or contusion). As a result, they can be venous, arterial, or mixed in origin. They carry a significantly worse prognosis than their spontaneous counterparts. Not all subdural hematomas require surgical evacuation. If they are small enough (eg, <30 mL volume) without midline shift and the patient is doing well clinically, the patient can be treated conservatively with careful follow-up, neurologic examination, and serial CT scanning. The majority of subdural hematomas will naturally resorb.

Within 7 to 14 days, the RBCs in the clot begin to lyze and the hematoma may appear as a mixed-density mass or even isodense compared with the brain. At this subacute

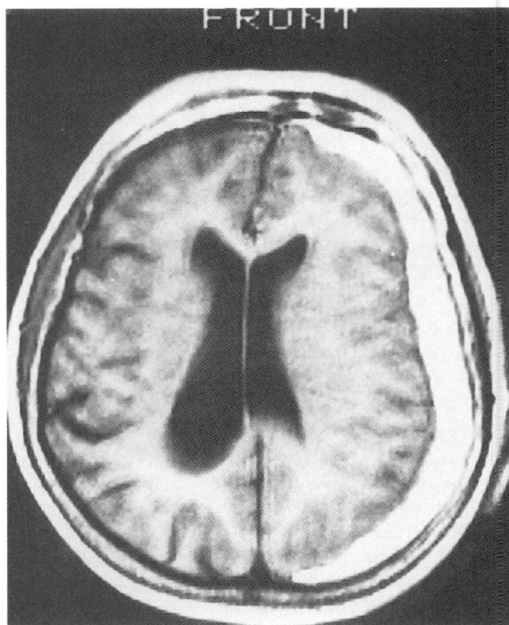

Figure 28-5. Magnetic resonance imaging of a subacute subdural hematoma. (From Lawrence PF. *Essentials of Surgical Specialties*. 3rd ed. Lippincott Williams & Wilkins; 2007.)

stage, the hematoma can sometimes be difficult to see on a CT scan, but its presence can usually be detected with careful image windowing, inferred from unilateral loss of gyral surface pattern, or inferred by mass effect on the ipsilateral lateral ventricle. If the hematoma has not been absorbed by approximately 4 to 6 weeks after formation, the body will have walled it off by forming an enclosing membrane of fragile neovascularity, which can easily rebleed with minor trauma. The clot itself is fully lysed, is liquid in consistency (either straw-colored fluid or crank-case-oil appearance grossly, depending on age), and can usually be effectively drained through burr holes.

Epidural Hematomas

Epidural hematomas are acute in origin. They occur between the skull and the dura (Figure 28-6). They are usually associated with adjacent skull fractures. On CT scans, they tend to appear biconvex (lenticular) in shape because they can extend only to the next point of dura attachment to the cranial vault (usually a suture line, ie, coronal or squamosal suture). In adults, fractures of the temporal squama are worrisome because they can be associated with epidural hematomas from damage to the MMA. Given the size of the artery involved and the direct lateral vector, and the associated clot places on the supratentorial temporal lobe, they are at great risk for rapid enlargement (even in a delayed fashion in a normal-appearing patient) and early herniation syndrome. Fractures in other locations and fractures in the vascular calvarium of children more commonly lead to venous epidural hematomas. Not all epidural hematomas require surgical evacuation, if they are small enough (eg, <30 mL volume) and the patient is doing well clinically. If the location and skull fracture

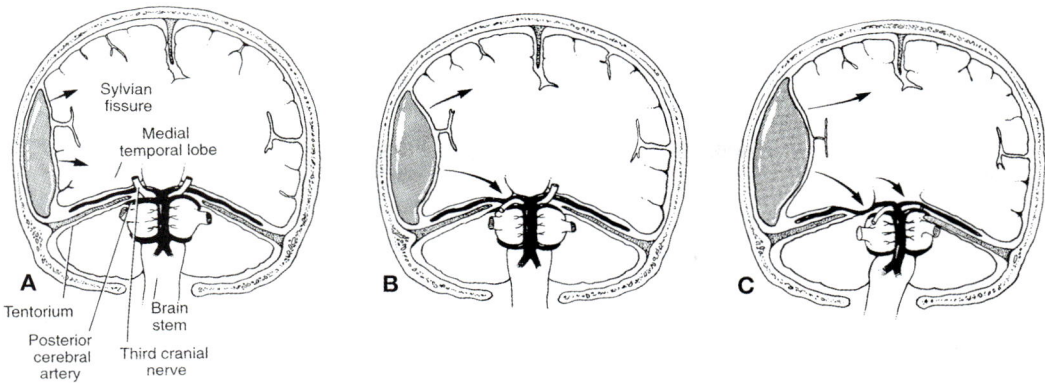

Figure 28-6. A. Extracerebral clot with local brain compression. B. Early transtentorial herniation. C. Late stage of herniation. (From Lawrence PF. *Essentials of Surgical Specialties.* 3rd ed. Lippincott Williams & Wilkins; 2007.)

do not suggest MMA involvement, they can be followed conservatively with careful neurologic examination and serial CT scanning. The majority will go on to naturally resorb. Given the fact that the dura remains intact as a protective layer and the fact that they are not routinely associated with the underlying direct brain, epidural hematomas carry a much better prognosis than subdural hematomas of the same size and location.

Contusions and Intraparenchymal Hematomas

Cerebral contusions are literally tissue bruises of the brain. Following acceleration-deceleration forces, they tend to occur on the inferior surface of the brain (inferior frontal lobes and inferior temporal lobes) because of abrasion of the brain against the irregular anterior cranial fossa and middle cranial fossa bony floor. The rapid acceleration-deceleration forces lead to translational brain movements within the CSF-filled cranial cavity. The forces also tend to act on the anterior poles of the brain (frontal pole, temporal pole, and occipital pole), because these surfaces impact against the inner surface of the cranium during the same translational brain movements. With direct blows to the head, they can occur directly underneath the point of impact (coup injury) as a result of an overlying skull fracture or transmission of percussive force. Coup injuries are often associated with contrecoup injuries involving the brain on the opposite side of the head. The injury occurs when that opposite area is suddenly translated against the inner skull surface as a result of translational brain movement or a fall to that side, leading to a second cranial impact on the opposite side. If the contusion is associated with disruption of a moderately large tissue blood vessel, a frank intraparenchymal hematoma can develop. Contusions can also lead to brain tissue homogenization and are thus at risk for causing coagulopathy from tissue thromboplastin release, which can lead to the conversion of a contusion into a hematoma or enlargement of the contusion. Most contusions can be managed conservatively without operation, and smaller traumatic hematomas can also be managed conservatively so long as the patient does not have a coagulopathy and is doing well clinically. Most contusions and intraparenchymal hematomas warrant a follow-up CT scan 12 to 24 hours later to rule out lesion evolution or enlargement.

Penetrating Head Injury

Penetrating head injury includes open skull fractures and projectile injuries. They are much more common in military conflicts than in peacetime and more common in urban than in suburban or rural civilian settings.

Open Skull Fractures

Open skull fractures require operative exploration if they are associated with brain herniation, significant underlying hematoma or other surgical mass lesions, CSF leak, substantial localized intracranial air on CT scan, or fragments of bone driven into the brain or if they are significantly depressed. The goal of these explorations is to restore dural integrity, debride intraparenchymal foreign bodies, deal with any associated brain injury or intracranial hematoma, and repair depressed or comminuted skull fractures. Simpler open skull fractures can be treated with local irrigation, antibiotics, and scalp closure in layers in the emergency department.

Cerebral Gunshot Wounds and Other Projectile Injuries

Cerebral gunshot wounds (GSWs) can be very serious injuries. Indicators of a very poor outcome even with surgical intervention include a GCS score of 8 or less, as well as bihemispheric involvement, transventricular passage, multilobar dominant hemisphere involvement, and brain stem involvement. These injuries often involve tremendous energy transmission to the brain, often associated with extensive cavitation and homogenization of brain tissue. They are also associated with a high incidence of disseminated intravascular coagulation and coagulopathy. The decision of whether to explore surgically is based on the patient's age, neurologic status, and the extent of anatomic damage. The goals of surgery include obtaining hemostasis, debriding obviously dead brain and hematomas, removing superficial and readily accessible bone fragments, and restoring dural integrity. Deeper explorations in an attempt to retrieve additional bone fragments or the bullet itself will not reduce the incidence of subsequent infection or posttraumatic seizures, may cause further brain damage, and are no longer generally recommended. The patient is treated with intravenous antibiotics and anticonvulsants.

A GSW is caused by high-velocity projectiles with tremendous force transmission. Shrapnel fragments or other foreign body projectiles may or may not have a larger mass than a bullet, but they are usually not traveling at a great velocity. As a result, the prognosis for patients injured with these projectiles is generally better than those with cerebral GSWs, and the surgical outcomes are usually better as well. The surgical principles and goals remain the same.

Traumatic Cerebrospinal Fluid Leak

Traumatic CSF leaks associated with open cranial injuries usually require surgical exploration for debridement and dural closure. CSF leaks associated with basilar skull fractures are another matter. These patients are kept on bed rest with their head elevated to 30° to 45°. Most of these CSF leaks will spontaneously cease and heal within 3 to 5 days. If they do not, a trial of lumbar drainage may allow the major subset of the remainder to go on to heal without surgery. Prophylactic antibiotics to prevent meningitis have not been shown to be effective and may select for resistant organisms. If the patient develops a fever, an LP is performed if safe according to associated injuries, and antibiotics are started only after the CSF culture has been sent to the laboratory. Broad-spectrum antibiotics are tailored by organism identification and antibiotic sensitivities once they are known. Only those who fail conservative management acutely or because of delayed recurrent CSF leaks require surgery to repair the defect. The goals of surgery include restoration of dural integrity with dural patch grafting and treatment of any predisposing hydrocephalus that may be present. Skull-base surgical techniques including vascularized, pedicled, pericranial grafts (for anterior cranial fossa leaks), endoscopic or microscopic trans-sphenoidal approaches (for sphenoid sinus leaks), or transmastoid temporal bone approaches (for temporal bone origin leaks) are often the most effective. The preoperative precise definition of the probable leak site by CT cisternography can be most helpful.

Scalp Lacerations

The scalp is very vascular, and scalp lacerations can lead to significant blood loss, particularly in children. All scalp blood vessels lie between the galea and the dermis. As a result, scalp bleeding can be easily controlled by placing the galea under tension by grasping it with a hemostat or a suture. Scalp lacerations require generous irrigation, occasional debridement, and careful closure. The scalp may be closed in a single layer. However, placing a few interrupted absorbable stitches to reapproximate the galea before closing the skin controls scalp bleeding, takes the tension off the epithelial closure, and leads to a more cosmetically acceptable scar.

Brain Attack and Cerebrovascular Disease

"Stroke" is a term that reflects a sudden ictus (being struck down). Strokes are sudden cerebrovascular events that can be classified as ischemic infarction or intracerebral hemorrhage (ICH). ICH can be further divided into spontaneous IPH and SAH. Ischemic infarction is the most severe and permanent form of symptomatic atherosclerotic cerebrovascular disease that also includes transient ischemic attacks (TIAs—reversible ischemic neurologic deficit lasting <24 hours) and reversible ischemic neurologic deficits (transient focal neurologic deficits that last >1 day but

<1 week). Risk factors for cerebral atherosclerotic disease include family history, hypertension, smoking, diabetes mellitus, and hyperlipidemia. Risk factors for IPH include hypertension, drug use (especially cocaine and methamphetamine), dementia, and coagulopathy. Risk factors for aneurysmal SAH include a family history and a prior history of a berry aneurysm.

Transient Ischemic Attacks

TIAs often precede the onset of permanent ischemic stroke, and they can serve as a warning sign to allow intervention to prevent a stroke. Seventy percent of TIAs last less than 10 minutes. Common symptoms include transient monocular visual obscuration (amaurosis fugax), unilateral motor weakness, unilateral sensory paresthesias or numbness, or speech deficit. Most TIAs result from either artery-to-artery emboli or cardiac-origin emboli. The most common source of artery-to-artery emboli is an atherosclerotic plaque at the carotid bifurcation. The MCA distribution is the one most commonly affected by both TIAs and ischemic infarctions. Patients with TIAs should be assessed for carotid bruits (2% per year stroke risk with a symptomatic carotid bruit, 0.1%-0.4% annual stroke risk for an asymptomatic carotid bruit). Their STA pulses should be assessed for asymmetry (increased STA pulse may indicate near occlusion of the ipsilateral ICA). Funduscopic examination should be done to assess for cholesterol plaques and central retinal artery occlusion. They should also be assessed for treatable cerebral atherosclerotic risk factors. In general, the risk of cerebral ischemic infarction after a TIA is approximately 5% per year. Rapid repetitive or clustering of TIAs (crescendo TIAs) is a particularly risky and ominous situation that should lead to an aggressive search for a treatable source with consideration given to anticoagulation with heparin until the workup can be completed. Initial workup for cause should include cervical carotid imaging (carotid duplex ultrasonography, MR angiography, CT angiography, or cerebral angiography), 12-lead electrocardiogram, 24-hour Holter monitoring, and echocardiography (transesophageal is superior to transthoracic). A vascular coagulopathy panel, lipid screening panel, and basic screening studies to assess for arteritis should be considered.

Ischemic Infarction

Ischemic infarction can occur from a loss of CBF caused by cervical vessel occlusion or cerebral embolus. Embolic infarction is overwhelmingly more common and can occur from artery-to-artery emboli (carotid bifurcation is the most common source), a primary cardiac source (due to atrial fibrillation, postmyocardial infarction mural thrombus, or cardiac valvular disease), or transmission of a venous embolus resulting from deep venous thrombosis through a patent foramen ovale. Small, flow-related strokes can occur from progressive hypertension-related arteriolar sclerosis affecting the small perforating end arteries of the diencephalon (basal ganglia, thalamus, and internal capsule), brain stem, and deep cerebellar nuclei. These lacunar strokes can be either silent or surprisingly symptomatic, given their small size relative to the eloquence and redundancy of function of the deep cerebral areas affected. Unlike patients with ICH, who usually present with sudden-onset headaches with or without alteration of consciousness, nausea, or vomiting, patients with ischemic infarction usually present with a rapid onset of neurologic deficit, with little or no headache and only rarely effects on the level of consciousness. CT scan may appear normal and is primarily obtained to rule out ICH or hemorrhagic conversion of an ischemic infarction, but MRI will show a diffusion defect in the area of intracellular cytotoxic edema. Medical workup is similar to that described for TIAs.

If the patient has an appropriate neurologic assessment, does not show blood on the CT scan, and presents for initiation of therapy within 3 hours of ictus, intravenous tissue plasminogen activator (tPA) has been shown in prospective randomized clinical trials to improve patient neurologic outcome with a finite but acceptable risk of ICH. For selective endovascular delivery of thrombolytics, this 3-hour therapeutic window can be extended to 6 hours for ICA distribution emboli or thrombosis and to 12 to 24 hours for posterior circulation vertebrobasilar disease.

A completed ischemic infarction contains a central area of irreversibly dead brain surrounded by an ischemic penumbra region of the brain with persisting marginal CBF. This ischemic penumbra region is susceptible to secondary ischemic injury with subsequent stroke enlargement if blood flow is not maintained to this region. Thus, overly strict blood pressure control is generally unwise in the setting of ischemic infarction, particularly for a patient whose brain is used to basal levels of hypertension. Generally, as long as coagulopathy is not present, and the spontaneous pressure levels are not malignant (roughly ≥200 mm Hg systolic), blood pressure should be allowed to seek its own desired level and hypotension should be avoided and treated.

The early mortality rate from completed and irreversible ischemic infarction is generally less than 20%, but can be as high as 33% for complete MCA distribution infarctions and as high as 50% for complete ICA distribution (ACA + MCA) infarctions. Death in these large strokes is usually from progressive edema, mass effect, elevated ICP, and herniation syndrome. Maximal edema and risk of death generally peak 3 to 5 days after the initial event. Decompressive craniectomy can be a lifesaving measure in these situations. All the previously mentioned methods of dealing with elevated ICP are employed.

Intraparenchymal Hemorrhage

IPH can result from hypertensive arteriolar disease, amyloid angiopathy, drug abuse, coagulopathy, AVM rupture, hemorrhage into a brain tumor, cerebral infection, or vasculitis. Hypertension, amyloid angiopathy, and drug abuse (especially cocaine and methamphetamine) are currently the most common causes. IPH usually presents with symptoms of headache, nausea, or vomiting associated with a sudden new neurologic deficit. Level of consciousness is much more likely to be affected in these patients than in patients with ischemic infarctions. The mortality rate for IPH is much higher than that for ischemic infarction and currently exceeds 50%, despite aggressive efforts at intervention.

Hypertensive Hemorrhage

Hypertensive hemorrhage typically occurs in patients with a prior history of hypertension. Patients usually have systolic blood pressures of 190 mm Hg or higher (often

≥200 mm Hg systolic). Common locations for hypertensive hemorrhage parallel the locations for lacunar infarctions and include, in decreasing order of frequency, the basal ganglia (putamen most common), thalamus, brain stem, deep cerebellar nuclei, and deep hemispheric white matter. Multiple prospective randomized clinical trials, including the recent surgical treatment for ICH trial, have shown that the neurologic damage is done by the tissue trauma caused by the initial hemorrhage and that routine surgical primary clot evacuation does not improve neurologic outcome or survival. Generally, most neurosurgeons currently reserve primary clot surgical evacuation for three special circumstances: (a) when the clot is in the cerebellum and is large enough to cause direct brain stem compression, as well as obstructive hydrocephalus; (b) when the patient has a normal level of consciousness, deteriorates while an inpatient, and can be in the operating room with surgery initiated in less than an hour; and (c) younger, healthier patients with good neurologic function who present with clots 300 mL or greater in volume. Short of primary clot evacuation, surgical insertion of a ventriculostomy is often indicated to relieve or prevent obstructive hydrocephalus in cases of smaller cerebellar clots and cases of IPH with intraventricular extension and to serve as an ICP monitor to guide best medical therapy. Unlike in ischemic infarctions, there is no significant at-risk ischemic penumbra area surrounding the IPH. The major risk is clot enlargement through rebleeding. Thus, careful blood pressure control with titrated intravenous infusions and strict control of coagulopathy are critical steps. Encouraging preliminary results are also being reported for using concentrated recombinant factor VII as a means of preventing clot enlargement over the first 24 to 48 hours after presentation.

Amyloid Angiopathy

Amyloid angiopathy is a vasculopathy characterized by fragile cerebral arteries resulting from amyloid protein deposition in the vessel wall, which appears as apple-green birefringence with polarized light under the microscope. It predominantly occurs in older adults and is positively associated with Alzheimer disease. Indeed, at least 50% of patients with amyloid angiopathy IPH have a prior history of symptomatic dementia. Amyloid hemorrhages tend to be subcortical and lobar in location. The parietal lobe at the parietal-occipital junction is most common, followed by the frontal lobe. The hemorrhages can be quite large but are often remarkably well tolerated because of preexisting cerebral atrophy. Surgical intervention is generally reserved for clots 30 mL or greater in patients with good neurologic condition. The best functional outcomes are achieved in patients who have clots in the nondominant hemisphere but who do not have any baseline dementia. Given the underlying vasculopathy present throughout the brain, it should not be surprising that amyloid hemorrhage resection cavities carry a much higher recurrent hemorrhage risk than other surgical resection (SR) cavities.

Arteriovenous Malformations

AVMs are usually congenital. They consist of multiple arteriovenous communications that form a knot of feeding arteries and draining veins within brain tissue (Figure 28-7). Because of the abnormal structure of the vessel walls and the direct communication between the feeding and

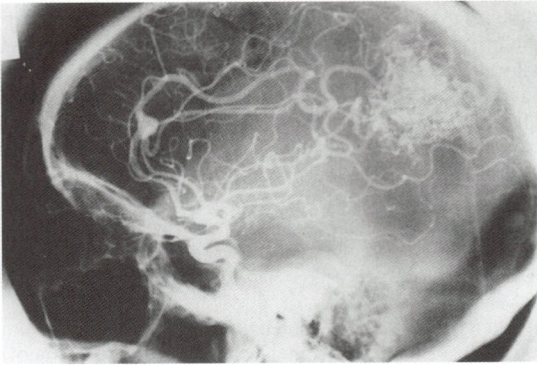

Figure 28-7. Lateral angiogram of a parietal arteriovenous malformation. An aneurysm is located proximally on an enlarged feeding vessel. (From Lawrence PF. *Essentials of Surgical Specialties*. 3rd ed. Lippincott Williams & Wilkins; 2007.)

draining vessels, clinical signs of rupture are common. The second most common presenting symptom is a seizure. Bleeding is typically intraparenchymal rather than subarachnoid and is approximately 2% to 3% per year for typical AVMs. Hemorrhage usually occurs from the thinner-walled venous portion of the malformation that still contains arterial pressure blood. AVMs with accentuated risks of hemorrhage include those with venous outflow obstruction and those with associated feeding artery aneurysms. Potentially curative treatment includes stereotactic radiosurgery, or microsurgical excision, and, rarely, endovascular embolization. Surgical morbidity and mortality for AVMs are related to the size of the lesion, the eloquence of the brain involved, and the presence or absence of deep venous drainage to the vascular nidus. Stereotactic radiosurgery leads to myointimal cell proliferation on the

vascular channel walls, eventually leading to complete nidus occlusion in approximately 75% to 80% of cases over a period of 3 years. Endovascular embolization of AVMs is only rarely curative. It can, however, serve a temporizing protective role against initial rehemorrhage, as well as assist in optimizing the safety and efficacy of subsequent radiosurgery or microsurgical excision.

Aneurysmal Subarachnoid Hemorrhage

Unruptured berry (saccular) aneurysms tend to occur at vascular bifurcations and tend to project in the direction that the blood would have gone without the bifurcation present. Much rarer forms of cerebral aneurysms include fusiform aneurysms (often atherosclerosis associated) and infectious aneurysms (mycotic aneurysms). Approximately 2% to 3% of people in the US general population are thought to have berry aneurysms at any given time. They are named after the main branch occurring at their point of origin. Anterior circulation aneurysms are more common (85%) than posterior circulation aneurysms (15%), and, depending on the series reporting, either aCom A or pCom A aneurysms are most common (Figure 28-8). Aneurysms are multiple in 20% of cases, with bilateral mirror aneurysms most commonly affecting the MCA, followed by the intracavernous ICA. The tendency for aneurysms can run in families, particularly for patients with multiple aneurysms. The annual rate of rupture for berry aneurysms greater than 9 mm in diameter is estimated to be 2% to 3% per year, but is estimated to be 1% or less per year for aneurysms less than 1 cm in diameter.

Aneurysmal SAH is characterized by a sudden onset of severe headache often associated with immediate loss of consciousness. In those with milder forms who do not lose consciousness, nausea, vomiting, stiff neck, photophobia, and drowsiness are common symptoms. Approximately

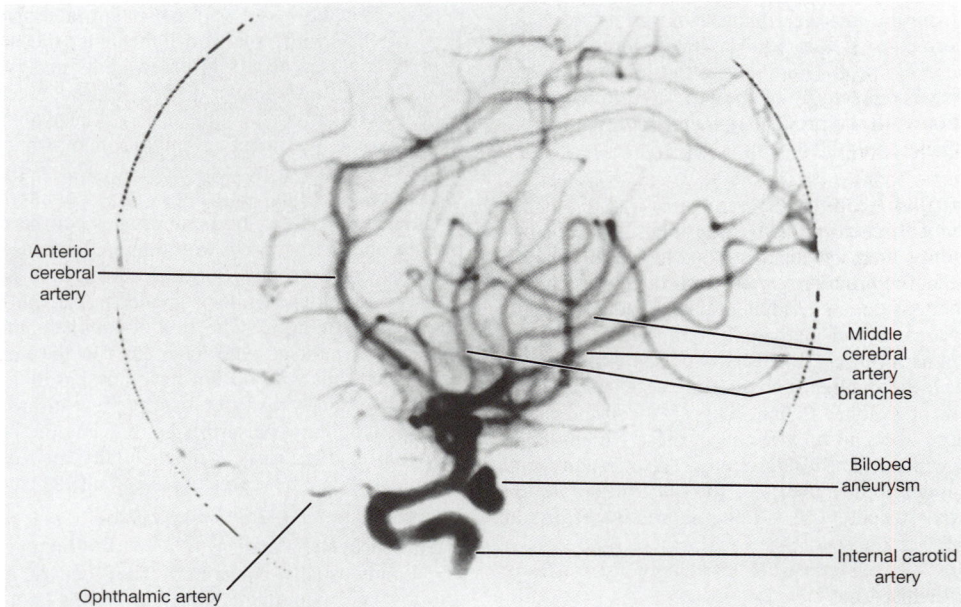

Figure 28-8. Internal carotid artery with an aneurysm in the posterior communicating artery. (From Lawrence PF. *Essentials of Surgical Specialties*. 3rd ed. Lippincott Williams & Wilkins; 2007.)

50% will have a history of a probable "sentinel bleed" marked by transient severe headache 1 to 2 weeks before their current SAH. The remaining patients presenting with normal level of consciousness may actually be presenting with their sentinel bleed. Examination may reveal meningismus, and funduscopic examination may reveal hemorrhages. Approximately 35% of patients with aneurysmal SAH die before they reach a hospital or before they can be stabilized. Another 40% will die or remain functionally dependent from a neurologic deficit as a result of rebleeding or ischemic vasospasm injury. Only 25% of patients will return to a functionally independent state after aneurysmal SAH. CT scanning is approximately 90% effective in detecting acute SAH, and sensitivity can be increased to approximately 95% to 98% by performing an LP in patients with a highly suggestive history but a negative or equivocal CT scan. CT angiogram can rapidly determine whether a cerebral aneurysm is present and guide subsequent treatment decisions. SAH is an extremely dangerous condition.

The initial risk of a ruptured aneurysm is the risk of rehemorrhage if the aneurysm is not sealed by either microsurgical clipping or endovascular coiling. Rehemorrhage is statistically maximal in the first 12 to 48 hours after initial hemorrhage. The mortality rate of a rehemorrhage is approximately 50%. The next risk after SAH is ischemic deficit from delayed vasospasm, which tends to begin 3 to 10 days after SAH and usually resolves by 2 weeks after SAH. The third risk is from the development of hydrocephalus from RBCs and subsequent CSF debris interfering with arachnoid villi CSF absorption. Clinical outcome after SAH and the subsequent risk of vasospasm are directly related to the patient's clinical condition on presentation (Hunt-Hess clinical grades 1-5) and the degree of blood present in the basal cisterns on CT scan (Fisher grades 0-3).

Patients diagnosed with SAH are admitted to the intensive care unit and are given phenytoin to prevent seizures and nimodipine (an oral calcium channel blocker) to help prevent vasospasm. An arterial line to monitor and strictly control blood pressure and a central line to monitor and optimize intravascular volume are usually needed. If hydrocephalus is present, consideration is given to placing a ventriculostomy without allowing rapid ventricular decompression. Until the aneurysm is protected by coiling or clipping, the patient is protected from anxiety, stress, or straining by being placed in a quiet environment and given anxiolytics, stool softeners, and analgesics as needed. If intubated, the patient is premedicated before any endotracheal suctioning.

Initial clinical decision making usually centers on deciding whether to take the patient urgently to surgery or to have an angiogram performed. Angiography provides a better determination of anatomic detail and information as to the technical possibility of endovascular coiling. Because microvascular clipping is known to be both definitive and permanent, patients who are young, with uncomplicated anterior circulation aneurysms, and who are in good clinical condition (Hunt-Hess grades 1-3) are more often treated with microsurgical clipping. Patients who are older, have significant medical problems, have complex or posterior circulation aneurysms, and who are in poor clinical condition (Hunt-Hess grades 4-5) tend to undergo endovascular coiling. In the future, an increasing number of aneurysms may be treated by endovascular means, thus avoiding craniotomy, if the early success rates prove to be durable over the long term. Endovascular coiling and stenting techniques continue to evolve and improve in this nascent field of aneurysm treatment.

Once the aneurysm is protected from rerupture, the focus shifts to preventing and detecting vasospasm. Nimodipine is continued while daily transcranial Doppler cerebral artery velocities are monitored for upward trends that would indicate vasoconstriction. Intravascular volume is expanded to optimize cardiac preload and to optimize blood viscosity for small-vessel rheology purposes through hemodilution down to a hematocrit of 30 to 32. If symptomatic vasospasm develops, the patient is treated with vasopressors to elevate systolic blood pressure to 160 mm Hg or greater. Vasospasm is best confirmed by cerebral angiography, which can also allow for endovascular treatment with either chemical (selective intra-arterial papaverine or a calcium channel blocker) or mechanical angioplasty with a soft balloon. Continued CSF drainage at this point can lower ICP and maximize CPP for a given MAP. Ultimately, approximately 20% of surviving patients will require a ventriculoperitoneal (VP) CSF shunt for persisting or delayed hydrocephalus. Delayed hydrocephalus usually presents 4 to 8 weeks after SAH and is characterized by a loss of cognitive and consciousness recovery milestones.

Brain Tumors

Brain tumors are classified as either primary (arising from the brain, cranial nerves, and surrounding meninges) or secondary (metastasizing to the brain from primary cancer elsewhere). Primary brain tumors can be further characterized by being either primary parenchymal tumors (either neuronal-glial or immune system in origin) or extraparenchymal. Pediatric primary brain tumors are also often considered a separate category. Symptoms from brain tumors can arise from brain tissue destruction, brain tissue mass effect, or dysfunction resulting from compression by the brain tumor mass or associated vasogenic edema. The latter two causes are potentially reversible with surgical decompression of mass effect and treatment of vasogenic edema with steroids, respectively. Symptoms from brain tumors usually arise either from generalized phenomena such as increased ICP from tumor mass, vasogenic edema, hydrocephalus (eg, headache, nausea, vomiting, papilledema, diplopia), or seizures (if the lesion is cortical and supratentorial). More specific symptoms relate to the area of the brain involved and commonly include motor weakness, sensory deficits or paresthesias, speech deficits, visual field cuts, ataxia, endocrine dysfunction, or deficits in other higher cortical functions. Seizures occur in 26% of cases of brain tumors, and a new-onset seizure in an adult should be considered to indicate a potential brain tumor until proven otherwise.

MRI is the test of choice for evaluating brain tumors. However, CT scanning and cerebral angiography can provide complementary information regarding the presence of calcium; bone or skull erosion, destruction, or involvement; tumor vascularity; and the relationship of the mass to important cerebral blood vessels. These neuroimages indicate whether the tumor is intrinsic or extrinsic to the brain, show its location, and suggest its histology (Figure 28-9). Stereotactic biopsy is often helpful in establishing the cell type and in confirming the diagnosis (Figure 28-10).

Secondary (Metastatic) Brain Tumors

Metastatic brain tumors are increasingly more common than primary brain tumors (see Figure 28-9C). They have an annual incidence of 36/100,000/y. There are more than 100,000 new patients with metastatic brain tumors diagnosed every year in the United States. At the time of clinical diagnosis, approximately 37% to 50% of patients present with a single lesion and 50% to 63% have multiple tumors. Lung cancer is the most common CNS metastasis, closely followed by breast cancer in women. Melanoma is the most common histology to present with multiple lesions, and renal cell is the most likely histology to present with a single lesion. Most patients present with brain metastasis within 6 months to 2 years of the diagnosis of their original primary tumor. Symptoms of the metastatic brain tumor led to the initial discovery of cancer in 15% of cases. Approximately 43% to 60% of these patients will have an abnormal chest x-ray film, either from a primary lung tumor or from additional pulmonary metastases. In 1% to 5% of cases, the primary source of the metastasis is not found in the initial workup. Melanoma, choriocarcinoma, renal cell carcinoma, and thyroid carcinoma are the

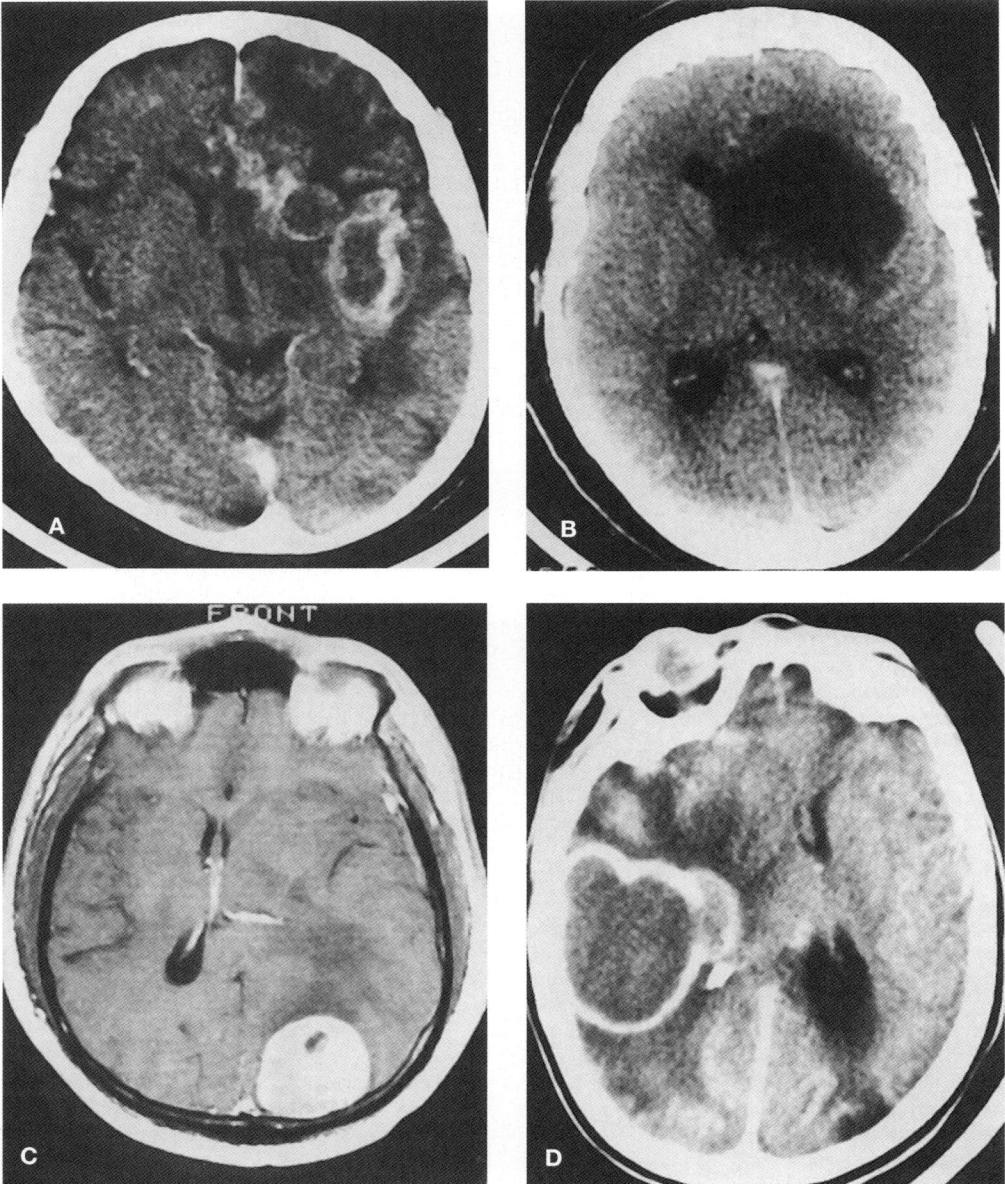

Figure 28-9. Enhanced computed tomography scans showing brain disorders. A. Glioblastoma multiforme. B. Low-grade astrocytoma. C. Metastatic melanoma. D. Brain abscess. E. Meningioma. (From Lawrence PF. *Essentials of Surgical Specialties*. 3rd ed. Lippincott Williams & Wilkins; 2007.)

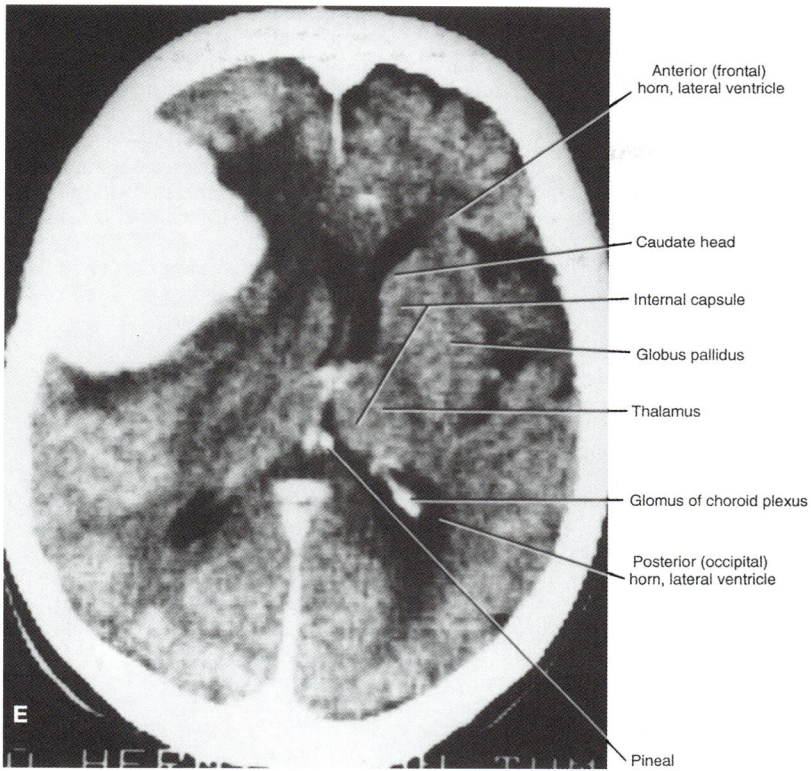

Anterior (frontal) horn, lateral ventricle

Caudate head

Internal capsule

Globus pallidus

Thalamus

Glomus of choroid plexus

Posterior (occipital) horn, lateral ventricle

Pineal

Figure 28-9. (*continued*)

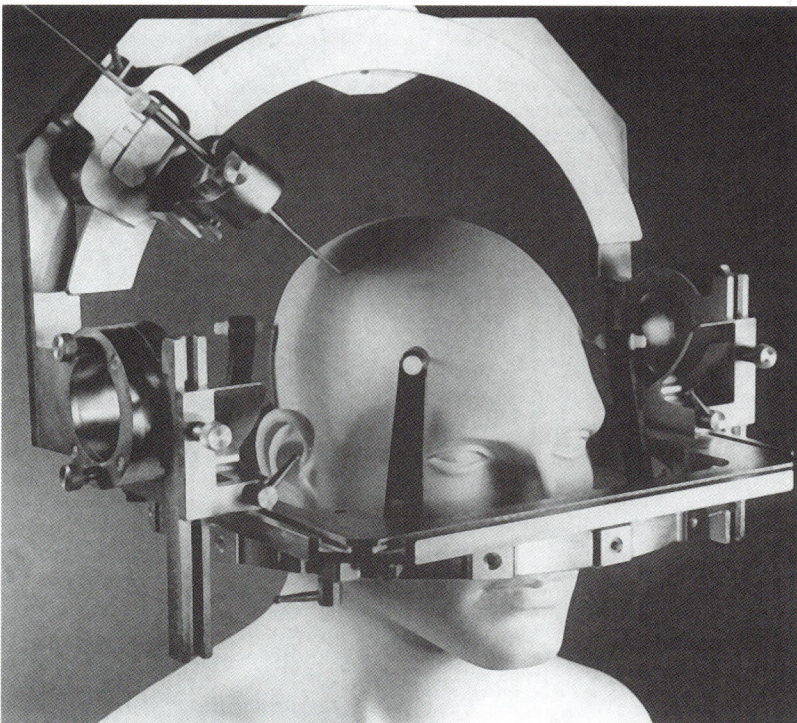

Figure 28-10. Stereotactic biopsy. (From Lawrence PF. *Essentials of Surgical Specialties*. 3rd ed. Lippincott Williams & Wilkins; 2007.)

most common histologies to present with an intratumoral hemorrhage. As systemic therapies for breast, lung, and skin cancers improve, the incidence of brain metastasis is likely to increase as patients with these cancers continue to survive longer in systemic therapies.

Primary Brain Tumors

Primary brain tumors have an annual incidence of 9.9/100,000/y. Primary parenchymal brain tumors constitute 63.6% of the total and primary extraparenchymal tumors 36.4%. Primary parenchymal tumors are predominantly malignant tumors and include tumors of glial origin (~97%) and primary CNS lymphoma (PCNSL ~3%). Glial-origin tumors are truly benign in only 18% of cases. The remaining tumors consist of low-, intermediate-, and high-grade glial malignancies. All PCNSLs are malignant. On the contrary, only approximately 5% of primary extraparenchymal brain tumors are malignant. The majority are benign tumors and include meningiomas (65%), cranial nerve schwannomas (18%), pituitary tumors (16%), and craniopharyngiomas (2%).

Benign brain tumors are often best treated with surgical excision, which can be curative. If they are small enough and have an appropriate relationship to surrounding sensitive structures, many benign tumors can be treated with stereotactic radiosurgery. Most malignant brain tumors can also be treated with varying combinations of fractionated radiotherapy and chemotherapy, with varying degrees of success. Long-term survival (>5 years) and cure are unfortunately rare for most malignant brain tumors.

Glial Tumors

Glia are the supporting cells in the CNS, and the overwhelming majority of primary parenchymal brain tumors are gliomas. Astrocytes are the structural scaffolding of the CNS neuropil. They serve as metabolic nurse cells for the neurons and help maintain extracellular ionic, neurotransmitter, and metabolic homeostasis. Oligodendrocytes manufacture myelin and provide electrical insulation for axons. Ependymal cells line the ventricular system. They are important in maintaining the CSF barrier and have a role in CSF physiology and homeostasis. Both neurons and glia originally derived from a common multipotential stem cell that went on to differentiate into a glial-restricted precursor cell and a neuronal-restricted precursor cell. Ependymal cells diverged earliest from the glial-restricted precursor cell, leaving oligodendrocytes and astrocytes to develop from a bipotential progenitor cell. Primitive neuroectodermal tumors (PNETs), medulloblastomas in the posterior fossa, and pineoblastomas in the pineal gland are believed to arise from a multipotential neuronal-glial stem cell.

Gliomas include astrocytomas (most common), oligodendrogliomas, mixed oligo-astrocytomas, and ependymomas. All categories are classified by the World Health Organization (WHO) into numeric grades of malignancy on the basis of histologic criteria: grades II to IV for astrocytoma and mixed oligo-astrocytoma and grades I to III for oligodendroglioma and ependymoma. It is thought to be the natural disease history for most low-grade gliomas to progress over time to a higher grade. Grade III histologic astrocytomas are often referred to as "anaplastic," and high-grade gliomas are termed "malignant." A grade IV malignant astrocytoma is also known as a "glioblastoma multiforme" (GBM; see Figure 28-9A).

In general, the prognosis for patients with gliomas is related to the histologic grade of the tumor, functional clinical status (Karnofsky Performance Status), and patient age (younger do better) in descending order of importance. GBM is one of the most malignant tumors of the brain. Median survival with surgery-fractionated radiotherapy and chemotherapy is only 12 to 13 months, with only 12% alive at 2 years and 2% to 5% alive 5 years after diagnosis. Recently, clinical trials of concomitant temozolomide chemotherapy during radiotherapy and continuous temozolomide chemotherapy after radiotherapy have been completed, and these have shown an improved median survival. Low-grade, anaplastic, and malignant oligodendrogliomas have now been shown to respond well to chemotherapy with either PCV (procarbazine, Lomustine, and vincristine) or temozolomide. For malignant gliomas, molecular biomarkers are becoming increasingly important for estimating prognosis as well as selecting therapy. Examples include isocitrate dehydrogenase mutation in glioblastoma, loss of heterozygosity on chromosomes 1p and 19q, which predicts chemo responsiveness of oligodendrogliomas, and methylguanine O'6'-methyltransferase promoter methylation, which predicts the accentuated responsiveness of anaplastic astrocytoma and GBM (WHO grades III and IV) to concomitant temozolomide and fractionated radiotherapy.

Unlike other malignancies in the body, gliomas rarely metastasize. They have a tendency to recur locally (95% recur within 2 cm of the original resection cavity) but also show a remarkable tendency for individual tumor cells to display impressive migratory and tissue invasion potential. Preferential pathways for invasion and migration include functional white matter connections of the area of the brain where the tumor developed as well as along the basement membranes of blood vessels and the ependymal lining of the ventricles. It is this tendency toward diffuse normal functional tissue invasion that frustrates surgical attempts at a more radical cure. CSF spread is most common with PNETs and ependymomas, but can rarely occur in other gliomas late in their clinical course.

Primary Central Nervous System Lymphoma

The incidence of PCNSL is rising, presumably because of the rising incidence of HIV infection in the world. In the United States, 50% of PCNSL is now associated with AIDS. The majority of PCNSL is B cell in origin. When it is diagnosed, it is important to check the patient's fundi, because up to 20% will have associated involvement of the eye. PCNSL is a nonsurgical disease that has an excellent and dramatic initial imaging response to either chemotherapy or fractionated radiotherapy. Unfortunately, this response is not durable over the long term. Surgery is usually limited to stereotactic needle biopsy. Currently, chemotherapy is usually tried first in an attempt to delay the potential cognitive side effects of radiotherapy, especially if intrathecal chemotherapy is used along with systemic chemotherapy. Intrathecal CSF therapy is indicated if CSF cytology is positive or if the ventricular lining or meninges is obviously involved on an MRI scan.

Extraparenchymal Benign Tumors

Meningiomas are benign tumors that arise from arachnoid cap cells (see Figure 28-9E). They are multiple in about 10% of cases and can rarely be associated with genetic conditions such as neurofibromatosis type 2 (chromosome 22) or meningiomatosis. They can arise from the dura of the convexity, the dura of the falx or tentorium, the dura of the skull base, or the arachnoid cap cells in the choroid plexus of the ventricles. They can directly involve adjacent bones (hyperostosis). Because they arise from the dura, meningiomas commonly have an ECA blood supply via meningeal branches. Meningiomas are benign 92% of the time, anaplastic 6% of the time, and malignant 2% of the time. Benign meningiomas can be treated with SR, ideally with resection of all the tumor, all the attached dura, and all the adjacent bone (Simpson grade 1 resection). Neuroimaging recurrence rates are 15% to 20% at 10 to 20 years for patients where Simpson grade 1 or 2 resection can be achieved. Recurrence rates are very high for Simpson grades 3 to 5 resections. Endovascular embolization preoperatively can assist with limiting surgical blood loss. Additional alternative therapies include stereotactic radiosurgery if the tumor is small enough and sufficiently distant from radiation-sensitive brain structures. Certain tumor locations and/or structural involvements limit the ability to achieve a Simpson grade 1 or 2 resection, including cavernous sinus involvement, involvement of the posterior two-thirds of the sagittal sinus, and involvement of the torcula or transverse sinus. In these cases, subtotal resection followed by stereotactic radiosurgery for the residual tumor in the high-risk area is an alternative treatment strategy that maximizes the preservation of neurologic and cranial nerve function. Radiation therapy is advisable in most cases of anaplastic and malignant meningioma, even after complete resection. Chemotherapy with hydroxyurea has been utilized for patients with malignant meningioma with some degree of success in a subset of responsive patients.

Vestibular schwannomas are the most common cranial nerve schwannoma and the most common tumor of the cerebellum pontine angle. Unilateral tumors are sporadic, whereas bilateral vestibular schwannomas are usually diagnostic for neurofibromatosis type 2. These tumors arise from Schwann cells of the vestibular nerve at or inside the internal auditory canal (Figure 28-11). The patient usually has a history of unilateral tinnitus with vertigo that disappears as the vestibular nerve is destroyed. As the tumor grows into the cranial cavity at the cerebello-pontine angle, pressure on the auditory nerve eventually leads to deafness, which usually begins as a preferential high-frequency hearing loss on the audiogram. The function of the adjacent, equally stretched facial nerve (motor) is preserved until very late in the course. Unilateral sensorineural hearing loss with impairment of taste on the same side is highly suggestive of vestibular schwannoma. As the tumor grows, it involves the fifth cranial nerve with facial numbness and eventual loss of the corneal reflex. Ultimately, cerebellar signs (staggering gait, veering toward the side of the lesion) and ninth and tenth cranial nerve deficits (ie, hoarseness, dysphagia, aspiration) occur. Microsurgical treatment options include resection by way of a retrosigmoid, translabyrinthine, or middle cranial fossa approach. Hearing can be spared only by way of the retrosigmoid or middle cranial fossa approach, but the latter approach is typically used only for very small tumors. Microsurgical cranial nerve preservation rates vary according to tumor size and the experience of the skull-base surgical team. Stereotactic radiosurgery is an alternative to micro SR for tumors 3 cm or less in diameter. Ten-year neuroimaging control rates for current tumor doses are 90% for unilateral vestibular schwannomas. Cranial nerve preservation rates exceed those of microsurgery for all, but the

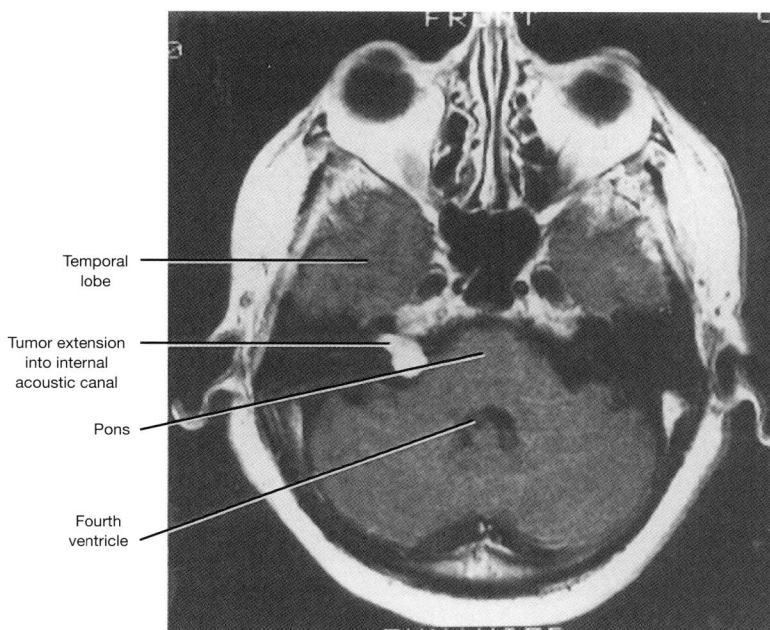

Temporal lobe

Tumor extension into internal acoustic canal

Pons

Fourth ventricle

Figure 28-11. Enhanced magnetic resonance imaging showing an acoustic neuroma. (From Lawrence PF. *Essentials of Surgical Specialties.* 3rd ed. Lippincott Williams & Wilkins; 2007.)

smallest intracanalicular, tumors. Fractionated stereotactic radiotherapy has been shown in the literature to be able to treat larger tumors with the likelihood of improved hearing preservation rates.

Pituitary adenomas can be functional (hormone secreting) or nonsecretory. They are classified as either microadenomas (<1 cm diameter) or macroadenomas (≥1 cm diameter). Most secretory adenomas are diagnosed while they are still microadenomas because of the presence of hormone-related symptoms such as menstrual irregularities, galactorrhea, frontal sinus bossing, enlargement of hands and feet, and coarseness of facial features. Most nonsecretory tumors are not diagnosed until they become macroadenomas and cause visual symptoms from downward pressure on the optic chiasm (bitemporal hemianopsia) or cranial nerve symptoms from invasion of the cavernous sinus (Figure 28-12). Rarely, pituitary tumors present with sudden-onset headache, visual loss, and Addisonian crisis from sudden pituitary infarction or hemorrhage (pituitary apoplexy).

The most common functional tumor of the pituitary is prolactinoma, which causes amenorrhea-galactorrhea syndrome in women and impotence in men. Somatotrophic tumors secrete excess growth hormone and cause acromegaly. In addition to coarsened features, prognathism, and hand and foot growth, patients have hypertension, diabetes mellitus, and myopathy, including cardiomyopathy. Corticotrophic tumors secrete adrenocorticotropic hormone (ACTH) and cause Cushing disease. In addition to truncal obesity, buffalo hump, striae, and easy bruising, these patients have hypertension, diabetes mellitus, and myopathy. These changes are caused by an excess of circulating cortisol because of an excess of circulating ACTH. Gonadotrophic tumors secrete follicle-stimulating hormone or luteinizing hormone. They are rare and cause sterility, loss of libido, and impotence.

Many secretory pituitary tumors can be treated medically (bromocriptine for prolactinoma, somatostatin for acromegaly, and ketoconazole for Cushing disease) with both hormone reduction and some tumor shrinkage. Unfortunately, because these tumors require lifelong therapy, some patients become intolerant of the drug and others are concerned with preserving fertility. In these settings, consideration should be given to either the microsurgical or endoscopic transsphenoidal approach for tumor resection. Apparent complete removal of the microadenoma is accomplished in approximately 85% of cases. The recurrence rate is approximately 20% after 5 years. Hormonal cure is less common and approaches only 50% to 60% at 5 years.

For macroadenomas, SR affords the opportunity to decompress the optic pathway, often leading to dramatic visual improvement, which can usually be accomplished transsphenoidally. Craniotomy is generally reserved for rare firm and adherent tumors and for extensions of the tumor lateral to the ICA or up into the root of the Sylvian fissure. For pituitary adenomas, stereotactic radiosurgery is usually reserved for cavernous sinus residual disease, recurrence, or cases in which the patient refuses open surgery and there is at least 2 mm of space separating the top of the tumor from the optic pathway. The risk of hypopituitarism varies according to the ability to visualize and spare the normal gland and stalk during stereotactic radiosurgery.

Cerebral Infection

Cerebral infection is quite common worldwide as a cause of cerebral mass lesions. Although the most common intracranial mass lesion in the United States is tumor, in Mexico, it is a parasitic infection known as "cysticercosis," and in India, it is tuberculoma. Even in the United States, infectious bacterial meningitis is common in the

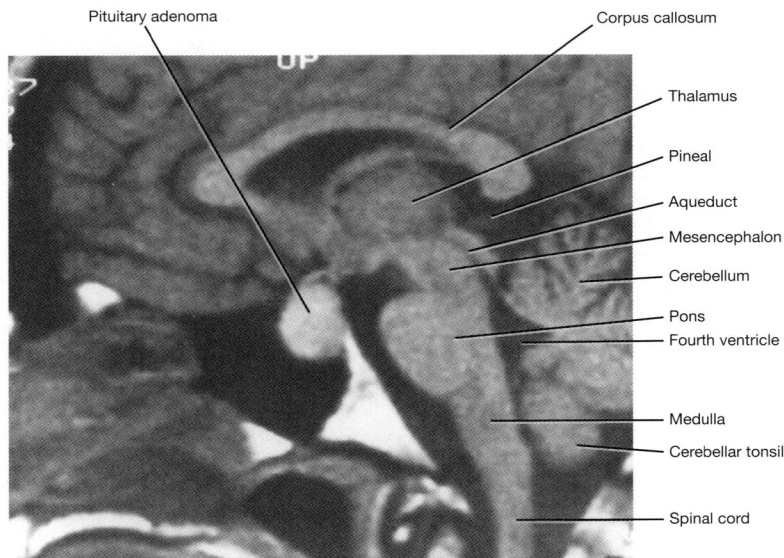

Figure 28-12. **Midsagittal enhanced magnetic resonance imaging showing pituitary adenoma.** (From Lawrence PF. *Essentials of Surgical Specialties.* 3rd ed. Lippincott Williams & Wilkins; 2007.)

pediatric age group and among young people clustered together for the first time (eg, schools, military barracks). Primary CNS viral infection is the rule rather than the exception in patients who are HIV positive. Infections can be characterized by their organism of origin (eg, bacterial, fungal, viral, parasitic, and prion). Although specific medical antimicrobial therapy is the mainstay of treatment, surgery occasionally plays a role in helping with confirming the correct diagnosis, as well as managing the complication that can arise from disease progression or evolution.

Meningitis, Tuberculosis, and Subdural Empyema

Community-acquired, infectious bacterial meningitis most commonly arises from *Streptococcus pneumoniae* (pneumococcus), *Haemophilus influenzae*, *Neisseria meningitidis,* and *Staphylococcus aureus*. The disease is most commonly seen in children, young adults newly collectively domiciled, and in older adults. *H. influenzae* is the most common organism in young children, *N. meningitidis* and *S. pneumoniae* are the most common in adolescents and young adults, and *S. pneumoniae* is the most common in older adults. Gram-negative bacilli such as *Escherichia coli* and *Klebsiella pneumoniae* should be considered in infants (<1 month of age). Acute suppurative meningitis can lead to an altered level of consciousness, cerebral edema, seizures, central and cortical venous thrombosis, and hydrocephalus. It can lead, rarely, to subdural empyema.

Tuberculosis can manifest as cerebral mass lesions (tuberculoma or tuberculous abscess) or tuberculous meningitis. Tuberculous meningitis tends to be much more clinically indolent and insidious than pyogenic bacterial meningitis. It tends to affect the basal arachnoid cisterns with basal meningitis and can also lead to hydrocephalus.

If postmeningitic hydrocephalus is bacterial in origin, it is treated with external ventricular drainage until the infection is cleared, at which time a permanent VP shunt may be necessary if the hydrocephalus has not resolved. Hydrocephalus from tuberculous meningitis usually requires the placement of a VP shunt even before the infection is cleared. Antituberculous agents are administered throughout the perioperative and postoperative period, and the infection can take 12 to 18 months to clear.

Subdural empyema is an emergent neurosurgical condition. These patients appear ill and febrile. They often have recurring or refractory seizures, despite antibiotics and anticonvulsants. CT scans and MR scans usually show an enhancing subdural fluid collection. MR is superior to CT for detecting subdural empyema because the volume of fluid collection can be subtle, and MR can directly image in the coronal plane. Treatment is urgent surgical evacuation of the purulent matter and continued antibiotics. Evacuation can usually successfully be performed with irrigation between strategically placed burr holes, and conversion to craniotomy for fenestration of loculations is occasionally necessary. Subdural empyema is a very serious clinical condition. Despite surgical intervention and aggressive medical therapy, mortality rates approach 21% to 35%. Seizures occur in the first few postoperative days in almost 50% of cases. The long-term, serious, disabling morbidity rate is reported to be approximately 20%.

Cerebral Abscess

Pyogenic brain abscesses evolve over approximately a 2-week period. At first, localized cerebritis occurs with the inoculation of bacteria into the brain. As polymorphonucleated white blood cells (WBCs) and lymphocytes invade, necrosis progresses concentrically. Initially, the process is not walled off, and cerebral edema is maximal. Approximately 10 days later, a reticulin matrix develops and walls off the central zone of necrosis (pus) and inflammation. Two weeks or more after inoculation, a mature collagen wall forms around the pus. Intracranial abscesses are usually found in the cerebrum, but may also be found in the cerebellum. In approximately 80% of cases, the source of infection is identifiable. Previous surgery and penetrating head trauma account for approximately 10%. Another 20% are extensions from adjacent localized cranial infections (eg, sinusitis, mastoiditis, dental infection). A further 20% have a cardiac source (eg, valvular or congenital heart disease). In congenital heart disease, right-to-left shunts and pulmonary AVMs are common predisposing causes because they bypass the filter of the lungs. Hematogenous spread from infected loci elsewhere in the body accounts for 30%. Another 5% of cases (rapidly increasing in number) occur in patients who are immunocompromised because of organ transplants or AIDS.

The cause of infection depends on the source. Multiple organisms are common. Abscesses that arise after surgery or penetrating trauma are usually caused by *S. aureus, Staphylococcus epidermidis,* or *Streptococcus*, although gram-negative infections are increasing. Brain abscesses that arise from distant hematogenous sources, as well as paranasal sinus, mastoid, or inner ear infections, are usually caused by anaerobic *Streptococci*, although *Bacteroides* or other species are often present as well. Many cerebral abscesses are polymicrobial (and should be assumed to be so) and treated with empiric broad-spectrum aerobic and anaerobic, as well as gram-positive and gram-negative, antibiotic coverage until disproven by aerobic and anaerobic cultures.

The classic symptoms of brain abscess are headache, fever, and focal neurologic deficits. However, this triad is found in fewer than 50% of patients. Headache is the most common symptom (70%-90%) and may be accompanied by nausea and vomiting. Fewer than 50% of patients have a fever, which is usually low grade. There is usually little elevation of the sedimentation rate or peripheral WBC count. An abscess acts like any other cerebral mass lesion with surrounding vasogenic edema. Increased ICP can cause obtundation or confusion. Focal neurologic deficits depend on the location of the abscess. Seizures occur in approximately 30% of cases. Symptoms are those of a brain tumor, but evolve more rapidly; 75% of patients have symptoms for less than 2 weeks. Intraparenchymal abscesses tend to extend toward the ventricles. Intraventricular rupture, increased ICP, and local brain destruction are the major causes of disability and death.

Evaluation of the patient with headache and neurologic change begins with the realization that the suspected mass lesion could be a brain abscess or tumor. A history or finding of sinus, middle ear, lung, or other infection; recent head trauma; or cranial surgery is sought. Inquiry and examination should include the possibility of rheumatic and especially congenital heart disease, previous cardiac surgery, hemoptysis, immune compromise, or drug abuse. The presence of one or more of these factors suggests a brain abscess rather than a brain tumor. Fever should alert the examiner to the possibility of brain abscess, but its absence should never lead the examiner to dismiss the diagnosis.

Brain scans have helped decrease the mortality rate from 30% to 40% to approximately 5% to 10%. CT or MRI scanning permits rapid diagnosis, localization, and identification of multiple abscesses. A uniform thin, enhancing wall surrounding a low-density core (see Figure 28-9D) suggests, but does not prove, the diagnosis. LP has little role in diagnosis or management because it decreases the pressure beneath a mass lesion and encourages infratentorial herniation, which could lead to disastrous outcomes. Further, the CSF is usually sterile, with few or no WBCs, unless the abscess is a secondary complication of bacterial meningitis (rare). In a significant number of patients, aggressive antibiotic therapy alone will resolve the infectious process in cerebritis, immature abscesses, and abscesses less than 1 cm in diameter. Trials of primary medical therapy should be carefully monitored by serial neurologic and neuroimaging examination to confirm evolution toward resolution. Surgical intervention is performed for patients with larger, mature lesions and for patients with small lesions or immature abscesses that progress despite aggressive primary medical management.

Stereotactic aspiration (see Figure 28-10) under local anesthesia has evolved into one of the main treatments for brain abscesses, particularly if the abscess is not readily accessible, is small, is associated with congenital heart disease that makes general anesthesia risky, or there are multiple lesions. Each lesion is punctured by a needle or catheter, and the contents are aspirated and sent for aerobic, anaerobic, fungal, and acid-fast bacilli cultures. Care is taken to aspirate slowly and gently and not to withdraw more than 50% of the preoperatively calculated volume of each lesion for fear of precipitating a hemorrhage from the collapsing wall, which contains fragile neovascularity. A drainage catheter is left in each abscess cavity and connected to gravity drainage to allow the abscess to spontaneously drain out any remaining pus over the next few days. The catheters are gradually withdrawn every day, over several days, once spontaneous drainage stops. Using this technique and culture-directed antibiotics, more than 90% of bacterial abscesses can be cured without disrupting the surrounding brain tissue. Open surgery is now usually reserved for cases of stereotactic failure, abscess recurrence, or those in which a skull-base defect with fistula is presumed to be the cause, thus requiring primary repair to prevent recurrence. Corticosteroids are usually reserved for patients who have significant and symptomatic mass effect and edema because steroids will also suppress the patient's immune response.

Chiari Malformations

Chiari malformations are congenital abnormalities of the posterior fossa. Cerebellar development is characterized by an extension of cerebellar tissue (the tonsils) through the foramen magnum to obstruct normal CSF flow, inhibit normal instantaneous equilibration of CSF pressures between the cranial and spinal CSF compartments, and place pressure on the dorsal medulla and upper spinal cord, which can

become symptomatic. Disruption of CSF flow and pressure equilibration dynamics can lead to secondary spinal cord or brainstem syrinx formation, which can also be symptomatic.

Chiari I malformation is characterized by tonsillar displacement greater than 5 mm through the foramen magnum into the spinal canal. In severe cases, the end of the tonsils can be as low as the C2 or C3 level. It is associated with a reduced posterior fossa compartment volume, a low insertion of the torcula onto the skull, and a steepened tentorial angle rising up to the tentorial incisura. Syringomyelia is common with significant caudal displacement of the tonsils but rare in minor cases (Figure 28-13). Chiari I malformations usually do not become symptomatic until adolescence or adulthood unless symptoms from an associated spinal cord syrinx (eg, scoliosis) or tethered cord syndrome supervene during a growth spurt. Symptoms are broad and can include varying combinations of posterior occipital headaches radiating upward (usually worse with Valsalva maneuvers), tinnitus, hearing loss, imbalance, oscillopsia from nystagmus, hiccups, nausea, dysphagia, hoarse voice, dysarthria, and bilateral hand numbness (presumably from dorsal pressure on the gracilis and cuneatus nuclei in the upper spinal cord at the top of the dorsal columns).

Chiari II (Arnold-Chiari) malformation is uniquely associated with myelomeningocele. In addition to the reduction in posterior fossa volume, this syndrome is associated with intrinsic congenital migrational abnormalities of the brain stem including tectal beaking and actual physical kinking of the medulla. The brain is maldeveloped, with hypoplasia of the lower cranial nerve nuclei as well as cerebellar and cerebral microgyria and heterotopias common. Hydrocephalus occurs because the fourth ventricular outlet foramina are obstructed and because aqueductal stenosis is common. Syringomyelia may occur as well. Both the tonsils and lower vermis of the cerebellum can descend down into the spinal canal and the caudal extent of descent can reach inferiorly as low as C3-C5. The onset of symptoms from Chiari II malformation may occur in infancy, childhood, or even adult life. In infants, symptoms include opisthotonos (extensor posturing with an arched spine), difficulty swallowing, regurgitation, stridor, and apnea. In children and adults, the manifestations are classified as brainstem (dysphagia, bulbar speech), cerebellar (nystagmus, oscillopsia), and upper motor neuron (hemiparesis, quadriparesis). In addition, syrinx, if present, can become symptomatic and cause lower motor neuron weakness in the upper extremities. The patient may also have a hanging sensory deficit over the shoulders that can extend to the arms and chest, sparing the lower body. With Chiari II malformations, surgery is often necessary to decompress the brain stem and reopen the foramen magnum CSF pathways as the patient develops the symptoms. Multiple studies have now shown that once patients become symptomatic, syndrome progression can be rapid, and once the function is lost, it is not likely to be recovered after subsequent decompression. Emphasis needs to be placed on preventing dysfunction in Chiari II patients, especially when they are infants and small children.

Epilepsy

Epilepsy is a condition involving repeated seizures over time. Idiopathic epilepsy usually presents in childhood. New-onset seizure in an adult should prompt a thorough

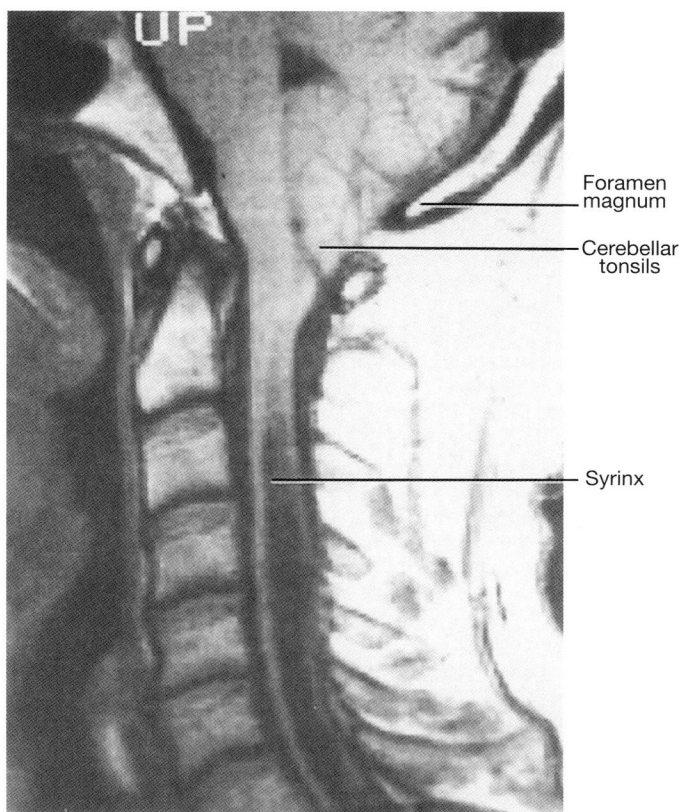

Figure 28-13. **Magnetic resonance imaging showing a Chiari I malformation.** (From Lawrence PF. *Essentials of Surgical Specialties.* 3rd ed. Lippincott Williams & Wilkins; 2007.)

workup to rule out cerebral mass lesions (eg, tumor, AVM, or abscess) or drug or alcohol abuse. Epilepsy can be considered to be lesional (ie, related to an image-defined mass lesion such as a tumor, heterotopia, AVM, or abscess) or idiopathic. Idiopathic epilepsy is usually associated with the primary neuronal focus that has developed a tendency toward electrical irritation and autonomous electrical activity. It can result from areas of prior brain injury where neurons become trapped in gliosis or scar (eg, prior head injury, encephalitis, meningitis, brain surgery) or can be an area of stunted CNS development (eg, mesial temporal sclerosis). Seizures can be simple partial, complex partial, partial with secondary generalization, or generalized (grand mal or petit-mal/absence). Most epilepsy is controllable with anticonvulsant therapy, and different medications work best for different types of seizures. Occasionally, multiple agents are required to control the disorder.

It is only when epilepsy becomes intractable and is significantly disabling to the patient that primary epilepsy surgery is considered. Intractability can be a slippery concept, but generally implies that adequate dose trials of at least three appropriate anticonvulsants for the particular seizure type have been tried, either solo or in combination, without success. Evaluation of a patient for potential epilepsy surgery involves standard diagnostic surface EEG and video-EEG monitoring to carefully confirm the type of seizure. MR neuroimaging is also used to assess anatomy

and rule out structural lesions. Functional testing is used to localize speech function and hemispheric dominance. Formal neurocognitive testing is often performed as a baseline for postoperative comparison. If seizure focus localization cannot be adequately assured with standard EEG, then invasive three-dimensional monitoring with subdural electrode grids, stereotactically implanted depth electrodes, or both may help confirm and define the precise point of seizure origin. The appropriateness of the patient for primary epilepsy surgery and the actual type of surgery attempted is usually decided by multidisciplinary epilepsy team consensus. Even if primary epilepsy surgery is not thought to be of help, some seizure control improvement can sometimes be obtained with the surgical insertion of a vagal nerve stimulator.

Primary epilepsy surgeries include standard temporal lobectomy, selective amygdalohippocampectomy, cortical resections guided by intraoperative electrocorticography, partial corpus callosotomy, subcortical disconnections, and functional hemispherectomy. Patients may undergo only one surgery or may receive a series of incrementally more invasive procedures in an effort to do the minimum necessary to control epilepsy. With carefully selected patients, a modern multidisciplinary epilepsy team can be expected to achieve epilepsy cure (no seizures, off all anticonvulsants) in up to 50% of patients. An additional group is either seizure free or significantly controlled with continued anticonvulsant use. Overall, at least 70% to 80% of selected patients can expect significant benefit from the process.

The effect on the quality of life, as well as subsequent cognitive function, is very significant. Unfortunately, it is estimated that less than 20% of patients who are potential candidates for epilepsy surgery are currently referred to an epilepsy center for surgical evaluation.

Movement Disorders

Movement disorders are usually related to abnormalities localized to the corpus striatum, the thalamus, and the subthalamic and red nuclei. Surgically treatable conditions include hemifacial spasm (HFS), Parkinson disease, other tremors of various types, dystonia, and athetosis.

HFS is a progressive disorder of the facial nerve and facial nerve nucleus that leads to unilateral rhythmic facial twitching of the facial musculature. It usually starts around the eye and then progresses over time to involve the lower face (in rare atypical situations, the reverse is true). Eventually, the spasms progress to involve the platysma and frontalis muscles. Tonus phenomenon occurs when the syndrome is severe. It consists of a titanic burst of repetitive muscle contractions without intervening relaxation that can grip the side of the face and hold it in a unilateral forced grimace smile while the eye is unable to open. Medications do not work for HFS. Peripheral injections of botulinum toxins can temporarily mask the muscle twitches in mild cases, but it does not prevent syndrome progression. Furthermore, chronic repetitive injections are required; there is a risk of epiphora; and injections in the lower face can lead to unwelcome facial weakness. Posterior fossa cerebellopontine angle exploration with microvascular decompression (both arteries and veins) of the centrally myelinated portion of the facial nerve as it leaves the brainstem (root entry zone) leads to a permanent cure of HFS in 80% of patients treated by an experienced surgeon.

With time, patients with Parkinson disease become refractory to pharmacologic agents and begin a progressive course of deterioration with worsened tremor, increased rigidity and bradykinesia, and changing on-off intervals. Stereotactic neurosurgical interventions can provide assistance when patients become refractory to medications. Stereotactic lesioning of select areas of the globus pallidus (pallidotomy) and thalamus (thalamotomy) can provide relief for both rigidity and tremor. More recently, efforts at selective thalamic stimulation after stereotactic insertion of stimulator electrodes have moved to the forefront for this condition. Stimulators have fewer complications, are reversible (they can be turned off), and are programmable in order to customize and titrate the desired response.

Dementia

Most causes of dementia are not surgically reversible. Normal pressure hydrocephalus (NPH) is an exception.

NPH is a clinical condition in which symmetric ventricular enlargement on CT or MR scan with normal ICP with diagnostic LP is associated with a triad of symptoms (gait disturbance, incontinence, and dementia) that improve or resolve with CSF diversion by VP shunting. They tend to occur in the order listed and tend to resolve in the same order. Once true dementia is present, the syndrome is advanced and complete resolution is rarely possible.

NPH must be distinguished from ex vacuo ventriculomegaly resulting from gradual brain loss (due to multiple ischemic insults, previous traumatic injuries, primary neurodegenerative disorder, or a combination of these three). This distinction is important because placing a VP shunt in an older patient with ex vacuo ventriculomegaly carries reported complication rates between 20% and 50%, with subdural hygromas and hematomas being the most common. Attempts to diagnose those who truly have NPH (symptomatic, shunt-responsive ventriculomegaly) from those with ventriculomegaly from other causes have included high CSF volume LP "tap tests," radionuclide CSF cisternograms, and MR CSF flow studies. None of these studies has proven to have an acceptable positive and negative predictive value. The situation is compounded by a very high placebo effect and anticipation bias for patients and families (particularly with the LP tap test), as well as a high evaluator bias on the part of the neurosurgeon or the neurologist.

The key to understanding patient selection with NPH is realizing that the syndrome must be shunt responsive. Therefore, the best test will either be a shunt or will accurately mimic a shunt. There are now two independent studies demonstrating that administering an ambulatory lumbar drainage test will correctly identify those patients who have a greater than 90% chance of therapeutic response with placement of a permanent shunt. The test involves placing a lumbar drain and setting it to withdraw CSF at VP shunt rates while the patient is independently evaluated for gait by a physical therapist (with video gait analysis and balance master objective testing) as well as for cognitive function by a speech therapist (using validated testing instruments) on a daily basis for 3 days. This test is currently the gold standard for assessing patients for NPH.

Although others have relied on empiric VP shunting, this practice is reported to have a high complication rate. Using a newer programmable shunt valve with the valve turned off at the time of insertion and then gradually turned on in an incremental manner over time may help reduce the risk over acute overdrainage with subdural hygroma and subdural hematoma formation.

SPINE AND SPINAL CORD DISEASE

Anatomy and Physiology

The spine develops segmentally from each somite during fetal development. It consists of seven cervical segments, 12 thoracic segments (each associated with a rib), five lumbar segments, and five sacral segments fused into one solid sacrum. It is composed of an anterior component that provides structural attachment for the axial skeleton and musculature, as well as the support necessary for upright ambulation. The posterior component serves a neural protective role. It consists of a spinal canal created by rings of bone extending posteriorly from each vertebral body (one pedicle and one lamina on either side) segmentally stacked upon one another (Figure 28-14). In between each segmental ring of bone is a neural foramen on each side through which passes the nerve root associated with each segment. Each vertebral segment can be considered a tripod with three joints. Anteriorly, the intravertebral disk serves as both a joint and an axial shock absorber. Posteriorly, paired facet joints on either side connect the pedicles and lamina above and below. The majority of cervical rotation occurs between C1 and C2 as well as between the occiput and C1. The majority of cervical flexion and extension occur between C2 and T1. The majority of thoracolumbar flexion occurs at T12-L2, whereas the majority of lumbar extension occurs at L4-S1. Both the cervical and lumbar segments have a natural lordosis, whereas the thoracic spine has a gentle kyphotic curve.

From a biomechanical stability standpoint, the spine can be considered to have three columns in the sagittal plane. The anterior column consists of the anterior longitudinal ligament and the anterior half of the vertebral body and disk. The middle column consists of the posterior half of the vertebral body and disk as well as the posterior longitudinal ligament. The posterior column consists of the paired facet joints and the interspinous ligament (extending between the spinous processes at each level). In general, a traumatic injury to the spine is considered to be unstable if it anatomically disrupts two of the three spinal columns.

The spinal cord continues down to the osseous L1-L2 level, at which point it ends in a terminal fibrous filum that

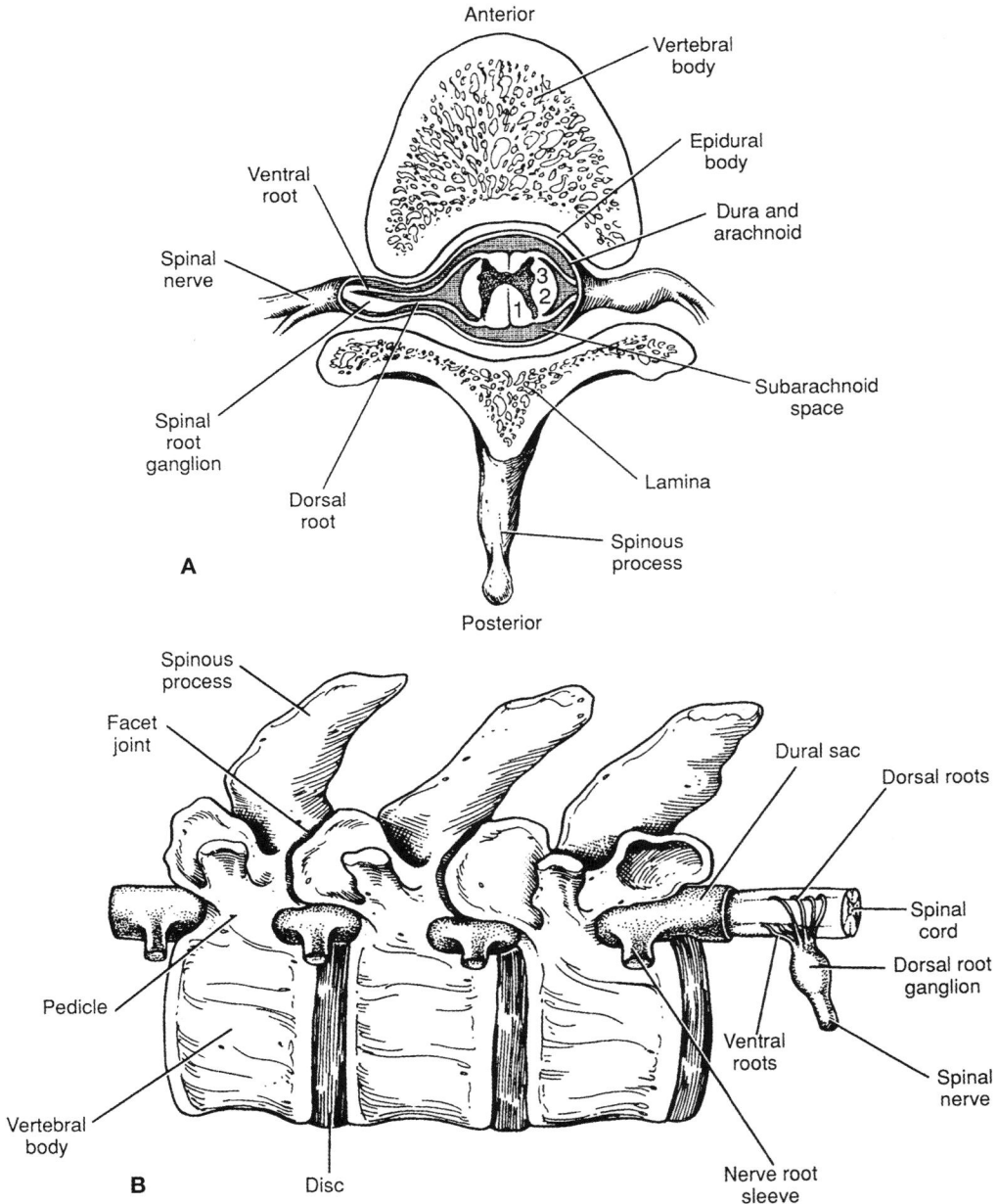

Figure 28-14. A. Spinal cross-section. *1*, Posterior column (position and vibration sense); *2*, posterolateral column (motor); *3*, anterolateral column (pain and temperature). B. Lateral view of the vertebral column and its contents. (From Lawrence PF. *Essentials of Surgical Specialties*. 3rd ed. Lippincott Williams & Wilkins; 2007.)

tethers it to the sacrum (filum terminale). From L2 down to S5, the lower spinal nerve roots continue downward within the dura of the spinal canal to the level of their foramen and exit as the cauda equina. The spinal cord extends from the foramen magnum to the lowest lumbar level in the newborn. As the child matures, the greater growth rate of the spinal canal causes relative ascent of the spinal cord within the canal. By adulthood, the tip of the cord reaches only as far as the top of L1-L2. If the cord is tethered at its distal end during development, it is stretched as the child grows. Neurologic deficit can result.

Unlike the brain, the spinal cord has white matter tracts on its outer surface with the gray matter internally. Each cord segment is bilaterally symmetric and innervates a specific body segment (dermatome, sclerotome, and myotome) through its paired segmental nerves. The lemniscal sensory pathway (vibration and joint position sense) runs dorsally in the dorsal columns. The pyramidal tracts run laterally, and the spinothalamic tracts (pain and temperature sense) run anterolaterally on either side. Each segment relays the sensory information that it receives from its dorsal nerve roots up to the brain, through ascending reticular and lemniscal systems. Correspondingly, the segmental motor output through the ventral roots is brought under voluntary control by descending suprasegmental systems to the motor neurons of each cord segment. The level and vector direction of any compressive spinal cord lesion can be determined from the relative involvement of these three tracts as well as the dermatome and myotome level determined by examination.

With degenerative spine disease (disk degeneration and herniation as well as facet arthropathy), symptoms can result from spinal canal stenosis, spinal foraminal stenosis, or a combination thereof. In the cervical and thoracic spine, **spinal stenosis** leads to symptoms of chronic partial spinal cord compression (myelopathy). In the lumbar spine, stenosis impinges upon the cauda equina and leads to a condition known as "neurogenic claudication." With neurogenic claudication, back pain, radiating leg pain, and other cauda equina nerve root symptoms manifest with ambulation and are relieved by rest and flexing at the waist to increase the lumbar canal midsagittal diameter. Foraminal stenosis, whether caused by compression by anterior disk herniation, anterior vertebral body osteophyte, and posterior facet joint osteophyte or by a combination of the three, leads to pain, sensory loss, reflex change, and weakness signs and symptoms originating from the one nerve root affected (radiculopathy).

The blood supply to the spine comes from paired segmental arteries that accompany the nerve roots through each spinal foramen. The branch to the osseous segment penetrates the bone at the pedicle and then branches ventrally to supply the posterior three-fourths of the vertebral body as well as dorsally to supply the lamina, transverse process, and spinous process. This osseous vascular arrangement helps explain why metastatic tumors to the spine, which arrive as arterial emboli, tend to establish themselves initially within the pedicle of the spinal segment. Vertebral body or lamina involvement usually occurs by secondary extension. Blood supply to the spinal cord continues on to pierce the dura along with the nerve roots to supply the single anterior spinal artery (which runs in the ventral midline and supplies the anterior two-thirds of

the spinal cord), as well as two smaller-paired dorsal spinal arteries that run over each dorsal column and together supply the posterior medial one-third of the spinal cord. The spinal cord segmental arteries are not symmetric at each level. Generally, several dominant radicular arteries provide the majority of the blood flow. In the cervical cord, the dominant contributors are the bilateral VA contributions to the anterior spinal artery, which come off after dural penetration and before they take off from the PICA. In the lower spinal cord, the dominant radicular artery is called the "artery of Adamkiewicz." It usually arises from the aorta on the left. It arises between T9 and L2 in 85% of patients. This artery is subject to injury with subsequent anterior spinal cord infarction during abdominal aortic aneurysm surgery. The vascular border zone between the major contributors to the anterior spinal artery (where the spinal cord is susceptible to ischemia in low-flow states) is usually located at T4-T5.

Evaluation

Spinal cord neurologic evaluation includes both long-tract and segmental assessments. Long-tract evaluations include the following: (1) assessing the integrity of the pyramidal tracts and noting any upper motor neuron findings (increased tone, spasticity, hyperreflexia, and upper motor neuron pathologic reflexes such as extensor plantar response or Hoffman sign); (2) evaluating the upper and lower-extremity distal joints for lemniscal pathway function (vibration—128-Hz tuning fork and position sense); (3) evaluating the upper- and lower-extremity distal joints for spinothalamic function (pain testing); and (4) evaluating for the presence of autonomic dysfunction (presence or absence of priapism as well as bowel bladder and sexual function). Segmental examination includes assessing the muscle groups, patches of skin sensation, and reflexes associated with each significant appendicular nerve root.

The brachial and lumbar plexuses mix nerve roots into peripheral nerves so that muscles and reflexes have some overlap in impulse origin. To assist with segmental examination, there are a few rules for major nerve root contributions. The C5 nerve root is the only root supplying the rhomboid muscle and is the dominant root to the deltoid. It is the dominant root to the biceps reflex and supplies the skin on the upper outside of the shoulder (shoulder patch). The C6 nerve root is the dominant root to the brachioradialis muscle and reflex and supplies sensation to the first two fingers (six shooters). The C7 nerve root is the dominant root to the triceps muscle and reflex and supplies sensation to the middle finger. The C8 nerve root is the dominant root supplying the intrinsic hand muscles (grip and finger abduction). It does not have a reliable reflex and provides sensation to the fifth finger (pinky). The L4 nerve root is the dominant root to the tibialis anterior (which dominates ankle dorsiflexion). It is the dominant root to the patellar reflex and supplies skin sensation on the medial calf down to the medial malleolus. The L5 nerve root is the dominant root to the extensor hallucis longus (great toe dorsiflexion). It does not have a reliably associated reflex and supplies skin sensation to the dorsal medial aspect of the foot (best tested in the first web space). The S1 nerve root is the dominant root supplying the gastrocnemius-soleus complex (controlling ankle plantar flexion). It is the dominant root to the Achilles reflex and supplies skin sensation to the ventral lateral aspect of the foot (best tested on the lateral aspect of the fifth toe).

Important clinical corollaries of these observations include noting that, with the exception of C5, all C6-C8 nerve roots extend below the elbow to the fingers for sensation. Therefore, with the exception of C5, arm pain should not be referred to as a "radicular pain" unless it extends down the arm to the fingers. Likewise, all L4-S1 nerve roots extend below the knee to the calf or foot for sensation. Therefore, leg pain should not be referred to as "radicular pain" unless it extends below the knee. Likewise, a straight leg raise test is not considered positive for L4-S1 nerve root stretch unless the pain produced radiates below the knee.

Anterior Spinal Cord Syndrome

Anterior spinal cord syndrome leads to bilateral dysfunction of the spinothalamic pathways and pyramidal tracts with sparing of the lemniscal pathways. This leads to upper motor neuron findings and pin sensation reduction or loss bilaterally below the level of the lesion with sparing of joint vibration and position sense bilaterally. The level affected is determined by the segmental dermatome, myotome, and reflex examination. The severity of compression and/or the depth of involvement are indicated by sparing versus dysfunction of the autonomic functions below the level of the lesion. Lesions that lead to variations of this syndrome include anterior spinal artery infarction, central disk herniation, ventral spondylotic myelopathy, spinal cord compression from a ventral meningioma, ventral compression from a spine tumor predominantly affecting the vertebral body, and ventral compression from an anterior canal burst fracture fragment.

Posterior Spinal Cord Syndrome

Posterior spinal cord syndrome leads to bilateral dysfunction of the lemniscal sensory pathways and pyramidal tracts with sparing of the spinothalamic pathways. This leads to upper motor neuron findings and vibration and joint position sense reduction or loss bilaterally below the level of the lesion with sparing of pin sharpness appreciation bilaterally. The level affected is determined by the segmental dermatome, myotome, and reflex examination. The severity of compression and/or the depth of involvement are indicated by sparing versus dysfunction of the autonomic functions below the level of the lesion. Lesions that lead to variations of this syndrome include posterior spondylotic myelopathy, dorsal epidural hematoma or abscess, spinal cord compression from a dorsal meningioma, dorsal compression from tumor metastasis to Batson plexus of epidural veins (eg, lymphoma), or in-driven lamina fragment after spinal fracture.

Lateral Spinal Cord Syndrome

Also known as Brown-Séquard syndrome, lateral spinal cord syndrome leads to unilateral dysfunction of the lemniscal and spinothalamic sensory pathways as well as the ipsilateral pyramidal tract. This leads to ipsilateral upper motor neuron findings and vibration and joint position sense reduction or loss below the level of the lesion along with contralateral pin sensation reduction or loss below the level of the lesion. The level affected is determined by the segmental dermatome, myotome, and reflex examination.

Careful pin examination may allow the detection of a thin band of a suspended sensory level to pin testing at the specific level of the lesion in the spinal cord. The severity of compression and/or the depth of involvement are indicated by sparing versus dysfunction of the autonomic functions below the level of the lesion. Lesions that lead to variations of this syndrome include lateral disk herniation, spinal cord compression from a lateral nerve root schwannoma, and compression from a spine tumor predominantly affecting the pedicle of the vertebra.

Central Spinal Cord Syndrome

Lesions in the center of the spinal cord (intramedullary tumors, syringomyelia) cause a loss of pain and temperature sensation at and just below the level of the lesion. An island of hypalgesia lies suspended between regions of normal sensation. This loss is caused by injury to second-order fibers that cross from the root entry zone to the contralateral anterior spinothalamic tract. As the lesion expands, the most medial aspects of the long fiber tracts are affected with spastic weakness, anesthesia, and dorsal column deficits that extend down from the level of the lesion.

Neuroimaging

The same general comments and observations noted about CT and MR scanning in the cranial and cerebrovascular regions (and discussed in that section) apply to the evaluation of the spine and spinal cord. MR is an excellent screening tool to assess the spine for canal mass, osseous spine tumor, disk herniation, spinal canal stenosis, and segmental foraminal stenosis. It is the imaging procedure of choice for assessing the spinal cord for diagnostic purposes, including syrinx, tumor, or tethering, and for assessing the spine for infection or ligamentous injury. It is good at showing changes in vertebral body bone marrow and paraspinal soft-tissue masses. CT scan is superior for assessing osseous fractures, facet joint alignment and integrity, and the presence of osteophytes, calcification of the posterior longitudinal ligament, or calcified spondylotic bars. CSF contrast myelography remains the best means of assessing nerve root sleeve CSF cutoff, confirming significant foraminal stenosis as well as assessing split spinal cord malformations. Spinal angiography remains the best means of detecting spinal AVMs or dural artery-venous fistulae. Each segmental spinal artery has to be individually and selectively sampled with the endovascular catheter in order to have a complete study. Plain spine films still have a role in the initial assessment of spine trauma and are a good screening tool for spine involvement with metastatic tumor. Bone scans are also an excellent screening tool for spine involvement with metastatic tumor as well as spine infection and compression fractures.

Spine Trauma

Spine trauma includes ligamentous injuries, spine fractures, fracture dislocations, acute disk herniations, and incomplete and complete spinal cord injury.

Trauma Evaluation

Patients with spinal cord injury should be assessed to determine whether their injury is complete or incomplete, according to the long tract and nerve root schemas outlined in Table 28-4. Careful sacral examination is very important because sacral sparing may be the only sign of an incomplete lesion and may go unnoticed if the sacral area is not carefully assessed. The presence or absence of priapism should be noted, and rectal tone, bulbocavernosus reflex, abdominal reflexes in all four quadrants, and the cremasteric reflexes should be carefully assessed. In addition to the neurologic examination, examination of the spinal column includes palpation for deformity, tenderness, and spasm as well as tests of mobility are performed only when radiographs confirm that no further injury would result from them. These tests include flexion, extension, rotation, and tilting of the neck and back.

Radiographs of the spine provide information about vertebral anomalies, displacement, destruction or remodeling, and disk space narrowing. Ninety percent of the diagnostic information gleaned from a simple A-P, lateral, and open-mouth trauma c-spine series is contained in the lateral view. It must have adequate technique and show the spine all the way down to the top of the T1 vertebral body. An additional swimmer's view is sometimes required to see this low. If no change is obvious, but the patient has significant symptoms or findings, or if some changes seem to merit further investigation, CT with coronal and sagittal reconstructions or MRI scan is performed. An alternate study is myelography, with or without a subsequent CT scan. Myelography requires LP and may increase a neurologic deficit if the spinal canal is significantly compromised because of tumor or abscess. In these cases, no CSF is removed, and the amount of contrast material injected is small. Trauma myelography is now only rarely performed at most medical centers. If the patient has normal imaging studies and a normal examination but still has neck pain, dynamic flexion-extension views are obtained. If the patient cannot perform an adequate flexion-extension study because of muscle spasm, the cervical collar is left in place for 7 to 10 days. The patient is restudied once the spasms have reduced.

Stabilization

Patients are kept in a hard cervical collar until their cervical spine can be officially cleared, both clinically and radiographically. Clearing of a cervical spine requires a normal radiographic study (trauma series plain films or a fine-cut CT scan with axial and coronal reconstructions), a normal exam, and a pain-free patient with a normal mental status, or a patient with persisting pain but with no abnormal motion on adequate dynamic films. Patients are kept on a long board until their thoracic and lumbar spines can be assessed with log rolling as well as screening A-P and lateral T-, and L-spine plain films.

Controversy currently exists as to whether patients with incomplete spinal cord injury should be treated with either 24- or 48-hour high-dose methylprednisolone infusions. Both have been shown to lead to marginally statistically significant improvement of an extremely small magnitude compared with the best supportive care without steroids in randomized clinical trials. However, the effect is very small in magnitude, barely reaches a significant level, and comes at the expense of a higher medical complication rate resulting from megadose steroid use. Currently, reasonable arguments can be made against high-dose steroid use for trauma, and the determination is left to the responsible licensed staff physician whether or not to employ them. There is no proven role for high-dose steroids in patients with complete spinal cord injury or a currently asymptomatic adult patient (despite a history of transient extremity paresthesias that previously resolved) with a normal examination. Additional stabilization measures include bladder decompression with a self-retaining catheter and maintaining oxygenation and systemic blood pressure. Systemic pressors such as dopamine are sometimes needed to maintain good spinal cord perfusion pressure in the face of a sudden loss of systemic vascular tone from neurogenic shock.

Spine Fractures

Spinal fractures include specialized fractures of the C1-C2 complex, fracture dislocations of the C3-C7 cervical spine, thoracic compression fractures, thoracolumbar compression and burst fractures, and lumbosacral fracture dislocations.

C1 (Jefferson) Fracture

A C1 Jefferson fracture is a fracture in two places of the atlas, usually caused by axial load injury. The fracture is inferred from lateral spreading of the lateral masses on open-mouth c-spine views. It is directly visualized on axial CT scan views. Forty percent of Jefferson fractures are associated with C2 fractures. Jefferson fractures rarely present with neurologic injury and usually heal with hard cervical collar immobilization for 3 months. After healing,

TABLE 28-4. Potential Complications of Spinal Cord Lesions at or Above Specific Levels

Level	Innervation	Potential Risks	Treatment
S2-S5	Sphincters	Retention, incontinence (urinary tract infection)	Bladder catheterization
L1-S2	Legs	Anesthesia and immobility (decubitus ulcers)	Careful, frequent positioning
T1-T12	Sympathetics	Temporary hypotension	Catecholamines
	Chest cage	Respiration (pneumonia)	Respiratory care
C5-T1	Upper extremities	Inability to perform self-care	
C3-C5	Diaphragms	Respiration (apnea, pneumonia)	Ventilatory assistance

the patient should be assessed with flexion-extension views to rule out C1-C2 instability from anterior C1-C2 ligamentous disruption.

C2 (Odontoid) Fracture

C2 odontoid fractures are transverse plane fractures through the stem of the axis that usually result from acute sudden extension as can occur when one falls forward like a tree trunk, with the forehead as the point of impact. Type II odontoid fractures occur right at the base of the odontoid peg. Type III fractures go down into the base of the body of C2, and type I fractures are avulsion fractures of the odontoid tip at the apical alar ligament insertion point. Type I and III lesions usually heal well with halo immobilization for 3 to 6 months. Type II odontoid fractures are more problematic. They have a high nonunion rate with halo immobilization because of tenuous vascular supply at this C1 and C2 somite fusion interface. Age plays an important role in determining the risk of nonunion. Generally, patients younger than age 40, who do not smoke and who have less than 4 mm fragment displacement, will likely heal with halo immobilization. For other patients, either halo immobilization or operative fusion can be employed. Surgical approaches for this lesion include anterior odontoid lag screw fixation (if the transverse check ligament is assessed to be intact), bilateral posterior transarticular screw fixation, or posterior C1-C2 interlaminar fusion.

C2 (Hangman) Fracture

C2 Hangman fracture (also known as C2 traumatic spondylolisthesis) is a bilateral pedicle fracture of C2, usually from acute hyperextension injury. Approximately 95% of these patients will be neurologically intact. The majority of these patients can be successfully treated with halo immobilization for 3 to 6 months. Rare cases with significant displacement and irreducible anterior angulation of the C2 on C3 may require operative fusion.

Subaxial C3-C7 Fractures

The majority of C3-C7 fractures are traumatic fracture dislocations (Figure 28-15). Exceptions are the clay shoveler's fracture, which is a stable isolated spinous process fracture resulting from hyperextension that usually heals well with a cervical collar. Another fracture dislocation is the anterior vertebral body corner tear-drop fracture, which also usually heals well with only collar immobilization.

Acute fracture dislocations usually result from hyperflexion injuries or hyperflexion injuries with axial loading. When an axial load is involved, there is usually an associated compression or burst fracture of the vertebral body, and there may be an associated fracture of the lamina. The flexion component often leads to disruption of the interspinous ligament posteriorly and can lead to either unilateral or bilateral jumped facets with anterior subluxation of the superior vertebral body in relation to the inferior vertebral body. Unilateral jumped facets can lead to a subluxation of up to a maximum of 25% vertebral body midsagittal width on lateral c-spine films. The A-P view is usually associated with misalignment of the spinous processes at this level because of the rotational component. Anterior subluxations greater than 25% of the vertebral body midsagittal width on lateral c-spine films should lead one to suspect bilateral facet dislocation.

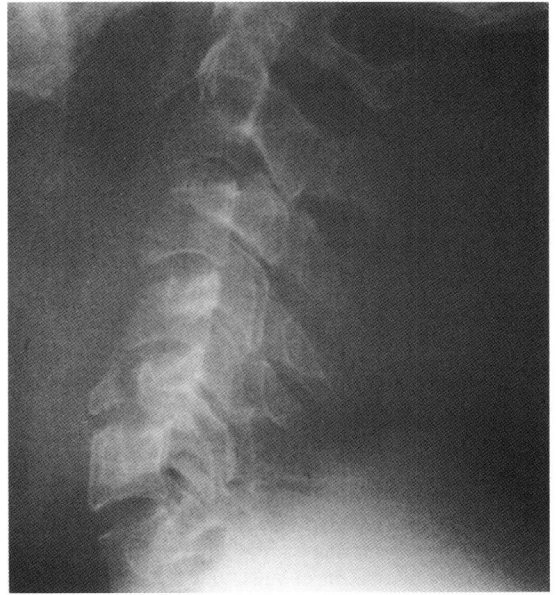

Figure 28-15. Fracture dislocation, C5 on C6. (From Lawrence PF. *Essentials of Surgical Specialties*. 3rd ed. Lippincott Williams & Wilkins; 2007.)

To rule out ventral herniated disc or hematoma with C3-C7 fracture dislocations, an MR scan is useful before the fracture is reduced. If there is no burst or compression fracture component likely to warrant intraoperative reduction through anterior corpectomy and cervical plate fusion, then an attempt at closed reduction may be made. After placing Gardner-Wells tongs percutaneously to pick-up the skull bilaterally above the ear canal, weighted in-line traction is gradually initiated along with muscle relaxants. It is customary to start with 5 to 10 lbs of traction and then proceed in 5-lb increments waiting for a minimum of 20 to 30 minutes between each weight change and checking a lateral c-spine film prior to each new weight increment to assess for the success of reduction or signs of overdistraction that might indicate ligamentous injury. Efforts continue until a maximum weight of 10 lbs per involved level is achieved or until reduction is successful. Successful reduction gains should be held by halo immobilization for 3 to 6 months. Failure to achieve reduction usually leads to surgical exploration and intraoperative reduction and fusion. This can be done anteriorly with an anterior cervical discectomy with plate fixation after reduction or posteriorly with lateral mass plating fusion and/or intralaminar fusion sometimes supplemented by an intraspinous process dorsal tension band reconstitution, depending on the anatomy of the associated fractures. Facet fracture is a common reason for the failure of closed reduction attempts. Very rarely, a C3-C7 three-column spinal fracture is so unstable as to require a 360° fusion both posteriorly and anteriorly.

Vertebral Artery With Cervical Fractures

Fractures involving the transverse foramen C2-C6 should raise the question of the status of the associated VA. Even cervical spine fractures not involving the transverse foramen can lead to VA occlusion or compromise caused by traumatic dissection. Although these injuries are rarely symptomatic because of the usual presence of a contralateral collateral VA, delayed embolization and posterior circulation stroke can occur. The VA should be examined for occlusion by means of a CT angiogram, MR angiogram, or cerebral angiogram before considering a posterior-lateral fusion with screws. Both C2-T1 lateral mass and C1-C2 transarticular screw fixation run a small risk of VA injury. If the VA injured is the only remaining VA supplying the brainstem, then significant problems could result.

Thoracic Compression and Burst Fractures

Vertebral body compression fractures are the most common mid-thoracic traumatic fractures. Because of the presence of the circumferential rib cage at T1-T10, these fractures usually heal well without surgery and only require an external thoracolumbar sacral orthosis (TLSO) to assist with pain control. Standing weight-bearing T-spine films should then be obtained. Surgical intervention should be considered for greater than or equal to 50% loss of body height and/or greater than or equal to 20° of kyphotic angulation, which are risk factors for progressive kyphotic angulation. Burst fractures are very rare in the T1-T10 thoracic spine, and operative indications include those for the compression fracture as well as greater than or equal to 50% spinal canal midsagittal canal compromise on axial CT scan.

Thoracolumbar Junction Compression and Burst Fractures

The thoracolumbar junction (T11-L2) is a point of maximum axial load as well as a pivot point for thoracolumbar flexion. As a result, it is particularly prone to compression and burst fracture resulting from axial load coupled with flexion. Compression fractures do not disrupt the posterior wall of the vertebral body, whereas burst fractures include the posterior wall and often lead to the retropulsion of bone fragments into the spinal canal. Surgical intervention should be considered for greater than or equal to 50% loss of body height and/or greater than or equal to 20° of kyphotic angulation, which are risk factors for progressive kyphotic angulation with either fracture type. An additional risk factor for progressive kyphotic angulation seen with burst fractures is greater than or equal to 50% midsagittal spinal canal compromise on axial CT scan. In the absence of these indications, additional surgical exploration considerations include three-column spinal disruption and canal compromise in a patient with an incomplete spinal cord injury. Surgical fusion can be done from the front with corpectomy and short-segment anterior-lateral plate; from the back with short-segment pedicle screw fixation with long-moment arm-chance screws utilized to maximize the chance of kyphotic correction, and anterior fragment reduction through ligamentotaxis (relying on the intactness of the posterior longitudinal ligament); from the back with long-segment fixation (two levels above and two levels below the injury); or from a combination of anterior and posterior approaches.

Thoracolumbar Junction Chance Fractures

More commonly, before the shoulder harness and airbags were added to the traditional lap belt in automobiles, the Chance fracture is the fracture that disobeys the three-column stability rule. It results from thoracolumbar hyperflexion and extension, leading to an axial plane fracture that goes through the pedicles and facet joints as well as either the vertebral body or the disk space. Paradoxically, these fractures are usually stable and can usually be treated with a TLSO brace for pain control followed by early mobilization. Surgical fusion can be considered if there is a need to explore the spinal canal for bone or disk fragments in the presence of a partial spinal cord injury, if the patient wishes to have more rapid active mobilization as part of a posttraumatic rehabilitation program, or if doubt remains about the fracture stability on the basis of anatomic concerns.

Lumbar-Sacral Fracture Dislocations

Lumbar-sacral fracture dislocations include traumatic L4-L5 or L5-S1 spondylolisthesis and combinations of vertebral body compression and burst fractures. These levels are below the level of the conus medullaris and thus do not risk spinal cord injury. The need for surgical fusion versus conservative management in a TLSO or lumbar-sacral corset is based on the same three-column injury anatomic criteria and progressive kyphosis risk criteria listed earlier. In addition, traumatic anterolisthesis greater than 25% as well as lateral plane and rotational dislocations are given careful consideration. Surgical fusion can be performed posteriorly, anteriorly, or in a 360° combination.

Spinal Cord Injury Sequelae

Patients with spinal cord injuries are very susceptible to urinary reflux, urinary infection, decubitus ulcers of the skin, pneumonia, deep venous thrombosis, and pulmonary embolus. They are also at risk for septicemia from pyelonephritis, pneumonias, or infected decubitus. Autonomic dysreflexia can be a dangerous cardiovascular reflex response to overly rapid or aggressive bladder decompression.

Patients with spinal cord injury must begin mobilization soon after stabilization. A proper bowel regimen is critical, and both bowel training with daily suppositories and bladder training with intermittent catheterization begin as soon as spinal shock resolves. Compression stockings, sequential compression devices, and subcutaneous heparin are used as prophylaxis against deep venous thrombosis. Careful pulmonary toilet is maintained (usually with the assistance of a Roto-Rest bed in patients with high quadriplegia). Regular nursing positioning, skin care, and special antidecubitus beds are utilized. Physical therapists and occupational therapists begin working with the patient at the bedside, as soon as possible. Ultimately, early transfer to an inpatient spinal cord injury facility is ideal.

Degenerative Spine Disease

Degenerative diseases of the spine include disk herniation, spinal osteoarthritis and stenosis, and spondylolisthesis.

Disk Degeneration and Herniation

The intervertebral disc is composed of the nucleus pulposus and the surrounding annulus fibrosis. Degeneration of the disk occurs when the nucleus pulposus becomes desiccated because of age or recurrent trauma. This can be readily detected as a "black disk" on a T2-weighted MR scan. In contrast, the herniation of a disk occurs when the nucleus pulposus is extruded through a tear in the annulus.

Extrusion usually occurs posterolaterally and often causes compression of a nerve root (radiculopathy). When it occurs centrally in the cervical or thoracic spinal canal, it can compress the spinal cord (myelopathy, anterior syndrome, lateral syndrome, or combination). Unlike disk herniation, disk degeneration is often asymptomatic.

Most symptomatic disk herniations occur in the lumbar or cervical regions. For the lumbar region, 95% occur at the L4-L5 and L5-S1 levels (point of maximal lumbar lordosis), with L3-L4 making up another 3% to 4%. Cervical disk herniation is also common, especially at the C5-C6 and C6-C7 levels (point of maximal cervical lordosis). C4-C5 and C7-T1 can also be affected. Symptomatic thoracic disks are uncommon, but may cause paraplegia. Bulging of a disk posteriorly beneath the posterior longitudinal ligament is often asymptomatic. Greater protrusion, with herniation and extrusion beneath or through the posterior longitudinal ligament, is likely to cause radicular pain and even neurologic deficit (Figure 28-16). Surgery for frank extrusion is more likely to relieve radicular pain than back or neck pain.

Symptoms of disk herniation almost always include pain, both in the spine and down one extremity. This pain is often exacerbated by straining, coughing, or sneezing, and by motion of the affected portion of the spine. Herniated discs and other cervical spine problems cause neck pain and often refer pain to in the scapular region, arm, and hand. Lumbar disk herniations produce low back and leg pain that is usually worse on weight bearing. This leg pain is characteristically sciatic. It radiates down the posterior or lateral leg into the calf or even to the foot. Signs of disk herniation include radicular numbness and weakness within the innervation of a single nerve root as well as reflex loss (Table 28-5).

Herniation of an L4-L5 disk usually compresses the L5 nerve root, although the L4 nerve root exits the spinal canal between the L4 and L5 vertebrae. Because the roots of the cauda equina leave the spinal foramina just above the corresponding disk, they escape compression by herniations of the disk. The root that begins to leave the dural sac at this level to exit the foramen below is at risk from the usual lumbar disk herniation.

The differential diagnosis of cervical disk disease (neck or arm pain) includes angina if the patient has left arm pain, cervical osteoarthritis and stenosis, upper limb nerve entrapment, tumor or infection within or adjacent to the spine, and shoulder and elbow disease. Corresponding considerations in the lumbar region include vascular claudication, hernia, gynecologic disease, abdominal aortic aneurysm, spinal or retropelvic tumor or infection, lumbar osteoarthritis and stenosis, lower limb nerve entrapment, and hip and knee disease.

Initial treatment of most patients is conservative. The exception is patients who present with foot drop, bowel or

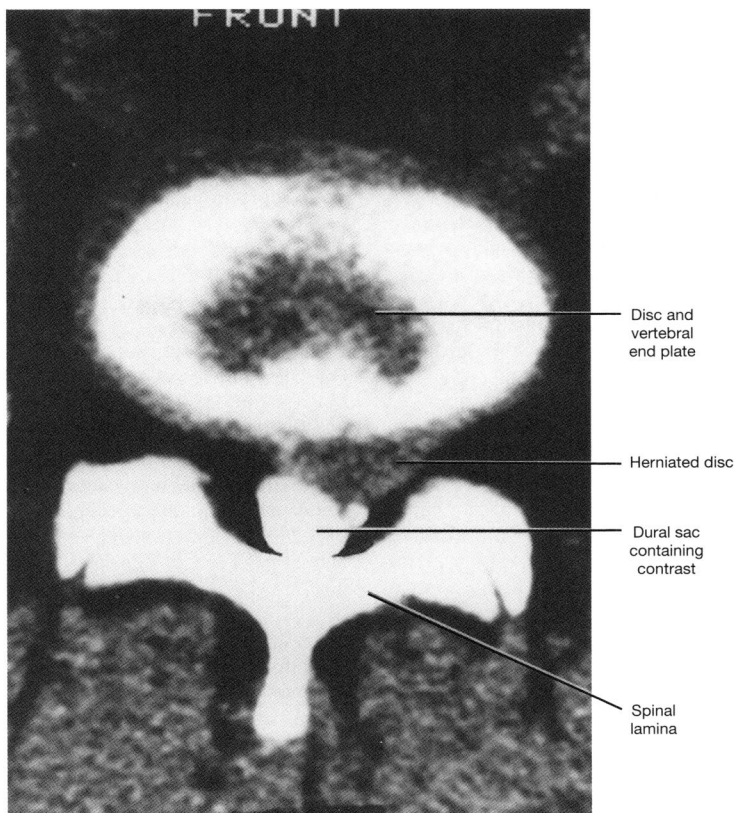

Figure 28-16. Positive contrast computed tomography showing a herniated nucleus pulposus at L5-S1. (From Lawrence PF. *Essentials of Surgical Specialties.* 3rd ed. Lippincott Williams & Wilkins; 2007.)

TABLE 28-5. Signs of Disk Herniation

Level	Root	Weakness	Reflex Loss	Numbness
C4-C5	C5	Deltoid	Biceps	Outer deltoid
C5-C6	C6	Brachioradialis	Brachioradialis	Thumb, index
C6-C7	C7	Triceps	Triceps	Middle
C7-T1	C8	Intrinsic hand	–	Pinky
L3-L4	L4	Tibialis anterior	Patella	Medial calf
L4-L5	L5	Extensor hallucis longus	–	Medial foot, first toe
L5-S1	S1	Gastrocnemius	Achilles	Lateral foot, left toe

bladder difficulties, or full-blown cauda equina syndrome or acute myelopathy. These patients should undergo urgent neuroimaging with consideration for early surgery if appropriate correlative abnormalities are identified. Initial conservative treatment consists of a short rest period for the symptomatic spinal segment, analgesics, anti-inflammatory agents, and possibly muscle relaxants. In the cervical region, treatment includes a collar to limit motion and may include traction. In the lumbar region, treatment consists of at least 24 to 48 hours of rest, followed by a gradual increase in activity and progressive physical mobilization as tolerated. As improvement occurs, the patient may resume normal activities, but should avoid excessive lifting or bending. If progress is slow, physical therapy may be added to the regimen. Surgery is considered only if the patient shows no further progress over a period of weeks, if the condition worsens, or if there is marked weakness.

Disk herniation is suspected when examination and history localize the lesion to a specific nerve root. Diagnosis is confirmed by an MR scan or myelo-CT scan. Back or neck pain with or without nonradicular arm or leg pain does not confirm that disk or foramen abnormalities seen on spine MR are the cause of the symptoms. Degenerative disk and spine abnormalities are seen in up to 70% of people in the United States over the age of 40. High confidence that the imaging abnormality is the source of the patient's symptoms requires clinical correlation with the correct affected nerve root.

Surgical treatment of disk herniation consists of microscopic or endoscopic excision. Standard techniques for lumbar or cervical discectomy include a posterior approach with limited removal of the adjacent lamina on the side of herniation, excision of the ligamentous flavum, gentle retraction of the nerve root, and removal of the underlying disk herniation. For cervical disk herniation, an anterior approach with or without spinal fusion with interposition bone graft and possible anterior cervical plate has become more common than posterior cervical discectomy. The disk is approached between the trachea and esophagus medially and at the carotid sheath laterally. The disk is excised through the anterior longitudinal ligament, back to and through the posterior longitudinal ligament. The herniated fragment is removed.

Good relief of radicular symptoms can be expected in more than 90% of patients with a clear radiculopathy that correlates with the lesion in question. Axial back and neck pain is less responsive, with complete relief in only 60% to 70% of patients. Surgery is successful less often if these conditions are not met or if the patient has had a previous operation.

Foraminal Compression Syndrome

Even without frank disk herniation, radiculopathy can develop from foraminal or lateral recess stenosis because of a combination of three-dimensional factors. Disk bulge or herniation as well as endplate osteophyte can compress from the front, whereas posterior compression from facet joint arthropathy compounds the situation from behind. Because of the common absence of frank disk herniation and the poor resolution of MR for bony anatomy, the extent of nerve root compression can be underestimated with isolated MR scanning. For this setting, plain CSF myelography with direct visualization of nerve root sleeve cutoff remains the most sensitive and specific test for confirming significant foraminal or lateral recess stenosis.

Treatment of this condition includes microscopic or endoscopic discectomy as described for disk herniation syndromes, but also critically depends on decompressive micro-foraminotomy to deal with the facet overgrowth and osteophyte compression. Results are equally effective so long as bony decompression is judicious and does not lead to spinal instability.

Cervical Stenosis

Cervical spinal canal stenosis leads to signs and symptoms of myelopathy. In cases of multilevel disk degeneration with chronic osteophyte formation, multiple segmental spondylotic "bars" can cause compression from a ventral vector. Degenerative thickening of the posterior ligamentum flavum often associated with ligamental folding and buckling with extension can lead to compression from a posterior vector. Ultimately, canal stenosis can be caused by a combination of ventral and dorsal factors. Patients are more susceptible to developing cervical stenosis with myelopathy if they are born with a congenitally tight cervical canal to start with, as a result of short pedicles bilaterally. Asians are particularly prone to a special stenotic syndrome known as "ossification of the posterior longitudinal ligament (OPLL)," which causes the posterior longitudinal ligament (PLL) to ossify (usually with the ventral dural incorporation into the bone formed).

Treatment of myelopathy from cervical stenosis involves enlargement of the cervical canal. For ventral vector spondylotic bar lesions, this can be done anteriorly with multilevel anterior discectomy and fusions or with vertebrectomy and strut graft instrumentation. Good results can be achieved with actual improvement in myelopathy in the majority of patients for segments extending up to three disks and two vertebral body lengths. Longer segments have a tendency to forfeit cervical lordosis and carry a higher incidence of graft and instrumentation failure. For posterior vector compression, a multilevel decompressive laminectomy with or without lateral mass fusion to prevent loss of cervical lordosis and subsequent swan-neck deformity can be done. Alternatively, a decompressive multilevel laminoplasty that reconstructs the posterior spinal canal with a larger diameter can be performed. Posterior decompressive operations can more easily be performed for disease affecting more than three motion segments (C2 or C3-C7 can be completed in the same sitting). Posterior decompressions usually stabilize the patient's clinical syndrome but are less likely than anterior decompressions to actually reverse the process. Patients with OPLL are now more commonly treated with posterior decompressions because of the relatively high risk of disabling anterior dural tears and subsequent CSF leak seen with an anterior approach to this difficult disease.

Preexisting cervical spinal stenosis can predispose patients to developing an acute central cord syndrome from sudden flexion-extension movements. If this occurs, the patient is immobilized in a hard cervical collar while the swelling of the spinal cord is allowed to resolve. Surgical decompression is performed in a delayed fashion to avoid the risk of further irritating an already damaged spinal cord.

Lumbar Stenosis

Lumbar stenosis develops from a progressive encroachment of the spinal canal from the ventral aspect (disk degeneration, disk bulge, and reactive osteophyte formation) as well as the two posterior-lateral directions (facet hypertrophy and arthropathy). These three compass points of encroachment can collectively so indent the dural sac that it comes to appear as a tricornered hat in cross-sectional diameter. The points of maximal compression are at the inferior level of each lamina, with interval widening between the rings of constriction. On lateral CSF myelogram, the thecal sac can come to look like a string of sausage links.

As the lumbar stenosis progresses, it puts pressure on the nerve roots at the level of the cauda equina. At rest, they may be asymptomatic, but with exertion such as walking, there is no room for the nerve roots to swell with increased blood flow necessary to meet their increased metabolic demands. This supply-demand mismatch leads to nerve root dysfunction and radicular symptoms (radiating radicular pain, numbness and tingling paresthesias, and myotomal weakness), which can affect multiple nerve roots bilaterally, and to lower back pain. These symptoms characteristically come on with walking and are relieved by rest, especially if the patient rests flexed at the waist (leaning over or sitting down) in such a way as to increase the midsagittal spinal canal diameter to provide the nerve roots with more room. With time and progression, the patient reports being able to walk shorter and shorter distances before having to stop to rest. This classic syndrome is called "neurogenic claudication" and must be distinguished from vascular claudication because of peripheral vascular disease.

Diagnosis is easily made on an MR scan or CSF myelogram/CT scan. Treatment consists of posterior decompression of the involved segments. Although simple multilevel decompressive laminectomy was the treatment of choice for many years, and usually led to dramatic immediate improvement, unintentional disruption of the large degenerated facet joints on one or both sides often led to subsequent need for lumbar fusion in approximately 10% of cases.

Spondylolysis and Spondylolisthesis

Forward slippage of one vertebral body on another (spondylolisthesis) most commonly occurs at the L4-L5 or L5-S1 level. Bilateral defects (spondylolysis) across the spinal lamina diagonally, just below the pedicle, allow the most rostrolateral part of each lamina, with the attached pedicle and vertebral body, to separate and shift anteriorly. The spinal canal is sometimes compromised. These shifts are most common in children and adolescents and tend to stabilize. Back pain and nerve root compression symptoms can occur in this younger age group. Adults, especially older adults, sometimes have spondylolisthesis without spondylolysis. In these patients, ligamentous laxity that accompanies osteoarthritic change permits slippage of adjacent vertebral bodies on one another to cause stenosis of the spinal canal. CT and MRI scans are extremely helpful in evaluating the patient and planning surgery. Operative stabilization and fusion may be necessary. Decompression is performed if there is a neurologic deficit or radicular pain. The nerve root involved is usually one above that is usually encountered for degenerative disk disease (L4 for L4-L5 and L5 for L5-S1 spondylolisthesis).

Vascular Spine Disease

Spinal Cord Arteriovenous Malformation and Dural Arteriovenous Fistula

Spinal vascular malformations are uncommon but are almost always AVMs, A-V dural fistulae, or cavernous malformations. Cavernous malformations occur within the cord, but AVMs may be located on the cord or within it. Dural A-V fistulae are always located adjacent to the spinal cord in intimate association with a segmental nerve root and its vascular pedicle. This relation to the cord defines the type and hazards of surgical treatment. Like tumors, lesions within the cord are more difficult to excise, and operation risks spinal paralysis to a far greater degree than operation on extramedullary AVMs. With dural A-V fistulae, the feeding arteries enter along the nerve root. Either surgical division of these feeders or, more recently, endovascular embolization of these feeders leads to cure. Vascular malformations of the cord often cause repeated attacks of spinal cord dysfunction or progressive spinal cord deficit. Spinal SAH is uncommon.

Spinal Cord Stroke

Stroke can affect the spinal cord from embolic occlusion of the anterior spinal artery or from border zone flow–related ischemia because of significant systemic hypotension or loss of a major segmental feeding artery such as the artery of Adamkiewicz. The cord is most susceptible to flow-related ischemia at the T4-T5 level. The artery of Adamkiewicz is most susceptible to sacrifice during surgeries to repair abdominal aortic aneurysms, but can also be lost during left-sided retroperitoneal approaches to the thoracolumbar junction to repair and stabilize thoracolumbar compression or burst fracture. The syndrome is an anterior cord syndrome that spares the dorsal lemniscal pathways. Recent evidence suggests that lowering ICP by continuous perioperative lumbar drainage can lower the risk of anterior spinal artery infarction and reduce the severity of any subsequent stroke. It may be that this phenomenon works by optimizing spinal cord perfusion pressure by lowering ICP.

Epidural Hematoma

Spontaneous spinal epidural hematomas are associated with ruptured aneurysmal bone cysts involving the osseous spine, the rupture of dural A-V fistulae, and iatrogenic coagulopathy. Iatrogenic epidural hematomas can be associated with LP, but are more commonly linked to the placement of epidural catheters for pain control and/or lower-extremity epidural anesthesia. In cases of abdominal aortic aneurysm repair performed under epidural anesthesia, neurosurgeons are often asked to distinguish catheter-related epidural hematoma from spinal cord infarction when the patient cannot move their legs postoperatively. The distinction is actually quite straightforward. Epidural hematomas lead to a posterior cord syndrome as opposed to the anterior syndrome seen with anterior spinal infarction. Even if the patient is intubated and sedated, somatosensory-evoked potentials will indicate whether dorsal lemniscal function is preserved. An MR scan should be able to distinguish a dorsal hematoma from edema within the substance of the spinal cord. Epidural hematomas are treated with urgent correction of any coagulopathy that may be present. If they are small and asymptomatic, they can be treated conservatively with observation. If they are symptomatic with cauda equina syndrome, conus medullaris syndrome, or any other cord compressive syndrome, they are surgically evacuated.

Spine Tumors

Spinal tumors are divided into three groups. These groups differ somewhat in age of presentation and prognosis. Extradural tumors arise from the osseous element of the spinal column (Figures 28-17 and 28-18). Intradural extramedullary tumors arise from the dural sheath around the spinal cord or from the Schwann cell sheath around the spinal roots. Intramedullary tumors arise from the glial element of the spinal cord or from trapped ectodermal elements. Presenting symptoms of spinal tumors can be a variation of any of the spinal cord syndromes described previously. Characteristically, they are also associated with back pain that is worse lying down, worse at night, and especially worse in the morning. A history of belt-like radiation of intercostal pain with the Valsalva maneuver is also highly suggestive.

Secondary (Metastatic) Extradural Tumors

The most common spinal tumors in adults are extradural and are usually metastatic (Figure 28-19). Metastases grow rapidly and usually cause symptoms of spinal cord compression that last from hours to a week. Most are carcinomas. Common primary lesions are located in the lung, breast, prostate, and kidneys. With the exception of lymphoma (which predominantly affects the dorsal and lateral epidural space), these tumors usually destroy the bone. They compress the spinal cord either by growing in the epidural space or by causing collapse of the involved vertebrae. This collapse causes distortion, narrowing, and instability of the spinal column. Radiologic evaluation starts with plain spine films. Extradural (metastatic) tumors destroy bony elements. X-rays may show vertebral collapse that spares the disk spaces, but not the cortical end plates. Often there is a loss of one or more pedicles (the winking owl sign—see Figure 28-19A). If plain x-rays appear

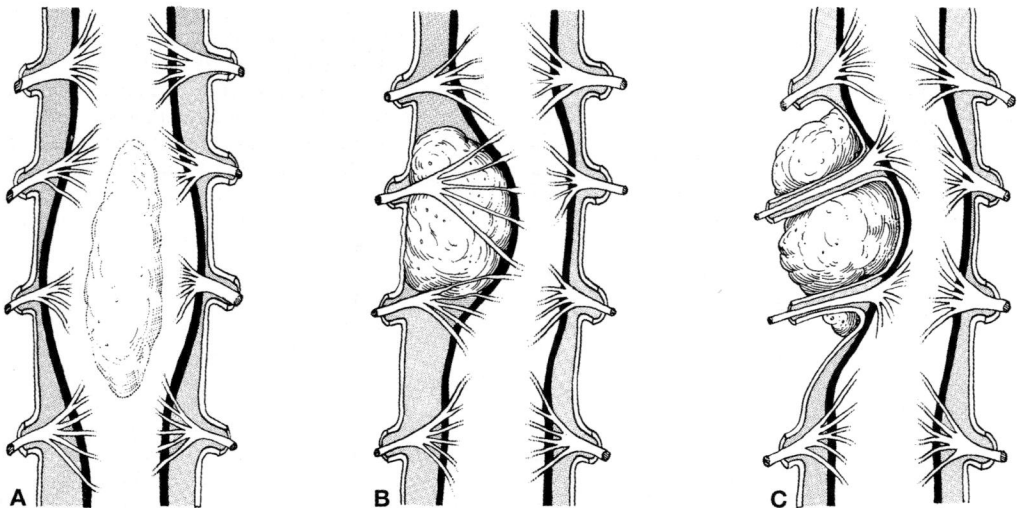

Figure 28-17. Spinal tumors. A. Intramedullary tumor causing bulging of the spinal cord. B. Extramedullary intradural tumor lying in the subarachnoid space, displacing and compressing the spinal cord, but not the dura. C. Extradural tumor lying in the epidural space, displacing the dural sac and the spinal cord. (From Lawrence PF. *Essentials of Surgical Specialties.* 3rd ed. Lippincott Williams & Wilkins; 2007.)

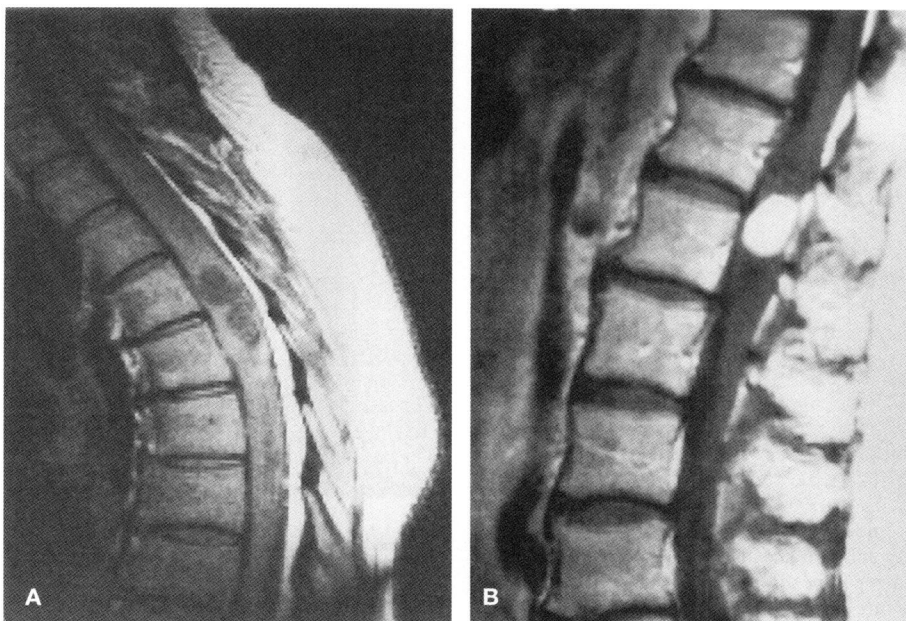

Figure 28-18. A. Enhanced magnetic resonance imaging showing spinal cord astrocytoma (intramedullary tumor). B. Enhanced magnetic resonance imaging showing spinal neurofibroma (extramedullary intradural tumor). (From Lawrence PF. *Essentials of Surgical Specialties*. 3rd ed. Lippincott Williams & Wilkins; 2007.)

normal but strong suspicion persists, a nucleotide bone scan can be very sensitive to subtle early lesions. Both CT myelography and MR scanning are used to evaluate these patients. MR scanning avoids the danger of LP and also visualizes the lesions, their effects on the spinal cord, and changes in the vertebrae. Gadolinium enhancement of MRI scan increases the definition of many spinal tumors. MRI scan is the most useful early step when a patient has spinal cord symptoms. It is especially urgent if the patient has a history of cancer.

As soon as spinal cord compression from metastatic tumor is suspected, the patient is treated with high-dose intravenous steroids. If the patient is in good clinical shape and the tumor is radiosensitive, then emergent radiotherapy is begun and the patient is observed closely for neurologic deterioration caused by tumor swelling in reaction to the radiation. In this setting, surgical decompression is reserved for evidence of neurologic deterioration. If the tumor is radio-insensitive, the patient is already on the verge of losing ambulatory function. If the imaging suggests significant kyphotic or pending kyphotic deformity, then decompressive surgery with or without fusion is performed, followed by postoperative radiotherapy. The location of the compression dictates the type of operation performed. If the compression is from the back of the spinal canal or in the lateral gutters, laminectomy with tumor removal from the extradural space should suffice. Fusion is seldom necessary. If the compression is from the front because of vertebral collapse with angulation or because of tumor anterior to the cord, the operation is more difficult. Although a lateral posterior (costotransversectomy or lateral extracavitary) approach is advocated, the most common approach is anterior decompression with subsequent fusion (see Figure 28-19C). Tumor surgery is most effective for patients who do not have a complete loss of

spinal cord function. The ability of the patient to walk prior to surgery is the single most important determinant of whether the patient will be ambulatory after surgery. The average survival after surgery for metastatic disease is generally 6 months.

Primary Spine Tumors

Primary spine tumors include both intradural extramedullary tumors and intradural intramedullary tumors.

Intradural Extramedullary Spine Tumors

Intradural extramedullary tumors lie within the dural tube but outside the confines of the spinal cord. In the cervical and thoracic spine, they lie adjacent to the spinal cord and the local nerve roots. They often distort and compress these structures and produce symptoms and signs of root or cord dysfunction. In the lumbar canal, they lie among the roots of the cauda equina and produce polyradicular symptoms and signs. These tumors are well circumscribed and do not extend over many segments. Because they are usually benign, the history is often long.

Neurofibromas are the most common intradural extramedullary tumors. They typically arise from a single dorsal sensory root. Multiple tumors are found in patients with neurofibromatosis. Neurofibromas can extend through an intervertebral foramen and grow out extradurally into the retropleural or retroperitoneal space. This dumbbell extension can become very large and may be the first portion of the tumor identified. For this reason, masses located near the spine require additional radiologic evaluation to determine whether they extend into the spinal canal.

Meningiomas are almost as common as neurofibromas and are based on the dura. They occur 4 times as often in women as in men. They are most common in the thoracic region and more commonly occur ventrally than dorsally.

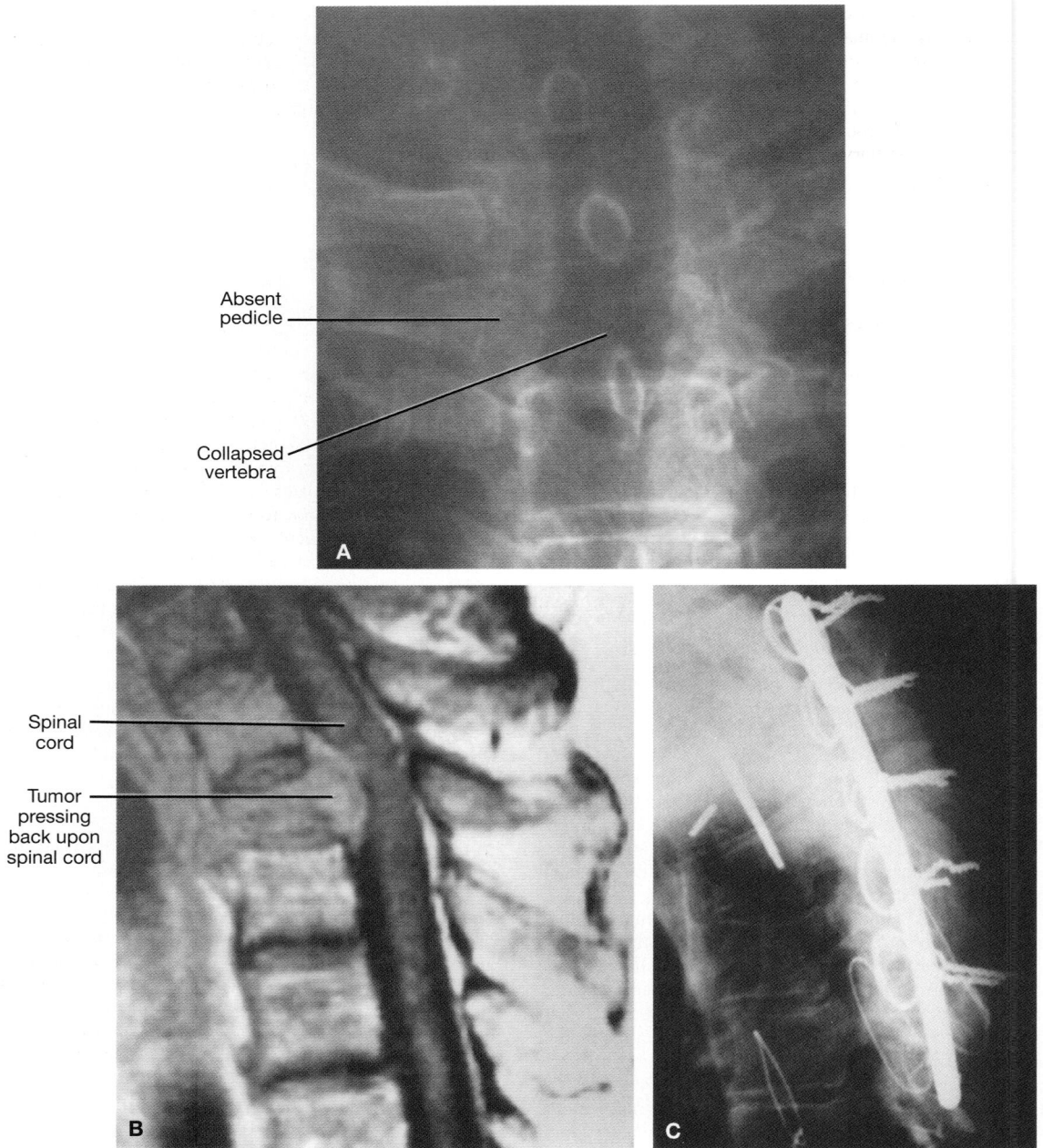

Figure 28-19. A. Metastatic tumor to the spine. B. Enhanced magnetic resonance imaging showing a metastatic spinal tumor. C. Lateral spine film after anterior decompression and fusion, with posterior stabilization and fusion, showing a metastatic spinal tumor. (From Lawrence PF. *Essentials of Surgical Specialties*. 3rd ed. Lippincott Williams & Wilkins; 2007.)

The filum terminale within the cauda equina contains a continuation of the ependymal lining of the central spinal canal. It is prone to develop a particularly benign form of ependymoma known as a "myxopapillary ependymoma."

Contrast-enhanced MR is the imaging procedure of choice for seeing the type and extent of the tumor as well as its relationship to the spinal cord. CT scanning is better able to assess the surrounding bone changes resulting from the tumor. Neurofibromas may cause widening of a neural foramen on x-ray.

Intradural extramedullary tumors can be cured because they can usually be removed completely. Before the dura is opened, real-time ultrasound can be utilized to localize the tumor and ensure adequacy of rostral-caudal exposure. The operating microscope and microsurgical techniques, including the laser and ultrasonic aspirator, are used to remove the tumor. Laser is particularly effective and useful for dealing with lipomas. Neurologic function is monitored by repetitive testing of somatosensory and motor-evoked responses. Lower-extremity and rectal electromyographic monitoring are useful for assisting with dissecting the cauda equina nerve roots free from a cauda equina schwannoma or myxopapillary ependymoma. A recurrence rate of only 6% after 15 years is reported for meningioma. Similar or better results are expected for neurofibroma. Of these patients, 80% improve and 50% become completely normal.

Intradural Intramedullary Spine Tumors

Intramedullary tumors lie within the substance of the spinal cord. They are more common in children than in adults. Some are associated with a large cyst and may be confused with simple syrinx. Astrocytoma of the spinal cord is the most common intramedullary tumor of childhood (see Figure 28-18A). The biologic behavior of this tumor resembles that of low-grade cerebral astrocytoma, including the common presence of a cleavage plane between the low-grade tumor and the spinal cord. Malignant forms are rare. In some regions, the tumors blend with the spinal cord and limit the extent of surgical excision.

Ependymoma of the spinal cord is the most common intramedullary tumor in adults. These tumors arise from the ependyma of the central canal. They are usually well demarcated, and gross total excision is feasible.

Hemangioblastomas of the spinal cord account for fewer than 10% of intramedullary tumors. These tumors are sometimes cystic, are fairly well circumscribed, and do not extend over many segments. Total removal is possible in most cases, although bleeding can be a problem. Just as with cerebellar hemangioblastomas, these tumors are often associated with von Hippel-Lindau syndrome and are often multiple.

Dermoids, epidermoids, and lipomas are also found within the spinal cord or cauda equina, usually at or below the conus. A dermoid is often associated with a dermal sinus tract in the skin overlying the spine. This tract leads to the intraspinal tumor. Likewise, a lipoma that involves the conus or filum is usually in continuity with an overlying subcutaneous extension. The skin overlying this region may contain a hairy patch or cutaneous hemangioma.

Contrast-enhanced MR is the imaging procedure of choice for delineating the type and extent of the tumor as well as its relationship to the spinal cord. CT scanning allows assessment of the surrounding bone changes resulting from the tumor. Intramedullary lesions can enlarge the spinal canal and increase the interpedicular distance.

Intramedullary tumors are treated surgically in an attempt to remove the tumor and prevent further neurologic deterioration. Unlike intracranial ependymomas, ependymomas of the spinal cord can often be removed completely. The lack of a clear cleavage plane between an anaplastic or malignant astrocytoma and the spinal cord hinders attempts at complete removal. Only approximately 50% of spinal astrocytomas can be removed relatively completely. Microsurgical techniques greatly facilitate resection. Even if gross total resection is not possible, spinal cord internal decompression as well as spacious dural patch grafting can maximize additional functional time until deterioration restarts. Although most patients improve after surgery, spinal cord astrocytomas tend to recur, with increasing disability and even death. Radiation

is an important adjunct in the management of chordoma. The role of radiotherapy in the treatment of intramedullary tumors (eg, incompletely removed intramedullary astrocytomas) is poorly defined to date, but it is probably helpful for residual ependymomas.

Spine Infection

Spinal infections include discitis, osteomyelitis, and epidural abscess.

Osteomyelitis and Discitis

Discitis is far more common than osteomyelitis of the spine. It usually occurs in patients with diabetes, those who are immunocompromised, intravenous drug abusers, and patients with previous disk surgery. Infection is pyogenic (usually staphylococcal). Patients usually have severe back or neck pain and occasionally radicular pain. Local tenderness to both palpation and percussion is often present. Spinal cord or cauda equina compromise is rare. Within several months, spinal x-rays show the dissolution of the vertebral end plates that define the disk space. Disk collapse and destruction follow. Ultimately, collapse and angulation of the adjacent vertebral bodies occur. MRI and CT scans show changes earlier than do x-rays. As with all types of spinal infections, the sedimentation rate is almost always elevated. Repeated studies provide a means to assess response to therapy. Fever and leukocytosis are uncommon because most cases are subacute or chronic and follow an indolent course.

Osteomyelitis can be bacterial, fungal, or tubercular in origin. Bacterial osteomyelitis often develops as a contiguous spread of an adjacent discitis. The most common fungal osteomyelitis is caused by coccidioidomycosis. Tuberculous osteomyelitis of the spine (Potts disease) is a chronic condition that usually begins beneath the two vertebral end plates that define a disk space and ultimately extends to involve both vertebral bodies. Unlike pyogenic osteomyelitis or discitis, in Potts disease, the disk architecture and endplates remain relatively well preserved. Collapse of the vertebral bodies can lead to angulation of the spine and kyphotic deformity. Infection may spread to form an epidural abscess. Angulation, epidural abscess, and even disk prolapse can compress the spinal cord and lead to paralysis. The associated paraspinal abscess is common and has a telltale radiographic appearance.

Discitis and osteomyelitis are treated with appropriate intravenous antibiotics for 6 to 8 weeks (which are best guided by culture results) and TLSO bracing to help control pain. Cultures can be obtained by CT-guided percutaneous needle biopsy but can be sterile in up to 50% of postoperative discitis cases. Advanced osteomyelitis requires operative debridement and bone grafting. Tuberculous infection requires 12 to 18 months of multiple anti-TB agents. Coccidioidomycosis of the spine can be very difficult to clear, despite aggressive medical and surgical therapy.

Epidural Abscess

Epidural abscess may be caused by hematogenous spread or direct extension from an abscess of the vertebral body, disk, or paraspinal tissues. These abscesses are usually pyogenic (mostly staphylococcal) and often occur in the thorax. Acute abscesses cause neck or back pain, fever, and spinal tenderness. Progression is similar to that of epidural tumors, with subsequent onset of radicular pain followed by spinal cord paralysis. Chronic abscesses progress more slowly and usually do not cause fever or leukocytosis. MRI scan is especially helpful in identifying the lesion. Treatment requires appropriate antibiotics and surgical drainage.

PAIN

The best strategy for treating most pain involves determining and removing its cause. Unfortunately, this is not always possible. Some causes of pain cannot be removed. In addition, there are situations and conditions where the upstream pain circuitry either becomes hypersensitive to even minor or trivial stimulation (eg, dysesthesia, causalgia, reflex sympathetic dystrophy) or becomes autonomous at a CNS level, with pain occurring even in the absence of a stimulus (eg, anesthesia dolorosa or phantom limb pain). Cancer pain in terminally ill patients remains a major problem in our health system. Although pain medications are the first line of defense for palliation in these situations, they do not always work (particularly for autonomous central pain), and patients can become refractory to relief even at supratherapeutic doses. Some chronic pain medications also come with unwanted end-organ (liver or kidney) side effects as well as physical and psychosocial dependence issues. When these situations are recognized, neurosurgeons can be of assistance. The best treatment for a given condition often varies with the specific requirements of the case and the surgeon's judgment. The issues can be complex and are not always straightforward or clearly defined. Attempting to treat a chronic pain syndrome from a purely organic or physical standpoint is not likely to work or lead to a durable response unless the psychosocial issues intimately related to the syndrome are also addressed simultaneously.

Specifically Treatable Syndromes

There are specific pain syndromes, usually related to the cranial nerves, that have a long history of successful treatment with neurosurgical procedures. With these syndromes, correct recognition and diagnosis of the syndrome and early referral to the neurosurgeon will often lead to the best outcome for affected patients.

Trigeminal Neuralgia

Trigeminal neuralgia is a facial pain syndrome that affects the distribution of the trigeminal nerve (cranial nerve V). It is usually unilateral, but in rare situations (2%-4%) can be bilateral. It is characterized by sudden shock or sharp-stabbing episodes of pain radiating down one or more trigeminal divisions. Early in the syndrome, the pain tends to last only seconds before ending just as abruptly as it started. Later in the syndrome, painful shocks can temporarily group or cluster in a string of repetitive tetanic jolts that may make the pain seem like it lasts for a few minutes before it resolves. Early in the syndrome, the patient experiences no pain or other trigeminal symptoms between episodes. The pain comes spontaneously in an unpredictable manner but also can be triggered by trigeminal tactile stimulation (eg, cold wind on the face, brushing teeth, washing the face, putting on makeup, talking, or even chewing). Through operant conditioning, the patient soon learns which activities to avoid. Neurologic examination is usually grossly normal, but very careful testing reveals subtle hypalgesia (10%-20%) in the medial distribution of V2 or V3 in up to one-third of patients. This incidence increases with chronicity of the syndrome and with surgical attempts at treatment. Spontaneous periods of remission lasting up to 6 months in length are common (up to 50% of patients), but recurrence is the rule, because the syndrome is slowly progressive in severity, frequency, and trigeminal nerve distribution. The pain of trigeminal neuralgia is so excruciating that patients will abruptly stop whatever they are doing and hold themselves immobile until it passes.

Differential diagnosis includes temporal-mandibular-joint syndrome, postherpetic neuralgia, cluster headache, and deafferentation facial pain. Approximately 98% of cases are considered idiopathic in origin, with vascular cross-compression of the nerve affecting myelin insulation at the nerve root entry zone considered to be the likely cause. The remaining 2% of patients include patients with multiple sclerosis (~2% of multiple sclerosis patients will develop trigeminal neuralgia), brainstem lacunar infarctions in the trigeminal system, or cerebellopontine or Meckel cave mass lesions (eg, tumors, cysts, aneurysms, or AVMs). MR scanning is useful to rule out these alternate causes. It does not, however, rule in or out vascular compression, given the size and multiplicity of vessels found to be involved at surgical exploration.

Initial therapy involves anticonvulsant medications to raise the threshold for electrical stimulation of the trigeminal system. Carbamazepine and oxcarbazepine have been proven to be the most effective agents in clinical trials and appear to be equivalent in terms of short-term efficacy. Oxcarbazepine is currently preferred because of its more favorable toxicity and side-effect profile but lacks the long-term follow-up data available for carbamazepine. Approximately 95% of trigeminal neuralgia patients will respond to initial anticonvulsant therapy. Unfortunately, some are intolerant of side effects, some have idiosyncratic drug reactions, and some tend to gradually become refractory to increasing doses as the syndrome progresses. Approximately 56% of patients will fail carbamazepine therapy for one of these reasons over a period of 16 years. Despite these observations, it remains a sad truth that most trigeminal neuralgia patients will have undergone several dental procedures over a period of several years before the correct diagnosis is made, and the average trigeminal neuralgia patient has suffered with the syndrome for more than 5 years and has seen two to four neurologists before they are finally referred to a neurosurgeon.

In well-trained and experienced hands, microvascular decompression of the trigeminal nerve leads to initial cure (no pain, no medications) in approximately 80% of patients, and this success remains durable at 70% up to 20 years. Other important palliative treatment options include procedures that selectively and partially damage the ganglion or nerve root with either heat (percutaneous radiofrequency lesion), chemicals (percutaneous glycerol rhizotomy), mechanical crush (percutaneous balloon compression) or highly concentrated radiation (gamma knife stereotactic radiosurgery). The latter four procedures do not address the purported cause of the syndrome and are designed to treat the symptom. As palliative procedures, they are all initially effective in about 65% to 80% of cases (pain free with or without medications at 1 year). However, they each have an annual recurrence rate of approximately 6% to 10% per year, so that by 5 years after treatment, this number drops to around 50%. The need for repeat palliative intervention is common. Currently, stereotactic radiosurgery appears to have the lowest rate of treatment-related numbness, and it avoids percutaneous needle placement from the cheek into the foramen ovale. Unfortunately, it is not immediately effective, with lesion maturation and therapeutic effect usually requiring 6 to 8 weeks (range, days to 6 months).

SUGGESTED READINGS

Jüttler E, Unterberg A, Woitzik J, et al; DESTINY II Investigators. Hemicraniectomy in older patients with extensive middle-cerebral-artery stroke. *New Engl J Med.* 2014;370(12):1091-1100.

Lawton MT, Vates GE. Subarachnoid hemorrhage. *New Engl J Med.* 2017;377(3):257-266.

Sanai N, Mirzadeh Z, Berger MS. Functional outcome after language mapping for glioma resection. *New Engl J Med.* 2008;358(1):18-27.

SAMPLE QUESTIONS

QUESTIONS

Choose the best answer for each question.

1. What percentage of stroke volume (from each heartbeat) does the brain receive?

   A. 5%
   B. 20%
   C. 40%
   D. 60%
   E. 80%

2. What is the first step in evaluating a patient with an acute head injury?

   A. CT scan
   B. Neurologic examination
   C. ABCs
   D. GCS score
   E. MRI scan

3. Which of the following is correct?

   A. Intravenous tPA cannot be given within 3 hours of the stroke onset.
   B. The maximum therapeutic window for tPA is usually 3 to 6 hours after ictus for ICA emboli or thrombosis.
   C. tPA should be given only after 12 hours after the stroke onset.
   D. tPA can be given up to 36 hours after infarction onset in the case of posterior circulation vertebrobasilar disease.
   E. tPA must be given for all TIAs.

4. A 27-year-old male is brought to the emergency department after surviving a motor vehicle accident where he fell and hit his head on the ground. A CT scan is taken and shows a fracture of the temporal bone and a lenticular hematoma. Which of the following is the most likely differential diagnosis?

   A. Subdural hematoma
   B. Epidural hematoma
   C. Subarachnoid hemorrhage
   D. Intraparenchymal hematoma
   E. Stroke

5. Which is the most common cancer to metastasize to the CNS?

   A. Lung cancer
   B. Prostate cancer
   C. Ewing sarcoma of the bone
   D. Renal cell carcinoma
   E. Glioma

ANSWERS AND EXPLANATIONS

1. **Answer: B**

   Twenty percent of blood flow is given to the brain, demonstrating its flow importance. Except for the heart, the first area of perfusion is also the brain. For more information on this topic, please see the section "Blood Supply."

2. **Answer: C**

   Even before neurologic examination and CT scans of a trauma scenario, it is important that the ABCs are evaluated and treated first in a head injury scenario. For more information on this topic, please see section "Evaluation of Acute Injuries."

3. **Answer: B**

   tPA can be given within the first 6 hours after an ischemic infarct in an attempt to reperfuse the brain. There are current trials to aim to extend this treatment window, but currently, less than 6 hours is the standard. That is why neurologic assessment and evaluation are of critical and time importance. For more information on this topic, please see section "Ischemic Infarction."

4. **Answer: B**

   A temporal bone fracture is most commonly associated with a laceration of the MMA, which results in an epidural hematoma. Epidural hematomas are surgical emergencies. For more information on this topic, please see section "Epidural Hematomas."

5. **Answer: A**

   The most common metastasis to the brain from other organs are lung, breast, skin, gastrointestinal, and kidney cancers. Because lung cancer is the most common of those, it is also the most common brain metastasis. For more information on this topic, please see section "Secondary (Metastatic) Brain Tumors."

Index

Note: Page numbers followed by "*f*" denote figures and "*t*" denote tables.